Audiology
Treatment

Second Edition

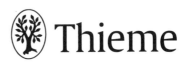

Audiology
Treatment

Second Edition

Michael Valente, Ph.D.
Professor of Clinical Otolaryngology
Director of Adult Audiology
Division of Audiology
Department of Otolaryngology—Head and Neck Surgery
Washington University School of Medicine
St. Louis, Missouri

Holly Hosford-Dunn, Ph.D.
Managing Member
Arizona Audiology Network, LLC
President
TAI, Inc.
Tucson, Arizona

Ross J. Roeser, Ph.D.
Lois and Howard Wolf Professor in Pediatric Hearing
Executive Director Emeritus
School of Behavioral and Brain Sciences
University of Texas at Dallas/Callier Center for Communication Disorders
Dallas, Texas

Thieme
New York · Stuttgart

Thieme Medical Publishers, Inc.
333 Seventh Ave.
New York, NY 10001

Editor: Birgitta Brandenburg
Associate Editor: Ivy Ip
Vice President, Production and Electronic Publishing: Anne T. Vinnicombe
Production Editor: Molly Connors, Dovetail Content Solutions
Vice President, International Marketing: Cornelia Schulze
Chief Financial Officer: Peter van Woerden
President: Brian D. Scanlan
Compositor: Thomson Digital Services
Printer: Maple-Vail Book Manufacturing Company

Library of Congress Cataloging-in-Publication Data

Audiology. Treatment / edited by Michael Valente, Holly Hosford-Dunn, Ross J. Roeser. — 2nd ed.
   p. ; cm.
Companion v. to Audiology : diagnosis, and Audiology : practice management.
Includes bibliographical references and index.
ISBN 978-1-58890-520-8 (US : alk. paper) — ISBN 978-3-13-116422-3 (rest of world : alk. paper)
   1. Audiology. 2. Hearing disorders—Treatment. I. Valente, Michael. II. Hosford-Dunn, Holly. III. Roeser, Ross J. IV. Title: Audiology treatment.
   V. Title: Treatment.
   [DNLM: 1. Hearing Disorders—therapy. 2. Hearing Aids. WV 270 A9125 2007]
RF290.A926 2007
617.8—dc22

                2007039508

Important note: Medical knowledge is ever-changing. As new research and clinical experience broaden our knowledge, changes in treatment and drug therapy may be required. The authors and editors of the material herein have consulted sources believed to be reliable in their efforts to provide information that is complete and in accord with the standards accepted at the time of publication. However, in view of the possibility of human error by the authors, editors, or publisher of the work herein or changes in medical knowledge, neither the authors, editors, nor publisher, nor any other party who has been involved in the preparation of this work, warrants that the information contained herein is in every respect accurate or complete, and they are not responsible for any errors or omissions or for the results obtained from use of such information. Readers are encouraged to confirm the information contained herein with other sources. For example, readers are advised to check the product information sheet included in the package of each drug they plan to administer to be certain that the information contained in this publication is accurate and that changes have not been made in the recommended dose or in the contraindications for administration. This recommendation is of particular importance in connection with new or infrequently used drugs.
Some of the product names, patents, and registered designs referred to in this book are in fact registered trademarks or proprietary names even though specific reference to this fact is not always made in the text. Therefore, the appearance of a name without designation as proprietary is not to be construed as a representation by the publisher that it is in the public domain.

Printed in the United States of America

5 4 3 2 1

US ISBN: 978-1-58890-520-8
GTV ISBN: 978-3-13-116422-3

Contents

Preface to the Second Edition

Harry Truman was a great leader and, some would say, an effective president. However, as is clearly evident in the second edition of our three volumes—*Audiology: Diagnosis, Audiology: Treatment,* and *Audiology: Practice Management*—he was off target when he said, "The only thing new in the world is the history you don't know." Since the publication of the first edition of our series just 7 years ago, there has been not only new information but also new technology, treatments, and trends in practice that have affected audiology in a way that has resulted in all areas of our profession growing exponentially. We now have better diagnostic procedures, more advanced technology and treatment programs, and additional practice strategies that allow audiologists to be more effective in diagnosing and treating their patients.

What's more exciting about the growth in the field of audiology that has occurred in the past few years is that we now have an expanding and maturing educational system for graduate students who choose to spend their lives in the profession. During the preparation of the first edition of our series, the doctor of audiology degree (Au.D.) was new. Yes, in 2000 there were programs in existence, and most universities at the time were in the planning stages of upgrading their programs to the doctoral level. However, at the time it was unclear how this shift in the educational model would impact the profession. Today, according to the Audiology Foundation of America, there are 70 university programs offering the Au.D. degree, 1500 residential students currently enrolled in Au.D. programs, and more than 3725 practicing doctors of audiology. So, we have an expanded body of knowledge that is being consumed by a growing and more sophisticated constituent body of professionals who have dedicated themselves to providing the best diagnosis and treatments to those with hearing disorders using more sophisticated practice procedures. All of these trends point to growth.

A novel thought is to consider the information in these three volumes as a mathematical equation:

$$X = D + T + P$$

where D is diagnosis, T is treatment, P is practice management, and X is the sum of all of the current knowledge in the three represented areas provided by the most knowledgeable experts in their respective fields. That is what we wanted these books to represent.

People don't just decide one day that because there's more information and more individuals to consume it, they will devote a couple years of their lives to putting it together in a bundle of books. The three of us jointly arrived at the decision to publish a second edition of the "trilogy," as it has become known colloquially, because we felt a need to pay back to our profession a modicum of what it has given to us. We each have been very fortunate to be exposed to some of the best mentors, have been provided with tremendous support both psychologically and financially, and have been rewarded greatly in many other ways by being audiologists. We feel that we have been fortunate to practice audiology during the period of growth that the profession has experienced. We want to share those positive experiences with our readers.

We owe a special debt of gratitude to the authors of the chapters in these three volumes, who were willing to contribute their knowledge and experience as well as their valuable time in preparing the material. We thank them not only for all of their hard work and diligence in meeting a demanding publication schedule, but also for their tolerance in putting up with what we considered "constructive editorial comments." We realize that criticism is easy, but it is the science and art that are difficult. They were quite tolerant and gracious.

Finally, Thieme Medical Publishers provided us with the support of Ivy Ip. Ivy was our front-line representative with our authors once they agreed to be part of our team. We thank her for all of her efforts in making the second edition of our books a reality.

Michael Valente—valentem@ent.wustl.edu
Holly Hosford-Dunn—tucsonaud@aol.com
Ross J. Roeser—roeser@utdallas.edu

Preface to the First Edition

This book is on the topic of treatment in audiology, and is one in a series of three texts prepared to represent the breadth of knowledge covering the multifaceted profession of audiology in a manner that has not been attempted before. The companion books to this volume are *Diagnosis* and *Practice Management*. The three books provide a total of 73 chapters covering current knowledge on the range of subjects audiologists must have to practice effectively. Because many of the chapters in the three books relate to each other, our readers are encouraged to have all three in their libraries so that the broad scope of knowledge in the profession of audiology is available to them.

A unique feature of all three books is the insertion of highlighted boxes (pearls, pitfalls, special considerations, and controversial points) in strategic locations. These boxes emphasize key points the authors are making and expand important concepts.

This volume is intended to provide a comprehensive overview of the numerous treatment options available to help relieve patients' clinical symptoms. The intended audience is either an audiology graduate student or a practicing clinician.

To accomplish this task, this volume is divided into three sections. The first section underscores the Principles of Treatment. This section is designed to provide the graduate student and practitioner with a solid background before going into the specifics of available treatment options. First, Dave Preves and Jim Curran provide an excellent overview of the instrumentation and procedures involved in measuring the *electroacoustic* performance of hearing aids. The chapter by Michael Valente, Marueen Valent, Lisa Potts, and Edward Lybarger illustrates the numerous ways that the amplified sound can be modified by the manner in which the hearing aids are connected to the coupler or real-ear. A chapter by Larry Revit follows on the instrumentation and procedures used to accurately measure the *real-ear* performance of hearing aids when worn on the individual ear(s) of the patient. Dawna Lewis provides the reader with an overview of the numerous issues to consider when fitting hearing aids to children, while Carol Sammeth and Harry Levitt provide similar information that must be considered when fitting the adult population.

Over the past few years there have been a large number of manufacturers introducing hearing aids whose performance technology created the need for new approaches for selecting, fitting, and verifying the performance of hearing aids. Prior to this, signal processing provided by hearing aids was predominantly linear; that is, the gain provided by the hearing aids remained constant as the level of the input signal changed. Thus, the early prescriptive formulas were appropriate when fitting hearing aids with linear signal processing. However, with the proliferation of hearing aids with nonlinear signal processing, new prescriptive procedures needed to be developed so that a different prescriptive target was available for different input levels. Francis Kuk presents an overview on recently introduced approaches to selecting and fitting nonlinear hearing aids.

The appropriate fitting of hearing aids is only one step in the rehabilitation/habilitation process. Once the hearing aids are fit, the patient requires counseling on realistic expectations and other important aspects of what amplification can and cannot provide. This information is provided in the chapter by Jane Madell. In addition, audiologists need to be aware of the numerous state and federal regulations dealing with dispensing hearing aids and assistive listening devices (ALDs). Holly Kaplan and John Hesse do a masterful job in providing this vital information.

The second section deals with the Applications in Treatment. The first three chapters provide information on current medical and surgical treatments available for patients with conductive (Elizabeth Dinces and Richard Wiet), cochlear, or neural hearing loss (J. Gail Neeley and Mark Wallace). Assuming that amplification is an appropriate treatment option for the hearing loss, Catherine Palmer, George Lindley, and Elaine Mormer provide information on the procedures to follow for selecting, fitting, and verifying the performance of conventional hearing aids. The chapter by Robert Sweetow provides similar information for those who are considering selecting, fitting, and verifying the performance of programmable (analog signal processing) and recently introduced digital hearing aids. Selecting, fitting, and verifying the performance of hearing aids is an important step in providing amplification. However, the patient needs to be counseled on the use and care of the hearing aids. This information is provided in the chapter by David Citron. A relatively recent trend in amplification is the surgical implantation of hearing aids for patients whose hearing loss is severe enough that they receive little or no benefit from conventional or digital hearing aids. Doug Miller and John Fredrickson provide an excellent chapter on the recent trend of implanting hearing aids into the middle ear or brainstem. A chapter by Pat Chute and Mary Eleen Nevins follows on cochlear implants in children, while Susan Waltzman and William Shapiro provide similar information for cochlear implantation in the adult population. As is well known by experienced dispensers, hearing aids alone cannot solve all the listening problems experienced by the user. This is especially true when the user is attempting to hear optimally in a noisy environment or when using a telephone. The chapter by Jean-Pierre Gagné and Mary Beth Jennings provides information on the role of aural rehabilitation in improving the listening skills of patients with reduced hearing. This is followed by the chapter by Peter Bengtsson and Preben Brunved which contributes a wealth of information on the numerous assistive listening devices that can be coupled to the patient's hearing aids or used alone. Another population to consider is those patients who have hearing sensitivity within normal limits, but are easily distracted by the environment surrounding them. Carl Crandell and Joe Smaldino provide the reader with an excellent chapter on methods to improve the acoustical environment within the classroom. Another patient population is those reporting dizziness and vertigo. Aside from the medical and surgical treatment options outlined in the chapter by J. Gail Neely and Mark Wallace, Alan Desmond reports on the relatively new treatment option of eliminating the sensations of dizziness through vestibular rehabilitation. For those patients whose hearing loss has been a result of excessive exposure to loud sounds (or for those who currently have normal hearing but are exposing themselves to loud sounds), Elliott Berger and John Casali offer insightful information on protective devices that are used to prevent hearing loss or further decrease in hearing. Still another population to consider are those who experience tinnitus or report hypersensitivity to typical environmental sounds. Robert Sandlin and Robert Olsson present an excellent chapter on the evaluation and treatment options for these patients.

The final section of this volume hopefully will serve to help the reader understand what may be arriving in the future in terms of treatment options. Christopher Schweitzer presents a wonderful chapter on what may lie ahead in amplification treatment options. His chapter leaves the promising impression that in the near future it will be possible for listeners with hearing loss to actually hear better in noisy environments than persons with normal hearing. Denis Byrne and Harvey Dillon present a thought-provoking chapter on what may lie ahead for the practitioner as he selects, fits, and verifies the performance of hearing aids. Finally, Brenda Ryals presents a fascinating chapter on procedures that may result in the regeneration of hair cells in the cochlea that will restore hearing to normal. If this approach proves successful, then much of the information presented in this volume concerning treatment options will become obsolete!

The three of us were brought together by Ms. Andrea Seils, Senior Medical Editor at Thieme Medical Publishers, Inc. During the birthing stage of the project Andrea encouraged us to think progressively—out of the box. She reminded us repeatedly to shed our traditional thinking and concentrate on the new developments that have taken place in audiology in recent years and that will occur in the next 5 to 10 years. With Andrea's encouragement and guidance, each of us set out what some would have considered to be the impossible—to develop a series of three cutting edge books that would cover the entire profession of audiology *in a period of less than 2 years.* Not only did we accomplish our goal, but as evidenced by the comprehensive nature of the material covered in the three books, we exceeded our expectations! We thank Andrea for her support throughout this 2-year project.

The authors who were willing to contribute to this book series have provided outstanding material that will assist audiologists in-training and practicing audiologists in their quest for the most up-to-date information on the areas that are covered. We thank them for their diligence in following our guidelines for preparing their manuscripts and their promptness in following our demanding schedule.

The consideration of our families for their endurance and patience with us throughout the duration of the project must be recognized. Our spouses and children understood our mission when we were away at editorial meetings; they were patient when we stayed up late at night and awoke in the wee hours of the morning to eke out a few more paragraphs; they tolerated the countless hours we were away from them. Without their support and encouragement we would never have finished our books in the timeframe we did.

Finally, each of us thanks our readers for their support of this book series. We would welcome comments and suggestions on this book, as well as the other two books in the series. Our email addresses are below.

Ross J. Roeser—roeser@utdallas.edu
Michael Valente—valentem@ent.wustl.edu
Holly Hosford-Dunn—tucsonaud@aol.com

Contributors

Shilpi Banerjee, Ph.D
Senior Research Audiologist
Department of Hearing Research
and Technology
Starkey Laboratories, Inc.
Eden Prairie, Minnesota

A. U. Bankaitis, Ph.D.
Vice President and General Manager
Oaktree Products, Inc.
Chesterfield, Missouri

Teri James Bellis, Ph.D.
Associate Professor and Chair
Department of Communication
Disorders
Adjunct Associate Professor
Division of Basic Biomedical Sciences
Sanford School of Medicine
University of South Dakota
Vermillion, South Dakota

Victor Bray, Ph.D.
Vice President and Chief
Audiology Officer
Sonic Innovations, Inc.
Salt Lake City, Utah

Marshall L. Chasin, Au.D.
Director of Audiology Research
Musicians' Clinics of Canada
Toronto, Ontario, Canada

Patricia M. Chute, Ed.D.
Professor and Chair
Division of Health Professions
and Natural Sciences
Department of Communication
Disorders
Mercy College
Dobbs Ferry, New York

David Citron III, Ph.D.
Director
South Shore Hearing Center
South Weymouth, Massachusetts

Carl C. Crandell, Ph.D. (deceased)
Professor, Director of Audiology
Department of Communication
Sciences and Disorders
Institute for the Advanced Study of
Communication Processes
University of Florida
Gainesville, Florida

Alan L. Desmond, Au.D.
Director
Blue Ridge Hearing and Balance
Clinic
Princeton, West Virginia

Elizabeth A. Dinces, M.D., M.S.
Assistant Professor
Department of
Otorhinolaryngology–Head
and Neck Surgery
Albert Einstein College of Medicine
Bronx, NY

Leisha R. Eiten, M.A.
Clinical Coordinator
Department of Audiology
Boys Town National Research Hospital
Omaha, Nebraska

Kristina M. English, Ph.D.
Associate Professor
Department of Speech Language
Pathology and Audiology
University of Akron
Akron, Ohio

Robert L. Folmer, Ph.D.
Associate Professor
Department of Otolaryngology
Oregon Health and Science University
Portland, Oregon

Kristina E. Frye
Project Manager
Frye Electronics, Inc.
Tigard, Oregon

Jean-Pierre Gagné, Ph.D.
Professor of Audiology
École d'Orthophonie et
d'Audiologie
Université de Montréal
Montréal, Québec, Canada

Holly Hosford-Dunn, Ph.D.
Managing Member
Arizona Audiology Network, LLC
President
TAI, Inc.
Tucson, Arizona

Mary Beth Jennings, Ph.D.
Assistant Professor
National Centre for Audiology
School of Communication Sciences
and Disorders
Faculty of Health Sciences
University of Western Ontario
London, Ontario, Canada

Andrew B. John, Ph.D.
Assistant Professor
Department of Communication
Sciences and Disorders
University of Oklahoma Health
Sciences Center
Oklahoma City, OK

Brian M. Kreisman, Ph.D.
Assistant Professor
Department of Audiology,
Speech-Language Pathology,
and Deaf Studies
Towson University
Towson, Maryland

Nicole V. Kreisman, Ph.D.
Assistant Professor
Department of Audiology,
Speech-Language Pathology,
and Deaf Studies
Towson University
Towson, Maryland

Francis K. Kuk, Ph.D.
Director of Audiology
Office of Research in Clinical
    Amplification
Widex Hearing Aid Company
Lisle, Illinois

Dawna E. Lewis, Ph.D.
Senior Research Associate
Department of Audiology
Boys Town National Research
    Hospital
Omaha, Nebraska

George A. Lindley IV, Ph.D., Au.D.
Manager of Distance Learning
Oticon, Inc.
Somerset, New Jersey

Robert Martin, Ph.D.
Private Practice Audiologist
La Mesa, California

William Hal Martin, Ph.D.
Professor
Department of Otolaryngology
Oregon Health and Science University
Portland, Oregon

Douglas A. Miller, B.S.E.E.
Technology Research Coordinator
Cochlear Americas
Englewood, Colorado

Elaine A. Mormer, M.A.
Instructor
Communication Science and Disorders
University of Pittsburgh
Pittsburgh, Pennsylvania

John Gail Neely, M.D.
Professor and Director of Otology/
    Neurotology/Base of Skull Surgery
Department of Otolaryngology–Head
    and Neck Surgery
Washington University School of
    Medicine
St. Louis, Missouri

Mary Ellen Nevins, Ed.D.
Director, Professional Preparation in
    Cochlear Implants
Independent Contractor to The
    Children's Hospital of Philadelphia
Philadelphia, Pennsylvania

Michael Nilsson, Ph.D.
Director, Auditory Research
Sonic Innovations, Inc.
Salt Lake City, Utah

Catherine V. Palmer, Ph.D.
Associate Professor
Communication Science and Disorders
University of Pittsburgh
Pittsburgh, Pennsylvania

David A. Preves, Ph.D.
Senior Staff Engineer
Starkey Laboratories
Eden Prairie, Minnesota

Ross J. Roeser, Ph.D.
Lois and Howard Wolf Professor in
    Pediatric Hearing
Executive Director Emeritus
School of Behavioral and Brain
    Sciences
University of Texas at Dallas/Callier
    Center for Communication
    Disorders
Dallas, Texas

Carol A. Sammeth, Ph.D.
Adjunct Associate Professor
Department of Speech, Language,
    and Hearing Sciences
University of Colorado at Boulder
Senior Regulatory/Clinical Specialist
Cochlear Americas
Englewood, Colorado

William H. Shapiro, M.A.
Clinical Associate Professor
Department of Otolaryngology
NYU School of Medicine
New York, New York

Joseph J. Smaldino, Ph.D.
Professor and Chair
Department of Communication
    Sciences and Disorders
Illinois State University
Normal, Illinois

L. Maureen Valente, Ph.D.
Director of Audiology Studies
Assistant Professor of Otolaryngology
Program in Audiology and
    Communication Sciences
Washington University School
    of Medicine
St. Louis, Missouri

Michael Valente, Ph.D.
Professor of Clinical Otolaryngology
Director of Adult Audiology
Division of Audiology
Department of Otolaryngology–Head
    and Neck Surgery
Washington University School of
    Medicine
St. Louis, Missouri

Susan B. Waltzman, Ph.D.
Professor
Department of Otolaryngology
NYU School of Medicine
New York, New York

Richard J. Wiet, M.D.
Professor of Clinical Otolaryngology
    and Neurosurgery
Feinberg School of Medicine
Northwestern University
Chicago, Illinois

Acknowledgments

For the Book Series

The three editors of this book series came together in late 1990. Prior to the first meeting we had all known of each other, but only casually. However, during the first meeting there was an immediate recognition among us that, although we had very different backgrounds and professional orientations, a professional magnetism drew us together. Long hours together flew by during the many sessions where we discussed contents, possible contributors, and logistics. When asked to produce a second edition, each of us was very reluctant, but agreed because we knew that this would provide us with an opportunity to work together once again. So, strange as it may seem, each of us would like to thank our two other editorial colleagues for making the second edition a reality. We each said that the main reason for taking on this gargantuan task was that we had the support of the two other editors.

Each of us would like to thank the authors for the considerable time and effort they took from their private and professional lives to produce chapters reflecting the highest scholarship.

The staff of Thieme Medical Publishers, Brian Scanlan, President, Birgitta Brandenburg, Editor, and Ivy Ip, Assistant Editor, who worked so many hours during the entire production process deserve special recognition. These key individuals keep the machines running at the Thieme headquarters in the background so that authors and editors can carry out their writing, recruiting, and editorial tasks.

Holly Hosford-Dunn—tucsonaud@aol.com
Ross J. Roeser—roeser@utdallas.edu
Michael Valente—valentem@ent.wustl.edu

For this Book

As primary editor for *Audiology: Treatment,* I want to thank the audiology staff at Washington University School of Medicine—Diane Duddy, Laura Flowers, Judy Peterein, Cathy Schroy, Jennifer Listenberger, Emily Adams, Kathy Swan, Toby Schuman, and Derrick Morris—for providing me the time to concentrate on the tasks required to complete the recruiting, communications, editing, and proofreading for the book.

I especially want to thank my wife, Dr. Maureen Valente, and daughters, Michelle and Anne. Their continued unselfish love, encouragement, and understanding helped minimize my enormous feelings of guilt for not being there to take on my responsibilities as a husband and father for so many evenings and weekends.

Michael Valente—valentem@ent.wustl.edu

Section I

Principles

Chapter 1

Hearing Aid Instrumentation, Signal Processing, and Electroacoustic Testing

David A. Preves and Shilpi Banerjee

The history of electronic hearing aids has been characterized by a reduction in the units' physical size accompanied by a constant quest for performance improvement. Completely-in-the-canal (CIC) hearing aids, the smallest models, now feature digital signal processing (DSP) with many automatic features that provide amplification with good sound quality. However, the total sales percentage of custom in-the-ear (ITE) hearing instruments, the most popular models since the late 1970s, has been decreasing in recent years because of the growing trend in small behind-the-ear (BTE) and over-the-ear open fittings.

Hearing aid designers continue to be challenged to produce small, high-performance models that require low-voltage, low-current capacity batteries. With batteries having a very limited life and off-the-shelf components required for good performance that use current at a relatively high rate, engineers have had to be inventive in the way signal processing and amplification are accomplished. The ability of hearing aid industry engineers to package better performance into smaller physical size has continued. Advances in technology come from many sources, including

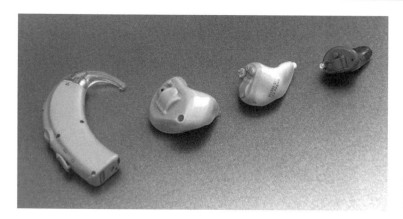

Figure 1–1 Types of hearing aid styles (*from left to right*): behind the ear, in the ear, in the canal, and completely in the canal.

hearing aid manufacturers' design teams and the various suppliers that provide components.

◆ Hearing Aid Styles

Whereas body-style and eyeglass hearing aids were popular in the 1940s and 1950s, respectively, these models now represent only a small percentage of total hearing aid sales.

Higher power BTE hearing aids have replaced much of the need for powerful body aids. Current BTE hearing aids offer the highest amount of gain and OSPL90 (output sound pressure level [SPL] with a 90 dB SPL input signal) available; they are capable of providing 2 cc coupler gain as high as 80 dB, with OSPL90 values up to 145 dB SPL peak.

Much of the rationale for custom hearing aids is based on the favorable microphone position they provide. A comparison of the average field-to-microphone transfer functions at 0 degree for four styles of hearing aids—BTE, ITE, in the canal (ITC), and CIC—shows a progressive increase in the high-frequency signal between hearing aid styles as the position of the microphone goes deeper into the outer ear. These response differences are due mainly to differences in the location of the hearing aid microphone.

Behind the Ear

The BTE style, shown at far left in **Fig. 1–1,** although first introduced in the 1950s, did not actually rise to prominence until the late 1960s. Popularity of BTE styles was eclipsed by custom hearing aids beginning in the mid-1970s. However, the BTE hearing aid style has experienced a resurgence in the last few years mainly due to two factors: (1) many audiologists prefer to fit BTE hearing aids because there are no remakes of the entire hearing aid for poor physical fit (in case of physical fit issues if a custom earmold is used, only the earmold needs to be remade) and (2) the popularity of "open fittings," an idea from the 1960s that is more viable with today's DSP feedback cancellation techniques and nearly invisible thin receiver tubing. Open fittings provide the equivalent of very large earmold vents, resulting in significant attenuation of low-frequency gain and occlusion reduction. They are thus appropriate particularly for those with normal or near-normal low-frequency hearing who have never worn a hearing aid. Most open-fitting BTE aids use a standard-size ear insert in place of a custom earmold (**Fig. 1–2**), eliminating one significant step in the traditional hearing aid fitting process. At the time of this writing, about one of every two hearing aids dispensed in the United States are BTE models (Strom, 2007).

> **Special Consideration**
>
> - BTE hearing aids are not new, having been widely used in the 1960s and 1970s. However, some of today's open-fitting models are packaged in extremely small housings and are relatively inconspicuous on the wearer.

The BTE style has many standard and optional features, including a telecoil in every hearing aid, some with automatic switching for telephone-proximity sensing, patient-operated controls that may be used to select memory and direct-audio input signal alternatives, and automatic directional and nondirectional microphone-switching capabilities. Some BTE hearing aids incorporate a frequency modulation (FM) receiver and antenna to facilitate using radio frequency (RF) classroom amplification and assistive listening systems. These features are being expanded by digital wireless capability utilizing Bluetooth and other RF transceivers, which provide increased immunity to interference as compared with analog FM systems (Yanz, 2006).

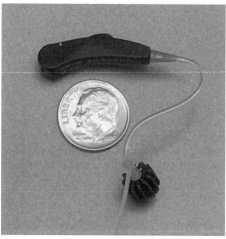

Figure 1–2 Open-fitting behind-the-ear hearing aid and standard earpieces.

Custom

When custom hearing aids were introduced into the mainstream hearing aid market, beginning with the ITE in the 1970s, the ITC in the 1980s, and the CIC in the 1990s, their sales rapidly grew to dominate the market. At the present time, custom hearing aids account for 50% of total hearing aid sales in the United States (Strom, 2007).

Early on, researchers showed that the custom ITE family of instruments provides several acoustic advantages over the other types of hearing instruments. Studies have shown that the position of the microphone in custom ITE hearing aids (second from left in **Fig. 1–1**) produces ~4 to 6 dB enhancement of the high frequencies compared with BTE aids with identical performance and components (Griffing and Preves, 1976). When a hearing aid receiver is installed in a custom ITE aid instead of a BTE, the tubing-related resonance in the BTE hearing aid at 1000 Hz disappears because the receiver is now contained within the ear shell, close to its medial tip, and only a very short length of tubing is needed (Madafarri and Stanley, 1996). The absence of the 1000 Hz peak allows the volume control to be turned higher for the many patients who have better hearing in the low and middle frequencies and greater loss in the high frequencies. Finally, by moving the receiver closer to the tympanic membrane, as is the case for deep-fitting CIC hearing aids (far right in **Fig. 1–1**), less coupler gain is required in the hearing aid itself to provide an appropriate gain–frequency response for a given hearing loss, compared with an equivalent BTE aid.

Special Consideration

- Even though the receiver tubing is much longer in BTE hearing aids than in custom hearing aids, their frequency responses can be made similar by inserting a damper in the BTE earhook. If the damper has the appropriate acoustic impedance, it suppresses the 1000 Hz peak in the BTE hearing aid frequency response, leaving only the higher frequency peaks that are characteristic of custom hearing aids.

◆ Hearing Aid Components

A hearing aid is comprised of a series of components, as shown in **Fig. 1–3**. An acoustic input signal first enters the microphone, which converts the incoming acoustic signals to electrical signals. These signals then go to the hearing aid amplifier, in which there are three separate stages: a preamplifier, a signal processor, and an output stage. The amplifier increases and selectively processes the electrical output of the microphone. From the amplifier, the signal is delivered to the receiver (or speaker), which converts the processed electrical signals from the amplifier output back to acoustic signals. The battery provides the power needed by all of the components.

Microphones

Directional Microphones

An omnidirectional microphone has equal sensitivity to sounds incident from all directions and, until recently, was the predominant type used in hearing aids. Directional hearing aids were first introduced to the marketplace in the 1970s. At that time, most were full-time directional, although a few could be switched between omnidirectional and directional modes using mechanical shutters that covered the rear port. During the 1980s and much of the 1990s, comparatively few directional aids were dispensed. Over the past decade, directional hearing aids became more popular again, principally because the wearer could switch them between omnidirectional and directional modes simply by changing programmable memories. In the latest directional hearing aids, the hearing aid itself switches between omnidirectional and directional modes automatically. (See the section Digital Signal Processing for more details.) Current estimates find that about one out of every three hearing aids dispensed is directional (Strom, 2007).

Making hearing aids directional may be accomplished in one of two ways: (1) using matched omnidirectional microphones combined with signal processing to make their summed output directional or (2) using acoustic or dedicated

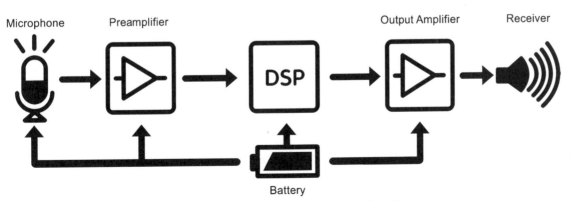

Figure 1–3 Block diagram of the components of a generic hearing aid. DSP, digital signal processing.

directional microphones. In either case, directionality may be switched on and off. Most directional hearing aids exhibit first-order pressure-gradient directionality, although there are a few examples of higher order directionality in the marketplace. Some hearing aids switch between omnidirectional and directional modes automatically by sensing which mode has the better signal-to-noise ratio (SNR; see the section Digital Signal Processing).

First-Order Directional Microphones The earliest directional microphones were bidirectional. A bidirectional microphone is normally made by creating an opening in an omnidirectional microphone (a rear port) in the rear cavity behind the diaphragm. Bidirectional microphones have equal output for sounds incident from the front and rear (0 and 180 degrees, respectively) and minimum output for sounds incident from the sides (90 and 270 degrees). The first unidirectional microphones (now called directional microphones) were made by summing the outputs of an omnidirectional microphone element and a bidirectional microphone element (Harry, 1940). For sounds originating from the front, the output voltages of the omnidirectional and bidirectional microphone elements are in phase and add. For sounds coming from the rear, the phase of the bidirectional element output is opposite that of the omnidirectional element, and the output voltages cancel. Thus, a greater microphone output results for sounds incident from the front than from the sides and rear.

Microphone inventors discovered more than 60 years ago that a bidirectional microphone can be converted to a directional microphone by covering the rear port opening with an acoustic resistance, such as a fine mesh screen. The acoustic resistance of the screen acts in combination with the compliance formed by the volume of air in the rear cavity of the microphone to produce a phase shift for sounds entering the rear port of the microphone (**Fig. 1–4**). The result of this phase shift is an acoustic delay for sounds entering the rear port of the microphone. The acoustic resistance of the screen is selected such that sounds incident from the rear of the hearing aid wearer are delayed so that they arrive at the back of the diaphragm simultaneously with their arrival at the front of the diaphragm. Equal sound pressure arriving on opposite sides of the microphone diaphragm simultaneously results in cancellation of sound from the rear because the diaphragm cannot move. Typical delays for ITE hearing aid applications depend on the distance between microphone ports and are in the order of 25 to 50 µs.

Use of a directional microphone in a hearing instrument is based on two assumptions: (1) the wearer will turn his or her head toward the direction of the desired signal (thus making the axis of directionality adaptive), and (2) undesired signals emanate from the back and sides of the wearer.

Some hearing aids also vary the location of nulls in their polar directivity patterns by estimating from which directions noises are emanating. This latter feature makes sense in a laboratory anechoic chamber or in nonreverberant environments, but it has questionable value in real-world listening situations that are quite reverberant (see the section Digital Signal Processing).

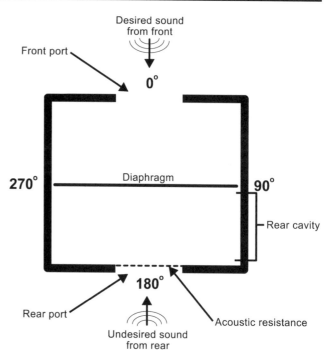

Figure 1–4 Schematic of the operating principle of a directional microphone.

During the development of the first directional microphones, acoustical engineers formulated several methods of measuring and expressing the amount of directivity provided by a directional microphone. Among these are the polar directivity pattern and the directivity index (DI; Preves, 1997). The polar directivity pattern is a graphical plot of the microphone (or hearing instrument) output as a function of angle of sound incidence (**Fig. 1–5**). Sound diffraction produced by the head of a directional hearing aid wearer alters the theoretical polar patterns shown in **Fig. 1–5**. Even hearing aids with omnidirectional microphones have a nonspherical polar pattern when on a hearing aid wearer. The DI, which is proportional to the ratio of frontal incident sound energy to random incident sound energy, predicts the amount of directivity provided by a directional microphone in a diffuse sound field environment. It is derived from the two-dimensional or three-dimensional polar directivity pattern measurements (see discussion of American National Standards Institute [ANSI] S3.35–2004 in the Standards section of this chapter).

Regardless of the type of hearing aid, in any directional hearing instrument the axis of directionality (normally the 0–180 degree axis in the polar pattern when the hearing aid is not on a wearer) is defined by drawing a line through the microphone inlet holes. It is important for good directional hearing aid performance to ensure in design that the axis of directionality lies in or near to the horizontal plane when worn by the hearing aid wearer.

Unless compensated for, a directional microphone usually has less low-frequency gain for sounds at 0 degree incidence than the same microphone with an omnidirectional polar pattern. The closer the microphone port openings are in the hearing aid case, the greater the reduction in low- and

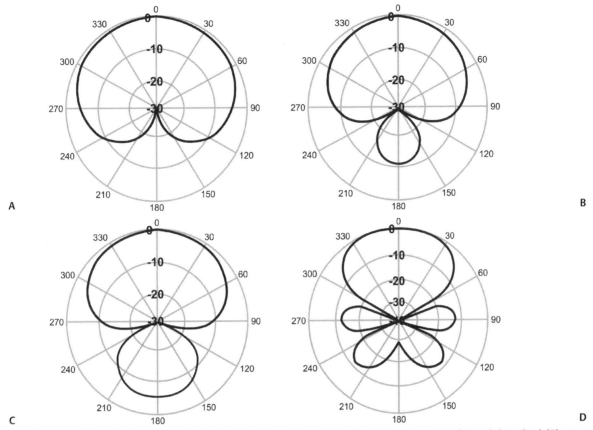

Figure 1–5 Schematized theoretical two-dimensional polar directivity patterns of directional microphones in isolation. **(A)** Cardioid, **(B)** supercardioid, **(C)** hypercardioid, **(D)** five-microphone beamformer showing multiple nulls.

midfrequency gain in directional mode. By boosting overall gain and reducing high-frequency gain, this loss of low-frequency gain can be compensated for, but this may raise the circuit noise level of the hearing aid in directional mode. Alternatively, the high-frequency gain of the hearing aid in directional mode can be normalized to that in the omnidirectional mode to prevent a circuit noise increase in directional mode.

Controversial Point

- A "front/back ratio" measurement in an anechoic chamber was used for the first directional hearing aids ~30 years ago to express the amount of directionality provided. This measurement was contrived by hearing aid manufacturers expressly for directional hearing aids with cardioid microphones. A front/back measurement on a coupler shows a cardioid microphone at its best because there is maximum sensitivity for sounds from the front and minimum sensitivity in the null of the cardioid for sounds from 180 degrees **(Fig. 1–5A).** If used to express directivity, the front/back ratio will unfairly penalize hearing aids with supercardioid or hypercardioid polar patterns, both of which have lobes at 180 degrees and nulls at other angles, resulting in a higher DI than the cardioid has.

Pitfall

- Assessment of directional microphone performance in conventional hearing aid test boxes is problematic because of the sound reflected from the walls inside the test chambers (Preves, 1975). The use of an anechoic chamber (or a simulated anechoic chamber made by selective time gating) is the one sure way to determine the directional performance of a hearing aid with sound coming from only one direction at a time. Roberts and Schulein (1997) present an overview of technical considerations in measuring the performance of directional microphones with various levels of reverberation in the test environment.

Pearl

- Without an anechoic test environment, the best that one can do is to approximate directional performance at 0 degree azimuth with hearing aid analyzers and test boxes by trying to align the axis of directionality (the line drawn through the two microphone ports) with the axis of the loudspeaker in the test chamber. See **Fig. 1–6** for examples of microphone port locations and axes of directionality on BTE and ITC directional hearing aids.

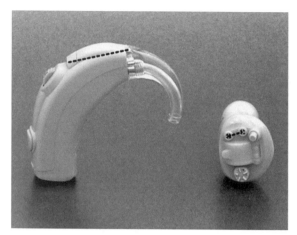

Figure 1–6 Directional behind the ear (*left*) and in the ear (*right*) hearing aids. Broken line indicates the connection of the microphone ports along the axis of directionality.

The amount of directivity actually achieved by a wearer of hearing aids with directional microphones depends on the degree of reverberation in the listening environment. Investigators discovered almost immediately that a moderate amount of reverberation can degrade the amount of directionality (Lentz, 1974). Investigators of the performance of hearing aids with directional microphones should be aware of the critical distance in the test environment (Hawkins and Yacullo, 1984). The critical distance is the distance from the sound source at which the level of direct sound is equal to the level of reverberant sound. At source-test point distances less than the critical distance, sometimes called the near field, the level of direct sound exceeds the level of reverberant sound. At distances greater than the critical distance, sometimes called the far field, the performance of directional microphones in hearing aids is degraded because the level of reverberant sound exceeds the level of the direct sound. For more information on the effect of the critical distance on directionality, readers are referred to Leeuw and Dreschler (1991).

Higher Order Directional Systems and Beamformers

Higher order directional systems can be made by combining the outputs of two or more directional microphones or more than two omnidirectional microphones. Such microphone arrays are called beamformers and have DIs several decibels higher than first-order gradient directional microphones. Beamformers have the ability to emphasize desired signals while filtering or nulling out one or more noise sources. Some beamforming arrays have nulls (a much reduced output) at fixed locations in their polar directivity patterns that do not change with time and are called fixed beamformers (**Fig. 1–5D**). Other beamformers sense adaptively the directions of undesirable noises and automatically move their nulls in their polar directivity patterns to the locations of these noises. These directional arrays are called adaptive beamformers. Adapting the locations of the nulls is accomplished by using an adaptive filter to "steer" the array. In general, a beamformer can produce up to $n - 1$ nulls in its

polar directivity pattern, where n is the number of microphones used.

Fixed beamforming with unchanging polar patterns can produce excellent performance for hearing aids because the wearer's head normally turns in the direction of the desired signal, thus making the fixed beamformer somewhat adaptive. Fixed polar pattern beamformers have the advantage in hearing aid applications of less signal processing and resulting power consumption as compared with adaptive beamformers.

Fixed beamformers are preferred in high levels of reverberation because of overall discouraging results in reverberant environments with adaptive beamformers (see, e.g., Maj et al, 2004).

A fixed beamformer has time-invariant processing that produces a fixed polar pattern. However, in a relatively non-reverberant environment, Greenberg et al (2003) found that an adaptive directional system provided a 6 to 12 dB improvement in speech reception threshold (SRT) compared with a four-microphone fixed directional system. Kates and Weiss (1996) compared the performance of several directional systems: (1) a delay and sum fixed beamformer using five nondirectional microphones in an endfire configuration, (2) two types of superdirective arrays, and (3) two types of adaptive arrays. A superdirective array has a fixed polar pattern over time and can be implemented by using greater delays in the delay and sum network than those produced by the physical space between the microphones in the array. Kates and Weiss (1996) evaluated the different systems in an office and a conference room with a male talker located at 0 degree and uncorrelated multitalker babble incident from five azimuths. They found that the number of microphones is not an important factor at low frequencies but is important at high frequencies. They recommended using an adaptive array at low-input SNR conditions but to convert to a superdirective array at high-input SNR conditions.

In acknowledgment of the deterioration in performance of adaptive beamformers in high levels of reverberation, investigators have also combined fixed and adaptive beamformers. These arrays normally operate adaptively; however, in high levels of reverberation and in high levels of SNR, the amount of adaptability is considerably reduced, and the array essentially becomes a fixed-pattern beamformer. For example, in Kates and Weiss (1996), the adaptive array converges to a superdirective array in a diffuse field.

Amplifiers

The hearing aid amplifier is usually composed of three parts: the preamplifier stage, the signal-processing stage, and the output stage (**Fig. 1–3**). The preamplifier stage provides enough gain to amplify incoming signals to a level above the circuit noise of the amplifier. The signal-processing stage manipulates the signal to enhance or extract the information it contains. The output stage amplifies the output of the signal-processing stage and drives the hearing aid receiver. Several illustrations of modern hearing aid amplifier packaging for custom (left and middle) and BTE (right) hearing aids are shown in **Fig. 1–7.**

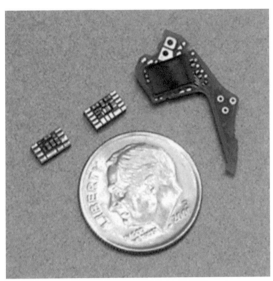

Figure 1–7 Typical circuitry packaged in hybrids and on PC boards for today's in-the-ear and behind-the-ear digital hearing aids, respectively.

Preamplifier Stage

The first stage of the hearing aid amplifier is a preamplifier, which provides gain to the microphone and telecoil output signals. Sometimes the preamplifier stage is packaged within the microphone, but it also may be packaged with the telecoil.

Signal-Processing Stage

The signal processing produced by the hearing aid amplifier is very important in determining how well a hearing-impaired person will function with hearing aids. The hearing aid amplifier selectively processes and amplifies the output signal from the microphone(s) and telecoil. All modern hearing aid amplifiers employ compression and expansion functions that are implemented digitally. Digital signal processing forms the basis for almost all currently marketed hearing aids and is covered in a later section in this chapter.

Receivers

The receiver is essentially a loudspeaker in miniature, converting the processed electrical signal from the hearing aid amplifier back to acoustic energy. Calling a subminiature loudspeaker a receiver seems wrong because it is the hearing aid microphone that receives acoustic energy. However, the term *receiver* is derived from the telephone, in which the speaker in the handset is referred to as a receiver because it receives the signal from the telephone line.

For extremely high gain applications, two receivers have been used back-to-back to cancel mechanical feedback caused by the vibrations produced by the receivers. The two receivers are essentially mounted tightly together, side by side, but with their orientations reversed so that their diaphragms move in opposite directions. The receivers are wired together to the same amplifier output terminals.

With dual receivers, mechanically induced feedback problems are reduced for high-level output signals because when the diaphragm of one receiver moves in one direction, the diaphragm of the other receiver moves in the opposite direction, thereby reducing the net vibration of the total assembly.

For more information on hearing aid receivers, the interested reader is referred to Madafarri and Stanley (1996).

Batteries

Present-Day Primary Batteries

Batteries provide power to the microphone, preamplifier, signal processor, output amplifier, and usually the receiver of the hearing aid. Almost all batteries used in today's hearing aids are the zinc air primary type.

Battery capacity is rated in milliampere-hours, the product of the number of hours a battery can deliver a particular current times the current. Battery companies have continued to increase the capacity of zinc air hearing aid batteries without increasing their size significantly by downsizing internal parts of the battery to allow room for more zinc. The instantaneous current a zinc air battery can provide, which may be a limiting factor for the highest power hearing aids, is determined in part by the number and size of its airholes.

The zinc air battery combines air from the environment with zinc inside the battery. Before use, the air intake hole(s) in zinc air batteries are covered to prevent the chemical reactions in the battery from starting while the batteries are stored. Once the tape tab is removed, the voltage rises quickly to ~1.3 V, and the expected life of the battery, if it not used at all or is lightly used, is typically ~6 weeks in many climates. This occurs because zinc air batteries are sensitive to the amount of humidity in the environment. Batteries must operate under widely varying climates, from the coldest winter day in Minnesota to the hottest and driest summer day in Arizona to the most humid summer day in Florida. In dry climates or when it is not being used, a zinc air battery may stop working when it experiences a "dry-out" phenomenon as water evaporates from the cell. In humid climates, a zinc air battery may stop working when water evaporates inside the cell.

In actual use of the battery, open circuit voltage (battery voltage without loading by the hearing aid) is less important than the operating voltage of the battery while it is being used. The operating voltage of a battery may actually fluctuate due to the hearing aid amplifiers demanding more or less current as the input signal varies. The operating voltage of a battery is determined by its open circuit voltage, the current being drawn by the hearing aid at a particular instant of time, and the output impedance of the battery, as represented by the following equation:

Instantaneous operating voltage = open circuit voltage

− (instantaneous current) × (battery output impedance)

Zinc air batteries have very low output impedance throughout the life of the battery. Output impedance of the

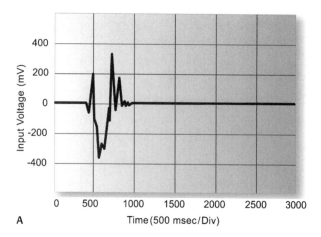

A

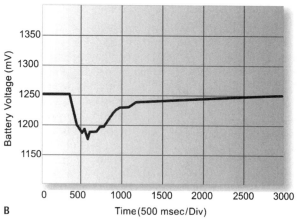

B

Figure 1–8 Effect of a high-level speech input on loaded battery voltage. **(A)** Input signal is /pa/ with an 88 dB peak sound pressure level. **(B)** Loaded battery voltage has up to a 60 mV dip during the speech segment.

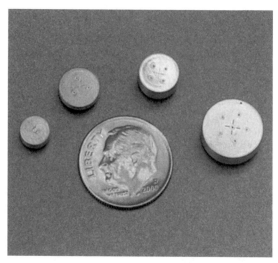

Figure 1–9 Four hearing aid battery sizes: 10A, 312, 13, and 675 (*left to right*).

battery is critical in some hearing aid circuits because of the pulsed inputs hearing aids are required to process. For example, the speech signals produced by hearing aid wearers are high-level, pulsing input signals, in the range of 75 to 80 dB SPL at the microphone inlet (Olsen, 1991). In hearing aid amplifier output stages, the current drain rises and falls as the input signal level to the hearing aid rises and falls. Excluding the effects of output-limiting compression, in general, the higher the input signal, the greater the peak current the output stage must draw. The voltage regulator, the part of the circuit that keeps the power supply voltage constant, could "drop out" (cease to function) because of insufficient loaded battery voltage.

If the battery cannot supply enough current to the output stage and signal-processing sections of the amplifier during peaks of the input signal, distortion results. **Fig. 1–8B** shows an example of the operating voltage of a hearing aid battery during a pulsed signal. Note that the voltage is significantly decreased during the peaks in the input signal **(Fig. 1–8A)**.

At the time of this writing, the most popular primary hearing aid battery sizes are the 10A, 312, 13, and 675 as shown left to right in **Fig. 1–9.**

Rechargeable Batteries

The hearing aid industry has known for many years that it is advantageous for hearing aid wearers not to have to keep changing batteries. Rechargeable batteries in sizes 13 and 675 have been used in hearing aids for many years. Early rechargeable systems for hearing aids used nickel cadmium(NiCd) batteries, which were known for their inability to continue charging after a few hundred cycles. Those custom hearing aids that incorporated a NiCd rechargeable battery inside the hearing aid rather than with a battery drawer had to be returned to the manufacturer for replacing the battery that could no longer be charged to provide near full capacity. More recently, nickel metal hydride (NiMH) batteries have become available in sizes 675 and 13, with greater capacity than that of the same-size NiCd cells. Also, the NiMH cells can be charged many more times than the NiCd cells without significant loss of capacity.

Current consumer electronics products such as digital cameras and laptop computers commonly use rechargeable lithium-based batteries. These have a higher voltage (> 3 V) than primary zinc air, NiCd, or NiMH hearing aid batteries. This technology is already incorporated in assistive listening devices for hearing aid wearers (Yanz, 2006).

Induction Coils

There are two problems in picking up acoustic signals with hearing aid microphones: (1) hearing aid wearers frequently have difficulty understanding telephone conversations in high ambient noise levels, and (2) when using the telephone, placing the telephone handset near the hearing aid, microphone inlet may cause acoustic feedback oscillation.

Although microphones are used most of the time in hearing aids to pick up acoustic signals, an induction coil pickup may be used alternatively to alleviate these two problems. Induction coils in hearing aids **(Fig. 1–10)** pick up magnetic signals from telephone receivers, neckloops, or room loops. The acoustic feedback path created by the telephone receiver

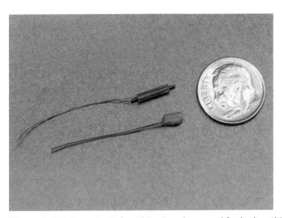

Figure 1–10 A passive telecoil (*top*) and an amplified telecoil (*bottom*).

cannot create an oscillation because signal pickup is inductive rather than acoustic, and the microphone is not used. Also, because only magnetic leakage from the telephone is picked up, environmental sounds are not transduced.

Alternating between microphone and telecoil traditionally has been achieved manually by the hearing aid wearer activating a switch. Most recently, switching between microphone and telecoil has become automatic, utilizing a tiny magnetic-sensing reed or silicon switch or a giant magnetoresistor (GMR) to sense the proximity of the direct current (DC) magnetic field in a telephone handset as it is brought close to the ear during phone use. The newest hearing aids have a fully programmable memory dedicated for telecoil use in which many parameters may be varied to optimize performance for individual wearers. During a telephone call, the hearing aid reacts to the magnetic field sensor by switching into a memory dedicated for telecoil. When the wearer is done with the telephone call and the telephone handset moves away from the hearing aid, these devices sense the drop in DC magnetic field and cause the hearing aid to switch back to a memory intended for microphone inputs. (Additionally, hearing aids with this feature are often programmed to switch the hearing aid back to the last memory used.) The magnetic sensing devices may also be used in hearing aids that do not have telecoils (e.g., CIC models) for switching them into a memory with parameter settings appropriate for acoustic telephone pickup via the microphone. These settings, for example, may provide most gain at lower frequencies (at which the speech signal level is highest) and less gain at higher frequencies at which the hearing aid may have acoustic feedback oscillation when the telephone handset is held over the ear. In this application, the magnetic sensing device could also signal the hearing aid DSP circuitry to recognize the nearby proximity of a telephone handset, thereby producing a feedback path change for the feedback cancellation algorithm.

Many induction coils have built-in preamplifiers to bring their output levels up to near that of hearing aid microphones. In addition, most modern hearing aid amplifiers contain an induction coil preamplifier (**Fig. 1–10**) whose gain and frequency response may be adjusted during programming for the individual hearing aid wearer.

To help ensure that adequate preamplification will be available for the induction coil, the hearing aid performance measurement standard ANSI S3.22–2003 recommends a procedure to determine differences in level between the microphone and induction coil in the hearing aid output. This measurement is called the Relative Simulated Equivalent Telephone Sensitivity (RSETS), which, if equal to 0 dB, indicates that the microphone and induction coil should produce about the same hearing aid output SPL at a given volume control setting (Teder, 2003).

Another important consideration is that the induction coil is sensitive to the direction from which the magnetic energy emanates. Good hearing aid design can alleviate this situation by orienting the induction coil in the hearing aid for the application(s) of most importance to the hearing aid wearer (e.g., telephone, audio room loops, or neckloops). Some hearing aids have their induction coils oriented horizontally to pick up sounds from telephones well but not sounds from audio room loops or neckloops. Other hearing aids have induction coils oriented vertically so they pick up sounds well from audio room loops and neckloops but not sounds from telephones. As a compromise, some hearing aids, especially BTE types, have their induction coils oriented at an angle so they can pick up sounds well from all three types of magnetic sources. It is important for those dispensing hearing aids to know how well a particular instrument will work in induction mode for the application(s) of most interest to the wearer. For more information on induction coils for hearing aids, refer to Madafarri and Stanley (1996).

Unfortunately, besides picking up the desired signal, an induction coil may transduce undesirable magnetic energy from sources such as power lines, computer monitors, transformers, fluorescent lights, and digital wireless telephones (Preves, 2003). If strong enough, these magnetic interference signals can make use of the induction coil very difficult because of the continuous hum or buzz produced in hearing aids.

Considerable attention has been focused on the interference signal generated in hearing aids by digital cellular and cordless telephones. The signal consists of an electrical field component and a magnetic field component. Hearing aid design engineers have attempted to prevent the magnetic component of the interference signal from getting into hearing aid induction coils, but the task is difficult because of the similar frequency range (audio baseband) of the desired and undesired signals. Hearing aid engineers have concluded that the magnetic audio frequency component of the interference signal is primarily the problem of the telephone companies to solve. One alternative being considered is to improve SNR by increasing the strength of the desired magnetic signal without increasing the noise signal emanating from telephones. As of this writing, hearing aid engineers are still working together with telephone company engineers in the ANSI C63 working group to evolve ANSI C63.19–2007 for cellular phones. Discussion about ANSI C63.19 appears in a later section of this chapter.

Hearing aid immunity to digital wireless telephone interference has improved by ~30 dB in the past 10 years (Victorian and Preves, 2004). To inform both hearing aid wearers and the dispensing community, the Hearing Industries Association has recently proposed language to the FDA for hearing aid manufacturers to voluntarily label their hearing aids with a digital cellular phone interference immunity rating per ANSI C63.19. (Most hearing aids now meet the M2 immunity rating). Adding this labeling value to the corresponding ANSI C63.19 cell phone emission rating label now required by the FCC predicts the degree of usability of the hearing aid with that cell phone. Although there are some exemptions, the FCC is now requiring a certain number of cell phones from each cell phone manufacturer and service providers to have at least an M3 rating for both radio frequency interference and induction coil coupling. An M2 hearing aid used with an M3 cell phone would have a total rating of 5, which would result in "normal usage" for the hearing aid wearer. At the time of this writing, there are indications that the number of cell phones required to be compatible for hearing aid telecoil coupling will be increased.

Additional efforts in the Telecommunications Industry Association's TIA-43.3 working group have resulted in standard measurement procedures for characterizing interference in hearing aids produced by digital cordless telephones (TIA-1083, 2007). Successful telecoil operation, in particular, is a serious challenge for many hearing aid wearers using digital cordless telephones. Currently, this working group is determining how to label cordless telephones per the TIA-1083 (2007) measurement standard.

◆ Compression and Expansion

The intact auditory system is capable of perceiving a wide range of sounds, from the quiet pitter-patter of rain to the loud boom of a clap of thunder. The most common complaint associated with hearing loss is the inability to hear weak sounds; average conversational speech may be barely audible,

whereas intense sounds are still perceived as being loud. It is tempting to try to alleviate a hearing loss by simply making sounds louder. Applying a fixed amount of amplification to all sounds makes weak sounds audible. However, average conversational speech may now be overly loud, and intense sounds are amplified beyond the loudness discomfort level (LDL), making them uncomfortably loud. Different amounts of gain must be applied to make weak sounds audible, average conversational speech comfortable, and intense sounds loud without being uncomfortable. As a result of such nonlinear amplification, the hearing aid user perceives the world of sounds in much the same way as a person with normal hearing. The exact manner in which nonlinear amplification, or compression, is applied depends on the goal of the hearing aid fitting as well as on the characteristics of the circuit.

Characteristics of a Compressor

The function and application of compression circuits are defined by their static and dynamic features. Static features, such as compression threshold and compression ratio, indicate the behavior of the circuit in response to steady input signals as illustrated by the input–output characteristic in **Fig. 1–11.** Dynamic features, such as attack time (AT) and release time (RT), describe the length of time required for the circuit to respond to a change in the level of the input signal (AT and RT in **Fig. 1–12**).

Compression Threshold

Compression threshold (CT) is defined as the input SPL (in dB) that, when applied to the hearing aid, reduces the gain by 2 (± 0.5) dB relative to the gain in the linear mode (International Electrotechnical Commission [IEC] 60118-2, 1983a). In other words, it is the point on the input–output (I/O) function at which the output first departs by 2 dB from the extension of the linear portion of the curve. Because it looks like the knee of a bent leg, the point at which the

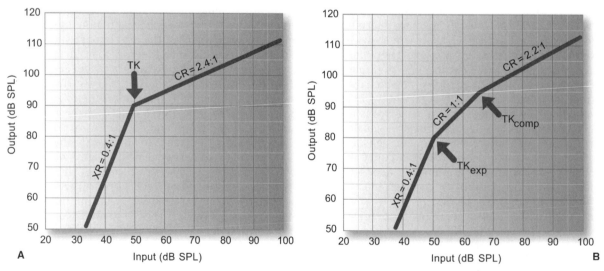

Figure 1–11 Static characteristics of compression and expansion. The threshold kneepoint (TK) for compression and expansion are the same in **(A)** but different in **(B)**. CR, compression ratio; SPL, sound pressure level; XR, expansion ratio.

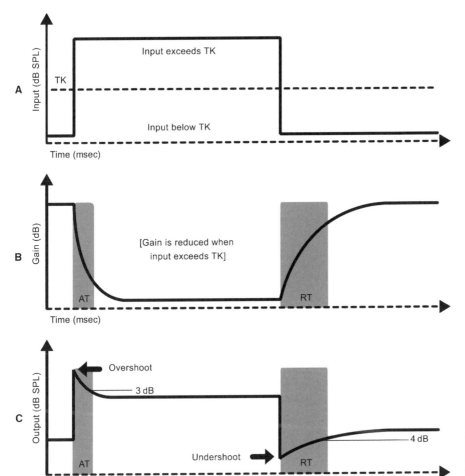

Figure 1–12 Dynamic characteristics of a compressor. **(A)** Changes in the input signal. **(B)** Changes in gain of the hearing aid. **(C)** Changes in output of the hearing aid. AT, attack time; RT, release time; SPL, sound pressure level; TK, threshold kneepoint.

slope of the I/O function changes is also referred to as the threshold kneepoint (TK) **(Fig. 1–11)**. The CT and TK are generally within a few decibels of each other, and the two terms are often used interchangeably.

Compression Ratio

Once the input signal has exceeded the TK, the compression ratio (CR) determines how much the signal will be compressed **(Fig. 1–11)**. Specifically, under steady-state conditions, it is the ratio of an input SPL difference (ΔInput) to the corresponding output SPL difference (ΔOutput; IEC 60118–2, 1983). CRs generally are expressed in terms of the number of decibels by which the input must change to effect a 1 dB change in output. Thus, for example, a CR of 2:1 indicates that a 2 dB change in input results in a 1 dB change in output. Because the reference condition is always a 1 dB change in output, the latter part of the ratio may be dropped (i.e., a CR of 2:1 may be expressed simply as 2).

Attack and Release Times

When the incoming signal changes significantly and abruptly, the gain of a hearing aid cannot react instantly. The dynamic characteristics refer to the length of time re-

quired for the compression circuit to respond to a sudden change in the input level.

Attack time is the time delay that occurs between the onset of an input signal above the TK and the resulting reduction of gain to its target value **(Fig. 1–12)**. Specifically, ANSI S3.22–2003 defines AT as the time between the abrupt increase in input level from 55 to 90 dB SPL and the point where the output level has stabilized to within 3 dB of the steady value for an input of 90 dB SPL. IEC standard 60118–2 defines AT as the time interval between the moment when the input signal level is increased abruptly by a stated number of decibels and the moment when the output SPL from the hearing aid stabilizes at the elevated steady-state level within ± 2 dB. According to IEC standard 60118–2, the AT for the normal dynamic range of speech is computed between input levels of 55 and 80 dB SPL, whereas the high-level AT is computed between 60 and 100 dB SPL. Because the gain of the hearing aid does not change immediately, the result is an overshoot in the output.

Release time is the time delay that occurs between the offset of an input signal below the TK and the resulting increase of gain to its target value **(Fig. 1–12)**. Specifically, ANSI S3.22–2003 defines RT as the interval between the abrupt drop in input level from 90 to 55 dB SPL and the point at which the output level has stabilized to within 4 dB of the steady value for an input of 55 dB SPL. IEC standard 60118–2 defines RT as the time interval between the moment when the input signal level is decreased abruptly by a stated number of decibels and the moment when the output SPL from the hearing aid stabilizes at the lower steady-state level within ± 2 dB. According to IEC standard 60118–2, the RT for the normal dynamic range of speech is computed between input levels of 80 and 55 dB SPL; the high-level RT is computed between 100 and 60 dB SPL. Because the gain of the hearing aid does not change immediately, the result is an undershoot in the output.

Some compression circuits incorporate adaptive or variable release times; that is, the RT is adjusted based on the duration and/or level of the triggering signal. Thus, if the input is a brief, transient sound, such as a door slam, the RT is short to have the least possible effect on the audibility of the speech that follows. A sustained input is indicative of a change in the overall level of sound in the environment. In this instance, a longer RT acts in much the same way as a manual adjustment of the volume control.

Pearl

- Although it is convenient to describe the static and dynamic characteristics of compression as discrete entities, they interact with each other in systematic ways. For example, CRs are determined from the response of the hearing aid to relatively steady signals, such as pure tones or speech-shaped noise. For time-varying inputs, such as speech, the CR is significantly affected by the AT and RT. When the AT and RT are short (i.e., shorter than the duration of a phoneme or syllable), the rapid gain changes amplify softer components more than louder components. The result is an effective CR for speech that is similar to that specified on the basis of steady signals. When the AT and RT are long (i.e., longer than the duration of a typical word or utterance), the gain does not change much between softer and louder phonemes. As a result, the effective CR for speech is much lower than would be expected for steady signals. Another example of the interaction between compression parameters is the observation that fast ATs and RTs are more detrimental to the perceived sound quality at high CRs than at low CRs (Neuman et al, 1998).

Types of Compression

At the present time, research offers no compelling reasons for setting a universally acceptable set of compression parameters. Thus, each must be adjusted to achieve a desired goal. Compression may be used to (1) limit the output of a hearing aid without distortion, (2) minimize loudness discomfort, (3) prevent further damage to the auditory system, (4) optimize use of the residual dynamic range, (5) restore normal perception of loudness, (6) maintain listening comfort, (7) maximize speech recognition ability, and (8) reduce the

adverse effects of noise. All of these applications can be achieved through compression limiting and wide dynamic range compression (WDRC).

Compression Limiting

Distortion, discomfort, and auditory system damage all have the same basis: intense sounds. Intense sounds force a hearing aid into saturation, causing distortion. They may be amplified beyond the individual's LDLs. Finally, if left unchecked, intense sounds entering a hearing aid may further damage the auditory system, causing amplification-induced hearing loss (Macrae, 1994). Although the latter two problems can be overcome simply by limiting the maximum output, compression limiting is the only way to prevent distortion. Desirable characteristics of a circuit designed for this purpose are as follows:

- A high TK (≥ 70 dB SPL) is used because the primary concern is with intense sounds.

- A high CR (> 8:1) is used to prevent the amplified sound from exceeding the LDL.

- A short AT minimizes the overshoot associated with a rapid increase in input level. Thus, ATs of 10 msec or less are generally used to limit the duration for which the output of the hearing aid exceeds the LDL.

- The RT is a less critical element because it is associated with decreasing input and output levels. That said, however, consider the situation where a pot dropping on a floor during a conversation forces the hearing aid into compression, resulting in a severe reduction in gain. If gain releases from compression limiting too slowly, the speech that follows may be inaudible. Thus, an RT of 100 msec or shorter would be preferred. A circuit with an adaptive release time may also be used.

- Single- or multichannel compression is suitable for this application.

Wide Dynamic Range Compression

As indicated earlier, hearing loss results in a loss of sensitivity for weak sounds, with little or no loss of sensitivity for intense sounds. Thus, for the range of environmental sounds to fit within the residual dynamic range of the individual, more amplification is required for weak sounds than for intense sounds. The net result is that weak sounds are audible, moderate sounds are comfortable, and intense sounds are perceived as loud without causing discomfort. This type of application is referred to as wide dynamic range compression. The following are some desirable characteristics of a circuit designed for this purpose:

- The TK is as low as possible to make weak sounds audible. Thus, the TK is typically set at or below 50 dB SPL. Hearing aids with TKs as low as 20 dB SPL are said to use full dynamic range compression (FDRC) because they aim to compress the entire gamut of sounds into the residual dynamic range of the individual.

- Low CRs of 4:1 or less can be used because compression acts over a wider range of inputs. Mueller (personal communication, 2005) gives the example that WDRC is akin to gentle braking as one approaches a stop sign while driving. (By the same token, compression limiting is more like screeching to a halt at the last minute.)

- Attack and release times may be short or long. When the ATs and RTs are shorter than the duration of a syllable (~40 msec), softer consonants are amplified more than the louder vowels. Increasing the consonant-to-vowel ratio (CVR)—i.e., the intensity of the consonant relative to that of the vowel—in this manner has been shown to improve speech understanding (Montgomery and Edge, 1988). However, several studies have shown that short ATs and RTs significantly degrade sound quality, especially if the TK is very low (Neuman et al, 1998; Woods et al, 1999). For such cases, ATs and RTs between 100 msec and 2 sec are known to cause a pumping sensation where the level of the background (or ambient) noise increases audibly during pauses and decreases when speech is present.

- Multichannel compression is used to accommodate a variety of audiometric configurations. Trine and van Tasell (2002) have shown that three or four channels are generally adequate to fit most audiometric configurations, provided that the crossover frequencies are adjustable.

Pitfall

- A word of caution against assumptions about the function of various compression controls. For example, consider the commonly held notion that the gain for weak sounds can be decreased by increasing the TK. Although this may be true in some cases, other compression schemes may result in decreased gain for all sounds. Yet other compression schemes may actually increase the gain for moderate to intense sounds when the TK is increased. Apart from not accomplishing the primary goal, this could give rise to a secondary complaint of sounds being too loud. The issue is not one of a right or wrong method of implementation, but rather an understanding of the underlying compression architecture.

Expansion

Issues Arising from Wide Dynamic Range Compression

Compared with linear amplification, WDRC provides additional gain for weak sounds. The advantage of this approach is increased intelligibility of soft speech and normalized loudness perception. The disadvantage is that other soft sounds, such as the drone of a refrigerator, the creaking of floorboards, and the hum of an air conditioner, are also amplified. How can this be a disadvantage when a person with normal hearing is able to hear these everyday sounds?

The onset of presbycusis, the most common cause of hearing loss in adults, is typically insidious. As a result, by the time the hearing loss becomes noticeable to the individual, many of the weaker sounds in the environment may not have been heard for some time. Because WDRC enables amplification of weak sounds to within the audible range, this can be overwhelming to an auditory system that has been deprived for a long period of time. On a different note, individuals who have good residual hearing at some frequencies may be able to hear the noise that is inherent to the hearing aid (i.e., circuit noise). Either of these scenarios may produce an unpleasant experience and result in hearing aids spending most of their time in a drawer. To avoid this rejection, the problem must be addressed.

Expansion is a viable alternative to simply reducing the amount of gain provided for weak sounds. Expansion is designed to make a hearing aid sound silent in quiet environments. One can think of it as a noise reduction strategy for quiet environments. The use of expansion can lead to greater listener satisfaction by reducing the intensity of weak environmental sounds and circuit noise, without sacrificing speech audibility and intelligibility. In hearing aids, expansion is applied only to weak sounds. The principle behind expansion is that the weakest of the weak sounds are amplified less than the more intense components. As a result, the weakest sounds are kept below the individual's dynamic range of hearing, and only the more intense components are audible.

Characteristics of Expansion

Expansion is characterized in much the same way as compression, by an expansion threshold, expansion ratio, and attack and release times. There are, however, a few key differences that will be highlighted here. (Note: At the time of this writing, there are no standards for defining the characteristics of expansion.) Attack and release times are defined, described, and used in the same way for both compression and expansion.

- *Expansion Threshold* Expansion threshold (XT) is the input level below which expansion operates **(Fig. 1–11)**. Because it looks like a bent knee in an input–output function, the XT is also referred to as a TK. The potential for confusion arises when expansion is coupled with compression, both of which are characterized by a TK. The TKs for both expansion (TK_{exp}) and compression (TK_{comp}) frequently occur at the same input level. However, the TK_{comp} may be higher than the TK_{exp}. In either case, expansion always acts below the TK (or TK_{exp}), and compression always acts above the TK (or TK_{comp}).

- *Expansion Ratio* Like its counterpart in compression, the expansion ratio (XR) is an indicator of the extent to which the input signal is expanded **(Fig. 1–11)**. The XR is calculated as a ratio of the change in input level (ΔInput) to the change in output level (ΔOutput). CRs are always > 1 when compression is applied, and a larger number indicates a greater degree of compression. In contrast, the application of expansion is signaled by XRs between 0 and 1. Furthermore, the smaller the XR (i.e., closer to 0), the greater the degree of expansion.

For a more detailed discussion of compression and expansion, the reader is referred to Banerjee (2006) and Dillon (2001).

♦ Digital Signal Processing

An advantage of digital processing is that very sophisticated manipulations of the input signal can be performed. Some algorithms implemented with DSP are not even possible using analog circuitry. However, one should keep in mind that DSP circuitry in itself does not guarantee better hearing performance for a hearing aid wearer than analog signal processing (see, e.g., Boymans et al, 1999; Valente et al, 1999). Although most state-of-the-art hearing aids are referred to as being digital or using DSP, they all still must have a minimum amount of analog circuitry to preamplify the analog signal inputs from microphones and telecoils.

There are two main types of DSP hearing aid circuits: (1) the open platform, in which new signal-processing algorithms may be implemented via firmware changes as they become available, and (2) the fixed platform types, in which algorithms designed for a restricted set of specific applications are implemented in hardware that cannot be changed. Different hearing aid manufacturers using the same open platform DSP circuitry can provide features distinguishing their hearing aids from other manufacturers' products by using different signal-processing algorithms.

Almost all DSP hearing aids are also digitally programmable, with the parameter settings for their digital filters stored in memory. Adjustable parameters that may be altered during a fitting session of DSP hearing aids include gain and crossover frequencies between channels and bands. A band is a portion of the entire frequency range of the hearing aid in which signal amplitude is adjustable. Most current DSP hearing aids have at least three bands, and some have up to dozens of bands. A channel is a portion of the entire frequency range of the hearing aid in which specific signal processing is performed. Parameters such as CR, CT, and RT may have one set of values in a particular channel and another set of values in an adjacent channel. A channel may consist of one or more bands.

In a DSP hearing aid, memories store algorithms as well as parameter values for the DSP circuitry. There can be several memories (or programs) that correspond to several acoustical listening environments. One memory is usually dedicated to listening in a quiet environment; another memory may be more suited for noisy situations, whereas still other memories store settings for using the telephone and other applications.

Current developments in hearing aid technology have used advancements made in fields such as semiconductors and wireless, as well as other fields outside the industry. For example, the latest DSP developments in hearing aids are possible because the feature sizes (smallest geometric spacing) on complementary metal oxide semiconductor (CMOS) integrated circuitry have been getting small enough to incorporate enough DSP circuitry to perform powerful algorithms such as noise reduction and feedback cancellation. As the feature size of integrated circuitry technology gets smaller, the amount of processing power and the speed of hearing aid DSP circuits continue to increase, while the current required from the hearing aid battery stays about the same or decreases.

Directionality

Directional processing in hearing aids is the only proven way to improve speech understanding in noise by increasing the SNR. This is done by reducing the sensitivity of the hearing aid to sounds coming from the rear and/or sides without affecting the sensitivity to sounds in front of the wearer. Although the basic principle of directionality is realized through acoustical or electronic means (discussed earlier), the use of DSP allows the implementation of advanced algorithms, such as dynamic, adaptive, and multiband directionality.

Dynamic Directionality

Although few would argue against the benefits of directional technology in hearing aids, Walden and colleagues (2004) reported that hearing aid users generally prefer the directional mode over the omnidirectional mode only in the presence of background noise and when the speech signal is located near and in front of the listener. These conditions account for ~33% of the total time that the hearing aid user is actively engaged in listening. Furthermore, ~25% of all users of directional hearing aids are unable or unwilling to appropriately use the directional mode (Cord et al, 2002). From these data, it can be concluded that directional technology is a desirable feature, although it is not appropriate for use under all listening conditions or by all individuals.

Dynamic, or automatic, directionality is an algorithm that allows the hearing aid to switch automatically between the omnidirectional and directional modes, depending on the characteristics of the environment. Although the details of implementation vary from one algorithm to the next, there are several general criteria to determine switching between the two modes: input level, SNR, and signal location. Not all of these criteria are necessarily used in all hearing aids with dynamic directionality, and they may be used in combination.

Quiet, indoor environments have ambient noise levels of 45 dB SPL or lower (Pearsons et al, 1977), whereas environments characterized as noisy are known to have long-term average levels upwards of 60 dB SPL (Keidser, 1995). If the purpose of a directional microphone is to reduce the amount of noise entering the device, then it follows that a hearing aid must be in the directional mode at moderate-to-high input levels. One reason for not switching to the directional mode at lower input levels is the presence of circuit noise. There is an inherent decrease in the sensitivity of directional microphones (typically in the low frequencies), relative to omnidirectional microphones, to sounds located at 0 degrees azimuth and elevation. Depending on the hearing loss, this low-frequency roll-off may be compensated for by increasing the gain of the hearing aid. However, this has the negative side effect of amplifying the internal noise of the hearing aid to within the audible range.

Pearsons et al (1977) also reported that the +10 dB SNR necessary for near-perfect intelligibility of sentences is maintained at and below noise levels of 45 dB SPL. For levels between 48 and 70 dB SPL, people begin to raise their voices at the rate of 0.6 dB per decibel increase in ambient noise level. In other words, at the upper end of the range, communication must occur at SNRs of −3 dB. Speech recognition is known to decrease as the SNR decreases. It follows that, at poor SNRs, any improvement that can be provided by directional microphones is sorely needed. Ricketts and colleagues (2005) showed greater directional benefit for poorer SNRs. Although +10 dB SNR yields 100% correct speech recognition in individuals with normal hearing, the same cannot be said of those with hearing impairment. Killion (2004) reported that ~50% of individuals with hearing loss have an SNR loss of at least 5 dB. Thus, there is benefit to be gained by switching to the directional mode even at relatively good SNRs.

The premise of directional design in hearing aids is that the signal of interest is always in the frontal hemisphere. It is not uncommon, however, for the signal to be located to the side or in the rear hemisphere. For example, at meetings, it is important to be able to hear comments made by a fellow participant who is seated adjacent to, or even behind, the hearing aid user. The dynamic directionality algorithm may be constrained to remain in the omnidirectional mode under such conditions. In contrast, the directional mode is preferred when the sound in the rear hemisphere is known to be noise.

Another design consideration for dynamic directionality is the time required to transition between the omnidirectional and directional modes. A rapid rate allows the hearing aid to respond quickly to changes in the environment, such as walking into a noisy restaurant. On the downside, rapid transitions cause the hearing aid to respond to brief transient sounds in the environment, such as a cough or a door slam. Indeed, this was the primary drawback of the first generation of algorithms, leading hearing aid users to complain about a sensation of motion sickness. Although there are no guidelines for the rate of switching between modes, it may be argued that slower is better.

The results of field trials from Olson et al (2004) indicate that dynamic directionality functions as desired for most people in most environments—that is, the mode (omnidirectional or directional) selected automatically by the algorithm—was the same as that preferred by the hearing aid user. There were exceptions to this rule, however. For example, one participant reported that, when she was at the playground, the hearing aid automatically switched to the directional mode, but she preferred the omnidirectional mode because wind noise was more tolerable in the latter. In summary, although the decision-making criteria are far from perfect, dynamic directionality appears to work well in most environments. Moreover, an individual's preference may be related to factors other than the acoustics of the environment. As an example, automatic switching is perhaps

most useful for individuals who are unable or unwilling to manually switch the hearing aid between the omnidirectional and directional modes.

Adaptive Directionality

The exact location of the null in a directional polar pattern depends on the relationship of the physical distance between the front and rear microphones (i.e., the external delay) and the internal delay at the rear microphone. Thus, for instance, a cardioid polar pattern (**Fig. 1–5A**) results when the internal and external delays are exactly equal. In contrast, the lack of an internal delay produces a bidirectional polar pattern. Whatever the underlying philosophy, directional technology places the null of the polar response at a fixed location. Unfortunately, noise sources in real environments do not occur conveniently in the same location all the time for all individuals. Even if it were possible, the average hearing aid user has neither the knowledge nor the understanding of the technology to enforce this requirement by adjusting the listening environment. Furthermore, one often encounters listening situations where there is relative motion between noise sources and the listener. Having a conversation with someone by the side of a busy street is an example of such a situation—every noisy truck that rumbles by virtually obliterates the sound of the speaker's voice.

Adaptive directionality refers to an algorithm that allows the polar pattern of the hearing aid to change depending on the environment. At the present time, this is achieved by using two omnidirectional microphones and by electronically altering the internal delay. The algorithm computes the polar pattern that provides the largest reduction in noise level. In theory, the azimuth/elevation of the null of the polar pattern selected should coincide with the location of the noise source. The only constraint on the location of the null is that it is never placed in the frontal hemisphere, because the target signal is assumed to be located in that area. Another practical consideration for selection of polar patterns is the time required to evaluate all possible solutions. Currently, hearing aids take anywhere from a few milliseconds to a few seconds to switch from one polar pattern to another. Although there are no guidelines for how long this should take, shorter time constants would appear to be advantageous in tracking a moving noise source.

Ricketts and Henry (2002) evaluated fixed and adaptive directionality under a variety of conditions in the laboratory. The speech signal was always located at 1.25 m in front of the listener. The stationary noise conditions included a diffuse noise field and a discrete noise to the side or behind the listener. In the panning noise conditions, the noise was panned between adjacent speakers over the course of a single sentence. Although testing was conducted in a relatively reverberant environment, the speech and noise sources were placed within the critical distance of the room. The results indicated a significant adaptive advantage, especially when the noise was located to the side. The authors concluded that adaptive directionality is advantageous for discrete noise sources and when reverberation is of minimal concern. Ricketts et al (2005) subsequently corroborated this finding. Furthermore, the latter study found comparable performance with two- and three-microphone implementations of adaptive directionality.

In summary, adaptive directionality is perhaps best described as being superior to fixed directionality only under very specific listening conditions: when a discrete noise source is located very close to the listener in an otherwise quiet environment. When the noise conditions are diffuse and/or the environment is reverberant, adaptive systems generally default to a hypercardioid polar pattern that provides the highest DI. Put differently, although it does not reduce speech understanding in noise, adaptive directionality probably does not improve it further (over fixed directionality) under most everyday listening conditions.

Controversial Point

- Although sound in principle, research has not shown adaptive directionality to be unequivocally superior to fixed directionality under realistic listening conditions. Indeed, Bentler and colleagues (2004) reported no perceptible advantage over fixed directionality in localization ability or perceived benefit during field trials. There are three primary factors affecting real-world utility of adaptive directionality.

- Ricketts and Hornsby (2003) showed that directional benefit is significantly reduced in moderate-to-high levels of reverberation (RT_{60} = 900 msec) when speech is located outside the critical distance of the test room.

- An adaptive system defaults to the hypercardioid pattern in reverberant environments (Woods and Trine, 2004) or when the noise is relatively diffuse (Ricketts et al, 2005).

- The difference in level between a diffuse noise field and a discrete noise source found in typical listening environments (~8 dB) is not sufficient to show an adaptive advantage (Bentler et al, 2004; Ricketts et al, 2005).

Multiband Directionality

Inherent to the premise of dynamic and adaptive directionality is the assumption that the selected mode or polar pattern is appropriate across the entire range of frequencies. There may be situations where the omnidirectional mode is better at some frequencies, whereas the directional mode is optimal at other frequencies. Wind is an example of one such environment. As a result of compensation for the loss of sensitivity at low frequencies, the noise generated by wind turbulence is louder in the directional mode than in the omnidirectional mode. Thus, despite the noise, the omnidirectional mode may be preferable to the directional mode under such conditions. Noise from wind is dominated by energy at low frequencies. It may be argued, then, that, whereas the omnidirectional mode is appropriate at low frequencies, the directional

mode may still offer some advantage at high frequencies and aid in speech understanding.

Multiband directionality is an algorithm that automatically selects the optimal mode, omnidirectional or directional, independently in various frequency regions. Theoretically, if speech is mixed with wind noise, for example, as is the case when having a conversation outdoors on a windy day, the omnidirectional mode minimizes the impact of wind noise at low frequencies, and the directional mode maximizes speech intelligibility (by improving the SNR) at high frequencies. Apart from its frequency-dependent nature, the parameters for multiband directionality are essentially the same as those for broadband adaptive directionality. This includes the decision criteria and the time constants for switching.

The premise of multiband directionality is that multiple noise sources are frequently present in everyday environments. Furthermore, these noises must occur in different regions of the frequency spectrum and are located at different azimuths/elevations. The main argument against realizing the hypothetical benefits of multiband directionality over broadband directionality is that the signals and noises that occur in our everyday environment cover a broad range of the frequency spectrum. Indeed, Kochkin (2002a) reports that hearing aid users are least satisfied with their ability to understand speech in restaurants and in large groups, where the background noise has much the same spectral characteristics as the speech signal. Thus, despite the theoretical advantages, there are few data to support the benefits of multiband directionality over broadband directionality in everyday life. Perhaps the most significant contribution of this technology lies in alleviating the loudness discomfort associated with wind noise.

The primary advantage of directionality comes from the multimicrophone technology itself. The role of directional DSP algorithms is to make the technology more user-friendly and, under certain conditions, optimize the parameters to improve speech recognition. The importance and relevance of these improvements vary across hearing aid users and depend on their individual needs. For a more detailed discussion of directionality, the interested reader is referred to Dillon (2001) and Ricketts and Dittberner (2002).

Feedback Reduction

Audible feedback oscillation is among the most prominent problems with hearing aids (Kochkin, 2002b). In some cases, the annoyance associated with the problem may be sufficient to negate the perceived benefits of amplification, resulting in nonuse of the hearing aid.

Feedback may be mechanical or acoustic. Mechanical feedback occurs when the mechanical vibrations from the receiver are picked up by the microphone of the hearing aid. The transmission of vibrations is direct when the two components are in close proximity to each other. Vibrations also may be transmitted indirectly through the shell or case of the device. The obvious solution to reducing mechanical feedback is physical isolation of the microphone and receiver from each other as well as from the shell or case of the hearing aid. Although hearing aid manufacturers are careful to ensure that mechanical feedback does not occur, everyday wear and tear may take a toll on the device. At the present time, the best way to address mechanical feedback is to return the hearing aid to the manufacturer for repair.

Acoustic feedback occurs when the output of the receiver leaks out of the ear canal and enters the microphone of the hearing aid. This acoustic leakage may be intentional, such as through a vent, or unintentional, in the form of slit leaks around the edges of the hearing aid or earmold. Together, these sources of leakage constitute the acoustic feedback path. Because it is virtually impossible to seal the ear canal hermetically with a hearing aid or earmold without causing discomfort, this leakage is a common occurrence. The acoustic leakage is often attenuated considerably by the physical presence of the hearing aid or earmold itself; that is, the feedback path is small. Each time the sound feeding back enters the microphone, it is reamplified along with all the other sounds entering the hearing aid. This does not pose a problem as long as the amount of attenuation is greater than the gain of the hearing aid. When the gain does exceed the amount of attenuation, the signal feeding back is amplified further each time it goes around the loop from the microphone to the receiver to the ear canal and back to the microphone. Ultimately, the feedback signal grows strong enough to become unstable and create an audible oscillation, commonly referred to as a ring, whistle, or squeal. The conditions necessary for audible feedback oscillation are met when the degree of attenuation is small (e.g., in the presence of a large vent or improperly fitting device) and/or when the gain of the hearing aid is high. A second requirement for audible feedback oscillation to occur is that the feedback signal must be in exactly the same phase (i.e., an integer multiple of 360) as the input signal at the microphone.

Traditionally, audible feedback oscillations have been addressed by plugging vents and reducing slit leaks, limiting the amount of gain at the time of the fitting, or manually reducing the volume control during hearing aid use. The drawback of either method is that it adversely affects the audibility and/or loudness of all sounds as well as the intelligibility of speech. Because audible feedback oscillations are most likely to occur at or near the peaks of the frequency response, another approach to alleviating this problem is to shift the primary peak of the frequency response. This technique is not always reliable for eliminating audible feedback oscillation because the problem may still occur at a different frequency.

With the advent of the DSP era, audible feedback oscillation can be minimized without significantly sacrificing gain, audibility, loudness, and speech intelligibility. DSP-based electronic methods for minimizing audible feedback oscillations are desirable for three reasons. First, they permit greater amounts of usable gain; this is especially important for individuals with severe or profound hearing loss or when a smaller style of device is desired. Second, they allow the provision of adequate gain with an open earmold or a shell with a large vent. Third, certain types of feedback controls can adapt to changing environments, such as when a telephone is placed close to the ear.

Dynamic Feedback Management by Gain Reduction

The primary shortcoming of the traditional gain limitation approach is that it is in effect at all times (or, at least, most of the time). That is, lower than optimal amounts of gain are provided to the listener even under conditions where audible feedback oscillations do not pose a problem. Dynamic feedback management is a variation on the gain limitation or reduction theme. Rather than limiting it at all times, gain is affected only when the system becomes unstable. An obvious implication is that the system must be monitored constantly for the presence of feedback oscillations. Although audibility, loudness, and speech intelligibility may still be affected when the feedback management algorithm is engaged (i.e., when the gain is reduced), the hearing aid amplifies as intended at other times. Variables affecting the effectiveness of the algorithm include the bandwidth, amount, and rate of gain reduction. In general, a large amount of gain reduction over a wide frequency range lowers the likelihood of audible feedback oscillation, but it may also affect audibility, loudness, and speech intelligibility. Highly flexible algorithms allow different amount of gain reduction simultaneously at multiple frequencies. Furthermore, the amount of gain reduction is proportionate to the magnitude of the feedback oscillation. Because the algorithm depends on the detection of oscillation, a small amount of audible feedback oscillation often occurs before the gain is reduced. Rapid reduction of gain minimizes the duration of this "whoop" of audible feedback oscillation.

Feedback Path Cancellation

One deficiency of many feedback reduction techniques is that they involve some amount of reduction in gain. Although often small, the effect of gain reduction can be significant. For example, in hearing aids with WDRC, audible feedback oscillations are most likely to occur for weak inputs when the gain is at its highest. Gain reduction under such conditions may severely affect audibility.

Rather than automatically manipulating the gain of the hearing aid, feedback path cancellation (FBC) algorithms introduce an additional feedback signal to cancel out the acoustic leakage. As shown in **Fig. 1–13A,** acoustic leakage that is sufficiently large mixes a significant amount of feedback with the input to the hearing aid. When feedback is detected at the output stage of the hearing aid, the feedback canceller generates another "cancellation" signal to mimic the feedback (i.e., with the same frequency, phase, and level [or magnitude] characteristics; **Fig. 1–13B**). The feedback is then canceled by subtracting the cancellation signal from the input. Because FBC algorithms simply cancel out the unwanted feedback, this technique of feedback reduction should result in an improvement or increase in the maximum stable gain (MSG) with the feedback canceller operating relative to the condition without a feedback canceller. MSG is the greatest

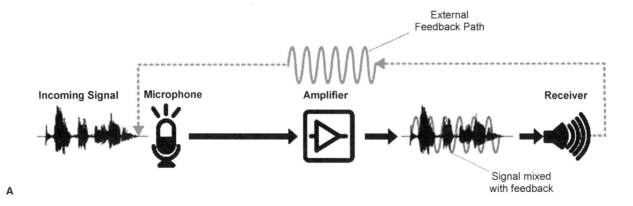

A

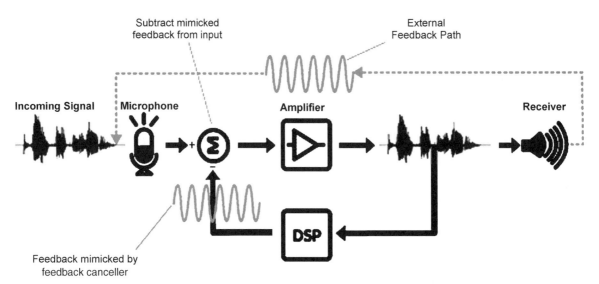

B

Figure 1–13 Schematic representation of the principle of feedback path cancellation. **(A)** Acoustic feedback mixed with the input to the hearing aid. **(B)** Feedback canceller that mimics the feedback signal and subtracts it from the input, resulting in no audible feedback oscillation at the output of the hearing aid. DSP, digital signal processing.

amount of gain that can be provided without interference from audible feedback oscillation. Practical considerations, such as the processing capabilities of the DSP chip in a hearing aid and environmental acoustics, limit the potential improvement in MSG to between 15 and 25 dB (Kates, 2001; Merks et al, 2006).

Although not essential, knowledge of the characteristics of the acoustic leakage improves the effectiveness of the feedback canceller. This information may be gathered by means of an "initialization" performed in the clinic. The principle of an initialization is simple: the external feedback path can be measured by comparing a known signal at the output of the receiver (i.e., in the ear canal) and at the microphone of the hearing aid. During an initialization, a broadband noise with a known spectrum (e.g., white noise) is played through the hearing aid. The frequency, level, and phase response of the initialization signal detected at the microphone of the hearing aid indicates the amount of attenuation provided by the physical presence of the hearing aid and the frequency regions in which feedback

is most likely to pose a problem. Initialization of the feedback canceller must be performed in a relatively quiet environment to avoid contamination of the signal detected by the microphone.

The threat of audible feedback oscillation remains a real possibility even after an initialization has been performed because the feedback path does not remain constant over time. Movements of the jaw and head, variations in insertion of the hearing aid or earmold into the ear canal, and the presence of objects such as a telephone near the hearing aid all change the characteristics of the acoustic leakage. Under such conditions, adaptive FBC is most effective because it can accommodate changing feedback paths. A negative side effect of some adaptive FBC algorithms may be the occurrence of entrainment artifacts. Entrainment occurs when the feedback canceller mistakenly attempts to cancel a tonal input to the hearing aid. This results in the addition of a tone to the original by the hearing aid itself. The hearing aid user may report hearing the additional tone, feedback after the original sound has stopped, or a modulation-type distortion of the sound. On a bright note, entrainment does not pose a problem for all hearing aid users; in fact, entrainment may be least problematic for those with larger acoustic leakages, who are most susceptible to feedback.

Pearl

- Adaptive feedback cancellation is essential to accommodate changes in the feedback path, such as placing a telephone by the ear or putting on a hat. However, as discussed above, because of the difficulty in differentiating a tonal signal from feedback, adaptive systems are prone to entrainment artifacts. Entrainment artifacts can be eliminated by using a static feedback canceller. Thus, the goals of adapting to a changing feedback path and minimizing the occurrence of artifacts are contradictory. It is relatively easy to achieve one goal or the other. The hallmark of a good feedback canceller is striking the right balance between the two extremes.

Although there are no standards for defining the performance of feedback reduction algorithms, efforts are currently under way to benchmark the effectiveness of such algorithms (Merks et al, 2006; Freed and Soli, 2006). Future improvements in such algorithms may include reliable prediction of system instability to prevent audible feedback oscillation and reduction of the undesirable artifacts associated with adaptive feedback path cancellation. For a more detailed discussion of feedback and the methods to reduce audible oscillation, the reader is referred to Dillon (2001).

Occlusion Management

The occlusion effect was originally described in the context of improved low-frequency bone-conduction thresholds when the ear was occluded with an earphone (Tonndorf, 1972). The hypothesis is that the bone conductor sets up vibrations within the ear canal. The low-frequency energy generated by these vibrations can escape through the ear canal of an unoccluded ear. However, in the occluded condition, this excess energy becomes trapped within the ear canal and is transmitted to the cochlea in much the same way as an air-conducted signal. A similar scenario occurs when the earphone is replaced by a hearing aid, and the bone conductor is replaced by the person's own voice. That is, occluding the ear canal with a hearing aid may result in a buildup of low- frequency energy every time the individual speaks as laryngeal vibrations are transmitted to the ear canal via bone conduction. This may result in complaints regarding a "hollow," "echoey," or "boomy" quality to the person's own voice.

Traditional methods for addressing occlusion include greater depth of fit, increased vent size, and decreased low-frequency gain. Vibration of the cartilaginous portion of the ear canal can be minimized by physically sealing the hearing

aid within the bony portion of the ear canal (Killion et al, 1988). However, this method has typically been unacceptable due to discomfort, especially with hard-walled earmolds and earshells. A second method, increasing vent size, is a common approach for dealing with own-voice problems; however, there is some evidence of a lack of relationship between acoustically measured low-frequency energy in the ear canal and the perception of occlusion (Kampe and Wynne, 1996). Furthermore, the largest vent size that can be used is limited by the potential for audible feedback oscillation. Finally, although reducing the amount of low-frequency energy in the ear canal by decreasing the gain of the hearing aid is an acceptable solution to the hollow-voice problem (Kuk et al, 1992), it may adversely affect the perception of speech and does not address the true cause of occlusion.

Pitfall

- Occlusion is only one of several sources of complaints related to the quality of one's own voice and hearing aid use. Too much or too little amplification, delays introduced by the DSP, distortion, and previous experience with hearing aids (or lack thereof) may give rise to similar complaints. Although each of these causes has a legitimate basis, none is truly related to the buildup of low-frequency energy that results from occluding the ear canal.

The word *open* is applied to hearing aid fittings that use a nonoccluding earmold (**Fig. 1–2**). One might think of it as a very large vent that allows low-frequency energy to escape from the ear canal. As such, the primary application of an open fitting is in the reduction of complaints associated with occlusion. Although this concept is not new, it has seen resurgence in recent years for several reasons, including improved cosmetics and the ability to instantly fit the device using one-size-fits-most eartips. However, the single most important advancement, related to signal processing, has been in the provision of greater amounts of gain with less risk of audible feedback oscillation. The feedback cancellation technology that enables this capability was discussed previously.

Dynamic Gain Reduction

Although reduction in low-frequency gain has long been used to counter the occlusion effect, it has an undesirable impact on the perception of all sounds. Because the primary complaint about occlusion is related to the perception of one's own voice, it follows that any low-frequency gain reduction should ideally be applied only when the talker is the hearing aid user. The critical assumption here is that it is possible to distinguish between a speaker's own voice and that of others. Speaker recognition techniques have been used in other fields for the purposes of automatic speech recognition, speaker verification, and biometric identification. Due to constraints on the processing speed

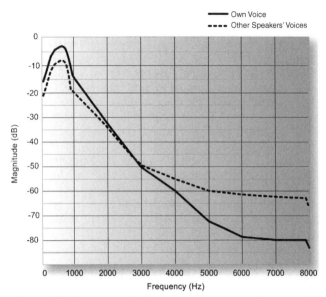

Figure 1–14 Representative long-term average speech spectra of a speaker's own voice and the voices of others.

and memory size, the analysis techniques typically used for these purposes may not be suitable for application in hearing aids in the near future.

Because the sound source is within a few inches of the hearing aid microphone as opposed to a few feet away, the hearing aid user's own voice has unique features related to the near-field effect. **Figure 1–14** shows the long-term average spectra of an individual's own voice and the voices of other speakers. The recordings were made at the listeners' ear, and the data are averaged across 13 individuals, 6 female and 7 male. Two differences are immediately noticeable. First, the individual's own voice contains significantly more low-frequency energy than other speakers' voices. Second, the spectral slope is much steeper for the individual's own voice (i.e., high-frequency energy drops off at a more rapid rate) than for the voices of others. At a rudimentary level, features such as these may be applied to identify the hearing aid user's own voice.

Once it has been determined that the detection of a speaker's own voice can be performed with reasonable accuracy, there remain a few unresolved issues: the magnitude and rate of low-frequency gain reduction and the training of the occlusion management algorithm. As mentioned previously, the subjective perception of occlusion appears to be unrelated to objective measurement. Thus, when a client reports a problem with occlusion, the clinician must arrive at the optimum settings mostly through trial and error. Reducing the gain by too much may result in sounds not being loud enough, whereas a small gain reduction may be imperceptible to the user. In most situations, speech occurs in the context of a discourse where the utterances are short and alternate between the speaking partners at a rapid rate. The process of detecting the speaker's own voice requires time, and there is bound to be a delay between the time that the person starts talking and the reduction of gain. Neuman et al (1998) showed that rapid

adaptation of gain, especially by large amounts, adversely affects sound quality. However, adapting too slowly may result in hearing aid users perceiving no relief from occlusion or, worse, inadvertent reduction of others' voices rather than their own. Finally, if the algorithm depends on the characteristics of a given talker, it follows that detection accuracy could be increased by training the algorithm. Training may take only a few minutes and may involve the individual reading a predetermined passage to provide the algorithm with a clean speech sample. In reality, because of time pressures in the clinic, this additional step may be overshadowed by more apparent issues, such as audible feedback oscillation.

Despite its potential for success, reduction of occlusion by dynamic reduction of low-frequency gain is a symptomatic treatment of the matter. The real problem is the buildup of low-frequency energy in the ear canal due to vibrations transmitted via bone conduction. Future improvements call for true occlusion cancellation, which involves eliminating the problem at its source without affecting the signal processing of the hearing aid itself. For example, much like a feedback canceller, the hearing aid may generate a signal to cancel out the excess energy in the ear canal. The trick lies in detecting the buildup of energy and determining its characteristics.

Environment Classification and Adaptation

Pattern classification is a scientific discipline with the goal of sorting inputs into various classes or categories. These inputs can take various forms, including images, odors, and sounds. Environment classification is the specific application of the principles of pattern classification to the acoustic inputs arriving at the microphone(s) of a hearing aid. Whereas speech is arguably the single most important signal in a listener's environment, amplification aimed at maximizing speech intelligibility may be less than optimal under certain conditions. Although many hearing aids offer the flexibility of manual adjustment at the push of a button or turn of a wheel, many individuals are unable or reluctant to "fuss" with their hearing aids. From the point of view of the hearing aid user, the goals are simple: maximum intelligibility for speech with minimum interference from background noise, and optimum listening comfort and sound quality in all environments. Prior to the advent of DSP, these goals were somewhat contradictory and difficult, at best, to achieve simultaneously.

The problems of separating speech from noise, or minimizing background noise, are being tackled in many areas of audio processing, such as cellular phones and music. Noise-canceling headphones are a popular application of noise reduction at the present time. There are several challenges unique to environment classification in hearing aids. First, the signal arriving at the ear is degraded by the presence of noise and/or reverberation in the environment. Second, it is difficult to isolate the desired signal from the undesirable noise. Third, DSP in hearing aids is severely limited in computational horsepower (because of the small size of the chip) and by current consumption. Fourth, there is considerable individual variability in listening preferences.

Nonetheless, algorithms are currently available in hearing aids to differentiate among various types of acoustic stimuli in the environment and to automatically apply this knowledge.

Single-Microphone Processing

The idea of adjusting processing parameters based on the characteristics of the environment is not new. Based on the premise that background noise is relatively intense and is dominated by low-frequency components, the traditional approach has been to reduce the low-frequency response of the hearing aid at high input levels. Advances in DSP capabilities have eliminated the need to rely on universal assumptions regarding the nature of the listener's environment. Although these processing techniques are independent of the number of inputs (from microphones), they are frequently referred to as single-microphone algorithms to distinguish them from methods that specifically require inputs from multiple microphones.

The primary objective of early classifiers was to differentiate speech from noise, a seemingly simple task. One obvious approach to making this distinction is on the basis of fluctuations—it only takes a few minutes of listening to realize that the intensity of speech from a single talker ebbs and flows, whereas the background noise stays relatively unchanged over time. The fluctuating nature of speech and constant characteristic of noise are reflected in the temporal envelopes of the two types of signals (**Fig. 1–15**). On this basis, the algorithm assumes that the incoming sound is noise if the envelope is relatively steady-state or speech if the envelope is time-varying. This determination may be performed continually in multiple channels across the frequency range of the hearing aid. The basis for this technique evolved from recommendations made by Graupe et al (1986), who designed the Zeta Noise Blocker, one of the first digitally based noise reduction circuits in hearing aids. In most realistic environments, speech and noise seldom occur in isolation. Fortunately, the mixing of the two signals does not pose a problem because the depth of fluctuation is systematically related to the SNR.

An alternate approach is to use the harmonic nature of speech to distinguish it from noise. The acoustic energy of speech is dominated by vowels that have a specific harmonic structure; that is, the vocal tract creates resonances, or formants, at frequencies that are integer multiples of the fundamental frequency. Furthermore, the energy at all of these formants changes synchronously with the shape of the vocal tract. Once the classifier determines that an incoming signal is speech, it provides the prescribed amount of gain to maximize speech intelligibility, regardless of whether or not noise is also present in the environment. If the algorithm is designed to also detect noise, it may provide varying amounts of gain depending on the amount of noise and/or the SNR.

None of the above-mentioned approaches is perfect. For example, a high-level input may be loud speech, and a music signal may have a steady temporal envelope similar to noise or may have a harmonic structure like speech. In both cases the desired sound (speech or music) may be mistakenly reduced. With increased DSP capabilities, the complexity of environment classification schemes has also increased. The ability to make use of multiple features of the input signal to make a decision dramatically decreases the error rate and improves the reliability and validity of the classification (**Fig. 1–16**). As a result, many of the algorithms currently available can detect the presence of speech, distinguish music from noise, and also differentiate among various types of noise. This capacity offers the potential for processing each of these signals differently. For example, amplification of speech may be optimized for maximum audibility, processing for music may be made less compressive for improved sound quality, and noise may be attenuated to maintain listening comfort.

The course of action to be taken once it is determined that noise is present in the environment depends on the underlying philosophy. At one extreme, if the primary goal is to maintain listener comfort, the gain of the hearing aid may be decreased any time that noise is detected. At the other end of the continuum, to preserve speech understanding, the gain may be decreased only if no usable speech is detected in the environment. Algorithms currently available in the marketplace typically strike a balance between these two boundaries. Studies on suppressing noise for hearing aid wearers (e.g., Alcantara et al,

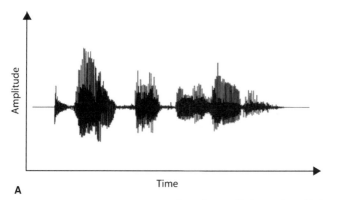
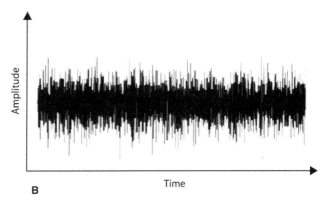

Figure 1–15 Representative temporal envelopes of **(A)** speech and **(B)** noise.

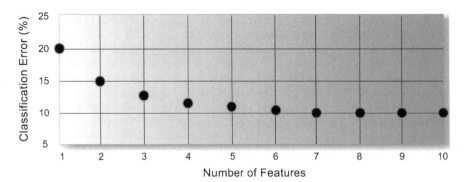

Figure 1–16 An example of changes in the rate of error as a function of the number of features used for classification.

2003) have demonstrated no significant improvement in speech intelligibility because reducing the noise within a channel also reduces the desired speech signal, leaving the SNR essentially unchanged.

Spectral subtraction is another technique for noise reduction that has recently made its way into the realm of hearing aids. It has been studied extensively in research laboratories as a method for enhancing noisy speech in single-microphone audio systems (Boll, 1979). An estimate of the noise magnitude is made during a nonspeech interval and is then subtracted from the noisy speech interval to obtain an estimate of the original speech. The outcomes of studies evaluating the performance of spectral subtraction algorithms have been mixed. For example, Levitt and colleagues (1993) demonstrated no improvement in speech intelligibility, although listening fatigue was considerably reduced from lowering the noise level. On the other hand, Tsoukalas et al (1997) reported a 40% improvement in speech intelligibility when parameters were adjusted on the basis of auditory masked thresholds.

In the future, we may see hearing aids performing speech recognition in conjunction with consonant enhancement algorithms to improve speech recognition in noise.

Multimicrophone Processing

The traditional application of multimicrophone technology in hearing aids is based on the premise that the spectral and temporal characteristics of the inputs at the two microphone ports are similar (i.e., they are correlated). This is true for most sounds entering the hearing aid, speech and noise (including multitalker babble at restaurants, vacuum cleaners, etc.), regardless of the azimuth/elevation from which they originate. Thus, the two inputs can be combined in various ways to alter the sensitivity of the hearing aid to sounds arriving from certain azimuths/elevations. The use of directional technology has been discussed previously.

Inputs from multiple microphones are also used for adaptive noise cancellation, a technique commonly applied in noise-canceling headphones. In this method, one microphone is used to pick up the desired signal (e.g., speech or music) as well as noise. The other microphone serves as a reference and senses the noise only. The desired signal is extracted by subtracting the outputs of the two microphones. Difficulty with this method arises if the reference microphone also picks up the desired signal, which results

in a part of the speech being canceled out along with the noise. This is a real concern with hearing aid applications.

Interference from wind is a common complaint related to the outdoor use of hearing aids. Noise is generated from wind blowing past an object and also from the turbulence created around the object. Wind noise can easily reach levels of 120 dB SPL, especially at low frequencies, thereby causing discomfort. The high input levels associated with wind noise frequently saturate the microphone or amplifier, and there is little hope for improving speech understanding. Traditional solutions are known to be unsuccessful; indeed, a scarf worn around the head is more effective in reducing wind noise than the typical microphone screen or hood. The best course of action, therefore, is to improve listening comfort. The adverse impact of wind noise varies by device style and becomes more problematic with directional processing. Compensation for the low-frequency roll-off inherent to directional processing exacerbates the discomfort and annoyance associated with wind noise. Because wind noise is primarily due to turbulence around the head, the input to one microphone port bears little or no resemblance to the input at the other port. When the two inputs are combined, the result is greater than either input alone. Thus, the lack of correlation between the two inputs can be used to detect the presence of wind noise. Using this information, the obvious solution is to switch the device into the omnidirectional mode. Additional gain reduction may be used to further alleviate the situation.

The MarkeTrak survey (Kochkin, 2002a) has shown that hearing aid users are least satisfied with their devices in noisy environments, both indoors and outdoors. Furthermore, satisfaction with benefit is strongly correlated with the number of listening situations in which benefit is perceived. It is, therefore, in the clinicians', as well as the consumers', best interest to increase user satisfaction in a variety of environments. Although noteworthy advances have been made in the environment classification algorithms available in hearing aids, little is currently done by way of adaptation beyond improving listening comfort. Additional research is required to guide the utilization of this information in adjusting processing parameters.

Dereverberation

In any confined environment, sounds heard by a hearing aid wearer are not simply the original emitted sounds, but also a combination of a large number of echoes from different surfaces. Persons with normal hearing can concentrate on the original sounds despite the presence of these echoes, but those with hearing loss often perceive degradation in speech sound quality, particularly in noisy and crowded listening areas (Hopgood, 2000).

Reverberation may be thought of as an acoustical noise that occurs from repeated reflections of sound on the walls and objects in an enclosed space. For example, when someone speaks in a reverberant room such as a lecture hall, multiple echoes add to the direct sound, resulting in a blurred sound signal and correspondingly reduced speech intelligibility. This reverberation causes the temporal variations of desired speech signals to be "filled in," making listening much harder for people with hearing loss.

Suppressing the undesirable effects of reverberation on speech intelligibility is perhaps more difficult than noise suppression because reverberation is often more transient in nature than environmental noise. Reverberation may be suppressed by a variety of DSP techniques when the characteristics of the acoustical environment are precisely known. Often, however, the room response surrounding the hearing aid wearer is not well known. Similar to its application for noise reduction, a kind of spectral subtraction may also be used for speech dereverberation. As with the noise reduction application, this method may result also in musical noise artifacts when the desired signal is absent. These artifacts may be eliminated by modifications of the spectral subtraction algorithm (Levert et al, 2001).

Blind signal separation is another technique for suppressing reverberation that is based on nonstationarity in signal processing (Hopgood, 2000). This method is difficult to implement in real-time situations because of the large amount of processing power required in the DSP engine.

Concept of Firmware

In the days of analog hearing aids, including the programmable analog type, instruments were known by the type of amplifier circuit they used (à la "Intel Inside"). If the analog circuitry was programmable, as almost all of the most recent were, the fitting software for programming the hearing aid usually selected "best fit" performance to a prescription target and enabled the dispenser to make parameter value changes for fine-tuning to individual preferences.

With DSP hardware, firmware and fitting software play a more significant role because of the added flexibility and features provided by the digital hardware. Firmware and fitting software for digital hearing aids enable several hearing aid manufacturers to distinguish between their products even with the same digital hardware. With most digital hearing aids, it is no longer possible (or interesting) to determine what type of amplifier circuitry is being used inside.

Firmware for software-based algorithms may be downloaded and stored into a reusable (erasable) memory in the most recent DSP hearing aids. This important feature enables digital hearing aids to become more general purpose and to last much longer. As new and improved signal-processing algorithms and features become available, they may be downloaded and stored in the hearing aid.

◆ Advanced and Emerging Technology

Wireless Technology

Some manufacturers have developed remote wireless devices for communicating with and controlling the hearing aid. The first remote devices many years ago used analog wireless transmission that controlled only a few parameters, such as volume and single-channel frequency shaping. More recently, remotes that transmit digital information wirelessly have been developed. These remotes can change variables such as gain, memory selected, and signal-processing parameters, and, in some cases, they can reprogram and load new signal-processing algorithms into hearing aids. The most advanced remote devices serve as a relay from external wireless sources such as cellular and cordless telephones (Yanz, 2006). Other applications of wireless for hearing aids include one hearing aid in binaural fitting controlling the hearing aid on the other side. These ear-to-ear wireless transmissions can change variables in the other hearing aid to achieve synchronization of gain via volume control, memory selected, and signal-processing methodology.

Currently, the NOAHlink hearing aid programming interface, developed by the Hearing Instrument Manufacturers' Software Association (HIMSA), provides Bluetooth wireless communication from a personal computer to the pendant worn by the patient. Although this is a significant achievement, at the time of this writing, wires are required from the NOAHlink to the hearing aids to be programmed **(Fig. 1–17)**. It would be desirable if all of the wires for programming hearing aids are eliminated. If this capability comes to pass, perhaps hearing aids could be adjusted under dispenser control wirelessly via the Internet or a cell phone.

Proliferation of Bluetooth wireless technology in headsets, cell phones, and computers has offered hearing aid wearers

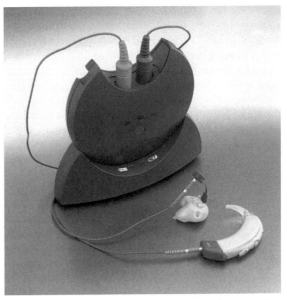

Figure 1–17 NOAHlink connecting with wires to hearing aids.

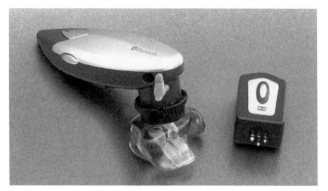

Figure 1–18 A Bluetooth headset with a custom earmold (*left*) and the ELI accessory device (*right*).

the same wireless connectivity that normal-hearing persons have. Wireless accessories, such as ELI (Starkey Labs) **(Fig. 1–18)**, BluePal (Starkey Labs), and SmartLink (Phonak), provide hearing aid wearers both hands-free cell phone operation and a means for improving SNR in noisy listening environments (Yanz, 2006). Future developments for hearing aid wearers will likely continue to include such assistive devices and use technologies developed in other fields.

Although Bluetooth accessories for hearing aid wearers are available in today's marketplace, currently they are limited in use because of Bluetooth size and battery current requirements. At the time of this writing, Bluetooth integrated circuits consume over 815 mA from a 3 V battery and are too large to package in custom hearing aids. Thus, accessories such as ELI and SmartLink require intermediate relay devices to convert the Bluetooth communication link to a hard-wired connection via an accessory shoe on the hearing aid or a lower power and smaller size wireless link, respectively. Having much smaller size wireless components that consume much less current would eliminate the need for accessory shoes and intermediate relay devices and permit wireless transmission from remote devices directly to all models of hearing aids, from CIC to BTE styles. Such capability would allow direct wireless programming from remote computers and mobile devices, eliminating the myriad sets of nonstandardized programming cables required in hearing aid dispensing offices. This capability would also facilitate ear-to-ear communication transmitting audio as well as control signals between ears. This ear-to-ear wireless capability would allow future hearing aids to implement binaural DSP noise reduction algorithms based on a signal input from a hearing aid on each side of the head.

Artificial Intelligence

The term *artificial intelligence* (AI) conjures up images from the science fiction genre—HAL, R2D2, and C3PO. In reality, it is a vital branch of science dealing with intelligent behavior, learning, and adaptation in machines. Research in AI is concerned with producing machines to automate tasks requiring intelligent behavior. Thus, AI systems may be involved in recognizing speech as well as emotion, planning and scheduling, responding to questions, or even assisting with

activities of daily living. There are several different types of AI, some characterized by statistical analysis and others involving learning based on empirical data.

Almost all DSP algorithms use some knowledge of the statistics of the incoming signal to adapt their performance. For example, many hearing aids currently available in the market can apply different amounts of gain depending on whether the incoming signal is determined to be speech or noise. The algorithm is provided with the information that speech is modulated, whereas noise is relatively constant. Furthermore, the criterion for modulation is defined, as is the amount of gain to be applied if the criterion is met. A more intricate algorithm may employ multiple criteria (e.g., modulation depth and signal level) or manipulate multiple features simultaneously (e.g., compression, directionality, and environment classification). Despite their complexity, current algorithms are unable to interact with the hearing aid user and use that input for future decisions, a key element of true artificial intelligence. The following are some realistic applications of AI to hearing aids.

Expert Systems

Expert systems are programs that analyze information about problems and recommend a course of action to resolve them. The "rules of thumb" for evaluating the problem are provided by real experts and use a similar process of reasoning. The rule base is made up of inference rules, which are interrelated but independent of the problem at hand. The system asks the individual requiring problem-solving assistance a series of questions to determine a suitable solution. Responses are not required for all of the questions posed; that is, the system can work with an incomplete dataset. One advantage of expert systems is the ability to provide the level of confidence associated with a recommended solution.

Addressing hearing aid user complaints is one practical application of expert systems. For example, if the individual indicates that his or her own voice sounds "boomy," the expert system might recommend turning down the gain of the hearing aid at low frequencies. In a survey of ~300 audiologists, Jenstad et al (2003) found a remarkable consistency in the recommended solutions to a variety of complaints. Additionally, the expert system may be only 75% confident in the solution, unless the individual indicates that other sounds in the environment are also too loud. Although some problem-solving systems are currently capable of recommending solutions, they are typically limited to addressing one problem at a time. In contrast, a true expert system may arrive at a solution by combining knowledge of the input signal, the settings of the hearing aid, and the individual user's preferences in various environments and for a host of different features.

Genetic Algorithms

Genetic algorithms are inspired by concepts from evolutionary biology, such as inheritance, mutation, crossover, and natural selection. For each problem, the solution, or gene, is represented by a set of parameters. The best solutions mutate and/or cross over from one generation to the next, whereas poorer solutions die off. The beauty of the genetic algorithm lies in its ability to manipulate multiple variables simultaneously and arrive at a solution quickly. Because each comparison takes the listener closer to the ideal solution, little time is wasted on less-than-optimal solutions.

Consider the application of the genetic algorithm in optimizing the frequency–gain settings of a two-channel hearing aid. The algorithm starts with a population of solutions representing the gain in each channel. The listener is asked to compare potential solutions and indicate a preference. Once the algorithm has sufficient data to rank the solutions, the lowest ranked solutions are dropped, fresh solutions are added (using the principles of mutation and crossover), and the evaluation is repeated with the new generation of solutions. This process continues until a termination condition is reached. The termination condition may involve a plateau in performance, an allocated period of time, a predefined number of generations, or some combination of these criteria. Despite the obvious appeal of genetic algorithms in fitting and fine-tuning the multitude of features currently available in hearing aids, much remains to be learned about the process. Durrant (2002) found considerable individual variability in optimizing feedback cancellation and expansion parameters. It is difficult to evaluate the reliability and validity of the algorithm when there is no universal best outcome.

Neural Networks

Once again, borrowing from biology, a neural network is a group of structurally and/or functionally connected neurons. Much like the human brain, though based on advanced mathematical models, learning occurs through exposure to stimuli and repetition of tasks that cause the connections to appear, strengthen, weaken, or even disappear altogether. To ensure true learning, rather than memorization, generalization is assessed on a different set of stimuli than the ones used for training. Neural networks are designed for pattern recognition: they identify trends and features, even when the information is complex and less than perfect. The ultimate goal of the system is to learn a particular task.

The principle of neural networks can be applied to self-learning in hearing aids. For example, based on the typical volume control setting, the hearing aid may learn over time that the user prefers less gain than prescribed. Settings for many advanced features may also be fine-tuned in a similar manner to meet the individual's needs.

Fuzzy Logic

Commonly used in household appliances such as washing machines and automatic-focusing cameras, fuzzy logic is a way to arrive at a decision based on ambiguous, imprecise, or "noisy" data. It allows a system to deal with degrees of truth (or membership in a set). For example, it does not require that height be described as tall or short, but rather tolerates the use of terms descriptors such as "fairly tall" and "somewhat short."

One example of implementing fuzzy logic in hearing aids relates to the perceived loudness of various sounds. That is, a hearing aid user may rate a desirable signal (e.g., music) presented at 90 dB SPL as relatively comfortable, whereas an undesirable signal (e.g., noise from a vacuum cleaner) at the same level may be considered uncomfortably loud. Based on this information, the gain of the hearing aid may be reduced to maintain listening comfort in noise but remain unchanged for listening pleasure in the presence of music.

As a scientific discipline, AI has the potential for solving real-life problems. The single biggest hindrance to implementation in hearing aids is the significant processing power required. Some applications are not as far out in the future as one might imagine, whereas others require significantly more digital processing power than is currently available. The potential of a hearing aid may be expanded by combining AI models. For now, the ability to log data about real-life situations and user preferences, a feature widely available in today's hearing aids, is both evidence and a solution that brings us one step closer to realizing AI.

◆ Standards for Electroacoustic Measurement of Hearing Aid Performance

Standards for hearing aid measurements provide those working with hearing aids methods for making electroacoustic assessments of specific performance parameters. For example, they provide an indication of how much gain and maximum output SPL (OSPL90) a hearing aid provides and what its frequency response is. They also show how much internal circuit noise and distortion a hearing aid has and how much current it draws from the battery. It is important for those making and using these measurements to understand what their purpose is, under what conditions they are valid, and what their limitations are.

The existence of such measurements implies that a consensus has been reached by those involved in the standardization process. In the development of an ANSI standard, all persons likely to be affected are invited to participate in formulating or modifying a standard. ANSI has defined the process to be followed for formulating standards and has organized the participants into committees and working groups.

Standardization is a living, ongoing process. Once an ANSI standard exists, every 5 years a decision is required by ANSI from the working group that formulated it to reaffirm it, modify it, or make it obsolete. Changes in ANSI standards are not made arbitrarily because their implementation may require considerable expenditure by hearing aid manufacturers and dispensers to modify test equipment. Recommended changes in standard measurement procedures must be proven viable. Frequently, round-robin testing on the same hearing aids is conducted at several different laboratories to try newly proposed procedures. Procedures recommended in ANSI standards are voluntary unless they are mandated by a regulatory agency. Such is the case with the measurements specified originally in ANSI S3.22 (1976), which were adopted by the Food and Drug Administration (FDA) as a set of product testing requirements for hearing aid manufacturers.

The IEC also has standardized hearing aid measurements in its 60118 series of documents. Up until recently, because of measurement procedural differences between ANSI and IEC hearing aid standards, manufacturers had to provide two sets of data: one set in accordance with ANSI S3.22 for use in the United States and Canada, and another set for use in countries requiring the IEC 60118 series of hearing aid standards. At this time, cooperation exists between IEC and ANSI working groups in an effort to harmonize the standards so that differences will be minimized. The entire series of IEC 60118 hearing aid standards is currently undergoing major revisions that may make several of them more compatible with ANSI standards. For example, in revising IEC 60118-7, the hearing aid quality control standard, the IEC hearing aid standards working group, TC29/WG13, adopted nearly entirely the latest revision of ANSI S3.22–2003 (IEC 60118-7, 2005). Other analogous ANSI and IEC standards, such as ANSI S3.35–2004 and IEC 60118-8 (1983b), have many aspects in common, but they are generally less well harmonized.

"The" ANSI Standard for Characterizing Hearing Aid Performance

From the first publication of ANSI S3.22–1976, measurements recommended in that document have been intended mainly for ensuring quality control, as mandated by the FDA. Parameters measured are not representative generally of the performance of hearing aids in real-world listening environments. Because this standard was adopted by the FDA, its measurements are required rather than voluntary. Measurements specified in ANSI S3.22–2003 are performed with the hearing aids mounted on metal couplers. S3.22 specifies using the 2 cc coupler, as has the corresponding IEC standard 60118-7 for about the past 10 years (IEC 60118-7, 2005). Couplers are not designed to represent the ear canal, but rather to ensure repeatable results between laboratories. Devices such as the modified Zwislocki occluded ear simulator and IEC 711 occluded ear simulator are available to be more predictive of performance under actual use conditions (ANSI S3.25–1989; IEC, 1981).

A typical data sheet showing the electroacoustic performance of a hearing aid in accordance with ANSI S3.22–2003 is reproduced in **Fig. 1–19.**

The FDA requires these data to accompany all new hearing aids shipped from hearing aid manufacturers, either as a preprinted specification (normally used for BTE hearing aids) or in a data sheet representing the actual performance of the hearing aid being tested (normally used for custom hearing aids). The frequency response with a 60 dB SPL input level with the volume control set at reference test position and output SPL with a 90 dB SPL input level (OSPL90) are both provided in the two top graphs. The

reference test position of the volume control is obtained with the hearing aid in linear mode by setting the high-frequency average (HFA) gain with a 60 dB input SPL to a level 77 dB below the HFA OSPL90. If the hearing aid does not have enough gain to reach a level 17 dB below the HFA OSPL90, the volume control is left full on. Reference test position for all hearing aids is determined in several steps. First, set the controls on the hearing aid or program the hearing aid so that it has the widest frequency response bandwidth and the highest OSPL90 and full-on gain. Where possible, the compression function of automatic gain control (AGC) hearing aids is set to have minimum effect except for the AGC tests shown at the bottom of **Fig. 1–19.** Other adaptive features, such as noise management and feedback cancellation systems, should be disabled. Second, calculate the HFA of the OSPL90 at 1000, 1600, and 2000 Hz (or the special purpose average [SPA] of the OSPL90 at three other preferred one-third octave frequencies that are separated by another one-third octave frequency). Third, lower the volume control setting, if required, until the average gain from the hearing aid at the same frequencies with a 60 dB input SPL is 77 ± 1.5 dB less than the HFA OSPL90 or SPA OSPL90. The reference test gain is the HFA OSPL90 or SPA OSPL90 – 77 dB or the HFA full-on gain if the volume control is left full on. SPA frequencies are used for extreme high-pass or low-pass hearing aids (Preves, 1988). An example of a set of SPA frequencies is 2000, 3150, and 5000 Hz.

Figure 1–19 shows several numerical specifications for the hearing aid being tested. These include HFA full-on gain, the three-frequency average of the output SPL with a 50 dB input SPL and full-on gain setting minus the 50 dB input level; reference test gain (RTG), the gain at the reference test setting (RTS) of the volume control; equivalent input noise, the output SPL with no input minus the RTG; battery current, the amount of current drawn by the hearing aid with a 65 dB 1000 Hz pure-tone input and the volume control set to RTS; low response limit F_1, the low-frequency intersection of a horizontal line 20 dB lower than the HFA full-on gain and the frequency response curve with the volume control at RTS; high response limit F_2, the high-frequency intersection of a horizontal line 20 dB lower than the HFA full-on gain and the frequency response curve with the volume control at RTS; induction coil sensitivity, the output of a hearing aid with telecoil activated (if present) using the Telephone Magnetic Field Simulator (TMFS) fixture; and total harmonic distortion produced by the hearing aid at 500, 800, and 1600 Hz (or at one half the SPA frequencies) with the volume control at reference test position with input levels at 70, 70, and 65 dB SPL, respectively.

Most currently produced hearing aids contain an AGC circuit. The bottom portion of **Figure 1–19** depicts a typical printout of AGC tests obtained in accordance with ANSI S3.22–2003. The bottom graph is the input–output characteristic, plotted for a 2000 Hz pure-tone input whose SPL is varied from 50 to 90 dB SPL in 5 dB steps. The ordinate shows the hearing aid output in dB SPL resulting from the input levels denoted by the abscissa.

The bottom left part of **Figure 1–19** also records the attack and release times for this hearing aid. The attack time (AT) is defined as the length of time taken for the output signal to settle to within 3 dB of the final value as a result of the 2000 Hz input level changing from 55 dB to 90 dB SPL. The release time (RT) is defined as the length of time taken for the output signal to settle to within 4 dB

of the final value as a result of the 2000 Hz input level changing from 90 dB to 55 dB SPL. Attack and release times provide an indication of how long it will take the circuit to react to fast transient signals.

Induction Coil Sensitivity Tests

To assess the maximum sensitivity of the hearing aid induction coil, place the gain control at full-on and the hearing aid set to the "T" (telephone input) mode, the hearing aid is placed in a sinusoidal alternating magnetic field having a root-mean-square (rms) magnetic field strength of 31.6 mA/m at 1000 Hz and is oriented to produce the greatest coupler SPL. The SPL in the coupler is recorded. A curve of the SPL in the coupler over the frequency range 200 to 5000 Hz, using a magnetic field strength of 31.6 mA/m, may also be provided.

To assess hearing aid induction coil performance with telephones, use the TMFS instead of an arbitrary-size radiating

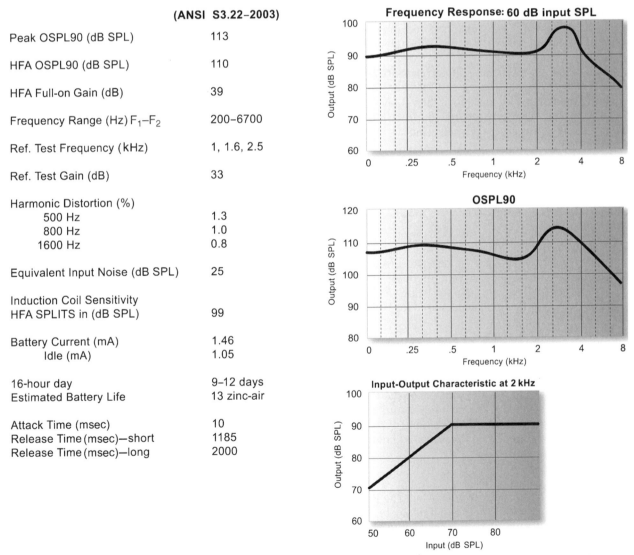

	(ANSI S3.22–2003)
Peak OSPL90 (dB SPL)	113
HFA OSPL90 (dB SPL)	110
HFA Full-on Gain (dB)	39
Frequency Range (Hz) F_1–F_2	200–6700
Ref. Test Frequency (kHz)	1, 1.6, 2.5
Ref. Test Gain (dB)	33
Harmonic Distortion (%)	
500 Hz	1.3
800 Hz	1.0
1600 Hz	0.8
Equivalent Input Noise (dB SPL)	25
Induction Coil Sensitivity HFA SPLITS in (dB SPL)	99
Battery Current (mA)	1.46
Idle (mA)	1.05
16-hour day	9–12 days
Estimated Battery Life	13 zinc-air
Attack Time (msec)	10
Release Time (msec)—short	1185
Release Time (msec)—long	2000

Figure 1–19 Typical data sheet for a hearing aid in accordance with ANSI S3.22–2003. HFA, high-frequency average; OSPL90, output sound pressure level with a 90 dB sound pressure level input signal; SPL, sound pressure level; SPLITS, SPL in an inductive telephone simulator.

coil used above for maximum induction coil sensitivity. The TMFS is a fixture with geometric shape representing the receiver portion of a telephone handset. It produces a magnetic field level of 31.6 mA/m when driven by the specified current. With the gain control at the RTS and the hearing aid switched to induction coil (telecoil) mode, position the hearing aid on the test surface of the TMFS and orient it for maximum output, subject to the following constraints: a BTE hearing aid should lie as flat as possible on the test surface. The faceplate of an ITE or ITC hearing aid should be parallel to the test surface of the TMFS and as close as possible to it. With the TMFS driven by the specified test current, record the coupler SPL as a function of frequency in the range 200 to 5000 Hz. The abbreviation for this parameter is SPLITS, which stands for SPL in an inductive telephone simulator. Calculate the HFA-SPLITS or the average of the SPLITS values at the 3 HFA frequencies (**Fig. 1–19**). Calculate the Relative Simulated Equivalent Telephone Sensitivity (RSETS) as the difference in decibels obtained by subtracting the RTG + 60 dB SPL from the HFA-SPLITS. RSETS is a figure of merit for how much the volume control will have to be moved when switching from microphone to telephone on a hearing aid when using it for telephone pickup.

To assess hearing aid induction coil performance with loop systems, calculate the Equivalent Test Loop Sensitivity (ETLS) for a figure of merit for how much the volume control will have to be moved when switching from microphone to telephone on a hearing aid when using it for room or neck loop pickup.

Other ANSI Standards for Hearing Aid Measurements

Coupler Calibration of Earphones (ANSI S3.7–1995)

ANSI S3.7–1995, Method for Coupler Calibration of Earphones, provides specifications for couplers and their use in calibrating hearing aid and audiometric earphones. (A hearing aid earphone pertains to the receiver.) All the HA series couplers except the HA-1 type incorporate an internal earmold simulator. Among the 2 cc couplers used for hearing aid testing are the following.

HA-1 Coupler This coupler allows direct coupling of an earmold of a postauricular hearing aid, a molded insert with an internal earphone, or a shell of an ITE hearing aid. Clay or putty is used to seal the earmold or shell into the coupler. The S3.22 standard recommends testing with the vent in the hearing aid closed. An example of a custom hearing aid mounted on an HA-1 coupler is shown in **Fig. 1–20A.**

HA-2 Coupler This coupler is used for earphones with nubs such as an external receiver of a body aid. The HA-2 coupler is sometimes used with an external tubing to connect an earphone in a hearing aid to an earmold or to an ear insert. For high-volume testing, the external tubing may be rigid for longer wear. Unless otherwise stated, the connecting tubing outside the coupler has a length of 25 mm and an inner diameter of 1.93 mm (no. 13 tubing). The length

and diameter may be specified by the manufacturer and simulate the actual tubing used in practice. The earmold simulator in the HA-2 coupler has a 3 mm bore diameter, which may produce a high-frequency boost compared with an actual earmold with 2 mm bore diameter tubing (Lybarger, 1985). An illustration of a BTE hearing aid mounted on an HA-2 coupler is shown in **Fig. 1–20B.**

HA-3 Coupler This coupler is intended for testing modular ITE hearing aids, as well as earphones and insert type receivers that do not have nubs. The entrance tubing may be either flexible or rigid and, unless otherwise stated by the manufacturer, has a length of 10 mm and a diameter of 1.93 mm (i.e., no. 13 tubing). A picture of a modular ITE hearing aid mounted on an HA-3 coupler is shown in **Fig. 1–20C.**

HA-4 Coupler The HA-4 coupler is a modification of the HA-2 coupler using entrance tubing. It is used for testing postauricular or eyeglass hearing aids in conjunction with a constant sound path bore of 1.93 mm diameter from the hearing aid output through the earmold. An illustration of an HA-4 coupler is shown in **Fig. 1–20D.** (The interested reader is referred to Lybarger, 1985, for further information on couplers.)

Occluded Ear Simulator (ANSI S3.25-R2003)

Ear simulators have been designed specifically to represent the characteristics of a normal real ear over a wide frequency range, unlike the various hearing aid couplers discussed earlier. This standard specifies the physical configuration and acoustical characteristics of the four-branch modified Zwislocki ear simulator (**Fig. 1–21A**). This ear simulator is used in the Knowles Electronics Manikin for Acoustic Research (KEMAR; GRAS Sound & Vibration A/S, Vedbæk, Denmark). The occluded ear simulator simulates the portion of the ear canal between the tip of an earmold and the eardrum and also the median acoustic impedance at the eardrum for persons with normal middle ears. A photograph of KEMAR is found in **Fig. 1–21B.**

The IEC 711 ear simulator (IEC, 1981) conforms to the specifications of the Brüel & Kjær (Nærum, Denmark) ear simulator. Because of slight differences in measurement data, the acoustical performance in the IEC 711 ear simulator standard does not quite meet the specifications of the four-branch modified Zwislocki ear simulator in ANSI S3.25-R2003. The formulation of separate ANSI and IEC ear simulator standards is an example of the difficulty ANSI and IEC have had in the past developing compatible standards for measuring hearing aid performance.

Manikin Measurements (ANSI S3.35–2004)

ANSI S3.35–2004, Methods of Measurement of Performance Characteristics of Hearing Aids under Simulated in situ Working Conditions, provides guidance on how to use KEMAR for estimating hearing aid performance, and in particular, directionality, for an average wearer. The standard simulates the acoustical effect, for example, of head and torso diffraction caused by a person wearing the hearing aid. Measurements in accordance with this standard are normally performed in an

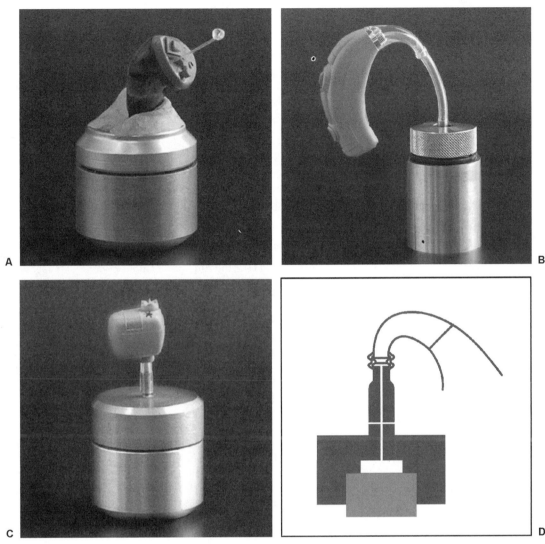

Figure 1–20 Examples of 2 cc couplers commonly used for electroacoustic assessment of hearing aids. **(A)** HA-1, **(B)** HA-2, **(C)** HA-3, and **(D)** HA-4.

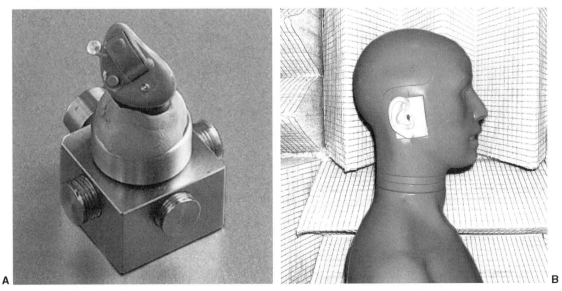

Figure 1–21 **(A)** Zwislocki coupler and **(B)** Knowles Electronics Manikin for Acoustic Research (KEMAR).

acoustical environment with excellent sound absorption and sound attenuation (i.e., an anechoic chamber). Because one objective is the calculation of DI from the polar pattern, an alternate is to attempt to find a diffuse sound field in a near totally reverberant environment in which to make the measurements. Theoretically, though difficult to prove in practice, the measures specified in ANSI S3.35–2004 in an anechoic environment should correlate to those made in a totally reverberant chamber.

Because of the relative ease in making measurements in the horizontal plane, until recently, polar directivity patterns were obtained only in two dimensions, assuming symmetry in the vertical plane. With the publication in 2004 of the latest revision of ANSI S3.35, whose measurements are described in a later section of this chapter, polar patterns in three dimensions were advocated. However, because of the relative difficulty of turning a hearing aid in a vertical arc, polar pattern data are frequently taken only in the horizontal plane, and symmetry is assumed in the vertical plane (i.e., the polar pattern in the vertical plane is assumed to be the same as that in the horizontal plane).

The standard includes the acoustical requirements for the test space and a coordinate system to specify loudspeaker position and direction of sound incidence relative to the manikin. Measurements and calculations defined in the standard are as follows:

♦ Manikin frequency response

♦ Simulated real ear gain

♦ Simulated insertion gain–frequency response

♦ Simulated real ear output SPL with a 90 dB input SPL

♦ Three-dimensional polar directivity pattern measurements

♦ Directivity index

During the formulation of the S3.35 standard, several round-robin series of measurements with various hearing aids were conducted in accordance with the procedures outlined in the S3.35 standard (Burns, 2005; Teder, 1984). The repeatability of the measurements on the same hearing aid between laboratories was reported in these studies. For more information on manikin measurements, consult the Manikin Measurements Conference Proceedings (Burkhard, 1978).

Whereas ANSI S3.35–2004 describes simulated real ear measurements on the manikin KEMAR, ANSI S3.46–1997 has been formulated to recommend methods of measurement of real ear performance of hearing aids using probe tube microphones on hearing aid wearers. This document specifies basic terminology (analogous to those terms and measurements used in ANSI S3.35) that are used in making and reporting real ear measures with probe microphone systems. Among these are the real ear unaided response (REUR), real ear aided response (REAR), real ear occluded response (REOR), and real ear insertion gain (REIG), which is a calculated quantity equal to REAR minus REUR. The S3.46 standard also recommends test equipment, test space, setup, and stimuli for performing real ear measures.

Assessing Interference from Cell Phones (ANSI C63.19–2007)

This document provides procedures to categorize the degree of usability of a hearing aid–telephone combination. To determine this categorization, the standard recommends procedures to assess the amount of immunity to electromagnetic interference provided by hearing aids and to measure the amount of electromagnetic radiation from telephones.

Procedures for measuring the degree of immunity to interference are also provided in IEC 60118–13 (2004) using a gigahertz transverse electromagnetic (GTEM) cell. The IEC method is incorporated in an annex of ANSI C63.19–2007.

Hearing Aid Standards Directions

Predicting Hearing Aid Sound Quality with Electroacoustic Measures The measurements specified in ANSI S3.22–2003 are mainly for quality control purposes, not for providing an indication of hearing aid performance on the wearer. For example, the harmonic distortion measurements cannot be used as a predictor of hearing aid sound quality. Subjective measures are the final answer, but they are time consuming and relatively difficult to perform. In the mid- to late 1990s, the S3-WG48 working group began discussing the possibility of finding electroacoustic measurements that correlate well to hearing aid sound quality. Such a tool could be very useful for hearing aid design engineers to improve signal processing algorithms and assist those dispensing hearing aids to select the best performing hearing aids. The methods considered included intermodulation distortion, difference frequency distortion, signal-to-distortion ratio, coherence function, modulation transfer function, speech transmission index, and auditory distance. However, after more than 3 years and many meetings discussing using possible existing methods, no consensus had been reached on a suitable method, and the working group abandoned this quest.

Recently, the ANSI S3-WG48 hearing aid standards committee has again attempted to find an objective metric for measuring hearing aids that predicts accurately the processed sound quality wearers would experience. With the proliferation of products that utilize compressed audio data such as MPEG-3, this has been a popular topic of articles presented and published, for example, by the Audio Engineering Society. Several perceptual metrics have been widely used in the telephone industry. Some of these are purely subjective, using five-category Mean Opinion Score ratings obtained from subjective listening tests with a wide variety of audio processing and data compression. Of the better known perceptual metrics, the Perceptual Speech Quality Measure (PSQM) and its replacement, the Perceptual Evaluation of Speech Quality (PESQ), which address listening quality, have been adopted by the International Telecommunication Union (ITU). An evaluation of the Perceptual Analysis Measurement System (PAMS), by S3-WG48 working group member Ron Scicluna, showed that sound quality had a good correlation to the percent of muted speech metric (speech activity). The PAMS method also takes into account both listening quality and listening effort, which were not found to correlate well to subjective sound quality assessments. The Perceptual Evaluation of Audio Quality (PEAQ), which has been adopted as ITU standard BS.1387, is an objective method that uses a neural network in combination with several psychoacoustic parameters. These sound quality measures have in common assessing the amount of signal degradation using a baseline reference signal for comparison to the processed signal. Although these metrics are of some interest, they may be useful only for speech signals, and they do not take into account the effects of spectral differences between the original reference signal and the processed hearing aid output signal. The accuracy score objective rating of fidelity used by Mead Killion, also a member of the working group, is another metric being examined by the group. Its fidelity ratings appear to correlate well to subjective sound quality assessments, particularly for those with a flat mild loss. The PErception Model based Quality estimation (PEMO-Q) objective method of predicting sound quality, advocated by Oldenberg University (Rohdenburg et al, 2005), has been proposed as a possible standard method. The method compares the unprocessed input signal to an internal representation of the processed hearing aid output signal, after passing both through a psychoacoustically based auditory model. Signal distortions below masked threshold levels are considered inaudible. Any perceptible differences are considered degradations of audio quality. But before PEMO-Q can be used for hearing aid wearers, it needs to be modified to factor in the effects of hearing loss.

Extending ANSI S3.42–1996   Similarly, considerable effort was made by the working group in the mid to late 1990s to extend ANSI S3.42–1992 to use a temporally modulating input signal instead of a steady-state speech-shaped noise. Some of the signals considered by the working group were RASTI (RApid Speech Transmission Index), ITU P50, ICRA (International Collegium of Rehabilitative Audiology), and IEEE (Institute of Electrical and Electronics Engineers) 1329 simulated speech generator and real speech segments. This work was also abandoned when no consensus was obtained, after several years of discussion, on which temporally modulating input signal to use. Recently, however, this topic has also been revisited in the S3-WG48 working group meetings because of work being done by others in these areas. For example, the IEC TC29/WG13 committee for hearing aid standards is considering revising and combining several of the IEC 60118 series of standards to utilize an actual speech signal as a temporally modulating input signal.

Effects of Time Delay through Digital Hearing Aids   There has been some concern within the S3-WG48 standards committee that the longer delays caused by digital signal processing, in comparison to those with analog processing, may be objectionable to hearing aid wearers. As a result, a proposal has been discussed to measure the group delay of hearing aids and report it on specification sheets so as to be available for those dispensing hearing aids. Group delay relates to how fast the hearing aid changes phase as a function of frequency, which, in turn, is usually directly proportional to the steepness of the frequency response. Thus, group delay can and does vary significantly across frequency range. If, for example, low frequency sounds are delayed more than high frequency sounds through a hearing aid, the basic characteristics of sounds may be altered enough to compromise identification of some sounds being processed. A related metric is processing delay, a term that has been used interchangeably with group delay. Processing delay refers to the delay between hearing aid input and output and is expressed as a single number of milliseconds, independent of frequency.

◆ Summary

Hearing aid technology has evolved and continues to evolve. Modern hearing aid transducers have improved performance while having experienced considerable miniaturization. Advancements in hearing aid amplifiers have been made possible by innovations in signal processing and dramatic downsizing of semiconductor technology. As a result, hearing aids of the future offer promise for continued technological advances and improved performance for hearing aid wearers. Hearing aid measurement standards evolve in reaction to hearing aid technology evolution.

Acknowledgments   We gratefully acknowledge the following individuals for their assistance in preparing this chapter: Karrie Recker (section on genetic algorithms), Natalie Breitung and Tom Burns (illustrations), James Curran (insightful comments), Patricia Argote-Muza (references), Ron Scicluna (sound quality information), and William Cole (hearing aid delay information).

References

Alcantara, J. L., Moore, B., Kühnel, V., & Launer, S. (2003). Evaluation of the noise reduction system in a commercial digital hearing aid. International Journal of Audiology, 42(1), 34–42.

American National Standards Institute. (1979). Occluded ear simulator (ANSI S3.25–1979). New York: Acoustical Society of America.

American National Standards Institute. (1989). For an occluded ear simulator (ANSI S3.25–1989). New York: Acoustical Society of America.

American National Standards Institute. (1992). Testing hearing aids with a broadband noise signal (ANSI S3.42–1992). New York: Acoustical Society of America.

American National Standards Institute. (1995). Method for coupler calibration of earphones (ANSI S3.7–1995). New York: Acoustical Society of America.

American National Standards Institute. (1997). Methods of measurement of real-ear performance characteristics of hearing aids (ANSI S3.46–1997). New York: Acoustical Society of America.

American National Standards Institute. (2007). Methods of measurement of compatibility between wireless communication devices and hearing aids (ANSI C63.19–2007). New York: Institute of Electrical and Electronic Engineers.

American National Standards Institute. (2003). Specification of hearing aid characteristics (ANSI S3.22–2003). New York: Acoustical Society of America.

American National Standards Institute. (2004). Method of measurement of performance characteristics of hearing aids under simulated real-ear working conditions (ANSI S3.35–2004). New York: Acoustical Society of America.

Banerjee, S. (2006). The compression handbook: Overview of the characteristics and applications of compression amplification. Eden Prairie, MN: Starkey Laboratories.

Bentler, R. A., Palmer, C., & Dittberner, A. (2004). Hearing-in-noise: Comparison of listeners with normal and (aided) impaired hearing. Journal of the American Academy of Audiology, 15, 216–225.

Boll, S. (1979). Suppression of acoustic noise in speech using spectral subtraction. IEEE Transactions on Audio, Speech, and Signal Processing (ASSP), 27, 113–120.

Boymans, M., Dreschler, W., Schoneveld, P., & Verschuure, H. (1999). Clinical evaluation of a full-digital in-the-ear hearing instrument. Audiology, 38(2), 99–108.

Burkhard, M. (1978). Manikin measurements. Itasca, IL: Knowles Electronics.

Burns, T. (2005, October). Round robin measurements of 3-D directivity using the ANSI S3.35 protocol. Paper presented at the meeting of the Acoustical Society of America, Minneapolis, MN.

Cord, M. T., Surr, R. K., Walden, B. E., & Olson, L. (2002). Performance of directional microphone hearing aids in everyday life. Journal of the American Academy of Audiology, 13, 295–307.

Dillon, H. (2001). Hearing aids. New York: Thieme Medical Publishers.

Durrant, E. (2002). Hearing aid fitting with genetic algorithms. Unpublished doctoral dissertation, University of Michigan, Ann Arbor.

Freed, D., & Soli, S. (2006). An objective procedure for evaluation of adaptive antifeedback algorithms in hearing aids. Ear and Hearing, 27, 382–398.

Graupe, D., Grosspietsch, J., & Taylor, R. (1986). A self-adaptive noise filtering system: 1. Overview and description. Hearing Instruments, 37(9), 29–34.

Greenberg, J. E., Desloge, J., & Zurek, P. (2003). Evaluation of array-processing algorithms for a headband hearing aid. Journal of the Acoustical Society of America, 113(3), 1646–1657.

Griffing, T., & Preves, D. (1976). In-the-ear aids. Part one. Hearing Instruments, 27, 22–24.

Harry, W. (1940). Six-way directional microphone. Bell System Technology Journal, 19, 10–14.

Hawkins, D. B., & Yacullo, W. (1984). Signal-to-noise ratio advantage of binaural hearing aids and directional microphones under different levels of reverberation. Journal of Speech and Hearing Disorders, 49, 278–286.

Hopgood, J. (2000). Non-stationary signal processing with application to reverberation cancellation in acoustic environments. Doctoral thesis, University of Cambridge, UK.

International Electrotechnical Commission. (1981). Occluded-ear simulator for the measurement of earphones coupled to the ear by ear inserts (IEC Pub. No. 711). New York: Author.

International Electrotechnical Commission. (1983a). Hearing aids with automatic gain control circuits (IEC Hearing Aids Pub. No. 60118-2). New York: Author.

International Electrotechnical Commission. (1983b). Measurement of hearing aids under simulated in-situ working conditions (IEC Hearing Aids Pub. No. 60118-8). New York: Author.

International Electrotechnical Commission. (2004). Hearing aids: 13. Electromagnetic compatibility (IEC Hearing Aids Pub. No. 60118-13). New York: Author.

International Electrotechnical Commission. (2005). Measurement of performance characteristics of hearing aids for quality inspection for delivery purposes (IEC Hearing Aids Pub. No. 60118-7). New York: Author.

Jenstad, L. M., Van Tasell, D., & Ewert, C. (2003). Hearing aid troubleshooting based on patients' description. Journal of the American Academy of Audiology, 14(7), 347–360.

Kampe, S., & Wynne, M. (1996). The influence of venting on the occlusion effect. Hearing Journal, 49(4), 59–66.

Kates, J. M. (2001). Room reverberation effects in hearing aid feedback cancellation. Journal of the Acoustical Society of America, 109(1), 367–378.

Kates, J. M., & Weiss, M. (1996). A comparison of hearing-aid array-processing techniques. Journal of the Acoustical Society of America, 99(5), 3138–3148.

Keidser, G. (1995). Long-term spectra of a range of real-life noisy environments. Australian Journal of Audiology, 17, 1–8.

Killion, M. (2004). Myths about hearing in noise and directional microphones. Hearing Review, 11(2), 14, 16, 18, 19, 72, 73.

Killion, M., Wilber, L., & Gudmundsen, G. (1988). Zwislocki was right: A potential solution to the "hollow voice" problem (the amplified occlusion effect) with deeply sealed earmolds. Hearing Instruments, 39(1),14–18.

Kochkin, S. (2002a). MarkeTrak VI: 10-year customer satisfaction trends in the US hearing instrument market. Hearing Review, 9(10), 14–25.

Kochkin, S. (2002b). MarkeTrak VI: Consumers rate improvements sought in hearing instruments. Hearing Review, 9(11), 18–22.

Kuk, F. K., Plager, A., & Pape, N. (1992). Hollowness perception with noise reduction hearing aids. Journal of the American Academy of Audiology, 3(1), 39–45.

Leeuw, A. R., & Dreschler, W. (1991). Advantages of directional hearing aid microphones related to room acoustics. Audiology, 30, 330–344.

Lentz, W. (1974). A summary of research using directional and omnidirectional hearing aids. Journal of Audiological Technique, 13, 42–46.

Levert, K., Boucher, J., & Denbigh, P. (2001). A new method based on spectral subtraction for speech dereverberation. Acustica, 87, 359–366.

Levitt, H., Bakke, M., Kates, J., Neuman, A., Schwander, T., & Weiss, M. (1993). Signal processing for hearing impairment. Scandinavian Audiology Supplementum, 38, 7–19.

Lybarger, S. (1985). The physical and electroacoustic characteristics of hearing aids. In J. Katz (Ed.), Handbook of audiology (pp. 849–884). Baltimore: Williams & Wilkins.

Macrae, J. H. (1994). A review of research into safety limits for amplification by hearing aids. Australian Journal of Audiology, 16, 67–77.

Madafarri, P., & Stanley, W. (1996). Microphone, receiver and telecoil options: Past, present and future. In M. Valente (Ed.), Hearing aids: Standards, options and limitations (pp. 126–156). New York: Thieme Medical Publishers.

Maj, J.-B., Wouters, J., & Moonen, M. (2004). Noise reduction results of an adaptive filtering technique for dual-microphone behind-the-ear hearing aids. Ear and Hearing, 25(3), 215–229.

Merks, I., Banerjee, S., & Trine, T. (2006). Assessing the effectiveness of feedback cancellers in hearing aids. Hearing Review, 13(4), 53–57.

Montgomery, A. A., & Edge, R. (1988). Evaluation of two speech enhancement techniques to improve intelligibility for hearing-impaired adults. Journal of Speech and Hearing Research, 31, 386–393.

Neuman, A. C., Bakke, M., Mackersie, C., Hellman, S., & Levitt, H. (1998). The effect of compression ratio and release time on the categorical rating of sound quality. Journal of the Acoustical Society of America, 103(5, Pt. 1), 2273–2281.

Olsen, W. (1991). Clinical assessment of output limiting and speech enhancement techniques. In G. Studebaker, F. Bess, & L. Beck (Eds.), The Vanderbilt hearing-aid report II (pp. 53–61). Timonium, MD: York Press.

Olson, L., Ioannou, M., & Trine, T. (2004). Appraising an automatically switching directional system in the real world. Hearing Journal, 57(6), 32–38.

Pearsons, K., Bennet, R., & Fidell, K. (1977). Speech levels in various noise environments (EPA Report No. 600/1–77–025). Washington, DC: Environmental Protection Agency.

Preves, D. (1975). Obtaining accurate measurements of directional hearing aid parameters. Hearing Aid Journal, 28(4), 13–34.

Preves, D. (1988). Revised ANSI Std. S3.22 for hearing instrument performance measurement. Hearing Instruments, 39(3), 26–34.

Preves, D. (1997). Directional microphone use in ITE hearing instruments. Hearing Review, 4(7), 21–27.

Preves, D. (2003). Hearing aids and digital wireless telephones. Seminars in Hearing, 24(1), 43–62.

Ricketts, T., & Dittberner, A. (2002). Directional amplification for improved signal-to-noise ratio: Strategies, measurements and limitations. In M. Valente (Ed.), Hearing aids: Standards, options and limitations. New York: Thieme Medical Publishers.

Ricketts, T., & Henry, P. (2002). Evaluation of an adaptive, directional-microphone hearing aid. International Journal of Audiology, 41, 100–112.

Ricketts, T. A., & Hornsby, B. (2003). Distance and reverberation effects on directional benefit. Ear and Hearing, 24(6), 472–484.

Ricketts, T., Hornsby, B., & Johnson, E. (2005). Adaptive directional benefit in the near field: Competing sound angle and level effects. Seminars in Hearing, 26(2), 59–69.

Roberts, M., & Schulein, R. (1997, September). Measurement and intelligibility optimization of directional microphones for use in hearing aid devices. Paper presented at the meeting of the Audiological Engineering Society, New York.

Rohdenburg, T., Volker, H., & Kollmeier, B. (2005, September). Objective perceptual quality measures for the evaluation of noise reduction schemes. Paper presented at the Ninth Annual International Workshop on Acoustic Echo and Noise Control, Eindhoven, Netherlands.

Strom, K. (2007). Hearing aids sales rise by 3.5% in first half of 2007. Hearing Review Insider, July 26. Retrieved August 2, 2007, from http://www.hearingreview.com/insider/2007-07-26_01.asp

Teder, H. (1984). Repeatability of KEMAR insertion gain measurements. Hearing Instruments, 35(10), 16–22.

Teder, H. (2003). Quantifying telecoil performance: Understanding historical and current ANSI standards. Seminars in Hearing, 24(1), 63–70.

Tonndorf, J. (1972). Bone conduction. In J. V. Tobias (Ed.), Foundations of modern auditory theory (pp. 195–273). New York: Academic Press.

Trine, T., & van Tasell, D. (2002). Digital hearing aid design: Fact vs. fantasy. Hearing Journal, 55(2), 36–42.

Tsoukalas, D., Mourjopoulos, J., & Kokkinakis, G. (1997). Speech enhancement based on audible noise suppression. IEEE Transactions on Audio, Speech and Language Processing, 5(6), 497–513.

Valente, M., Sweetow, R., Potts, L., & Bingea, B. (1999). Digital versus analog signal processing: Effect of directional microphone. Journal of the American Academy of Audiology, 10, 133–150.

Victorian, T., & Preves, D. (2004). Progress achieved in setting standards for hearing aid/digital cell phone compatibility. Hearing Journal, 57(9), 25–29.

Walden, B. E., Surr, R., Cord, M., & Drylund, O. (2004). Predicting hearing aid microphone preference in everyday listening. Journal of the American Academy of Audiology, 15, 353–364.

Woods, W., Frush, R., & Van Tasell, D. (1999, October). "Preference space" for parameters of two-channel speech compression. Poster presented at the IEEE Workshop of Applications of Signal Processing to Audio and Acoustics, New Paltz, NY.

Woods, W., & Trine, T. (2004). Limitations of theoretical benefit from an adaptive directional system in reverberant environments. Acoustics Research Letters Online, 5, 153–156.

Yanz, J. (2006). The future of wireless devices in hearing care: A technology that promises to transform the hearing industry. Hearing Review, 13(1), 18–20.

Chapter 2

Earhooks, Tubing, Earmolds, and Shells

Michael Valente and L. Maureen Valente

The electroacoustic characteristics of hearing aids, measured according to American National Standards Institute (ANSI) S3.22–2003 specifications (ANSI, 2003) in either HA-1 or HA-2 couplers, can be significantly altered by the manner in which the hearing aids are coupled to the ears. Some alterations of the electroacoustic characteristics (i.e., head diffraction, concha and ear canal resonances, head shadow, body baffle, residual ear canal volume, and the impedance of the eardrum and middle ear) may be unpredictable and are beyond the control of the audiologist. The audiologist, however, can alter, in a fairly predictable way, the electroacoustic characteristics of hearing aids via changes in the transmission line (i.e., earhook, tubing, and earmold or custom shell), relative to the electroacoustic characteristics originally measured in the coupler.

This chapter will provide a comprehensive overview of how altering the earhook, tubing, earmold, or custom shell may affect the electroacoustic characteristics of the delivered signal to the eardrum. The goal of this chapter is to provide readers with some of the tools necessary to provide a hearing aid fitting that has the following qualities:

1. Allows aided performance in quiet to be significantly better than unaided performance in the same listening situation.

2. Allows aided performance in noise to be significantly better than unaided performance in the same listening situation. It is important, however, for the patient to understand that aided performance in noise will not be as

satisfactory as aided performance in quiet. Even normal listeners experience greater difficulty listening in noise compared with listening in quiet.

3. Allows "soft" input signals to be judged as soft but audible, "average" input signals to be judged as comfortable, and "loud" input signals to be judged as loud but not uncomfortably loud.

4. Provides excellent sound quality and good intelligibility of speech.

5. Is relatively distortion free (≤10%) at high input levels.

6. Is free of feedback throughout the useable range of amplification.

7. Preserves the balance between the low- and high-frequency regions of the average speech spectrum.

8. When appropriate, extends the high-frequency range of the hearing aid.

9. When appropriate, minimizes excessive gain at around 1500 Hz.

10. When appropriate, maintains a gently rising frequency response.

11. Creates a comfortably fitting earmold or custom shell.

12. Reduces or eliminates the sensation that the patient's head is "at the bottom of a barrel."

As mentioned earlier, the primary goal of this chapter is to provide a comprehensive overview of the transmission line from the earhook to the earmold. Because little has changed over the years regarding the acoustics of the transmission line, the authors do not feel it necessary to "rewrite" this information. Interested readers should consult Cox (1979).

◆ Dimensions of the Typical Transmission Line

The tubing from the receiver encased in behind-the-ear (BTE), in-the-ear (ITE), or in-the-canal (ITC) hearing aids is typically 8 to 15 mm long and has an inner diameter of 0.5 to 1.5 mm wide (Cox, 1979). The sound bore of the earhook is typically 20 to 30 mm long and 1.2 to 1.8 mm wide (Cox, 1979). The tubing from the earhook to the tip of the earmold is usually 40 to 45 mm long and 1.93 mm wide (Cox, 1979). This latter dimension should be compared with the ANSI S3.22–2003 standard that requires 25 mm of 1.93 mm tubing connected to an HA-2 coupler, which is designed to simulate the average earmold with a bore length of 18 mm and inner diameter of 3 mm. Thus, the transmission line of a typical BTE is ~75 mm long. In an eyeglass fitting, the transmission line is ~20 to 30 mm shorter, due to the absence of an earhook. Finally, the dimensions of the typical

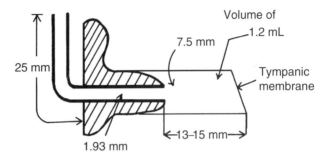

Figure 2–1 An earmold coupled to the ear canal.

ear canal from the earmold tip to the eardrum is 13 to 15 mm long and 7.5 mm wide (Cox, 1979). **Figure 2–1** is a schematic of the typical dimensions of the transmission line from the tubing to the eardrum.

◆ Earhook

An earhook is a semirigid acoustic connector used to retain a hearing aid over the ear and to conduct sound to tubing that is connected to the earhook. Earhooks are available in a variety of shapes (e.g., quarter, half moon) and materials. The bore diameter of the earhook usually tapers at the tubing end, although some earhooks have minimal tapering (i.e., 2.25 mm at the start and 1.83 mm at the end). Cox (1979) compared the output of a hearing aid–earmold system with a variety of earhooks ranging in length from 20 to 30 mm and with constant diameters of 1.2 to 1.5 mm. She reported 1 to 2 dB greater high-frequency output when using the shorter and wider earhooks.

Some earhooks come with dampers, whereas others allow the audiologist to add or change the damper. Some are threaded, and others are of the snap-on variety. ANSI S3.37–1987 (ANSI, 1987) specifies a preferred earhook nozzle thread (5–40 UNC-2A; modified and unmodified) to reduce the number of different earhook styles currently stocked by audiologists in their clinics.

Tubing Resonances

As stated earlier, one of the goals of a successful fitting is to deliver a smooth, gently rising frequency response to the eardrum of the listener. Unfortunately, many hearing aids (particularly undamped BTEs) provide a frequency response that is characterized by numerous sharp resonant peaks that can hamper a successful hearing aid fitting.

The typical length of the transmission line from the receiver to the tip of the earmold is ~75 mm, with an inner diameter ranging from 1.0 to 1.93 mm. In a tube open at both ends, a length of 75 mm and a diameter of 1.93 mm will produce a half-wave resonance at ~2300, 4600, and 6900 Hz (Cox, 1979). A half-wave resonance will occur at

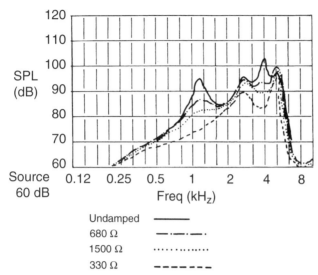

Figure 2–2 Frequency responses of a hearing aid with an undamped and damped earhook. For the damped conditions, a 680, 1500, and 3300 Ω (ohm) fused mesh damper was placed at the earhook. SPL, sound pressure level.

frequencies that are twice the effective wavelength of the tubing. In a hearing aid fitting, the tube is closed at the receiver end, with relatively low acoustic impedance in the ear canal and eardrum. The presence of the closed tube and the impedance mismatch will create a quarter-wave resonance, where the wavelength of the incoming signal is 4 times the effective length of the tube. Additional resonances will occur at odd-number intervals of this fundamental frequency. Thus, for a 75 mm effective length tube closed at both ends, a quarter-wave resonance will produce resonances between 1000 and 10,000 Hz at ~1100, 3300, and 5500 Hz. **Figure 2–2** illustrates the presence of these resonances for a BTE hearing aid when damping was not placed in the earhook (solid line).

Damping

Fused Mesh Dampers

To reduce the sharp resonant peaks in the frequency response, several types of damping materials have been introduced. Damping allows the user to increase the volume control setting with less probability of feedback and thus achieve greater usable gain and output. In addition, the reduction of gain at 1000 Hz will reduce the upward spread of masking and improve word recognition in noise.

These peaks are undesirable because they degrade sound quality, introduce transients, and may allow the output to exceed the listener's loudness discomfort level. Knowles Electronics LLC (Itasca, IL) introduced fused mesh dampers to reduce the gain and output to acceptable levels and smooth the frequency response (Gastmeirer, 1981). A fused mesh damper is a finely woven plastic screen held in place by a stainless steel screen and encased in a 2.5 mm long by 2 mm wide metal ferrule. The damper provides pure acoustic resistance and negligible reactance and, therefore, does not attenuate the high-frequency region of the

frequency response; this was one of the problems with earlier materials used for damping. The Knowles Electronics dampers were originally designed to fit snugly inside no. 13 tubing with an inner diameter of 1.93 mm. They are available in five discrete resistances of 680, 1500, 2200, 3300, and 4700 Ω (ohms), which are color coded as white, green, red, orange, and yellow, respectively. These dampers allow greater high-frequency output and a smoother frequency response. **Figure 2–2** illustrates the smoothing of the frequency response and increased low-frequency attenuation by adding 680, 1500, or 3300 Ω dampers to the earhook. From **Fig. 2–2**, it can be seen that the 3300 Ω damper decreased output at 4000 Hz, which may be considered undesirable, depending on the magnitude of hearing loss in this frequency region.

Currently, the most common position for the damper is at the tip of the earhook. Inserting the damper farther along the transmission line will increase its ability to dampen the peaks, but it also will increase the probability of the damper becoming clogged with moisture and/or debris. In fact, if a patient reports that a BTE is "dead," the first troubleshooting response should be to remove the earhook (after checking the battery). If the hearing aid produces feedback, the damper is clogged. Simply replace the earhook with a new damper (most manufacturers provide damped and undamped earhooks at no charge), and the patient will be satisfied that the problem has been solved.

The effectiveness of dampers is determined by the density (i.e., resistance in acoustic ohms) of the material and the number and location of the damper(s). Killion (1988) reported using two fused mesh dampers, one at the tip of the earhook and another at the threaded end, to reduce the gain and output by ~15 dB and provide a smoother frequency response. As a cautionary note, if resonances do not appear when electroacoustically analyzing a BTE hearing aid, the manufacturer has probably provided damping; inserting additional dampers will further reduce the gain and output of the hearing aid.

Briskey (1982) reported that a 680 Ω damper reduces average full-on gain and saturation sound pressure level (SSPL) with a 90 dB SPL input (SSPL90) by 3 dB; the remaining four dampers reduce the gain and output by 4, 5, 6, and 9 dB, respectively. Teder (1979) reported that by reducing the peak in the frequency response, the audiologist can increase the "headroom" (i.e., output) of the aid and expand the range of linear amplification. Furthermore, Teder (1979) reported that a peak in the SSPL curve can cause a "volume expansion effect" when high-intensity sounds (e.g., dishes clattering and car horns) occur at the peak frequency. These sounds are then limited by the output but are higher in intensity than the remainder of the output curve, which is relatively flat.

Other Dampers

Star Damper Made of flexible silicone, the star damper allows drainage of moisture, thereby preventing buildup. It provides some gain at 2700 Hz to compensate for the loss of ear canal resonance. The star damper must be cut to different lengths, and electroacoustic measures must be made to ensure the desired effect has been achieved.

Dampers in Custom Products   A variety of dampers are now available in custom hearing aids that reduce the peak ~2000 Hz. These include, from one manufacturer, a white damper that reduces the output by 3 to 5 dB; a green damper, which reduces the output by 7 to 8 dB, and a red damper, which reduces the output by 10 dB.

Effect of Dampers on Speech Intelligibility and Clarity

Research has suggested that improved speech intelligibility, greater clarity of speech, and increased user satisfaction will result when using dampers (Cox and Gilmore, 1986). Decker (1975), however, reported no significant differences in word recognition scores (W-22) for 10 subjects who listened to the monosyllabic words using broadband and high-frequency emphasis hearing aids with and without the insertion of sintered filters.

Cox and Gilmore (1986) reported that damping could improve speech intelligibility and/or sound quality by reducing the effects of the upward spread of masking. Suppression of the peaks by damping should reduce these effects and improve the overall fidelity of amplification. Using a paired comparison paradigm, Cox and Gilmore (1986) analyzed 10 subjects with sensorineural hearing loss who evaluated $1^1/_2$ minutes of male-connected discourse embedded in multitalker babble presented at 55 and 70 dB equivalent continuous (sound) level (Leq). In general, they reported that damping the frequency response did not provide improved clarity of speech or a more advantageous preferred listening level. However, they found that reducing resonant peaks by damping could be useful in reducing feedback.

◆ Tubing

Characteristics and Materials

NAEL Tubing Sizes

Table 2–1 outlines the system used by the National Association of Earmold Laboratories (NAEL) to identify various tubing sizes. As can be seen, as the tubing number increases, the inner diameter decreases. For example, no. 9 tubing has an inner diameter of 2.4 mm, and no. 13 tubing has an inner diameter of 1.93 mm. The outer diameter can be thin, standard, medium, thick, or double-walled. The thick and double-walled tubing sizes are often used for power BTEs to reduce the probability of feedback and vibration.

Table 2–1 Inside and Outside Diameters of Tubing Sizes as Standardized by the National Association of Earmold Laboratories

Tubing Size	Inside Diameter		Outside Diameter	
	(inches)	(mm)	(inches)	(mm)
9	0.094	2.4	0.160	4.1
12	0.085	2.2	0.125	3.2
13 standard	0.076	1.9	0.116	2.9
13 medium	0.076	1.9	0.122	3.2
13 thick wall	0.076	1.9	0.130	3.3
13 double wall	0.076	1.9	0.142	3.6
14	0.066	1.7	0.116	2.9
15	0.059	1.5	0.166	2.9
16 standard	0.053	1.3	0.166	2.9
16 thin	0.053	1.3	0.085	2.2

Tubing Styles

Tubing can be ordered as bulk, preformed, quilled, or single-, double-, or triple-bend. It can also be ordered as clear or tinted or with a cut-tapered end for easier insertion into the earmold sound bore. Also available is Libby horn Dri-Tube. This type of tubing is made from a denser, more rubbery material that helps to eliminate or reduce condensation. It is available as 3 or 4 mm horn, no. 13 medium, and thick walled.

Tubing Adapters

Several variations of adapters are available to connect to tubing. For example, male and female adapters (large and miniature sizes) can be used with receiver earmolds. These fit onto the tubing to allow direct snap-in connectors to the receiver earmold. In addition, elbows made of hard vinyl with gradual or sharp right-angle bends can be ordered that are threaded or cemented into a hole in a Lucite earmold for easier changing of tubing. Another possibility is a hard plastic, stepped-bore permanent elbow that creates an acoustic effect similar to the Libby 4 mm horn, which will be discussed in a later section.

Tubing Cement

Generally, cementing tubing into the bore of an earmold is a relatively simple task when using hard Lucite earmolds. For polyvinyl and other soft earmolds, however, the dispenser should use "sheer" tubing cement. Another solution is to use tube lock, tube lock plus, and tubing retention systems, which have recently been introduced. These use a small 14-carat gold–coated brass ring containing a small flange. It is assembled and permanently affixed by the earmold laboratory. Using this system, the tubing can never be loosened or pulled out. It is available in two sizes, regular and double walled, and requires a special tool for insertion and removal of the tube lock. The tube lock can be used with any size tubing and is highly recommended for materials where glue will not easily adhere. More recently, several earmold manufacturers introduced a special tube lock, EZ Tube, for soft earmolds designed for patients with severe to profound hearing loss. This is a permanently installed nozzle in the sound bore of the earmold; the audiologist can remove the old tubing from the nozzle and replace it with new tubing. Another possibility is the continuous flow adapter (CFA) for earmolds, which will be explained in greater detail in a later section.

Pearl

- Never use Super-Glue (Super Glue Corp., Rancho Cucamonga, CA) or similar cyanoacrylate product to glue tubing into the sound bore of an earmold. The use of this product makes it very difficult to replace tubing.

Tubing Length

Recall that ANSI S3.22–2003 (ANSI, 2003) requires BTE hearing aids to be electroacoustically analyzed using 25 mm of no. 13 tubing coupled to an HA-2 coupler. In reality, changing tubing length is limited because tubing length is related to anatomical dimensions of the head. As **Fig. 2–3** illustrates, however, if the length is increased to 37 mm (re 25 mm), the primary resonant peak will shift downward, and the output will increase in the lower frequencies and

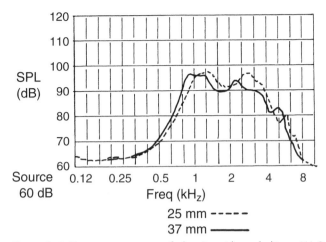

Figure 2–3 Frequency response of a hearing aid coupled to an HA-2 coupler with 25 and 37 mm of no. 13 tubing.

decrease in the middle and high frequencies. Also, the amplitude of the second and third peaks will be reduced. If the tubing is shortened to 25 mm (re 37 mm), the primary and secondary peaks will shift upward in frequency. Also, the output will decrease in the low frequencies and increase in the middle and high frequencies. **Table 2–2** summarizes the

Table 2–2 Effect of Various Modifications on Four Regions of the Frequency Response

	Frequency Region (Hz)			
Change	**< 750**	**750–1500**	**1500–3000**	**> 3000**
Tubing length				
Short	Slight decrease	Moves peak to higher Hz	Moves peak to higher Hz	Minimal
Long	Slight increase	Moves peak to lower Hz	Moves peak to lower Hz	Decrease
Tubing diameter				
Wider	Minimal	Moves peak to higher Hz	Moves peak to higher Hz	Increase
Narrower	May decrease	Moves peak to lower Hz	Reduces height of peak and moves to lower Hz	Decrease
Bore length				
Short	Slight decrease	Moves peak to higher Hz	Moves peak to higher Hz	Increase
Long	Slight increase	Moves peak to lower Hz	Moves peak to lower Hz	Decrease
Bore diameter				
Wider	Minimal	Moves peak to higher Hz	Moves peak to higher Hz	Increase
Narrower	Minimal	Moves peak to lower Hz	Moves peak to lower Hz	Decrease
Belling	Minimal	Minimal	Minimal	Increase
Tubing insertion				
Medial	Minimal	Minimal	Shifts peak to lower Hz	Decrease
Lateral	Minimal	Minimal	Shifts peak to higher Hz	Increase
Venting				
Small (0.8 mm)	Minimal	Minimal	Minimal	Minimal
Medium (1.6 mm)	Decrease	Increases peak height	Minimal	Minimal
Large (2.4 mm)	Decrease	Increases peak height	Minimal	Minimal
Parallel	Less attenuation of low-frequency SPL than diagonal venting, but no attenuation of high-frequency SPL			
Diagonal	Greater attenuation of low-frequency SPL than parallel venting, and greater attenuation of high-frequency SPL			

SPL, sound pressure level.
Source: Adapted from Microsonic, Inc., with permission.

effect changing tubing length may have on four regions of the frequency response curve.

Tubing Diameter

ANSI S3.22–2003 (ANSI, 2003) also requires BTE hearing aids to be electroacoustically analyzed using 25 mm of no. 13 tubing, which has an inner diameter of 1.93 mm. Using tubing with a wider diameter (no. 9, 11, or 12 tubing) will increase the gain between 1000 and 2000 Hz and decrease the gain in the lower frequencies. Using tubing with a narrower diameter (no. 14–16 tubing) will increase the gain in the lower frequencies and decrease the gain in the higher frequencies. **Table 2–2** summarizes the effect changing tubing diameter may have on four regions of the frequency response curve.

Tubing Length and Diameter

Changes in length and diameter are consistent when either length or diameter is varied independently. That is, a long tube with a narrow inner diameter will shift the frequency peaks downward. Using a short tube with a wider diameter will shift the frequency peaks upward.

Minimal Insertion of Tubing

Up to this point, the discussion has assumed that the audiologist has inserted the tubing to the tip of the earmold. Another strategy is to insert the tubing minimally into the sound bore and create a "dual-tube" fitting. This strategy takes advantage of the fact that when there is a significant step-up in diameter toward the ear canal, there is a quarter-wave open-end resonance in the larger bore section that exits into the ear canal. This can result in considerable high-frequency amplification above 2000 Hz.

An example of such a strategy would be inserting no. 13 tubing only 3 mm into the sound bore. **Figure 2–4** illustrates 2 cc coupler measures of a BTE hearing aid when no. 13 tubing was inserted 3, 9, and 16 mm (tip) into the sound bore. Notice the improved high-frequency output when the tubing was inserted only 3 mm (solid line) into the sound bore when compared with the tubing inserted to the tip (dashed line). In this case, there is 10 to 12 dB greater output at 5000 to 6000 Hz than when the tubing was cemented to the tip. **Table 2–2** summarizes the effects insertion of tubing in the sound bore has on four regions of the frequency response curve.

Special Consideration

- When using the strategy of minimal insertion of tubing into the sound bore, it is very important that a high-quality cement be used to anchor the tubing into the bore.

Figure 2–5 reveals that the effect of minimal insertion of the tubing is directly related to the length of the sound bore. That is, as the bore length increases, the effect of minimal

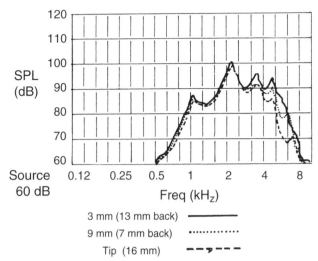

3 mm (13 mm back) ————
9 mm (7 mm back)   ·············
Tip (16 mm)   — — ⸌ — — —

Figure 2–4 Change in output when inserting no. 13 tubing 3 mm, 9 mm, and to the tip of an earmold when the bore length is 16 mm.

insertion becomes greater. As bore length is reduced, the advantage of this strategy is diminished. Finally, the magnitude of the effect is dependent upon the length and diameter of the second segment. The longer and wider the second segment, the greater the high-frequency boost.

Pearl

- If the goal of the hearing aid fitting is to achieve as much high-frequency gain as possible, do not order earmolds with no. 13 tubing cemented to the tip. Instead, order an earmold with a "horn" design or tubing only slightly inserted into the sound bore.

Open Canal Fittings

Tube Fitting

One of the most significant advances in hearing aid technology has been the open fitting. This type of fitting is covered in great depth in Chapter 1.

One method of tube fitting is to use a free-field mold that is adjusted in varying lengths to create the desired change in the frequency response and then cemented in place to a nonoccluding earmold (**Figs. 2–6** and **2–7**). When used with a conventional BTE, this would be classified as an ipsilateral routing of signals (IROS) fitting. Another method is using a tube fitting (**Fig. 2–6**) in which the tubing is not cemented. The rationale is to achieve maximum high-frequency gain without feedback, obtain maximum low-frequency attenuation (up to 30 dB at 500 Hz), and provide maximum comfort. This type of tube fitting will not occlude the ear canal, which can reduce the transmission of low-frequency sounds by as much as 15 to 30 dB, depending on the magnitude of occlusion by the earmold. This type of tube fitting also takes

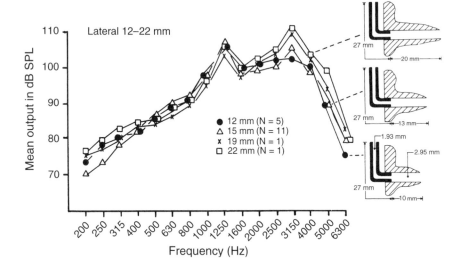

Figure 2–5 Change in output when inserting no. 13 tubing 2 mm into the sound bore for four earmolds in which bore lengths are 12, 15, 19, and 22 mm.

advantage of the natural resonance of the ear canal, which is around 17 dB at 2800 Hz. For some patients, greater retention of a nonoccluding earmold may be necessary. A design offering the benefits of a nonoccluding earmold, but with greater retention, is illustrated in **Fig. 2–7C.**

In the past, tube fittings were not considered when the patient has a ski-slope audiometric configuration with hearing loss up to 50 dB above 2000 Hz. At that time, it was recommended that if the hearing loss was >50 dB, the audiologist should not consider using a tube fitting but, instead, use a conventional earmold with some degree of venting because of acoustic feedback. As a result of advances in feedback management in current digital hearing aids, the upper range of hearing loss that can be fitted with modern digital open-fit hearing aids is in excess of 70 to 80 dB without the presence of feedback.

A tube fitting may be considered when an earmold is contraindicated due to middle ear drainage, irritations in the ear canal, allergic reactions to earmold materials, psoriasis, eczema, and scars. It should not be used with a high-frequency emphasis hearing aid but, instead, should be used with a broadband hearing aid. Furthermore, for tube fittings to provide adequate high-frequency gain, insertion of the tubing must be > 15 mm beyond the orifice of the ear canal. As the tubing is moved closer to the eardrum, the frequency response below 1500 Hz is shifted downward, producing a broader response. As the tubing is placed farther away from the eardrum, there is greater low-frequency attenuation. Also, its use in smaller ear canals will produce greater high-frequency gain than in longer canals, with tubing length held constant.

Currently, numerous open-fit hearing aids incorporate "links," that is, very thin tubing of varying discrete lengths that are attached to the hearing aid and act as a means to send the amplified sound to the ear canal. At the termination of the link, a soft plastic "dome" that is preset in varying diameters is coupled to the end of the link to keep the link comfortably placed and retained in the ear. The use of this very thin link provides the user with a very cosmetically appealing BTE fit.

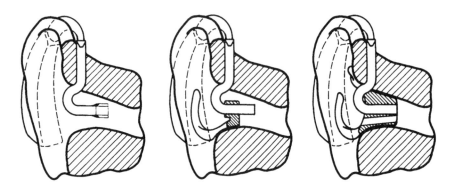

Figure 2–6 Three nonoccluding earmold designs: tube fitting, free field, and full mold with a large vent. (From Microsonic, Inc., with permission.)

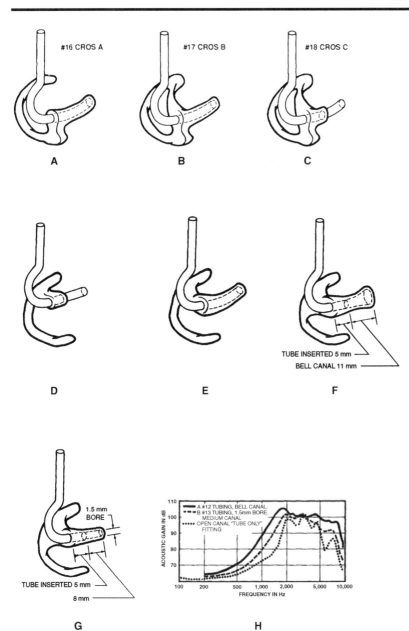

Figure 2–7 Examples of seven nonoccluding earmolds: **(A)** Contralateral routing of signals (CROS) A, **(B)** CROS B, **(C)** CROS C, **(D)** free field, **(E)** Janssen, **(F)** extended range earmold, **(G)** another extended range earmold, and **(H)** frequency response of three nonoccluding earmolds. (From Microsonic, Inc., with permission.)

To properly fit tube fittings, it is suggested that the audiologist first use no. 15 tubing (inner diameter = 1.5 mm) and then try tubing with a wider diameter (no. 9) to achieve even greater high-frequency emphasis. To achieve maximum comfort, it is necessary to bend the tubing to comfortably fit in the ear canal. To do this, wipe isopropyl alcohol over solid core solder wire whose outer diameter is sufficiently wide enough to fit snugly inside the tubing. Next, bend the tubing to the desired configuration and add heat via an air blower with a heat-directing shield. Cool the tubing in alcohol or water to preserve the configuration, then remove the solder. At this point the tubing will maintain its shape.

Traditional CROS Open Mold

Harford and Barry (1965) introduced the contralateral routing of signals (CROS; **Fig. 2–7A-C**) earmold for unilateral and high-frequency hearing loss. It must be noted that CROS amplification is most effective if the aided (better) ear has a mild to moderate high-frequency hearing loss. If the hearing thresholds in the better ear are within normal limits, the prognosis for success with CROS amplification will be greatly diminished. For these patients, a transcranial CROS should be considered as an option (Valente et al, 1995). In a transcranial CROS, a power BTE, ITE, or CIC is fitted to the "dead" ear. Valente et al (1995) demonstrated that, in half their subjects, the transcranial fitting provided significant benefit. The authors believe that success with transcranial CROS fittings can occur if the patient (1) has lower transcranial thresholds, and (2) is fitted with a power BTE with a tightly fitting earmold with a long bore and pressure vent. Success is less likely if the fitting is attempted with a power ITE or CIC.

Harford and Barry (1965) reported that the CROS mold can improve aided word recognition scores in noise due to significant low-frequency reduction. Courtois et al (1988) advocated use of CROS molds for patients with mild to moderate hearing loss to attenuate low frequencies, thereby reducing both the amplification of ambient noise and the occlusion effect. They measured the SPL in closed and open molds and found differences of 30 to 40 dB below 125 Hz; these differences disappeared at ~2000 Hz. They also reported that a 2 mm vent reduces the occlusion effect at 250 to 500 Hz, and a 3 mm vent reduces the occlusion effect to 750 Hz.

The CROS mold is similar to a parallel-vented earmold, which has a vent so large that only a small piece of earmold is left to hold the tubing in place. Cox (1979) reported that the acoustic difference between a CROS mold and a tube fit is minimal, providing the ear canal is not so small as to be occluded by the small retention portion of the open mold fitting. If retention does occlude the ear canal, a tube fitting is preferred to obtain the desired acoustic effect. The tube fitting will significantly reduce low-frequency amplification and provide some high-frequency emphasis above the vent-associated resonance. This effect is dependent upon the depth of insertion, the inner diameter of the tubing, and the size of the ear canal. As insertion depth is closer to the eardrum, less low-frequency energy will escape, but, more importantly, greater high-frequency amplification will occur. As tubing diameter is reduced, there will be an overall reduction in output and a shift of the first peak to a lower frequency. If no gain is required below 2000 Hz, the audiologist should use tubing with a narrower inner diameter for greater user satisfaction. This strategy, however, will reduce the overall SPL and provide less high-frequency gain. Low-frequency attenuation will be less for a tube fit when fitted to a small ear canal than if the ear canal is of average length.

Controversial Point

- Should a hearing aid ever be placed in a "dead" ear? Valente et al (1995) demonstrated that in half of their subjects, a transcranial CROS was viewed by the subjects as providing significant benefit. The authors believe that success with transcranial CROS fittings can occur if (1) the patient has reduced transcranial thresholds and (2) is fitted with a power BTE; also, the earmold must be tight fitting and have a long bore and pressure vent. Less success will be achieved if the fitting is attempted with a power ITE or CIC.

Pearl

- CROS amplification is most effective if the better (aided) ear has a mild to moderate high-frequency hearing loss. If the hearing thresholds in the better (aided) ear are within normal limits, the prognosis for success with CROS amplification will be greatly diminished. For these patients, a transcranial CROS should be considered as an option (Valente et al, 1995).

Libby 3 and 4 Millimeter Horns

Libby (1981) designed injection-molding techniques to obtain a one-piece 3 and 4 mm tapered horn. The 4 mm design is comprised of 21 mm of no. 13 tubing, enlarged to 22 mm of tubing 4 mm wide. The 3 mm horn has 21 mm of no. 13 tubing, enlarged to 22 mm of tubing 3 mm wide. The 3 mm horn will provide 5 to 6 dB less gain at 2500 to 3000 Hz in comparison to the 4 mm horn. Both styles are designed to work best with a 1500 Ω fused mesh damper at the tip of the earhook. Libby (1981) advocated that the stepped diameter earmold should be used with a hearing aid having a wideband receiver to obtain high-fidelity sound quality, an extended frequency response, and reduced battery drain. **Table 2–3** reports the relative changes in the output of a

Table 2–3 Changes in Gain/Output (dB) for Several Acoustically Tuned Earmolds Relative to the Response Obtained Using an HA-2 Coupler or No. 13 Tubing to the Tip of the Earmold Measured in an HA-1 Coupler

Earmold Design	250 dB	500 dB	1000 dB	2000 dB	3000 dB	4000 dB	6000 dB
No. 13 tubing to the tip (HA-1 coupler)							
Libby 4 mm*	−1	−2	−3	−2	−6	10	6
Libby 3 mm	−1	−2	−2	0	6	8	2
3 × 18 mm (HA-2 coupler)							
Libby 4 mm*	−1	−1	−2	0	2	3	0
Libby 3 mm	0	0	0	1	3	2	−4

* Dimensions of Libby 4 mm: 680 Ω damper at earhook tip.
Source: Data from Dillion, H. (1985). Earmolds and high-frequency response modification. Hearing Instruments, 36(12), 8–12; and Dillon, H. (1991). Allowing for real ear venting effects when selecting the coupler gain of hearing aids. Ear and Hearing, 12, 404–416.

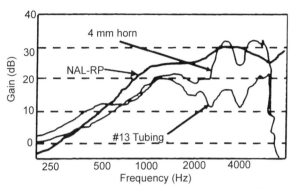

Figure 2–8 Real ear insertion gain (REIG) measured with no. 13 tubing and a 4 mm Libby horn for National Acoustic Laboratories–Revised Profound (NAL-RP) prescriptive target.

hearing aid produced by the Libby 3 and 4 mm designs relative to the output measured in an HA-1 or HA-2 coupler.

Figure 2–8 illustrates an important point concerning the benefits of the Libby horn. In this case, the first author was fitting a patient who had arrived at the clinic from another facility with a BTE coupled to the earmold with no. 13 tubing. Initial real ear insertion gain (REIG) measures were performed to verify if the measured REIG reasonably matched the prescribed National Acoustic Laboratories–Revised Profound (NAL-RP; solid curve) target. The initial REIG (lower curve) with the no. 13 tubing revealed that the measured REIG was significantly below the prescribed NAL-RP. Rather than attach the hearing aid to the programmer to increase the gain to match the target, it was decided to remove the no. 13 tubing and drill the bore to make it wider to accept the wider outer diameter of the 4 mm horn. A repeat REIG with the 4 mm horn (upper curve in **Fig. 2–8**) clearly indicates that the REIG with the 4 mm horn arrives much closer to the prescribed REIG than was possible with the no. 13 tubing. More importantly, the amplifier in the hearing aid was not programmed to achieve the greater required gain (i.e., maintained greater headroom). This leaves the amplifier available for future increases in gain should the patient's hearing loss decrease. In addition, by not programming the amplifier to provide greater amplification, there was probably less distortion at the output of the hearing aid, and the amplified sound was crisper. Thus, it is the strong belief of the authors that almost all patients should be fit with a 3 or 4 mm horn unless the hearing loss is of a rising configuration. In our clinics, virtually all patients are fit with a 3 or 4 mm horn.

In its original development, the Libby 3 or 4 mm horn was ordered without a vent. Pedersen (1984), however, reported that a 2 mm diagonal vent intersecting near the end of the earmold did not affect the high-frequency gain provided by the 3 or 4 mm horn. The mean difference was less than 1 dB at six discrete frequencies between 250 and 4000 Hz. To reduce the likelihood of inducing the occlusion effect, the authors suggest that 3 and 4 mm horns be ordered with some degree of venting. The authors of this chapter routinely order Select-A-Vent (SAV) or Positive Venting Valve (PVV) vent "trees" for all horn fittings. The advantage of this strategy will be presented in a later section.

Burgess and Brooks (1991) reported that the sound quality from a hearing aid using the Libby horn was rated clearer, more natural, undistorted, and more acoustically comfortable when compared with an earmold where the tubing was cemented to the tip of the earmold. Objectively, real-ear and functional gain measures reported greater gain (mean of 8 dB) in the higher frequencies (1500–6000 Hz). They also reported improved recognition of phonemes, especially the fricatives and affricates. Mueller et al (1981) compared the Libby 3 mm horn to a free-field mold for 24 subjects with high-frequency sensorineural hearing loss. Functional gain measures revealed 5 to 10 dB greater functional gain at 3000 Hz with the Libby horn in comparison to the free-field earmold. There were no significant differences in word recognition scores, however, or subjective ratings between the two earmold designs. Robinson et al (1989) compared the performance of 21 inexperienced users with the Libby 4 mm horn and an earmold where no. 13 tubing was cemented to the tip of the earmold. Aided scores for speech in noise (+5 dB signal-to-noise ratio [SNR]) using consonant-vowel-consonant (CVC) words were, on average, only 2.4% better with the Libby 4 mm horn. Two thirds of the subjects, however, preferred the sound quality of the 4 mm horn. After a 4-week trial period, the 4 mm horn was preferred by those subjects who had poorer hearing above 2000 Hz. The researchers concluded that improved word recognition could be achieved with a hearing aid providing a smooth rising frequency response in which the response extended the higher frequencies.

Bergenstoff (1983) reported that the real-ear gain above 2000 Hz for a hearing aid coupled to an earmold in which no. 13 tubing is inserted to the tip was as much as 20 dB lower than the gain reported in a 2 cc coupler whose dimensions are 18 mm long and 3 mm wide. When using a 4 mm horn coupled to a hearing aid having a narrow frequency range, the frequency response was extended by almost an octave, the gain was increased by 10 to 15 dB, and the midfrequency resonant peak was reduced by 4 dB. When the same earmold was coupled to a hearing aid providing a wideband response, the 4 mm horn extended the frequency response by almost two octaves, increased high-frequency gain by 20 dB, and reduced the midfrequency resonant peak by 8 dB. Sung and Sung (1982) compared the performance of the Libby 3 and 4 mm horns to a conventional earmold with no. 13 tubing to the tip on 28 subjects with sensorineural hearing loss. Word recognition scores (Northwestern University 6 [NU-6] and high-frequency word lists) presented in quiet at 70 dB SPL and noise (SNR of +6 dB) were improved only 0.9 to 4.9%. Functional gain increased by 0.5 dB at 1500 Hz to 6.4 dB at 4000 Hz. For some subjects, the improvement was as large as 15 dB. In addition, 54% of the subjects expressed a preference for the Libby designs. Finally, some audiologists might question the feasibility of the average ear canal being wide enough to accommodate an earmold requiring a 4 mm bore and venting. However, in the experience of the authors, an earmold requiring an inner diameter of 4 mm is feasible for a majority of adult subjects. Clearly, this may be a viable concern when providing services to a pediatric population.

Finally, it is the opinion of the authors that if a patient has hearing thresholds no greater than ~70 to 75 dB at 2000 to 4000 Hz, use of a 3 or 4 mm Libby horn is essential for improving speech recognition. It is not in the best interests of the patient to order no. 13 tubing. If the hearing thresholds above 2000 Hz are >75 dB, no. 13 tubing or a reversed horn is recommended. These are recommended because it is unlikely for a patient with this magnitude of hearing loss to gain any benefit from the amplification provided in the high-frequency region. In addition, the amplification required to "correct" this hearing loss is likely to cause feedback. If feedback occurs, the patient is forced to turn down the volume control, resulting in underamplification in the frequency region where hearing thresholds are better.

Pearl

- If a patient has hearing thresholds no greater than 75 to 80 dB at 2000 to 4000 Hz, use of a 3 or 4 mm Libby horn is essential. It is not in the best interests of the patient to use no. 13 tubing. If the hearing loss is greater than 80 dB, a reversed horn is recommended to reduce the chance of feedback. If feedback occurs, the patient may be forced to reduce the volume control. This will reduce the gain in the frequency region where hearing thresholds are better.

Reverse Horn

Libby (1981) designed injection molding techniques to obtain a one-piece reverse tapered horn (i.e., the diameter of the tube at the tip is narrower than the diameter of the tube at the earhook) for patients with severe to profound hearing loss, to reduce the likelihood of feedback for BTE fittings caused by peaks in the high-frequency region of the frequency response. The reverse horn reduces the gain above 2000 Hz and shifts the energy toward the lower frequencies (8–10 dB shift in low-frequency gain). This is appropriate for patients who cannot achieve sufficient gain prior to feedback and must reduce the volume control to eliminate feedback. When feedback is reduced via a reverse horn, patients can achieve sufficient low-frequency gain where their hearing is typically better.

♦ Earmolds

Early earmold selection in the United States was rather simple. The hearing aid fitter poured plaster of paris to cast the impression, and the completed earmold was fabricated from a black hard rubber material. The only style available was a "regular" earmold and a large button receiver, painted in a bright pink and optimistically called "flesh," which was attached to the earmold. An alternative fitting used a flat 2-inch-diameter earphone, which covered most of the pinna and was held in place by a 19 mm wide spring steel headband. By World War II, plastic technology grew to include thermosetting acrylic impression materials and methyl methacrylate (Lucite) earmolds.

Currently, audiologists have a wide range of material and style options available to them. Earmolds are designed to seal the ear canal, correctly couple the hearing aid to the ear from an acoustical viewpoint, retain the hearing aid to the pinna, be comfortable for an extended period of time, modify the acoustic signal produced by the hearing aid, be able to be easily handled by the patient, and be cosmetically appealing.

Use of Scanning Technology to Manufacture Earmolds

One of the most significant advances in earmold technology is the manner in which impressions for earmolds and custom products are being processed after the impression has been made. In the past, the impression was made, placed in a box with the order form, and forwarded to the hearing aid manufacturer or earmold laboratory. This process is still followed, but with one major change. In the past several years, advances in computer and software technology have allowed the audiologist to make the impression, place it a box with the order form, and send it to the manufacturer, where the impression is now scanned and stored electronically (Lesiecki, 2006). The scanned impression is then modeled, and decisions are made by the software. Initially, scanning technology was available only from the leading hearing aid manufacturers—GN ReSound A/S (Ballerup, Denmark), Siemens Hearing Instruments Inc. (Piscataway, NJ), Phonak AG (Stäfe, Switzerland), Oticon A/S (Smørum, Denmark), Widex A/S (Vaerloese, Denmark), and Starkey Laboratories Inc. (Eden Prairie, MN)—for the purpose of modeling custom products. In fact, Siemens recently introduced technology allowing the audiologist to scan an impression in the clinic and download the scanned image to the manufacturer via the Internet. Now, several earmold laboratories provide similar technology. One of the obvious advantages of this method is that it is no longer necessary to remake impressions when a problem is present with the initial impression; instead, the remake can be manufactured from the scanned image. The day is not far off when this method of scanning will be replaced by the ability of audiologists to directly scan the ear and ear canal and send the scanned image over the Internet. In the not too distant future, the concerns and issues of placing eardams and impression material into the ear canal will be a thing of the past.

Changing Earmold Bore to Change Frequency Response

Changing Bore Length

Lybarger (1979) reported that changing the bore length from minimum to maximum will increase or decrease the overall gain by no more than 2 dB in either direction. Increasing bore length, however, will increase low-frequency gain, and decreasing bore length will increase high- frequency gain. **Table 2–2** summarizes how changing the bore length may affect four regions of the frequency response curve.

Changing Bore Diameter

Lybarger (1979) reported that the wider the diameter of the bore, the greater the high-frequency emphasis; the narrower the diameter of the bore, the greater the low-frequency emphasis. **Table 2–2** summarizes how changing the bore diameter may affect four regions of the frequency response curve.

Changing Bore Length and Diameter

Changes in length and diameter are consistent when either length or diameter is varied independently. That is, a long bore with a narrow inner diameter will shift the frequency response downward. Using a short bore with a wider diameter will shift the frequency response upward.

Belling the Bore

Another method of increasing high-frequency amplification is to drill, or "bell," the last segment of the earmold with a bur to create a wider diameter than at the entrance of the earmold. Cox (1979) reported that belling the end of the earmold effectively produces a limited horn effect that can increase high-frequency amplification, but its effectiveness depends on the length of the bore. **Figure 2–9** illustrates a belled bore with minimal insertion of tubing and a parallel vent. **Figure 2–10** illustrates such an earmold that was prepared for a patient with a gently sloping audiogram. **Figure 2–11** illustrates the performance of a BTE hearing aid measured in an HA-1 2 cc coupler under two conditions. First (dotted line), the hearing aid was measured using no. 13 tubing and a 1000 Ω damper at the tip of the earmold. Second, the same hearing aid was measured using a config-

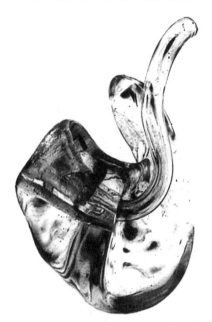

Figure 2–10 Example of an earmold with a belled bore, parallel vent, and minimal insertion of tubing ordered for a patient with a gently sloping audiogram.

uration described in **Figs. 2–9** and **2–10,** but with the vent closed with putty. Notice how the belled bore increased high-frequency output and extended the high-frequency response (dashed line).

Taking Earmold Impressions

To develop the skills required to take an acceptable impression of the ear, it is necessary for the audiologist to become familiar with the anatomy of the external ear and to have a working knowledge of the vocabulary used to identify key anatomical sites (**Fig. 2–12**). The audiologist must become

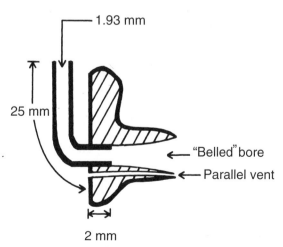

Figure 2–9 An earmold with a belled bore and parallel vent, with tubing inserted 2 mm into the sound bore.

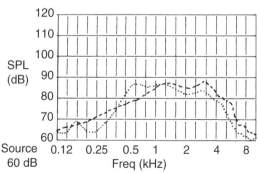

Belled bore and 3 mm insertion of tubing
with 1000 Ω damper   -----
#13 tubing to tip of earmold with 1000 Ω damper   ....

Figure 2–11 Frequency response using an earmold with a belled bore, 3 mm insertion of tubing, and a 1000 Ω damper at the tip of the earhook. Also illustrated is the frequency response generated when using an earmold with no. 13 tubing to the tip of the earmold and a 1000 Ω damper at the tip of the earhook.

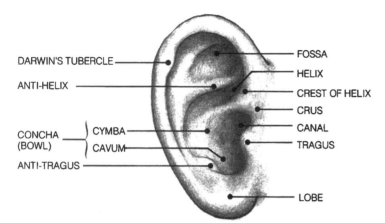

Figure 2–12 Anatomical sites of the outer ear. (From Microsonic, Inc., with permission.)

familiar with the terminology used by earmold manufacturers to describe important segments of the earmold in relation to the anatomy of the ear **(Fig. 2–13)**. Alvord et al (1997) recommended nomenclature that should be used when describing the parts of an earmold. For example, they suggest using the term *canal stalk* instead of *canal*. In addition, these authors divide the canal stalk into superior, anterior, inferior, posterior, and medial surfaces. They go on to suggest 13 other terms to be used in describing the segments of an earmold.

Examination of the Ear Canal

The first step is to perform an otoscopic observation. For an adult, pull the pinna upward to straighten the ear canal; for a child, pull the pinna downward. Be sure the ear canal is free of cerumen and foreign objects. Inspect the ear canal to determine if deformities (i.e., atresia), pathologies (warts, moles, and tumors), infections (drainage, irritations, and redness of the canal wall or eardrum), or abnormalities of the ear canal (stenosis, prolapsed canal, and surgically altered canal) are present. If any of these conditions are present, do not proceed with the impression but instead refer the patient to an otolaryngologist for consultation.

Selection and Placement of an Otoblock

One of the first decisions made when preparing an earmold impression is selecting the appropriate otoblock, which is placed in the ear canal to prevent the impression material from coming into contact with the eardrum. Attached to the otoblock is thread or dental floss, which helps in the removal of the impression from the ear canal. It is important, however, to remember that the removal of the impression from the ear canal is achieved primarily by pulling back on the impression and not by pulling the thread. This thread should be placed along the floor of the ear canal and draped over the intratragal notch of the pinna.

Morgan (1994) reminded us of the importance of selecting the correct otoblock. An undersized otoblock will allow impression material past the otoblock or push the otoblock too deep into the ear canal. An oversized otoblock will abnormally expand in the ear canal or prevent the otoblock from being placed sufficiently deep. Morgan suggests that the otoblock be correctly placed, using an ear light, beyond the first bend of the ear canal and optimally to at least the second bend. The authors highly recommend deep impressions (i.e., beyond the second bend) for all patients regardless of type of fit. The rationale for this suggestion will be presented in greater detail in a later section.

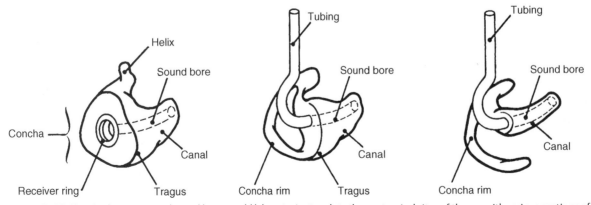

Figure 2–13 Terminology commonly used by earmold laboratories to relate the anatomical sites of the ear with various sections of three common earmolds. (From Microsonic, Inc., with permission.)

Another option is the pressure relief otosystem (PROS), which are soft-form otoblocks with a silicone tube running through the center. They ease pressure buildup that occurs while injecting impression material into the ear canal and eliminate the sensation of a vacuum reported by many patients when removing the impression.

Choice of Impression Materials

The audiologist can choose either powder (polymer)/liquid (monomer) or silicone impression materials. In recent years, the advantages and disadvantages of these materials have become the focus of debate, and no uniform agreement seems imminent. However, there is agreement that, whichever material is chosen, it is imperative that the audiologist carefully follow the instructions provided by the earmold laboratory.

Procedure for Taking an Earmold Impression

Figure 2–14 illustrates the step-by-step procedure for taking an earmold impression. Using the syringe technique, carefully mix the impression material and place in the syringe, with the nozzle of the syringe in the ear canal. Gently press the plunger and gradually withdraw the nozzle as the material fills the ear canal and begins to flow into the concha. Finally, fill the entire outer ear, especially the helix area. Keep the nozzle submerged in the impression material at all times for better filling of the ear.

Do not press the outer surface of the impression, because any pressing may lead to distortion of the impression. At this point, it is our practice to allow the patient to exercise jaw movement while the impression material is setting in the ear canal. We find this practice results in less chance of feedback and a greater chance for providing a more comfortable earmold or custom shell. Allow at least 15 minutes with powder/liquid material and 5 minutes for silicone for the impression to set. Gently break the seal by asking the patient to yawn or use exaggerated facial expressions. Remove the impression by grasping the pinna firmly with one hand and the impression with the other. Rotate the impression slowly with an upward and outward motion. The otoblock should remain on the tip of the impression.

Figure 2–15 provides several illustrations of correct and incorrect earmold impressions. Inspect the ear canal with an otoscope to be sure no impression material remains in the canal.

Morgan (1994) reported that silicone impression material retains a highly accurate and dimensionally stable impression of the ear canal from the clinic to the earmold laboratory. Many audiologists are hesitant to use silicone impression material because it is relatively messy in that it requires the proper mixing of two "pastes." One paste is a base material (silano-terminated gum) that is measured in a scoop; the second is an activator agent that is spread over the base material. The two pastes are mixed together by hand for 20 to 30 seconds until an even, consistent color is reached (see **Fig. 2–16** on p. 52); the mixture is then inserted into a syringe that is specially designed for silicone impressions. Trade names for some silicone impression

material across earmold laboratories include Yellow Stuff I and II, XL-80, X-SIL, Otoform A/K, XL-100, XL-200, Micro-SIL, Blue Velvet, Gold Velvet II, and Silicast. Prepackaged silicone is available. This material is delivered in prepackaged, self-mixing cartridges and is injected into the ear canal using an injection gun (see **Fig. 2–17** on p. 52).

Staab and Martin (1995) recommend using silicone material with a relatively low viscosity rating (20 Shore) for the bony section of ear canal and a higher viscosity rating (40 Shore) for the cartilaginous section of the ear canal. Hosford-Dunn (1996) suggest making two impressions, one with the jaw closed and a second with the jaw open. She suggests having the patient insert five tongue depressors between the teeth for the open-jaw impression. At our clinic, we have patients hold 10 to 15 tongue depressors between their teeth for the open-jaw impression. For patients who cannot accept 10 to 15 tongue depressors, we reduce the number to 5. The need for making open- and closed-jaw impressions becomes more critical when the impression is taken for a CIC hearing aid.

Although there is a growing consensus on the advantages of silicone impression material, it is the opinion of the authors that powder and liquid can provide an excellent impression if the audiologist uses the proper proportions and the resulting mixture is correctly syringed into the ear canal in a timely fashion. If the mixture of powder and liquid is incorrect and not properly cured (at least 15 minutes), the impression can stretch during removal. If the mixture is too dry (too much powder or too little liquid), it will be difficult to push through the syringe and will cause voids. Too much liquid will make the impression susceptible to melting.

To reinforce these points, ethyl methacrylate will shrink if the powder and liquid are poorly mixed. The magnitude of shrinkage can be 2 to 3% in 24 hours, 4 to 5% in 48 hours. One cause of increased shrinkage is increased use of liquid in proportion to the amount of powder. Other reasons are not shaking the liquid and/or powder before using and loss of liquid via evaporation due to a poorly sealed container.

A key factor in providing a good impression of the ear canal is "gel time" or "set-up time." This is the time it takes for the mixing of the powder and liquid to become solidified, or "cured," in the ear canal. As a rule, silicone time is 5 minutes and gel time is at least 15 minutes. Gel time decreases with increased temperature and humidity. Thus, the impression will gel faster on a hot, humid summer day than in winter. To retard gel time, some audiologists increase the amount of liquid. To evaluate this strategy, Agnew (1986) increased the liquid amounts by 10 and 20% and found that shrinkage increased by 12 and 22%, respectively, in comparison to when the correct mixture ratio was used.

Excessive heat (e.g., created when the impression is placed in an outdoor mailbox) will increase warpage and distortion of the impression. It may cause the tip of the impression to distort toward the body after 5 days. For this reason, it is important to keep the impression in a cool place. Also, it is important not to use excessive force during the impression. This will "balloon" the ear canal, and the resulting earmold will cause the ear canal to become sore.

Morgan (1994) also reminded us to encourage patients to talk, turn their head in all directions, smile, and chew while

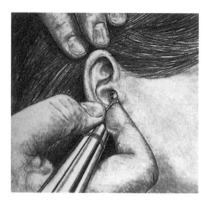

Step 1
A cotton or foam block is an ABSOLUTE NECESSITY when using the syringe. Set a tight block just past the second bend. Foam blocks MUST be compressed to insure proper results. Be sure to use the correct size foam block even though it may appear to be larger in diameter than the ear canal.

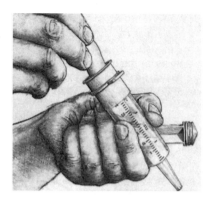

Step 2
Mix the impression material according to instructions and place in the barrel of the syringe. The quicker you can use the material the better the impression.

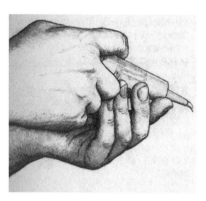

Step 3
Insert the plunger and gently push the material into the nozzle to remove air pockets.

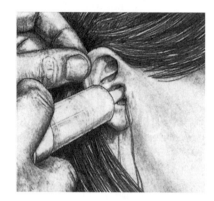

Step 4
Place the nozzle into the canal and fill the canal.

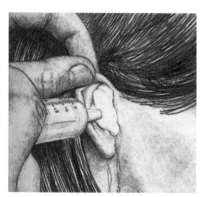

Step 5
As the material fills the canal, slowly withdraw the syringe and fill the helix and concha areas completely. Then cover the tragus.

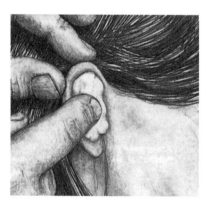

Step 6
When the external ear has been filled completely, press your finger GENTLY in the concha and helix areas. BE CAREFUL NOT TO PRESS HARD AS IMPRESSION WILL DISTORT.

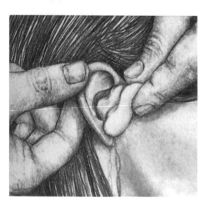

Step 7
Allow a FULL 10 MINUTES of curing time before removing. The impression can be distorted if removed too soon. To remove, gently press ear away from the impression. Remove helix curl slightly. Bring impression straight out while holding thread. Take your time. Don't strain the impression with a long steady pull.

Helpful Tips For Better Impressions
- If the client wears glasses or dentures, make sure these are in place while taking the impression.
- NEVER flatten or smooth out the finished impression with the palm of your hand while impression material is in the client's ear.
- Ask your client to talk and chew after the impression material is in place. This is to help assure a comfortable fitting custom earmold which will not unseat when the jaw muscles constrict the ear canal.
- Children are sometimes fearful and can be hard to work with. Let the child watch you take an impression of mother's ear to alleviate his fears. Let him play with a piece of the "dough". NOTE: It is difficult to use a block with SOME children. The impression may be better formed without it in these cases.

Figure 2–14 Syringe techniques for making an earmold impression. (From Microsonic, Inc., with permission.)

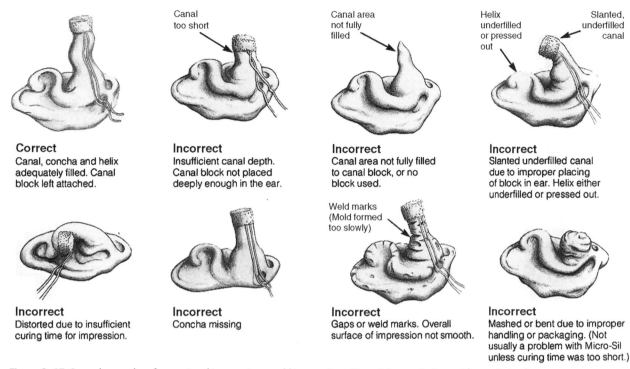

Figure 2–15 Several examples of correct and incorrect earmold impressions. (From Microsonic, Inc., with permission.)

impression material is setting in the ear canal. This will result in a more accurate impression of the dynamics of the ear canal and reduce the probability of feedback when patients move their jaw while wearing hearing aids.

When shipping, it is necessary to secure the powder and liquid impression; a silicone impression can be shipped loose in the box. Also, it is important that the order form does not come in contact with the impression, because this may cause distortion of the impression.

Procedure for Taking an Earmold Impression on a Surgically Altered Ear Canal

Taking an earmold impression on a surgically altered ear canal can present a significant challenge to the dispensing audiologist. **Figure 2–18** illustrates the potential problem. First, a foam dam is inserted into the ear canal at the position of the second bend **(Fig. 2–18A)**. Medial to the dam is the significantly larger than usual surgically altered ear canal. Next, silicone material is injected into the ear canal, stopping at the position of the dam **(Fig. 2–18B)**. **Figure 2–18C** illustrates the dam moving because of the force of the injection of the silicone material (silicone is typically denser than powder and liquid) combined with the poor "staying" power of the foam dam and the larger than usual canal size medial to the dam. The movement of the dam has now allowed the impression material to bypass the dam and fill up the ear canal space between the foam dam and the remaining canal wall. When this occurs, removal of the impression material is nearly impossible. If

there is any resistance to the removal of an impression, stop and immediately seek the assistance of an otologist. Depending on the status of the space beyond the dam, this event can lead to very serious problems and is something all audiologists should avoid. To prevent this from occurring, the following precautions should be followed. First, we highly recommend that cotton dams be used instead of foam dams. It has been our experience that properly sized cotton dams are more likely to adhere to the canal wall when impression material is injected. Second, it is often necessary to use numerous cotton dams instead of just one. An otologist should be consulted on the placement of the dams in a surgically altered ear canal. Also, the otologist should remove the impression from the ear canal. Third, powder/liquid material (or the least dense silicone material) should be used because of its reduced viscosity, thus being less likely to cause the dam to move.

To support this concern, Wynne et al (2000) reported on 10 cases where taking earmold impressions resulted in significant external trauma (cerumen impaction on the eardrum), as well as middle ear trauma (hematoma or perforation of the eardrum; perforation with the injection of impression material into the middle ear; perforation with perilymph fistula).

Earmold Materials

Earmolds are available in both hard and soft materials, and it is not a simple task to select the appropriate earmold material for a patient. For example, if the pinna is hard, then a soft earmold material may be more appropriate.

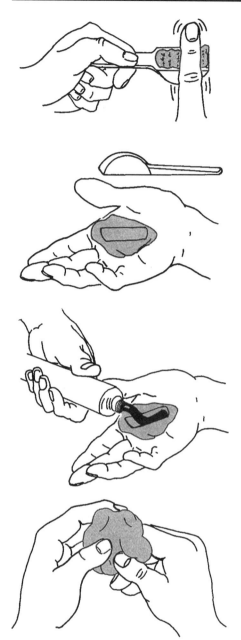

Figure 2–16 The base material and activator agent must be mixed when making an impression using silicone material. (From Microsonic, Inc., with permission.)

Conversely, if the pinna is soft, then a hard earmold material may be more appropriate. If the gain/output requirements of the hearing aids are high (usually 70 dB of gain and 125 dB SPL of output), then the audiologist might consider ordering a hard Lucite body with a soft canal or a material that softens to the heat of the ear canal, which provides a better seal to prevent feedback. For mild to moderate gain aids, a Lucite earmold might be considered. If there is any indication of an allergic reaction to the earmold material, then the audiologist might consider polyethylene (hard) or silicone (soft) material. If the patient indicates difficulty with inserting an earmold, then a Lucite material may be considered, because it is easier to

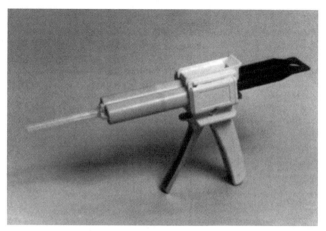

Figure 2–17 An impression gun used when making earmold impressions with premixed silicone material.

insert earmolds made of hard material. If the audiologist prefers the flexibility of having the ability to make modifications (venting, changing bore length or diameter, and belling), then ordering a Lucite material may be better because of its greater ease in allowing for such modifications. Finally, the audiologist needs to be familiar with the terminology used by the earmold laboratory because there is quite a variance in terminology across laboratories. The following are some of the more common earmold materials:

Lucite Polymethyl methacrylate is a hard material that is easily modified, easy to insert and remove, and very durable. Lucite can be clear, tinted, or opaque. It is also available as a nontoxic material. The canal portion is rigid and may lead to sound leakage during chewing or other facial movement if applied to a high-gain hearing aid.

Lucite Body with Vinylflex Canal This type of earmold combines a Lucite body with a canal made of vinylflex (see Vinylflex). This combination of materials is designed for patients who want the comfort and increased sealing capacity of the vinylflex material when fit with hearing aids having greater gain and output.

Vinylflex This polyethyl methacrylate material is a heat-cured semisoft plastic that will soften with body temperature. It is available in clear, beige, and tint. It is not easy to modify.

Semisoft This is a fairly rigid vinyl material that softens at body temperature. It is typically used for additional comfort, while maintaining ease of insertion. It is fairly easy to modify.

Soft Vinyl This is the most common soft material used for earmolds when allergies are not a concern. The material will shrink with body contact and age, but it can become discolored over time. Cementing tubing can cause problems; therefore, a tube locking system is recommended.

Silicone This is a flexible, inert rubber material. It is available in clear, opaque, pink, beige, and brown. Silicone has very little shrinkage and is good for high-power aids; it is not easy to modify. Silicone material will solve most

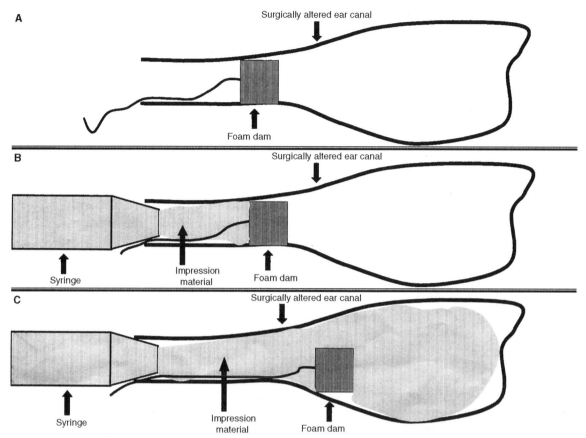

Figure 2–18 Earmold impression on a surgically altered ear canal. **(A)** Placement of the foam dam. **(B)** Injection of the impression material can **(C)** result in dislodgment of the foam dam.

allergy problems. A tube locking system is required because cement does not adhere to silicone.

Soft Silicone This material is recommended for the highest gain requirements. It is most effective when used in a canal or canal-shell earmold design, but it is not easy to modify. This material also requires an accurate impression to at least the second bend of the ear canal.

Polyethylene This is a hard material that is appropriate for severe cases of allergy; it is easy to modify. It is available only in opaque white and pink.

DisappEar This material, offered by Westone Laboratories Inc. (Colorado Springs, CO), features embedded microfibers that allow the earmold to have minimal outline and reflection. It is available in hard acrylic or silicone.

Earmold Styles

Two-Stage versus One-Stage Impression Earmolds

Custom earmolds require two stages. First, there is the impression of the ear by the audiologist. The impression is then mailed to an earmold laboratory, where it is wax dipped and invested in a matrix medium that is either silicone or plaster. A polymeric material is cured in plaster or silicone; it is then drilled, tubed, and polished. Many problems may arise that will not allow the finished product to "duplicate" the ear. These include poor impression-taking techniques, shrinkage of the impression and/or earmold, incorrect trimming of the impression, and changes in the dimensions of the ear canal between the time of the impression and the fitting.

Single-stage earmolds (i.e., the impression is the earmold) include such commercially available products as Instamold, Silisoft, and Otozen. These earmolds have been used in our clinic as temporary earmolds to allow patients to continue using their hearing aids while waiting for a custom mold to be delivered. The authors have also used single-stage earmolds instead of stock earmolds for evaluating benefit from amplification during a hearing aid evaluation.

Some single-stage earmolds have reportedly presented problems, such as producing a high degree of heat related to setting reaction that may cause burns to the ear; a high degree of shrinkage; too great a degree of hardness; and poor resistance to tearing, which may lead to difficulties in removal of the earmold.

Disposable Foam Earmolds

Another option is disposable foam earmolds. Smolak et al (1987) reported on seven subjects who used the 3M Comply

(3M, St. Paul, MN) disposable foam earmold. This earmold incorporates retarded recovery foam technology to provide a comfortable fit and eliminate the need for an earmold impression. Venting is provided by the use of four trench vents in the foam to control the low-frequency response. Smolak et al found that differences between a custom earmold and foam earmold were, at its greatest, < 2 dB. The four vents provided by the disposable foam earmold yielded an average reduction of 3.1 to 6.0 dB at 250 to 1000 Hz. Twenty-five percent of subjects, however, did not achieve as satisfactory a fit with the disposable foam earmold as they did with the custom earmold. These differences were attributed to the inability of the disposable foam earmold to adequately address ear canals that were unusually narrow or tortuous. These types of ear canals reduced retention and provided inadequate venting. Finally, it was found that the disposable foam earmold was more effective in reducing feedback due to the adaptive sealing capabilities of the disposable foam and the excellent sealing capability that prevents acoustic signals from reentering the ear canal via a vent or slit leak.

Oliveira et al (1992) reported on results with the Comply disposable foam earmold versus custom earmolds at 15 test sites. They reported significantly better performance of the disposable foam earmold in providing greater comfort and in reducing feedback. However, the disposable foam earmold did present some problems with retention and proper insertion for patients over 75 years of age.

Another option for a disposable earmold is the ER-13 generic BTE earmold kit, which is delivered with small, medium, and large disposable foam eartips and no. 13 or 3 mm CFA elbows.

NAEL Types According to Earmold Design

The nomenclature for earmold designs as agreed to by the NAEL are the following:

Regular, receiver, or standard earmold (**Fig. 2–19A**) This earmold design is typically used for fitting body aids and BTEs. It is usually ordered with a vinyl or metal snap ring that is either $^1/_4$- or $^1/_{16}$-inch wide. In a body aid fitting,

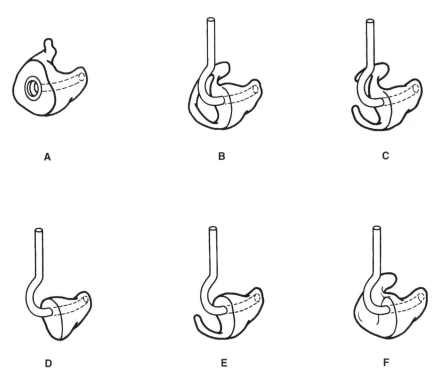

A   B   C

D   E   F

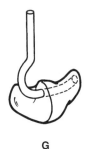

G

Figure 2–19 Examples of several earmold designs: **(A)** regular, **(B)** skeleton, **(C)** semiskeleton, **(D)** canal, **(E)** canal lock, **(F)** shell, and **(G)** canal shell. (From Microsonic, Inc., with permission.)

the external receiver from a body aid fits into the snap ring. For a BTE fitting, a plastic nub attached to tubing from the earhook fits into the snap ring, or it can be ordered with glued tubing. The plastic nub over which the tubing from the earhook slips can be ordered in several sizes (standard, D90, 8080, etc.). An alternative is a regular earmold with a wire hook for cases where the pinna has little cartilage (e.g., in a young child); this style will hold the weight of the receiver and earmold in place.

For a regular earmold, bore dimensions of 18 by 3 mm will produce a relatively flat frequency response to 3400 Hz. When the bore length is longer and the diameter narrower (23.4 × 2.4 mm), a loss in the high-frequency response occurs. Actually, a long bore may be better for patients with severe hearing loss. This is because attenuating the high-frequency response reduces the possibility of feedback. In addition, the benefits from high-frequency amplification are questionable in patients with profound high-frequency hearing loss. Lybarger (1979) reported that regular earmolds containing a snap ring can reduce the high-frequency gain by 8 to 10 dB above 2800 Hz and increase gain around 1000 Hz by ~4 dB relative to when no. 13 tubing is inserted to the earmold tip. The magnitude of the high-frequency reduction is related to the volume of the cavity in front of the receiver, which has been denoted as V2 by Lybarger (1979). The smaller the V2, the less the reduction of high-frequency gain. Again, as noted earlier, the reduction in high-frequency gain for patients with severe to profound hearing loss may be desirable.

Skeleton (**Fig. 2–19B**) This is similar to the shell (see Shell), but the center of the concha section is removed to provide less bulk and greater comfort.

Semiskeleton (**Fig. 2–19C**) This earmold is the same as the skeleton, but the upper portion of the concha ring is removed. It is appropriate for patients who have reduced manual dexterity or hardened ear texture.

Canal (**Fig. 2–19D**) This design is for mild to moderate gain hearing aids. It is easy to insert, but retention may be poor, and it is prone to problems with feedback. This is also available in canal lock (**Fig. 2–19E**).

Shell (**Fig. 2–19F**) This earmold fills the concha completely. It can be ordered with or without the helix segment. Adding the helix improves retention of the earmold to reduce the possibility of feedback. However, the addition of the helix increases the probability of discomfort in the helix region. It usually is selected for high-gain hearing aids.

Special Consideration

• Should the helix segment be included with the earmold? It is the experience of the authors that including the helix will often result in patient discomfort and greater difficulty in correctly inserting the earmold. Currently, the authors routinely exclude the helix when ordering earmolds.

Half-shell or canal shell (**Fig. 2–19G**) The entire helix area is removed, and the earmold covers the bottom half of the concha bowl. This design is recommended for patients with reduced manual dexterity.

Nonoccluding earmolds As noted earlier in the sections discussing tubing and earhooks, there are a variety of nonoccluding earmolds. These include tube fitting, free-field, CROS, Janssen, Lybarger dual-diameter, Lybarger 1.5LP, and extended range earmolds.

Extended Range Earmold

This is a specially designed earmold that provides a smooth frequency response between 2000 and 5000 Hz and extends the effective frequency response to 9000 Hz. It is available in two versions from several earmold laboratories. In the first version, no. 13 tubing is inserted to within 5 mm from the lateral end of the earmold; this is followed by a wide-diameter belled canal that is 11 mm long. The second version features a narrower, shorter sound bore that has no. 13 tubing inserted 5 mm into the sound bore followed by a bore length of 8 mm, which is reduced in diameter to 1.5 mm. This version provides slightly less high-frequency amplification than the first version. Because it is a nonoccluding design, it provides a fair degree of low-frequency attenuation. It is very similar in performance to the Janssen earmold, which is very similar to a CROS mold, except that the canal portion of the mold runs along the top of the ear canal.

Wide Range Earmolds (WRM)

This is a special resonator earmold that is designed to provide maximum gain at 5000 Hz. It uses no. 13 double-walled tubing inserted 3.2 mm into the sound bore, followed by a short bore 3.4 mm wide. If the audiologist wants a smoother response, the WRM can be ordered with two dampers in the sound bore that are placed between the end of the no. 13 tubing and the beginning of the 3.4 mm sound bore. The WRM also has a vent, which is 1.35 mm in diameter.

Frequency Gain Modifier Earmold

This earmold is available in numerous occluding and nonoccluding designs. Its construction is highlighted by using a stepped bore, a belled canal, and a plastic elbow for efficient changing of tubing. Some designs use venting, and others do not. This earmold is designed to damp the low-frequency region and amplify the high-frequency region.

Vogel Earmold

This is designed for severe to profound hearing loss and for patients who illustrate "excessive" mandibular jaw movement. It is comprised of a Lucite base for rigid retention in the outer ear and a soft, flexible silicone section in the ear canal portion that moves with the ear canal to maintain a constant acoustic seal.

CFA Earmolds

These earmolds (e.g., CFA 1 and CFA 2) feature a single snap-in/snap-out elbow that has a constant internal diameter to incorporate the earmold designs of Killion, Libby, and Janssen. The advantages of CFA are the ease of changing tubing and the elimination of damping in the earhook or tubing to smooth the frequency response. Another advantage is the inability of the tubing to become crimped or pinched, which is a common problem when inserting Libby 3 or 4 mm tubing inside the sound bore.

It is important for the audiologist to consult the earmold laboratory manual to determine the dimensions and purpose of the various CFA designs, because the nomenclature can vary from manufacturer to manufacturer. For one manufacturer, for example, CFA 1 has a small bore of 1.93 mm that provides high-frequency emphasis at 2000 to 5000 Hz and a smooth frequency response. CFA 2 has a belled bore of ~4.0 mm, which also provides high-frequency emphasis at 2000 to 5000 Hz and a smooth frequency response. CFA 3 has a sound bore between 1.93 and 4.75 mm to provide greater high-frequency emphasis.

CFA 4 also has a large open bore of 4.75 mm to provide even greater high-frequency emphasis. CFA 5 is designed for rising configurations and uses venting and a short-wide bore that removes 8 to 10 dB of gain at 2000 to 5000 Hz. For all CFA designs, it is not necessary to remove the damaged tubing. The audiologist simply needs to pull out the old CFA (with the attached tubing) and snap the new CFA (with the attached tubing) into the seating ring above the sound bore.

Earmolds Used with Stethoscopes

In our clinic, based in a large medical center, it is common for physicians, nurses, and anesthesiologists to request an earmold that can be used concurrently with their hearing aids or stethoscope because they report difficulties due to their hearing loss or the presence of excessive ambient noise. One earmold is designed for simultaneous use with a stethoscope and BTE. The earmold (Lucite or soft) accepts the plastic tips (i.e., lug) of stethoscopes. For this earmold design, the rubber tips of the stethoscope are removed, and the ends of the stethoscope are inserted into 6.4 mm holes drilled in the earmolds. Another option is a "stethomold," which does not require the stethoscope's plastic tip to be removed.

Other Issues with Earmolds

Attenuation or Sealing Capacity

As stated earlier, earmolds are designed to provide (1) an adequate seal, (2) comfort, (3) appropriate gain throughout the entire frequency range, (4) prevention of feedback, and (5) prevention of the sensation that the earmold is "blocking" the ear (i.e., occlusion effect). The seal provided by earmolds and shells has become increasingly important as the microphone has gotten closer to the receiver.

Sound can propagate through the earmold; vibrate the earmold as a whole; radiate through tissues, cartilage, or bone surrounding the ear canal; and pass through the air pathway between the earmold and the walls of the ear canal via unintentional slit leaks. Some of these paths of propagation can cause feedback. The presence of feedback results in the need for the patient to reduce the volume control setting, which results in inadequate amplification. Another outcome of these problems may be unintentional attenuation of low-frequency amplification, which is necessary for patients with severe to profound hearing loss who need as much low-frequency amplification as possible. For these patients, there is a need for earmolds with minimal pathway for leaks between the sides of the earmold and walls of the ear canal. The ability to achieve this goal depends on the impression material and technique, as well as the earmold material and style.

To evaluate static pressure seal, Macrae (1990) used an immittance meter attached to the tubing and earmold. With the air pump and manometer connected to the tubing of the earmold, pressure was increased to 200 daPa and maintained for 5 seconds. During this time, the subject was encouraged to talk to determine if jaw movements broke the seal. If there was no loss of pressure in 5 seconds, it was concluded that the earmold created an adequate static pressure seal. Macrae evaluated two impression materials (silicone and dental impression) and four earmold materials (hard acrylic, silicone rubber, polyvinyl chloride, and Microlite). For 16 subjects, he found that 12 of the 128 earmold combinations provided an adequate seal; for those earmolds that did provide an adequate seal, the average length and width of the ear canal were larger. Thus, he felt that the dimensions of the ear canal may be a better predictor of maintaining an adequate seal than the impression or earmold materials. Macrae concluded that, because only 12 earmolds provided an adequate seal, the chance of sealing the ear with a two-stage earmold process with only a general buildup of the earmold was small. Also, using different impression material or earmold materials did not significantly improve the chances.

In another experiment, Macrae (1991) ordered two earmolds for one impression. He concluded that this method did not improve the chances of maintaining a static seal. In a final experiment, he "patted down" the surface of the impression material after it was syringed into the ear, but before the impression set. He then asked the earmold laboratory to apply a wax buildup to the impression with a hot wax knife. The results of this experiment revealed that "patting down" the impression did not increase the probability of a seal, but the special buildup did increase the probability of maintaining an adequate seal. In fact, in 55% of the cases, a buildup applied to the impression at the earmold laboratory resulted in an adequate seal. Macrae also found that earmolds with round tips are more likely to seal than those with more elliptical tips.

As mentioned earlier, unintentional leaks can occur around the periphery of the earmold. Some researchers estimate that the average leak is equivalent to the presence of a 1.4 mm vent. Lybarger (1979) reported that a vent this wide will have minimal effect on the output of a hearing aid coupled to an unvented earmold. However, when an unintentional leak is presented around an already vented earmold, low-frequency transmission is increased, and the effectiveness of the vent is diminished (Cox, 1979).

Frank (1980) compared the performance of Lucite and vinylflex earmolds (shell and skeleton) with and without the presence of a tragus lock against the performance of an E-A-R disposable foam earmold (Etymotic Research Inc., Elk Grove Village, IL). In 20 subjects, he found that the custom earmolds provided ~17 dB less attenuation than the E-A-R disposable foam earmold. In addition, he warned against the commonly held belief that an earmold provides adequate hearing protection. The custom earmolds revealed a mean noise reduction rating of 3.3 dB, whereas the E-A-R disposable foam earmold had a mean noise reduction rating of 18.2 dB.

Maximum Real-Ear Gain

For patients with severe to profound hearing loss, the audiologist wants to select an earmold that will provide the greatest usable gain prior to feedback. Madell and Gendel (1984) reminded us that hearing aids, at that time, were available that provided maximum gain in excess of 60 dB and SSPL90, which was greater than 130 dB. For these patients, these authors believe that a soft (vinyl or silicone) earmold used with double-walled tubing is the most suitable because it provides the tightest fit and offers the greatest retention and, therefore, the greatest usable gain.

Kuk (1994) reported on the maximum usable real-ear gain for 10 occluding earmolds (regular with helix lock and no. 13 tubing; shell with helix lock; canal; skeleton without helix lock; skeleton with helix lock; CROS with extended canal; CROS with partial IROS vent; tube mold; and the Oticon E43 earmold designed for patients with hearing loss above 2000 Hz). Kuk reported there is a tendency among audiologists to believe that a bulkier earmold (regular or shell) will result in greater user gain than those with less bulk (canal or skeleton). His findings revealed that the greatest real-ear gain was achieved by the skeleton and shell earmolds, followed by the canal and regular earmold. Kuk also reported that the average high-frequency gain was 44 dB for the skeleton and canal earmold, 46 dB for the shell earmold, and 40 dB for the regular earmold. In addition, he reported little advantage of using the helix lock, because this addition resulted in increased difficulty in correctly inserting the earmold into the ear canal, increased user discomfort, and increased possibility of feedback.

Earmold Design and Word Recognition

Past research has suggested that earmold designs may have an effect on improved word recognition scores. However, Hodgson and Murdock (1972) could not demonstrate significant differences in word recognition scores between unvented and vented earmolds in 18 subjects with high-frequency hearing loss.

If greater gain is desired, then the following suggestions may be helpful. First, if the pinna is hard, use a softer earmold material. Second, usable gain can be increased with a Lucite body with a soft canal. Third, consider one of the newer earmold materials that expand in response to the

heat of the ear canal. Examples include the JB1000, MSL-90, Audtex, and M2000 earmolds, available from several earmold manufacturers. Fourth, order an earmold with a long bore that will reduce the likelihood of the occlusion effect and feedback, while, at the same time, allowing the patient the opportunity to achieve greater usable gain. Fifth, be sure the earmold design allows the tip of the earmold to be round and face the eardrum, not the canal wall. If the tip of the earmold faces the canal wall, it will reflect sound back and cause feedback.

Problems with Earmolds

Impressions and the Presence of Perforations

Occasionally, an audiologist will discover an eardrum perforation during otoscopic observation in the process of taking an earmold impression. This should present major concerns for at least two reasons. First, the audiologist clearly needs to select the appropriate otoblock so that the impression material does not pass through the perforation into the middle ear space or expand the width of the perforation. Either event would cause discomfort and increase the possibility of middle ear infection. The second concern is that the presence of the earmold in the ear canal will enhance the probability of creating middle ear infections. Alvord et al (1989) reported that placement of earmolds in the ear canal will increase the risk of infection because the earmold reduces normal ventilation by creating a warm and moist environment for infectious growth. They also found that bacteria may be introduced by the earmold, or the earmold can induce allergic, irritating, or foreign body reactions. Alvord et al evaluated six subjects with perforations. Four of the six had a regular earmold with no vent, and two had a regular earmold with a 2 mm vent. The researchers' greatest success was with subjects with smaller perforations and vented earmolds. Also, they reported that pressure vents of ≤1 mm did not solve the problem and often became plugged. They suggested counseling patients not to use earmolds full time in order to provide ventilation.

Allergies to Impression and Earmold Materials

Occasionally, patients will report that use of the earmold or shell will cause discomfort to the ear or ear canal. Cockerill (1987) reported on patient allergic reactions to earmold materials. He wanted to determine if patient complaints of allergic reactions to earmolds were related to "true" allergic reactions or were due to irritation caused by a tight fit, surface roughness, lack of hygiene, or simple inflammation resulting from constant tissue coverage.

Often, the acrylic resins used in the manufacture of earmolds are in the form of a powder (polymer) and liquid (monomer). Polymerization is the process whereby the monomer is converted into a polymer, or the solid end product. The main component of both the polymer and monomer is methyl methacrylate, with other ingredients, including hydroquinine, dibutylphthalate, and benzoyl peroxide, acting as inhibitors, activators, and catalysts. Nonallergic materials may be vulcanite, silicone rubber, gold, and polyvinyl chloride (PVC), which is usually in the form of a thin coating brushed over the earmold or shell.

Cockerill (1987) evaluated 25 subjects who were subdivided into three subgroups. Group 1 included subjects who reported other skin problems but did not report problems relating to the earmold. Group 2 subjects had a history of external otitis or seborrheic dermatitis. Subjects in group 3 had or encountered otorrhea and had persistent reactions to earmolds. Cockerill performed skin patch tests and found reactions to eight substances specifically related to the ingredients used in earmolds. Reactions ranged from dry, itchy skin with a slight inflammation of the concha to painful edema of the pinna, cheek, or neck area, which prevented the use of the earmold. Fourteen subjects (55%) showed a reaction to methyl methacrylate. One subject (4%) had a reaction to vulcanite, and two subjects (8%) had a reaction to PVC.

Meding and Ringdahl (1992) reported 22 subjects who had long-standing severe dermatitis in the ear canal. Patch testing indicated that nine subjects had 15 positive reactions in the standard series. Six patients (27%) had contact allergy to the earmold materials. Four of these six patients had a reaction to methyl methacrylate (sensitizer), and two also had a reaction to ethylene glycol dimethacrylate and triethylene glycol dimethacrylate. The diagnosis was allergic contact dermatitis in seven cases and seborrheic dermatitis in six cases. For the remaining nine subjects, the diagnosis was not obvious, although irritation from occlusion was probable. These authors recommended making another impression using less monomer (liquid) or silicone material. They also recommended consideration for a bone-conduction hearing aid and patch testing in cooperation with dermatologists.

When a patient reports an allergic reaction to earmold or shell materials from previous experiences or due to current soreness of the ear, a polyethylene earmold should be ordered in either white or pink opaque colors.

Fitting the Elderly

Fitting the elderly can create some special concerns. One of these concerns is manual dexterity and its effect on ease of insertion of the earmold. Meredith and colleagues (1989) evaluated three groups of elderly patients, with 20 subjects per group. For each group, they compared ease of handling, comfort, and the general effectiveness of the half-shell, skeleton, and skeleton without the tragus notch. Results indicated that the skeleton with the tragus notch removed provided the greatest benefit in all three areas. However, the removal of the tragus notch did increase the possibility of feedback, and it was suggested that this mold would only be appropriate for low-gain hearing aids. Other generic problems in this study associated with inserting earmolds included (1) placing the tragus notch outside the crus of the tragus rather than underneath; (2) the presence of the concha rim, heel, and helix lock preventing easy insertion into the antitragus and antihelix areas; (3) inserting earmolds back to front or upside down; and (4) incorrect placement of the BTE hearing aid over the ear.

Feedback

In the beginning of the chapter, the authors stated that a successful hearing aid fitting was one where there was no feedback present in the usable range of the volume control wheel.

Reducing Feedback   There are several solutions available to combat the problem of feedback. Some that have been discussed earlier are checking the sealing ability of the earmold, using special earmold designs and materials, employing dampers, and adjusting the depth of insertion of the sound bore. To combat feedback, the audiologist might also consider the following:

1. Using antifeedback kits with sleeves (available in four sizes) that fit snugly over the earmold or shell and are cemented in place. This strategy has disadvantages because the sleeves are often uncomfortable, develop "ripples," fall off, or cause allergic reactions.

2. Applying a "soft seal" liquid around the surface of the shell or earmold to reduce or eliminate the spaces between the earmold or shell and the canal wall. Other types of sealing compounds are ADCO (ADCO Hearing Products Inc., Englewood, CO) Addon, for minor buildup of soft or hard earmolds; AdcoBuild, for a major buildup; and Adco Sheen, which is applied over AdcoBuild as a sealer to prevent discoloration.

3. Applying ER-13R E-A-R Ring Seal Kit (Etymotic Research) with tetrahydrofuran in small quantities around the shell or earmold. Seal rings are available in sizes 8, 10, 12, 14, 16, 20, and 22 mm.

4. Using an ER-13MF (Etymotic Research) microphone filter kit, which reduces gain by 10 to 15 dB at 5000 to 10,000 Hz.

5. Remaking the impression for a new earmold or shell because the original earmold or shell was too loose.

6. Narrowing the diameter of the vent if using any of variable venting schemes, which will be discussed later.

7. Decreasing the overall gain and/or output.

8. Placing a damper along the transmission line or in the vent.

9. Electronically reducing high-frequency gain via a high-cut potentiometer, feedback reduction circuit, or feedback notch filter, all of which are available from several ITE and ITC manufacturers. One additional possibility is using digital feedback suppression, which is available with virtually every digital hearing aid currently available on the market.

10. Making sure the opening from the receiver of the ITE or ITC is not facing the canal wall. This will result in reflection of the amplified sound off the canal wall and induce feedback. The same can be suggested as a cause for feedback with an earmold in a BTE fitting.

11. Ordering all ITE and ITC hearing aids with receiver extension tube (**Fig. 2–20**). This places the output closer

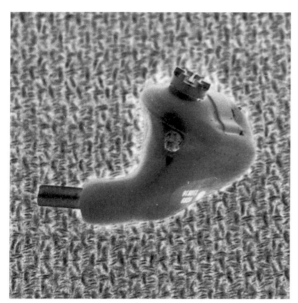

Figure 2–20 Use of extended receiver tube on an in-the-canal hearing aid.

to the eardrum and typically results in a lower volume control setting. The lower setting typically results in the patient's using less overall gain and thus reduces the chances for feedback. In our clinic, receiver extension tubes are ordered on all ITE and ITC hearing aids. An additional benefit of using receiver extension tubing is less possibility that the receiver will be clogged with cerumen, because the opening of the tubing is farther away from the receiver.

12. Dispensing any number of digital signal processing (DSP) hearing aids that incorporate feedback management algorithms.

13. Performing an otoscopic examination. Often, the cause of the feedback is the presence of excessive cerumen in the ear canal. This is typically the case for patients who do not have a history of feedback. In these cases, the cause is typically the presence of excessive cerumen. Having the cerumen removed typically solves the problem. It is also a good idea to counsel patients on the need to see a physician every few months to check for the buildup of cerumen.

Occlusion Effect

One of the goals of a successful hearing aid fitting is eliminating the occlusion effect, the sensation that the patient's head is "at the bottom of a barrel." Revit (1992) reported that placing an earmold or shell in the ear canal can amplify the patient's own voice by 20 to 30 dB in the lower frequencies. Furthermore, Revit reminded us that only a 10 dB increase results in a doubling of the perceived loudness of a signal. In this case, inserting the earmold or shell in the ear canal can cause the perceived loudness to be 4 times as great as when the hearing aid is not in the ear canal. This perceived increased in loudness is especially true for the closed vowels /i/ and /u/.

In the past, the only tool the audiologist had in dealing with the occlusion effect was subjective reports by patients, because objectively measuring the effect was a challenge. Revit (1992) reported on how a real-ear analyzer could perform spectrum analysis of externally generated signals, with and without the hearing aid in place, to objectively measure the occlusion effect. First, the patient is asked to vocalize a sustained vowel (e.g., the sound of *eee*), which is self-monitored at 70 dB(A) on a sound level meter held 1 m from the lips (see the thicker line in the upper graph of **Fig. 2–21**). With the hearing aid in place but turned off, the procedure is repeated (see the thin line in the upper graph

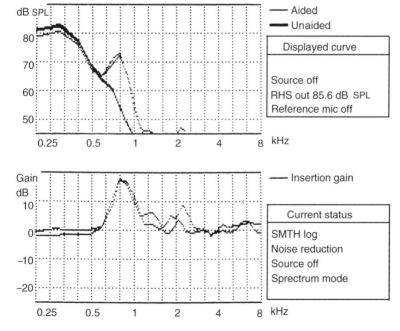

Figure 2–21 Measurement of the occlusion effect using a real-ear analyzer. The upper graph displays the spectrum of /ou/ measured in the ear canal without the hearing aid in place (*dark line*). The light line displays the spectrum of the same sound, but with the hearing aid in place and the volume control turned off. The lower graph displays the resulting occlusion effect.

of **Fig. 2–21**). The difference between the two measures, or the occlusion effect, is displayed as "insertion gain" in the lower graph of **Fig. 2–21**. For this patient, ~15 dB of occlusion effect is seen at 800 to 900 Hz. At this point, the audiologist can attempt several steps described below and repeat the measures to determine if the lower graph can be reduced to as close to 0 dB as possible.

Reducing the Occlusion Effect   One way to reduce or eliminate the occlusion effect is to apply venting of the earmold or custom shell to reduce low-frequency amplification. For example, a 2 mm vent can decrease the measured SPL at 200 Hz by 8.5 dB. Dempsey (1990) reported that venting options to reduce the occlusion effect in ITCs are limited due to space restrictions and the close proximity of the microphone and receiver and the resulting problems of feedback. Usually, vent diameter in ITCs is limited to 2 to 3 mm; therefore, reducing the occlusion effect via venting is limited. In this study, shells for ITEs and ITCs were manufactured for 10 subjects, and 1.5 to 3 mm vents were introduced. The mean occlusion effect was 5.4 dB for the ITEs and 8.6 dB for the ITCs with the vents in place.

Another method for reducing the occlusion effect is making a silicone impression and placing a cotton otoblock beyond the second bend of the ear canal in the osseous segment to provide the patient with a deep canal fitting. It is important to allow jaw movement during the impression and to ask the patient to yawn when removing the impression to reduce the effect of the vacuum created by the deep impression technique. Also, the audiologist should request a parallel pressure vent of 0.05 to 1.5 mm. Revit (1992) reported a 15 dB reduction in the occlusion effect at 200 Hz when the patient was fitted with a deeply inserted foam tip in comparison to a medium-length bore that was seated in the cartilaginous portion of the ear canal.

◆ Venting

It is the belief of the authors that virtually every hearing aid fit should have some degree of venting. Dillon (1991) reminded us of the many roles of venting. First, the vent allows some of the low-frequency amplified sound to dissipate outside the ear canal instead of contributing to the SPL buildup at the eardrum. The vent will reduce low-frequency gain and output relative to a closed earmold fitting. Second, the vent allows unamplified signals to enter the ear canal through the vent. This results in less attenuation of the low frequencies and greater attenuation of the higher frequencies. Third, the volume of the vent tube combines with the cavity of the ear canal to produce a Helmholtz resonator, creating a vent-associated resonant frequency at 250 to 1000 Hz. At the vent-associated resonant frequency, the vented mold provides greater gain than would have been present if the vent were blocked. Fourth, the vent can reduce or eliminate the occlusion effect. Other advantages of venting include providing pressure release to prevent a sensation of pressure buildup near the eardrum

and ventilation to minimize the buildup of moisture in the ear canal.

On a negative note, the presence of a vent can allow the amplified sound in the ear canal to pass back to the hearing aid microphone and lead to suboscillatory (heard by the patient as a "ringing," but not heard by the audiologist) or oscillatory (heard by the audiologist, family members, and, perhaps, the patient) feedback. As vent size increases, the amount of acoustic leakage increases, and the probability of feedback heightens. Oscillatory feedback will occur at any frequency when the attenuation along the feedback path is less than the gain of the hearing aid in the ear canal. In BTE fittings, the gain has to be greater or the attenuation along the path less, because the length of the path from the ear canal to the microphone of the hearing aid is greater than it is for an ITE or ITC fitting. Even for vents slightly smaller than this critical size, feedback will produce an additional peak in the frequency response and add a "ringing" or transient tone to the sound quality. For many low- to medium-gain hearing aids, it is necessary to specify a vent large enough to minimize the occlusion effect, yet small enough to avoid feedback.

Effect of Vent Diameter

Pressure Equalization

As a general guideline, a pressure vent is ~0.06 to 0.8 mm, and it will have no measurable effect on the frequency response. Kuk (1994) reported that the pressure vent changed the low-frequency real-ear response by 1 to 6 dB. For a medium-length bore (16.6 mm), Lybarger (1979) suggested a pressure equalization vent diameter of 0.64 mm (no. 72 drill). A 1.0 mm vent will be too wide because it will change the low-frequency response for earmolds with a short bore length (**Table 2–4**). Even "tight" earmolds will provide some degree of "slit leak," which will attenuate the frequency response around 100 Hz by 6 dB and be reduced to 0 dB of attenuation at 250 Hz (Lybarger, 1979).

Low-Frequency Enhancement

Lybarger (1979) reported that measurements of venting on 2 cc couplers have shown an increase of low-frequency gain as vent diameter increases. When the measurements were performed on a Zwislocki coupler, however, the increase in low-frequency gain was not as apparent (Lybarger, 1979). As seen in **Table 2–4**, with the same 16.6 mm bore length described above, a 1.0 mm vent will increase gain at 250 to 300 Hz with little effect on the frequency response above 500 Hz. A 2.0 mm vent will result in greater low-frequency attenuation below 500 Hz and increased gain between 500 and 700 Hz. A 3.0 mm will not provide amplification above the vent-associated resonance but will provide greater attenuation below 550 Hz. Similar low-frequency enhancement is seen for long (22.0 mm) and short (12.2 mm) bore lengths.

Moderate Low-Frequency Reduction

A 2.0 mm vent will provide considerable low-frequency reduction below 500 Hz, depending on the length of the

Table 2–4 Vent Minus Unvented Response (dB) for Simulated Earmolds Using Parallel and Diagonal Vents (1–3 mm) with Bore Lengths of 6.0, 12.2, 16.6, and 22 mm and Bore Diameters of 1.0, 2.0, and 3.0 mm as Measured in a dB 100 Coupler

	Parallel Vents											
Bore Length	6.0			12.2			16.6			22.0		
Vent Diameter	1	2	3	1	2	3	1	2	3	1	2	3
Frequency (Hz)												
200	−8	−22	−29	−2	−17	−25	0	−15	−23	2	−14	−22
250	—	—	—	4	−13	−20	6	−11	−19	6	−10	−18
315	—	—	—	7	-8	−16	6	−6	−14	5	−4	−13
400	8	−9	−16	5	−2	−12	4	0	−10	3	3	−8
500	6	−2	−11	3	6	−6	2	9	−4	2	9	−2
630	—	—	—	2	9	1	1	5	5	1	5	6
800	1	5	1	1	3	4	1	2	3	0	1	1
1000	1	4	1	1	3	3	1	3	3	0	2	2
1250	1	3	4	0	2	4	0	2	4	0	1	3
1600	0	2	3	0	1	3	0	1	2	0	1	2
	Diagonal Vents*											
Bore Length							16.6			22.0		
Vent Diameter							1	2	3	1	2	3
200							−6	−15	−21	−8	−17	−23
250							0	−11	−17	−2	−13	−20
315							6	−4	−11	4	−6	−13
400							6	3	−5	5	1	−7
500							3	6	2	2	4	2
630							1	2	3	0	0	−1
800							0	0	−1	−1	−2	−3
1000							−1	−1	−2	−1	0	−4
1250							−1	−2	−4	−2	−4	−6
1600							−1	−2	−5	−3	−5	−8

For the two diagonal configurations, vent length was 11.9 mm, and the bore length medial to the intersection was 6.3 and 11.7 mm, respectively, for the 16.6 and 22 mm conditions.

Measured sound pressure level (SPL) is greater. Measured coupler SPL is less.

Source: Data from Lybarger, S.F. (1985). Earmolds. In J. Katz (Ed.), Handbook of clinical audiology, 3rd ed (pp 885–910). Baltimore: Williams & Wilkins; Mueller, H. G., Hawkins, D. B., & Northern J. L. (1992). Probe microphone measurements: Hearing aid selection and fitting. San Diego: Singular Press.

sound bore **(Table 2–4)**. Also, as the vent size increases, there will be an increase in the height of the vent-associated resonance. To reduce or eliminate the undesired peak, Lybarger (1979) recommended placing light cloth damping over the lateral end of the vent.

Strong Low-Frequency Reduction

As a general rule, a medium size vent is 1.6 to 2.4 mm wide. A vent this wide will reduce amplification below 500 Hz and result in a vent-associated resonance that will increase amplification at 500 to 1000 Hz. As a general rule, a large-size vent is 3.2 to 4.0 mm, which will reduce amplification below 500 Hz, and its vent-associated resonance will increase amplification at 500 to 1000 Hz **(Table 2–4)**. A wide-

short vent will provide strong low-frequency reduction. Extreme low-frequency reduction will occur with an open or nonoccluding earmold. The magnitude of low-frequency reduction will be 25 dB at 250 Hz with a cutoff at 500 Hz. For a long bore (22 mm), there will be an 18 dB reduction at 250 Hz, and the cutoff frequency begins at 800 Hz (Lybarger, 1979).

Extreme Low-Frequency Reduction

For patients with normal hearing up to 1500 Hz, the use of a tube fitting would be very appropriate because it provides the greatest low-frequency reduction and greatest high-frequency enhancement. For maximum benefit of this strategy, the diameter of the tubing should be wide and the depth of insertion minimal.

Effect of Vent Length and Diameter

The length of the vent is related to the length of the bore and is not really the critical factor in decisions concerning vents. However, as a general rule, as bore length increases, there is less low-frequency attenuation when vent diameter is held constant **(Table 2–4)**. The crucial decision is usually the diameter of the vent. Chasin (1983) reported that venting can create a high-frequency antiresonance (notch) that may fall within the frequency range of the hearing aid. All vents have a characteristic vent-associated antiresonance frequency that produces a decrease in gain and whose frequency depends on the length and volume of the vent. The frequency of this vent-associated antiresonance is inversely related to the effective length of the vent. Shortening the effective length of the vent may increase the frequency of the antiresonance until it is above the frequency response of most hearing aids. As a general rule, for each 1.0 mm decrease in vent length, the frequency of the vent-associated antiresonance is increased by 400 Hz. One effective way to eliminate the vent-associated antiresonance is to bell the vent at the medial side of the earmold.

Another issue related to vent diameter is how much gain is available as the diameter is increased before feedback is present. Lybarger (1979) measured the SPL at a point 2.5 cm from the tip of the earmold in which the length of the sound bore was described as "short." He reported that maximum gain before feedback using a 0.8 mm vent was 43 dB, with a reserve gain of 10 dB. For a 3.2 mm vent, maximum gain before feedback was reduced to 36 dB, with a reserve gain of 10 dB.

Finally, as vent length is decreased, there will be a segment of the frequency response at which there is no further reduction in gain caused by the presence of the vent. This is referred to by some as the high-frequency cutoff. For example, in **Table 2–4**, when the vent length is 22 mm, the high-frequency cutoff for a 2 mm vent is ~315 Hz. However, when the vent is shortened to 6 mm, the high-frequency cutoff is increased to ~500 Hz. Also, as the vent length is decreased, there is increased attenuation of the low-frequency response. This latter effect also occurs when the vent is widened.

Types of Venting

Diagonal versus Parallel Venting

Aside from deciding the length and/or diameter of the vent, the audiologist needs to inform the earmold laboratory if the vent should run parallel (lower example in **Fig. 2–22**) to the sound bore or if the vent needs to intersect (i.e., diagonal; see upper example in **Fig. 2–22**) the sound bore at some point between the lateral and medial end. Most research indicates that the primary choice should be a parallel vent because a diagonal vent, relative to a parallel vent, will decrease high-frequency gain by as much as 10 dB, and the effect increases as vent diameter increases **(Table 2–4)**. Most researchers recommend diagonal venting only if space limitations (i.e., narrow ear canal) prevent the use of a parallel vent. If a diagonal vent is the only choice, minimizing high-frequency reduction can be achieved by ordering a

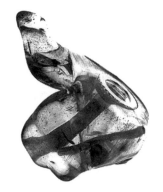

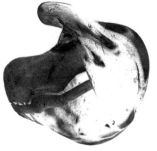

Figure 2–22 Example of diagonal (*top*) and parallel (*bottom*) venting.

shorter bore length or having the vent intersect the sound bore as close to the medial end as possible and then belling the final section of the sound bore (Cox, 1979).

> **Pitfall**
>
> • Always order an earmold or shell with a parallel vent. A diagonal vent or intersecting vent will reduce the high-frequency response.

Cox (1979) reported the results of measuring the effects of parallel versus diagonal venting on three earmolds measured in a Zwislocki coupler and the real ear. One earmold had a parallel vent of 16.8 mm. The second earmold had a diagonal vent that was 13.2 mm long and intersected the sound bore 7.6 mm from the tip of the earmold. The third earmold had a diagonal vent 8.5 mm long and intersected the sound bore 9.5 mm from the tip of the earmold. Results for the parallel vent showed the expected reduction in low-frequency output below 400 Hz, and a vent-associated resonance was seen between 300 and 700 Hz with little high-frequency attenuation. For the first diagonal condition, there was the same low-frequency reduction below 400 Hz, and a vent-associated resonance as was measured with the parallel vent. However, above the vent-associated resonance, there was a 3 to 5 dB attenuation of 3000 Hz. For the second diagonal condition, there was greater low-frequency reduction and a similar vent-associated resonance. However, there was a 10 to 11 dB attenuation in output between 2000 and 3000 Hz. Thus, the three venting conditions yielded similar low-frequency

Table 2–5 Custom Venting

Frequency (Hz)	Vent Diameter (mm)	Vent Length (mm)
250	1.1	17.8
	0.8	8.9
	0.5	4.4
500	2.2	17.8
	1.5	8.9
	1.1	4.4
750	3.0	17.8
	2.3	8.9
	1.6	4.4
1000	4.3	17.8
	3.0	8.9
	2.1	4.4
	1.5	2.2

Source: Adapted from Microsonic, 2003, with permission.

reduction and vent-associated resonances, but the diagonal vent revealed high-frequency attenuation that increased as the point of intersection moved more laterally in the sound bore. Above the vent-associated resonant frequency, the parallel vent did not reduce high-frequency gain, whereas the diagonal vent did yield greater reduction in high-frequency transmission as the point of intersection was moved more laterally. The magnitude of the high-frequency loss in diagonal vents is related to the diameter of the vent in relation to the diameter of the sound bore. As seen in **Table 2–5**, reduction in high-frequency gain increases as the vent diameter increases when vent length is held constant. Furthermore, the loss of high-frequency transmission can be as great as 15 to 20 dB if the diagonal vent intersects the main sound bore at a very lateral position and the diameter of the vent is large (≥ 3 mm).

Studebaker and Zachman (1970) reported that as the diameter of the diagonal vent increased (0.75, 1.5, and 3.0 mm), there was (1) greater low-frequency attenuation, (2) a shift in the vent-associated resonance to a higher frequency, (3) greater amplitude of the vent-associated resonance, and (4) greater reduction in high-frequency transmission. During real-ear measures, there was the same low-frequency reduction as was measured in the 2 cc coupler, but the height of the vent-associated resonances was smaller or was not present.

External or Trench Venting

Occasionally, the dimensions of the ear canal will be so small that neither parallel nor diagonal venting can be used. In these cases, a V-shaped groove can be cut into the bottom surface of the earmold from the outside to the tip. This method of venting is also suggested in cases where the ear may be draining.

Custom Venting

For audiologists who prefer to specify the exact length and diameter of venting, **Table 2–5** can be used for ordering vent sizes to specify the vent cutoff frequency at 250, 500, 750, or 1000 Hz. For example, if the audiologist wants the low-frequency attenuation to extend to 1000 Hz (i.e., greater low-frequency reduction because the patient has normal or near-normal hearing at 1000 Hz and below), he or she could specify that the bore length should be 8.9 mm, and the vent diameter should be 3.0 mm. To achieve the same degree of low-frequency attenuation in an earmold with a shorter bore (i.e., 4.4 mm), the vent diameter would be reduced to 2.1 mm. For example, let us assume the patient has some hearing loss in the lower frequencies, and the audiologist wants less low-frequency attenuation. In the case of the patient with the longer bore (8.9 mm), the audiologist would order a vent diameter of 0.8 mm. In the case of the patient with the shorter bore length (4.4 mm), the audiologist would order a vent diameter of 0.5 mm.

Pearl

- The authors routinely order "trench venting" for most CIC fittings. This has significantly reduced the occlusion effect in many of our fittings. In addition, it is much easier to remove cerumen from a groove vent than the pressure vent available in most CIC fittings.

Adjustable Venting

As mentioned earlier, it is the strong belief of the authors that virtually all earmolds/shells should be delivered to the patient with some degree of venting. An issue to consider is, should the diameter of the vent be fixed, or should the audiologist order a method of adjustable venting to better meet the needs of the patient as well as the audiologist? The next section will discuss several methods to vary the vent diameter at the time of the hearing aid fitting.

Select-A-Vent

In the past, audiologists often drilled their own vents on a trial-and-error basis. **Table 2–6** provides guidelines for readers who may wish to drill their own vents and the drill size required to accomplish the task. **Figure 2–23** illustrates examples of drill sets used in our facility to vent and modify earmolds and shells. Currently, however, most audiologists order earmolds or shells with either SAV, Select-A-Tube (**Fig. 2–24**), or Mini-SAV changeable venting systems, which eliminate the trial-and-error methods associated with drilling vent holes. For one manufacturer of ITE hearing aids, the inner diameter of the Select-A-Tubes are 1.9, 1.6, 1.3, and 0.77 mm, and a plug. Variable venting techniques provide the audiologist with greater flexibility to experiment with different vent diameters and their effect on (1) reducing low-frequency gain, (2) reducing or eliminating

Table 2–6 Common Drill Sizes and the Resulting Vent Diameter

Drill Size	Vent Diameter (mm)
31	3.17
33	2.93
47	2.00
53	1.57
61	1.00
65	0.89
68	0.79
70	0.72
75	0.54
76	0.51
80	0.35

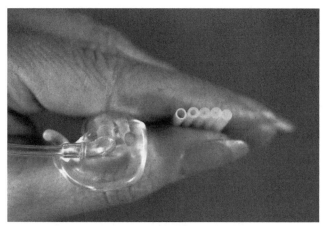

Figure 2–24 Examples of Select-A-Tube venting.

the occlusion effect, (3) yielding better sound quality, and (4) reducing or eliminating feedback. This flexibility is permitted by merely using different-sized vent plugs (no. 1–5) or tubes that vary in inner diameter and are inserted in a predrilled vent channel.

The SAV comes with a permanently installed clear styrene seating ring and a removable polyethylene venting plug, available in a "tree" of five sizes along with a solid plug. The insert channel for the SAV is 4.7 mm deep and 3.6 mm wide. For one manufacturer, the diameters of the SAV inserts are 0.8, 1.6, 2.4, 3.2, and 4.0 mm for inserts no. 1 to 5, respectively. There is also a no. 6 insert that is used as a plug to close the vent. The SAV is also available from some earmold and hearing aid manufacturers in a Mini-SAV format when the sound bore is unusually narrow. For one manufacturer, the diameters of the Mini-SAV inserts are 0.5, 0.8, 1.0, 1.6, and 1.9 mm for inserts no. 1 to 5, respectively. There is also a no. 6 insert that is used as a plug to close the vent **(Table 2–7)**. It is important for the reader to understand that the relationship between insert number

and the corresponding diameter may be different across manufacturers. In addition, the relationship between insert number and width of the vent may be the reverse of the one described above. That is, in our clinic, the no. 1 insert has the narrowest diameter, and the no. 6 insert plugs the vent. However, for another manufacturer, the no. 1 insert may plug the vent, and the no. 6 insert may provide the widest diameter vent.

Table 2–7 Dimensions of Select-A-Vent (SAV), Mini-SAV, and Positive Venting Valve (PVV)

Type	(inch)	(mm)
SAV Plug		
1	0.031	0.8
2	0.062	1.6
3	0.095	2.4
4	0.125	3.2
5	0.156	4.0
6	closed	closed
Mini-SAV Plug		
1	0.020	0.5
2	0.030	0.8
3	0.040	1.0
4	0.060	1.6
5	0.075	1.9
6	closed	closed
PVV Plug		
1	0.020	0.5
2	0.030	0.8
3	0.060	1.6
4	0.095	2.4
5	0.125	3.2
6	closed	closed

Source: Adapted from Microsonic, 2003, with permission.

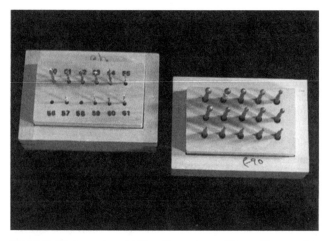

Figure 2–23 Examples of drill and bur sets used to modify earmolds and shells.

Positive Venting Valve

The PVV comes with a permanently installed clear styrene seating ring and a removable polyethylene venting plug that is available in a "tree" of five sizes along with a solid plug. In comparison to the SAV, the PVV has an insert channel that is shorter and wider (2.5 mm deep and 4.0 mm wide). For one manufacturer, the diameters of the PVV inserts are 0.5, 0.8, 1.6, 2.4, and 3.2 mm for inserts no. 1 to 5, respectively. There is also a no. 6 insert, which is used as a plug to close the vent (**Table 2–7**). Again, the audiologist needs to be careful because earmold laboratories may offer PVV inserts where the order is reversed (i.e., the smallest number insert has the widest vent size, and the largest number insert has the narrowest vent size), and the vent diameters may vary slightly from the diameters provided above.

Select-A-Vent versus Positive Venting Valve

For both the PVV and SAV systems, there is little change in the low-frequency response between inserts no. 1 to 3. However, some differences in low-frequency reduction will occur between inserts no. 4 and 5 (Cox, 1979; Lybarger, 1979). These same researchers favored using the PVV because the PVV uses a shorter and wider insert cup for the vent inserts. They believed that for variable venting systems to work properly, the vent channel must be short and wide so that the vent response will be controlled by the vent hole in the insert rather than the vent channel itself. If the vent channel is long and narrow (i.e., SAV), then changing from one vent insert to another will make little difference in the low-frequency response. It appears that the PVV offers greater low-frequency attenuation because of its shorter and wider insert channel.

Austin et al (1990a,b) reported in separate articles on the differences in real-ear versus 2 cc coupler responses for 47 earmolds with 157 different modifications. They reported that the PVV and SAV revealed very small differences in low-frequency reduction between any insert size, and the midfrequency vent-associated resonant peak measured in the coupler was not observed in the real ear. Finally, in agreement with past findings, Austin et al (1990a,b) concluded that the PVV provides greater low-frequency attenuation than the SAV.

Additional Issues with Venting

Intentional versus Unintentional Vents

The level of the signal reaching the eardrum is a result of combining two paths of sound. One is the unaided path, in which the signal passes through the vent (intentional vent) and leaks (unintentional vent) and reaches the eardrum unaided. The second is the aided path, in which the intensity level of the signal at the eardrum is provided by the hearing aid. Concurrently, these two paths have some of the amplified sound passing to "the outside" through the same vent and leaks to reduce the SPL at the eardrum in a narrow frequency region. At any frequency in which the intensity of one path exceeds the intensity of the other path by 20 dB or more, the path with the lesser intensity has an insignificant effect on the total intensity at the eardrum (< 1 dB). At any frequency where the two intensities are within 20 dB of each other, however, the manner in which the two intensities combine depends on the phase relationship between the two paths. At a frequency where the two paths have equal intensity (often at 250–750 Hz), the in-phase addition of the two paths will yield an intensity level that is 6 dB higher than the intensity within each path. At frequencies where the two paths are 180 degrees out of phase, there will be a strong attenuation of the signal. The magnitude of the vent effect is dependent upon the dimensions of the vent, the properties of the ear canal and eardrum, and the phase response of the hearing aid. In addition, the presence of vents can sharpen high-frequency resonant peaks so that a rounded response measured in a coupler, with the vent closed, can appear as a sharp peak in the real-ear aided response (Revit, 1994). The degree of "sharpening" of the vent-associated resonant peak from suboscillatory feedback is dependent upon the dimensions of the vent and the ear canal as well as the impedance of the eardrum. One method to reduce the height of the vent-associated resonant peak is to reduce the diameter of the vent.

Suboscillatory Feedback

Cox (1979) reported that vented earmolds may cause feedback at lower volume control settings than closed molds. This can prevent the user from achieving the desired gain due to the interference of feedback. In addition, one common practice used by many hearing aid users to adjust the volume control wheel is to rotate the volume control until audible feedback occurs and then "back off" slightly. This strategy may create suboscillatory feedback, which creates a frequency response marked by numerous peaks and troughs. It is clear that the practice of setting the volume control just below the point of audible feedback can have a significant deleterious impact on the frequency response of the hearing aid. If a patient complains that the hearing aid "echoes" or "rings," he or she is probably experiencing suboscillatory feedback.

Pitfall

- A common practice is to adjust the volume controls at a position just below where feedback is heard. However, suboscillatory feedback may be present at this setting, which can lead to reduced sound quality and speech intelligibility. It is best to counsel the patient to adjust the volume controls to where speech is comfortably loud.

Acoustic versus Electronic Low-Frequency Attenuation

Audiologists can control the low-frequency response via (1) a tone control in combination with a closed mold (electronic tuning) (**Fig. 2–25**); (2) use of venting in combination with a hearing aid having a wideband frequency response (acoustical tuning); or (3) combining strategies 1 and 2,

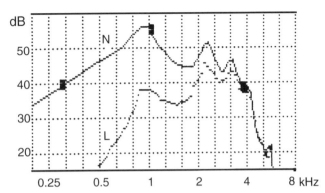

Figure 2–25 Frequency response of a hearing aid when the tone control was rotated for the broadest response (N) and the greatest low-frequency attenuation (L).

where low-frequency output is controlled by the tone control, and the vent may or may not provide additional low-frequency attenuation. The first strategy provides a very efficient way to predict low-frequency attenuation. The second strategy is not as strong in predicting low-frequency attenuation. This second method, as mentioned earlier, adds a midfrequency vent-associated resonant peak and the possibility of altering the frequency response due to audible and suboscillatory feedback, which does not occur with a closed mold.

Cox and Alexander (1983) recorded speech in KEMAR (Knowles Electronics Manikan for Acoustic Research) with a hearing aid coupled to closed molds, vented molds, and open molds, with the output from KEMAR matched for the different mold conditions. The researchers used a paired comparison paradigm of sound quality and speech intelligibility judgments for connected discourse presented at 65 dB with signal-to-noise ratios (SNRs) of +5 and +20 dB. They evaluated nine hearing aids, which were divided into 3 groups, depending on the cutoff frequency (i.e., below 750 Hz, between 750 and 1000 Hz, and above 1000 Hz). They evaluated 15 subjects who had normal hearing in the low frequencies and greater hearing loss in the higher frequencies. Results revealed that the subjects had a slight preference for the electronic modification strategy if the cutoff frequency was < 750 Hz. They had a strong preference, however, for the acoustic tuning strategy (venting) when the cutoff frequency was between 750 and 1000 Hz and an even greater preference for venting when the cutoff frequency was greater than 1000 Hz. These findings were the same for both SNR conditions and for sound quality or speech intelligibility judgments.

Mackenzie and Browning (1991) evaluated 83 inexperienced subjects with mild to moderate severe sensorineural hearing loss. When subjects had normal hearing to 1000 Hz, they generally preferred combining venting and high-frequency emphasis to achieve the desired balance between low- and high-frequency amplification rather than relying only on the tone control. For subjects having a flatter audiometric configuration from 250 to 4000 Hz, no consistent preferences were present.

Mackenzie and Browning (1989) reported on real-ear measures in 43 ears and found that adjusting the tone con-

trol between normal and high-frequency emphasis has less effect in the real ear than in the 2 cc coupler. Adding a 2 mm vent and returning the tone control to the normal position reduced the output by an average of 8 dB at 750 to 1000 Hz. By turning the tone control to high-frequency emphasis and using an earmold with a 2 mm vent, the low-frequency reduction was extended to 10 dB in the same frequency region.

Perceptual Consequence of Vents

Lundberg et al (1992) evaluated nine subjects with normal hearing. They reported no difference in sound quality for vented and unvented earmolds while listening to male and female recordings of connected discourse in quiet and noise. Four subjects reported that the unvented earmolds sounded louder than the vented earmolds, and there was an overall tendency of preferring the sound quality produced by the vented condition.

Kuk (1991) reported higher word recognition scores in noise when venting was introduced to the earmold. However, Hodgson and Murdock (1972) did not report significant improvement in word recognition scores with the introduction of venting. Kuk (1991) evaluated nine subjects with mild to moderate severe sensorineural hearing loss using unvented and vented (2.2 mm parallel vent) earmolds. Using a paired comparison strategy and a programmable hearing aid, the subjects shaped their preferred REIG while listening to connected discourse presented at 70 dB SPL. Results indicated that the preferred REIG was similar for the two earmold conditions. Sound quality for the "clarity" judgment, however, was significantly better for the vented condition. When reading aloud, most subjects preferred the vented condition. No significant differences were found in word recognition scores for W-22 word lists presented at 70 dB SPL. Kuk (1991) concluded that although electronic tuning can help to ensure that measured REIG matches prescribed REIG, venting is necessary to improve user satisfaction.

Venting in Custom Hearing Aids

Up to this point, the issue of venting has been presented in terms of venting an earmold. Similar decisions need to be made by the audiologist when fitting custom hearing aids. In a custom product, the length of tubing from the output of the receiver to the tip of the shell is typically 10 to 12 mm long and 1 to 2 mm wide. Preves (1980) described a dual-tubing, or stepped bore, arrangement for an ITE that increased the high-frequency response. In this design, the tubing at the receiver is 6.4 mm long and 1.4 mm wide, which increases to a width of 3.6 mm for the second section. In addition, a 2200 Ω fused mesh damper is placed at the receiver to smooth the frequency response. For short-bore shells, the 3.6 mm segment of tubing is extended beyond the tip of the shell to maintain the desired acoustic effect. Further increases in the high-frequency response can occur as the diameter of the tubing of the second segment is increased. To accommodate the damping needs for ITEs, Knowles Electronics has four dampers that fit into cups with outside diameters of 1.12, 1.25, 1.37, and 1.78 mm to fit

Table 2–8 Mean and Standard Deviation (in parentheses) of the Real-Ear Vent Effects (dB) for Three Vent Diameters (mm) Relative to the Occluded Condition for ITE Hearing Aids when No Sealing or Sealing Was Placed around the Shell of the ITE*

Diameter	Frequency				
	200 Hz	500 Hz	1000 Hz	1500 Hz	2000 Hz
No sealing					
1.3 mm	−7.1 (3.1)	0.3 (2.9)	1.5 (0.7)	0.5 (0.6)	0.1 (0.5)
2.0 mm	−11.1 (3.9)	−0.9 (3.6)	1.9 (0.9)	0.7 (0.7)	0.2 (0.8)
3.0 mm	−21.9 (4.0)	−10.5 (3.2)	3.1 (2.8)	2.6 (1.7)	1.9 (0.9)
Sealing with E-A-R rings					
1.3 mm	−6.8 (2.2)	2.8 (1.3)	0.8 (0.6)	0.3 (0.4)	−0.2 (0.9)
2.0 mm	−12.1 (2.5)	2.2 (3.5)	1.7 (0.7)	0.6 (0.7)	0.3 (0.9)
3.0 mm	−25.0 (2.6)	−9.8 (3.2)	5.1 (2.0)	2.9 (1.4)	2.0 (0.7)
Diameter (mm) × length (mm)†					
0.45 × 22	−4.9 (2.6)	0.5 (2.0)	0.7 (0.8)	0.1 (0.9)	0.0 (0.8)
0.95 × 22	−9.2 (2.0)	2.8 (2.5)	1.7 (0.7)	0.6 (1.1)	0.5 (0.7)
1.45 × 22	−12.1 (2.1)	1.5 (3.9)	2.3 (1.0)	1.0 (1.1)	0.8 (0.7)
2.0 × 22	−13.9 (1.7)	0.6 (4.0)	2.9 (1.3)	1.4 (1.1)	1.0 (0.7)
2.0 × 16	−15.8 (2.3)	−3.7 (4.5)	2.5 (1.4)	0.9 (1.2)	0.3 (1.0)
2.0 × 10	−18.9 (2.5)	−7.9 (3.7)	1.8 (1.7)	1.0 (1.2)	−0.1 (1.5)
2.0 × 4	−22.6 (2.9)	−11.4 (4.7)	0.7 (2.0)	1.5 (2.0)	0.3 (1.4)
3.0 × 4	−24.6 (1.8)	−13.4 (3.0)	0.1 (2.6)	2.2 (2.2)	0.9 (1.2)

* Data from Tecca, J. E. (1991). Real-ear vent effects in ITE hearing instrument fittings. Hearing Instruments, 30(4), 22–23, 38.
† Date from Tecca, J. E. (1992). Further investigation of ITE vent effects. Hearing Instruments, 43(12), 8–10.
Mean and standard deviations are given for real-ear vent effects (dB) for five bent diameters (mm) and four lengths (mm).
ITE, in the ear.

inside the narrow inner diameter of tubing used in custom hearing aids from the receiver to the tip of the shell. Dampers are available in acoustic resistance of 330 to 3300 Ω for the 1.78 mm diameter cup and 680 or 1500 Ω for the 1.25 mm diameter cup. They have a greater effect on smoothing the second peak instead of the first peak, which is common for BTE fittings.

Tecca (1991) believes that most of the research on venting for ITEs carefully eliminated slit-leak effects. In actual use, slit leaks are quite common in ITE fittings. Tecca found that the effect of slit leaks is predominantly at 200 Hz (**Table 2–8**). He performed real-ear measures on 10 subjects whose ear canals had an average length of 22.6 mm and a mean bore length of 8.2 mm. He used vent diameters of 1.3, 2.0, and 3.0 mm. For the 1.3 and 2.0 mm vents, the attenuation was restricted to below 1000 Hz (**Table 2–8**). The attenuation provided by the 3 mm vent extended 1 octave higher (**Table 2–8**). When E-A-R seal rings were used to minimize the effect of slit leak, there was only a slight attenuation of low-frequency gain (**Table 2–8**). In addition, the standard deviation shown in **Table 2–8** (0.4–4.0 dB) reveals minimal intersubject variability. Therefore, the ability to predict vent effects for a particular individual is rather good. Finally, as reported before, as vent diameter is increased, there is greater low-frequency attenuation, and the vent-associated resonant frequency increases. **Table 2–8** indicates that the vent-associated resonance increased for the 1.3 and 2 mm vent between the sealed and unsealed

conditions, but the effect of sealing was minimal for the 3 mm vent.

In another study, Tecca (1992) reported that most variable venting systems for custom hearing aids use vent inserts, of different inner diameters, which are inserted into the lateral end of the vent channel. He evaluated 10 subjects whose shells were manufactured having a bore length of 22 mm and vent diameters of 0.45, 0.95, and 1.45 mm. A second condition was where the vent diameter was a constant 2 mm and vent lengths were 4, 10, 16, and 22 mm. A final condition was where there was a vent diameter of 3 mm and vent length of 4 mm. Results revealed (**Table 2–8**) that the degree of attenuation at 200 Hz increased as vent diameter increased from 0.45 to 1.45 mm and length was held constant at 22 mm. Minimal attenuation occurred above 200 Hz. When vent diameter was held constant at 2 mm, attenuation increased as bore length decreased, and the vent-associated resonance increased in frequency. Also, differences in the magnitude of low-frequency attenuation between adjacent vent diameters were 3 to 5 dB at 200 Hz, and the effect was predominantly below 500 Hz. Recall that Cox and Alexander (1983) suggested using electronic tuning instead of acoustic tuning to enhance user satisfaction when the cutoff frequency was below 750 Hz for venting to result in greater user satisfaction. Finally, Tecca (1992) reported that the vent-associated resonance shifted to a higher frequency as vent diameter increased and the mean amplitude varied between 2.0 and 5.1 dB.

Vent diameters for custom hearing aids can also be changed by inserting silicone tubes of different inner diameters into the vent channel. This, for example, is the method used by GN ReSound for its custom hearing aids. With this method of venting, the audiologist has the advantage of knowing that the diameter of the selected vent tube is uniform from the lateral to the medial end of the vent channel.

♦ Problems with Hearing Aids and Fitting Hearing Aids

Cerumen Buildup

One of the most common problems in custom hearing aids is the buildup of cerumen in the tubing from the receiver. The presence of cerumen will change the electroacoustic characteristics of the hearing aid or attenuate the output so the hearing aid appears "dead." Several methods have been introduced to help audiologists address this problem.

One solution has been the introduction of the Ad-Hear wax guards (Oliveira and Rose, 1994). These are easy-to-apply disposable filters that stick onto the shell of the hearing aid; they are available in four sizes: ultra-slim, slim, standard, and large. Between the two adhesive strips is a filter that is placed over the tubing opening from the receiver to prevent cerumen from entering the tubing. The Ad-Hear wax guards do not change the frequency response of the hearing aid and will last for 1 week before they need to be changed (Oliveira and Rose, 1994). Another solution is the cerumen filter system. In this case, a small plastic "lid" is pressed into place over the receiver opening. These filters arrive in a pack of 10, and each filter lasts ~1 week.

Audiologists must understand that it is expensive for manufacturers to replace receivers due to contamination from cerumen. Thus, manufacturers offer numerous wax guard options. These include wax baskets, spring dampers, and element dampers, which are placed in the receiver opening to prevent cerumen from reaching the receiver. These devices are acoustically transparent in that they do not change the frequency response. However, REIG responses at our facility revealed that using a wax basket from one manufacturer decreased the real-ear gain around 3000 Hz by nearly 6 dB. Therefore, this facility routinely orders translucent receiver tubing and has it extend 3 to 4 mm past the tip of the shell (see **Fig. 2–19**). This allows the patient to "see" the cerumen and remove it with a wax loop before a buildup creates a problem. In addition, the extended receiver tube places the output from the hearing aid slightly closer to the eardrum. This reduces the volume control necessary to achieve a comfortable setting and also reduces the likelihood of feedback.

Solutions to Hearing Aid Fitting Problems

Fitting hearing aids can bring pride and satisfaction because of the opportunity to make life more enjoyable and satisfactory for patients. Successful fittings, however, are challenging. **Table 2–9** lists problems commonly brought to our attention by our patients. Also given are some solutions that

Table 2–9 Troubleshooting Chart

Problem	Possible Solutions
1. Soreness/ discomfort	a. Canal/shell modifications b. New impression c. Hypoallergenic material d. Allergy coating
2. Allergic reaction	a. Coat shell with hypoallergenic nail polish b. Remake impression for Lucite earmold c. Order hypoallergenic material
3. Too tight	a. Grind/buff areas that may be causing the tightness b. New impression
4. Too loose	a. Build up shell with ADCO Addon (soft or hard) b. New impression
5. Hole/crack in shell	a. Patch with polymer-monomer mix
6. Occlusion effect	a. Widen vent diameter b. Provide a deep canal fit c. Bell the bore d. Reduce low-frequency gain e. Use MCT material f. Increase crossover frequency

(Continued)

Table 2–9 (*Continued*) Troubleshooting Chart

Problem	Possible Solutions
7. Tinny or harsh	a. Insert filter in receiver or microphone
	b. Shift high frequencies with a resonant peak control
	c. Reduce vent and add filter
	d. Reduce low-frequency gain
	e. Reduce crossover frequency
	f. Reduce high-frequency output
	g. Increase compression ratio
	h. Reduce high-frequency gain
8. Too much bass	a. Widen vent
	b. Reduce low-frequency gain
	c. Increase crossover frequency
9. Too loud	a. Reduce output with output control
	b. Reduce gain
	c. Insert filter in receiver
	d. Widen vent
	e. Reduce compression ratio
	f. Reduce compression kneepoint
10. Too soft	a. Check battery
	b. Excessive cerumen
	c. Defective microphone
	d. Increase overall gain/output
	e. Increase low-frequency gain
	f. Increase compression kneepoint
	g. Decrease compression ratio
	h. Reduce vent diameter
	i. Check for excessive battery drain
	j. Check ear canal for debris
	k. Check receiver tube for debris
	l. Clean/replace filter in receiver tube
	m. Check for moisture
11. Wind noise	a. Use windscreen or windhood
	b. Place foam in the microphone port
	c. Decrease high-frequency gain or output
12. Internal feedback	a. Check for loose receiver tube
	b. Check for hole in vent
	c. Check for pushed-in receiver tube
	d. Send for repair
13. External feedback	a. Check for excessive cerumen
	b. Reduce vent size with SAV, PVV, or REVV (tube vents)
	c. Build up or lengthen canal
	d. Coat shell with non-petroleum-based oil ("soft seal")
	e. Use receiver extension tubing
	f. Add damping
	g. Reduce canal length because tip may be against canal wall
	h. Reduce high-frequency output/gain
	i. Remake the earmold/shell
	j. Use ER-13R (Etymotic Research) ring seals
	k. Use ER-13MF (Etymotic Research) microphone filter
	l. Consider receiver extension tube

(*Continued*)

Table 2–9 (*Continued*) Troubleshooting Chart

Problem	Possible Solutions
14. Distortion	a. Increase high-frequency output
	b. Lengthen high-frequency release time
	c. Replace microphone
	d. Repair circuit
15. Intermittent	a. Replace receiver/microphone
	b. Replace volume control
	c. Check for moisture buildup and recommend Dri-Aid kit
	d. Repair circuit
16. Excessive drain	a. Request lower battery drain from manufacturer
	b. Reduce gain or output
	c. Repair circuit

MCT, minimal contact technology; PVV, Positive Venting Valve; REVV, Real Ear Variable Venting; SAV, Select-A-Vent
Source: From Riess, J., L., & Guthier, J. D. (1986). In-the-ear modification cookbook. Hearing Instruments, 37(4), 18–24, with permission.

have been used successfully to address and correct these problems. Sometimes these solutions eliminate the problem and result in greater user satisfaction. Other times they only partially solve the problem, but the degree of improvement is sufficient to make the problem less troublesome. On more occasions than we care to admit, the solutions do not solve the problem, and the patient discontinues use of amplification. Also, the solution to one problem can create a new problem. For example, one solution for eliminating the occlusion effect is to widen the vent. It is entirely possible, however, that this solution will result in feedback.

♦ Summary

It has been suggested more than once that fitting hearing aids is an art as well as a science. It is the belief of the authors that greater knowledge of the transmission line's role in shaping the electroacoustic characteristics of hearing aids will help improve the skills of audiologists. It is hoped that the information in this chapter will provide readers with some of the tools necessary to become better "artists" and "scientists."

References

Alvord, L. S., Doxey, G. P., & Smith, D. S. (1989). Hearing aids worn with tympanic membrane perforations: Complications and solutions. American Journal of Otology, 10(4), 277–280.

Alvord, L. S., Morgan, R., & Cartwright, K. (1997). Anatomy of an earmold: A formal terminology. Journal of the American Academy of Audiology, 8, 100–103.

American National Standards Institute. (1987). Preferred earhook nozzle thread for postauricular hearing aids (ANSI S3.37–1987). New York: Author.

American National Standards Institute. (2003). Specifications of hearing aid characteristics (ANSI S3.22–2003). New York: Author.

Austin, C. D., Kasten, R. N., & Wilson, H. (1990a). Real-ear measures of hearing aid plumbing modifications, part 1. Hearing Instruments, 43(3), 18–22.

Austin, C. D., Kasten, R. N., & Wilson, H. (1990b). Real-ear measures of hearing aid plumbing modifications, part 2. Hearing Instruments, 43(4), 25–30.

Bergenstoff, H. (1983). Earmold design and its effect on real-ear insertion gain. Hearing Instruments, 34(9), 46.

Briskey, R. J. (1982). Smoothing the frequency response of a hearing aid. Hearing Aid Journal, 3, 12–17.

Burgess, N., & Brooks, D. N. (1991). Earmoulds: Some benefits from horn fitting. British Journal of Audiology, 25, 309–315.

Chasin, M. (1983). Vent modification for added high-frequency sound transmission. Hearing Journal, 6, 16, 17.

Cockerill, D. (1987). Allergies to earmoulds. British Journal of Audiology, 21, 143–145.

Courtois, J., Johansen, P. A., Larsen, B. V., et al. (1988). Open molds. In J. H. Jensen (Ed.), Hearing aid fittings: Theoretical and practical views (pp. 175–200). Copenhagen: Stougaard Jensen.

Cox, R. M. (1979). Acoustic aspects of hearing aid-ear canal coupling systems. Monographs in Contemporary Audiology, 1(3), 1–44.

Cox, R. M., & Alexander, G. C. (1983). Acoustic versus electronic modifications of hearing aid low-frequency output. Ear and Hearing, 4, 190–196.

Cox, R. M., & Gilmore, C. (1986). Damping the hearing aid frequency response: Effects on speech clarity and preferred listening level. Journal of Speech and Hearing Research, 29, 357–365.

Custom earmold manual. (2003). Cambridge, PA: Microsonic Earmold Laboratory.

Decker, T. N. (1975, Summer). The relationship between speech discrimination performance and the use of sintered metal inserts in the hearing aid fitting. Audecibel, 118–123.

Dempsey, J. J. (1990). The occlusion effect created by custom canal hearing aids. American Journal of Otology, 11(1), 44–46.

Dillon, H. (1991). Allowing for real ear venting effects when selecting the coupler gain of hearing aids. Ear and Hearing, 12, 406–416.

Frank, T. (1980). Attenuation characteristics of hearing aid earmolds. Ear and Hearing, 1, 161–166.

Gastmeirer, W. J. (1981). The acoustically damped earhook. Hearing Instruments, 32(10), 14–15.

Harford, E. R., & Barry, J. A. (1965). A rehabilitative approach to the problem of unilateral hearing impairment: The contralateral routing of signals (CROS). Journal of Speech and Hearing Disorders, 30, 121–138.

Hodgson, W., & Murdock, C. (1972). Effect of the earmold on speech intelligibility in hearing aid use. Journal of Speech and Hearing Research, 13, 290–297.

Hosford-Dunn, H. (1996). A basic primer for fitting CICs. Hearing Review, 3(1), 8–12.

Killion, M. C. (1988). Earmold design: Theory and practice. In J. H. Jensen (Ed.), Hearing aid fittings. Theoretical and practice views (pp. 155–172). Copenhagen: Stougaard Jensen.

Kuk, F. K. (1991). Perceptual consequences of vents in hearing aids. British Journal of Audiology, 25, 163–169.

Kuk, F. K. (1994). Maximum usable real-ear insertion gain with ten earmold designs. Journal of the American Academy of Audiology, 5, 41–51.

Lesiecki, W. (2006). Does the in-office electronic scanning of the impression really change everything? Hearing Review, 13(1), 32–35.

Libby, E. R. (1981). Achieving a transparent, smooth, wideband hearing aid response. Hearing Instruments, 32(10), 9–12.

Libby, E. R. (1982a). In search of transparent insertion gain hearing aid responses. In G. A. Studebaker & F. Bess (Eds.), The Vanderbilt hearing aid report (pp. 112–123). Upper Darby, PA: Monographs in Contemporary Audiology.

Libby, E. R. (1982b). A reverse acoustic horn for severe-to-profound hearing impairments. Hearing Instruments, 41(12), 29.

Lundberg, G., Ovegard, A., Hagerman, B., et al. (1992). Perceived sound quality in a hearing aid with vented and closed earmould equalized in frequency response. Scandinavian Audiology, 21, 87–92.

Lybarger, S. F. (1979). Controlling hearing aid performance by earmold design. In V. D. Larson, D. P. Egolf, R. L. Kirlin, & S. W. Stile (Eds.), Auditory and hearing prosthetics research (pp. 101–132). New York: Grune & Stratton.

Lybarger, S. F. (1985). Earmolds. In J. Katz (Ed.), Handbook of clinical audiology, 3rd ed (pp. 885–910). Baltimore: Williams & Wilkins.

Mackenzie, K., & Browning, G. G. (1989). The real-ear effect of adjusting the tone control and venting a hearing aid system. British Journal of Audiology, 23, 93–98.

Mackenzie, K., & Browning, G. G. (1991). Randomized crossover study to assess patient preference for an acoustically modified hearing aid system. Journal of Laryngology and Otology, 105, 405–408.

Macrae, J. H. (1990). Static pressure seal of earmolds. Journal of Rehabilitation Research and Development, 27, 397–410.

Macrae, J. H. (1991). A comparison of the effects of different methods of impression buildup on earmolds. British Journal of Audiology, 25, 183–199.

Madell, J. R., & Gendel, J. M. (1984). Earmolds for patients with severe and profound hearing loss. Ear and Hearing, 5, 349–351.

Meding, B., & Ringdahl, A. (1992). Allergic contact dermatitis from earmolds of hearing aids. Ear and Hearing, 13, 122–124.

Meredith, R., Thomas, K. J., Callaghan, D. C., et al. (1989). A comparison of three types of earmoulds in elderly users of post-aural hearing aids. British Journal of Audiology, 23, 239–244.

Morgan, R. (1994). The art of making a good impression. Hearing Review, 1(3), 10–14.

Mueller, H. G., Hawkins, D. B., & Northern, J. L. (1992). Probe microphone measurements: Hearing aid selection and assessment. San Diego, CA: Singular Press.

Mueller, H. G., Schwartz, D. M., & Surr, R. K. (1981). The use of the exponential acoustic horn in an open mold configuration. Hearing Instruments, 32(10), 16–17.

Oliveira, R. J., Hawkinson, R., & Stockton, M. (1992). Instant foam versus traditional BTE earmolds. Hearing Instruments, 43(12), 22.

Oliveira, R. J., & Rose, D. E. (1994). Keep your wax guard up. American Journal of Audiology, 3, 7–10.

Pedersen, B. (1984). Venting of earmoulds with acoustic horn. Scandinavian Audiology, 13, 205–206.

Preves, D. A. (1980). Stepped bore earmolds for custom ITE hearing aids. Hearing Instruments, 31(10), 24–26.

Revit, L. J. (1992). Two techniques for dealing with the occlusion effect. Hearing Instruments, 43(12), 16–18.

Revit, L. J. (1994). Using coupler tests in the fitting of hearing aids. In M. Valente (Ed.), Strategies for selecting and verifying hearing aid fittings (pp. 64–87). New York: Thieme Medical Publishers.

Robinson, S., Cane, M. A., & Lutman, M. E. (1989). Relative benefits of stepped and constant bore earmoulds: A crossover trial. British Journal of Audiology, 23, 221–228.

Smolak, L. H., Iserman, B. E., & Hawkinson, R. W. (1987). Disposable foam earmolds. Hearing Instruments, 38(12), 24–27.

Staab, W. J., & Martin, R. L. (1995). Mixed-media impression: A two-layer approach to taking ear impressions. Hearing Journal, 48(5), 23–27.

Studebaker, G. A., & Zachman, T. A. (1970). Investigation of the acoustics of earmold vents. Journal of the Acoustical Society of America, 47, 1107–1115.

Sung, G. S., & Sung, R. J. (1982). The efficacy of hearing aid–earmold coupling systems. Hearing Instruments, 33(12), 11–12.

Tecca, J. E. (1991). Real-ear vent effects in ITE hearing instrument fittings. Hearing Instruments, 42(12), 10–12.

Tecca, J. E. (1992). Further investigation of ITE vent effects. Hearing Instruments, 43(12), 8–10.

Teder, H. (1979). Smoothing hearing aid output with filters. Hearing Instruments, 30(4), 22–28.

Valente, M., Potts, L. G., Valente, M., & Goebel, J. (1995). Wireless CROS versus transcranial CROS for unilateral hearing loss. American Journal of Audiology, 4, 52–59.

Wyme, M., Kahn, J., Abel, D., & Allen, R. (2000). External and middle ear trauma resulting from ear impressions. Journals of the American Academy of Audiology, 11, 351–360.

Chapter 3

Real Ear Measurements

Kristina E. Frye and Robert Martin

Audiologists have long struggled to incorporate objectivity into the art of fitting hearing aids. Until the mid-1980s, audiologists relied on functional gain (i.e., the difference between unaided and aided sound field thresholds) and 2 cc coupler measurements, combined with subjective responses to such questions as How does that sound? Is that too loud? Is that too soft? There were few objective measurements available that could help audiologists verify and improve the hearing aid fitting. This changed in 1984 with the development of the first commercially available clinical real ear analyzer, the Rastronics CCI-10, now GN Otometrics A/S (Taastrup, Denmark) (Nielsen and Rasmussen, 1984).

Since that time, real ear analyzers have greatly advanced with improved test signals, analysis routines, techniques, and prescriptive targets that have necessarily adapted to the significant changes that have been made in hearing aid technology over the years.

Using real ear measurement (REM), the audiologist has an accurate tool that shows how much amplification the patient is receiving from the hearing aid fitting when it is exposed to different input levels and signals. In the hands of an experienced audiologist, REM can help the audiologist verify output, verify adequate amplification across the frequency range, and troubleshoot the hearing aid fitting. REM should be the primary hearing aid assessment tool in hearing aid fitting clinics.

So, what is meant by REM? Most objective hearing aid measurements can be classified as coupler or real ear. Coupler measurements are performed in a test box, also called a sound chamber, using an airtight metal coupler to simulate the human ear. Coupler measures typically are used for quality control to identify defective microphones and receivers and determine when the hearing aid is operating incorrectly (i.e., whether the hearing aid is operating within the manufacturer's specifications). Coupler measurements typically require minimal training of the audiologist and produce test results that are easily repeatable. However, when a hearing aid is fitted to an ear, the gain, output, and bandwidth of the amplifier may change markedly from its performance when attached to a coupler. Therefore, coupler measurements do not relate to how the hearing aid is performing in the real world. See Chapter 1 in this volume for more information on coupler measures.

REMs are performed with a very narrow probe tube inserted inside the ear canal. This probe tube, attached to a probe microphone, allows the measurement of the sound pressure level (SPL) near the eardrum. For this reason, REMs are often referred to as probe microphone measurements. Devices that perform REMs may also be referred to as real ear analyzers or REM machines.

REMs typically require more training on the part of the audiologist than coupler measurements. Test results are affected by the placement of the probe tube and sound field configuration, but when performed correctly, REMs provide the most accurate assessment of the performance of the hearing aid.

Traditionally, REMs have been used to report how much improvement the hearing aid provides the patient. Because hearing aids with linear amplification provide the same amount of gain for any input level (until the circuit is saturated), and because many hearing aids being fit had only linear amplification, REMs were typically performed with medium-level input signals (e.g., 65 dB SPL). However, as hearing aid circuitry has advanced from using single-channel linear analog circuitry to multichannel digital signal processing (DSP) with sophisticated software algorithms that can reduce environmental noise, enhance speech, and suppress feedback, REMs have also advanced. Clinicians now need to verify how much amplification the hearing aids provide at multiple input levels corresponding to soft (50 dB SPL), average (65 dB SPL), and loud (80 dB SPL). In addition, clinicians now have at their disposal real ear prescriptive targets to verify the fitting at these input levels. (See Chapter 7 in this volume for more information on prescriptive formulas for linear and nonlinear signal processing.) Real ear analyzers must be able to produce sophisticated test signals capable of providing measurements that are accurate and useful in verifying the hearing aid fitting. This chapter will focus on REM techniques and how these techniques can be used to troubleshoot and improve the hearing aid fitting.

◆ Real Ear Terminology

Any discussion of REM is usually accompanied by several acronyms that may be confusing to the clinician just starting to learn about REM. In this section, the authors will describe the most common acronyms. Later, the authors will use these acronyms to describe the different real ear techniques. It is hoped that this combination will provide the reader with a good understanding of real ear terminology.

Most REMs are referred to as gain or response measures. Gain and response are two ways of viewing the same information. The term *response* (also known as *output*) indicates the clinician is observing the absolute measurement of SPL generated in the ear canal. The response measurement is expressed as dB SPL. Some suggest the user envision a small person, deep in the ear canal, holding a sound level meter and measuring the SPL.

The term *gain* indicates the clinician is viewing a measurement that is relative to the level of the input signal. That is, the input level, as measured by the reference microphone placed outside the ear, has been subtracted from the output level as measured by the probe microphone placed near the eardrum. A gain measurement is expressed as dB gain. When gain is a positive number, the input signal has been amplified. When gain is a negative number, the input signal has been attenuated and is sometimes referred to as loss.

Almost all real ear acronyms begin with the letters *RE* for *real ear* and are followed by two more letters that describe the type of measurement being made and how the measurement is displayed (usually *G* for *gain* or *R* for *response*).

Figure 3–1 illustrates a measurement of an unaided ear canal resonance using a 65 dB SPL speech-weighted input signal. **Figure 3–1A** shows the gain provided by the ear canal resonance. The ear canal provides little amplification until 1500 Hz and has a maximum peak of 21 dB gain at 3500 Hz. **Figure 3–1B** shows the output (or response) of the measurement. This curve has a similar shape as the gain curve in **Fig. 3–1A,** but the input signal used to measure the response is also included in the test result. This affects both the amplitude of the response (with a maximum peak of 48 dB SPL) and the shape of the curve. The clinician should be able to identify whether a test curve is displayed in gain or in output by examining the overall amplitude or the maximum peak of the curve. These values should be significantly larger in an output curve than in a gain curve.

Many real ear tests have been standardized in American National Standards Institute (ANSI) S3.46–1997 (ANSI, 1997). The real ear saturation response (RESR), real ear-to-coupler difference (RECD), and real ear-to-dial difference (REDD) are not standardized measurements. The overall theory and procedure behind these measurements are described below, but the details may vary according to how the manufacturer of the real ear analyzer has implemented these procedures.

REUR/REUG

The acronyms REUR and REUG stand for *real ear unaided response* and *real ear unaided gain*, respectively. The unaided response is a measurement of the ear in its natural state. The acoustical dynamics of the outer ear, the natural amplification without a hearing aid in place, is measured. The unaided response is also sometimes referred to as the *ear canal resonance.* It is a sound field measurement that is

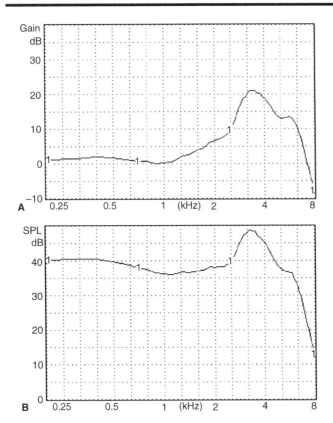

Figure 3–1 These two graphs indicate the unaided response measured with a 65 dB sound pressure level (SPL) American National Standards Institute (ANSI) speech-weighted composite signal. **(A)** Real ear unaided gain (REUG). **(B)** The same measurement in real ear unaided response (REUR).

made by placing the probe tube in the ear canal without the hearing aid or earmold. REUR is the absolute measurement of the unaided response (i.e., in dB SPL). REUG is the frequency response curve when the input signal has been subtracted from REUR, showing only the gain produced by the shape of the ear canal.

Figure 3–1 illustrates a measurement of an unaided ear canal resonance using a 65 dB SPL speech-weighted composite signal displayed as REUG **(Fig. 3–1)** and REUR **(Fig. 3–1)**.

REAR/REAG

The acronyms REAR and REAG stand for *real ear aided response* and *real ear aided gain*, respectively. The aided response is a measurement of the SPL in the ear canal created by the hearing aid when it is turned on, adjusted to a comfortable listening level, and placed on or in the ear. It is a sound field measurement made by placing the probe tube and the hearing aid (or hearing aid attached to an earmold) inside the ear. REAR is the absolute measurement of the aided response (i.e., dB SPL). REAG is the gain of the frequency response when it is compared with the response of the input signal outside the ear. That is, REAG is REAR minus the input signal.

Figure 3–2 is a measurement of an aided response using a 65 dB SPL speech-weighted composite signal. **Figure 3–2A** illustrates REAG, and **Fig. 3–2B** illustrates REAR.

REIG

The acronym REIG stands for *real ear insertion gain*. Insertion gain is not a direct measurement; instead, it describes a calculation: REIG = REAG − REUG. That is, the insertion gain is the difference in decibels, as a function of frequency, between the REAG and the REUG taken with the same measurement point and the same sound field conditions. Insertion gain describes the amount of sound added or inserted into the ear. It is always displayed and discussed in terms of gain and not response or output. Clinicians use REIG to verify how much amplification the hearing aid contributes to the ear in reference to prescriptive target(s).

Figure 3–3 illustrates REUG (curve 1), REAG (curve 2), and resulting REIG (curve 3). Both REUG and REAG were measured with a 65 dB SPL speech-weighted composite signal. Notice that REIG shows only the difference between REUG and REAG measures.

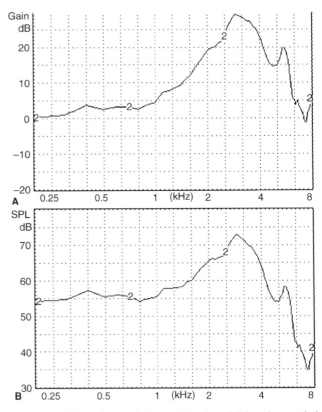

Figure 3–2 (A) Real ear aided gain (REAG) and **(B)** real ear aided response (REAR). Both graphs show the same measurement made with a 65 dB SPL ANSI speech-weighted composite signal.

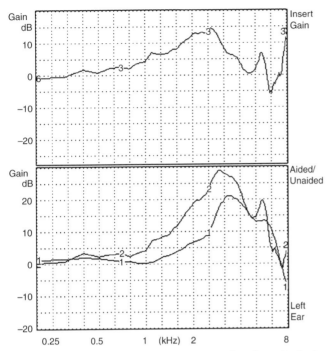

Figure 3–3 Real ear unaided gain (REUG, curve 1), real ear aided gain (REAG, curve 2), and real ear insertion gain (REIG, curve 3). REIG is the difference between REAG and REUG. Both the unaided and aided measurements were performed using a 65 dB SPL ANSI speech-weighted composite signal.

The reason insertion gain is considered important is that part of the amplification provided by a conventional hearing aid is used to compensate for the loss of the natural ear canal resonance. Said differently, placing a hearing aid on or in an ear changes the mechanical transform function of the ear. Amplified sound is not simply added to the REUR. The amplifier must first "work itself out of the hole" it created—the destruction of the natural amplification of the ear—before the amplified levels are greater than the unaided levels. Insertion gain describes only the amount of amplification provided by the hearing aid after it has compensated for loss of the natural ear canal resonance.

Pitfall

- Many clinicians confuse REAG and REIG. Both curves are referred to as "gain," but the measurements that are subtracted to obtain REAG and REIG are different. Remember that REAG is the difference between the sound field measured by the reference microphone outside the ear and the hearing aid response measured by probe microphone in the ear canal. REIG is the difference between REAG and REUG. That is, REIG is the difference between the aided and the unaided response.

There are a variety of hearing aid fitting formulas called "real ear targets." Numerous investigators have published

hearing aid fitting formulas. Most real ear targets are expressed in terms of insertion gain. Theoretically, audiologists will achieve better results in fitting hearing aids if they fine-tune the amplification so the measured REIG curve closely matches the prescribed insertion gain target. These real ear targets have undergone considerable research and modification over time. Current prescriptive formulas now yield targets that depend on the input level of the signal. See Chapter 7 in this volume for more information on prescriptive targets for linear and nonlinear signal processing.

RESR

The acronym RESR stands for real ear saturation response. This measurement is not defined in ANSI S3.46, but it is usually referred to as the measured REAR using a pure-tone sweep with a 90 dB SPL input signal. That is, it is the output of the hearing aid when the input signal is loud enough to saturate the circuit of some hearing aids. RESR is analogous to the output SPL at 90 dB (OSPL90) measurement described in ANSI S3.22 (ANSI, 2003).

RESR is especially useful when it is compared with the patient's loudness discomfort levels (LDLs). It is used to verify that the output of the hearing aids to a loud input level does not exceed the patient's LDL. **Figure 3–4** illustrates a comparison between the RESR (curve 1), the patient's LDLs (curve U), and the patient's thresholds (curve T). The authors recommend

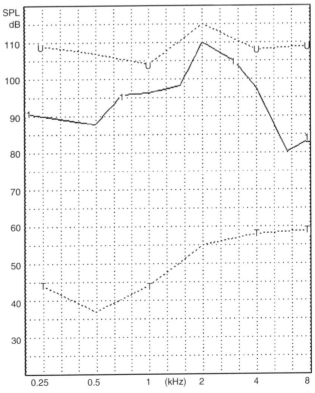

Figure 3–4 Real ear saturation response (RESR, curve 1) to a patient's loudness discomfort levels (curve U). The patient's thresholds (curve T) are shown. The RESR was measured with a 90 dB short pure-tone sweep.

that the hearing aid be programmed so that there is at least 5 dB between the measured RESR and the LDLs at all frequencies.

REOR/REOG

The acronyms REOR and REOG stand for real ear occluded response and real ear occluded gain, respectively. The occluded response is the measured SPL in the ear canal when the hearing aid or earmold is inserted with the hearing aid turned off.

The natural resonance of the unaided ear is an efficient amplifier that provides significant gain at ~2800 Hz and above. When a hearing aid is placed in the ear canal, such as an earmold attached to a behind-the-ear (BTE) aid or the case of an in-the ear (ITE) aid, in-the-canal (ITC) aid, or completely-in-canal (CIC) aid, the ear canal is occluded, and the natural amplification provided by the physical shape of the ear is eliminated. In some cases, this occlusion can be as great as 40 dB SPL (Martin, 2005). REOR is a measurement of this occlusion.

Figure 3–5A illustrates a comparison of REUG (curve 1) and REOG (curve 2). Both measures used a 65 dB SPL speech-weighted composite signal. REOG was measured with a vented earmold attached to a BTE placed in the ear with the aid turned off. REUR (curve 1) and REOR (curve 2)

are displayed in **Fig. 3–5B.** The difference between REUG and REOG illustrates to the clinician how much amplification the hearing aid needs to provide to restore hearing to the level it was before the hearing aid was inserted. No beneficial amplification is provided to the patient until REOR is compensated for and the hearing aid amplifies above the unaided response. For this reason, overcoming REOR can be considered "preliminary" or "preparatory" amplification (i.e., amplification that is needed before the amplification becomes "useful" or "productive" for the patient). In the example in **Fig. 3–5**, the hearing aid would need to provide up to 20 dB of gain above 2000 Hz to overcome the insertion loss caused by the insertion of the earmold into the ear canal.

Some devices that occlude the ear (e.g., CIC hearing aids) operate more efficiently than other devices. When CIC hearing aids are placed deeply in the ear canal, the volume of air between the instrument and the eardrum is very small. The output of the hearing aid is significantly higher because the amplifier is working more efficiently in this small volume. If the ear canal is open, and the volume of air is much larger, the amplifier needs to work much "harder" to produce amplification. Thus, although REOR is useful in determining the minimum amount of amplification needed by the hearing aid, it need not be overly emphasized.

Sometimes the term *occluded response* is confused with the term *occlusion effect*. Although the terms sound very much alike, these terms have significantly different meanings. The occluded response is the frequency response of the aid when it is in the ear and turned off. The occlusion effect, described later in this chapter, is the distortion the patient hears of his or her own speech when something, such as a hearing aid, is placed in the ear.

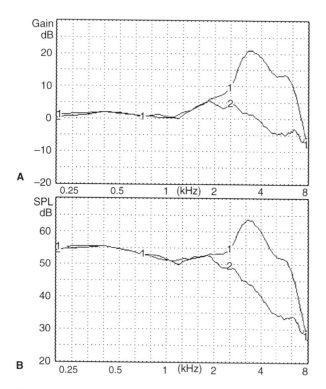

Figure 3–5 Comparison of the unaided and occluded responses. **(A)** Real ear unaided gain (REUG, curve 1) and real ear occluded gain (REOG, curve 2). **(B)** The same measurements as real ear unaided response (REUR, curve 1) and real ear occluded response (REOR, curve 2). The two measurements were performed with a 65 dB SPL ANSI speech-weighted composite signal. The REOG/REOR measurement was made with the hearing aid inserted into the ear canal but turned off.

RECD

The acronym RECD stands for *real ear-to-coupler difference* and is the difference between the occluded response in the ear canal and in a 2 cc coupler. To obtain RECD, the clinician must make two measures using the same transducer. This transducer is usually an insert earphone, but it can also be a linear hearing aid, as long as the volume control of the aid is in the same position for both measurements. One measure is performed in the occluded ear, and the other measure is performed with a 2 cc coupler. RECD is obtained by subtracting the coupler measure from the real ear measure. A procedure for measuring RECD is explained later in this chapter.

RECD is most commonly used to predict the real ear response of a hearing aid from the 2 cc coupler response. For this reason, RECD is usually referred to as a *transform* because it transforms one type of data (usually a coupler response) into another type of data (usually predicted real ear response). This is useful for testing infants, young children, and other patients (e.g., those with dementia or elderly patients who are not able to travel to a clinic) who may be difficult to test with typical real ear procedures. Once RECD has been measured, all other REMs can be predicted by measuring the hearing aid with a coupler.

Special Consideration

- One problem with RECD is there is no recognized standard method for measuring it. It has been left to manufacturers and researchers to develop the methods independently. This has led to the use of different transducers, couplers, and tubing lengths when measuring RECD. RECD measurements can therefore be inconsistent from analyzer to analyzer. There has been some research into determining the most accurate method for measuring RECD. Munro and Toal (2005) determined that using the patient's hearing aid when measuring RECD may be more accurate than using an insert earphone, although the insert earphone method is widely used in the profession. It is hoped that future research will eventually lead to a professional standard for measuring RECD.

REDD

The acronym REDD stands for real ear-to-dial difference. REDD is the difference between the output measured in dB SPL using a probe microphone near the eardrum to the measure made in dB hearing level (HL) from a calibrated audiometer. It usually requires an audiometer to produce the signal in dB HL and a real ear analyzer to measure the response near the eardrum in dB SPL.

In the SPL method described later in this chapter, the patient's thresholds measured in dB HL are converted into dB SPL so that they can be directly compared with the REM. REDD is used in this conversion formula. Measuring the patient's REDD instead of relying on average REDD values can make this conversion more accurate.

During the REDD measurement, a continuous pure-tone signal is usually produced from the audiometer at 70 dB HL using headphones or insert earphones as the transducer (the transducer should be that used to measure the patient's threshold values). The real ear analyzer measures the response near the eardrum with the probe microphone. The difference between the SPL value measured by real ear analyzer, and the amplitude produced by the audiometer in dB HL is the REDD at that frequency.

♦ Real Ear Techniques

Real Ear Equipment

At the simplest level, most REMs require an input signal (pure-tone, broadband, modulated, or speech), which usually arrives from a calibrated sound field loudspeaker, and a method to measure the intensity level of the signal generated in the ear canal. Real ear analyzers typically use two microphones for performing REM. A reference microphone is placed outside the ear, either over the pinna or under the earlobe. The probe microphone usually consists of a housing placed under the ear that is connected to a disposable slender silicone tube that is carefully placed in the ear canal.

Calibration and Preparation

The first step in performing REM usually consists of a calibration procedure. Two microphones are typically used in the measurement process: a reference microphone that measures the sound field outside the ear, and a probe microphone that measures the response near the eardrum in the ear. The sensitivity and frequency response of each microphone can vary. Therefore, it is important that these microphones be equalized or calibrated. This allows the difference between the probe and reference microphones to be recorded and later used during the REM. Some real ear analyzers only require this procedure to be completed occasionally during the year as part of typical equipment maintenance, whereas other real ear analyzers require that this procedure be completed before each use.

The sound field loudspeaker also needs to be calibrated (leveled) so the analyzer can adjust the input signal with the intended input intensity. Typically during the leveling process, the patient is positioned in the sound field. This will ensure that any changes in the sound field caused by the patient's body, clothes, and hair are accounted for in the leveling process. With some real ear analyzers, leveling is stored and used in the measurement process. Other analyzers perform leveling in real time as the measurement is completed. Measurements that use stored leveling are typically faster than measurements that include leveling in the measurement process. However, if the patient moves during REM, or if the sound field is otherwise disturbed during the measurement process, a measurement that uses real-time leveling can be more accurate.

When preparing the patient for REM, the loudspeaker is placed 12 inches (30 cm) to 39 inches (1 m) from the patient, using either a 0 degree azimuth (with the loudspeaker in front of the patient) or a 45 degree azimuth (with the loudspeaker pointed at an angle toward the patient). If the loudspeaker distance to the patient is too close, measurement results may be affected by distortions in the sound field. If the distance is too far, the real ear analyzer may not be able to produce signals as loud as the clinician may want them to be at the patient's ear. It is important for the clinician to refer to the operator's manual for details, as this procedure can vary widely from manufacturer to manufacturer.

It is also important for the clinician to take into account all the different items in the testing area that can affect the sound field. Walls, ceilings, chairs, and desks can affect measurement results because the signal from the loudspeaker will reflect off surfaces and rebound upon itself. Leveling can usually take care of most of the inconsistencies in the sound field caused by these surfaces, but it is best if the clinician maintains the testing area as uncluttered as possible. It is especially important to point the sound field loudspeaker toward an open area in the room and away from nearby walls. According to ANSI S3.46, the distance from the nearest surface to the patient or loudspeaker should be at least twice the distance between the loudspeaker and the patient (ANSI, 1997). For this reason, small enclosed sound booths are usually not the optimum environment to perform REMs.

ANSI S3.46 also states that the ambient noise in the testing environment should be at least 10 dB lower than the signal used in the REM. For example, if the clinician performs the REM using a 50 dB SPL input signal, the ambient noise in the testing environment should be less than 40 dB SPL. This should ensure that the ambient noise in the room has minimal effect on test results.

Inserting the Probe Tube

Once the clinician has prepared the patient in the sound field and completed all the necessary calibration procedures, the next step is to insert the probe tube into the ear canal. As with many audiological procedures, inserting the probe tube requires a fair amount of manual dexterity, and the clinician will need to practice this procedure before being able to do this easily. This process, combined with inserting the hearing aid without dislodging the probe tube, sometimes takes longer than the actual REMs. However, once it has been learned, it is fairly easy to incorporate into the hearing aid fitting process.

Before inserting the probe tube into the ear canal, the clinician should complete an otoscopic examination to determine if there is excess cerumen in the ear canal or if the patient has a pathological condition that may need a referral for medical care. Any excess cerumen should be removed, as it can block the probe tube and significantly affect measurement results.

The next step is to determine the probe tube insertion depth from the intertragal notch, illustrated in **Fig. 3–6.** Ideally, the end of the probe tube will be placed within 6 mm of the eardrum. This will usually occur with an insertion depth of ~31 mm for adult males, 28 mm for adult females, and 20 to 25 mm for children. Measure this length from the tip of the probe tube and mark it with a pen, as illustrated in **Fig. 3–6A,** or with the sliding marker that is part of some probe tubes.

Correct placement of the probe tube is especially critical in obtaining accurate measurements of frequencies above 2000 Hz. This is because sound enters the ear canal, reflects off the eardrum, and then bounces back into the ear canal. This reflection interferes with the incoming signal to create a standing wave in the ear canal at a distance from the eardrum equal to one quarter the wavelength of the frequency of the signal. In short, the higher the frequency the clinician wants to measure, the closer to the eardrum the probe tube must be placed. A 6 mm distance from the eardrum generally will provide measurement results of an accuracy of ± 2 dB at 6000 Hz and ± 4 dB at 8000 Hz (Dirks and Kincaid, 1987).

When performing insertion gain measurements, the probe tube insertion depth is slightly less important than it is when using the SPL method (i.e., REAR) as long as the depth is consistent for both the unaided and aided measurements. (The insertion gain and SPL methods will be explained later in this section.) This is because errors that may occur because of insertion depth will be present in both the unaided and aided measurements, and thus will be subtracted during insertion gain measures.

For insertion gain measurements, an easy method to determine the insertion depth is to hold the probe tube next to the hearing aid or earmold. The probe tube should be 5 mm past the part that is inserted into the ear **(Fig. 3–6A).** This technique should not be used when measuring with the SPL method because it generally does not place the probe tube close enough to the eardrum. When measuring with the SPL method, the clinician should use otoscopic inspection to verify that the probe tube is within 6 mm of the eardrum.

Insert the probe tube into the ear canal, twisting it gently to ease it past the hairs in the ear canal. The mark on the probe tube should rest on the intertragal notch, as shown in **Fig. 3–6B.** A fiberoptic otoscope is useful to ensure the end of the probe tube is placed correctly. In fact, an otoscopic

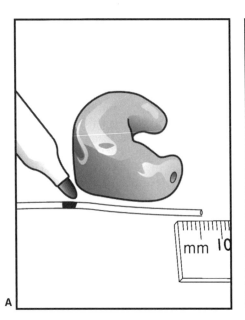

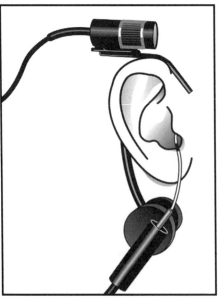

Figure 3–6 (A) Probe tube marked several millimeters longer than the length of the ear mold. **(B)** A typical real ear setup. The reference microphone is place above the ear, and the probe microphone is placed below the ear, with the attached probe tube inserted into the ear canal. The mark on the probe tube is placed at the intertragal notch, indicating how deep the probe tube should be inserted. Some real ear manufacturers place the reference microphone below the ear in the same housing as the probe microphone. (From Frye Electronics Inc., with permission.)

A
B

view of the ear canal can be considered absolutely necessary when performing REMs on children or ear canals of unusual size or length. A piece of medical tape on the cheek can be used to secure the probe tube in place.

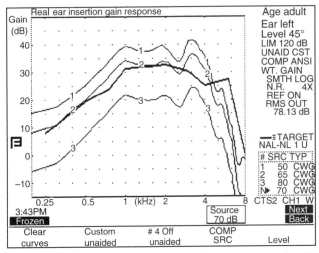

Figure 3–7 Real ear insertion gain (REIG) curves measured at 50 (curve 1), 65 (curve 2), and 80 (curve 3) dB SPL. The bold line indicates the NAL-NL1 REIG prescribed target for a 65 dB SPL input signal. All measurements were made with an ANSI speech-weighted composite signal.

Pearl

- An easy way to determine if the probe tube has been placed correctly in the ear canal is to examine the REUG. The REUG typically has a maximum peak between 2 and 3 kHz and returns to 0 dB between 6 and 8 kHz. A maximum peak before 2 kHz, or a negative response between 6 and 8 kHz, is usually an indication that the probe tube is not inserted deeply enough into the ear canal.

The Insertion Gain Method

The insertion gain method is currently the most popular approach to performing REMs. Insertion gain measures, however, are rapidly losing favor as clinicians are turning to the SPL method explained in the next section. During an insertion gain measurement, REUG and REAG are measured to obtain REIG, which is then compared with the insertion gain prescriptive target. See Chapter 7 in this volume for more information on prescriptive targets for linear and nonlinear hearing aids.

After the probe tube is inserted and the real ear analyzer is leveled (if required), the unaided response (i.e., REUG) is measured. This is usually completed using a 65 dB SPL input signal (**Fig. 3–1A**). Notice the −5 dB gain at 8000 Hz. This could be an indication that the probe tube is not inserted deeply enough into the ear canal.

Next, the hearing aid is inserted carefully into the ear canal. The clinician must hold the probe tube in place when inserting the hearing aid because it is important for the probe tube to be in the same position for both the unaided and aided conditions. The clinician must also be careful to avoid pushing the probe tube into the eardrum. Once the aid is inserted, REAG is measured. The real ear analyzer will use the measured REUG and REAG to calculate REIG (i.e., REIG = REAG − REUG). REIG can then be compared with the selected insertion gain prescriptive target. Adjustments to the hearing aid can be made, and subsequent measurements can verify the changes.

If the hearing aid uses linear signal processing, it is only necessary to measure REIG with an input level of 65 dB SPL. If the hearing aid has nonlinear signal processing, it is recommended to perform insertion gain measures at soft (50 dB SPL), average (65 dB SPL), and loud (80 dB SPL) input levels. This will ensure the hearing aid fitting will be appropriate for different input levels. Current real ear prescriptive targets, such as NAL-NL1 (National Acoustic Laboratories' nonlinear fitting procedure, version 1), are nonlinear. This means that the prescriptive target will change according to the input source amplitude so that soft sounds are provided

with more gain than loud sounds. **Figure 3–7** illustrates three REIG measurements. Curves 1, 2, and 3 were measured with 50, 65, and 80 dB ANSI speech-weighted composite signals, respectively. The bold line indicates the NAL-NL1 prescriptive target for a 65 dB SPL input signal.

Controversial Point

- Revit (2002) has theorized that it may be more accurate to use an average REUG than a measured REUG when performing REMs to a prescribed insertion gain target. The basic reasoning is that the individual REUG is an extraneous variable. Insertion gain targets are based on audiometric thresholds. Yet audiometric threshold testing is typically done in dB HL with insert or supra-aural earphones, which occlude the ear and destroy the natural ear canal resonance, and which are calibrated with the assumption of an acoustically average ear. In other words, every ear canal is different, so the dB SPL value at the eardrum for one person for a given signal from the audiometer can be markedly different from the dB SPL value for another person being exposed to the same signal, depending further on the transducer used (Valente et al, 1994). However, the recorded dB HL threshold assumes a fixed SPL at the eardrum of an average ear. Because these average ear–based threshold values are used by the fitting formula to generate real ear targets, the measured REUG will only introduce extraneous information to the REM verification process. Revit (2002) includes a mathematical justification in his reasoning, which is consistent with the use of REAG instead of REIG during verification, such as with the desired sensation level (DSL) and NAL-NL1 strategies.

The SPL (REAR) Method

The Desired Sensation Level (DSL) i/o fitting rule has popularized the SPL-O-Gram method of performing REMs. The concept behind the SPL-O-Gram is to convert all relevant measurements into real ear SPL, including audiometric measurements, REMs, and real ear targets. This allows the clinician to compare the patient's dynamic range (residual hearing between threshold and LDL) and the output from the hearing aid with a wide input (50–80 dB SPL). Using this method, the patient's dynamic range becomes the target. The clinician ensures that the output from a soft input level is above threshold, and the output from a loud input is below the LDL.

In a typical SPL-O-Gram, the patient's threshold, LDL, and real ear target(s) are displayed on the same graph in dB SPL. Real ear aided measurements are typically measured for soft (50 db SPL), average (65 dB SPL), and loud (80 dB SPL) levels. This ensures that soft input signals reach above the patient's threshold, average input signals meet the prescribed target, and loud input signals are below the LDL. This is referred to as normalizing the hearing aid fitting. In the SPL-O-Gram method, measuring the unaided response is not typically required. However, the unaided response is still a useful measurement in that it will allow the clinician to be sure the insertion loss created by inserting the hearing aid will be overcome with the hearing aid amplification.

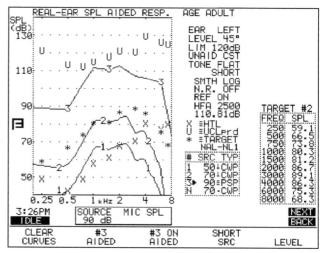

Figure 3–8 Real ear SPL-O-Gram. Curve 1 was measured with a 50 dB SPL ANSI speech-weighted composite signal. This curve can be compared with the patient's thresholds (*X*). Curve 2 was measured with a 65 dB SPL ANSI speech-weighted composite signal. This curve can be compared with the NAL-NL1 target for a 65 dB SPL input (*). It is apparent here that, by observing curve 1 and curve 2, additional amplification should be applied above 2000 Hz. Curve 3 was measured with a 90 dB SPL short pure-tone sweep. This curve is compared with the patient's loudness discomfort levels (*U*). This curve reports that the output of the hearing aid can be increased below 1000 Hz and above 2000 Hz.

- The DSL fitting method prescribes that soft input levels should exceed the patient's threshold (Seewald, 1992). This normalization philosophy will always lead to REAR targets that are above threshold. The NAL-NL1 fitting method uses an equalization philosophy in which the goal is to provide equal amplification across all the frequency regions of speech. On the other hand, NAL-NL1 may not always prescribe amplification above the patient's hearing thresholds. As explained in Ching et al (2001), the developers of NAL-NL1 believe that amplifying high frequencies in patients with severe or profound high-frequency hearing loss may decrease speech intelligibility instead of increasing it. Therefore, the clinician should not be alarmed to discover NAL-NL1 targets below the patient's hearing thresholds when performing REM with an SPL-O-Gram.

Figure 3–8 illustrates a real ear SPL-O-Gram. Adding amplification to the hearing aid at 3000 Hz so that the REM exceeds threshold at that frequency may improve the patient's speech recognition at soft speech levels. Curve 1 was measured with a 50 dB SPL ANSI speech-weighted composite signal. It exceeds the patient's thresholds, indicated by the *X*s, from 500 to 2000 Hz. Curve 2 was measured with a 70 dB SPL ANSI-speech weighted composite signal. It matches the 70 dB SPL prescriptive target, indicated by the asterisks,

from 500 to 2000 Hz. (Notice the NAL-NL1 target does not exceed the patient's threshold values at 6000–8000 Hz.) Additional amplification at this level, especially between 2000 and 4000 Hz, may also improve the hearing aid fitting. Curve 3 was measured with a 90 dB SPL pure-tone sweep. All measured frequencies are below the patient's LDLs, indicated by the *U*s. However, special care may be necessary at 1000 Hz, where curve 3 approaches the LDLs.

◆ Types of Input Signals

The type of input signal used during REMs will have a significant effect on the measured results. The input signal can activate signal-processing characteristics of the hearing aid, such as compression, noise suppression, and feedback suppression. Different types of input signals can affect these characteristics in different manners. Therefore, understanding the input signal and how it may affect test results are essential in understanding test results.

When measuring REAR (e.g., during the SPL method), the input signal is included in the test results. Changing the speech weighting or amplitude of the input signal will affect the test results even if the gain produced by the hearing aid does not change. Thus, the input signal will have an even greater effect on REAR results than it will on REAG or REIG results. This is something for the clinician to remember when using the SPL (REAR) method.

Pure-Tone Sweeps

The most traditional test signal used in REMs is the pure-tone sweep. A pure-tone sweep is a series of tones presented one at a time, increasing in frequency. Pure-tone sweeps are usually flat-weighted; that is, each tone in the sweep has the same amplitude.

Pure-tone sweeps generally are not recommended in REMs, except when testing the RESR, because most modern hearing aids will respond differently to a pure-tone sweep than they would to a more speech-like signal. In particular, the compression characteristics of the hearing aid can cause an effect known as artificial blooming in the low frequencies that can distort test results. In other words, low frequencies will show higher measurement results than the aid will probably produce when exposed to speech. In **Fig. 3–9,** curve 1 shows the aid's response to a speech-weighted composite signal (the speech weighting used is specified by ANSI S3.42), and curve 2 shows the hearing aid's response to a pure-tone sweep. Notice the greater gain between 200 and 2000 Hz in the measurement obtained using the pure-tone sweep in comparison to the measurement obtained when using the broadband signal. Notice the higher amplification shown by curve 2. Curve 1 is a more realistic representation of the hearing aid's response to a speech signal.

Pure-tone sweeps, however, are recommended when testing the patient's RESR. This is explained in the section below on the short pure-tone sweep.

Composite Signal

Most current real ear analyzers contain some sort of broadband continuous signal with multiple frequency components that are presented simultaneously. These signals are usually speech weighted; that is, the higher frequencies of the signal have less energy than the lower frequencies of the signal. This characteristic is so named because in a long-term average of speech, there is more energy in the lower frequencies than in the higher frequencies. The amount of high-frequency roll-off can vary from signal to signal, so it is important to know what type of speech weighting the signal uses to understand the test results it will produce.

The most common speech weighting is defined in ANSI S3.42–1992 (ANSI, 1992). The amplitude of the signal at 900 Hz is 3 dB down from its amplitude at 200 Hz. Higher frequencies continue to decrease in amplitude at a rate of 6 dB per octave. See curve 1 in **Fig. 3–10,** which illustrates this type of speech weighting. Notice that, although the overall energy of the signal is 65 dB SPL, the energy of each individual frequency component is significantly less, starting at 54 dB SPL at 200 Hz and decreasing to 37 dB at 8000 Hz. However, when summed, the overall input is 65 dB SPL. Curve 2 in **Fig. 3–10** shows the speech weighting of the male ICRA (International Collegium of Rehabilitative Audiology) signal, another common speech weighting used in real ear measures. See the section below on ICRA for more information.

This energy distribution can be explained by envisioning a single loudspeaker producing a signal. Next, add a second

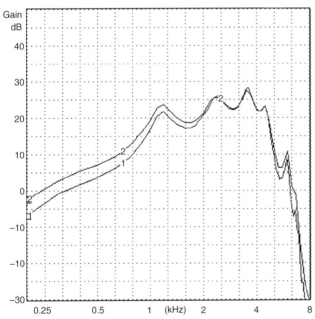

Figure 3–9 This is an illustration of the "blooming effect" (i.e., great output in the lower frequencies by using a pure-tone signal) on a non-linear hearing aid. Curve 1 was measured with an ANSI speech-weighted composite signal. Curve 2 was measured with a pure-tone sweep. The pure-tone signal activates the compression circuit of the hearing aid differently than the composite signal does.

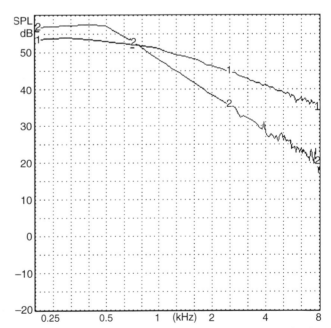

Figure 3–10 Curve 1 illustrates the speech weighting standardized in ANSI S3.42, and curve 2 illustrates the speech spectrum of the male ICRA (International Collegium of Rehabilitative Audiology) speaker. Although the root-mean-square (average) of the two signals is 65 dB SPL, the amplitude of the individual frequency components are significantly less for the ICRA signal above ~750 Hz.

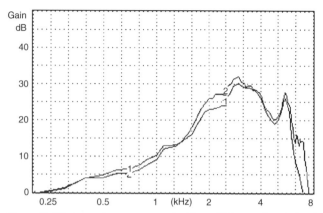

Figure 3–11 Curve 1 was measured with an ANSI speech-weighted composite signal. Curve 2 was measured with an ICRA speech-weighted composite signal. Note the slight differences in measured gain as a result of using the two different signals. See **Fig. 3–10** for an illustration of the speech weightings used in these measurements.

loudspeaker producing the same signal. The combined energy of the two output signals is 3 dB higher than the energy from each individual loudspeaker. Now imagine a broadband signal as an array of loudspeakers. The more frequency components that are available in the signal, the less energy each individual component will have to generate the specified overall energy. This is something to keep in mind when viewing REAR measurements.

The output of a broadband signal at a particular frequency will be much less than the output of the same frequency of a pure-tone sweep when both signals are set to the same

overall amplitude. **Figure 3–11** illustrates this difference. Curve 1 reports the REAR to a speech-weighted broadband signal, while curve 2 reports the REAR to a flat-weighted pure-tone sweep. Both curves were measured with a 65 dB SPL input level. This significant difference is why it is critical for the clinician to understand the speech weighting used in the input signal before interpreting test results in dB SPL.

The speech weighting of the input signal will also affect the compression characteristics of the hearing aid. **Figure 3–12** shows two REAG measurements. Curve 1 was measured with an ANSI speech-weighted signal. Curve 2 was measured with an ICRA speech-weighted signal. Beyond 750 Hz, the frequencies of the ICRA speech-weighted signal are of lower amplitude than the frequencies of the ANSI speech-weighted signal. This lower amplitude likely caused the compression circuit of the DSP hearing aid to increase the amplification of the ICRA speech-weighted signal more than it increased the amplitude of the ANSI speech-weighted signal. So, although one may expect for a signal with low amplitude in the high frequencies to result in a measurement with low amplitude in the high frequencies, the compression characteristics of the hearing aid caused the opposite to be true.

The speech weighting of the input signal has a significant impact on both the view of the test results in dB SPL (output) and the compression characteristics of the hearing aid. Therefore, it is always important for the clinician to understand the input signal before interpreting test results.

Modulated Signal

Digital hearing aids use noise suppression or speech enhancement processing that is designed to amplify the parts of the input signal that are speechlike (modulated) and suppress the

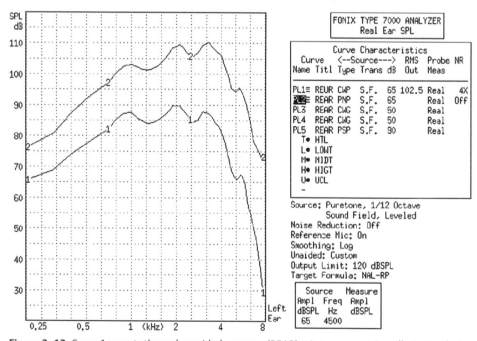

Figure 3–12 Curve 1 reports the real ear aided response (REAR) using a 65 dB SPL ANSI speech-weighted composite signal, and curve 2 reports the REAR using a 65 dB SPL flat-weighted pure-tone sweep. This comparison illustrates the importance of understanding the test signal used with REAR measures.

parts of the signal that are noiselike (continuous). Although different hearing aids have different techniques to determine which part of the signal is speech and which is noise, most work on the principal that speech is modulated (i.e., it varies in intensity and duration), and noise is constant.

Unfortunately, most conventional real ear analyzer test signals are continuous. Pure-tone sweeps vary in frequency as the test completes, but the amplitude of the tones is constant. Broadband signals may use a speech-weighted frequency spectrum but are presented continually to the hearing aid. Thus, most digital hearing aids with speech suppression technology enabled will treat conventional pure-tone and broadband signals as noise. For this reason, most modern real ear analyzers have been enhanced to use a modulated speech-like signal that can be used to test digital hearing aids while leaving the noise suppression algorithm on. One example of this is the FONIX Digital Speech signal (Frye Electronics, Tigard, Oregon), which is a broadband signal that is temporally modulated. The signal is turned on for 50 to 150 msec (configurable by the user) and turned off for a random 100 to 300 msec, repeating in this manner while the test runs. This has the effect of "tricking" the hearing aid into responding as it would to speech. Curve 1 in **Fig. 3–13** demonstrates a digital hearing aid measured with a modulated signal. Curve 2 demonstrates the same hearing aid measured with a continuous noiselike signal. The hearing aid is suppressing the amplification of the noiselike signal by 8 dB overall.

ICRA

The International Collegium of Rehabilitative Audiology (ICRA, 1997) has produced a compact disc (CD) that contains sound tracks of samples of the long-term average speech spectrum (LTASS). The CD has a variety of speakers (e.g., male, female, and child). Some current hearing aid test systems use these sound tracks as input signals or provide broadband signals with the speech weighting obtained from analyses of these tracks.

Live Speech

Recently, "live speech" has become a popular input signal. The clinician's voice, the voice of a family member, or a prerecorded voice can be used as the input to the hearing aid. This can be an effective counseling tool that can demonstrate to the patient how the amplification of the hearing aid can affect an actual speech signal and how that amplification compares with the patient's dynamic range. The disadvantage of using this type of speech signal is that its characteristics are not constant; the amplitude and frequency responses of speech vary as the test continues. Therefore, to use live speech as an input signal, the REM needs to be run long enough to obtain an average that can be compared with the real ear prescriptive target. Speech that is not prerecorded or calibrated is questionable for use as an input signal when adjusting the hearing aid to a prescribed target because test results from such speech signals are generally not repeatable, and the speech itself may have different characteristics than assumed by the prescriptive formula.

Some real ear analyzers also keep track of the minimum and maximum peak responses of the aid to the speech signal as a function of frequency and graph the resulting region. **Figure 3–14** is an SPL graph that includes a shaded

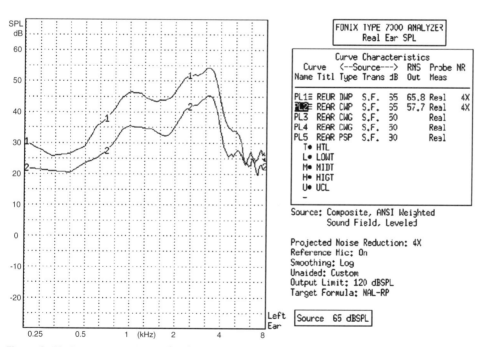

Figure 3–13 Curve 1 was measured with a 65 dB SPL modulated ANSI speech-weighted digital speech signal, and curve 2 was measured with a 65 dB SPL constant ANSI speech-weighted composite signal. The root-mean-square difference between the two curves is 8 dB, although the difference between the curves at some frequencies (e.g., 1700 Hz) is as great as 12 dB.

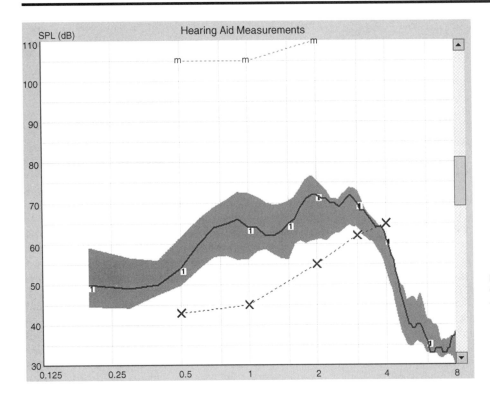

Figure 3–14 Example of live-speech SPL-O-Gram. The upper and lower boundaries of the shadowed region represent the maximum and minimum response of the hearing aid to the speech signal over time. Curve 1 indicates the last measurement, curve *X* indicates the patient's thresholds, and curve *m* indicates the patient's loudness discomfort levels.

region. The upper and lower limits of that region are the maximum and minimum responses of the hearing aid to the speech signal. The patient's hearing thresholds (*X*), the last measured frequency response of the hearing aid (curve 1), and the patient's LDLs (*m*) are also displayed, showing the clinician how the hearing aid's response compares with the dynamic range of the patient.

The live speech test is especially useful as a counseling tool. In one possible exercise, the clinician can instruct the patient's spouse (or other family member, loved one, or care-taker) to read a written passage. The REAR is measured using this speech passage as the input signal. The clinician can then have the spouse move several feet away and read the passage again while a second measurement is taken. The two measurement results can then be compared. This method can be used to demonstrate to both the patient and the spouse how close the two need to be in order for speech to be audible.

Short Pure-Tone Sweep

When performing a hearing aid fitting, it is important to be sure the hearing aid will not produce amplification that will exceed the patient's LDLs. When the LDLs are displayed on the SPL-O-Gram (converted from dB HL to dB SPL, if necessary), the RESR test can be measured to verify if the input signal plus the gain provided by the hearing aid exceeds the patient's LDLs.

Although it is recommended to use broadband signals for most REMs, when verifying maximum output, it is more desirable to use a pure-tone sweep. This is because when using a pure-tone sweep, the input of each frequency to the hearing aid is the same. As discussed earlier, when using a broadband signal, the energy of the individual frequency components of the signal is significantly less at each frequency than the overall energy of the signal. Using a pure-tone sweep presents the hearing aid with more energy at each frequency component, making it a more desirable signal type to use when verifying LDLs.

Obviously, it is important for the clinician to be very careful when presenting such loud input levels (i.e., 90 dB SPL in this case) to the patient. If the compression circuit in the hearing aid is not programmed correctly, the audiologist may run the risk of presenting the patient an output level that is above the LDL. The patient may become very irritated, and the clinician may run the risk of injuring the patient's hearing. High-intensity input levels (i.e., ≥ 80 dB SPL) have the potential of creating very loud output levels.

Some analyzers have a version of a pure-tone sweep designed just for testing the RESR. This short pure-tone sweep uses tones that are presented long enough to obtain an accurate measurement, but short enough in duration (a few milliseconds) that the ear does not hear the sound at its true input or output level. This type of signal actually sounds softer than the actual SPL.

♦ Performing Real Ear Measurements on Children

Performing REMs on children can present the clinician with some challenges. To obtain accurate and repeatable results, the patient must sit still and remain relatively stationary during the real ear test procedure. This, unfortunately, is often not possible with infants and young children. At the same time, REMs are even more important for children than for adults, because a child is less able to communicate to the clinician about the accuracy or sound quality produced by the hearing aid fitting. Refer to Chapter 4 in this volume on verifying hearing aid fittings in children.

Coupler Approach

To overcome difficulties in performing REMs on children, researchers at the University of Western Ontario popularized the coupler approach in their DSL fitting method (Moodie et al, 1994). The coupler approach uses the RECD transformation to convert data from real ear to coupler and back again. That is, if the clinician performs a coupler measurement on a hearing aid, then the RECD can be used to approximate what the REM would be for that child. These real ear approximations are known as simulated REMs. The RECD can also be used to convert a real ear target into one that is appropriate to be compared with coupler measurements. This type of target is known as a coupler target. The idea is that, if the clinician can perform an RECD on the child, then all other measurements can be performed in the sound chamber, minimizing discomfort for the child and frustration for the clinician. It is important for the clinician to remember than the ear canal of a child younger than 2 years changes rapidly. Therefore, the RECD of the child should be retested if there is more than 1 or 2 months between appointments.

Measuring the RECD

Most real ear analyzers have a special operational mode for measuring the RECD that simplifies the procedure. However, it is instructional to consider the following RECD procedure that uses the insertion gain mode on a real ear analyzer.

1. *Perform the coupler measure*   The first step in obtaining the RECD is performing the coupler measure. Enter the insertion gain mode on the real ear analyzer and disable the reference microphone. Insert the probe microphone into the 2 cc coupler using a probe microphone adapter. Configure the real ear analyzer to drive the signal through an insert earphone and attach the insert earphone to the 2 cc coupler. **Figure 3–15** illustrates this configuration. If possible, place the assembly in a sound chamber or sound-occluding environment. Configure the real ear analyzer to measure an unaided (REUG) frequency response, maintaining the setup described above. Set the analyzer to use a 50 dB SPL speech-weighted composite signal and perform the measurement. The unaided curve is the coupler part of the RECD.

2. *Perform the real ear measure*   The next step is to measure the real ear response. Configure the analyzer to measure an aided (REAG) frequency response. The reference microphone should still be disabled, and the real ear analyzer should be configured to drive the input signal using an insert earphone (the insert earphone used for the coupler measure should also be used for the real ear measure). Insert the probe microphone into the patient's ear canal. Carefully place the insert earphone

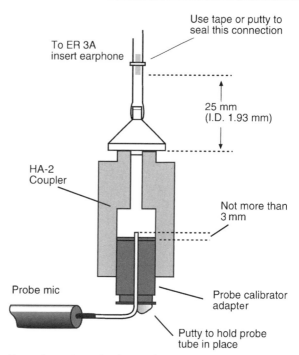

Figure 3–15 Setup for the coupler part of the real ear-to-coupler difference (RECD) measurement. The probe microphone is inserted into the coupler with the use of an adapter. The coupler is attached to an insert earphone, which is connected to the real ear analyzer. This allows the real ear analyzer to measure the response of the probe microphone inside a 2 cc coupler from a signal delivered with the ER3A insert earphone. (From Frye Electronics Inc., with permission.)

into the patient's ear canal using a custom earmold or foam eartip (**Fig. 3–16**). Using an input signal of the same type and amplitude used for the coupler measure (50 dB SPL speech-weighted composite), measure the aided response.

3. *Calculate the RECD*   In the real ear analyzer's insertion gain mode, the REIG is the difference between the REUG and the REAG. Because the coupler part of the RECD was performed as the REUG measure, and the real ear part of the RECD was performed as the REAG measure, the resulting REIG is actually the RECD.

Prescriptive Targets for Children

Another issue with real ear tests on children is that the traditional insertion gain method does not work very well with young children because the size of their ear canals changes so rapidly. When the hearing aid is fitted on the ear, the output level at the eardrum depends on the amplification capacity (output) of the hearing aid, but it also depends on the volume of air into which this amplification is routed. The volume of air between the end of the earmold and the eardrum is called the *residual volume.*

Children have small ear canals and small residual volumes. Children with severe to profound hearing loss are often fitted with BTE instruments and earmolds that have long canals and no vents. The residual volume of air in this type of

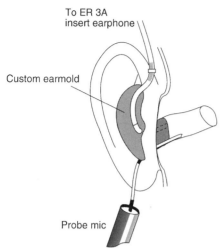

Figure 3–16 Setup for the real ear part of the real ear-to-coupler difference (RECD) measurement. The probe tube is inserted in the ear canal as usual. The insert earphone is connected to the custom earmold or a foam eartip and to the real ear analyzer. This allows the real ear analyzer to measure the occluded response at the ear canal from a signal delivered with the ER3A insert earphone. (From Frye Electronics Inc., with permission.)

hearing aid fitting is minimal, and the output may be 10 dB or more than those values seen on 2 cc coupler tests. To make things more difficult, the residual volume changes rapidly as the child ages, especially before the age of 2 years.

When it is determined that a certain amount of output is appropriate at the eardrum given the child's hearing loss, then the clinician would need a different insertion gain target for a 6-month-old than what would be needed for a 24-month-old. This is because the residual volume of the child's ear canal changes rapidly, affecting the natural amplification produced by the ear. An older child with a larger ear canal will need more power from the hearing aid to produce the same amount of output at the eardrum than a younger child with a smaller ear canal (Ching et al, 2002).

If the clinician can instead compare the REMs to targets in gain or SPL, then the targets do not need to change as the ear canal resonance changes, removing a complication from the fitting process. For this reason, current fitting rules (DSL i/o and NAL-NL1) use gain or SPL targets for fitting children instead of the traditional insertion gain targets. The amount of amplification produced by the hearing aid will need to change as the child ages, but the target can remain relatively constant.

♦ Special Tests

Open Ear Hearing Aids

In the past few years, so-called open ear or over-the-ear (OTE) hearing aids have increased in popularity. Hearing aids of this style are usually worn behind the ear with a thin tube extending from the top of the ear into the ear canal.

BTE hearing aids are attached to the ear with earmolds that occlude the ear and eliminate most of the natural resonance of the ear canal. OTE aids, in contrast, minimize occlusion of the ear and preserve the natural ear canal resonance. Modest high-frequency gain provided by the hearing aid is added to the high-frequency resonance of the ear canal, producing amplification of high-frequency emphasis with little or no occlusion effect. Feedback suppression features are also included in OTE aids to prevent the feedback that may result from the open-fitting style of the hearing aid.

OTE hearing aids present new challenges for REM. The amplified signal that is output from the hearing aid may escape from the ear canal and affect the sound field just outside the ear. Also, the feedback suppression software employed by the OTE aids may suppress some frequencies of the test signal outside the ear. In both cases, the reference microphone measurement may be affected, and the resulting REAG could be either artificially high or artificially low. Disabling the reference microphone and forcing the real ear analyzer to use only the calibration of the sound field loudspeaker performed before the measurement to calculate the REAG will produce more accurate results. See **Fig. 3–17** for an example of two REAR measurements of the same hearing aid using the same input signal.

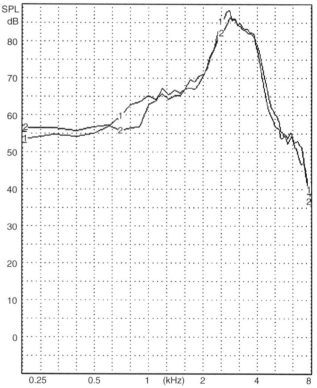

Figure 3–17 Real ear aided response (REAR) of a behind-the-ear (BTE) hearing aid measured with and without the real ear analyzer reference microphone. Curve 1 was measured with the reference microphone enabled, and curve 2 was measured with the reference microphone disabled. The feedback suppression of the BTE artificially inflates the REAR when the reference microphone is enabled.

Curve 1 was measured with the reference microphone of the real ear analyzer turned on. Curve 2 was measured with the reference microphone turned off. When measuring OTE hearing aids, the reference microphone of the real ear analyzer should be disabled.

Digital Processing Delay

When digital hearing aids process sound, they work like miniature computers, turning the analog signal into digital information, altering the signal according to its algorithm, and, finally, changing it back into an analog signal that is delivered into the ear canal. An artifact of digital processing technology is that this process always takes time. The amount of time it takes to process sound is called the *digital processing delay* of the hearing aid, also known as *group delay*. The digital processing delay depends on the type of signal-processing algorithm employed by the hearing aid.

When the patient wears only one hearing aid, or when the fit is binaural with open fit hearing aids or hearing aids with vents, sound can travel to the unaided ear or through the vent faster than through the hearing aid, creating an echoing effect. This effect can be perceived as a type of distortion and can possibly cause problems with localization and speech recognition. Research has shown that the group delay present in most hearing aids probably does not cause adverse affects when the patient is fit with an occluded binaural set of hearing aids. Unfortunately, not enough research has yet been done to determine how much group delay is acceptable for other types of hearing aid fittings. It is the opinion of the authors that group delay of less than 6 msec is probably acceptable for most patients, especially if both hearing aids of a binaural set have the same group delay. The clinician may want to avoid replacing one hearing aid of a binaural set if the new hearing aid has a significantly different group delay than the other hearing aid the patient will be wearing.

See **Fig. 3–18** for an example of a test of the group delay of the hearing aid. During this test, an impulse signal is delivered to the hearing aid, and the hearing aid's response is recorded. Notice the time domain is used to display the test results instead of the usual frequency domain. The hearing aid responds to the impulse signal with a series of peaks. In the example, the first peak with at least half the amplitude of the maximum peak is used as the delay of the hearing aid. The dotted line on the left side of the graph indicates the group delay of the hearing aid analyzer. The delay of the hearing aid is subtracted from the delay of the analyzer to obtain the final result of 5.6 msec.

Testing Noise Suppression

As mentioned earlier in the section on modulated signals, many hearing aids have special digital processing algorithms that suppress noise or enhance speech. Typically, the hearing aid monitors the input signal for signals that are constant in frequency and/or amplitude. These signals are suppressed. Signals that are modulated (like speech) are amplified. Some real ear analyzers have the ability to test noise suppression in the hearing aid when the noise is present in the signal at

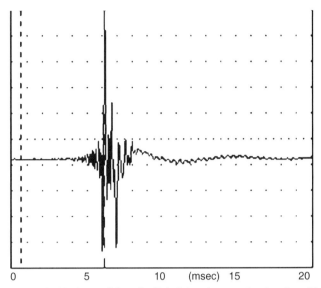

Figure 3–18 Group delay of a digital signal processing hearing aid. The hearing aid analyzer delivered an impulse signal to the hearing aid, and the results were graphed as a function of time. The first peak with at least half the amplitude of the maximum peak was determined to be the group delay of the hearing aid. The dotted line on the left side of the graph indicates the system delay of the hearing aid analyzer. The delay of the hearing aid is subtracted from the delay of the hearing aid analyzer to achieve the final result of 5.6 msec of digital processing delay for the hearing aid.

specific frequencies. This can demonstrate to the clinician how noise in one channel may affect the amplification of the signal in other channels. The real ear analyzer performs this test by inserting a noise signal into the modulated signal at a particular frequency. That is, while most of the signal is modulated, causing the hearing aid to respond to it as it would to speech, at a particular frequency the signal is constant, producing a noise for the hearing aid to suppress.

In **Fig. 3–19,** all three curves were measured with a 65 dB SPL modulated ANSI speech-weighted signal. Curve 1 included a 500 Hz bias signal, curve 2 included a 1000 Hz bias signal, and curve 3 included a 4000 Hz bias signal. In this example, the 500 Hz signal had little effect on the frequency response of the hearing aid, but the bias signals at 1000 and 4000 Hz decreased the amplification provided by the hearing aid in the channel at which the bias was present. This test can provide a valuable troubleshooting tool that allows the clinician to determine the performance of the noise suppression feature of the hearing aid.

Verifying Directionality

Over the past few years, the technology used to control directional microphones on hearing aids has advanced greatly. Most manufacturers of hearing aids provide a polar plot of the directionality of the hearing aid and values labeled DI (directivity index) and AI-DI (articulation index–directivity index). (See Chapter 1 for more information on this topic.) Unfortunately, these values and plots are measured by the manufacturers in an anechoic chamber and using an elaborate testing setup that is not practical for most clinics. However, the clinician can use REM to determine whether or not the hearing aid

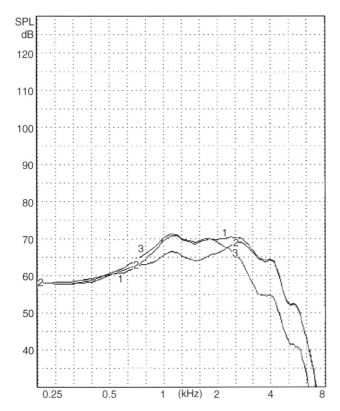

Figure 3–19 Real ear aided response (REAR) using a 65 dB SPL modulated ANSI speech-weighted signal. Curve 1 included a 500 Hz bias signal, curve 2 included a 1000 Hz bias signal, and curve 3 included a 4000 Hz bias signal. Although the 500 Hz bias tone had little effect on the amplification of the hearing aid, the 1000 and 4000 Hz bias signals decreased the amplification of the signal in the channel of the hearing aid in which the bias signal was present.

forward measurement with the patient facing the real ear loudspeaker and a reverse measurement with the patient pointed away from the loudspeaker. Together, these measurements can verify that the patient is provided with more amplification when the signal is in front and less amplification when the signal is behind.

Most hearing aid analyzers do not have a separate mode specifically designed for directionality measurements. However, the insertion gain mode that is available on most real ear equipment is well suited for the directionality measurement. That is, the insertion gain curve in the real ear mode is a subtraction curve created from the unaided and the aided response measurements. If the clinician uses the "unaided" curve slot for the directional reverse measurement and the "aided" curve slot for the directional forward measurement, the resulting insertion gain will actually be the directional advantage of the hearing aid. This response curve is the difference between the forward and reverse measurements.

The following procedure assumes the clinician is using the real ear analyzer's insertion gain test mode to test directionality and that the clinician has calibrated its microphones and/or leveled the real ear loudspeaker (**Fig. 3–20**). The directionality test is easiest if the real ear loudspeaker is on a swing arm, allowing the clinician to move the loudspeaker around the patient. The clinician can also place the patient in a swivel chair and turn the patient around in relation to the loudspeaker.

The first step is to do the reverse measurement. Position the loudspeaker behind the patient. Ideally, the clinician will want the loudspeaker at the azimuth of the null of the directional hearing aid, that is, the azimuth at which the input signal is the most suppressed by the hearing aid. This can be at 180 degrees, directly behind the patient (a cardioid pattern), but it can also be at a different azimuth, usually 130 or 230 degrees (a hypercardioid pattern; **Fig. 3–20B**).

Set the hearing aid analyzer to perform an "unaided" measurement, but place the probe tube and the hearing aid in the ear. Use a modulated signal with ANSI speech weighting with an amplitude of 40 or 50 dB SPL, if possible, so as

is providing a directional advantage and to obtain a good estimation of the quality of this advantage.

To determine the directional advantage of the hearing aid, the clinician must perform at least two measurements: a

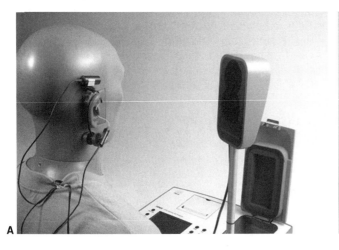
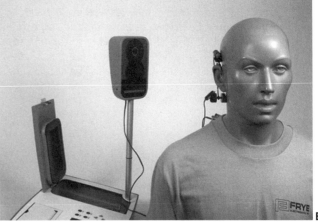

Figure 3–20 **(A)** Setup for the forward measurement of a real ear test of directionality. The manikin is facing the loudspeaker at a 0 degree azimuth. **(B)** Setup for the reverse measurement, with the speaker at a 130 degree azimuth. (From Frye Electronics Inc., with permission.)

not to activate the compression circuit of the hearing aid. Start the measurement and, while the signal remains on, adjust the azimuth of the loudspeaker until the frequency response of the aid is at its lowest point (i.e., the clinician will see the REUG decrease when the directional microphone is in the null). Once the clinician has determined this azimuth, stop the measurement and save the response curve.

Next, position the loudspeaker in front of the patient or at the angle that produces the greatest amplification. This is usually at 0 degree, directly in front of the patient. Set the hearing aid analyzer up to do an "aided" measurement, leaving the probe tube and the hearing aid in the ear. **Figure 3–20A** illustrates this position. Be sure the signal is programmed to the same type and amplitude used for the reverse measurement. Perform the real ear aided measurement in the usual way.

The real ear analyzer should now be able to provide three curves. First, there is the "unaided" curve of the reverse measurement of the directional test. Next, there is the "aided" curve of the forward measurement of the directional test. Finally, there is the "insertion gain" curve that is the directional advantage of the microphones, or the difference between the reverse and forward measurements. In **Fig. 3–21,** curve 1 shows the reverse measurement, curve 2 shows the forward measurement, and curve 3 shows the difference between the two, which is the improved gain provided by the directional microphones when noise is presented from the rear. Finally, it is imperative that the distance between the loudspeaker and the microphons remain the same for both measurements.

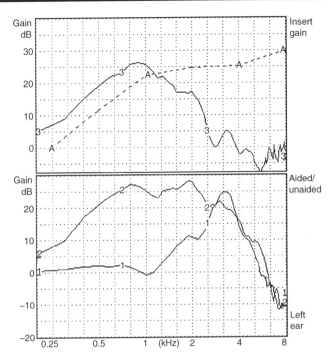

Figure 3–22 Real ear insertion gain (REIG) measurement indicating poor high-frequency amplification. Curve 1 is the real ear unaided gain (REUG), curve 2 is the real ear aided gain (REAG), curve 3 is the real ear insertion gain (REIG), and A is the linear NAL-RP target. The clinician should add at least 10 to 15 dB of gain between 2000 and 6000 Hz and then perform another REIG measurement to verify the change in amplification.

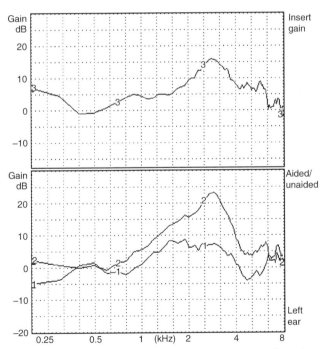

Figure 3–21 Curve 1 shows the reverse measurement of a real ear test of directionality. Curve 2 shows the forward measurement. Both curves were performed using a 50 dB SPL modulated ANSI speech-weighted signal. Curve 3 indicates the directional advantage of the hearing aid (curve 2 – curve 1).

◆ Using Real Ear Measurements to Improve Fittings

REMs are primarily tools that can be used to improve the hearing aid fitting process. However, the clinician needs to know how to use REM effectively, or they will not be able to serve their purpose. This section attempts to explain some basic situations in which REMs may be helpful in troubleshooting problems with hearing aid fittings.

Word Recognition

When a patient says he or she can hear but does not understand the words, REMs can provide insight into the observation. Glaring errors are often observed when REAR curves are compared with target curves. There may be little or no useful amplification in a specific frequency region, the output may be far below or far above the patient's LDLs, or the frequency response may be jagged and irregular across the frequency range.

When the gain in the high frequencies is reduced to avoid feedback, the REM will often show the patient getting little or no useful amplification in the high-frequency region. This is frequently the area most critical to speech recognition. **Figure 3–22** illustrates a typical hearing aid fitting where the REIG (curve 3) is low, in the 2000 to 6000 Hz region,

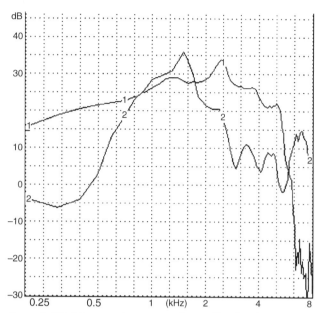

Figure 3–23 A 2 cc coupler response (curve 1) and real ear insertion gain (REIG) response (curve 2) of the same hearing aid. Both measurements were formed with a 65 dB SPL ANSI speech-weighted composite signal. Notice the REIG curve shows little amplification below 750 Hz and above 3000 Hz, although the coupler response shows considerably more gain at those frequencies. This illustrates the importance of examining real ear measures instead of relying on data provided by coupler measures.

when compared with the prescriptive target (i.e., *A*). The REM can provide the initial baseline for reprogramming the hearing aid so that the hearing aid frequency response arrives closer to the prescribed target. In this example, 10 to 15 dB of gain will need to be added to the hearing aid amplification. A repeated REIG should be measured to verify that the reprogramming was successful.

When a hearing aid with a large vent is fitted, much of the low-frequency amplification escapes through the vent. Remember, REMs show the clinician the SPL near the eardrum, and these values often differ greatly from measurement results made using a coupler. Curve 1 in **Fig. 3–23** reports the gain response curve of a hearing aid measured in a test box, and curve 2 shows the insertion gain response of the same hearing aid with the same settings, but measured in the ear. Observe the 19 dB difference in amplification at 500 Hz between the two measurements. An inexperienced clinician might observe the frequency response curve obtained using a coupler measurement and unwisely believe the hearing aid was contributing much more than 20 dB of gain in the low frequencies. Clearly, in this case, the hearing aid is adding little amplification in this region in the ear.

Figure 3–23 also demonstrates the difference in the REM and coupler responses of the hearing aid in the mid- and high-frequency regions. The maximum peak of the coupler response (curve 1) occurs at 2500 Hz and shows 20 to 35 dB of gain between 2000 and 4000 Hz. The maximum peak of the REM (curve 2) occurs at 1500 Hz and shows only 5 to 20 dB of gain at those frequencies. The REM reveals that the

hearing aid is not producing as much amplification as the clinician may believe it to be producing based on the coupler response.

REMs allow the clinician to determine how much amplification the hearing aid is providing in different frequency regions. This, in turn, can help the clinician determine which frequency regions may need more amplification to provide the patient with the brightness and clarity needed to improve speech recognition.

Working with Real Ear Targets

The information obtained by comparing the measured REIG to the REIG prescriptive target is invaluable. However, this tool requires experience and clinical judgment. The second author (RM) suggests the clinician use REIG targets as a "guide" to program the hearing aids so that the measured REIG is reasonably close to the prescribed target (5–10 dB).

Errors in poor fittings can be substantial, with 10 to 30 dB deviations between the measured and targeted REIG. When the clinician modifies the amplification to better match the target, other problems are often created, such as feedback or excessive amplification, that may be uncomfortable for the patient. If the measured and targeted REIG comparison indicates the fitting is markedly weak in a specific frequency region, the authors suggest the clinician increase gain in the frequency region where more gain is needed, then remeasure the REIG to determine if it arrives closer to the target. At this point, it may be necessary to reevaluate the patient's word recognition and comfort levels, before spending more time trying to match the target. The concept is to use the measured REIG to target comparison as a guide that helps the clinician move the fitting in the correct direction, while constantly watching all other aspects of the fitting (feedback and patient comfort).

When the gain and output for the fitting are appropriately adjusted, it is important to remember that patients who have never experienced hearing aids will need considerable time using amplification before they may be able to accept the fit at the prescriptive target.

It is also important to remember that prescriptive target recommendations may not be appropriate for all patients. Some patients (and some types of hearing loss) may need more amplification than the target prescribes. For example, nonrecruiting hearing loss may require substantially higher levels of amplification than recommended by the target. Conversely, some patients cannot tolerate or accept the amount of amplification recommended by a prescriptive target. Clinicians need to interact with patients to determine whether or not the fitting is providing the patient excessive or inadequate amplification in specific frequency regions.

Typically, however, the measured REIG to target comparison will show the clinician ways to improve the fitting. Excessive amplification in one frequency region may deteriorate the quality of the fitting and result in inadequate amplification in other frequency regions. The fitting illustrated in **Fig. 3–24** reveals excessive amplification in the midfrequency region (1000–1500 Hz) and inadequate amplification in the lower (250–750 Hz) and higher (3000–8000 Hz) frequency

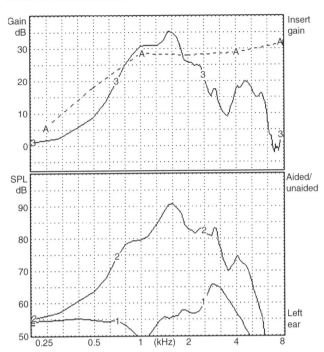

Figure 3–24 Real ear measures reporting less than prescribed amplification in the low and high frequencies and excess amplification in the midfrequencies. Curve 1 is the real ear unaided response (REUR), and curve 2 is the real ear aided response (REAR). Both measurements were performed with a 65 dB SPL ANSI speech-weighted composite signal. Curve 3 is the real ear insertion gain (REIG), and A is the NAL-RP prescribed target.

regions. Correcting these regions by programming greater gain in the low and high frequencies and less gain in the midfrequencies may markedly improve the hearing aid fitting and help improve the patient's word recognition scores and sound quality judgments.

Troubleshooting the Hearing Aid Fitting

One of the most practical uses of REM is in troubleshooting and fine-tuning the hearing aid when a patient reports problems with amplification in specific listening situations. This may happen after a patient obtains a pair of new hearing aids or after the patient has worn the aids for several years. Consider the patient who was satisfied with the hearing aids when first fitted. Then, after 12 months, the patient returns to the clinic, reporting, "I am just not hearing as well as I did when I first received the aid."

Moisture and debris can take their toll on hearing aids. After 12 months of use, the microphone and receiver in the hearing aid may start to deteriorate, causing distortion and loss of fidelity. The patient's hearing loss or perception of amplification may also change over time, requiring an adjustment to the hearing aid. The authors suggest the following troubleshooting sequence to determine the possible causes of errors with the hearing aid fitting.

1. *Obtain a new audiogram* This will determine if the patient's hearing loss has changed since the last clinic visit.

It may be necessary to adjust the hearing aid amplification to account for any deterioration in the patient's thresholds.

2. *Inspect the patient's ears with a fiberoptic otoscope* If excess cerumen or dry skin is present in the ear canal, it may be affecting the ability of the hearing aid to produce amplification. If necessary, clean the patient's ear canal, and vacuum and dehumidify the hearing aid(s).

3. *Listen to the hearing aid with a listening scope* This step is used by the clinician to judge the quantity and quality of the sound produced by the hearing aid. If the hearing aid has completely ceased to function or is producing a signal with high distortion, using the listening scope may allow the clinician to determine that the hearing aid is in need of repair or replacement.

4. *Measure the use-gain of the hearing aid in the test box* After a hearing aid has been adjusted, it is useful to establish a baseline for the adjustment by measuring it in the text box using a broadband modulated signal at 50, 65, 80, and 90 dB SPL. During the troubleshooting process, this test sequence is repeated to determine if the frequency response of the hearing aid has changed. The clinician can adjust the hearing aid to its previous amplification level, if necessary. Also, if there is a question concerning the clarity or cleanness of the amplification, the clinician can study the frequency response for intermodulation distortion. Intermodulation distortion is visible as "peaks" and "wrinkles" in a frequency response curve measured with a broadband signal. The presence of intermodulation distortion could be an indication the hearing aid needs repair or replacement.

5. *Measure harmonic distortion at 90 dB SPL* If the patient is experiencing problems with the sound quality of the hearing aid in noisy environments, such as that found in a loud restaurant, harmonic distortion should be measured on the hearing aid at loud levels (90 dB SPL). In the ANSI S3.22 standard, harmonic distortion is only measured at 65 and 70 dB SPL. This test is not always sufficient to detect distortion that may occur at levels of higher amplitude. Therefore, this measurement will need to be performed outside the usual ANSI test sequence. If harmonic distortion above 5% is measured with a 90 dB SPL input signal, the clinician should attempt to minimize it by changing how the hearing aid is programmed to compress the signal at loud levels. Some hearing aids may be programmed to "peak clip" loud signals instead of compressing the signal. This may cause harmonic distortion. If changing the compression characteristics of the hearing aid does not lessen its harmonic distortion, the hearing aid may be in need of repair or replacement.

6. *Verify directionality (if applicable)* One or more of the microphones in a directional hearing aid may deteriorate, affecting the directionality feature of the hearing aid. Therefore, it is necessary to verify directionality as part of the troubleshooting procedure. The real ear procedure for testing directionality is described earlier in this chapter. If a problem with the directionality of the hearing aid

is found, the clinician can attempt to reprogram the hearing aid to restore directionality. If that procedure does not improve directionality, one of the microphones of the hearing aid may need replacement.

7. *Perform REMs* REMs should be performed to determine the amplification the hearing aid is providing at soft (50 dB SPL), average (65 dB SPL), and loud (80 dB SPL) levels. The REMs are used to see how much useful amplification the patient is receiving in all frequency regions. Over time, the real ear gain in the higher frequencies may decrease due to deterioration in the microphone and receiver. REMs provide the clinician with an opportunity to reassess the fitting. Sometimes, custom hearing aids need to be recased so additional amplification can be provided without feedback. Other times the vent diameter needs to be increased to make the patient more comfortable with his or her own voice. In these cases, substantial gain and output are lost in the low and midfrequencies, and the fitting may need to be reprogrammed. Patients who have worn the instruments for many months are usually ready for a change, especially if the modification provides improved clarity and word recognition.

Managing Feedback

When an amplifier goes into feedback, the shape of the frequency response curve changes from smooth to peaked. REMs help the clinician manage feedback problems by allowing the feedback to be visualized.

Figure 3–25 illustrates a hearing aid fitting that has excessive feedback. Curve 1 shows the fitting with the hearing aid placed securely in the ear. Notice the smoothness of the frequency response. Curve 2 illustrates the fitting after the patient has moved his or her jaw while chewing gum. Notice the peak in the frequency response at around 2000 Hz. Clearly, this instrument is producing feedback.

Feedback can occur at any point along the frequency range, but most feedback is typically observed in the higher frequencies. REMs like those illustrated in **Fig. 3–12** show the clinician the precise frequency region when the feedback is occurring. Sometimes feedback is seen in a high-frequency region where the patient has little or no useful hearing. In these cases, simply reducing the high-frequency gain helps to control the feedback and not reduce speech recognition. Other times, feedback occurs in a frequency region where the patient has good auditory function, and other approaches to reducing feedback must be found, for example, recasing the instrument, adding a helix lock to the aid, and exchanging this hearing aid style for a style less prone to feedback or one with better feedback management software.

Measuring the Occlusion Effect

When patients receive their first pair of hearing aids, they often say, "My voice sounds 'funny,' different, like I am in a

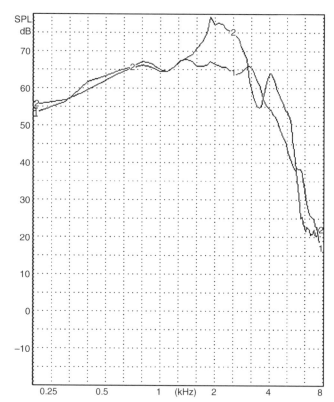

Figure 3–25 Curve 2 illustrates a hearing aid with excessive feedback that occurs when the hearing aid has shifted position in the ear canal when the patient has moved his or her jaw. Curve 1 shows the same hearing aid when placed correctly in the ear.

barrel." This is especially true if the patient has normal or near normal hearing in the lower frequencies and is fitted with occluding hearing aids. This reaction is referred to as the occlusion effect. There are two reasons the patient's own voice may sound unusual. First, the hearing aids or earmolds may be trapping the patient's voice in the ear canal, causing an artificial elevation of the voice level. Second, the hearing aids may be amplifying the patient's voice.

Gailey (2005) reports that this problem can be resolved by answering two questions: (1) Is the patient's voice disturbing because of changes due to amplified sound? and (2) Is it disturbing because of occlusion of the ear from a device introduced into the patient's ear canal? He notes that the effects of the amplification issue may disappear if the hearing aid is left in the ear but turned off. However, if the effect is from occlusion, it will persist if the hearing aid is in the ear, even if the hearing aid is turned off.

Revit (1992) described a method to measure the occlusion effect. The patient is evaluated using REMs, and the real ear analyzer is placed into "spectrum analysis" mode. That is, the real ear analyzer is prepared to measure the frequency response of the hearing aid to an external stimulus (in this case, provided by the patient) instead of responding to one of the test signals. The patient is instructed to vocalize and sustain the vowels *ee* or *uu,* and a measurement is taken. The clinician can improve the accuracy of this measurement by using a signal level meter. Set the signal level meter to 60 dB SPL, and ask the patient to vocalize the sounds while keeping his or her voice at the 0 on the signal level meter.

Next, the hearing aid is inserted into the ear but turned off. The patient is instructed to vocalize the same vowel while another measurement is taken. The difference between these two measurements is the measured occlusion effect. It is usually seen in the low frequencies around 500 Hz. When this measure is above 10 dB, the fitting is often unacceptable to patients.

When the ear is open, the energy created by the patient's voice passes out of the ear canal. When the ear is occluded by a hearing aid, the trapped sound of the patient's voice can produce an additional 10 to 30 dB. The primary effect of the occlusion effect is in the lower frequencies. The occlusion effect may be an irritation to a wide range of patients, but patients with good hearing in the lower frequencies are especially bothered by it.

There are many clinical procedures used to resolve the occlusion effect, but the primary tool used by most clinicians to resolve this problem is venting. The wider the vent, the more low-frequency voice energy escapes from the ear.

REMs are the primary clinical tool used to evaluate the magnitude of the occlusion. Successive measurements can reveal the success or failure of clinician attempts to reduce or eliminate occlusion effects.

◆ Summary

New advancements in hearing aid technology are being made with increasing frequency as hearing aid manufacturers are growing closer to the ultimate goal of restoring audibility for the hearing impaired. Hearing health-care professionals have more tools today than they ever did in the past to help them add brightness and clarity to the hearing aid fitting. These advances include noise suppression, speech enhancement, feedback suppression, and complex directionality. Indeed, it is tempting for the clinician to allow the computer to control the fitting and trust that the adjustments being made are the best ones for the patient. However, as hearing aid technology advances, REMs become even more critical as a tool to ensure that all of these new features on the hearing aid are working properly. They are also used to ensure that the hearing aid fitting is appropriate for the patient. Finally, REMs can establish a baseline that can be used in future visits to determine if and how the frequency response of the hearing aid has changed.

Acknowledgments Much of the funding, test equipment, and graphical support used in the creation of this chapter were provided by Frye Electronics Inc. of Tigard, Oregon. Special thanks to Alan Rose for assistance with many of the graphics and to Larry Revit, who wrote the chapter in the first edition upon which much of this chapter was based.

References

American National Standards Institute. (1992). Testing hearing aids with a broad-band noise signal (ANSI S3.42). New York: Acoustical Society of America.

American National Standards Institute. (1997). Methods of measurement of real-ear performance characteristics of hearing aids (ANSI S3.46). New York: Acoustical Society of America.

American National Standards Institute. (2003). Specification of hearing aid characteristics (ANSI S3.22). New York: Acoustical Society of America.

Ching, T. Y., Britton, L., Dillon, H., & Agung, K. (2002). RECD, REAG, NAL-NL1: Accurate and practical methods for fitting non-linear hearing aids to infants and children. Hearing Review. 9(8), 12–20.

Ching, T. Y. C., Dillon, H., Katsch, R., & Byrne, D. (2001). Maximizing effective audibility in hearing aid fitting. Ear and Hearing, 22(3), 212–224.

Dirks, D. D., & Kincaid, G. (1987). Basic acoustic considerations of ear canal probe measurements. Ear and Hearing, 8(Suppl 5), 60S–67S.

Gailey, C. (2005). Amplification issues with the patient's own voice. Mount Pleasant: Central Michigan University.

International Collegium of Rehabilitative Audiology. (1997, February). ICRA noise signals version 0.3 (CD). International Collegium of Rehabilitative Audiology, Hearing Aid Clinical Test Envirionment Standardization Work Group.

Martin, R. (2005). Introduction to real ear measurements and totally open hearing aid fittings. Westport, CT: Vivatone Hearing Instruments.

Moodie, K. S., Seewald, R. C., & Sinclair, S. T. (1994). Procedure for predicting real-ear hearing aid performance in young children. American Journal of Audiology, 3, 23–31.

Munro, K. J., & Toal, S. (2005). Measuring the real-ear to coupler difference transfer function with an insert earphone and a hearing instrument: Are they the same? Ear and Hearing, 26(1), 27–34.

Nielsen, H. B., & Rasmussen, S. B. (1984). New aspects in hearing aid fittings. Hearing Instruments, 35(1), 18–20.

Revit, L. (1992). Two techniques for dealing with the occlusion effect. Hearing Instruments, 43(12), 16–18.

Revit, L. (2002). Real-ear measures. In M. Valente (Ed.), Strategies for selecting and verifying hearing aid fittings (pp. 66–124). New York: Thieme Medical Publishers.

Seewald, R. (1992). The desired sensation level method for fitting children: Version 3.0. Hearing Journal, 45(4), 26–41.

Valente, M., Potts, L. G., Valente, M., Vaas, W., & Goebel, J. (1994). Intersubject variability of real-ear sound pressure level: Conventional and insert earphones. Journal of the American Academy of Audiology, 5(6), 390–398.

Chapter 4

Hearing Instrument Selection and Fitting in Children

Dawna E. Lewis and Leisha R. Eiten

As the title suggests, this chapter will focus on the selection and fitting of amplification in children. One might wonder why this topic is presented in a separate chapter, given that other chapters in this volume also address amplification. Although it has been said before, it bears repeating that children are not miniature adults. Several factors distinguish children from adults, including physical size, speech and language levels, cognition, and listening environments. These factors must be addressed in the selection and fitting process. The process begins with the selection of appropriate instrument and signal-processing options for the child. Once these options have been determined, the next step is to select gain and output targets for the hearing instrument. Prescriptive methods that are appropriate for infants and young children are necessary to develop targets. Once it has been determined that the hearing instruments meet prescribed targets, verification of performance is completed. The next step in the process is the validation of auditory function. Any discussion of hearing instruments for the pediatric population would be incomplete without addressing the practical issues involved in use of amplification. Because hearing instruments alone do not provide access to acoustic information in all environments, assistive technology should also be considered. This chapter will address each of these issues in the selection and fitting of amplification for children.

When discussing the selection and fitting of hearing instruments for children, it is important to remember that amplification is just one aspect of the total (re)habilitation program. A review of hearing loss identification issues and how they relate to the amplification process will help set the stage.

♦ Identification of Hearing Loss

Evidence suggests that children whose hearing loss was identified before 6 months of age had significantly better language development than those whose hearing loss was identified after 6 months of age (Yoshinaga-Itano et al, 1998). In addition, Moeller (2000) found that children with hearing loss who were identified before 11 months of age exhibited stronger vocabularies and verbal reasoning skills at 5 years of age than children who were identified later. In a review article, Ruben (1997) reported on numerous studies indicating that the critical period for development of phonology is up to 12 months of age. These studies confirm the importance of early identification and remediation of hearing loss.

Given the accepted importance of early identification of hearing loss, what are the statistics regarding newborn hearing screening and follow-up? **Figure 4–1,** from the National Center for Hearing Assessment and Management (2006),

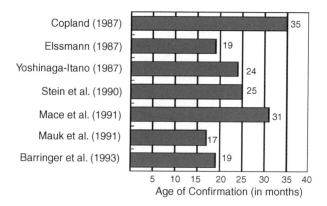

Figure 4–1 Age of confirmation of hearing loss in the United States, 1987–1993. (From infanthearing.org, with permission.)

reports that the average age of confirmation of hearing loss in the United States from 1987 to 1993 ranged from 17 to 35 months. As these findings indicate, the recommendation that all infants with hearing loss be identified and intervention begun by 6 months of age (Joint Commission on Infant Hearing, 2000) was not being met. Harrison et al (2003) studied the age of identification and age of hearing instrument fitting for children who had received Universal Newborn Hearing Screening (UNHS) and contrasted that with children who had not received screening. They reported a significant trend of earlier identification and fitting of amplification in children who received UNHS. Children with mild to moderate hearing loss who had received UNHS were identified between 4 and 10 months and received hearing instruments by 6 to 12 months. In contrast, in children who had not received UNHS, the age of identification was 25 to 32 months, and age of hearing instrument fitting was 30 to 33 months.

With the advent of newborn hearing screening, recommended ages for identification of hearing loss as well as habilitation have declined (American Academy of Pediatrics, 1999). Across the United States, Early Hearing Detection and Intervention (EHDI) programs recommend that hearing be screened before 1 month of age. For infants who fail initial hearing screening, diagnostic audiologic evaluation is recommended before 3 months of age. The reader is referred to Chapter 23 in *Audiology: Diagnosis* for further information on neonatal screening and diagnostic test protocols. Infants who are identified with hearing loss should be enrolled in early intervention services by 6 months of age. As of March 2005, at least 85% of babies born in 47 states and the District of Columbia were screened for hearing loss at birth (National Center for Hearing Assessment and Management [NCHAM], 2007). Of the remaining three states, none had a screening rate below 75%.

As the age of identification of hearing loss is lowered, audiologists encounter new challenges when selecting and fitting amplification. The amount of audiologic information available varies depending on the age or developmental level of the child. For infants from birth to approximately 6 months of age, the audiologist will be relying primarily on auditory

brainstem response (ABR), auditory steady-state response (ASSR), otoacoustic emission, and immittance test results. After a developmental age of approximately 6 months, behavioral tests can be performed. However, depending on factors such as age, developmental status, attention, and/or middle ear dysfunction, behavioral results can vary from one test session to another. As a result, numerous visits may be required to obtain complete audiologic information.

Formal tests of speech recognition generally are limited for children younger than 3 years of age. Boothroyd (2005) presents information on a series of tests being investigated for infants and children beginning as young as 9 months of age. For further information on methods of assessing hearing in infants and young children, including speech perception, the reader is referred to Chapters 15, 16, and 23 in *Audiology: Diagnosis.*

Once hearing loss has been identified and confirmed, the next step is to determine whether amplification should be worn. According to the Pediatric Working Group (1996), "thresholds equal to or poorer than 25 dB HL would indicate candidacy for amplification in some form. For children with unilateral hearing loss, rising or high-frequency hearing loss above 2000 Hz, and/or milder degrees of hearing loss (< 25 dB HL), need should be based on the audiogram plus additional information including cognitive function, the existence of other disabilities, and the child's performance within the home and classroom environment" (p. 54). Similar recommendations were made by the American Academy of Audiology (2004), which also expanded the recommendations for use of amplification to include some children with normal hearing sensitivity. For these children (e.g., those with auditory processing disorders), the goal often is simply to maintain the level of a speaker's voice at an optimal signal-to-noise ratio (SNR) relative to background noise.

Controversial Point

• Many questions remain about the use of amplification for infants and children identified with auditory neuropathy or auditory dys-synchrony. No single solution has been found because the individuals who have been identified represent a heterogeneous group. Decisions about the use of amplification should be made on an individual basis with input from a team of individuals, including, but not limited to, the child's family, audiologist, speech-language pathologist, and educational and medical personnel.

◆ Selection of Amplification Systems

Differences between Children and Adults

When selecting any amplification system, it is necessary to define specific goals and then develop a strategy for achieving those goals. For most degrees of hearing loss, with the possible exception of profound loss, the goal of amplification is to make speech audible, comfortable, and intelligible without allowing sounds to be uncomfortably loud. As stated previously, children are different from adults in many ways. These differences must be considered in the process of achieving amplification goals. Research has shown that infants and young children have poorer thresholds for the detection of speech and tonal stimuli in the presence of background noise than adults. For example, Allen and Wightman (1994) measured the ability of 3- to 5-year-olds to detect tones in the presence of noise. Results indicated that, on average, children's thresholds were 13 dB higher than adults, and the slopes of the psychometric functions were shallower. Individual differences across children were large. The authors suggested that the differences in threshold and slope may be related to listening strategies and/or control of selective attention. In a study of infants' speech-sound discrimination in noise, Nozza et al (1990) reported that infants required a greater SNR than adults ($\sim$6 dB) for comparable levels of performance.

Another important difference between children and adults is that children are learning speech and language. Children do not have the same knowledge base that adults have when attempting to make sense of auditory signals that may be distorted, incomplete, or affected by noise. In a study of perception with high and low predictability sentences in noise, Elliott (1979) concluded that lack of knowledge about language rules may have affected the performance of the youngest group tested (9-year-olds). In a study on the effects of context on speech perception in noise, Nittrouer and Boothroyd (1990) reported that young children were unable to use semantic information as effectively as adults.

Using spectrally reduced speech, Eisenberg et al (2000) evaluated speech recognition for children (younger: 5–7 years; older: 10–12 years) and adults. Stimuli included words, sentences, and phonemes. Results revealed that younger children required greater spectral resolution to perform at the same level as older children and adults on speech recognition tasks. In addition, results indicated that younger children were less able to use context to recognize words in sentences. The authors concluded that younger children's immature speech pattern recognition as well as more limited linguistic and cognitive skills played a role in the results.

Johnson (2000) investigated the effects of reverberation and noise on listeners' (ages 6–7, 10–11, 14–15 years, and adults) abilities to identify vowels and consonants in nonsense words presented at a variety of sensation levels. Results indicated that children's maximum performance varied by listening condition and age, with some conditions not achieving adultlike performance until the late teenage years. For example, identification of vowels reached adult levels by 10 years of age in all conditions, whereas consonant identification scores in noise plus reverberation remained significantly lower than adults even for the oldest group of children. Thus, children's abilities to perceive speech in noise and reverberation appears to develop over a wide age span.

In addition to linguistic and processing differences, there are physical and practical limitations encountered when working with children. The fact that children are physically smaller than adults must be taken into account when selecting amplification. The small size of infants' and children's ear canals means that the sound pressure level (SPL) delivered to their ears will be greater than that measured in adult ears. The real ear-to-coupler difference (RECD) is defined as the difference, in decibels, between the SPL measured in a real ear versus a 2 cc coupler. Feigin et al (1989) measured RECDs in children (ages 4 weeks–5 years) and adults. Results indicated that children's mean RECD values were higher than adults' across all frequencies except 250 Hz. The RECD values decreased with increasing age, and the authors predicted that values would fall within one standard deviation of the adult mean by $\sim$7.7 years of age. Westwood and Bamford (1995) measured RECDs in infants younger than 12 months of age. Their findings also revealed higher RECD values than adults'. In both studies, high intersubject variability was reported. To provide detailed normative RECD data, Bagatto et al (2002) collected RECDs from 392 infants and children from 1 month to 16 years of age using personal earmolds and acoustic immittance tips. The results allowed examination of RECD values in 1-month intervals. As with the earlier studies, intersubject variability was large, reaching as much as 15 dB at 500 Hz for subjects younger than 6 months of age who were tested with personal earmolds.

The external ear canal resonance peak also has been shown to vary as a function of age in children. Kruger and Ruben (1987) measured the average external ear canal resonance (also referred to as the real ear unaided response [REUR] or real ear unaided gain [REUG]) in infants from birth to 37 months of age. Results indicated that the peak resonance frequency decreased as a function of age, approaching adultlike values by the second year of life. Bentler (1989) measured REUR for children ages 3 to 13. Although results were similar to previously reported data for adults, a large degree of intersubject variability was present. Thus, it was recommended that individual values be used whenever possible. Westwood and Bamford (1995) measured REUR over an 18-month period for infants from $\leq$ 3 to 21 months of age. Their results also indicated the mean peak resonance frequency decreased during the first year of life.

Another difference between children and adults is the amount of audiologic and medical information that is available at the time of the hearing instrument fitting. Audiologic information for infants and young children may be limited. Delaying amplification until complete information is available may mean the child is without amplification during critical periods of language development. At the time hearing instruments are being selected for infants and young children, audiologic information might only consist of ABR thresholds for clicks and a few frequency-specific tones. With older infants (older than 6–7 months), behavioral thresholds from either sound field or individual ears may be available at only a few frequencies. In addition, the child's ability to participate in the selection and fitting process may be limited by cognitive and language levels.

Subjective measures of most comfortable level (MCL) and loudness discomfort level (LDL) often are used in adult hearing instrument selection. These measures are not possible with infants and toddlers. Kawell et al (1988) tested children (7–14 years) and adults using a modification of an LDL procedure reported by Hawkins et al (1987). Results suggested that children with hearing loss who were as young as 7 could perform the task. Another LDL procedure was developed by MacPherson et al (1991) using the concept of "too much." After training, children with normal hearing who had mental ages of 5 years were able to perform the task. No techniques for establishing LDL in younger children have been reported.

Children have less control over their listening environments than adults. Depending on age, the position of the child relative to another speaker may vary considerably. Consequently, the intensity level of speech reaching the child's ear also will vary. Stelmachowicz et al (1993) evaluated the effects of distance and postural position on the long- and short-term characteristics of speech produced by parents of children ages 2 months to 2 years. Results indicated that the overall level of the long-term average speech spectrum (LTASS) varied with position and was 10 to 18 dB higher in close conditions (cradle position, hip position) when compared with the reference condition (1 m). In addition, the spectral shape of the LTASS was affected by position. As the child gets older and the distance between the person speaking and the listener increases (e.g., on the playground), the expected level reaching the child's ear will be significantly lower. It may not be feasible for the child to change positions to make speech more audible or to adjust the listening environment to enhance visual cues or reduce noise levels.

Children also may not be able to adjust the volume control of their hearing instruments. In noisy or reverberant listening situations, adults may reduce the volume control on hearing instruments. Children, in comparison, may have covers on their volume controls or have the volume controls deactivated, ensuring the settings remain fixed regardless of the listening environment. If the hearing instruments use multiple memories to provide different processing for different listening environments, an adult caretaker usually is responsible for selecting the memory that will be used in a particular setting.

General Hearing Instrument Options

When making choices about hearing instruments for children, an audiologist has important practical and performance decisions to make. The need to make speech audible across a wide range of input levels is the major factor to consider when fitting children. In addition, durability and safety of the hearing instruments should be important considerations in the fitting process.

Hearing Instrument Style

In general, behind-the-ear (BTE) hearing instruments are the style of choice for infants and young children for many reasons, including comfort, safety, fit, and durability (American Academy of Audiology, 2004). Ear size changes dramatically in infants and young children over time. When BTE instruments are used, only the earmolds need replacement as the child grows. In addition, most BTE hearing instruments are compatible with hearing assistance technology (HAT), the importance of which will be discussed later in this chapter. The hearing instruments selected for infants or young children should be small enough to fit comfortably on their ears. This is especially important for infants, whose pinnas may not support the weight of larger, heavier hearing instruments.

Earhooks

Use of pediatric-sized earhooks is especially helpful in positioning hearing instruments comfortably on the ears of young children (**Fig. 4–2**). Often, the change from an adult- to pediatric-sized earhook is all that is needed to help retain a hearing instrument that had been constantly falling from behind a child's ear. Filtered earhooks can be helpful in smoothing the frequency response of a hearing instrument, providing a better fit to gain and output targets across frequencies. **Figure 4–3** illustrates the change in output for a hearing instrument with three earhooks. Reducing the peak in the response using a 1000 Ω filtered earhook (dashed line) would allow an increase in the maximum output setting of the hearing instrument without exceeding targets.

Volume Controls

Volume controls allow caregivers to increase or decrease the gain of the instruments, within a range specified by the

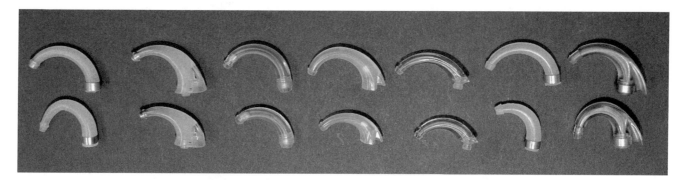

Figure 4–2 Adult (*top row*) and pediatric-sized (*bottom row*) earhooks.

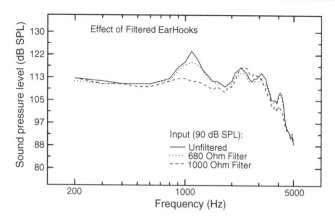

Figure 4–3 Effect of three different earhooks on maximum output of a hearing instrument[Q34].

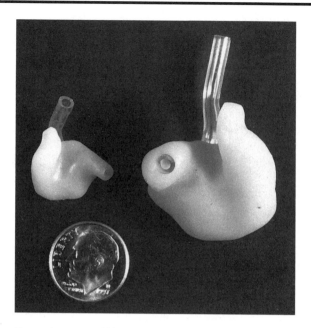

Figure 4–4 Earmold for a 3-month-old infant compared with an earmold for an adult.

audiologist. Current technology provides several choices relative to hearing instrument volume controls. In many hearing instruments, the volume control can be deactivated or set to be adjustable over a predetermined range. In the latter case, if the child reacts negatively to sounds or experiences feedback, caregivers may decrease the volume. If the child does not appear to be responding to sounds as well as expected, the volume could be increased. Limiting the range of available volume reduces inadvertent changes in output that might result in either overamplification or inaudibility, at least until internal controls can be adjusted by the audiologist. If hearing instrument volume controls have been deactivated, manually covered, or locked, caregivers will be unable to make adjustments to the instruments when they may be needed. During periods of rapid growth, feedback may occur when earmolds become loose. If the caregivers cannot adjust the volume to control feedback temporarily, the child may not be able to wear the instrument(s) until new earmolds are obtained.

acoustic modifications such as parallel vents, belled bores, and open molds, which are commonly used in adult hearing instrument fittings, may not be possible with children's molds because of size. In small ears, the only type of venting that may be available is diagonal. The acoustic effect of diagonal venting is a reduction in high-frequency gain, which makes this a poor choice for most children (Leavitt, 1986). Any type of venting will increase the chances of experiencing feedback. The reader is referred to Chapter 2 of this volume for additional information about earmolds and earhooks.

Pearl

• Many earmold manufacturers make earmolds in colors that are particularly attractive to motivate young children to use their hearing instruments consistently. Allowing children to select the color schemes for their earmolds is a relatively low-cost way to give them input into decisions about their amplification. In addition, color choices can be changed as often as new earmolds are made.

Pitfall

• Predicting changes in frequency/gain characteristics of hearing instruments on the basis of potential earmold modifications will often be inaccurate for infants and young children. The small size of their earmolds compared with adult earmolds may preclude modifications such as parallel vents, belled bores, and extended canals.

Tamper-Resistant Battery Doors

For the safety of younger children, it is important that tamper-resistant battery compartments be available for their hearing instruments. The durability of the device also must be considered, given that hearing instruments worn by children may experience greater wear and tear than those worn by adults. Extended loss and damage warranties

Earmolds

Earmolds made of soft material will enhance comfort, retention, and safety. Because children are still growing, their earmolds may need to be replaced more often than adults' earmolds to ensure a good fit (**Fig. 4–4**). In addition,

Table 4–1 Reasons to Wear Binaural Hearing Aids

1. Better understanding of speech
2. Better understanding in groups and noise
3. Better directionality
4. Better sound quality
5. Smoother tone quality
6. Binaural loudness summation
7. Better sound identification
8. Prevention of sensory deprivation
9. Improved ease of listening
10. Balanced hearing
11. Greater comfort when loud noises occur
12. Reduced feedback and whistling
13. Tinnitus masking
14. Consumer preference
15. Consumer satisfaction

Source: Adapted from Kochkin, S. (2000). Binaural hearing aids: The fitting of choice for bilateral loss subjects. Retrieved July 30, 2007, from http://www.betterhearing.org/research/ with permission.

should be recommended, as well as insurance coverage once the manufacturer's warranty expires.

Monaural versus Binaural

Kochkin (2000) summarized results of research studies and consumer surveys/questionnaires supporting the advantage of binaural hearing and use of binaural hearing instruments. He concluded with 15 reasons why individuals with hearing loss should wear two hearing instruments **(Table 4–1)**. Hawkins and Yacullo (1984) reported a significant SNR advantage for binaural over monaural hearing instruments when they evaluated speech recognition in noise and reverberation. Research also has suggested that children using monaural amplification may experience a reduction in speech perception in the unaided ear (Gelfand and Silman, 1993). In addition, studies of children with unilateral hearing loss indicate poorer performance in noise and reverberation and a higher risk of academic and psychosocial difficulties (Bess et al, 1998). Because monaural hearing instruments result in a unilateral listener (not to mention that the one ear is impaired), similar problems could be experienced. Binaural hearing instruments are recommended for children unless it can be demonstrated that a particular child performs more poorly with two hearing instruments than with one.

Circuitry and Signal-Processing Options

Given that limited audiologic information may be available at the time of the fitting, hearing instruments having flexible electroacoustic characteristics and compatibility with a variety of earhooks are essential. As with adults, it is important that the amplified signal children receive be clear and undistorted across a variety of listening environments. As stated previously, children may have more difficulty

detecting and understanding auditory signals in the presence of noise than adults. In addition, they cannot use linguistic cues and world knowledge in the same ways as adults to fill in missing information in a message. Flexibility in the adjustment of gain, output, and frequency response of hearing instruments allows audiologists to fine-tune the devices as more information becomes available about the degree and configuration of the child's hearing loss and his or her auditory responsiveness. Advances in hearing instrument technology and signal processing have greatly improved the flexibility of hearing instruments. (See Chapter 1 for additional information regarding signal processing.) A variety of options may be appropriate, including compression circuits, multimemory systems, directional microphones, and frequency modulation (FM) systems.

Several practical issues must be addressed when selecting amplification for a child with hearing loss. Because children are learning speech and language, it is especially important they receive auditory signals that are audible, clear, and not uncomfortably loud. When making circuitry and signal-processing decisions, it may be helpful to refine the amplification goals, making them more specific to the individual child and his or her particular listening environments. Examples of possible goals include the following:

- Make speech audible across a wide range of input levels
- Ensure that speech is undistorted for high-level inputs and acoustic conditions
- Increase speech recognition in background noise
- Accommodate a progressive or fluctuating hearing loss
- Amplify an unusual audiometric configuration

Advances in signal processing have resulted in a wide variety of options. Studies investigating advanced signal-processing options with children are limited. A list of readings and references on advanced signal processing with children is included in Appendix 4–1.

Bandwidth

Results of research examining the benefit of high-frequency amplification in adults have been equivocal. Several studies have suggested that some adults with moderate to severe sensorineural hearing loss may not benefit from, and may actually be negatively affected by, high-frequency amplification (Ching et al, 1998). In contrast, Simpson et al (2005) have demonstrated continued improvement in speech understanding as bandwidth is increased. For children who are still developing speech and language, audibility of high-frequency components of speech may be more important. Stelmachowicz and colleagues have demonstrated that bandwidth may have an impact on perception and production of fricatives as well as development of morphological rules for young children. For example, Stelmachowicz et al (2002) examined fricative perception in normal-hearing (NH) and hearing-impaired (HI) children and adults at several low-pass cutoff frequencies from 2000 to 9000 Hz. Results revealed that children performed more poorly than adults, and HI subjects performed more poorly than NH subjects across bandwidths. In addition, a significant speaker effect was noted for the phoneme /s/ in that the bandwidth for optimal performance for a male speaker was much lower (4000–5000 Hz) than for a female speaker (9000 Hz). These findings have implications for hearing instrument fitting in young children. Although the bandwidth of current hearing instruments (4000–5000 Hz) may be adequate for adults and older children, wider bandwidths may be needed for infants and younger children who are still developing speech and language. Further research in this area is needed.

Multiple Memories

Multimemory hearing instruments allow the use of different signal-processing strategies that can be programmed for different listening environments and selected from the memories available in the instrument (see Chapter 1). Some multimemory hearing instruments use a remote control device to access the various memories, whereas others use switches or push buttons on the hearing instruments. From a practical standpoint, if a caregiver (not the child) will be selecting the memories for various situations, then a device that uses a remote control may be easier to use than a memory toggle on the hearing instrument itself. Those in control of selecting the appropriate memory must understand how and when this should be done.

Deciding which memories to program into the hearing instrument and when to use a particular memory raises other issues. It has been suggested that, for very young children, available memories be programmed on the basis of the expected speech input levels to the hearing instrument. Thus, one memory might be programmed on the basis of high input levels when an infant or young child is close to caregivers and a second memory on the basis of low input levels when the child is farther away from the speaker. Another possibility is to program the first memory with certain frequency/gain characteristics and vary the relative gain in subsequent memories (e.g., a second memory could be set with more gain and a third with less gain than the first). Caretakers would observe the child's responses using the different memories in similar listening situations. Fine-tuning the hearing instruments would be done on the basis of those observations. Once a desired response is achieved in the first memory, other memories could be set for particular situations, such as in the car, at a playground, or while watching television.

No studies have been designed to evaluate the ages at which children can independently use multimemory devices. Studies evaluating different sound-processing strategies in older children and adolescents have commented that children were able to change memories and preferred having the ability to adjust hearing instrument processing for different environments (Christensen, 1999). Further studies are needed in this area to determine when and how multiple memory devices should be used.

Controversial Point

- An important concern when considering multimemory hearing instruments is whether routinely changing the way the hearing instruments operate will be beneficial or detrimental to a child who is learning language. It is possible to argue this point both ways. If selecting different memories makes it easier for the child to hear and understand speech in a greater variety of listening situations, theoretically, at least, multiple memories should provide benefit. On the other hand, if dramatically different signal processing is used in each memory, acquisition of speech and language could potentially be affected. To date, no tools to determine the efficacy of multiple memories in children are available. Systematic methods of gathering efficacy information, which are sensitive to the possible effects of processing, need to be developed.

Directional Microphones

Single-microphone directional technology has been available for many years. More recently, directional microphones using dual- and even triple-microphone technology have become available. Because hearing instruments in the directional mode of operation attenuate sounds from the sides and rear (i.e., off-axis), a person speaking directly in front of the listener should be easier to hear. The amount of attenuation provided for off-axis sounds when using a directional microphone can vary across devices and listening situations. There are several issues related to this technology that should be considered when fitting amplification for infants and young children.

Currently, directional technology may allow users to switch from omnidirectional mode to various levels and patterns of directionality. In addition, the hearing instrument can be set to require manual switching between omnidirectional and directional modes, or to automatically activate the directional microphone when the hearing instrument detects particular levels/types of noise. For young children who do not understand the rules of communication, directional microphones may hinder interactions that do not take place when the speaker and listener are facing one another. In addition, hearing instruments operating in the directional mode may reduce the amount of overhearing a child experiences, hindering learning that takes place incidentally. As such, a directional microphone may not be appropriate for use with infants and young children. If hearing instruments with directional microphones are chosen, it is important they be switchable from directional to omnidirectional operation depending on communication needs. Being able to alter the directionality also is important for those instances when, for safety, it is necessary that the user hear sounds from all directions. For infants and young children, adult caregivers will be responsible for determining when the hearing instruments will be used in directional versus omnidirectional mode. Thus, it is important they understand how and when to select the appropriate mode for a given situation. It also is important the person in charge of the device remember to change modes as the environment changes, such as when a child goes from a single talker situation in the home to a game of soccer on the playground.

As children reach school age, there may be more situations when it would be useful for them to be able to switch their hearing instruments to the directional mode. Ricketts and Tharpe (2005) suggest that directional microphones may be useful in some multitalker environments such as lunch, the bus, or the playground. To investigate the benefit of directional microphones in the classroom, Ricketts and Tharpe examined head angle in classroom environments for 20 NH and HI children from 5 to 12 years of age. Results revealed that, on average, NH and HI children across the age range tested were able to accurately orient their heads toward a speaker of interest. However, there were considerable individual differences. The authors hypothesized these differences might be related to the listening task. For example, they reported students who are taking notes may be focusing down and away from the speaker. They also reported on younger children who, during story time, sat on the floor with their heads tilted back and their eye gaze lowered toward the teacher. In this latter case, directional microphones would be pointed up toward the ceiling rather than directly at the person speaking. In addition, in any classroom where the listening situation changes from one main talker (e.g., a lecture) to talkers speaking from a variety of locations (e.g., a classroom discussion), it is important the listener be able to change from a directional to omnidirectional mode of operation. These examples remind us of the importance of understanding the listening environment as well as the listener when recommending use of directional microphones.

Although the research examining children's benefit from directional microphones is limited, there are some studies suggesting improvement in degraded listening environments. Gravel et al (1999) reported that a group of HI children from 4 to 11 years of age, on average, received an additional 4.7 dB SNR advantage when using hearing instruments with directional versus omnidirectional microphones. Large individual differences were noted. Results also revealed that younger children required a more favorable SNR than older children for the same level of performance and that these differences were related to receptive vocabulary skills. In addition, large individual differences across subjects highlight the importance of examining benefit on an individual basis.

Special Consideration

- Directional microphones should be used with caution for children with visual impairments who need to be aware of sounds from all locations within their environments.

Noise Reduction

In addition to directional microphones, many hearing instruments include noise reduction signal processing. Several studies with adults have demonstrated improved comfort and/or ease of listening but have failed to show improved word recognition in noise (e.g., Boymans and Dreschler, 2000). No studies of the efficacy of single-microphone noise reduction have been conducted with children. Because this circuitry can reduce gain, and thus audibility, of speech and important environmental sounds, it may be detrimental for infants and young children who are learning speech and language. The ability to deactivate noise reduction signal processing is an important consideration when selecting hearing instruments for young children.

Compression Circuits

Even a cursory examination of current hearing instrument technology would reveal that wide dynamic range compression (WDRC) circuits are employed more often than linear circuits. In general, WDRC circuits apply more gain to less intense signals than to more intense signals (**Fig. 4–5**). As such, these circuits should provide audibility over a wider range of input levels than linear processors, allowing the listener to hear speech across a greater range of listening environments. On the negative side, the potential for feedback with WDRC circuits is greater than for linear devices because of the increased gain for low input levels. In single-channel instruments, gain and compression characteristics are the same across all frequencies. In multichannel instruments, gain and compression characteristics can be adjusted independently across channels, providing greater fitting flexibility.

For children whose ears are smaller and are still growing, feedback may be more of a concern than it would be for adults. It is important that caregivers understand the importance of replacing earmolds when feedback occurs rather than simply adjusting the volume control to reduce gain of the hearing instrument. If hearing instrument gain is consistently reduced because of feedback, the amplification

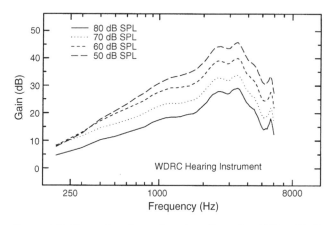

Figure 4–5 Change in gain as a function of input level (50 to 80 dB SPL) for a wide dynamic range compression (WDRC) hearing instrument. SPL, sound pressure level.

the child receives may be inadequate. Currently, the issue of feedback with WDRC instruments often is addressed by increasing the compression threshold or through the use of feedback reduction circuits (see below).

Research had suggested that compression-limiting circuits may not provide enough gain and output to make speech cues and environmental sounds audible for some children with severe to profound hearing loss. Boothroyd et al (1988) used a master hearing instrument with and without amplitude compression to evaluate speech pattern perception for 9 children (ages 11–16 years) with severe to profound hearing loss. All but one child showed small but significant decreases in performance with compression. The authors suggested that changes in time/intensity cues may have caused the decrement. Dawson et al (1990) measured maximum output for pure-tone (90 dB SPL) and speech (86.5 equivalent continuous level [Leq]) signals through hearing instruments using peak clipping and compression limiting. Although output SPL with a 90 dB SPL input signal (OSPL90), measured using pure-tone signals, differed by only 3 to 5 dB, output for speech stimuli differed by 6 to 9 dB, with the compression instruments demonstrating lower output levels. As Dawson et al (1990) reported,

> undoubtedly this is because such signals have a high crest factor (ratio of instantaneous peak level to Leq), and if the low distortion possible with compression limiting is to be obtained, the instruments must be designed so that clipping of the peaks does not occur to a significant degree. This implies that the (compression limiting) instrument will have a lower long term equivalent output level than would a similar instrument employing peak clipping. (p. 4)

Such differences in output may render all or parts of the speech signal inaudible for some individuals with severe to profound hearing loss when using compression-limiting hearing instruments.

More recently, Marriage and Moore (2003) examined speech recognition for 15 children with severe to profound hearing loss wearing bilateral high-power hearing instruments incorporating peak-clipping, compression-limiting, or WDRC circuits. The children wore each circuit for at least 1 week prior to testing. Improvements with the WDRC circuit were found only for one task (closed set monosyllabic words). On all other tasks, no statistically significant differences were seen among the three circuits. Thus, unlike the results of Boothroyd et al (1988), listeners with severe to profound hearing loss were not negatively impacted by compression circuitry. One important difference noted by Marriage and Moore (2003) was that the digital hearing instrument used in their study "may result in less distortion of the envelope shape of speech than the analog compression processing used by Boothroyd et al" (p. 45).

Feedback Reduction

Feedback reduction is an important feature to consider when fitting amplification to infants and young children. As stated previously in this chapter, periods of rapid growth will result in the need for frequent earmold remakes during infancy and early childhood. Families may not return for

remakes as often as needed, and the result may be loose-fitting earmolds and potential feedback problems. Infants and young children also may be more likely to be in close proximity to other objects such as when they are being held or are sitting in infant seats or car seats. Recall that WDRC processing in hearing instruments may result in greater potential for feedback than is the case with linear amplification.

Historically, gain reduction, through internal controls or the volume control, was the primary means of reducing feedback. Although this may temporarily alleviate the annoying "whistling" from hearing instruments, it can have negative consequences for hearing and understanding speech. In single-channel hearing instruments, reducing gain because of feedback from one frequency region reduces gain in all frequency regions. In hearing instruments with multiple channels and those that use notch filters to reduce feedback, the effect of gain reduction is less extensive. However, even narrow-channel gain reduction may have negative consequences for someone who is learning speech and language. Currently, many digital hearing instruments use a phase-shifted signal to eliminate feedback without reducing gain. The ability to nullify feedback without sacrificing gain is a useful feature to consider when fitting infants and young children.

Frequency Compression

A signal-processing strategy that is being used for individuals with limited or unusable high-frequency hearing is frequency compression. This strategy proportionally compresses high-frequency speech information into lower frequency ranges by reducing the bandwidth and frequency of this information. Doing so allows higher frequency information that may not be audible with conventional amplification to be moved into a range with better hearing. Proportional frequency compression attempts to preserve the relationships of the high-frequency energy peaks while leaving low-frequency information uncompressed but amplified. The amount of compression applied varies with the degree and configuration of hearing loss.

Few studies have been conducted examining the effectiveness of this type of processing. Miller-Hansen et al (2003) investigated the use of frequency-compression processing on HI listeners from 1 to 21 years of age. A subgroup of 16 children had previously worn conventional hearing instrument amplification. For this subgroup, word recognition scores improved by a mean of 12.5% with the use of frequency compression. As a processing option, frequency compression should be considered as a means of providing audibility of high-frequency sounds that might otherwise be inaudible.

When signals are degraded by noise, distance, and reverberation, the benefits that can be achieved by even the most advanced hearing instrument technology will have limits. In classrooms where children are learning new information, the effects of noise, distance, and reverberation can be especially detrimental (see Chapter 18). With the RApid Speech Transmission Index (RASTI), Leavitt and Flexer (1991) evaluated the integrity of speechlike signals at different locations in a classroom. Perfect reproduction of the transmitted signal would result in a score of 1.0. Results indicated that this score was achieved only at the location of the reference microphone (6 inches from the loudspeaker). At other distances, scores ranged from 0.83 in the center of the front row to 0.55 in the back row of the class. These findings indicate a decrease in the fidelity of the signal as a function of distance. Thus, even if a hearing instrument were able to perfectly reproduce the signal received at its microphone, distance and interfering noise in the environment would result in an imperfect signal at the listener's ears. Hicks and Tharpe (2002) reported that HI children expended more listening effort than NH children in both easy and difficult classroom listening situations. These results suggest that children with hearing loss are at a disadvantage compared with their NH peers when listening in a classroom environment.

In many listening environments, hearing instruments alone may not be sufficient to overcome the deleterious effects of noise, distance, and reverberation. Thus, hearing instruments should have direct audio input (DAI) and telecoil capabilities that allow hearing instruments to be compatible with other assistive technology, such as FM systems (see Chapter 17).

Pitfall

- Some individuals incorrectly assume that the use of advanced technology precludes the need for additional HAT in difficult listening environments. In reality, a degraded signal, even if perfectly reproduced, is still a degraded signal. For example, digital hearing instruments cannot substitute for FM in a classroom or other high noise environment.

FM Systems

Frequency modulated systems take advantage of microphone placement close to a talker's mouth to overcome the effects of noise, distance, and reverberation. They have long been used in educational settings and are also being integrated into daily home use (Gabbard, 2005). The signal is sent by means of FM radio transmission from a system's transmitter/microphone to a listener's receiver. Ongoing advances in FM technology and design have produced increasingly smaller receivers that are worn at ear level and either fully integrated into the hearing instrument case or easily switched between hearing instruments. Universal receivers can be used with a variety of hearing instruments and even cochlear implant processors as long as the appropriate coupling or processor connection is available. The miniaturization of the receiver means that FM should be considered part of an amplification system that children can use in a variety of listening and communication situations.

Some FM receivers allow the FM level to be adjusted. Thus, the audiologist is able to determine and set the optimal relationship between the FM signal and other signals arriving from the local (hearing instrument) microphone. In addition, FM channel synthesis in some instruments provides a means of changing FM channels on receivers that are in close proximity to a given FM transmitter at the push of a button or by passing close by a wall unit set to the FM channel of choice.

FM systems are also increasingly being recommended for use with very young children (Gabbard, 2005). As infants become mobile, distance and background noise effects may interfere with optimal audibility, even with well-fitted hearing instruments. Many communication situations, both inside and outside the home, may benefit from the remote microphone of an FM system. The small size of FM receivers and audio boots may pose a choking hazard for young children, and care should be taken if the devices are not tamper proof. Small ear-level receivers may not have "Low battery" or "No FM signal" lights, making parental monitoring critical.

Pearl

- As ear-level FM receivers become more popular, loss of FM receivers has become more common. Ear Gear (Lake Country, British Columbia, Canda) makes a neoprene hearing instrument sleeve that is designed to cover a hearing instrument with a universal FM receiver and boot attached. In addition, insurance policies exist to cover loss and damage of these instruments.

Ear-level FM receivers also are available for children diagnosed with auditory processing or attention deficits. These types of receivers have minimal amplification power and no local microphone. Older systems used with this population required a body-worn receiver with headphones or earbuds that were uncomfortable for long-term use and were themselves a source of distraction for some children. The ear-level system is used to provide a consistent, audible transmission of the teacher's voice through the FM microphone to overcome distraction or interference from background noise and reverberation in a typical classroom environment. In some cases, this FM-only receiver may also be used for children with temporary or fluctuating hearing related to chronic middle ear effusion.

Body-style FM systems are still available in some classroom settings but are not often used outside of educational settings. Such systems may operate in conjunction with a student's personal hearing instruments via DAI or neckloop coupling, or may operate independently from hearing instruments via button or ear-level receivers.

If an FM system is coupled to a child's personal hearing instrument, it is important to ensure that the instrument allows appropriate coupling and that electroacoustic characteristics are maintained. It also is important to ensure that the FM signal is audible, comfortable, and safe, requiring electroacoustic verification in all modes of operation.

- In a longitudinal study of FM use in nonacademic settings, Moeller et al (1996) reported that, despite training, FM systems often were used inappropriately. Some parents used the FM system as an intercom or pager to introduce behavioral control beyond a typical listening range. Some families reported this to be a positive aspect of home FM use, as children reported increased feelings of security, especially in public settings. Another misuse was when the FM transmitter was used in situations where there was not a primary talker, such as group situations with multiple talkers. The authors concluded that extensive training regarding proper FM system use and ongoing monitoring by an audiologist would be important to the success of an FM fitting.

When selecting any amplification system, especially for children, the cost/benefit ratio of the technological choices must be considered. The same amount of money could purchase hearing instruments with the most sophisticated and expensive technology or could purchase two basic instruments with fewer processing choices and an FM system. It is the responsibility of the audiologist to choose devices that will best meet the auditory needs of the child. If expensive hearing instrument technology is chosen, that expense should be justified by improved ability to meet the amplification goals for that child. As discussed previously, even the most sophisticated hearing instrument processing may not overcome problems with distance, background noise, and reverberation in the same way that an FM system can. A critical need still exists for current efficacy studies of advanced technology with children.

♦ Selecting Amplification Targets

The research as well as practical and technological considerations discussed above must be considered for every hearing instrument fitting. The audiologist then specifies the gain and output characteristics for an individual child's hearing loss. When selecting a prescriptive method for use with young children, it is important to choose one that requires only threshold information, because many children initially will be limited in their ability to perform additional measures, such as speech recognition, MCL, or LDL. Although many prescriptive methods have been developed (e.g., Byrne et al, 2001; Libby, 1986), only a few have been developed specifically for use with children (Seewald et al, 2005).

The Desired Sensation Level Approach

Desired sensation level (DSL) is a computer-based formula approach developed by Seewald and colleagues (Neuman, 2005). The DSL procedure was originally designed for children,

although the most recent versions also can be used for adults. This approach is based on a habilitative amplification philosophy, that is, a assumption that children will learn to use the audibility that is provided to them. DSL targets are based on several assumptions regarding fitting amplification to children:

1. Children typically wear hearing instruments at fixed settings.

2. Amplification characteristics that are selected are important in speech and language acquisition.

3. Limited audiometric data may be available at the time of hearing instrument selection.

4. Several factors important for hearing instrument selection will vary with age.

The DSL program allows the clinician to enter thresholds that have been obtained using a range of signal transducers (e.g., TDH earphones, insert earphones, loudspeakers) and appropriate average transforms are used to convert all information to dB SPL in the ear canal. The individual child's RECD and REUR can be measured, or the program will use age-appropriate average transforms. With the data that are entered and appropriate transforms, the program provides targets for various real ear and coupler measures. Corrections are made for hearing instrument microphone location (i.e., BTE, in-the-ear [ITE], in-the-canal [ITC], and completely-in-the-canal [CIC]), and numerous options for verification are provided. The most recent version of the DSL program, DSL v5.0 $m[i/o]$, provides an algorithm for fitting multichannel WDRC hearing instruments in addition to linear circuitry. For further details regarding the history and current implementation of the DSL prescriptive approach, the reader is referred to a series of articles by the group from the University of Western Ontario (Bagatto et al, 2005; Scollie et al, 2005; Seewald et al, 2005). **Figure 4–6** is a graphic display—Verifit by Audioscan (Dorchester, Ontario)—of target values from DSL [i/o] for a child with a mild to moderate hearing loss. The open circles represent the child's hearing thresholds converted to dB SPL in the ear canal. The plus signs (+) represent targets for the amplified long-term average speech spectrum (70 dB SPL), and the asterisks (*) represent targets for maximum output (90 dB SPL).

NAL-NL1

NAL-NL1 (National Acoustic Laboratories' nonlinear fitting procedure, version 1) is a prescriptive approach for fitting nonlinear amplification that was developed at the National Acoustics Laboratory (Byrne et al, 2001). Current versions of NAL-NL1 use appropriate acoustic corrections for children, including measured RECD and/or age- related averages. Targets for gain are based on an effective audibility philosophy. Effective audibility assumes that additional high-frequency gain may degrade word recognition performance in adults (Ching et al, 1998). Consequently, NAL-NL1 calculations

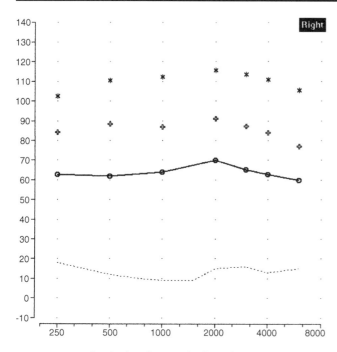

Figure 4–6 Graphic display of targets for desired sensation level (DSL [i/o]) using Audioscan Verifit (version 2.4.27). The *dashed line* at the bottom of the graph represents normal thresholds in dB sound pressure level (SPL). Open circles represent thresholds in ear canal SPL. The plus signs (+) represent targets for the amplified long-term average speech spectrum (70 dB SPL), and the asterisks (*) represent targets for maximum output (90 dB SPL).

generally result in lower target levels than those prescribed by DSL (Byrne et al, 2001). **Figure 4–7** illustrates targets for real ear amplified speech and real ear aided gain (50, 65, and 80 dB SPL) for a child with a moderate hearing loss, using the NAL-NL1 computer program.

◆ Verification of Amplification Performance

Once a decision about a specific manufacturer and model of hearing instrument is made, verification is the critical next step to ensure that the child receives appropriate audibility and output.

Behavioral Measures

Traditionally, amplified sound field thresholds (ASFTs) have been used to verify amplified performance in children. Because sound field behavioral testing is familiar to both patients and audiologists and requires only the test equipment that is available in most audiological settings, it might seem that these measures would be the method of choice for verifying amplified performance. However, several limitations are associated with ASFT.

First, these measures are behavioral and thus require both cooperation from the individual being tested and the ability to produce the desired behavioral response. If a child cannot or will not respond behaviorally to the test stimuli or responds inconsistently, little information is obtained. Multiple sessions may be required to complete testing. Because of time constraints, ASFT measures typically provide data only at a few frequencies. This limited sample of frequencies may not give an accurate picture of the performance of the instrument.

Second, these threshold measures may not provide an accurate estimate of hearing instrument performance under typical use conditions.

◆ In regions of normal hearing, amplified threshold measures may be affected by the noise floor of the hearing instrument and/or noise in the test environment. Thus, the gain of the hearing instrument in those regions may be underestimated.

◆ Because ASFT measures are made at relatively low input levels to the hearing instrument microphone, they may overestimate the amount of gain available from the hearing instrument for higher inputs, such as normal conversational speech. This discrepancy will occur whenever the hearing instrument is functioning in its nonlinear operating range (e.g., WDRC hearing instruments and linear hearing instruments with low maximum output). **Figure 4–8** from Lewis (1997) illustrates this issue. In this figure, input/gain curves are shown for three hypothetical hearing instruments. At low input levels (10–40 dB), the gain of the instruments is the same. As the input level increases, however, the amount of gain begins to differ across the three instruments. At input levels comparable to raised voice (70 dB SPL), the gain is 25, 35, and 40 dB for hearing instruments C, B, and A, respectively. If ASFTs had been used for verification, these devices would have been judged to have similar responses. In reality, however, the amplification of speech would be very different.

◆ Amplified thresholds will not provide information about the maximum output of the hearing instrument, which is critical when fitting hearing instruments to children and adults.

Third, if ASFT measures are being considered as a means of comparing one hearing instrument to another, it is important to know what differences will be needed to determine that an actual difference in performance exists between the two instruments. Hawkins et al (1987) investigated test–retest variability of amplified sound field thresholds. Their results indicated thresholds would have to differ by > 15 dB to be significantly different at the 0.05 confidence level. Stuart et al (1990) determined the critical difference in amplified thresholds for children ages 5 to 9 and 10 to 12 years. They found no statistically significant differences between the two groups and reported differences in amplified thresholds would need to be greater than 10 dB to be statistically significant at the 0.05 confidence level. One cannot assume the results from

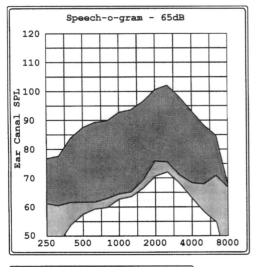
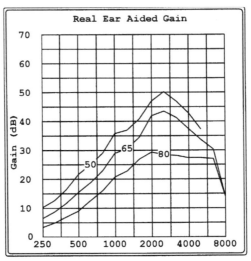

REAG Speech Level parameters

Channel:	1	2
Crossover Frequency:	2000	
Test Frequency:	630	3150
Compression Threshold:	52	52
Compression Ratio:	1.76	1.57
Gain (50):	25	47
Gain (65):	19	41
Gain (80):	13	28

Figure 4–7 Graphic display of target amplified speech at 65 dB SPL (*left curve*) and real ear aided gain (REAG) for three input levels (*right curve*) for NAL-NL1 (version 1.24).

these two studies would hold true for younger children who would likely show even greater variability.

Pediatric Amplification Guidelines (American Academy of Audiology, 2004) also stresses the limitations of ASFT as a verification method. These measures are useful for evaluating the audibility of soft sounds and, as such, are a useful cross-check of hearing instrument performance.

There are instances where behavioral threshold testing may be the verification method of choice. Stelmachowicz and Lewis (1988) reported that behavioral threshold measures may provide a more accurate picture of amplified performance in cases where unamplified thresholds represent vibrotactile rather than auditory responses. In this case, amplified thresholds are subtracted from unamplified re-

sponses to calculate functional gain. Functional gain is then compared with expected electroacoustic gain of the hearing instrument. If functional gain is significantly less than the electroacoustic gain, vibrotactile responses are suspected. ASFT measures are the only clinically feasible method available for verifying performance of bone conduction hearing instruments or cochlear implants. Even in these latter cases, it must be remembered that results represent the softest level at which signals can be detected and may not represent performance with higher level input signals. ASFT may be the best verification method available to evaluate the performance of frequency compression devices in the range where compression is occurring. For the last situation, however, real ear measures are needed for those frequency

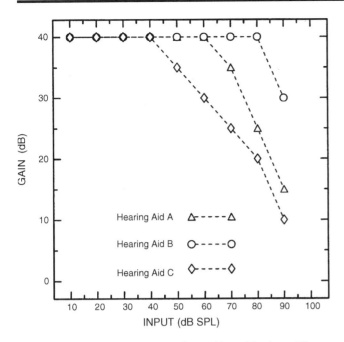

Figure 4–8 Gain (dB) as a function of input (dB SPL) for three different hearing aids. (From Lewis, D. [1997]. Selection and assessment of classroom amplification. In W. McCracken & S. Laoide-Kemp (Eds.), Audiology in education (pp. 323–347). Hoboken, NJ: John Wiley & Sons, Ltd., with permission.)

regions without frequency compression and for assessment of maximum output.

Objective Measures

Probe microphone measures are a necessary means of assessing the amplification provided by a child's hearing instrument. They can be performed with input levels comparable to those that will be encountered in use conditions, providing an accurate estimate of the audibility of signals. Probe microphone measures also provide information about gain in regions of normal hearing and about maximum output of the hearing instrument. They are less time consuming and require less cooperation from the child as compared with AFSTs, allowing more measures to be obtained in a single session. They also provide greater frequency resolution than available with AFSTs.

Given the benefits of probe microphone measures, one would expect they would be the verification method of choice for infants and children. However, in a survey of pediatric hearing instrument fitting practices in the United States, Tharpe et al (2001), reported that behavioral measures of verification, such as ASFT, amplified speech recognition thresholds (SRTs), and speech awareness thresholds (SATs), were used by more than 50% of respondents for children ages 12 years and younger. Sound field amplified thresholds were used much more frequently than probe microphone measures to verify hearing instrument performance with children younger than 2 years of age.

- The type of input signal used to evaluate amplified audibility will affect the measured results. Advanced circuits react differently to speechlike signals than they do to signals processed as noise. Some circuits process broadband speech-shaped signals as noise, resulting in noise reduction activation and gain changes. Live speech inputs can use the voices of family members and other familiar speakers to evaluate audibility "online" for the instrument user. If performance is being compared with prescriptive targets, the variability of live speech may be too great to judge how well the instrument performs when compared with those targets. Using calibrated and recorded speech provides a repeatable representation of speech for hearing instruments with complex digital signal processing (Scollie et al, 2002). There is no current standard for the test signals used to evaluate amplified performance. As such, it may be difficult to compare measurements obtained using different test systems.

Let us assume that at least part of the reason probe microphone measures are not used routinely with children is that audiologists are concerned about the difficulties they may experience when attempting these measures. That being the case, how can the ability to obtain real ear measures with children be improved? It may be helpful if the child is drowsy or asleep during the test procedure. If awake, visual distracters can be used to keep his or her attention focused without increasing activity levels. If the hearing instrument settings have been carefully selected and preset ahead of time with coupler measures and RECD, the amount of time needed for real ear testing will be greatly reduced. Probe tube insertion depths of 10 mm past the ear canal entrance for children younger than 5 years of age and 15 mm for older children (not adult sized) may increase comfort during testing. In all cases, it is desirable that the probe tube extend at least 5 mm past the tip of the earmold (Hawkins and Mueller, 1992).

Pearl

- Mirrors, puzzles, or toys used for distraction during testing and even videos without sound can be used to improve cooperation during real ear probe microphone testing.

Pearl

- Use of a sealing substance, for example, Otoferm (Hal-Hen, Garden City Park, NY) or Otoease (Western Laboratories, Inc., Colorado Springs, CO), on the earmold and probe tube may prevent the probe from moving during insertion of the earmold and may reduce feedback when testing high-gain hearing instruments.

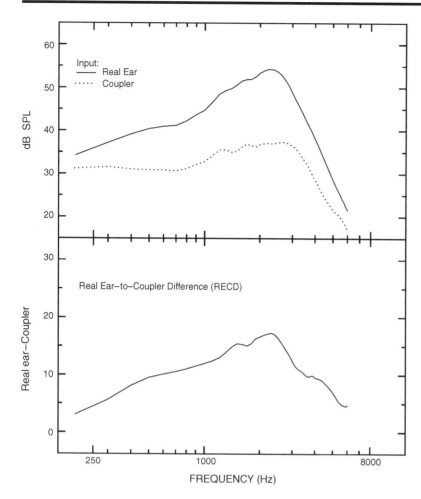

Figure 4–9 Real ear-to-coupler difference (RECD) measurement. In the *top panel*, the *dotted line* represents response in a 2 cc coupler, and the *solid line* represents response in the real ear using the child's custom earmold. The difference between the two curves (*bottom panel*) is the RECD.

A procedure that can greatly enhance real ear measurements is the RECD method developed by Seewald and colleagues (Moodie et al, 1994). In this quick procedure, a measurement is made in a 2 cc coupler. Using the same transducer and stimulus, a measurement is then repeated in the child's ear using his or her own earmold. Results of a typical measurement are shown in **Fig. 4–9.** In this graph, the dashed line represents the coupler response, and the solid line represents the real ear response. The difference between the two curves is the child's RECD. Once the RECD has been measured, subsequent measures can be made in the hearing instrument test box. The RECD is added to the coupler response to predict real ear aided response (REAR) and real ear saturation response (RESR). Bagatto (2001) provides a step-by-step guide to improve RECD measures. **Table 4–2** summarizes Bagatto's practical suggestions.

Special Consideration

- RECD results will be affected by the size of the child's ear, middle ear status, the style and fit of the child's earmold, and the insertion depth of the probe tube during measurements. Measurements should be repeated whenever the child receives a new earmold or at least annually.

Table 4–2 Optimizing the RECD Measurement

What to Do	Why
Measure and mark probe tube	Ensure appropriate probe insertion depth
Use otoscopy and look	Check canal shape and probe placement
Lubricate	Lubrication keeps probe tube in place and eases earmold insertion
Coordinate	Stabilize probe tube during earmold insertion
Don't hesitate	Have all distractor toys ready for child; practice with equipment before testing child
Troubleshoot	Evaluate real ear portion of measure for unusual negative or positive values; be familiar with what a typical RECD looks like

RECD, real ear-to-coupler difference.

Source: Adapted from Bagatto, M. P. (2001). Optimizing your RECD measurements. Hearing Journal, 54(9), 34–36 with permission.

The validity of the RECD was assessed by Seewald et al (1994). These authors compared the RECD plus coupler measures and microphone location effects to measurements of REAR and RESR on 15 subjects. Results indicated that REAR and RESR were predicted with a high degree of accuracy using the RECD measures. Sinclair et al (1994) evaluated the repeatability of the RECD for children from birth to 6.9 years of age. Results indicated that the RECD is repeatable as a function of both age and frequency.

When verifying hearing instrument performance using RECD plus coupler measures, several practical issues must be remembered. Because real ear performance is predicted from measurements made in a coupler, problems with feedback preventing the use of the instrument at the recommended volume control setting will not be indicated. Therefore, it is important to place the instrument on the child at use settings, coupled to the personal earmold. If feedback occurs, the hearing instrument and/or earmold may require adjustment. After adjustment, coupler measures should be repeated to provide an estimate of performance at the new settings. It is recommended that RECD measures be repeated whenever the earmold is replaced or at least annually. Adjustments in hearing instrument settings may be needed on the basis of new RECD values.

Most real ear test systems allow in situ verification of hearing instrument performance in relation to predetermined targets. *Pediatric Amplification Guidelines* (American Academy of Audiology, 2004) recommends the use of REAR rather than real ear insertion gain (REIG) responses for verification. When using insertion gain as the target response, an adult ear canal resonance (REUR) is often assumed and could differ significantly from an individual child's ear. Insertion gain targets often exist outside the context of speech audibility; therefore, REAR targets are preferred for verification.

REAR measures using real ear or RECD plus 2 cc coupler responses can be compared with age-specific targets generated by DSL [i/o]. Many real ear test systems have incorporated DSL [i/o] applications to allow the audiologist to make "online" adjustments in the hearing instrument response to meet audibility targets. Verifying speech audibility at several input levels (e.g., soft, moderate, and loud) provides the audiologist a more comprehensive picture of expected audibility in different listening situations. **Figure 4–10** illustrates results of verification using DSL [i/o]. The open circles represent hearing sensitivity of the right ear. The plus signs (+) represent the recommended (target) hearing instrument output for amplified long-term average speech as prescribed by the DSL procedure. The shaded region shows the +12/–18 dB (i.e., 30 dB) range of speech after being amplified by the hearing instrument. The solid line through the shaded region is intended to meet the DSL targets (+). The line at the top of the graph plots the maximum output of the hearing instrument at the eardrum. The measured maximum output is intended to meet, but not exceed, the targets (*). In this example, the hearing instrument response meets targets from 250 to 4000 Hz, and all but the softest components of speech are above threshold at 6000 Hz. It is probable that real ear test system manufacturers will continue to promote in situ verification for children and adults by implementing future DSL and NAL-NL1 updates in their test systems.

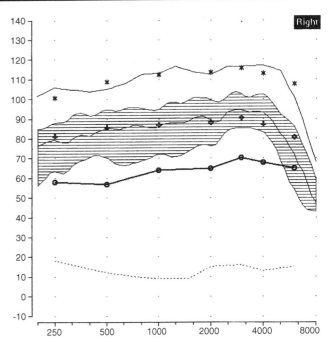

Figure 4–10 Hearing instrument verification using DSL [i/o] targets and Audioscan Verifit (version 2.4.27).

The ability to evaluate the audibility of different speech levels is helpful because in real life, speech does not occur at a single level. Differences in talker-to-listener distances and vocal effort affect the level of speech reaching the hearing instrument microphone. For children who are learning speech and language, it is especially important to ensure that speech will be audible to them across many different listening situations. **Figure 4–11** illustrates audibility of amplified soft (55 dB SPL) and loud (75 dB SPL) speech. For this instrument, all but the softest components of soft speech (horizontal hatched area) are above threshold. As expected, loud speech (vertical hatched area) is higher on the graph, but the peaks are well below the maximum output of the instrument.

Hearing instrument manufacturers often display simulated in-ear performance for instruments in their software fitting applications. It is important to note that these values are simulations based on average or expected performance and do not reliably predict the actual instrument response. Hawkins and Cook (2003) recommended that verification measures be made in situ and not simulated due to findings of large variability between simulated and measured performance across manufacturers and models.

FM System Evaluation

Verification of an FM system presents further considerations due to the nature of how the FM microphone/transmitter is used and how it is designed to function. Input compression is an important part of the design of FM microphone/transmitters to assist with the FM transmission and to control distortion from high input levels at such a closely placed microphone. The reader is referred to Platz (2004) for a complete discussion of the issues. Although

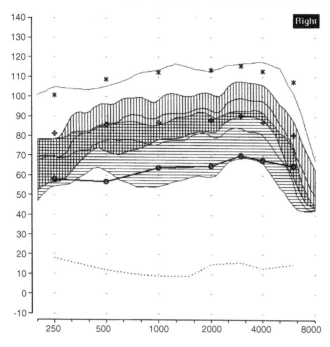

Figure 4–11 Hearing instrument verification of the range of soft speech (*horizontal hatched area*) and the range of loud speech (*vertical hatched area*) inputs, using Audioscan Verifit (version 2.4.27).

hearing instrument/FM amplification systems are most typically used in the FM + hearing instrument or simultaneous input setting, all current verification protocols and test systems allow only sequential measurements. That is, although these systems typically function with sounds arriving at both the FM microphone and the hearing instrument microphone at the same time, the response of the hearing instrument and the FM are measured separately. This is an important issue in verification, as hearing instrument processing becomes increasingly complex and typically incorporates some type of compression. With compression in the hearing instrument processor and compression in the FM microphone/transmitter, results obtained with sequential testing may differ significantly from how the system operates in response to simultaneous inputs (Lewis and Eiten, 2005).

When setting and verifying an FM system, the goal is to ensure audibility of the talker wearing the FM microphone, the user's own voice, and others who are not wearing the FM microphone. FM system guidelines from the American Speech Language Hearing Association (ASHA, 2002) recommend that a 10 dB advantage of the FM signal over other signals be maintained. This is a reflection of the higher input levels that are achieved when placing a microphone close to the speaker's mouth.

With widespread use of ear-level FM receivers, the hearing instrument acts as the local microphone. The hearing instrument provides audibility of the user's own voice and all other signals or speech in the local environment not transmitted by the FM system.

The first step in any FM verification is to ensure that the local microphone is providing appropriate gain and output, because all other measures are based on this assumption.

Second, the local microphone should be evaluated with the recommended FM coupling in place (FM+ boot, DAI, or neckloop) to determine if any changes in the microphone response are occurring due to impedance effects.

Third, FM transparency should be evaluated by comparing inputs to the FM microphone to the response of the local microphone, as above. Transparency of the FM signal assumes that no alteration of the frequency or amplitude characteristics of the audio signal occurs when the FM signal is received by the hearing instrument (Platz, 2004). Systems that allow FM level changes can be adjusted to ensure transparency.

◆ Validation of Amplification Performance

Once the hearing instrument has been selected and set, and testing has verified the performance of the instrument, the next step is validation. According to the Pediatric Working Group (1996), "The purpose of validating aided auditory function is to demonstrate the benefits/limitations of a child's listening abilities for perceiving the speech of others as well as his or her own speech" (p. 56).

Boothroyd (2005) addressed the importance and goals of measuring young children's capacity to perceive speech.

> The wide range of unassisted, aided, and implanted auditory capacity in young children with hearing loss creates a need for assessment. The goals include:
>
> 1. To describe and quantify impairment and disability before intervention.
>
> 2. To guide decisions about sensory intervention.
>
> 3. To evaluate the outcome of sensory intervention.
>
> 4. To guide decisions about educational intervention.
>
> 5. To monitor and evaluate the outcome of that intervention.
>
> 6. To provide the evidence needed for an evolving evidence-based practice.
>
> The current lack of effective tools is of special concern because inappropriate decisions, based on inadequate data (or unquestioned optimism), can have far-reaching implications for language development, general development, psychosocial development and, ultimately, quality of life. (p. 129)

With infants and children, validation requires input from many sources, including parents/caregivers, educational personnel, audiologists, and other professionals who may be working with the child. Validation is affected by a variety of factors, including the age of the child, the age of onset of the hearing loss, the type and degree of hearing loss, and additional conditions such as physical or cognitive developmental concerns. For infants and children, validation is assessed in a variety of ways:

◆ Observable benefit

◆ Informal observation

◆ Direct measures

The term *observable benefit* refers to observed behaviors that suggest the child is or is not responding in some way to the amplified signal provided by the hearing instruments. These behaviors might include alerting, increased vocalizations, or comments from the parents that the child "seems better" when wearing the instruments. Informal observation might include situations where the child's auditory responses are observed in a natural environment. Parents/caregivers could be instructed to observe and document the child's behavior in various environments. Though valuable, these are difficult to quantify. Direct measures of amplified auditory function would be used to assess behavioral responses when the hearing instruments are being worn. These might include amplified sound field responses (e.g., music and environmental sounds) and speech perception measures. The position statement "Amplification for Infants and Children with Hearing Loss" (Pediatric Working Group, 1996) includes a list of speech recognition materials used with children. Appendix 4–2 provides a partial list of currently available validation resources.

Boothroyd (1991) developed a computer-based game (Video Speech Pattern Contrast [VidSPAC]) to evaluate the perception of acoustic contrasts (e.g., vowel height and initial and final consonant voicing) in children. Children as young as 3 to 4 years of age select a colorful character who presents test stimuli. The child responds to changes in a string of stimuli (e.g., *doo, doo, doo* vs *doo, doo, daa*). The program includes animated scenes that are displayed as a reward after a certain number of trials. Boothroyd (2005) describes further investigations of a visual reinforcement audiometry (VRA) task being developed to evaluate speech pattern recognition for use in infants as young as 9 months of age.

The Functional Listening Evaluation (FLE) was developed by Johnson and Von Almen (1997) and revised by Johnson (2001). It is designed to simulate actual listening conditions and to evaluate the effects of noise, distance, and visual input in a child's listening and learning environments. Because it is designed to be administered in a specific classroom, it is more representative of a child's real-world listening performance than testing completed in a sound booth. Recorded speech and noise materials, as well as a sound level meter, are required for test administration.

Indirect validation includes functional performance measures. With infants and young children, responses most often are obtained from parents/caregivers and/or educational personnel. One such measure, the Screening Instrument for Targeting Educational Risk (SIFTER, Anderson, 1989) was developed to identify children at risk for educational problems caused by hearing loss. Teachers are asked to rate the child compared with other students in five areas: academics, attention, communication, classroom participation, and social behavior. On the basis of positive feedback from those using the SIFTER, Anderson and Matkin (1996) developed a preschool version of the test, which assesses the same basic areas of concern. Anderson (2004) also developed an adolescent version of the test (Secondary SIFTER) based on the more complex academic and classroom demands placed on HI students in secondary academic settings.

Anderson and Smaldino (2000) created the Children's Home Inventory of Listening Difficulties (CHILD) to be used by parents and children 3 to 12 years of age. The measure represents typical family communication situations in quiet and in noise and at different listening distances. An 8-point scale uses the illustration of an "Understand-O-Meter" to judge the child's ability to listen and understand. A child's format of the scale can be completed by children as young as 7 to 8 years of age. Results from the CHILD can be used to evaluate the effectiveness of amplification, indicate the need for assistive devices, or serve as a counseling tool with parents and children regarding difficult communication situations.

The Listening Inventory for Education (LIFE) was developed by Anderson and Smaldino (1997) to determine amplification benefit or effectiveness of an intervention strategy for elementary school students. It is composed of three inventories. The student inventory uses cartoonlike pictures to identify difficult classroom listening situations. The teacher inventory is used to evaluate the student's attention, classroom participation, and learning. The third inventory, also completed by teachers, uses open-ended questions to gather more information regarding the teacher's observations and opinions. The inventories are intended to be completed before and after classroom intervention, such as amplification or acoustic modifications.

Kopun and Stelmachowicz (1998) modified the Abbreviated Profile of Hearing Aid Performance (APHAP) (Cox and Alexander, 1995) for use with children ages 10 to 16 years. The purpose of the CA-APHAP is to allow comparison of amplified and unamplified performance in a variety of situations. Children with mild to severe hearing loss and their parents were given the test. Results indicated that for children with moderate to severe hearing loss, patterns of responses were similar to amplified adult data from Cox and Alexander (1995). Correlations between scores for children and parents were very low, indicating that they did not agree about the communication difficulties the children were experiencing. This latter finding suggests that the results may have value as a counseling tool.

The Meaningful Auditory Integration Scale (MAIS, Robbins et al, 1991) was developed for use with children with profound hearing loss. The scale evaluates three aspects of the child's ability to use sound meaningfully in everyday situations—bonding to device, alerting to sound, and deriving meaning from auditory phenomena. An interview format, based on 10 "probes," is used with parents to obtain information about their child's behavior in specific situations. An infant/toddler version, IT-MAIS (Zimmerman-Phillips et al, 2000), was developed to evaluate a young child's spontaneous responses to sounds in his or her environment using the same interview and probe format.

The Client Oriented Scale of Improvement (COSI, Dillon et al, 1997) was developed as a self-report tool for measuring hearing instrument benefit and satisfaction. With this tool, the individual with hearing loss selects up to five listening situations where he or she is experiencing hearing difficulty. After rehabilitation, the situations are reviewed relative to improvements. Although the scale was developed using situations encountered by adults, it can be modified to include categories that would be pertinent to infants and children with hearing loss. Examples of categories for young children include the following:

- Changes in behavior (e.g., quiets, smiles in response to sound)

- Increased vocalization

- Requests hearing instrument

- Awareness of loud environmental sounds

- Awareness of soft environmental sounds

- Awareness of voice

- Response to music

- Localization to sound/voice

Parents would complete the form before and after specific rehabilitation, such as the introduction of amplification. As the child develops, goals would be changed to reflect developmental changes and expectations. A pediatric-focused version of the COSI, called the Children's Outcome Worksheet (COW), was developed and is distributed through Oticon (Somerset, NJ; www.oticonusa.com).

The Early Listening Function (ELF), by Anderson (2002), is appropriate for infants and toddlers. It uses the illustration of the "sound bubble" to describe responses to quiet, average, and loud sounds. The parent or caregiver monitors the child's responses to sounds originating from different distances and rates the child's responses on a 3-tier scale. The questionnaire was designed to be completed at home to elicit and observe the child's responses. Results can be shared with the early interventionist and audiologist for ongoing monitoring of amplification benefit.

The Functional Auditory Performance Indicators (FAPI), by Stredler-Brown and Johnson (2003), evaluates seven categories of auditory skills in a hierarchical order, from sound awareness through linguistic auditory processing. A profile of a child's functional auditory skills can be generated from the results. The tool was designed to be used in a variety of ways, including direct observation or parent report. Because children are usually working on many auditory skills at the same time, the scale takes an integrated approach to validation. No age limits are stated for this tool, and many different skills can be evaluated over time.

Professionals at the University of Pittsburgh have developed a set of tools to be used to assess listening needs and evaluate efficacy of intervention (Palmer and Mormer, 1997, 1999). The first tool is the Developmental Index of Audition and Listening (DIAL). The DIAL provides a table of auditory and listening skills that are to be expected at specific ages for children with normal hearing. The HI child's current auditory skills are determined as a "starting point" for auditory skill development. The pediatric Hearing Demand, Ability, and Need Profile (HDAN) allows the clinician to assess communication difficulties with and without amplification, current compensations for those difficulties, and recommendations for solutions. Finally, the information from the DIAL and HDAN is incorporated into the Family Expectation Worksheet (FEW). FEW is similar to COSI in that the family, with input from the child when possible, develops goals for (re)habilitation. Using FEW, the family rates how the child functions currently (before intervention) and

how they expect the child to function after intervention. Expectations, based on a variety of factors (e.g., hearing loss, amplification, and age), may be addressed by the audiologist. After intervention, the family rates their perception of the child's performance. Thus, a goal could be that the child will respond to his or her name. Current levels of success may be "hardly ever" if the child has a severe to profound hearing loss and has not yet been fit with amplification. The family's goal for the child might be that he or she will respond "almost always." The goal might be changed to "most of the time" or "half of the time" to account for situations where noise, distance, attention, or the talker's vocal effort would interfere with the child's ability to respond appropriately.

Special Consideration

- As children mature and can begin to understand hearing and hearing loss, it is incumbent upon audiologists to include them in discussions about their hearing loss. It is important that, within the constraints of their developmental levels, children understand audiologic and management issues so that they can participate in and eventually make their own decisions about hearing health and amplification.

Especially with the youngest children, developing appropriate validation methods is difficult. In addition, several questions will remain regardless of the validation tools used to assess performance. For example, what is optimal performance as opposed to observable improvement? Is "optimal" performance even feasible, or is "better" good enough, and, if so, how do we quantify either? These are questions that do not have easy answers and will require continued discussion and evaluation as attempts are made to develop tools to demonstrate the effectiveness of intervention strategies.

♦ Practical Issues in Facilitating Adjustment

Pearl

- Products such as Super Seals (Just Bekuz Products Co., Castle Rock, CO), Hearing Aid Sweatbands (Van B Enterprises, West Valley, NY), or Ear Gear (Ear Gear, Lake Country, British Columbia) can be used to protect the battery compartment and/or volume control on hearing instruments without tamper-resistant features. Care should be taken to ensure that the child cannot remove these products because they may be choking hazards.

To achieve goals related to amplification use, consistent use of the hearing instruments must be established. Because caregivers are in charge of the instruments, it is important they have a clear understanding of how each device functions, how to use the device correctly, and how to troubleshoot and maintain the device. Families need a "hearing instrument kit" to assist in instrument maintenance. The kit should consist of the following items:

♦ Listening tube

♦ Battery tester

♦ Batteries

♦ Retention devices (**Table 4–3**)

♦ Drying devices (e.g., Dri-Aid, Hal-Hen, Garden City Park, NY, and Dry-N-Store, Ear Technology Corporation, Johnson City, TN)

♦ Earmold blower

♦ Printed instructions

Several hearing instrument manufacturers produce troubleshooting/maintenance kits for children. Some have

Table 4–3 Strategies to Assist in Hearing Instrument Retention and Acceptance

♦ Huggie Aids (Huggie Aids Ltd, Oklahome City, OK)
♦ Fishing line/dental floss and safety pin
♦ Otoclips/Critter Clips (Westone Laboratories, Inc. Colorado Springs, CO)
♦ Ear Gear (Ear Gear, Lake Country, British Columbia, Canada)
♦ Hearing Aid Sweatbands (Van B Enterprises, West Valley, NY)
♦ Pediatric tone hooks
♦ Doublestick or toupee tape
♦ Bonnet with hole cut out for hearing instrument microphone
♦ Pilot caps by Hanna Andersson (www.hannaandersson.com)
♦ Ribbon with loops for behind-the-ear (BTE) instruments
♦ Eyeglass holders
♦ Sweatbands to hold hearing instruments/earmolds in place
♦ Orthodontic rubber bands to hold BTE instruments to eyeglasses
♦ Vests with pockets for body-worn instruments
♦ Colored hearing instrument cases
♦ Colored earmolds
♦ Colored beads on earmold tubing (be aware of choking hazard for young children)
♦ Decorating hearing instruments with stickers
♦ Colored Super Seals (Just Bekuz Products Co., Castle Rock, CO)
♦ EarWear hearing instrument covers (EarWear, Inc., Toronto, Ontario, Canada)
♦ Safe N Sound security straps and clips (Safe N Sound, Havelock, NC)
♦ It Stays! body adhesive (Decollete Enhancement, Warren, ME)

programs for children that may include special kits that include care and maintenance tools, stickers, booklets, and information for parents and educators. In addition, many family-friendly Web sites provide support and information (Appendix 4–3). Including information about these sites during hearing instrument orientation and follow-up allows the audiologist to direct parents to helpful information.

In the typical scenario for hearing instrument fitting and follow-up, caregivers are instructed in the care and use of the hearing instruments at the initial fitting, and instructions are reviewed at subsequent visits. Families are encouraged to call with any questions or concerns. With children, frequent follow-up is important to monitor hearing, hearing instrument function, and earmold fit and to allow discussion with families about adjustment, emerging questions, or concerns and changing needs.

Hearing instrument retention is a concern that is often raised by families of infants and children. Retention is affected by the size of the child's head and ears relative to the hearing instruments or by behavioral issues related to keeping the hearing instrument in place. Pediatric audiologists often must be creative as they assist families with this challenging issue. Because no single strategy works with all children, a variety of options can be tried to select the ones that work best for the individual child and his or her family. **Table 4–3** lists several strategies to assist in hearing instrument retention and acceptance.

Pearl

♦ When bone-conduction hearing instruments are chosen for infants and very young children, it may be difficult to find headbands that will fit well. Rigid headbands limit bone-conduction placement, and changes in skull shape can occur. Alternatively, a sweatband, made smaller to fit the child's head, can be used. Both the bone-conduction transducer and the hearing instrument are held in place on the band with Velcro.

Hearing instrument adjustment also is enhanced by close and regular communication between the audiologist and educational personnel who work with the child. It is helpful to discuss goals and expectations for amplification (e.g., what is expected to be audible and at what distances), to review progress and concerns so modifications can be made when needed, and to provide in-service training regarding use and care of hearing instruments. The child wearing hearing instruments should participate in his or her care and maintenance to the extent possible for his or her developmental level.

Even when the hearing instruments selected for a child meet targets and when goals and expectations for everyday listening are met, situations will occur where additional assistive technology is necessary to allow the child to participate more fully in his or her environment. Hearing assistance technology is addressed more fully in Chapter 17 in this volume. The next section will focus specifically on selection and use of additional assistive technology with children.

◆ Choosing Hearing Assistance Technology for Children

As when choosing hearing instruments, selection of other HAT begins with goals. The goals may change over time as the child develops, as needs change, and if hearing loss changes. One of the first goals of HAT may be to help the child be aware of auditory events in his or her environment. Children with normal hearing may learn cause–effect relationships incidentally. For example, the doorbell rings, Mom goes to the door, and someone is there. After this happens over time, the child begins to make the association between the doorbell sounding and the presence of someone at the door. Now, think of a child with hearing loss who cannot hear the doorbell. The child is playing on the floor; suddenly, Mom goes to the door and someone is there. How did she know to go to the door? How will the child learn to understand and interpret these events? By use of a visual alerting device, such as a doorbell/doorknock indicator, the family can help the child to begin to make associations between the flashing light and the presence of someone at the door.

Another goal of HAT is to foster independence. As children get older, it is important for them to develop independence. Fostering independence helps prepare children for the time when they will be living away from their families. One example is helping a child find the most successful method for waking himself or herself up in the morning. Visual, amplified, or vibrating alarm clocks are available. When evaluating options, it is important to consider family members with normal hearing. For example, a sibling sharing the bedroom may tolerate a flashing or vibrating alarm much better than a more intense auditory signal.

Independence also means increasing degrees of privacy. The ability to have phone conversations without assistance from parents or siblings is especially important as children get older. Use of amplified handsets or telecommunications devices for the deaf (TDDs) used with or without telephone relay services will allow the child to talk to family and peers, make appointments, and even order pizza. Privacy also extends to the child's own room in the home. For a child with hearing loss, someone knocking at the bedroom door may be inaudible, especially if the child is not wearing his or her hearing instruments. Consequently, family members may get into the habit of entering the room unannounced, an especially distressing event during adolescence. Door-knock devices are available that will flash whenever someone knocks on the door. These devices are portable and can be moved around the house as needed.

Pitfall

- When evaluating HAT equipment, particularly alerting or alarm devices, it is important to know whether the child will be wearing his or her hearing instruments whenever the device will be used, to determine whether the signal should be auditory, visual, or vibrotactile. Choosing alarms and signaling devices that are auditory only may create problems if the child cannot hear the signal without his or her hearing instruments.

As children get older, they also are more likely to stay home alone or to care for other, younger siblings while parents are away. In these cases, safety also becomes an issue. It is important that the child with hearing loss be aware when someone is at the door or the phone is ringing, be able to use the phone when needed, and be aware of alarms such as smoke detectors in the home. Again, selecting assistive technology before the child is in a situation requiring its use is prudent.

Assistive technology also may be chosen to improve the child's communications skills. Devices for the telephone will enable the child to communicate with a variety of individuals and improve telephone skills. Assistive technology also may help the child communicate in a variety of listening environments where hearing instruments alone are inadequate because of distance, noise, and reverberation. Access to television, radio, tapes and compact discs, and computers also may be enhanced with assistive technology. Communications technologies change constantly. Children and youth with hearing loss are able to take advantage of many of the options available. Text messaging and Bluetooth connections make telephone communications more accessible regardless of the degree of hearing loss. Webcam access makes it possible to have real-time face-to-face communications.

Pearl

- Remember that assistive technology that is available at home may not be available in other locations. If a child is staying with friends or relatives, it is helpful to have portable assistive devices that the child can take along. For travel, the Americans with Disabilities Act requires that hotels have assistive technology available for guests.

When choosing assistive technology for a child, individual characteristics should be considered. These include the child's age, degree of hearing loss, hearing instruments and their compatibility with assistive technology, any physical limitations, the child's and family's lifestyle, and the family budget. As the child matures, his or her needs will change. For example, a very young child may only need to know that the telephone is ringing. Soon, however, an amplifier or TDD may need to be added to home telephones to enhance communication with family and friends. As the child gets older, cell phones or pagers with text messaging, portable phone amplifiers, or portable TDDs can provide communications accessibility when the child is away from home.

◆ Summary

Infants and children present a challenge to audiologists during the selection, fitting, and management of amplification. However, it is not an insurmountable challenge. Many options and resources are needed to help audiologists meet this challenge. Sources are available that will assist the audiologist in making informed decisions about appropriate amplification from among the myriad of choices that are available today. As the child matures, and as available audiologic information increases, amplification needs and priorities change. The process from identification of hearing loss to fitting of amplification is a continuous loop: steps are repeated, goals and fittings are adjusted, and management changes to meet the ever-changing needs of the child and his or her family.

Appendix 4–1

Hearing Instrument Technology and Children

Bamford, J., McCracken, W., Peers, I., & Grayson, P. (1999). Trial of a two-channel hearing aid (low-frequency compression, high-frequency linear amplification) with school-age children. Ear and Hearing, 20, 290–298.

Christiansen, L. A., & Thomas, T. E. (1997, September). The use of multiple memory programmable hearing aid technology in children. Paper presented at the Second Biennial Hearing Aid Research and Development Conference, Bethesda, MD.

Condie, R., Scollie, S., & Checkley, P. (2001, November). Children's performance with analog vs a digital, adaptive dual-microphone hearing aid. Poster presented at A Sound Foundation through Early Amplification Conference, Chicago. Retrieved July 31, 2007, from http://www.dslio.com/condie%20et%20al%20poster.pdf

Fabry, D. A. (1991). Signal processing hearing aids with the pediatric population. In J. A. Feigin & P. G. Stelmachowicz (Eds.), Pediatric amplification: Proceedings of the 1991 National Conference (pp. 49–60). Omaha, NE: Boys Town National Research Hospital.

Flynn, M. C., Davis, P. B., & Pogash, R. (2004). Multiple-channel non-linear power hearing instruments for children with severe hearing impairment: Long-term follow-up. International Journal of Audiology, 43, 479–485.

Gravel, J., Fausel, N., Liskow, C., & Chobot, J. (1999). Children's speech recognition in noise using dual microphone hearing aid technology. Ear and Hearing, 20, 1–11.

Kuk, F. K., Kollofski, C., Brown, S., Melum, A., & Rosenthal, A. (1999). Use of digital hearing aids with directional microphones in school-age children. Journal of the American Academy of Audiology, 10(10), 535–548.

Marriage, J. E. & Moore, B. C. J. (2003). New speech tests reveal benefit of wide-dynamic-range, fast-acting compression for consonant discrimination in children with moderate to severe hearing loss. International Journal of Audiology, 42, 418–425.

Marriage, J. E., Moore, B. C. J., Stone, M. A., & Baer, T. (2005). Effects of three amplification strategies on speech perception by children with severe and profound hearing loss. Ear and Hearing, 26, 35–47.

Miller-Hansen, D. R., Nelson, P. B., Widen, J. E., & Simon, S. D. (2003). Evaluating the benefit of speech recoding hearing aids in children. American Journal of Audiology, 12, 106–113.

Palmer, C. V., & Grimes, A. M. (2005). Effectiveness of signal processing strategies for the pediatric population: A systematic review of the evidence. Journal of the American Academy of Audiology, 16, 505–514.

Ricketts, T., & Tharpe, A. M. (2005). Potential for directivity-based benefit in actual classroom environments. In R. C. Seewald & J. M. Bamford (Eds.), A sound foundation through early amplification (pp. 143–154). Stäfa, Switzerland: Phonak.

Stelmachowicz, P. G., Lewis, D. E., Hoover, B. M., & Keefe, D. H. (1999). Subjective effects of peak clipping versus compression limiting in normal and hearing impaired children. Journal of the Acoustical Society of America, 105(1), 412–422.

Stelmachowicz, P. G., Pittman, A. L., Hoover, B. H., & Lewis, D. E. (2001). Effect of stimulus bandwidth on the perception of /s/ in normal- and hearing-impaired children and adults. Journal of the Acoustical Society of America, 110(4), 2183–2190.

Stelmachowicz, P. G., Pittman, A. L., Hoover, B. M., & Lewis, D. E. (2002). Aided perception of /s/ and /z/ by hearing-impaired children. Ear and Hearing, 23(4), 316–324.

Stelmachowicz, P. G., Pittman, A. L., Hoover, B. M., Lewis, D. E., & Moeller, M. P. (2004). The importance of high-frequency audibility in the speech and language development of children with hearing loss. Archives of Otolaryngology Head and Neck Surgery, 130, 556–562.

Zorowka, P. G., & Lippert, K. L. (1995). One-channel and multichannel digitally programmable hearing aids in children with hearing impairment. Annals of Otology Rhinology Supplement, 166, 159–162.

Appendix 4–2

Validation Resources

Children's Home Inventory for Listening Difficulty (CHILD): Anderson, K., & Smaldino, J. (2000). Children's home inventory for listening difficulty. Retrieved July 31, 2007, from http://www.kandersonaudconsulting.com

Client Oriented Scale of Improvement (COSI): National Acoustics Laboratory. Available for download from http://www.nal.gov.au/nal-products%20front%20page.htm

Children's Outcome Worksheets (COW): Available for download from Oticon, http://www.oticonusa.com/SiteGen/Uploads/Public/Down-loads_Oticon/Pediatrics/cow.pdf

Developmental Index of Audition and Listening (DIAL): Available as a downloadable file to members of the Educational Audiology Association from http://www.edaud.org

Early Listening Function (ELF): Anderson, K. (2002). Early listening function. Retrieved July 31, 2007, from http://www.kandersonaudconsulting.com

Family Expectation Worksheet (FEW): Available as a downloadable file to members of the Educational Audiology Association from http://www.edaud.org

Functional Auditory Performance Indicators (FAPI): Stredler-Brown A, & Johnson, C. (2004). Functional auditory performance indicators. Retrieved August 9, 2007, from http://www.csdb.org/chip/resources/docs/fapi6_23.pdf

Functional Listening Evaluation (FLE): Johnson, C. (2001). The functional listening evaluation. Retrieved August 9, 2007, from http://www.cde.state.co.us/cdesped/download/pdf/s4-FunListEval.pdf

(Pediatric) Hearing Demand, Ability, and Need Profile (HDAN): Available as a downloadable file to members of the Educational Audiology Association from http://www.edaud.org

Infant/Toddler version of MAIS (IT-MAIS): Zimmerman-Philips, S., Osberger, M. J., & McConkey Robbins, A. (2000). Assessing cochlear implant benefits in very young children. Retrieved August 9, 2007, from http://www.cochlearimplant.com/printables/it-mais-brochure.pdf

Listening Inventory for Education (LIFE): Anderson, K., & Smaldino, J. (1997). Listening inventory for education. Retrieved July 31, 2007, from http://www.kandersonaudconsulting.com

Meaningful Auditory Integration Scale (MAIS): Robbins, A. M., Renshaw, J. J., & Berry, A. S. Evaluating meaningful auditory integration in profoundly hearing-impaired children. Retrieved August 9, 2007, from http://medicine.iu.edu/documents/Otolaryngology/mais.pdf

Preschool Screening Instrument for Targeting Education Risk (SIFTER): Anderson, K., & Matkin, N. (1996). Pre-school screening instrument for targeting education risk. Retrieved July 31, 2007, from http://www.kandersonaudconsulting.com

Secondary SIFTER: Anderson, K. (2004). Screening instrument for targeting education risk in secondary students. Retrieved July 31, 2007, from http://www.kandersonaudconsulting.com

SIFTER: Anderson, K. (1989). Screening instrument for targeting education risk. Retrieved July 31, 2007, from http://www.kandersonaudconsulting.com

Appendix 4–3

Family-Friendly Web Sites

Deaf Education

Beginnings (http://www.beginningssvcs.com/)

Electronic Deaf Education Network (http://www.bradingrao.com/)

Hands and Voices (http://www.handsandvoices.org/)

John Tracy Clinic (http://www.jtc.org/)

Laurent Clerc National Deafness Education Center (http://clerccenter.gallaudet.edu/)

Listen-Up Web (http://www.listen-up.org/)

Marian Downs National Center for Infant Hearing (http://www.colorado.edu/slhs/mdnc/)

My Baby's Hearing (http://www.babyhearing.org)

National Center for Hearing Assessment and Management (http://www.infanthearing.org/index.html)

Where Do We Go from Hear? (http://www.gohear.org/link/link.html)

Manufacturers

Oticon (http://www.otikids.oticon.com/)

Phonak (http://www.phonak.com/consumer/parents.htm)

Siemens (http://www.siemens-hearing.com/hearing_Aids/children/index.aspx?w=c)

Unitron (http://www.unitronhearing.us/ccus/people/childrenparents.htm)

Widex (http://www.widex.com/children)

References

Allen, P., & Wightman, F. (1994). Psychometric functions for children's detection of tones in noise. Journal of Speech and Hearing Research, 37, 205–215.

American Academy of Audiology. (2004). Pediatric amplification guidelines. Audiology Today, 16(2), 46–53.

American Academy of Pediatrics. (1999). Newborn and infant hearing loss: Detection and intervention. Pediatrics, 103, 527–530.

American Speech-Language-Hearing Association. (2002). Guidelines for fitting and monitoring FM systems. In ASHA Desk Reference. Rockville, MD: Author.

Anderson, K. (1989). Screening Instrument for Targeting Educational Risk (SIFTER). Retrieved July 31, 2007, from http://www.kandersonaudconsulting.com

Anderson, K. (2002). Early Listening Function (ELF) instrument for infants and toddlers with hearing loss. Retrieved July 31, 2007, from http://www.kandersonaudconsulting.com

Anderson, K. (2004). Screening Inventory for Targeting Educational Risk in Secondary Students (Secondary SIFTER). Retrieved July 31, 2007, from http://www.kandersonaudconsulting.com

Anderson, K., & Matkin, N. (1996). Screening Instrument for Targeting Educational Risk in Preschool Children (Preschool SIFTER). Retrieved July 31, 2007, from http://www.kandersonaudconsulting.com

Anderson, K., & Smaldino, J. (1997). Listening Inventory for Education (LIFE). Retrieved July 31, 2007, from http://www.kandersonaudconsulting.com

Anderson, K., & Smaldino, J. (2000). Children's Home Inventory of Listening Difficulties (CHILD). Retrieved July 31, 2007, from http://www.kandersonaudconsulting.com

Bagatto, M. P. (2001). Optimizing your RECD measurements. Hearing Journal, 54(9), 34–36.

Bagatto, M. P., Scollie, S. D., Seewald, R. C., Moodie, K. S., & Hoover, B. M. (2002). Real-ear-to-coupler difference predictions as a function of age for two coupling procedures. Journal of the American Academy of Audiology, 13, 407–415.

Bagatto, M., Moodie, S., Scollie, S., Seewald, R., Moodie, S., Pumford, J., & Liu, K.P.R. (2005). Clinical protocols for hearing instrument fitting in the Desired Sensation Level Method. Trends in Amplification, 9(4), 199–226.

Bentler, R. A. (1989). External ear resonance characteristics in children. Journal of Speech and Hearing Disorders, 54(2), 265–268.

Bess, F. H., Dodd-Murphy, J., & Parker, R. A. (1998). Children with minimal sensorineural hearing loss: Prevalence, educational performance, and functional status. Ear and Hearing, 19(5), 339–354.

Boothroyd, A. (1991). Assessment of speech perception capacity in profoundly deaf children. American Journal of Otology, 12, 67–72.

Boothroyd, A. (2005). Measuring auditory speech-perception capacity in young children. In R. C. Seewald & J. M. Bamford (Eds.), A sound foundation through early amplification (pp. 129–140). Stäfa, Switzerland: Phonak.

Boothroyd, A., Springer, N., Smith, L., & Schulman, J. (1988). Amplitude compression and profound hearing loss. Journal of Speech and Hearing Research, 31, 362–376.

Boymans, M., & Dreschler, W. A. (2000). Field trials using a digital hearing aid with active noise reduction and dual-microphone directionality. Audiology, 39, 260–268.

Byrne, D., Dillon, H., Ching, T., Katsch, R., & Keidser, G. (2001). NAL-NL1 procedure for fitting nonlinear hearing aids: Characteristics and comparisons with other procedures. Journal of the American Academy Audiology, 12(1), 37–51.

Ching, T. Y., Dillon, H., & Byrne, D. (1998). Speech recognition of hearing-impaired listeners: Predictions from audibility and the limited role of high-frequency amplification. Journal of the Acoustical Society of America, 103, 1128–1140.

Christensen, L. A. (1999). A comparison of three hearing-aid sound processing strategies in a multiple-memory hearing aid for adolescents. Seminars in Hearing, 20(3), 183–196.

Cox, R. M., & Alexander, G. C. (1995). The abbreviated profile of hearing aid benefit. Ear and Hearing, 16(2), 176–186.

Dawson, P., Dillon, H., & Battaglia, J. (1990). Output limiting compression for the severe-profoundly deaf. Australian Journal of Audiology, 13(1), 1–12.

Dillon, H., James, A., & Ginis, J. (1997). Client oriented scale of improvement (COSI) and its relationship to several other measures of benefit and satisfaction provided by hearing instruments. Journal of the American Academy of Audiology, 8(1), 27–43.

Eisenberg, L. S., Shannon, R. V., Martinez, A. S., Wygonski, J., & Boothroyd, A. (2000). Speech recognition with reduced spectral cues as a function of age. Journal of the Acoustical Society of America, 107, 2704–2710.

Elliott, L. L. (1979). Performance of children aged 9 to 17 years on a test of speech intelligibility in noise using sentence material with controlled word predictability. Journal of the Acoustical Society of America, 66(3), 651–653.

Feigin, J. A., Kopun, J. K., Stelmachowicz, P. G., & Gorga, M. P. (1989). Probe-microphone measures of earcanal sound pressure levels in infants and children. Ear and Hearing, 10, 254–258.

Gabbard, S. A. (2005). The use of FM technology for infants and young children. In R. C. Seewald & J. M. Bamford (Eds.), A sound foundation through early amplification (pp. 155–162). Stäfa, Switzerland: Phonak.

Gelfand, S. A., & Silman, S. (1993). Apparent auditory deprivation in children: implications for monaural versus binaural amplification. Journal of the American Academy of Audiology, 4(5), 313–318.

Gravel, J. S., Fausel, N., Liskow, C., & Chobot, J. (1999). Children's speech recognition in noise using dual microphone hearing aid technology. Ear and Hearing, 20, 1–11.

Harrison, M., Roush, J., & Wallace, J. (2003). Trends in the age of identification and intervention for deaf and hard-of-hearing infants. Ear and Hearing, 24, 89–95.

Hawkins, D. B., & Cook, J. A. (2003). Hearing aid software predictive gain values: How accurate are they? Hearing Journal, 56(7), 26–34.

Hawkins, D., & Mueller, H. G. (1992). Procedural considerations in probe-microphone measurements. In H. G. Mueller, D. B. Hawkins, & J. L. Northern (Eds.), Probe microphone measurements: Hearing instrument selection and assessment (pp. 67–89). San Diego, CA: Singular Publishing.

Hawkins, D. B., Walden, B. E., Montgomery, A., & Prosek, R. A. (1987). Description and validation of an LDL procedure designed to select SSPL90. Ear and Hearing, 8, 162–169.

Hawkins, D. B., & Yacullo, W. S. (1984). Signal-to-noise advantage of binaural hearing instruments and directional microphones under different levels of reverberation. Journal of Speech and Hearing Disorders, 49, 278–286.

Hicks, C. B., & Tharpe, A. M. (2002). Listening effort and fatigue in school-age children with and without hearing loss. Journal of Speech, Language and Hearing Research, 45(3), 573–584.

Johnson, C. D. (2001). The functional listening evaluation. Retrieved August 9, 2007, from http://www.cde.state.co.us/cdesped/download/pdf/s4-FunListEval.pdf

Johnson, C. D., & Von Almen, P. (1997). The functional listening evaluation. In C.D. Johnson, P.V. Benson, & J.B. Seaton (Eds.), Educational audiology handbook (pp 336–339). San Diego, CA: Singular Publishing Group.

Johnson, C. E. (2000). Children's phoneme identification in reverberation and noise. Journal of Speech, Language and Hearing Research, 43, 144–157.

Joint Committee on Infant Hearing (JCIH). (2000). Year 2000 position statement. Pediatrics, 106(4), 798–817.

Kawell, M. E., Kopuun, J. G., & Stelmachowicz, P. G. (1988). Loudness discomfort levels in children. Ear and Hearing, 9, 133–137.

Kochkin, S. (2000). Binaural hearing aids: The fitting of choice for bilateral loss subjects. Retrieved July 31, 2007, from http://www.betterhearing.org/research/

Kopun, J. G., & Stelmachowicz, P. G. (1998). Perceived communication difficulties in children with hearing loss. American Journal of Audiology, 7(1), 30–38.

Kruger, B., & Ruben, R. J. (1987). The acoustic properties of the infant ear: A preliminary report. Acta Otolaryngologica, 103, 578–585.

Leavitt, R. (1986). Earmolds: Acoustic and structural considerations. In W. R. Hodgson (Ed.), Hearing aid assessment and use in audiologic habilitation (3rd ed., pp. 71–108). Baltimore: Williams & Wilkins.

Leavitt, R., & Flexer, C. (1991). Speech degradation as measured by the rapid speech transmission index (RASTI). Ear and Hearing, 12, 115–118.

Lewis, D. (1997). Selection and assessment of classroom amplification. In W. McCracken & S. Laoide-Kemp (Eds.), Audiology in education (pp. 323–347). Hoboken, NJ: John Wiley & Sons, Ltd.

Lewis, D., & Eiten, L. (2005). Proposed protocol for setting FM advantage levels with MLx-S FM receivers. In R. C. Seewald & J. M. Bamford (Eds.), A sound foundation through early amplification (CD-ROM). Stäfa, Switzerland: Phonak.

Libby, E. R. (1986). The 1/3–2/3 insertion gain hearing instrument selection guide. Hearing Instruments, 37, 27–28.

Macpherson, B. J., Elfenbein, J. L., Schum, R. L., & Bentler, R. A. (1991). Thresholds of discomfort in children. Ear and Hearing, 12, 184–190.

Marriage, J. E., & Moore, B. C. J. (2003). New speech tests reveal benefit of wide-dynamic-range, fast-acting compression for consonant discrimination in children with moderate to severe hearing loss. International Journal of Audiology, 42, 418–425.

Miller-Hansen, D. R., Nelson, P., Widen, J., & Simon, S. (2003). Evaluating the benefit of speech recoding hearing aids in children. American Journal of Audiology, 12(2), 106–113.

Moeller, M. P. (2000). Early intervention and language development in children who are deaf and hard of hearing. Pediatrics, 106, E43. Retrieved August 9, 2007, from http:/www.pediatrics.org/cgi/content/full/106/3/e43

Moeller, M. P., Donaghy, K. F., Beauchaine, K. L., Lewis, D. E., & Stelmachowicz, P. G. (1996). Longitudinal study of FM system use in nonacademic settings: Effects on language development. Ear and Hearing, 17(1), 28–41.

Moodie, K. S., Seewald, R. C., & Sinclair, S. T. (1994). Procedure for predicting real-ear hearing instrument performance in young children. American Journal of Audiology, 3(1), 23–31.

National Center for Hearing Assessment and Management (NCHAM). (2006). Reported average ages of confirmation of significant hearing loss in the U.S. in the absence of universal newborn hearing screening. Retrieved July 27, 2007, from http://infanthearing.org/background/ageid/html

National Center for Hearing Assessment and Management (NCHAM). (2007). State summary statistics: Universal newborn hearing screening. Retrieved July 27, 2007, from http://infanthearing.org/status/ unhsstate.html

Nittrouer, S., & Boothroyd, A. (1990). Context effects in phoneme and word recognition by young children and older adults. Journal of the Acoustical Society of America, 87, 50–57.

Nozza, R. J., Rossman, R. N. F., Bond, L. C., & Miller, S. L. (1990). Infant speech-sound discrimination in noise. Journal of the Acoustical Society of America, 87, 339–350.

OTICON. (n.d.). Children's outcome worksheet. Retrieved August 10, 2007 from http://www.oticonusa.com/SiteGen/Uploads/Public/Downloads_Oticon/Pediatrics/cow.pdf

Palmer, C., & Mormer, E. (1997). A systematic program for hearing aid orientation and adjustment. High Performance Hearing Solutions, 1(Suppl.), 45–52.

Palmer, C. V., & Mormer, E. (1999). Goals and expectations of the hearing aid fitting. Trends in Amplification, 4(2), 61–71.

Pediatric Working Group of the Conference on Amplification for Children with Auditory Deficits. (1996). Amplification for infants and children with hearing loss. American Journal of Audiology, 5(1), 53–68.

Platz, R. (2004). SNR advantage, FM advantage, and FM fitting. In D. Fabry & C. Deconde Johnson (Eds.), Achieving clear communication employing sound solutions (pp. 147–154). Stäfa, Switzerland: Phonak.

Ricketts, T. A., & Tharpe, A. M. (2005). Potential for directivity-based benefit in actual classroom environments. In R. C. Seewald & J.M. Bamford (Eds.), A sound foundation through early amplification (pp. 143–154). Stäfa, Switzerland: Phonak.

Robbins, A. M., Renshaw, J. J., & Berry, S. (1991). Evaluating meaningful auditory integration in profoundly hearing-impaired children. American Journal of Otology, 12(Suppl.), 144–150.

Ruben, R. J. (1997). A time frame of critical/sensitive periods of language development. Acta Otolaryngologica, 117, 202–205.

Scollie, S., Seewald, R., Cornelisse, L. Moodie, S., Bagatto, M., Laurnagaray, D., et al. (2005). The Desired Sensation Level multistage input/output algorithm. Trends in Amplification, 9(4), 159–197.

Scollie, S. D., Steinberg, M. J., & Seewald, R. C. (2002). Evaluation of electroacoustic test signals: 2. Development and cross-validation of correction factors. Ear and Hearing, 23(5), 488–498.

Seewald, R., Moodie, S., Scollie, S. & Bagatt., M. (2005). The DSL method for pediatric hearing instrument fitting. Historical perspective and current issues. Trends in Amplification, 9(4), 145–157.

Seewald, R. C., Sinclair, S. T., & Moodie, K. S. (1994, April). Predictive accuracy of a procedure for electroacoustic fitting in young children. Paper presented at the convention of the American Academy of Audiology, Richmond, VA.

Simpson, A., Hersbach, A., & McDermott, H. (2005). Improvements in speech perception with an experimental nonlinear frequency compression hearing device. International Journal of Audiology, 44(5), 281–292.

Sinclair, S. T., Beauchaine, K. L., Moodie, K. S., & Feigin, J. A. (1994, April). Repeatability of a real-ear to coupler difference measurement as a function of age. Paper presented at the convention of the American Academy of Audiology, Richmond, VA.

Stelmachowicz, P. G., & Lewis, D. E. (1988). Some theoretical considerations concerning the relation between functional gain and insertion gain. Journal of Speech and Hearing Research, 31, 491–496.

Stelmachowicz, P. G., Mace, A. I., Kopun, J. G., & Carney, E. (1993). Long-term and short-term characteristics of speech: Implications for hearing instrument selection for young children. Journal of Speech and Hearing Research, 36(3), 609–620.

Stelmachowicz, P. G., Pittman, A. L., Hoover, B. M., & Lewis, D. E. (2002). Aided perception of /s/ and /z/ by hearing-impaired children. Ear and Hearing, 23(4), 316–324.

Stredler-Brown, A., & Johnson, D. C. (2003). Functional auditory performance indicators: An integrated approach to auditory development. Retrieved from http://www.csdb.org/chip/resources/docs/fapi6_23.pdf

Stuart, A., Durieux-Smith, A., & Stenstrom, R. (1990). Critical differences in aided sound field thresholds in children. Journal of Speech and Hearing Research, 33, 612–615.

Tharpe, A. M., Fino-Szumski, M. S., & Bess, F. H. (2001). Survey of hearing aid fitting practices for children with multiple disabilities. American Journal of Audiology, 10(1), 32–40.

Westwood, G. F. S., & Bamford, J. M. (1995). Probe-tube microphone measures with very young infants: Real-ear to coupler differences and longitudinal changes in real-ear unaided response. Ear and Hearing, 16(3), 263–273.

Yoshinaga-Itano, C., Sedey, A., Coulter, D., & Mehl, A. (1998). Language of early- and later-identified children with hearing loss. Pediatrics, 102(5), 1161–1171.

Zimmerman-Phillips, S., Robbins, A. M., & Osberger, M. J. (2000). Assessing cochlear implant benefit in very young children. Annals of Otology, Rhinology and Laryngology Supplment, 185, 42–44.

Chapter 5

Hearing Aid Selection and Fitting in Adults

Catherine V. Palmer, George A. Lindley IV, and Elaine A. Mormer

The purpose of this chapter is to teach students how to select and evaluate assistive technology, including hearing aids, in adults. To meet that goal, students must be provided with a framework within which to think about fitting amplification, because fitting hearing aids is both an art and a science. This chapter has been approached in the same manner (see Palmer, 1998, for a complete description of a hearing aid curriculum). The basic framework consists of what audiologists need to measure, up-front decisions that have to be made regarding the hearing aids, ordering/selecting the hearing aids, verification of the selection, orientation, follow-up and fine-tuning of the hearing aid response, and outcomes assessment. It is essential to interrelate the various components. For instance, measurements related to the patient must be used to order the hearing aids and to verify performance. Audiologists will always need to measure something about the auditory system or decide to use average data. Hearing aids will have to be obtained and preset in some fashion. Some sort of verification is necessary to ensure that the audiologist has done what was planned. Finally, an evaluation will be necessary to establish that the use of hearing aids has made an impact on the individual in some positive way. The following information describes a reasonable way to approach selecting, fitting, and evaluating hearing aid technology in adults.

This framework is consistent with and expands upon the various hearing aid fitting guidelines that have been published by experts over the years. Valente et al (2006), in particular, have produced a comprehensive evidence-based hearing aid fitting guideline. This text is consistent with the general outline of that guideline and provides details on accomplishing goals set forth there. In addition, wherever possible, the authors have highlighted evidence that supports the recommendations made in this chapter.

In the first edition of this text, the fitting and selection of conventional hearing aids and programmable/digital hearing aids were discussed in separate chapters. This distinction has become erroneous, and therefore the selection and fitting of hearing aids are now discussed in one chapter. There are, however, distinctions in the ordering and presetting process between these technologies, and these differences will be pointed out when necessary throughout the chapter.

For the purposes of this text, conventional hearing aids are defined by what they are not. Conventional hearing aids are not programmable by means of a computer interface or handheld programmer. The difference between programmable hearing aids and conventional hearing aids is that one must choose desired hearing aid responses before receiving the conventional hearing aid. Programmable hearing aids, however, offer room for error because one can manipulate various parameters (compression ratio [CR], gain, crossover frequency, etc.). Thus, conventional hearing aids can be thought of as less flexible and in need of more precise ordering specifications. In addition, conventional hearing aids differ from programmable hearing aids in how the audiologist interacts with the hearing aid specifications and the manufacturer.

If one is unsure how to manipulate various programmable parameters, the approach outlined for conventional technology may serve as a good starting point whether ordering conventional technology or programming digitally programmable technology.

♦ Goals of the Hearing Aid Fitting

The goals of hearing aid fittings do not change whether one is fitting conventional or programmable technology. Most audiologists can agree on the following major set of goals for a hearing aid fitting: sounds are audible but not uncomfortable, the hearing aids provide good sound quality and a safe listening environment, and amplification meets the patient's communication needs and expectations. Most also would add that hearing aids should improve speech recognition in quiet and noise, but this most likely is included in the patient's communication needs and expectations. The goals do not change depending on the technology chosen. How these goals are met may change slightly.

The goals of each fitting (some will apply to all fittings, and some will be specific to the individual) should be defined before hearing aid selection in that they should dictate much of the selection and measurement procedures. They should dictate how the hearing aids ultimately will be assessed. In other words, if sound quality is essential, selection is impacted (one might want circuitry that demonstrates low distortion, including compression output limiting), and the individual's perception of sound quality should be incorporated into the verification procedure. If audibility is important, circuitry that can make a wide range of input signals audible (e.g., wide dynamic range compression [WDRC]) might be selected, and the individual's ability to hear soft, average, and loud sounds might be assessed during the hearing aid fitting. In addition, if a feature has been deemed important enough to order for the individual (e.g., telecoil, noise reduction, directional microphones, or feedback management), then the feature's performance should be verified. A mechanism should be available for measuring each of the goals of the hearing aid fitting whether the goal is physical (fit of the earmold) or subjective (improving the quality of an individual's life).

♦ Evaluation and Measurement of the Auditory System, Environment, and Individual

At a minimum, one must document an individual's ear-specific thresholds as a function of frequency to start the fitting process. However, there is more about the auditory system, the listening environment, and the individual that may assist in the selection and fitting of hearing aids.

Evaluation of the Auditory System

At present, some clinicians and researchers are advocating measurement of an individual's loudness growth to assist in the selection of a hearing aid's response. Loudness growth may be interpolated by measuring an individual's threshold and uncomfortable loudness level. This assumes a fairly linear growth of loudness between the two end points. These data are not mandatory but can be used in selection programs such as National Acoustic Laboratories' Revised (NAL-R; Byrne and Dillon, 1986) and desired sensation level input/output (DSL [i/o]; Cornelisse et al, 1994). Individual loudness growth curves do not assume that individual loudness growth functions are linear from the threshold of detection to the threshold of discomfort and, perhaps more importantly, that comfortable loudness is halfway between the threshold of detection and the threshold of discomfort (see also Pascoe, 1989; Valente et al, 1997).

The amount of auditory data that one collects will depend on one's interest in individual-specific measures and which hearing aid fitting program is being used. One may be comfortable using a hearing aid fitting program with average data as a starting point with programmable instruments because the hearing aids can be fine-tuned through a variety of verification procedures. One may become less comfortable with this protocol when using conventional instruments that cannot be manipulated to such a large extent. Unfortunately, there are no carefully controlled studies that provide clear evidence as to whether using individual loudness growth data improves the outcome of a hearing aid fitting.

Additional measures can be employed to define auditory function more specifically, predict aided performance, and help in the selection of appropriate hearing aid features. For example, the primary complaint of most individuals with hearing loss, both when unaided and aided, is speech recognition in the presence of background noise. The standard diagnostic audiologic evaluation typically includes word recognition ability in quiet. Testing in noise often is not completed. Although poor performance in quiet is likely associated with poor performance in noise, the reverse cannot be said for those with normal word recognition ability in quiet. Performance in quiet is often not a good predictor of performance in noise.

Current technology provides the audiologist and patient with several options to address speech recognition in noise, including directionality and digital noise reduction schemes. Measurement of speech recognition ability in noise up-front may be a useful measure in determining candidacy for these options and realistic expectations. Fewer than 25% of audiologists indicated they routinely measure speech recognition ability in noise prior to the hearing aid fitting (Lindley, 2005). Of those who do, most conduct the testing unaided using a conversational presentation level, thus limiting usefulness as a predictor of aided ability.

Two popular commercially available speech-in-noise tests are the Hearing in Noise Test (HINT; Nilsson et al, 1994) and the QuickSIN (Killion et al, 2004) test. Both are easily administered via an audiometer and compact disc (CD) player. With some experience, a measure can be obtained in approximately 5 minutes. The test metric is a signal-to-noise ratio (SNR). The QuickSIN determines the SNR at which a patient performs at a predetermined level (e.g., SNR at which the patient correctly repeats half the target words or sentences). This can be compared with normal performance, and an SNR "loss" can be determined. For example, a patient with an SNR loss of 5 dB would need the target speech 5 dB louder to perform at the same level as a normal hearing individual. This SNR loss is useful in determining whether an option such as a directional microphone may be beneficial or whether hearing assistive technology (HAT) would be more appropriate. HINT provides an SNR value that is determined through a bracketing procedure that adjusts the level of the noise until 50% of the sentences are repeated correctly. Like QuickSIN, these data can be compared with normal performance for this measure.

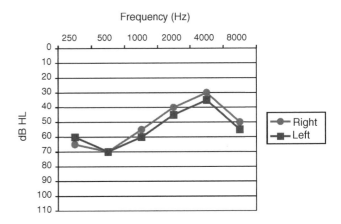

Figure 5–1 Patient with poor speech recognition ability in noise and a low-frequency dead hair cell region. Signal-to-noise ration (SNR) loss: left, 13 dB; right, 12 dB. Dead region at 500 Hz bilaterally. HL, hearing level.

The testing protocol may vary depending on the goal. If the purpose is to assess how much difficulty a patient will have once audibility is restored, then an elevated presentation level is employed. The idea is to minimize audibility as a contributor and assess the degree of suprathreshold damage.

Consider the audiometric findings from a patient in **Fig. 5–1.** Given the relatively mild degree of high-frequency hearing loss coupled with good word recognition ability in quiet, one might expect this patient to perform adequately in background noise when properly aided. Testing using the QuickSIN at an audible presentation level, however, revealed a large SNR loss bilaterally (left = 13 dB, right = 12 dB). Current hearing aid technology alone would not likely overcome this deficit. Although the patient may notice some improvement in noise, it would be unrealistic to expect functioning close to normal, and a frequency modulation (FM) system could be considered if understanding in noise is a goal.

Testing for cochlear "dead regions" has been proposed as an additional measure that can aid in determining realistic expectations, appropriate technology, and appropriate hearing aid settings. A cochlear dead region is typically defined as a region of the cochlea with extensive inner hair cell damage. A "disconnect" between the peripheral auditory system and the central auditory system may exist, and the patient may not be able to make use of an audible signal in this region. The results of several studies have shown that, as a group, individuals with confirmed or suspected dead regions may perform poorer than expected when aided, especially in difficult listening situations (Baer et al, 2002; Mackersie et al, 2004; Preminger et al, 2005).

The Threshold Equalizing Noise (TEN) test has been proposed as a clinical measure for determining if cochlear dead region(s) are present in a given patient (Moore et al, 2000). With the TEN test, a specially shaped broadband masking noise is introduced to the ear to create equal masked thresholds. If 80 dB sound pressure level (SPL) of noise is introduced to the ear, and thresholds are retested, they should fall at ~80 dB hearing level (HL). In cochlear dead regions, the masked thresholds are often at least 15 dB poorer than the level of the masking noise because areas adjacent to the dead region no longer respond to the tone (as was the case during audiometric testing). Summers et al (2003) compared the TEN test to psychophysical tuning curves and reported fair to poor agreement. These results led Preminger et al (2005) to suggest updated criteria for interpreting the TEN test results. The TEN test is a relatively new tool, and the implications of finding cochlear dead regions with regard to the hearing aid fitting protocol have not been fully realized. Although some of these individuals may benefit from amplification in the dead region, others may not. Summers (2004) provided data illustrating that experienced clinicians generally could judge the severity of hearing loss at which the individual was unlikely to receive amplification benefit without administering the TEN test. The clinician must pick and choose tests that will inform the hearing aid selection and verification process and must be cognizant of time constraints related to all of the procedures used.

The presence of dead regions does have implications with regard to realistic expectations and may have value concerning adjustment of the hearing aid. For example, consider the patient data in **Fig. 5–1** discussed earlier. TEN testing revealed a low-frequency dead region bilaterally. This could help explain why the patient was more satisfied with less low-frequency gain than initially prescribed. In addition, the patient noted significant benefit from the digital noise reduction scheme in his hearing aids, likely due to attenuation of low-frequency noises.

This type of evaluation might assist the clinician in deciding which frequencies should be amplified. For instance, if a clinician knows that making sound audible at 4000 Hz will not assist a particular patient, the time in the hearing aid fitting will focus on audibility at the lower frequencies. In addition, an individual who cannot benefit from audibility at most of the high frequencies might become a reasonable candidate for a frequency transposition hearing aid (a hearing aid that transposes the inaudible high frequencies to low-frequency sound).

Pearl

• Research has shown that individuals with cochlear dead regions as a group do not benefit as much from amplification as do individuals without dead regions. There is significant variability, however, and some patients achieve additional benefit from amplification into the dead region. A conservative approach may be appropriate. The patient could be given the opportunity to benefit from amplification in these regions. However, if provision of significant amplification in a dead region elicits sound quality complaints, loudness issues, and other problems, one may be more aggressive in reducing gain early in the fitting process.

As mentioned earlier, understanding in noise is a concern for most patients with hearing loss. The ability to tolerate background noise also is a concern. Nabelek and colleagues (Nabelek, 2005; Nabelek et al, 2004) have suggested the

acceptable noise level (ANL) as a premeasure that may help determine needed hearing aid features and that may predict ultimate hearing aid success. The patient adjusts running speech to most comfortable level (MCL) and then adjusts the background noise level (BNL) to the highest level that is considered acceptable while listening to the speech. The smaller the ANL, the smaller the SNR that the subject found acceptable. Nabelek et al (2004) have reported that ANLs do not change over time, are not related to speech recognition scores, are unaffected by amplification, and are related to hearing aid use (i.e., individuals who use their hearing aids more had smaller ANLs). Audiologists will want to follow the data related to this technique to determine if it will aid in hearing aid selection and/or predicting amplification success.

It is evident that a variety of tests are available with the goal of assisting in hearing aid selection, presetting, and verification. It is incumbent upon the clinician to select a test that will provide critical data in a reasonable time frame. Clinicians continue to await scientific evidence related to tests that will enhance the hearing aid selection and fitting process.

Evaluation of Individual Communication Needs and the Listening Environment

Palmer and Mormer (1997) provide a systematic approach to hearing instrument orientation and adjustment. As part of that program, several forms for gathering patient information are presented. Specifically, the Hearing Demand, Ability, and Need Profile (**Fig. 5–2**) is used as a systematic interviewing tool that should define the patient's current communication abilities and demands, as well as the patient's communication needs. Communication needs are identified as a function of situation (alerting, one-to-one communication, etc.), hearing aid use, and listening environment. This worksheet allows data to be collected and analyzed easily. The results of the worksheet should lead directly to hearing solutions. These might include hearing aid features and/or assistive technology. For instance, difficulty in one-to-one communication because of background noise might lead one to consider directional microphone technology for the hearing aids, whereas difficulty in large group situations caused by distance might lead to coupling HAT to hearing aids that are equipped with direct audio input (DAI) or telecoil technology (see Chapters 1 and 17 in this volume). This type of measurement is used extensively in making up-front decisions regarding the hearing aid. The form is revisited after the hearing aid has been fit and worn for several months to evaluate whether all of the individual's communication needs have been met or whether further technology and/or communication strategies need to be pursued.

At the same time the clinician is investigating the patient's auditory abilities and communication needs, it is essential to establish realistic expectations as to the benefit that can be expected from the selected intervention. In a survey assessing the hearing aid fitting practices of audiologists, "unrealistic expectations" was chosen as the most common reason patients return their hearing aids

| Age | Description of Communication Milestone/Activity | Communication Problem is Present With Hearing Aid... | | | | | | The Problem Is Due to... | | | | Current Compensation |
| | | Home | | Work | | Travel | | | | | | |
		ON	OFF	ON	OFF	ON	OFF	Hearing	Noise	Distance	Visibility	(describe)
	Alerting											
	Telephone bell											
	Doorbell											
	Door knock											
	Alarm clock											
	Smoke alarm											
	Siren											
	Turn signal											
	Peronal pager											
	Personal Communication											
	Telephone											
	TV/stereo/radio											
	One-to-one (planned)											
	One-to-one (unplanned)											
	Group											
	Large room											
	Other Activities											
	Clubs/games											
	Lessons											
	Sports											
Further information (e.g., status of hearing aids, telecoil, DAI, communication environment):												
Recommendations (assistive technology, communication strategies, environmental manipulation)												

Figure 5–2 Hearing Demand, Ability, and Need Profile. DAI, direct audio input. (Adapted from High performance hearing solutions. (1997). Hearing Review, 1 (Suppl), with permission.)

(Lindley, 2005). One goal of the hearing aid selection process should include determination, to the extent possible, of how a patient can expect to perform when aided.

The Patient Expectation Worksheet (PEW, **Fig. 5–3**) is used to document the patient's expectations of the forthcoming intervention (hearing aids, HATs, communication strategies, etc.). This form is similar to the Client Oriented Scale of Improvement (COSI) developed by Dillon et al (1997). On the COSI, the listener rates his or her degree of change in hearing ability with use of the hearing instruments after hearing aid use; with the PEW, the listener rates current level of ability unaided, expected level of aided ability, and final aided ability. The patient generates two specific expectations. The clinician may have to assist the patient in creating specific expectations as opposed to general goals. For example, "hearing better in noise" is too general a comment. The patient should be questioned until a specific situation can be identified (e.g., "understanding what my 5-year-old daughter says at the dinner table"). The patient then indicates how he or she is performing currently and how he or she expects to perform after intervention. The clinician uses a check mark to indicate what would be considered a reasonable expectation given the patient's audition and the technology being pursued. This creates a

forum for assisting the patient in forming realistic expectations if the clinician's check mark and the patient's expectation are not in agreement. It also can provide a meaningful discussion of some of the up-front decisions regarding the hearing aid(s) that the patient has made. For instance, if the patient insists on pursuing monaural amplification when binaural amplification is indicated, the clinician can demonstrate that the level of success expected in noisy situations will be lower as a result of this decision. This helps all parties to understand that the up-front decisions made regarding hearing aid features will directly affect the outcome of the hearing aid fitting.

PEW is used to further assist in up-front decision making on the basis of the patient's communication goals. The expectations are used as an outcome measure in that the patient will indicate how he or she is performing after the intervention (short period of hearing aid use). If the patient is not meeting or exceeding the realistic expectations that were recorded on the sheet, the clinician and patient work to understand what further remediation needs to be implemented. Again, this can be a valuable counseling tool. If the patient indicates that dinner conversation is still a problem, and the clinician's interview reveals that the television is on during dinner, an obvious recommendation would be to

I am successful in this situation…

Goal (list in order of priority)	Hardly Ever	Occasionally	Half the Time	Most of the Time	Almost Always
1.					
2.					
3.					
4.					
5.					

C = how the client functions currently (pretreatment or with current technology/strategies)

E = how the client expects to function post intervention (HA, ALD, strategies, etc.)

√ = level of success that the audiologist realistically targets

A = how the client/family actually perceives level of success postfitting

Figure 5–3 The Patient Expectation Worksheet. HA, hearing aid; ALD, assistive listening device. (From High Performance Hearing Solutions. (1997). Hearing Review, 1 (Suppl), with permission.)

eliminate the television. If the individual is doing everything according to plan, and dinner conversation is still difficult, a directional microphone (if not already included) or an assistive device might be considered. Once all the individual's communication goals are met, the individual may generate new goals that he or she had not thought of until communication began to improve.

The Cleveland Clinic Group recently created the Characteristics of Amplification Tool (COAT; Sandridge and Newman, 2006), which provides a paper-and-pencil questionnaire that explores the patient's personal preferences and expectations. Expectations related to style of the hearing aid and price are included, as well as performance expectations, which are the primary focus of FEW and COSI.

Because a lack of speech recognition tasks that will be sensitive enough to document change before and after hearing aid fitting exists, and it is questionable whether one speech recognition task could measure all the possible benefits of wearing appropriate amplification, the clinician may want to use a measurement of hearing handicap or hearing aid benefit as an outcome measure. The authors routinely use the Abbreviated Profile of Hearing Aid Benefit (APHAB; Cox and Alexander, 1995) to further assess communication needs that may be addressed by the variety of up-front decisions made in the hearing aid selection process. Perhaps more importantly, the before and after APHAB scores are compared with a benefit score that can be used to document the hearing aid fitting outcome. Alternatively, the absolute post-APHAB scores can be compared with results from normal-hearing individuals (Cox, 1997). Demonstrating a return to normal performance can be very powerful for the individual seeking amplification.

Evaluation of Individual Physical Measurements

Real ear measures play a role in both diagnostic measures made before ordering the hearing aids and verification measures. (See Chapter 3 in this volume for a detailed description of real ear measures.) The amplification goal must be established at the time of measurement to realistically expect success in the verification process. For example, if one intends to verify the fitting with insertion gain measurements [real ear aided response (REAR) minus the individual's real ear unaided gain (REUG)], one would want to measure the REUG to be included in the selection of the hearing aid and select a fitting protocol allowing for its incorporation. In addition, the fitting protocol should include insertion gain targets for use in verification. The hearing aid fitting goal should be consistent across procedures and must be understood early on for the correct measurements, selection procedure, and verification measures to be used.

Compromises are made each time average data are used regarding a patient's responses or regarding individual ear characteristics. These compromises may be worth making for the sake of time management, but it is important to understand that a choice is being made. With conventional fittings, time may be better used up-front to obtain accurate measures because the conventional hearing aid may not be flexible enough to correct for deviations in response from targets as a result of individual ear differences from average. The real-ear measurements that may add to the accuracy of the hearing aid fitting are described later in this chapter, and case examples are provided to illustrate what may be gained from inclusion of individual-specific data in the hearing aid ordering process.

Armed with the evaluation data (auditory system, communication environment, and the individual's needs), the clinician is ready to make the up-front decisions required before selecting and ordering a hearing aid.

♦ Up-front Decisions

Up-front decisions are decisions that must be made in the selection process of any hearing aid(s). The difference between conventional and programmable hearing aids may be in when the decision can be made. For instance, with many programmable hearing aids, the clinician can create a linear or WDRC response depending on how the clinician manipulates the CR parameter. Peak clipping (PC), output compression limiting (OCL), and WDRC may be programmable parameters, so the decision of how to output limit the hearing aid(s) does not have to be made before selection of the hearing aid(s). With conventional technology, these decisions will have to be made up-front, or the decision of what potentiometers to order to allow these choices must be made up-front. The up-front decisions are made through a combination of information gleaned from the Hearing Demand, Ability, and Need Profile **(Fig. 5–2)**, PEW **(Fig. 5–3)**, APHAB, audiometric data, speech-in-noise testing, clinical experience, and empirical data. The patient will be involved in making some of these decisions. The realistic expectations that were documented on the PEW may have to be modified on the basis of some of the up-front decisions that are dictated by the patient. This provides a meaningful format for discussion of an individual's preferences.

In addition, various up-front decisions will impact other decisions. Based on the configuration of a patient's hearing loss, the audiologist may have chosen a behind-the-ear (BTE) model with a large vent (i.e., to allow natural low-frequency hearing in light of normal low-frequency thresholds). Other test results may have indicated the need for automatic/adaptive microphones (e.g., difficulty in noise and difficulty manipulating memory buttons). In this case, directional microphone technology will be implemented by digital signal processing (DSP). A large vent may reduce the effectiveness of directional microphones, and the electronic delay caused by DSP may be more noticeable when some hearing is achieved directly through an open vent. In this case, the need for better hearing in noise will most likely outweigh the desire for natural hearing in the low frequencies, and the venting option will be changed.

The list of up-front decisions is constantly changing in view of new technology and new research. Items are deleted and items are added. **Table 5–1** provides a current list of up-front decisions and a line to record the decision made (or action taken). Although the experienced clinician may not fill out this list every time hearing aids are dispensed, the wise clinician will review this list periodically to make sure that conscious decisions backed by patient and/or empirical data are made for every item. Decisions related to signal processing are considered up-front as well. These specific decisions are discussed in greater detail below.

Signal-Processing Requirements

Signal-processing decisions include expansion/compression, number of channels, bandwidth, type of microphone technology, noise reduction algorithms, and active feedback control.

Table 5–1 Decisions To Be Made before Ordering a Hearing Aid

Decision	
Air versus bone conduction	
Style/type/spare	
Routing of the signal (e.g., conventional, CROS, BICROS, BAHA, CI, middle ear implantable)	
Frequency transposition	
Monaural versus binaural	
Earmold material/type/color	
Earmold length and venting	
Sound channel/earhook	
Bandwidth	
Volume control (lock)	
Receiver type (class A or B)	
Output limiting	
Battery door lock	
Ability to fine-tune	
Multiple memories	
Remote control	
Telephone access	
Coupling to HATs	
Previous experience	
Signal processing	

BAHA, bone-anchored hearing aid; BICROS, bilateral contralateral routing of signals; CI, cochlear implant; CROS, contralateral routing of signals; HAT, hearing assistive technology.

Current signal-processing techniques are described in detail in Chapter 1 in this text. These techniques are described below to illustrate the decisions that must be made during the hearing aid selection process. Some choices will deal with whether a feature is desired, and some choices will affect how flexible that feature needs to be. In digital hearing aids, analog signals received by the microphone and sent through the preamplifier are converted to a series of binary digits (represented by 0s and 1s). Numerous mathematical calculations can be applied to the signal represented in this way. These manipulations generally are referred to as algorithms and may be dictated by the manufacturer or may be impacted by the audiologist programming the hearing aid(s). A new set of binary digits is created and then reconverted to an analog signal, which the receiver (loudspeaker) of the hearing aid produces as a sound in the ear canal. Although certain signal-processing schemes require digital processing, this text will focus on the strategies, not whether a clinician needs digital versus analog processing to implement them. The audiologist needs to determine what signal-processing strategies are appropriate for a given patient. In some cases, the desired signal processing will require the use of a digital hearing aid, whereas in other cases, it will not. It is likely that all hearing aids will be digital in the near future because that is the state of technology. In that case, the audiologist must continue to identify the desired processing strategies because it is likely that different "levels" of digital technology will provide different signal-processing strategies. Conventional (nonprogrammable) digital hearing aids already exist. The choice of appropriate features and signal-processing strategies is paramount, and determining how these are implemented (digital or analog) is relatively easy. The various signal-processing choices will be highlighted below, and the evidence base for these features will be provided. The technology hierarchy versus style breakout in **Table 5–2** can be used when counseling technology levels with a patient. (Various prices would replace the dollar signs.) The technology levels are described according to flexibility and features. Level of technology and style largely drive the cost of hearing instruments, so this becomes a reasonable way to discuss features and pricing. If the patient has responded to COAT (described earlier), his or her views on style, technology, and cost will already be known to the clinician.

Signal-Processing Induced Delays

Most hearing aids now feature DSP between the microphone and the receiver; this has opened up a seemingly endless number of manipulations that can be performed on the signal that enters the microphone. The computations performed on the digitized signal by these devices introduce a delay between the arrival of the signal at the hearing aid microphone (the ear) and the delivery of the signal to the ear canal. This is referred to as digital delay and is defined as the amount of time necessary for an acoustic signal to pass through the microphone, the DSP circuit, and the receiver of the hearing aid. A potential problem exists when there is a difference in arrival of the undelayed signal (through a vent path) and the delayed signal (through the hearing aid). Hearing aid users may describe an "echo" perception. In addition, DSP delays may be asynchronous in instruments making use of multiple frequency channels, which means that part of the bandwidth may be delayed relative to another part of the bandwidth (e.g., low vs high frequencies). An asynchronous delay will vary the formant relationships within a sound and alter the perception. The literature regarding the quantitative effects of digital delay on speech perception and production has grown substantially in recent years (see Stone and Moore, 2005). Digital delay is mentioned in the context of this text to remind the reader that, although an endless number of digital signal manipulations may be possible, manufacturers ultimately are constrained by the detrimental delay that is introduced in perceiving the original signal. Although there are variations in the reported amount of acceptable delay due to differences in research methodology, it appears that more than 15 msec of delay would begin to interfere with the listener's ability to process signals comfortably. Currently, no commercially available hearing aids are reporting >15 msec average delay. Research is only beginning to investigate the consequences of these delays on speech perception.

Table 5–2 Technology Hierarchy and Hearing Aid Styles

Technology	Behind the Ear	In the Ear	In the Canal	Completely in the Canal
Greatest flexibility, many frequency channels, automatic volume control, noise reduction, automatic/adaptive directional microphones, adaptive feedback control. Adjust gain for quiet and loud inputs independently, ability to custom arrange order and use of memories, many custom features available	$	$	$	$
Many adjustable frequency channels, automatic volume control, noise reduction, adaptive directional microphones, multiple memories, adjust gain for quiet and loud inputs independently	$	$	$	$
Several adjustable frequency channels, automatic volume control, direction microphones, adjust gain for quiet and loud inputs independently	$	$	$	$
Some flexibility, one frequency channel, user-operated volume control	$	$	$	$

The audiologist would fill in the dollars amounts.

Compression and Expansion

The most common signal-processing technique to provide audible signals across a wide range of input levels (soft, moderate, and loud) is WDRC (Jenstad et al, 1999; Marriage et al, 2005). Ideally, the programmable amplification system chosen for a patient will allow the manipulation of the CR. This is implemented by many manufacturers by allowing the independent manipulation of gain for soft and loud sounds. Manipulation of these parameters is the same as the manipulation of the CR (e.g., if the gain for soft sounds is increased without changing the gain for loud sounds, the CR is increased).

In an attempt to make the quietest sounds audible, some hearing aid users complain they are hearing too many soft sounds (e.g., the sound of a refrigerator motor) that are annoying or interfere with other listening tasks. Expansion provides increasing gain as a function of input level (the opposite of compression where gain decreases as a function of input level) and can be implemented to reduce these very quiet, unwanted sounds. The latest hearing aids come with software that allows for the implementation of several levels of expansion. Expansion has always been used by manufacturers to reduce microphone noise that can be noticeable to hearing aid users with good low-frequency hearing.

The components other than compression threshold (CT) and CR that define compression are the attack and release times. These are the time constants applied to transitioning the circuit from linear (or expansion) to compression (attack time) or transitioning from compression to linear (or expansion; release time). Although most commercially available hearing aids are designed with fast attack times ($\leq$ 10 msec), debate continues over the best use of fast and slow release times. There are data to support a fast release time to maintain audibility for speech that can vary from syllable to syllable by as much as 30 dB, but there also are proponents of slower release times to ensure that unwanted noise does not fill quiet gaps in speech (Bentler and Nelson, 1997; Hansen, 2002; Neuman et al, 1995). The newer technology is implementing both fast and slow release times based on the sampling of the signal that is conducted by the DSP. Different manufacturers have produced different algorithms to implement this decision making. The audiologist may choose to use amplification systems that allow programming of attack and release times, although there are few published data to assist in knowing how to adjust these times based on patient preferences.

Number of Channels

The useful dynamic range for a hearing-impaired individual often changes across frequencies (e.g., much wider dynamic range in the low frequencies, with a narrower dynamic range in the midfrequencies, and an extremely narrow dynamic range in the higher frequencies for a typical sloping sensorineural hearing loss). With the advent of multiple frequency channels in hearing aids, different compression characteristics can be applied to the different frequency regions. A channel is a bandwidth in which an independent amplifier is assigned to control the compression characteristics.

There is evidence that two to four channels is adequate for speech recognition (Keidser and Grant, 2001). More channels may be useful for resolving complaints other than speech intelligibility that impact acceptability of the hearing aid. These include the sound of one's own voice when wearing hearing aids and the problem of acoustic feedback. Currently, the number of channels is an up-front decision that the audiologist will make based primarily on the configuration of the hearing loss and other signal-processing goals (e.g., adaptive feedback control).

Bandwidth

Audibility as a function of input level has been discussed, but audibility as a function of bandwidth is critical as well. Current microphone and receiver technology provides a fairly flat frequency response from 100 to 16,000 Hz. Commercially available hearing aids, however, provide a frequency response from ~500 to 5000 Hz. This reduced bandwidth does not adequately represent essential formats for higher pitched consonants (e.g., /s/ and /z/) or music. Stelmachowicz et al (2002) revealed that pediatric listeners required audibility through 8000 Hz to perceive the /s/ sound that is essential to language development and speech recognition in English (possessives, verb tense, and plurals). Adults with language experience may not need quite as robust a representation of the speech signal because of their use of context, but whenever audibility is lacking, individuals are using more effort to comprehend. In addition, speech is not the only input signal to the hearing aid. Bandwidth limitation is attributed to the DSP and the resulting battery drain. The audiologist should be aware of the available bandwidth in the selected hearing aids.

Type of Microphone Technology

All hearing aids are equipped with omnidirectional microphones that collect sound from all directional sources to be amplified without relative delay. Directional microphones employ the use of (an) additional rear-facing microphone(s) or microphone port(s). The input signal arriving from behind the listener enters the back microphone (port) slightly before entering the front microphone port. An internal circuit delay is added to the path of the rear microphone (port), so that the two signals meet at the same time and cancel each other. Thus, microphone sensitivity to sounds arriving from behind the listener is reduced (e.g., sounds arriving from behind are attenuated). The directional sensitivity pattern of the microphones is determined by the ratio of the external delay (microphone port spacing) to the internal delay (a mechanical or electrical filter in the rear microphone). With the use of directional microphones, the signal at the null(s) (generally to the sides or behind the user) is provided with less microphone sensitivity and therefore is reduced relative to other signals.

Effective use of directional microphone technology requires the user to position himself or herself correctly within the environment. Ideally, the signal of interest should be to the front, the listener should not be beyond the critical listening distance, and the room should have a relatively low reverberation time (Ricketts and Hornsby, 2003). The farther the listener is from the wanted signal source or the more reverberation that is present, the less effective this technology will be for assisting with communication in noise.

Directional microphone technology is continually evolving with the implementation of three microphones, adaptive directional settings where the polar pattern changes depending on the acoustic environment being sampled by the digital circuit, and automatic directional devices that switch from the omnidirectional polar plot to a fixed or adaptive directional setting. Bentler (2005) provided an evidence-based review of the clinical use of directional microphones and concluded that directional microphones offer additional advantages over amplification alone.

Noise Reduction Algorithms

Digital noise reduction (DNR) circuitry also has been promoted for alleviation of difficulties in noise. Bentler (2005) reviewed the evidence base for use of DNR systems and concluded that there is no evidence to support the use of this signal processing as currently implemented for improving communication in noise, but that DNR may provide improved listening ease in select environments. The principle of the noise reduction (NR) algorithm is to reduce ambient noise in the environment by analysis of the acoustic properties of the incoming signal. The temporal and spectral characteristics of noise consist of a steady-state or constant level with a broad frequency bandwidth. In contrast, the acoustic properties of conversational speech are frequency specific and dynamic. By capitalizing on these contrasting properties, acoustic engineers design algorithms that reduce only the steady-state signals. The difficulty lies in the frequency overlap of the competing and desired signals. Once gain is reduced to decrease the interference of noise, the gain for the needed audibility of speech is decreased as well (i.e., does not improve the SNR). The most recent implementations of DNR make use of the numerous frequency channels (discussed earlier) that are now available in amplification systems. Reducing gain in narrower frequency channels may elicit more promising results.

Figure 5–4 provides an electroacoustic analysis of the NR algorithm implemented in a DSP hearing aid. The figure shows the difference in gain between noise reduction off and noise reduction on. Values around zero indicate that the NR had no impact. Three signals identified by listeners as annoying (Bakke et al, 1995) were presented. The NR algorithm aid does not treat dinner party sounds as noise (no reduction in gain), implements a moderate gain reduction for traffic with sirens, and implements the maximum gain reduction for traffic noise. It is evident from the graph that the gain reductions are implemented differently in discrete channels (different gain reductions across frequency). One lesson from these data is that just because a listener thinks a signal is annoying noise, the hearing aid algorithm may not (i.e., no reduction for restaurant noise).

Active Feedback Control

The best solution for eliminating feedback (amplified sound leaking out of the ear from the receiver and reaching the microphone) is a well-fitted earmold/hearing aid shell. Even

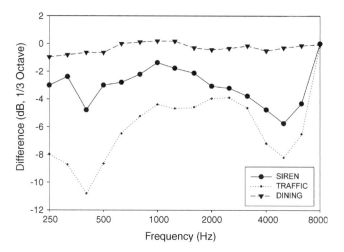

Figure 5–4 Electroacoustic evaluation of a noise reduction algorithm. (Courtesy of Ruth Bentler, University of Iowa.)

with an excellent fit, however, the hearing aid user still may experience feedback temporarily with jaw movement or when something is close to the ear (e.g., a hat). Recently, many manufacturers have introduced adaptive feedback reduction algorithms into their more advanced hearing aids. Generally, these circuits work in one of two ways. In both circumstances, the digital circuit is sampling the incoming signal. When the circuit identifies a signal as a pure tone, it assumes the signal is feedback. In one implementation of feedback management, the circuit will reduce the gain in the frequency channel that matches the feedback "signal." In an ongoing test, the circuit reintroduces the gain until no feedback is detected. For example, if a hearing aid user puts on a hat, the brim of the hat may cause feedback to start, the gain in the offending channel will be reduced, and the circuit will attempt to reintroduce the gain but will continue to find feedback until the hat is removed, at which time full gain can be reintroduced. The other implementation of feedback management consists of introducing a matched pure-tone signal that is 180 degrees out of phase (phase canceling). In either circumstance, the goal of the circuit is to allow maximum gain in the circuit while dealing with intermittent situations that might cause feedback rather than permanently reducing the gain in that frequency range. The audiologist may select adaptive feedback control as an option depending on the patient's needs, listening environment, lifestyle, degree of hearing loss, and hearing aid style preference.

Once the up-front decisions and signal-processing choices are made, the audiologist will know what type of hearing aid must be ordered. The two main differences between conventional and programmable technology relate to how much effort goes into selecting/ordering the instrument and then the subsequent flexibility of the instrument to be programmed to meet the individual needs of the patient. Within the general category of "programmable instruments" there is a wide range of flexibility **(Table 5–2)**. The next section will focus on the steps required to select/order conventional technology.

◆ Selecting Conventional Hearing Aids

Regardless of the type of circuitry fit, the audiologist must derive appropriate fitting targets that can be used to determine the electroacoustic characteristics before ordering the hearing aid(s) and to preset the aid(s). With conventional hearing aids, it becomes important to identify how the hearing aids should function before fitting, as less flexibility for adjustment will be available on the day of the fitting. Fortunately, the audiologist has a large number of fitting strategies from which to choose. Unfortunately, little research is available comparing the relative aided performance of individuals fit using these strategies. Therefore, the audiologist must choose the appropriate fitting strategy on the basis of past experience, amount of time available, and available resources.

Choosing a Prescriptive Strategy

The interaction among the patient's auditory and cognitive status, hearing aid signal-processing scheme, and prescribed hearing aid settings is not fully understood. The fact that no single combination of signal-processing scheme and prescriptive strategy yields the best performance in a majority of patients addresses the complexity of this issue. However, a starting point for the fitting is required, and to that extent, the audiologist must choose (or have chosen for him or her) an initial prescription for the hearing aid settings. See Chapter 7 in this volume for a detailed review of the prescriptive formula.

The underlying assumptions of the various prescriptive strategies differ. As a result, rarely will the targets derived from a set of prescriptive strategies be identical given the same hearing loss. How much the prescribed settings differ will depend on several factors, including the degree, type, and configuration of hearing loss, the age of the patient, previous experience, and audiometric data employed. At their core, however, most prescriptive strategies share the goal of making some degree of speech signal audible while maintaining an acceptable comfort and sound quality level. Prescriptive strategies differ on several dimensions. There is generally a core belief (e.g., restoration of normal loudness perception) that is the foundation for the strategy. The underlying theory behind many prescriptive strategies can be described as a loudness normalization (LN) or a loudness equalization (LE) rationale. With an LN rationale, the overall goal is to restore normal loudness perception for the patient wearing hearing aids. For example, the speech presentation levels judged to be "soft," "comfortable," and "loud" by normal-hearing individuals also should be judged "soft," "comfortable," and "loud" by the hearing aid wearer.

In addition, the normal relative loudness across frequency bands in a complex signal should be maintained. With a speech signal, for example, this means that at a given presentation level, the lower frequencies will be perceived at a greater loudness than the higher frequencies (i.e., vowels have more acoustic power than consonants). In its "purest" form, this rationale will necessitate low CTs and collection of individual-specific loudness ratings. The LN rationale is based on the assumption that restoration of normal loudness perception will lead to a more successful fitting and greater acceptance by the hearing aid user.

With an LE rationale, the goal is to equalize loudness across frequency bands. This occurs while normalizing overall loudness. Thus, the patient should perceive the overall speech levels in a manner similar to individuals with normal hearing. It is the relation between frequency bands within the signal that differs. At a conversational input level (i.e., 65 dB SPL), for example, the various frequency bands would be perceived as being equally loud. The development of the NAL fitting procedure has stimulated considerable research, the results of which suggest that hearing aid settings that equalize perceived loudness across frequency bands are preferred by many patients with hearing loss (Byrne, 1986). One assumption of this rationale is that speech recognition will be higher than that obtained with an LN rationale. **Figure 5–5** provides insertion gain for an LE (NAL's nonlinear fitting procedure, version 1 [NAL-NL1]) and LN (Independent Hearing Aid Fitting Forum [IHAFF]) fitting algorithm. The difference in recommended low- and high-frequency gain to achieve the two fitting rationales is evident.

Even strategies that share a similar underlying rationale can differ in how that rationale is implemented or be affected by other rules incorporated in the strategy. Some strategies recommend the use of individual-specific measures of loudness, whereas others employ average-based data. Different assumptions can be made with regard to how output limiting is incorporated, how (or if) the number of channels is taken into account, what CT is ideal, and so on. **Figure 5–6** demonstrates how one such "rule" can result in dramatically different prescriptions. In this figure, the targets derived for a severe, sloping sensorineural hearing loss are provided for both NAL-NL1 and DSL [i/o]. Note the greater amount of prescribed high-frequency gain with DSL [i/o]. Much of this difference can be attributed to the densensitization factor incorporated by NAL-NL1. This "rule"

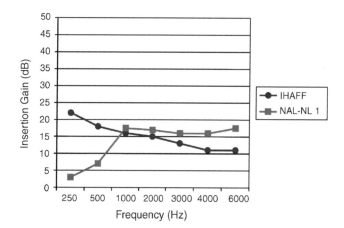

Figure 5–5 Example of differences in insertion gain between one prescriptive formula advocating loudness normalization (Independent Hearing Aid Fitting Forum [IHAFF]) and loudness equalization (National Acoustic Laboratories' nonlinear fitting procedure, version 1[NAL-NL1]) as applied to a flat 40 dB hearing loss.

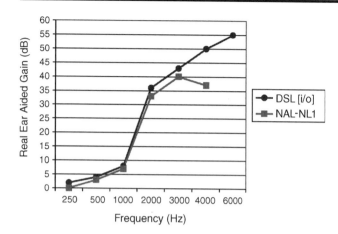

Figure 5–6 Example of difference in real ear aided gain between NAL-NL1 and DSL input/output (DSL [i/o]) indicating the desensitization factor applied to NAL-NL1 for a sloping hearing loss.

addresses the assumption that as the degree of loss increases, the ability of the individual to extract useful information with provision of audibility in the region decreases.

Based on their incorporation within the software of many hearing aid and real ear equipment manufacturers, NAL-NL1 and DSL [i/o] are the two most popular fitting strategies currently in use. At the time of writing, new versions of DSL

[i/o] (version 5) and the NAL strategy (NAL-NL2) have been released. Information provided by the authors of the newer versions has been included in **Table 5–3,** which compares certain features between the two strategies, and in the brief descriptions below.

Desired Sensation Level [Input/Output]

The initial goal of DSL [i/o] was to prescribe amplification characteristics so the wide range of acoustic signals available to a normal-hearing patient are placed within the dynamic range of the hearing-impaired patient (Cornelisse et al, 1994). The underlying rationale, with regard to relative loudness across frequency bands, has been described as a loudness normalization approach. Several significant revisions have been made to the most recent version (version 5) in accordance with research findings, necessitating some changes in how these goals are implemented. Advances in hearing aid signal processing (e.g., multichannel compression and expansion) also have been addressed.

Two major changes to DSL [i/o v5] include the generation of different targets according to age and the presence/absence of background noise. Different targets can now be generated for an adult versus pediatric patient and for quiet versus background noise. In general, less amplification is prescribed for adults. In noise, a higher CT is prescribed, leading to less gain

Table 5–3 A Comparison of Prescriptive Methods

Prescriptive Strategy	DSL 5.0	NAL-NL1
Audiometric data that can be used to derive targets	Thresholds obtained via headphones, insert earphones, sound field, and electrophysiologic measures	Headphones and insert earphones
Adjustment for conductive/mixed loss	Yes	Yes
Adjustments for binaural fitting	Yes	Yes
Individual-specific data can be entered and used in deriving targets	Yes, RECD, REDD, and REUR	Yes, RECD
Desensitization factor	No	Yes
Accounts for number of channels	Yes	Choose between 1 and 4 channels
Underlying rationale/goal	Loudness normalization, placement of acoustic cues available to normal-hearing listener into dynamic range of listener with hearing loss (given certain constraints)	Prescription designed to amplify speech such that at a given level, intelligibility is maximized with the constraints of normalizing overall loudness. Resulting targets similar to those of an LE approach
Allows for choice of CT	Yes, but recommends CT based on degree of loss	Yes, but recommends midlevel CT
Adjustment for venting/tubing	Yes	Yes
Age-related adjustments for ear canal characteristics	Yes	Yes
Age-related adjustments for audibility	Yes	No (for NAL-NL1)
Adjustment for hearing aid experience	No	No (for NAL-NL1)
Fitting information provided	Coupler targets, real ear aided targets, real ear gain targets, aided threshold targets, SPL-O-GRAM, and HA parameters (e.g., CT, CF, CR)	Coupler targets, real ear gain targets, REIG, aided thresholds, Speech-O-Gram and HA parameters

CF, crossover frequency; CR, compression ratio; CT, compression threshold; DSL [i/o], desired sensation level input/output; HA, hearing aid; LDL, loudness discomfort level; LE, loudness equalization; LN, loudness normalization; NAL-NAL1, National Acoustic Laboratories' nonlinear fitting procedure, version 1; RECD, real ear-to-coupler difference; REDD, real ear-to-dial difference; REIG, real ear insertion gain; REUG, real ear unaided gain; REUR, real ear unaided response.

Data from National Center for Audiology (Canada), www.uwo.ca/nca; National Acoustic Laboratories (Australia), www.nal.gov.au

for lower input levels. Changes in the frequency response also occur. In general, changes to the algorithms are the result of research findings of patients fitted using the older version of DSL [i/o]. For example, studies have shown that some adults prefer less gain than prescribed by older versions of DSL [i/o], whereas many pediatric patients are tolerant of the same prescription given a similar hearing loss.

NAL-NL1

The NAL nonlinear fitting procedure, version 1 is an extension of the NAL-R fitting strategy for linear amplification (Byrne et al, 2001). NAL-NL1 was designed for nonlinear signal processing and provides different prescriptive targets as a function of input level. With NAL-NL1, the goal is to maximize speech recognition for a given speech input level within the constraint that the hearing aid wearer should perceive the overall level of speech no louder than an individual with normal hearing.

A modified version of the Speech Intelligibility Index (SII) was used in conjunction with a loudness model to meet the goals of maximizing intelligibility while maintaining normal overall loudness perception (American National Standards Institute [ANSI], 1997; Byrne et al, 2001). At a given input level, however, the relative loudness across frequency regions is prescribed with the goal of maximizing intelligibility. The resultant frequency responses are more similar to an LE versus an LN approach. In general, NAL-NL1 prescribes less amplification than DSL [i/o] for several reasons, including incorporation of a desensitization factor discussed earlier and differing assumptions regarding the ideal CT (i.e., NAL-NL2 supports a CT of ~65 dB SPL). Future versions of NAL-NL1 will likely include refinement of rules related to the gain prescribed for loud sounds and different targets based on the experience level of the hearing aid user.

The importance of the "choice" of a particular strategy varies in accordance with how the targets are incorporated within the fitting process. For example, the targets can simply serve as a starting point. With a cooperative adult and flexible technology, the targets can provide a benchmark for verifying audibility within the constraints of comfort. After some aided experience, the patient can provide judgments that the audiologist can use to help fine-tune the response. In a sense, the starting point is not critical, as it is assumed that in many patients, changes will be made at a later date. In other cases, greater dependence may be placed on the targets derived from a prescriptive strategy. The usefulness of the prescriptive strategy is limited by the appropriateness of the verification procedures employed to ensure that the targets have actually been approximated.

♦ Deriving a Custom 2 cc Coupler Response

The focus of this section will be on methods that can be used with many fitting strategies in customizing the hearing aid order. This type of customization is necessary when conventional or less flexible hearing aid responses are ordered. With a fully programmable hearing aid, this upfront work will not be necessary because the programmable hearing aid can be configured for a variety of responses. When determining appropriate hearing aid characteristics, it is important to have a good estimate of how the hearing aids will function in a given individual's ear. A 2 cc coupler response is required when selecting and ordering conventional hearing aids. This is the only way to communicate the desired response of the hearing aids to the manufacturer. Because the fitter will have limited flexibility to change the response of the conventional hearing aids, the process of identifying the 2 cc coupler target takes on special importance when fitting conventional technology. By determining, a priori, what 2 cc coupler response will lead to the desired response in the individual's ear, the need for significant potentiometer adjustment at the time of the fitting may be avoided. See Chapter 1 in this volume for a detailed description of coupler measurements.

There are several points in the prefitting process where either average- or individual-based data can be used in deriving appropriate coupler targets. Average-based data work well when an individual is close to average; however, if an individual differs significantly from average, as most individuals do, the derived fitting targets may not be accurate. This may not be a problem with programmable hearing aids because a great deal of adjustment flexibility is available to the audiologist. A conventional hearing aid, however, may not accommodate significant changes that may be necessary at the fitting if the hearing aid is not functioning in the real ear as predicted (Feigin et al, 1989; Hawkins et al, 1990; Lewis and Stelmachowicz, 1993).

It is not clear if inclusion of individual measures will provide more satisfied patients. It is clear, however, that a lack of individual measures incorporated in target generation can produce the need for greater manipulation of the selected hearing aid during the fitting process. Therefore, the clinician fitting conventional technology may want to consider inclusion of individual measurements in generating 2 cc coupler targets to minimize the need for hearing aid adjustments to match real ear verification targets at the time of fitting.

The first column of **Table 5–4** lists measures that can be applied at various stages of the hearing aid fitting process. Depending on the fitting strategy, some or all of these measures are used when deriving appropriate hearing aid fitting targets, although the audiologist may not realize this because average-based values are often automatically applied. Individual-specific measures can be applied instead either by direct entry into the actual fitting protocol software applications (e.g., DSL [i/o]) or through the use of some simple calculations. These measures are not time consuming and can be obtained in most clinical settings using available hardware. The potential benefits for incorporating these measures into the various fitting strategies will be discussed. Case examples will be provided to show how these measures can be applied in clinical situations.

Audiometric Data

All fitting strategies require entry of various audiometric measures (i.e., thresholds, loudness discomfort levels [LDLs],

Table 5–4 Transformations that May Be Applied during Selection of an Appropriate 2 cc Coupler Response*

Measure	Definition	Application	Clinical Example
Audiometric information in real-ear dB SPL	Intensity value measured using a probe microphone near the eardrum at threshold, LDL, etc.	Eliminates need for average-based corrections in deriving real-ear targets.	Data obtained in this format can be entered directly into fitting software.
REDD	Difference between the intensity in dB HL on the audiometer dial and the intensity level in dB SPL measured near the eardrum.	Can be applied to audiometric data obtained in dB HL (i.e., thresholds, LDLs) to transform to real-ear dB SPL.	Can be entered directly into DSL[i/o], NAL-NL1, or real ear equipment to transform data in dB HL to real-ear SPL
REUR	Outer ear canal resonance as measured using probe microphone.	Can be used in deriving individual-specific insertion gain or coupler gain targets.	Can be entered directly into NAL-NL1 fitting software. As a result, individual-specific coupler targets can be created. Used in DSL [i/o] to customize sound field threshold results that might be used with children.
RECD	Difference between the output of a hearing aid, insert earphone, or earmold measured in the ear canal and the output in a coupler with an identical input signal	Can be applied to insertion gain targets or real-ear output targets in deriving appropriate 2 cc coupler targets. Can be used to transform dB HL threshold to dB SPL threshold.	Allows for verification of hearing aid settings in the coupler while accounting for individual ear canal characteristics.
Coupler response for flat insertion gain (CORFIG)	REUR-RECD-microphone location (i.e., BTE, CIC)	Correction factor that is added to REIG targets to obtain appropriate 2 cc coupler target.	Adding CORFIG value to NAL-NL1 REIG target to derive 2 cc coupler target.
Measure of dynamic range	Loudness discomfort levels, loudness contour	Determination of appropriate maximum output values and/or compression ratios for the hearing aid	These data can be entered into a real-ear system and used for verifying that maximum output of the hearing aid is set appropriately

* Transformations can be average-based or individual-specific data.

BTE, behind the ear; CORFIG, coupler response for flat insertion gain (CORFIG); DSL [i/o], desired sensation level input/output; HL, hearing level; LDL, loudness discomfort level; NAL-NL1, National Acoustic Laboratories' nonlinear fitting procedure, version 1; RECD, real ear-to-coupler difference; REDD, real ear-to-dial difference; REIG, real ear insertion gain; REUG, real ear unaided gain; REUR, real ear unaided response; SPL, sound pressure level.

loudness contour data, etc.) to derive appropriate fitting targets. Traditionally, these measures have been obtained with insert or supra-aural series earphones in dB HL. When thresholds are plotted on an audiogram, they are plotted in dB HL. Hearing aid data, however, are presented in dB SPL referenced to a 2 cc coupler. Somehow, the audiometric information obtained in dB HL not only must be transformed to dB SPL, but it must be dB SPL re a 2 cc coupler. This allows identification of appropriate 2 cc coupler and real-ear verification targets.

Typically, transformations based on average data are used. Using this method, the real-ear dB SPL value near the eardrum is predicted from the measured dB HL value on the basis of mean values obtained from large numbers of individuals. Valente et al (1991), however, have shown that at a given dB HL value, the actual real-ear dB SPL value recorded in the ear can vary considerably among individuals, sometimes by as much as 30 dB. This variance is related to individual differences in ear canal size and shape and differences in tympanic membrane compliance. See Chapter 3 in this volume for a full review of real-ear measures related to hearing aid fitting.

If an individual differs significantly from average, problems at the fitting may be encountered. For example, if LDLs are obtained in dB HL, an average-based transformation will be used to change those values into dB SPL. These predicted dB SPL values may be substantially higher or lower than the "true" dB SPL value in the individual's ears. As such, the prescribed saturation sound pressure level (SSPL) with a 90 dB SPL input (SSPL90) for the hearing aid may be too high or too low, both of which could have a negative impact on the success of the fitting. The clinician may meet the coupler target for SSPL90, yet have a patient who cannot tolerate a 90 dB SPL input. Conversely, the SSPL90 may be set too low, and a 90 dB SPL input may not be perceived as too loud. In this case, the individual's full dynamic range is not taken advantage of because the maximum output has been set too low.

The audiologist can use two methods to remove the need for average-based data at this point. With both methods, a probe microphone system is necessary. By placing a probe microphone near the eardrum during audiometric testing, individual-specific real-ear dB SPL values can be measured. With this method, the audiologist can continue to plot threshold values in dB HL on the audiogram. For the purposes of hearing aid fitting, however, the audiologist can record the threshold values in real-ear dB SPL by noting the level measured by the probe microphone in the real ear. The difference between the audiometer HL dial reading and the measured dB SPL at the eardrum is the real ear-to-dial difference (REDD). Remember that the reference microphone of the real-ear system should be disabled during measurement. This same setup can be used when obtaining LDLs or loudness contour data.

Another option would be to determine the REDD across frequencies and apply this to the threshold measured in HL. As the name implies, this measure is the difference between the audiometer dial in dB HL and the real-ear value in dB SPL obtained using a probe microphone. With a probe microphone near the eardrum, the REDD is determined by subtracting the audiometer dial reading in dB HL from the intensity value recorded in the ear canal. By presenting a series of tones across frequency at a given intensity level, the audiologist can quickly determine frequency-specific REDD values. A suprathreshold intensity level is used to determine REDD to avoid interference from the noise floor, which would be the case if thresholds are fairly low. The measure to obtain the frequency-specific REDD can be suprathreshold because REDD remains the same regardless of the patient's level of hearing loss (assuming the attenuator of the audiometer is linear). Once obtained, the REDD can be applied to all audiometric data (e.g., threshold and LDLs) obtained in dB HL when converting to dB SPL. Again, this removes the need for average-based transformations. Remember, these two methods have provided real-ear dB SPL data. Ultimately, the threshold in dB SPL becomes the target for verifying audibility of the hearing aid response during probe microphone measures. Hearing aids, however, are ordered using data obtained in 2 cc couplers; therefore, the final target data must still be referenced to a 2 cc coupler through further real-ear measures or by using average-based conversions.

The two procedures described above should provide identical data. For the first, every response is measured in dB SPL. In the second, individual-specific correction values are obtained and then applied to all dB HL results. These measures can be performed with a separate audiometer and real-ear system. Depending on the clinic layout, placement of the systems may be awkward. Some newer audiometers combine these systems and automatically record data both in dB HL and dB SPL.

◆ Clinical Example of Real Ear-to-Dial Difference

DSL [i/o] allows for entry of audiometric data in dB HL or in real-ear dB SPL. When entered in dB HL, average, age-appropriate transformation data are used to convert the audiometric data to dB SPL. Other programs may use adult average data at all times. This is why entry of an individual's birth date is required with DSL [i/o]. In addition, the audiologist can enter the individually measured REDD, and these values will be applied instead of the average values. DSL [i/o] uses audiometric values such as thresholds and upper limits of comfort in determining an individual's dynamic range. Verification and coupler targets are then generated with the goal of keeping soft, average, and loud speech within the individual's dynamic range.

Table 5–5 reports the 2 cc coupler data of a hearing aid derived with DSL [i/o] software. In the top half of **Table 5–5**, the transformation from dB HL to dB SPL was made on the basis of average data. In the bottom half of **Table 5–5**, individual-specific REDD values were entered and applied in transforming audiometric data from dB HL to dB SPL. The REDD values entered are +/− two standard deviations (SD) from the mean REDD values obtained in the Valente et al (1997) study for insert earphones. When the dB HL to dB SPL transformation is predicted, the data recommend a more powerful hearing aid and greater compression than would have been recommended when the individual-specific REDD is considered. This points to the advantage of using individual-specific data instead of relying on average transformations.

In this case, had the dB HL to dB SPL been predicted, output targets would have been considerably higher than needed, and the patient likely would have complained that the hearing aid was too loud. Looking at the hearing aid recommendation data, substantial differences exist in desired SSPL90, full-on gain, use gain, and CR. Thus, manipulation of a volume control would not necessarily rectify the differences between these two recommendations for the same individual, and many hearing aids are fit without volume controls. A conventional hearing aid may not be flexible enough to make these modifications, making incorporation of these real-ear peculiarities in the derivation of the coupler target an efficient use of time and energy.

Table 5–5 Hearing Aid Recommendation Data When an Average-based versus an Individual-specific REDD Is Used

	500 Hz	1000 Hz	2000 Hz	3000 Hz	4000 Hz
Average-based					
SSPL90	101.0	103.0	106.0	110.0	108.0
Full-on gain	20.0	26.0	32.0	38.0	37.0
Use gain	10.0	16.0	22.0	28.0	27.0
Compression ratio	1.5	1.8	2.0	2.7	3.0
Individual-specific					
SSPL90	98.0	100.0	100.0	101.0	97.0
Full-on gain	10.0	21.0	25.0	27.0	22.0
Use gain	−1.0	11.0	15.0	17.0	12.0
Compression ratio	1.1	1.6	1.6	1.9	1.8

REDD, real ear-to-dial difference; SSPL90, saturation sound pressure level with a 90 dB SPL input.

◆ Real Ear-to-Coupler Differences

The preceding section described obtaining individual-specific measures that can be used to gather data in dB SPL at the eardrum or converting data in dB HL to dB SPL at the ear canal through the use of individual-specific REDD values. Hearing aid targets and electroacoustic data, however, are provided in dB SPL referenced to a 2 cc coupler, not to an individual's eardrum. Therefore even with these individual measures applied, a conversion must still take place to create data referenced to a coupler for hearing aid ordering purposes. The output of a hearing aid is typically greater in an individual's ear than in a coupler in the middle to high frequencies. However, substantial intersubject variation exists. Individual real ear-to-coupler differences (RECDs) are affected by factors such as ear canal volume and middle ear immittance characteristics that have an impact on eardrum impedance (Feigin et al, 1989; Fikret-Pasa and Revit, 1992). The output of a hearing aid will be greater in an individual with a smaller ear canal versus an individual with a larger ear canal. As such, it becomes necessary to determine what 2 cc coupler response will lead to the desired output in the individual's ear canal. Unless entered directly, average-based data rather than individual-specific data are used in predicting an appropriate 2 cc coupler response. As with the dB HL to dB SPL transformation, the transformation from dB SPL in the ear canal to dB SPL in the coupler is derived from mean data obtained on a large number of individuals. This may lead to problems when an individual deviates significantly from average (Fikret-Pasa and Revit, 1992). One way to avoid this potential problem is through the use of two measures, the RECD and the real ear unaided response (REUR). The need to use one or both of these measures will depend on what type of targets will be used during the verification stage.

When output measures (i.e., real ear aided response [REAR]) will be used for real-ear verification, the audiologist needs to know what 2 cc coupler response a hearing aid should exhibit to achieve the desired REAR. The RECD is a measure that serves to quantify the difference in the hearing aid response obtained in a 2 cc coupler versus the response obtained in a real ear as measured using a probe microphone. Some real-ear systems can automatically calculate the RECD. For those that do not, it is a relatively simple measure to obtain. The 2 cc coupler response of an insert earphone (or hearing aid) is determined in the test box. Using probe microphone measures, the audiologist determines the frequency response of the same insert earphone in an individual's ear. The RECD is then determined by subtracting the response obtained in the coupler from the response obtained in the real ear. See Chapter 3 in this volume for examples of obtaining RECD and for an outstanding review of transformations.

Note that in the spirit of being efficient, the audiologist may use RECD to convert dB HL thresholds to real-ear dB SPL thresholds as well as using RECD to convert eardrum dB SPL data to coupler data. The dB HL threshold data are converted by first adding the reference equivalent threshold sound pressure levels (RETSPLs) and then the RECD. RETSPL is not an individual measurement; rather, it is a calibration value related to the calibrated testing equipment that is used clinically (ANSI, 1996b).

Clinical Example of Application of Real Ear-to-Coupler Differences

Using the DSL [i/o] software, it becomes relatively easy to incorporate individual-specific RECD values. DSL [i/o] offers the audiologist the option of using predicted or custom RECD values. **Table 5–6** reports the hearing aid recommendations for a WDRC hearing aid for a patient when RECD is predicted and when the individual-based RECD was entered. As can be seen, prescribed gain is higher, most notably at 500, 3000, and 4000 Hz, when the patient's measured RECD is entered.

◆ Real Ear Insertion Gain

When real ear insertion gain (REIG = REAR − REUG) targets are used, the RECD can be used in conjunction with the REUG to determine an appropriate 2 cc coupler response. The REUG is a probe microphone measure that represents

Table 5–6 Hearing Aid Recommendation Data When an Average-based versus an Individual-specific RECD Is Used

	250 Hz	500 Hz	1000 Hz	2000 Hz	3000 Hz	4000 Hz
Average-based						
SSPL90	91.0	98.0	97.0	100.0	102.0	95.0
Full-on gain	11.0	9.0	15.0	21.0	28.0	23.0
Use gain	1.0	−1.0	5.0	11.0	18.0	13.0
Compression ratio	1.2	1.1	1.3	1.3	1.7	1.6
Individual-specific						
SSPL90	95.0	97.0	101.0	105.0	112.0	111.0
Full-on gain	15.0	19.0	20.0	26.0	38.0	40.0
Use gain	5.0	9.0	10.0	16.0	28.0	30.0
Compression ratio	1.2	1.1	1.3	1.3	1.7	1.6

SSPL90, saturation sound pressure level with a 90 dB SPL input.

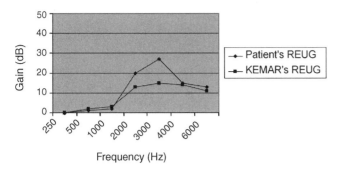

Figure 5–7 Knowles Electronics Manikin for Acoustic Research (KEMAR) median real ear unaided gain (REUG) versus individual REUG.

the resonance characteristics of the outer ear without a hearing aid inserted. This natural resonance is lost when a hearing aid is inserted and needs to be accounted for when deriving appropriate gain targets. For example, if an NAL-R REIG target prescribes 20 dB of gain at 3000 Hz, and the individual's REUG is 10 dB at 3000 Hz, the hearing aid itself would need to provide 30 dB of gain at 3000 Hz (NAL prescription [20 dB] + gain lost with insertion of hearing aid [10 dB]).

The importance of incorporating individual-specific REUG measures into the fitting process is demonstrated in **Fig. 5–7.** Here, the REUG obtained from the left ear of a patient is shown along with a median REUG obtained using Knowles Electronics Manikin for Acoustic Research (KEMAR; GRAS Sound & Vibration A/S, Vedbæk, Denmark). For this patient, if average-based data (KEMAR) had been used, prescribed coupler gain would have been ~10 dB less than required by the patient to meet the REIG target. When deriving an appropriate 2 cc coupler response that allows the audiologist to arrive close to meeting the REIG target, there is a need to account for both the REUG and the RECD.

♦ Coupler Response for Flat Insertion Gain

To account for an individual's REUG and RECD, the coupler response for flat insertion gain (CORFIG) is determined and applied to the prescribed REIG target to derive an appropriate 2 cc target (Killion and Revit, 1993). The CORFIG is determined by subtracting the individual's RECD and an appropriate microphone correction factor from the individual's REUG. This is completed at all frequencies for which the audiologist wants a target gain value.

In essence, it is unfair to the manufacturer of the conventional hearing aid if one plans to verify the hearing aid's response with REIG if the individual's REUG was not accounted for in the original coupler targets. The hearing aid could match the requested coupler targets (the only data the manufacturer has) and yet be far off from the REIG targets if average REUG is used to create the coupler targets, whereas individual REUG is used when obtaining REIG for verification.

Clinical Example of Application of Coupler Response for Flat Insertion Gain

A patient **(Fig. 5–8)** was fit binaurally with behind-the-ear (BTE) hearing aids using data from the FIG6 prescriptive formula (Gittes and Niquette, 1995). By entering this individual's thresholds into the FIG6 software, insertion gain targets (table in center of **Fig. 5–8**) and coupler targets (graphs to the left of **Fig. 5–8**) for a BTE instrument were derived for both ears. The hearing aids were adjusted to the coupler targets before the verification portion of the hearing aid fitting **(Fig. 5–9)**. Verification consisted of real-ear measurement and subjective ratings of loudness. Using probe microphone measures, REIG was determined at several input levels. As can be seen in **Fig. 5–10,** REIG fell short of the target in the higher frequencies, most notably at 4000 Hz (this was true for the soft and loud REIG targets as well). Thus, even though the hearing aids were adjusted to the prescribed coupler targets, when real-ear measures were performed, the real-ear targets were not met. Therefore this individual likely has an REUG and/or an RECD that differs significantly from normal.

In this case, the hearing aids were not sufficiently flexible to allow for the manipulation to the frequency response necessary to meet the target. In addition, loudness judgments of continuous discourse by the patient revealed that speech was not being perceived as sufficiently loud. In **Table 5–7,** the patient's CORFIG was determined by subtracting the RECD and BTE microphone response from the individual REUG. The difference between the individual's CORFIG and the average CORFIG is shown in **Fig. 5–1** (p. 138). Note the large difference in the high frequencies that led to insufficient prescribed gain when the average-based CORFIG was used. At this point, the individual's CORFIG values could be added to the insertion gain targets to derive the appropriate coupler gain response (see **Table 5–8**, p. 138). The resultant values represent the desired coupler gain target for a 65 dB input with the individual-specific CORFIG values incorporated. Substantial differences exist between the original coupler target and the individual-specific coupler target, most notably in the high frequencies (see **Fig. 5–12**, p. 138). By ordering a hearing aid that will arrive close to meeting the new coupler targets, it is likely that the REIG targets will be met as well. Indeed, that was the case for this patient. Loudness judgments also revealed appropriate loudness perception for comfortable and loud continuous discourse with the new fitting.

The preceding example can be applied to any insertion or coupler gain targets provided by insertion gain–based fitting strategies (e.g., NAL-R). All that is needed are insertion gain targets, the individual's REUG and RECD, and appropriate microphone correction values (see Appendix 5-1; personal communication, Killion, 1988).

Dynamic Range Measures

The preceding sections have shown how individual-specific measures can be used in transforming values obtained in dB HL to real-ear dB SPL and 2 cc dB SPL coupler data. Another aspect of the hearing aid fitting in which either average-based or individual-based data can be used concerns dynamic range

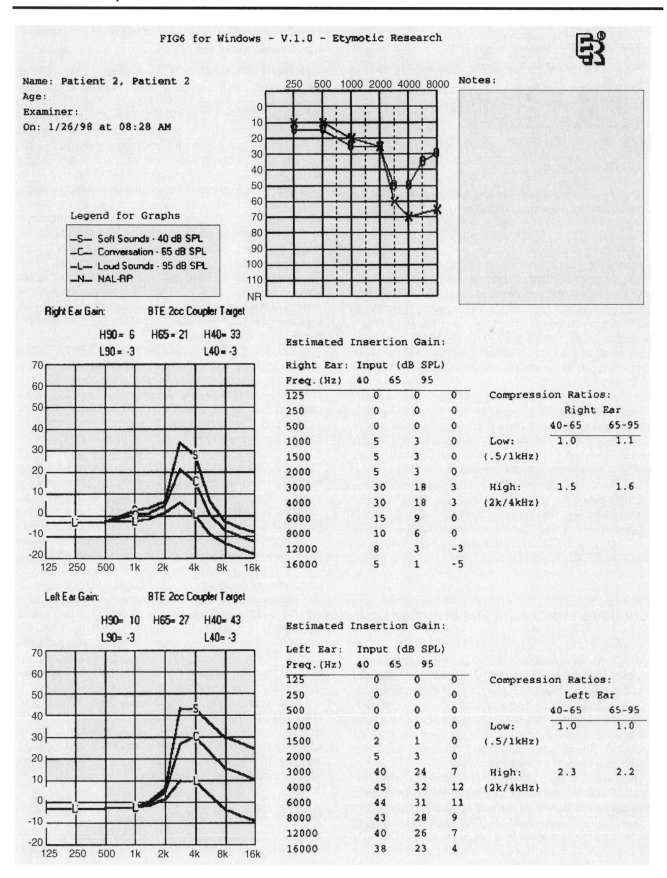

Figure 5–8 Data for a patient with real ear unaided gain (REUG) and real ear-to-coupler difference (RECD) different from average.

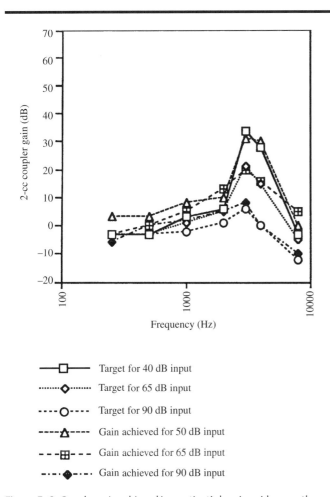

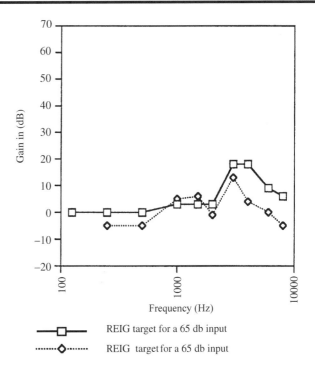

REIG target for a 65 db input

REIG target for a 65 db input

Figure 5–10 Real ear insertion gain (REIG) obtained from the patient versus the target REIG.

Target for 40 dB input

Target for 65 dB input

Target for 90 dB input

Gain achieved for 50 dB input

Gain achieved for 65 dB input

Gain achieved for 90 dB input

Figure 5–9 Coupler gain achieved in a patient's hearing aid versus the target coupler gain at three input levels.

(DR) measures. For many fitting strategies, measures of DR are used in deriving fitting targets. For WDRC hearing aids, depending on the fitting strategy used, loudness contour data or LDLs are used in determining appropriate CRs. DSL [i/o] determines an appropriate CR using threshold and LDLs. With linear hearing aids, LDLs are typically used in deriving an appropriate SSPL90.

When DR information is not obtained, this information is often predicted on the basis of threshold data. This can

lead to problems on the day of the fitting if an individual's DR differs substantially from average. The audiologist needs to consider the adjustment capability of the hearing aids to be ordered when deciding on an appropriate fitting strategy and whether individual-specific DR measures are necessary. When adjustment flexibility is limited, individual-specific DR measures easily can be justified, assuming the individual can perform the task. DR measures, just as threshold data, can be customized through the use of individual-specific transformations, as described previously. Mueller and Bentler (2005) presented an evidence-based review using LDLs in hearing aid fittings. Although the level of evidence was low, these authors concluded that there is sufficient evidence to support the use of unaided LDLs for selecting the maximum real-ear output of hearing aids.

Table 5–7 Calculating Individual CORFIG

Frequency (Hz)	Patient's REUG	Patient's RECD Response	BTE Microphone	Resulting Individual CORFIG
250	0.0	0.0	0.8	−0.8
500	2.0	−5.0	1.6	5.4
1000	0.0	−0.0	1.6	−1.5
2000	14.0	−1.8	2.8	13.0
3000	18.0	−2.9	2.8	18.1
4000	20.0	−7.2	3.2	24.0
8000	10.0	−5.0	3.9	11.1

BTE, behind the ear; CORFIG, coupler response for flat insertion gain; RECD, real ear-to-coupler difference; REUG, real ear unaided gain.

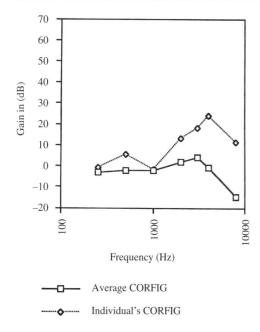

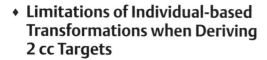

Figure 5–11 Average coupler response for flat insertion gain (CORFIG) versus the individual's CORFIG.

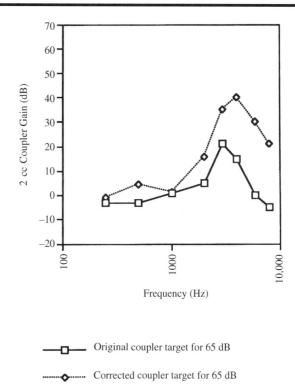

Figure 5–12 Coupler target based on average data versus the coupler target based on individual data.

♦ Limitations of Individual-based Transformations when Deriving 2 cc Targets

Most of the transformations described previously do not take into account venting characteristics (i.e., diameter, length, and parallel vs intersection), nor do tranformations account for canal length. Thus, when individual-specific REURs and RECDs are obtained and the 2 cc targets are met, real-ear targets may not be precisely matched without further adjustment to the hearing aid. When RECD is measured with the individual's earmold, the vent response will be included. By using individual-specific transformations, the audiologist can reduce, but not eliminate, differences between performance in the coupler

and performance in the real ear. When possible, it is always beneficial to verify using real-ear measures. In cases where this is not possible, however, the individual-specific 2 cc targets represent the best starting point. The new versions of DSL [i/o] and NAL-NL2 allow for entry of various earmold characteristics and provide the predicted effect on the real-ear response. Audiologists can consult published data that provide correction factors for various earmold characteristics. See Chapter 2 in this volume, which provides detailed information regarding earmold acoustics.

Armed with 2 cc coupler data, hearing aid circuitry, and other options (e.g., compression output limiting, telecoil) identified in the patient evaluation, the clinician is ready to order a conventional hearing aid. Once the clinician has chosen one or more manufacturers, it is time to examine the specification sheets to see whether one of the hearing aids in the product line will meet the patient's needs. Many specification sheets are now online. Even though conventional technology is being used, many manufacturers include their conventional technology along with their programmable hearing aids in their software. In this way, the audiologist can view the hearing aid parameters and coupler response as well as recommended potentiometer settings for the desired coupler response. The result, of course, would have to be verified in the coupler and/or real ear. The next section introduces the use of manufacturers' specification sheets, which is essential when ordering conventional hearing aids.

Table 5–8 Determining Desired 2 cc Coupler Gain Target Using CORFIG

Frequency	REIG Target	Individual's CORFIG	Desired 2 cc Gain Target
250	0.0	−0.8	−0.8
500	0.0	5.4	5.4
1000	3.0	−1.5	−1.5
2000	3.0	13.0	16.0
3000	18.0	18.1	36.1
4000	18.0	24.0	42.0
8000	6.0	11.1	17.0

Abbreviations: CORFIG, REIG, real ear insertion gain; REIG, real ear insertion gain.

◆ Understanding Manufacturers' Specification Sheets

Components of the Specification Information

Because conventional hearing aids are often chosen from a review of an individual manufacturer's specification information, it is important to correctly interpret the data that are presented. The information itself is usually compiled in a binder referred to as the specification book or in a software format that can be accessed by computer disc, CD, or online. The data provided serve as the means by which the audiologist understands the physical and electroacoustic capabilities of each instrument. The data usually begin with general information on features of the instrument, such as the number of channels, type of signal processing, range of hearing loss covered, and types of available potentiometers. The ANSI (1987, 1996b, 2003) technical summary will be included. This summary can be somewhat misleading because its data may reflect the combined available responses of a group of hearing aid matrices. It is, however, a good starting point from which one can further evaluate the suitability of the instrument in meeting the fitting goal. The specification data typically report gain and frequency response curves, and input/output curves as measured in a 2 cc coupler, using given source signals and input levels, potentiometer, and volume control settings when appropriate. Thus, these data show a sampling of the responses available from the instrument. With any adjustment to one or more of the variable controls (e.g., volume control, CR, and tone control), the response will be different from that shown in the data sheet. An example of hearing aid specification data are shown in **Fig. 5–13.**

Labeling of Specification Data

Labeling of the specification data is critical to the accurate interpretation of the hearing aid characteristics. When reviewing the gain and input/output curves presented by the manufacturer, the audiologist should first look for labels identifying the values represented on the vertical and horizontal axis, the frequency and intensity of the source signal, the volume control setting (usually full on), and the position of any settings. In this manner, target fitting data may be more easily compared with that displayed by the manufacturer.

The Matrix Approach

With the increased popularity of custom in-the-ear (ITE) hearing aids in the 1980s, it became possible for manufacturers to provide a variety of hearing aid responses available in a few different shell styles in conventional technology. Thus, audiologists could become more involved in the fitting process by actually choosing parameters of the hearing aid, such as the gain, output, and slope of the response. These response parameters were organized into groups called matrices. One matrix would be specified by the audiologist or manufacturer as the response most likely to meet the fitting target. The matrices available for a given hearing instrument are usually represented by a series of three numbers corresponding to the gain, output, and slope, respectively (**Table 5–9**). When ordering a hearing aid for a patient, the audiologist can specify the matrix to be used, or the manufacturer will make the choice for the audiologist. Some manufacturers include matrix selection in the computer software that is supplied with their hearing aids. Thus, the audiologist is able to enter patient data and a desired fitting formula, and a recommendation for the most appropriate instrument and matrix is automatically generated. Matrices also are used to describe programmable hearing aids to provide guidelines related to the gain and output that can be achieved.

◆ Prioritizing Potentiometers

Potentiometers on conventional hearing aids are controls that can be manipulated by a screwdriver to change the response of the hearing aid. BTE hearing aids usually are delivered with a preselected number of screw-set potentiometers. In some BTE instruments, the fitter may request alternate potentiometers. In ITE and smaller custom-type shells, size limitations often dictate the number of possible potentiometer options. For this reason, it is necessary to prioritize the capabilities that are desired for the instrument. The potentiometer capabilities are important to consider because potentiometers will dictate the electroacoustic flexibility in the hearing aid/earmold system. Other electroacoustic flexibility will come from options in the shell or earmold plumbing system (see Chapter 2 in this text). For example, the use of a select-a-vent (SAV) system will allow the audiologist to manipulate the low-frequency response without requiring placement of a low-cut potentiometer. Aside from the volume control, screw-set potentiometers often provide the only electroacoustic flexibility in the conventional hearing aid circuitry. In addition, potentiometers serve as the vehicle through which fine-tuning of the fitting can be achieved.

Thus, caution and attention to detail are advised when choosing which potentiometers to order and the positions at which the potentiometer should be set. Each manufacturer uses terminology that is not necessarily consistent with other manufacturers' terms when referring to available potentiometers. For example, one company may refer

SOUND F/X CUSTOM / MINI CANAL • CANAL • HALF SHELL • FULL SHELL

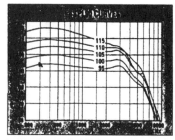

Input sound pressure level: 90 dB   Volume Control: full on
G_L Parameter: +   G_H Parameter: +   F Parameter: –
TK Parameter: –   P Parameter: +

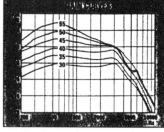

Input sound pressure level: 50 dB   Volume Control: full on
G_L Parameter: +   G_H Parameter: +   F Parameter: –
TK Parameter: –   P Parameter: +

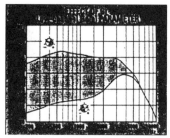

Input sound pressure level: 50 dB   Volume Control: full on
G_H Parameter: +   F Parameter: +
TK Parameter: –   P Parameter: +

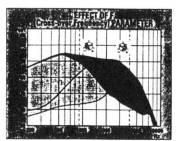

Input sound pressure level: 50 dB   Volume Control: full on
G_L Parameter: +/–   G_H Parameter: +/–
TK Parameter: –   P Parameter: +

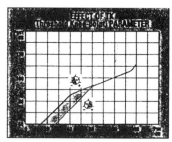

Input sound pressure level: 50 dB   Volume Control: full on
G_L Parameter: +   G_H Parameter: +
F Parameter: –   P Parameter: +

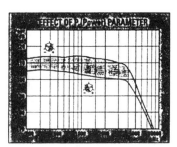

Input sound pressure level: 100 dB   Volume Control: full on
G_L Parameter: +   G_H Parameter: +
F Parameter: –   TK Parameter: –

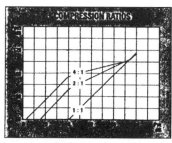

Input at 2000 Hz   Volume Control: full on
G_L Parameter: +   G_H Parameter: –/+   F Parameter: –
TK Parameter: –   P Parameter: +

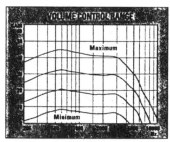

Input sound pressure level: 50 dB   Volume Control: as shown
G_L Parameter: +   G_H Parameter: +   F Parameter: –
TK Parameter: –   P Parameter: +

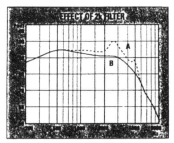

Input sound pressure level: 50 dB   Volume Control: full on
"A" unfiltered, not recommended   "B" filtered, standard

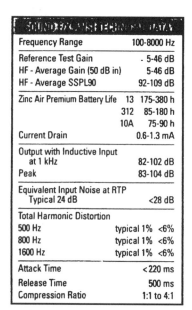

SOUND F/X CUSTOM TECHNICAL DATA	
Frequency Range	100-8000 Hz
Reference Test Gain	- 5-46 dB
HF - Average Gain (50 dB in)	5-46 dB
HF - Average SSPL90	92-109 dB
Zinc Air Premium Battery Life 13	175-380 h
312	85-180 h
10A	75-90 h
Current Drain	0.6-1.3 mA
Output with Inductive Input at 1 kHz	82-102 dB
Peak	83-104 dB
Equivalent Input Noise at RTP Typical 24 dB	<28 dB
Total Harmonic Distortion	
500 Hz	typical 1% <6%
800 Hz	typical 1% <6%
1600 Hz	typical 1% <6%
Attack Time	< 220 ms
Release Time	500 ms
Compression Ratio	1:1 to 4:1

CUSTOM PRODUCTS

SOUNDF/X

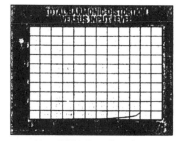

Input at 1600 Hz   Volume Control: full on
G_L Parameter: +   G_H Parameter: +   F Parameter: –
TK Parameter: –   P Parameter: +

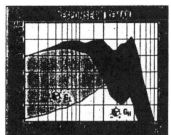

Input sound pressure level: 50 dB   Volume Control: full on
This insertion gain is similar to the functional gain for an
average adult with a closed earmold.

Figure 5–13 Example of a hearing aid specification sheet.

Table 5–9 Matrix Options on a Specification Sheet

	Custom Matrix Selections	
	FX	FX H
Mini canal	95/30–5/F/X	95/30–5/F/XH
	100/35–10/F/X	100/35–10/F/XH
	105/40–15/F/X	105/40–15/F/XH
Canal	95/30–5/F/X	95/30–5/F/XH
Half-shell	100/35–10/F/X	100/35–10/F/XH
	105/40–15/F/X	105/40–15/F/XH
	110/45–20/F/X	110/45–20/F/XH
Concha	95/35–5/F/X	95/35–5/F/XH
	100/40–10/F/X	100/40–10/F/XH
	105/45–15/F/X	105/45–15/F/XH
	110/50–20/F/X	110/50–20/F/XH
	115/50–25/F/X	115/50–20/F/XH
	115/55–25/F/X	115/50–25/F/XH

to a potentiometer increasing or decreasing the SSPL90 as the maximum power output (MPO) control, whereas another may call it the "P" control. At present, no standard format exists for referring to such controls. The audiologist needs to understand what parameter of the response will be affected by a given adjustment. In addition, different manufacturers choose different approaches to achieve the intended response adjustments from a potentiometer. For example, a potentiometer labeled "H" may suggest a high-frequency emphasis that is incorporated in the response when set to maximum. However, a variety of ways exist that such an emphasis could be achieved. One way would be to decrease the low-frequency gain. Another option is to increase the gain for high-frequency input or to broaden the response to include higher frequencies. To effectively use potentiometers, one needs to understand how the adjustment in the response is achieved. This information should be explained in the specification sheets provided by the manufacturer. Coupler or real-ear verification is the only way to know what has changed in the hearing aid response after a potentiometer is manipulated.

The setting of the potentiometer becomes a factor at the point when the audiologist is ready to compare the 2 cc coupler targets to the response of a hearing aid that has been ordered and received in the office. Some manufacturers include a potentiometer adjustment guide in their computer software, showing the audiologist the recommended settings for the given hearing loss and hearing aid. This assumes that the manufacturer is using the same fitting protocol (e.g., DSL [i/o] or NAL-NL1) to yield targets. That may not always be the case. Most likely, the audiologist will need to consult the manufacturer's product information for guidance as to the operation of the potentiometers. Once again, each manufacturer may use its own convention for such descriptions. For example, a potentiometer labeled "TK" is often designated as the compression threshold kneepoint (TK) control. The labeling on such a potentiometer is often shown as – for minimum and + for maximum. Without reading the product literature carefully, one could have difficulty understanding whether the minimum TK position actually refers

to the lowest available TK value or the minimum available amount of compression (actually the maximum TK value). Certainly, one can alleviate some of this confusion by implementing adjustments in the potentiometers and observing changes in the response, as measured in the coupler. When available, the manufacturer's computer software often will illustrate the electroacoustic changes taking place with potentiometer adjustments. These graphic simulations do not eliminate the need for objective verification of the actual hearing aid response, but they do illustrate the general direction of the change.

◆ Making Use of Data from the Fitting Formula in Selecting Conventional Instruments and Options

As noted previously, the outcome of a hearing aid fitting formula is a prescribed hearing aid response measured in a 2 cc coupler. Once derived by means of the formula, the clinician must identify an appropriate hearing aid that will closely approximate this prescribed response. For a BTE, the hearing aid is either ordered from the manufacturer by telephone or chosen from a stock of previously purchased instruments. For a custom product, a detailed order form unique to each manufacturer is completed. The process of selecting and ordering an appropriate instrument with which the targets will be met will be examined in this section.

The data presented in **Fig. 5–14** will be used in this description. On the basis of individual listening needs, cosmetic preferences, and financial resources, the audiologist has decided to fit binaural conventional in-the-canal (ITC) hearing aids. Although the fitting is binaural, the data from the right ear will be presented for the purposes of this example. Fitting targets will be derived using the DSL [i/o] procedure. This will be used to determine the suitability of a given hearing aid and to fill out an order form. To complete this process, one must (1) understand the data obtained from the formula, (2) understand the descriptions and data on circuits and options shown in the manufacturers' product literature, and (3) order an instrument with options that will allow execution of the fitting strategy by characteristics and/or controls on the hearing aid and meet any additional needs identified through our assessment (Hearing Demand, Ability, and Needs Profile; PEW; and APHAB).

Figure 5–13 illustrates the manufacturer's specifications on the hearing aid model and circuit chosen. This particular hearing aid was chosen for several reasons. Having two separate channels with some controls will allow the audiologist to address different gain as a function of input in the low- and high-frequency regions of this patient's audiogram. The parameters within these channels can be controlled independently, allowing for good flexibility in the instrument. In addition, the responses displayed on the specification sheet are very well labeled, avoiding the confusion of guessing where the potentiometers are set or at what level the volume control is adjusted.

University of Western Ontario
Canada

Patient Information

Patient ID : Patient 1	Street :
Name : ,	City :
Birth Date : 11-dec-1928	State/Prov. :
Professional :	Country :
Today's Date : 15-Jul-1998, 17:05:40	Phone :

ASSESSMENT DATA (dB HL)

RIGHT EAR		.25	.50	.75	1.0	1.5	2.0	3.0	4.0	6.0
	Threshold	20	35	37	40	50	55	65	70	80
	Upper Limit									
	Exponent									
	RECD									
	REUR									
	REDD									

HEARING AID RECOMMENDATION

RIGHT EAR
Selection Method : DSL [i/o]

HEARING AID | *OTHER* | *OTHER*
Style : ITC	Transducer : ER3	Speech : Cox/Moore
Make :	HL to SPL : Predicted	Compr. Thresh : 40
Model :	HA Style : ITC	Loudness : Predicted
Serial # :	Circuit : WDRC (fixed CR)	
	RE to 2cc : Predicted	Max. Out : Predicted

		.25	.50	.75	1.0	1.5	2.0	3.0	4.0	6.0
	SSPL-90	92	102	102	102	104	108	110	108	106
	Full-On Gain (Reserve 10 dB)	15	22	23	24	29	35	38	37	40
	User Gain (Input 65 dB)	5	12	13	14	19	25	28	27	30
	Comp. Ratio	1.4	1.6	1.6	1.7	2.0	2.2	2.7	3.0	4.2

VERIFICATION DATA

RIGHT EAR
Hi-Level (Coupler Output)

		.25	.50	.75	1.0	1.5	2.0	3.0	4.0	6.0
	Target 90 dB	88	93	93	93	97	101	103	100	101
	Measured 90 dB									

Mid-Level (Coupler Gain)

		.25	.50	.75	1.0	1.5	2.0	3.0	4.0	6.0
	Target 80 dB	1	7	7	8	11	17	19	17	18
	Measured									
	Target 65 dB	5	12	13	14	19	25	28	27	30
	Measured									
	Target 50 dB	9	18	19	20	26	33	38	37	41
	Measured									

Low-Level

		.25	.50	.75	1.0	1.5	2.0	3.0	4.0	6.0
	Aided SF 0°	8	13	12	15	18	21	25	25	25
	Measured									

Figure 5–14 The DSL [i/o] coupler target recommendations for the patient's right ear.

Figure 5–14 shows a printout of the DSL [i/o] targets derived for the right ear. The data that are most useful for comparing with manufacturers' specifications are the SSPL90, the full-on gain (reserve 10 dB), and the CR. Begin by comparing the SSPL90, shown from 250 Hz to 6000 Hz on the printout, to that displayed in the manufacturer's specification sheet. The corresponding curve appears in the upper left-hand corner of **Fig. 5–13.** Because the hearing aid recommendation DSL [i/o] targets are generated assuming a full-on volume control, it would be tempting to make a direct comparison between the values in the DSL [i/o] printout (**Fig. 5–14**) and those displayed in the specification sheet (**Fig. 5–13**). This would be misleading, however, because the positions of the adjustable parameters, such as the low-channel gain (GL), TK, crossover frequency (F), and high-channel gain (GH), must be considered (gain is changed through manipulation of the CR). The SSPL90 curve assists in assessing the suitability of this instrument for the target, and it also will help select the matrix number, as the lines labeled with matrix maximum output designators across the SSPL90 curves are examined.

It may appear that low-frequency gain is too high when selecting the manufacturer's gain curve. However, the curve labeled "Effect of GL Parameter" (**Fig. 5–13**) shows that an adjustment made to reduce the low channel gain could result in a reasonable approximation of the target.

Pitfall

- When comparing manufacturer's frequency-response curves to desired coupler targets, be sure to consider the volume control setting and the input level of the source signal.

In **Fig. 5–14**, DSL [i/o] shows CRs for each test frequency (1.4:1 to 4.2:1). It would be unusual to find a conventional hearing aid capable of this many different CRs. Thus, this information can be averaged across frequencies or frequency bands and the results compared with the hearing aid under consideration. In this case, all the CR values, except that found at 6000 Hz (4.2:1), fall within the capability of the hearing aid chosen. This is illustrated by the manufacturer in the graph labeled "Compression Ratios" in **Fig. 5–13**, showing that the CR can vary from 1:1 (linear) to 4:1 for a 2000 Hz input. Manufacturers typically display an input/output curve (where CRs can be viewed/calculated) only for 2000 Hz. With a multichannel instrument, it is important to know the CR for the low- and high-frequency channel and perhaps, more importantly, whether they can be manipulated independently. The CR range for the low-frequency channel is not provided in the specification for this hearing aid and would have to be obtained by contacting the manufacturer or testing the hearing aid in the test box.

Controversial Point

- Audiologists and manufacturers may tout the benefits of targeting the CR in the hearing aid. This parameter is intimately tied into the gain and output characteristics of a nonlinear hearing aid. Some would argue that by first targeting the appropriate gain and output values, the CR will necessarily fall at the appropriate value.

The adjustment of the CRs in this hearing aid is accessed by means of the GL parameter. This is a good illustration of how the gain in a channel is directly related to the CR. The DSL [i/o] printout (**Fig. 5–14**) for this patient specifies a 40 dB SPL CT. Compression threshold is selected from a list of possibilities by the clinician using the DSL [i/o]. The graph labeled "Effect of TK" in **Fig. 5–13** illustrates that such a TK should be possible. Once again, considering the function of each potentiometer, it would appear that the F (crossover) and GL parameters will assist in reaching the targets.

Special Consideration

- Never shy away from contacting the manufacturer for further clarification or information on product features. Often, product features or custom modifications are possible that are not described in the specification materials.

The manufacturer's software for the example hearing aid does allow the audiologist to enter a choice of hearing aid fitting formulas, including the DSL [i/o]. The resulting computerized recommendation for the patient's hearing loss includes the F and GL potentiometers, with a 110/45–20/FX matrix. As noted previously, the numbers in the matrix (**Table 5–9**) refer to peak output and gain of the hearing aid response. In the case of this patient, the DSL [i/o] SSPL90 (**Fig. 5–14**) recommendation shows a peak output of 110 dB at 3000 Hz in the right ear. Thus, the matrix option that begins with the number 110 is chosen. The second number in the matrix refers to the peak gain of the response. In an instrument such as the one that has been chosen, this value may vary greatly, depending on the adjustments that are made by means of the potentiometers. Thus, this manufacturer designates the gain value by showing the range of peak gain that is possible (**Fig. 5–13**). The peak value shown in the DSL [i/o] full-on gain recommendation (**Fig. 5–14**) is 40 dB at 6000 Hz. Realistically, the hearing aid that has been chosen only responds to ~5000 Hz, so the peak value below 5000 Hz would be more appropriate (38 dB at 3000 Hz). The canal matrix showing the range of 45 to 20 dB of gain would be appropriate for this fitting (**Table 5–9**). In this particular hearing aid, the slope is not designated in the matrix because it is so variable with the potentiometer adjustments. The company refers to the slope as F/X when listing the matrix options. Therefore, the matrix selected would be 110/45–20/F/X (**Table 5–9**).

Special Consideration

- Some audiologists choose to let the manufacturer select the matrix for the ordered fittings. Audiologists argue that, given the 2 cc coupler target, the manufacturer can best understand the ability of the product to meet the target. Others feel strongly that the audiologist should select the matrix and should not leave this role to the manufacturer.

As illustrated, the intent of the hearing aid fitting formula used in this example is not to select a particular hearing aid, but rather a particular electroacoustic response. One is limited to hearing aids that are commercially available. The chosen fitting formula serves as a guide by which to select a hearing aid that will later be fine-tuned to produce the desired response. Even when choosing conventional hearing aids, the manufacturer's fitting software can further serve as a guide to choosing a particular model, potentiometer, and potentiometer settings. Once the clinician is comfortable that the hearing aid described in the specifications contains all the needed features and can provide the required electroacoustic response, the hearing aid must be ordered.

If the audiologist is selecting programmable technology, the selection largely is based on number of channels and range of amplification because the audiologist knows a programmable hearing aid can be programmed to meet the amplification needs of many hearing losses. It is the signal-processing capabilities, features, and flexibility that will drive the selection decision for programmable hearing aids because the amplification response is expected to have a wide range. Currently there are two levels of gain/output when selecting programmable responses (i.e., adequate for mild to moderately severe and adequate for severe to profound hearing loss).

Special Consideration

- Some fitting strategies assume no volume control is included because the hearing aid is adjusting gain as a function of input so targets are in use gain. Add 10 dB (reserve gain) to obtain targets that can be compared with manufacturers' full-on gain specifications.

◆ Facing the Order Form

When a custom hearing aid is ordered, the final link from the audiologist to the hearing aid manufacturer is the order form. The authors recommend that order forms be previewed while the patient is still in the office. This will reduce the need to telephone patients later, wondering whether items such as removal notches or windscreens should be included. This same type of order form is used when ordering custom (completely-in-the-canal [CIC], ITC, or ITE) programmable hearing aids. In that case, the audiologist does not have to prioritize the choice of potentiometers because of the programmability. The audiologist, however, does have to choose all of the other options (e.g., shell color, telecoil, volume control, and memory buttons).

Pearl

- The audiologist should preview the order form before the patient leaves the office so that questions relevant to special options or features on the instruments can be asked.

As noted earlier, each manufacturer's order form features a different layout and design. It is critical to review all product literature, including specification sheets and general product information, before attempting to complete a given manufacturer's order form. Before filling in any information, examine the entire form. Determine first the circuit type, potentiometers, and other options. Then determine the nomenclature by which these features are referred to by that company. For example, the order form for the Starkey Sequel (Starkey Laboratories Inc., Eden Prairie, MN) lists the Starcoil with Switch as a control option. One would have to refer to the circuit option guide, a booklet distributed along with the specification book, to know that the Starcoil is Starkey's product name for a telecoil. For another example, look at the order form shown in **Fig. 5–15.** A section of the form in **Fig. 5–15** allows for entry of a desired matrix. If 2 cc target data are being supplied (e.g., DSL [i/o]), the manufacturer is left with the decision of which is the most appropriate matrix. In this example, the values were taken directly from the DSL [i/o] printout. The authors currently send the desired 2 cc targets (the printout from the fitting protocol can be used) because manufacturers may be able to create 2 cc responses closer to the actual targets than what are displayed in the specification book.

Pearl

- When sending a target to a manufacturer, the audiologist should inform the manufacturer what type of target it is (e.g., 2 cc vs real ear; use vs full-on gain). In addition, do not worry about filling out the patient's audiogram, speech testing results, and specifications of previous hearing aids on the order form. Provide the manufacturer with the 2 cc coupler targets. If audiologists are confident in target selection, they do not need to supply all the other supporting data.

In the end, the goals of the fitting process are to order instruments that meet the electroacoustic, cosmetic, and financial needs of the patient and to communicate these requirements in the most effective and efficient manner to the manufacturer. The impressions and order form are sent to the manufacturer; the next step will be evaluating and presetting the hearing aids upon receipt.

◆ Presetting the Hearing Aids

Whether one is fitting conventional or programmable hearing aids, time working with the patient is saved if the hearing aids are preset before arrival of the patient. If the presetting is accurate, time in the verification session can be spent on minimal fine-tuning and maximal counseling.

Programmable Technology

Presetting programmable technology implies ensuring that the hearing aids can be connected to the computer and the

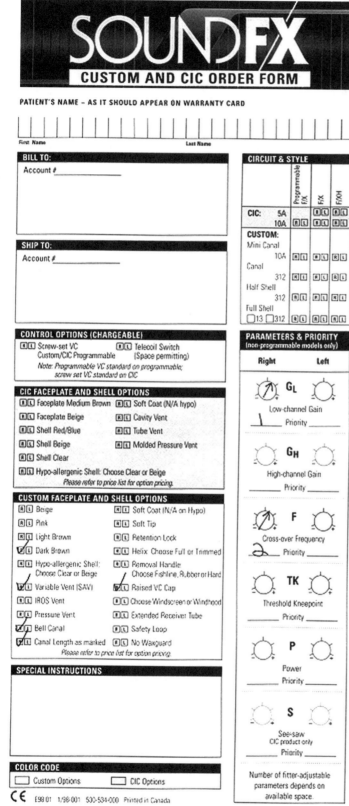

Figure 5–15 Custom product order form.

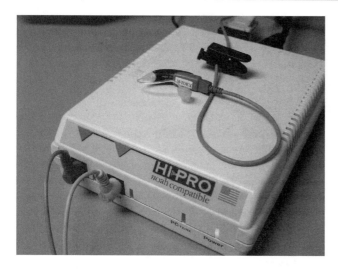

Figure 5–16 Hi-Pro box connecting the hearing aid to the computer (via cable) and programming software (via serial cable). (Courtesy of GN Otometrics A/S, Taastrup, Denmark.)

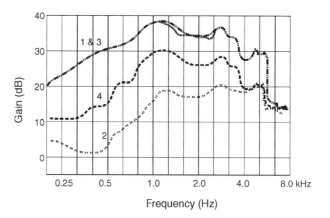

Figure 5–17 Coupler response for "first fit" for four memories in a programmable instrument.

program can be saved to the hearing aids. **Figure 5–16** illustrates the Hi-Pro box (GN Otometrics, Taastrup, Denmark) that connects the hearing aids by cable to the computer for programming. The NOAHlink (Hearing Instrument Manufacturers' Software Association) provides a wireless connection to the computer. Although not necessary for presetting the hearing aids, a wireless setup may be helpful if the patient needs to be mobile. Programmable hearing aids arrive with a "first fit" option that takes the threshold (and uncomfortable loudness level [UCL] if included) data and presets the hearing aids based on a known fitting formula (e.g., NAL-NL1 or DSL [i/o]) or a manufacturer's proprietary algorithm. Many proprietary algorithms vary significantly from the two most accepted fitting rationales, DSL [i/o] and NAL-NL1. Remember that the purpose of "first fit" is to create a starting place from which the audiologist will use real-ear verification to program final settings.

The manufacturer's screen for a programmable instrument will display both "coupler" and "insertion gain" or REAR estimates based on the current hearing aid settings. It is critical that the audiologist does not use these estimated values to verify programmed hearing aid performance. These estimates do not account for any of the individual characteristics of the patient's ear (described earlier), and in the case of custom (ITE, ITC, and CIC) hearing aids, these data are based on average hearing aids, not the hearing aids connected to the computer. Manufacturers' graphs should only be used to gain an estimate of what impact particular programming changes make (e.g., increasing or decreasing gain).

The audiologist must consider all of the features that have been selected when preprogramming the hearing aids. If the programmable hearing aids were ordered with multiple memories, a starting response must be selected for each. The audiologist should think twice before simply using a manufacturer's default setting for multiple memories. **Figure 5–17** illustrates the coupler gain response for four memories of a

programmable hearing aid when "first fit" was selected. It is difficult to imagine how each of these memories might be employed with the current responses. The audiologist will have selected a multimemory instrument for a reason and will want to individualize the memories accordingly. For instance, it may be desirable to have an omnidirectional microphone response fit to DSL [i/o] or NAL-NL1 in memory 1 and a directional response in memory 2.

Prior to the patient's arrival, the audiologist may want to equalize the low-frequency response for the directional microphone memory based on data from Ricketts and Henry (2002) that indicate that the natural loss of low-frequency amplification due to the directional microphone may be detrimental to listeners with low-frequency thresholds of 40 dB HL or poorer.

Memory 3 may have been designed for use with the telecoil. If a programmable telecoil has been ordered, the audiologist will want to preset this by increasing the gain in the low and middle frequencies if the default setting is matched to the microphone response. Because of the nature of the telephone signal, most users require more low- to midfrequency amplification.

Perhaps memory 4 will be deactivated until a specific listening environment is identified for the patient, or perhaps the audiologist plans to use DNR in memories 1 and 2 and therefore plans to program memory 4 for listening to music. It would be preferable to have noise reduction (NR) off for the music program because there is a good chance the NR algorithm will process music as noise and reduce the gain (perhaps differentially across frequencies), making the music distorted.

The audiologist should be aware of the default setting that a given manufacturer uses. Does the presetting account for binaural summation by reducing gain in both hearing aids? Does the program assume the user should start with less gain and then adapt over time? **Figure 5–18** illustrates four levels of adaptation in a hearing aid. The lower curve in **Fig. 5–18** (least gain) is meant for the newer hearing aid user, whereas the upper curve (most gain) is meant for an experienced hearing aid use. In a review of gain preferences and prescriptive fittings, Mueller (2005) reported that there

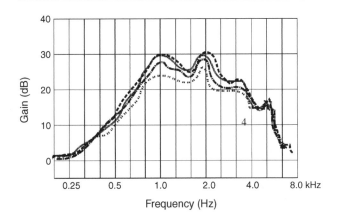

Figure 5–18 Coupler response for four levels of adaptation implemented by one manufacturer.

is a lack of evidence to support this type of gain adaptation for most users. The audiologist should be aware of the program automatically reducing gain and should decide if this is desired. Does the manufacturer preset DNR and expansion to maximum in all memories? Is this desired?

In addition, the tones that indicate switching between programs can be customized by level and frequency, low battery warning indicators can be implemented, the order of memories can be rearranged, volume controls can be deactivated, memories can be deactivated, and the use of NR and expansion can be manipulated. The audiologist will want to be very familiar with the instrument that he or she is fitting and will want to have a plan as to what should be left to the manufacturer's default settings, what should be preprogrammed, and what controls are better used for fine-tuning.

Presetting programmable hearing aids generally consists of obtaining a "first fit" response for memory 1, then tailoring the other memories to the needs of the patient identified earlier. Special features should be tested prior to the patient's arrival (e.g., telecoil response and directional microphones), but the final verification will be in the real ear for the adult patient. Conversely, with conventional technology, the hearing aid should be manipulated until the measured coupler response matches previously determined coupler target values.

Conventional Technology

Presetting conventional technology implies having a set of coupler targets that will guide the setting of the hearing aids and will serve to verify whether the hearing aids are functioning as desired in a coupler. The final verification will take place in the ear and will be dictated by the original goals of the hearing aid fitting.

Depending on the manufacturer, the hearing aids may have arrived with data for presetting. The manufacturer will have based these settings either on the targets that were provided with the order or by entering the audiometric data into a fitting protocol to which the particular manufacturer prescribes. Either way, these settings are probably a good

starting place. Review the requested potentiometers by examining the specification sheet or by using the manufacturer's software to see how changes in the potentiometer are expected to impact the response of the hearing aids.

Pearl

- With WDRC hearing aids, do not be overly concerned with the actual values of the CT and CR. If the audiologist can adjust the hearing aid to meet level-dependent targets, the CT and CR must be close enough.

At a minimum, with WDRC hearing aids the following should be measured in the coupler: (1) frequency response (gain or output depending on how the chosen fitting protocol provides target data) for three input levels (whatever levels were used to generate the targets), (2) SSPL90 curve (to check the limiting), (3) total harmonic distortion for a quiet (50 dB SPL) and loud (85 dB SPL) input, (4) circuit noise (equivalent input noise level), and (5) telecoil response. The audiologist may want to obtain input/output curves for a low (500 Hz) and high (3000 Hz) frequency to document CT and CR. If the three input level targets match, this measure is redundant. If the three input level targets do not match, the input/output data may help identify the problem. These measures are meant to be compared directly to the coupler targets provided by the fitting protocol that was used to order the hearing aid. Manipulate the available potentiometers until the targets are matched as closely as possible. Agreement within $+/-3$ dB is excellent. More than 7 dB difference between the hearing aid's response and the original targets is cause for concern and perhaps for return of the hearing aid if the response cannot be manipulated.

Pearl

- Use a hearing aid test box that allows for the selection of a variety of input levels and types of signals and provides input/output curves for a range of frequencies (not just 2000 Hz).

A linear hearing aid should be evaluated with the following coupler measures: (1) frequency response (gain or output) for a moderate input level (65–70 dB SPL), (2) SSPL90, (3) total harmonic distortion for a quiet (50 dB SPL) and loud (85 dB SPL) input, (4) circuit noise, and (5) telecoil response. A linear response implies that gain does not change as a function of input level, but a high- and low-frequency input/output curve still may be useful in identifying the input level that engages the output limiting of the hearing aid.

In the following sections, the example hearing aid has been adjusted using the GL and F potentiometers that were ordered and the volume control to match the coupler targets generated by DSL [i/o]. **Figure 5–14** provides all the coupler data needed to preset the hearing aids. Measure the output of the hearing aid with a 90, 80, 65, and 50 dB SPL input signal. In addition, test signal choices will interact with the hearing aid signal processing (e.g., gain may be reduced for a noise test signal by NR circuitry). See Stelmachowicz et al (1996) for a review of appropriate test signals. Make sure that the type of signal used in the coupler measures is the same as was used in creating the targets. In DSL [i/o], the user selects these parameters and will see the selections on screen. **Figure 5–19** illustrates the coupler measurements made with the example hearing aid. The measured values are compared with the prescribed values. In this case, the actual values obtained are in good agreement with the prescribed values. This provides an ideal documentation of the coupler response. Some of the coupler measurement systems will calculate the target for the fitting protocol that is being used or will allow entry of particular targets, which saves time because the measured values can be compared on screen to the targets. An alternative is to compare the coupler data to simulated real-ear measures (S-REM, AudioScan, Dorchester, Ontario, Canada; **Fig. 5–20**). The hearing aid is preset based on the manufacturer's recommended settings and then attached to the coupler. The AudioScan measurement system is set to S-REM, and the thresholds are entered. RECD is entered to provide an appropriate conversion from dB HL to dB SPL thresholds so that the coupler measures can be converted to estimated SPL at the eardrum. Now the hearing aid potentiometers are manipulated until the soft signal is above threshold and the loud signal is below UCL (indicated by asterisks in **Fig. 5–20**). As can be seen in **Fig. 5–20**, the output for the moderate signal is matching the targets.

If the level-dependent gain or output targets are matched, and the hearing aids are being limited at the appropriate output, the combination of CT and CR is appropriate. If the gain or output targets are not met, the CT and CR that can be deduced from an input/output curve may be instructive in what needs to be manipulated.

♦ Assessing the Function of Special Features

Telecoils

In the beginning of this chapter, assessing the telecoil response was included in the list of items to check using the 2 cc coupler. If a telecoil has been ordered, its frequency

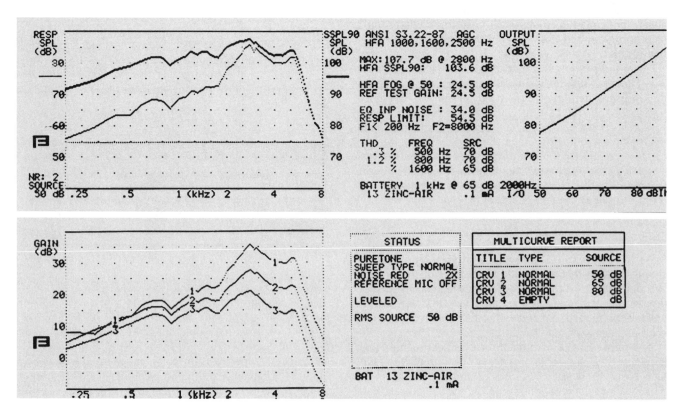

Figure 5–19 Coupler data used to preset the hearing aid according to a fitting protocol.

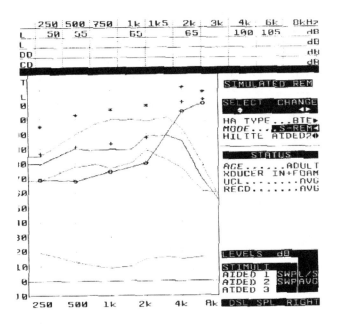

Figure 5–20 Simulated real ear measurement (S-REM).

response should be documented. Chapter 1 in this volume provides a detailed description of 2 cc coupler measurement of the telecoil. Although the clinician does not have any method of changing the telecoil response in the conventional hearing aid, a weak response should motivate the clinician to return the hearing aid until a reasonable telecoil response is obtained. The telecoil should produce the same response as the microphone with some additional low-frequency emphasis. A weak telecoil response would provide significantly less gain than the microphone response. Including a telecoil option is not useful if the telecoil is not functioning. The ANSI 1996 and 2003 standards include a measurement of telecoil response across frequency in the test box. **Figure 5–21** illustrates the resulting graph from this measurement. The sound pressure level in an inductive telephone simulator (SPLITS) compares the microphone

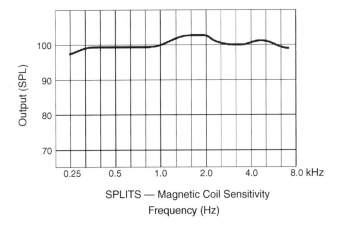

Figure 5–21 Telecoil response measured in a coupler. SPL, sound pressure level; SPLITS, SPL in an inductive telephone simulator.

response and telecoil response. In **Fig. 5–21,** the result is a SPLITS of −4.4 dB, suggesting the telecoil overall gain is 4.4 dB softer than the microphone response. In a programmable instrument, the audiologist may want to increase the gain so the standard threshold shift (STS)–SPLITS arrives closer to 0 dB. In a conventional instrument, the audiologist might use this information to counsel the patient about manipulating the volume control to increase the output of the telecoil.

If the audiologist does not have the capability of measuring the gain–frequency response of the telecoil directly in the hearing aid test box, the following procedure can be used. Set the telecoil for testing with a HAT using a neckloop. Place the hearing aid (set to telecoil) in the middle of a neckloop (positioned as if it were on an ear and neck) connected to the receiver of a HAT, and connect the hearing aid to the 2 cc coupler. The test box microphone is inserted into the 2 cc coupler. The HAT can be sitting outside the test box on a padded surface. Inside the test box, connect the microphone of the HAT to the transmitter. This is the unit that will pick up the signal generated inside the test box. The FM signal will be transmitted to the receiver coupled to the hearing aid, and the test box microphone will pick up and record the response. Make sure the hearing aid, HAT transmitter, and receiver are all turned on and have good batteries. An 80 dB SPL signal is reasonable because it mimics the input level at the microphone of a HAT. This will not necessarily mimic a telephone signal, but the measurement will document the frequency response of the telecoil. Returning inadequate telecoils will assist in educating manufacturers about the importance of this component of the hearing aid. A DAI or built-in FM receiver could be tested in the same manner.

Hearing Assistive Technology

If a HAT will be used with the hearing aids, it is essential to measure the hearing aid response when the HAT provides the input signal, whether that is via neckloop/telecoil, FM boot, internal FM receiver, DAI, Bluetooth, or some other coupling technology. The HAT and the coupling method may impact the final hearing aid response. Some HATs have potentiometers that can be manipulated to achieve an appropriate response; programmable hearing aids also may be manipulated to ensure an appropriate response when coupled to the HAT. See Chapter 17 in this text for a detailed description of HA/HAT measurement.

Directional Microphones

It is essential that the audiologist verifies that the directional microphones are functioning properly. The goal is for the output to be greater if the signal is presented in front while in the directional setting and less (at least by 3 dB) when the signal is behind. When this type of measurement is completed with a probe microphone in the patient's ear and the speaker is moved from in front to behind the individual, it is called a front-to-back ratio. Although this is a reasonable measurement, the drawback is that the patient has already arrived, and if the clinician determines that the

Table 5–10 Definitions of Terms Used to Describe Directional Microphone Settings

Term	Definition
Fixed directional	When functioning in the directional setting, one polar pattern is implemented
Adaptive directional	When functioning in the directional setting, multiple polar patterns are available and are implemented based on the algorithm that is imposed on the basis of digital sampling of the incoming signal
Automatic directional	The fixed directional polar plot or omnidirectional response is implemented automatically based on the algorithm that is imposed on the basis of digital sampling of the incoming signal
Automatic adaptive directional	Multiple polar patterns, including omnidirectional, are implemented automatically based on the algorithm that is imposed on the basis of digital sampling of the incoming signal

directional microphones are not functioning properly (e.g., reverse response or no difference), then the hearing aid(s) must be returned to the manufacturer. Frye (2006) presents step-by-step instructions for measuring the directional response in a test box and with a probe microphone with the hearing aid mounted on a pole. With one of these methods, the audiologist can assess this feature prior to the patient's fitting appointment. With the advent of automatic directionality, adaptive directionality, and automatic adaptive directionality (see **Table 5–10** for definitions), it is important to be sure the hearing aid actually is in the directional mode during measurement. Setting the hearing aid to fixed directionality for testing will ensure evaluation of the directional microphone in an appropriate setting.

Whether presetting and evaluating conventional or programmable hearing aids, listen to the hearing aids through a personal listening mold or listening stethoscope before the patient arrives. The ANSI (1987, 1996b, 2003) electroacoustic analysis does not provide a measure of all types of distortion and will not necessarily identify hearing aids with some intermittent problems. Move the hearing aid around and listen.

♦ Verification of the Selection

The conventional hearing aids that were ordered have arrived and have been preset to approximate the coupler targets supplied through the fitting protocol of choice. Programmable hearing aids will have been set to "first fit," and parameters discussed earlier will have been preset. The patient is scheduled for the hearing aid fitting and arrives expecting to leave with new hearing aids. It is time to verify the hearing aids' responses in the patient's ears and to verify any other features that were part of the original goal of the fitting. The goal of the hearing aid fitting and the data collected for ordering the hearing aids will dictate how the hearing aid verification should be conducted. If the audiologist has chosen to fit linear technology, assessing loudness ratings across input levels to verify the fitting is not appropriate and may be unfair to the manufacturer from whom the hearing aids were ordered. If the original goal was to ensure audibility of soft, moderate, and loud sounds or to restore normal loudness perception, some sort of evaluation to determine whether this has been achieved would seem to be essential.

The first item to verify is adequacy and comfort of the physical fit. There is no point in proceeding with verification measurements if there is a poor physical fit. This must be corrected. Although the patient may not consider the new sensation of having hearing aids in his or her ears comfortable, it should not be painful.

Real-ear verification should follow the procedures used to create the prescriptive target(s). If the measurement system includes the selected fitting algorithm, target(s) will appear on the same screen where the individual real-ear data are presented. This is ideal because the clinician is not looking back and forth between papers to see if the data appear to be the same. Some measurement systems will allow the audiologist to enter the actual targets even though the system does not calculate these. Either method provides good documentation in terms of matching the real-ear target. Regardless of the coupler data, the real ear is where the hearing aids work.

Pearl

- For easier verification and good record keeping, purchase a coupler and real-ear system that produce targets using the preferred fitting algorithm or, at a minimum, allow the audiologist to enter absolute targets for several input levels. Check to see the manufacturer's record of updating target selections as new fitting protocols are introduced and/or modified.

During real-ear measurements, the audiologist fitting conventional hearing aids will require a screwdriver to manipulate available potentiometers. Audiologists fitting programmable technology will connect the hearing aids to either the Hi-Pro box (**Fig. 5–16**) or the NOAHlink, which allows more movement because the patient is not wired to the computer.

For most individuals with mild, moderate, or moderately severe hearing loss, the essential goal of the hearing aid fitting will be to return audibility across input levels (soft, moderate, and loud) and frequency (as wide a bandwidth as possible). Auditory mapping provides a reasonable verification technique if this is the goal. For this technique, the individual's thresholds and LDLs (if measured) are entered into the probe microphone equipment. The HL data are converted

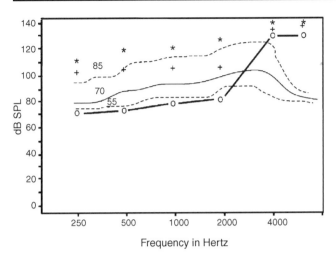

Figure 5–22 Auditory mapping without real ear-to-coupler difference (RECD) used to convert hearing level (HL) to sound pressure level (SPL) thresholds. Circles represent thresholds, plus signs (+) are desired sensation level (DSL) targets for moderate inputs, asterisks (*) represent the uncomfortable loudness level (UCL), broken lines represent the real ear aided response (REAR) for 50 dB input (*lower curve*) and REAR for 85 dB input (*upper curve*), and the solid line represents REAR for moderate inputs.

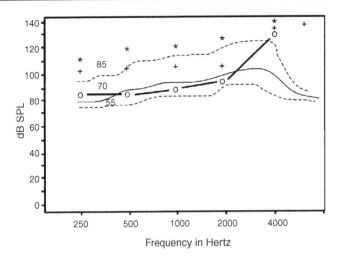

Figure 5–23 Auditory mapping with individual RECD used to convert HL to SPL thresholds. Circles represent thresholds, plus signs (+) are DSL targets for moderate inputs, asterisks (*) represent UCL, broken lines represent REAR for 50 dB input (*lower curve*) and REAR for 85 dB input (*upper curve*), and the solid line represents REAR for moderate inputs.

to dB SPL, and the DR is displayed on the REAR output screen (**Fig. 5–22**). Once again, the use of RECD is critical. If the verification will be based on a soft input level being just above thresholds, a moderate input level being well above thresholds, or matching an REAR target, such as DSL [i/o] values (represented by plus signs in **Fig. 5–22**), and a loud input level being just below LDL (asterisks in **Fig. 5–22**), then the accurate conversion from HL to SPL is essential. **Figure 5–22** illustrates threshold and LDL SPLs obtained by applying an average RECD to dB HL thresholds. The hearing aid response appears to return audibility through 3000 Hz across input levels and would be an adequate hearing aid fitting, considering the individual's hearing loss. **Figure 5–23** illustrates the same data when the individual's RECD was used to convert dB HL thresholds and LDLs to dB SPL. Now it is clear that the output for soft sounds is inadequate (below threshold). For severe hearing losses, one may find that soft sounds cannot be made audible across the frequency range. In this case, auditory mapping can be a good counseling tool to instill realistic expectations.

Some clinicians prefer to use real ear insertion gain (REIG) targets for verification of the hearing aid fitting. Although this technique does indeed verify that gain achieved by the hearing aids matches the derived targets, it does not guarantee that soft, moderate, and loud sounds are audible, which most likely was the minimum goal of the fitting. **Figure 5–24** provides an example of hearing loss to illustrate this point. **Figure 5–25** reports that the audiologist has carefully manipulated the left and right hearing aids to match the REIG targets for three input levels. **Figure 5–26** provides the REAR curves for the soft input level compared with the patient's actual dynamic range in SPL. It is evident that the hearing aid is underamplifying the high-frequency signals for a soft input level. The level of the thresholds may

preclude audibility, but the information still will be useful in counseling the patient.

The audiologist also must be cognizant of the signal being used in verification measures (this is true for presetting as well). Stelmachowicz et al (1996) reported that swept pure tones and speech-weighted composite noise underestimated the high-frequency gain for real speech. Speech-modulated noise and simulated speech (e.g., International Collegium of Rehabilitative Audiology [ICRA] noise) provide the closest approximation of continuous discourse. The test signal and hearing aid signal processing will interact as well. If the test signal is considered "noise" by the hearing

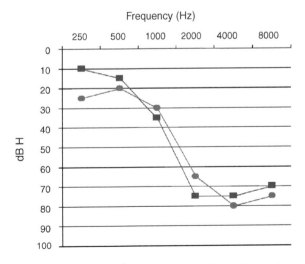

Figure 5–24 High-frequency sloping sensorineural hearing loss.

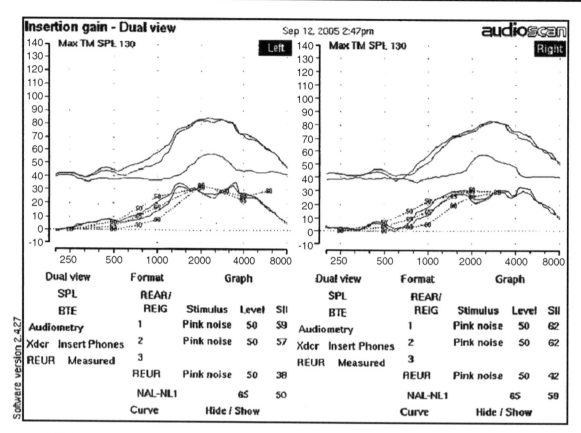

Figure 5–25 Insertion gain measurements compared with insertion gain targets.

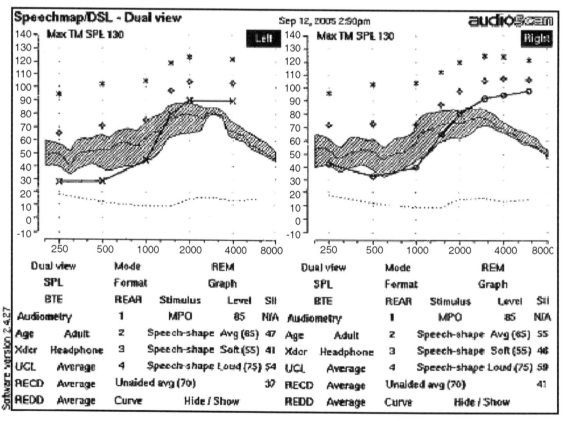

Figure 5–26 Auditory mapping showing inadequate audibility.

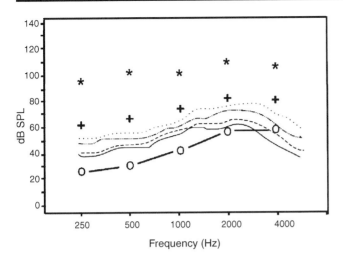

Figure 5–27 Coupler measurements for four levels of noise reduction using a pink noise as the input signal. The top curve (highest output) was measured with noise reduction off; the second curve from the top illustrates the response with "low" noise reduction, and the third with "moderate" noise reduction; the lowest output illustrates "maximum" noise reduction. o, individual patient's thresholds; *, uncomfortable loudness; +, target for moderate outputs.

aid, and noise reduction is being implemented, the output and/or gain response will be reduced compared with the amount that might be achieved when the hearing aid was processing speech. To solve this problem, NR can be turned off during verification, or the audiologist can use a signal that the hearing aid will treat as speech (e.g., ICRA noise). The audiologist may want to verify what NR is doing and therefore may choose a noiselike signal to test this feature. **Figure 5–27** illustrates the hearing aid response to pink noise with the four different NR levels available in this particular hearing aid.

♦ Orientation

Once responses have been modified, if necessary, and verified in some meaningful way (meeting fitting strategy generated targets, establishing audibility, etc.), it is time to orient the patient to the instrument. Palmer and Mormer (1997) provide a detailed process for hearing aid orientation. The details will not be repeated here, but the essential items will be outlined. See also Chapters 8 and 12 in this volume for a comprehensive discussion of hearing aid orientation.

The patient must be comfortable with the operation of the hearing aid(s) before leaving the session: removal, insertion, volume control wheel, telecoil switch, on/off switch, and battery. During orientation, the audiologist should play some continuous discourse (in quiet and noise at varying levels) for the patient to experience the hearing aid and to learn to rotate the volume control wheel, if one is provided. This testing environment also can allow the patient to practice

locating himself or herself appropriately (signal in front) for directional microphone use.

The authors' approach is to not elicit a great deal of input from the patient during the orientation session. For example, hearing aid response rarely is modified at this time. Other clinicians take a different approach and make modifications based on patients' initial reactions. The decision of whether to make modifications during orientation is a matter of individual judgment. Palmer et al (1998) offer a review of data that may shed light on which approach to take. New hearing aid users, who may not have heard a variety of sounds at different input levels in particular frequency regions for more than a decade, may not be capable of assessing sound quality, and previous users may be used to different signal processing (e.g., going from linear to WDRC). Trying to modify the hearing aid's response to the patient's wishes at this stage may result in a hearing aid that provides no gain for quiet sounds and no gain for any high frequencies (the authors have witnessed this). Several studies (e.g., Lindley et al, 2001; Mueller and Powers, 2001) have found that patients adapt to quiet sounds over time, so the audiologist would not necessarily want to reduce amplification for quiet sounds. Other studies (e.g., Kawell et al, 1988; Lindley et al, 2001) have found that individuals do not adapt to uncomfortably loud sounds. Therefore, during orientation, the output should be adjusted until loud sounds are tolerable to the patient. The venting or low-frequency response may need to be adjusted to make the individual's voice tolerable. Thus, minor adjustments may need to be made to make the sound tolerable, but the patient should be encouraged to wait for more fine-tuning (with programmable instruments) until a period of adaptation has been completed. Patient-specific modifications (other than discomfort) are better left to the 2-week follow-up appointment, unless these modifications are so important to the patient that he or she will not try the hearing aid(s). In these cases, the clinician may want to attempt to fine-tune the instrument during orientation. This entails providing less gain initially (especially in the high frequencies), then slowly adding the gain as the patient adjusts to the hearing aid.

A hearing aid wearing schedule should be created for the patient. The audiologist will suggest how many hours and in what types of situations (e.g., 2 hours the first day of use in the home) the patient should start using the hearing aid(s). This type of schedule may not be appropriate for the experienced user. The patient is instructed to increase the wearing time and to test the aid(s) in more difficult listening experiences. The audiologist also may encourage the patient to keep a journal of listening successes and difficulties over the next several weeks. The patient should be reminded of the situations from the PEW (**Fig. 5–3**) so he or she can focus on performance in these situations. Before leaving the orientation session, the patient should be scheduled for a 2- to 3-week follow-up visit. The patient is instructed to contact the clinic before this time if questions or concerns arise. Whenever possible, the patient should be contacted 1 or 2 days after fitting to inquire about success or difficulty.

♦ Follow-up/Fine-tuning

The checklist provided in **Fig. 5–28** guides the clinician through the follow-up appointment. This type of form provides excellent documentation of what has been discussed and recommended with a patient. Action plans are made for any areas that are not satisfactory; these plans will dictate when the patient needs to be seen next.

The clinician may want to make some additional measurements at the follow-up appointment based on the patient's comments. For instance, if the patient is complaining that soft sounds are too loud, the audiologist may want to measure loudness growth to decide what changes to make to a programmable hearing aid.

If the goal of the fitting was to restore a normal loudness growth (soft sounds are perceived as soft, moderate sounds are perceived as comfortable, and loud sounds are perceived

Checklist for 1 to 2 Week Follow-Up Visit

ITEM	OUTCOME	ACTION PLAN	✓
Hearing Aid Commentary			
Hours Worn Per Day			
Able to Insert Aid			
Able to Remove Aid			
Cleaning & Maintenance			
Situations of Best Success			
Situations of Least Success			
Assistive Devices			
Aural Rehab Follow-up			
Review Telephone Use			
Memory/Features Options			
Warranty Expiration			
Insurance Information			
Consent Form Signed			

✓ = Check off item if outcome is positive or when action plan is successfully completed.

_____   _____
Patient Signature   Date

_____   _____
Dispenser Signature   Date

Figure 5–28 Checklist for 1- to 2- week follow-up visit.

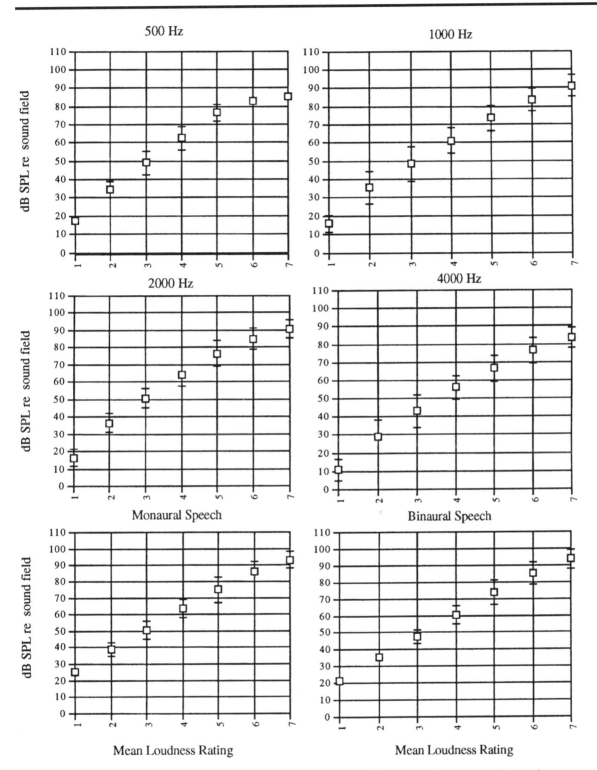

Figure 5–29 Loudness growth functions (500, 1000, 2000, and 4000 Hz warble tones and monaural and binaural continuous discourse) from normal-hearing subjects for purposes of verification.

as loud but not uncomfortable), a loudness growth test would be a reasonable procedure to assist with fine-tuning. **Figure 5–29** provides the data the authors use for this purpose. If the goal is to return a normal growth of loudness, one would want to compare the perception of the hearing aid user to the average perception of individuals with normal hearing. The graphs in **Fig. 5–29** represent the mean loudness ratings for warble tones presented monaurally and continuous discourse (speech) presented monaurally and binaurally. These data are in dB SPL and were obtained in the sound field. In the monaural condition, the nontest ear must be occluded and/or masked. The patient's ratings are marked on each graph. The clinician may want to verify with all available warble tone test frequencies (500, 1000, 2000, and 4000 Hz) or may just assess speech. At a minimum, it is useful to verify the monaural and binaural conditions of speech. In a case where the REIG or family of REAR curves was not within the prescriptive target and further manipulation of a conventional hearing aid was not possible, loudness perception verification may lead the clinician to accept the compromise in response or provide data that the compromise is unacceptable.

The graphic display can be very helpful when deciding what needs to be changed regarding the hearing aid response. The separation of frequencies allows the clinician to identify if a change is needed in a low or high channel. The input levels at which targets are met will enable the clinician to identify if CT, CR, or expansion needs to be adjusted. Remember that a change in gain without a change in limiting is a change in CR in a WDRC circuit. The normative data in **Fig. 5–29** were collected using 10 normal-hearing adults listening in the test booth that is used for hearing aid verification. Each test site or clinic should collect comparable data in its own booths and with its own equipment, because differences in results may occur.

Participation by the patient, particularly a first-time user, in the follow-up session can be a powerful counseling tool. Additionally, by recording data during the follow-up appointment, the clinician can show that the goal of the initial fitting has been met (i.e., the patient perceives a range of input levels). These data may encourage the individual to continue to adjust to the hearing aid(s).

Although it is tempting to evaluate speech recognition in quiet and noise in the sound booth, it is clear that this type of testing does not "mimic" real life and is unlikely to provide valuable information for fine-tuning or counseling. This type of testing can even be misleading in evaluating the benefit of directional microphones: the appropriate setup of the signal in front and noise in back at a close distance with little reverberation generally will produce a much improved score compared with omnidirectional listening, but it is unlikely that this benefit will be realized in real listening situations.

Whether adjustments will be based on interview or some type of measurement, the clinician needs a plan for fine-tuning that links complaints or loudness judgments to the parameters of the signal processing that can be manipulated. The key is to identify the area (input level and frequency region) the individual is complaining about, then determine what parameters in that particular hearing aid change that region (which channel, gain for soft sounds, CR, CT, maximum output, expansion, etc.). For instance, if the loudness judgment test reveals that the patient provides a rating of 4 at 35 dB for a 500 Hz warble tone with normal ratings for the louder input levels (e.g., a rating of 6 at 80 dB and 7 at 85 or 90 dB), then the clinician needs to decrease the gain for soft sounds in at least the low frequencies. Presumably, this same test would be done at a high frequency, and those results would be considered as well. In this example, a normal perception of loudness is

identified for the high frequencies. Considering these findings, it would be advantageous to have a programmable hearing aid that allowed manipulation of gain for soft sounds separately from moderate or loud sounds, and it would be essential to have at least two frequency channels to manipulate the low-frequency response separately from the high-frequency response (which was found to be accurate with the current hearing aid settings). Once the input level and frequency channel that need to be changed have been identified, the next decision is how to make the change. In this case, the gain for soft sounds in the low frequencies could be reduced, the CT could be increased, or expansion could be increased.

When the clinician is satisfied that the hearing aid is performing appropriately and any changes in response have been made (and verified), a final set of coupler measurements should be obtained, and the hearing aid settings should be documented. This documentation will serve as a basis for future troubleshooting.

♦ Outcomes Assessment

Just because all prescriptive targets have been achieved does not necessarily mean that a patient is satisfied. At present, the authors depend on post-test measures of the PEW and APHAB for outcome assessment. The PEW **(Fig. 5–3)** has strong validity for the patient who is recording his or her perceived level of success. An audiologist can feel confident in the methods of hearing aid fitting when he or she can report that the patient's clearly defined expectations have been met.

The APHAB can be readministered to determine a benefit score. The subsection results can be used to document the outcome of the hearing aid fitting. Perhaps more importantly, reactions to individual questions on the APHAB can guide the audiologist to further solutions that may be necessary for the hearing aid user.

The audiologist may prefer an absolute measure of satisfaction rather than a post-test that establishes benefit. The Satisfaction in Daily Life (SADL; Cox and Alexander, 1999) and the International Outcome Inventory for Hearing Aids (IOI-HA; Cox et al, 2003) are appropriate self-report inventories with good psychometric data that will establish satisfaction. These measures also may be valuable quality assurance measures for a clinic.

Palmer and Mueller (1999) introduced the Profile of Aided Loudness (PAL) to be used as an outcome assessment for a hearing aid fitting, when the goal was to return normal loudness perception. The loudness restoration verification procedure **(Fig. 5–29)** may document that the hearing aid user perceives warble tones and continuous discourse in a sound booth similarly to individuals with normal hearing. This does not necessarily translate into a restoration of loudness in the individual's listening environment. It also does not address the individual's reaction to loudness restoration. The PAL provides a list of sounds that have been judged as "very soft," "soft," "comfortable but slightly soft," "comfortable," "comfortable but slightly loud," "loud but OK," or "uncomfortably loud" by a large group of normal-hearing individuals. The items included in the profile revealed good test–retest reliability and consistency in loudness rating across subjects (differing by gender and age). The audiologist has the hearing aid wearer rate the perceived loudness of each of the listed sounds and the satisfaction with the loudness of the sound. For instance, the sound of a refrigerator motor could be perceived as soft, but the individual could be displeased with that perception. The results of the loudness rating are plotted against the perceptions of normal-hearing individuals. This allows the audiologist to judge whether the patient's perception is in a comparable range and indicates appropriate modifications. The satisfaction results are used for counseling purposes. For instance, if the loudness perception for an item is in agreement with the normative data, yet the individual is not satisfied, the normative data are useful in counseling the patient that most normal-hearing individuals perceive the sound the same way.

It is important for clinicians to choose outcome assessments that relate directly to the original goals of the hearing aid fitting. For example, if the goals were related to individual expectations, a final evaluation of whether the expectations were met makes greater sense. However, if the goal is related to hearing in background noise, the background noise subscale of the APHAB may provide the most appropriate data. Finally, if the goal was to equalize loudness perception (i.e., all input signals should be perceived as comfortable), it is not appropriate to compare the hearing aid user to normal-hearing individuals. See Chapter 6 in this volume for a full review of outcome measures.

♦ Summary

The individual with hearing loss enters into a process with the audiologist. The outcome does not focus on whether the individual will be a hearing aid wearer or not. Instead, it focuses on what will be the right combination of technology and other interventions for the individual, and these solutions will be found through the hearing aid fitting process. The process continues as the individual's needs change, as the communication environment changes, and as technology changes.

Acknowledgments   Thanks to the professionals at Unitron, in particular Ted Venema and Carol Zaccatto, for their assistance with the figures related to conventional technology. Thanks to Gus Mueller and Tom Powers of Siemens for their support (intellectual and financial) for a project that supplied the data in **Fig. 5–29**. Thanks to Randall Kesterson of the Eye and Ear Institute, University of Pittsburgh Medical Center, for assistance with many of the figures. The authors would like to acknowledge the students in the Amplification II (fall 2005) course at the University of Pittsburgh who provided the evidence-based reviews for the signal-processing section of this chapter. The authors also would like to thank Amanda Ortmann for her assistance on several sections of this work. Thanks to Harvey Dillon and Susan Scollie for advanced information about the changes for NAL-NL2 and DSL version 5, respectively. Finally, thanks to all of our students and the professionals in the Pittsburgh and Philadelphia areas who push us to systematically think about hearing aid evaluation, selection, fitting, and verification.

Appendix 5–1

Correction factors for microphone location used in **Fig. 5–7.** Data were obtained in a diffuse field and are courtesy of Killion (personal communication, 1988). Some additional sources for average-based values are Bentler and Pavlovic (1989) and Killion and Revit (1993).

Frequency (Hz)	BTE	Avg. ITE	Full ITC	Small ITC
250	0.4	0.5	0.5	0.5
500	1.0	1.3	1.5	1.2
1000	1.6	1.6	2.0	2.0
2000	2.8	2.7	3.4	3.8
3000*	2.9	3.7	4.9	6.3
4000	3.2	5.4	7.7	9.5

* Values actually obtained at 2918 Hz.

BTE, behind the ear; ITC, in the canal; ITE, in the ear.

References

American National Standards Institute. (1987). Specification of hearing aid characteristics (ANSI S3.22–1987). New York: Author.

American National Standards Institute. (1996a). Specification for audiometers (ANSI S3.6–1996). New York: Author.

American National Standards Institute. (1996b). Specification of hearing aid characteristics (ANSI S3.22–1996). New York: Author.

American National Standards Institute. (1997). Methods for calculation of the speech intelligibility index (ANSI S2.5–1997). New York: Author.

American National Standards Institute. (2003). Specification of hearing aid characteristics (ANSI S3.22–2003). New York: Author.

Baer, T., Moore, B. C., & Kluk, K. (2002). Effects of low-pass filtering on the intelligibility of speech in noise for people with and without dead regions at high frequencies. Journal of the Acoustical Society of America, 112, 1133–1144.

Bakke, M. H., Neuman, A., & Levitt, H. (1995, March). Evaluation of a hearing aid rating procedure. Poster session presented at NODCD/VA Conference on Hearing Aids, Washington, DC.

Bentler, R. A. (2005). Effectiveness of directional microphones and noise reduction schemes in hearing aids: A systematic review of the evidence. Journal of the American Academy of Audiology, 16(7), 473–484.

Bentler, R. A., & Nelson, J. A. (1997). Assessing release-time options in a two-channel ABC hearing aid. Ear and Hearing, 6(1), 43–50.

Bentler, R. A., & Pavlovic, C. V. (1989). Transfer functions and correction factors used in hearing aid evaluation and research. Ear and Hearing, 10(1), 58–63.

Byrne, D. (1986). Effects of frequency response characteristics on speech discrimination and perceived intelligibility and pleasantness of speech for hearing-impaired listeners. Journal of the Acoustical Society of America, 80(2), 494–504.

Byrne, D., & Dillon, H. (1986). The National Acoustics Laboratories' (NAL) new procedure for selecting the gain and frequency response of a hearing aid. Ear and Hearing, 7, 257–265.

Byrne, D., Dillon, H., Ching, T., Katsch, R., & Keidser, G. (2001). NAL-NL1 procedure for fitting nonlinear hearing aids: Characteristics and comparisons with other procedures. Journal of the American Academy of Audiology, 12, 37–51.

Cornelisse, L. E., Seewald, R. C., & Jamieson, D. G. (1994). Wide-dynamic-range-compression hearing aids: The DSL[i/o] approach. Hearing Journal, 47(10), 23–29.

Cox, R. M. (1997). Administration and application of the APHAB. Hearing Journal, 50(4), 32–48.

Cox, R. M., & Alexander, B. (1995). The abbreviated profile of hearing aid benefit. Ear and Hearing, 16, 176–183.

Cox, R. M., Alexander, G., & Beyer, C. (2003). Norms for the international outcome inventory for hearing aids. Journal of the American Academy of Audiology, 14(8), 403–413.

Cox, R. M., & Alexander, G. (1999). Measuring satisfaction with amplification in daily life: SADL. Ear and Hearing, 20, 306–320.

Dillon, H., James, A., & Gims, J. (1997). Client oriented scale of improvement (COSI) and its relationship to several other measures of benefit and satisfaction provided by hearing aids. Journal of the American Academy of Audiology, 8, 27–43.

Feigin, J. A., Kopun, J. G., Stelmachowicz, P. G., & Gorga, M. P. (1989). Probe-tube microphone measures of earcanal sound pressure level in infants and children. Ear and Hearing, 10(4), 254–258.

Fikret-Pasa, S., & Revit, L. J. (1992). Individualized correction factors in the preselection of hearing aids. Journal of Speech and Hearing Research, 35(2), 384–400.

Frye, G. (2006). How to verify directional hearing aids in the office. Hearing Review, 1, 48–54.

Gittes, T., Niquette, P. (1995). FIG6 in ten. Hearing Review, 2(10), 28–30.

Hansen, M. (2002). Effects of multi-channel compression time constants on subjectively perceived sound quality and speech intelligibility. Ear and Hearing, 23(4), 369–380.

Hawkins, D. B., Cooper, W. A., & Thompson, D. J. (1990). Comparisons among SPLs in real-ears, 2 cc and 6 cm^3 couplers. Journal of the American Academy of Audiology, 1, 154–161.

Jenstad, L. M., Seewald, R., Cornelisse, L., & Shantz, J. (1999). Comparison of linear gain and wide dynamic range compression hearing aid circuits: 2. Aided loudness measures. Ear and Hearing, 20, 117–126.

Kawell, M. E., Kopun, J., & Stelmachowicz, P. (1988). Loudness discomfort levels in children. Ear and Hearing, 9, 133–136.

Keidser, G., & Grant, F. (2001). The preferred number of channels (one, two, four) in NAL-NL1 prescribed wide dynamic range compression (WDRC) devices. Ear and Hearing, 22, 516–527.

Killion, M. C., Niquette, P. A., Gudmundsen, G. I., Revitt, L. J., & Banerjee, S. (2004). Development of a quick speech-in-noise test for measuring signal-to-noise ratio loss in normal-hearing and hearing-impaired listeners. Journal of the Acoustical Society of America, 116(4), 2395–2405.

Killion, M. C., & Revit, L. J. (1993). CORFIG and GIFROC: Real ear to coupler and back. In G. A. Studebacker & I. Hochberg (Eds.), Acoustical factors affecting hearing aid performance (pp. 65–85). Boston: Allyn & Bacon.

Lewis, D. E., & Stelmachowicz, P. (1993). Real-ear to 6 cm^3 coupler differences in young children. Journal of Speech and Hearing Research, 36, 204–209.

Lindley, G. (2005, September). Is your hearing aid fitting protocol in need of an extreme makeover? Paper presented at the annual meeting of the Pennsylvania Academy of Audiology, State College, PA.

Lindley, G. A., Palmer, C. V., Durrant, J. D., & Pratt, S. (2001). Audiologist-versus patient-driven hearing aid fitting protocols. Seminars in Hearing, 22(2), 139–160.

Mackersie, C. L., Crocker, T. L., & Davis, R. A. (2004). Limiting high-frequency hearing aid gain in listeners with and without suspected dead regions. Journal of the American Academy of Audiology, 15, 498–507.

Marriage, J. E., Moore, B., Stone, M., & Baer, T. (2005). Effects of three amplification strategies on speech perception by children with severe to profound hearing loss. Ear and Hearing, 26(1), 35–47.

Moore, B. C., Huss, M., Vickers, D. A., Glasberg, B. R., & Alcantara, J. L. (2000). A test for the diagnosis of dead regions in the cochlea. British Journal of Audiology, 34, 205–224.

Mueller, H. G. (2005). Fitting hearing aids to adults using prescriptive methods: An evidence-based review of effectiveness. Journal of the American Academy of Audiology, 16, 448–460.

Mueller, H. G., & Bentler, R. A. (2005). Fitting hearing aids using clinical measures of loudness discomfort levels: An evidence-based review of effectiveness. Journal of the American Academy of Audiology, 16(7), 461–472.

Mueller, H. G., & Powers, T. (2001). Consideration of auditory acclimatization in the prescriptive fitting of hearing aids. Seminars in Hearing, 22(2), 103–123.

Nabelek, A. E. (2005). Acceptance of background noise may be key to successful fittings. Hearing Journal, 58(4), 10–15.

Nabelek, A. K., Tampas, J. W., & Burchfield, S. B. (2004). Comparison of speech perception in background noise with acceptance of background noise in aided and unaided conditions. Journal of Speech, Language and Hearing Research, 47, 1001–1011.

Neuman, A. C., Bakke, M. H., Mackersie, C., Hellman, S., & Levitt, H. (1995). Effect of release time on compression hearing aids: Paired-comparison judgments of quality. Journal of the Acoustical Society of America, 98(6), 3182–3187.

Nilsson, M., Soli, S. D., & Sullivan, J. A. (1994). Development of the Hearing in Noise Test for the measurement of speech reception thresholds in quiet and in noise. Journal of the Acoustical Society of America, 95(2), 1085–1099.

Palmer, C. V., & Lindley, G. (1998). Reliability of the contour test in a population of adults with hearing loss. Journal of the American Academy of Audiology, 9, 209–215.

Palmer, C., & Mormer, E. (1997). A systematic program for hearing aid orientation and adjustment. Hearing Review, 1(Suppl.), 45–52.

Palmer, C. V., & Mueller, H. G. (1999). Profile of aided loudness: A validation procedure. Hearing Journal, 52(6), 34–41.

Palmer, C. V., Nelson, C., & Lindley, G. (1998). The functionally and physiologically plastic adult auditory system. Journal of the Acoustical Society of America, 103(4), 1705–1721.

Pascoe, D. (1989). Clinical measurements of the auditory dynamic range and their relation to formulas for hearing aid gain. In J. H. Jensen (Ed.), Hearing aid fitting: Theoretical and practical views (pp. 129–152). 13th Danavox Symposium: Stougaard Jensen.

Preminger, J. E., Carpenter, R., & Ziegler, C. H. (2005). A clinical perspective on cochlear dead regions: Intelligibility of speech and subjective hearing aid benefit. Journal of the American Academy of Audiology, 16, 600–613.

Ricketts, T., & Henry, P. (2002). Gain equalization in directional hearing aids. American Journal of Audiology, 11(1), 29–41.

Ricketts, T. A., & Hornsby, B. (2003). Distance and reverberation effects on directional benefit. Ear and Hearing, 24, 472–484.

Sandridge, S., & Newman, C. (2006). Improving the efficiency and accountability of the hearing aid selection process. Retrieved August 7, 2007, from http://www.audiologyonline.com/articles/article_detail.asp?article_id=1541

Stelmachowicz, P. G., Kopun, J., Mace, A., & Lewis, D. (1996). Measures of hearing aid gain for real speech. Ear and Hearing, 17(6), 520–527.

Stelmachowicz, P. G., Pittman, A., Hoover, B., & Lewis, D. (2002). Aided perception of /s/ and /z/ by hearing-impaired children. Ear and Hearing, 23, 316–324.

Stone, M. A., & Moore, B. C. J. (2005). Tolerable hearing aid delays: 4. Effects on subjective disturbance during speech production by hearing-impaired subjects. Ear and Hearing, 26, 225–235.

Summers, V. (2004). Do tests for cochlear dead regions provide important information for fitting hearing aids? Journal of the Acoustical Society of America, 115(4), 1420–1423.

Summers, V., Molis, M., Musch, H., Walden, B., Surr, R., & Cord, M. (2003). Identifying dead regions in the cochlea: Psychophysical tuning curves and tone detection in threshold-equalizing noise. Ear and Hearing, 24(2), 133–142.

Valente, M., Abrams, H., Benson, D., et al. (2006). Guidelines for the audiological management of adult hearing impairment. Retrieved January 12, 2006, from www.audiology.org

Valente, M., Potts, L., & Valente, M. (1997). Differences and intersubject variability of loudness discomfort levels measured in sound pressure level and hearing level for TDH-50P and ER-3A earphones. Journal of the American Academy of Audiology, 8, 59–67.

Valente, M., Valente, M., & Goebel, J. (1991). Reliability and intersubject variability of the real-ear unaided response. Ear and Hearing, 12(3), 216–220.

Chapter 6

Outcome Measures in the Fitting of Hearing Aids

Victor Bray and Michael Nilsson

Outcome measures quantify the results of intervention. With respect to audiology and hearing aid fittings, outcome measures determine the success, or failure, of the interaction between a medical professional and a patient. The process of using outcome measures has many subtleties that affect the accuracy, usefulness, and ease with which outcome measures are used. For example, to determine how something turns out, the audiologist must also have a measurement of how things began. Therefore, outcome measures should be accompanied by an evaluation of how the patient begins, as well as ends, his or her interaction with the audiologist. This chapter will look at the who, what, where, when, how, and why of outcome measures to clarify the use and importance of these measures in audiological rehabilitation (Bray, 1997).

Pearl

- Outcome measures should include an evaluation of how the patient begins and ends his or her interaction with the audiologist.

The audiological rehabilitation process concerns three domains: impairment, activity limitations, and participation restrictions. Identification and measurement of all three must be accomplished before intervention can begin. **Table 6–1** assigns each of the health condition domains (how an individual is affected) to the part of the auditory processing system that is affected by a hearing disability (what is affected).

Table 6–1 will be used as the nucleus in this chapter for discussions about outcome measures so audiologists can learn when certain measures should be made and where the measures are best obtained. The questions of who is to provide the measures and who benefits from them will lead to a discussion of why outcome measures are important.

The objectives of this chapter are twofold. The first is to help audiologists establish an outcome measures protocol for their clinical practice using a battery approach. The battery will provide assessment of treatment effects in all three auditory processing systems and health condition domains. The second objective is to help audiologists and their patients set realistic, achievable, individual expectations and goals for intervention that use the outcome measures protocol as both a road map (where the intervention is headed) and a yardstick (what the intervention has accomplished).

As audiologists, the vast majority of clinical intervention will require the fitting of hearing aids as an audiological rehabilitation tool. For this reason, this chapter puts an emphasis on outcome measures as they pertain to the fitting and benefit of amplification systems. The audiologist must use an outcome measures battery (OMB) approach to (1) identify impairment in the physiological system and assess amplification with respect to prescriptive targets, (2) identify activity limitations in the communication system and assess changes in speech recognition, and (3) identify participation restrictions in the psychological system and assess benefit and/or satisfaction.

As the involved auditory processing system moves from the physiological to the psychological level, several realities should be observed: (1) the systems become increasingly complex; (2) the effects of intervention become increasingly latent; and (3) communication assessments, then psychological assessments, are performed later in the audiological rehabilitation process.

◆ The "What" of Outcome Measures

Outcome measures are tools used by audiologists to assess performance, or a change in performance, that results during the course of audiological rehabilitation. Change in and of itself, whether measured or perceived, should be, but is not always, beneficial to the patient.

Because audiological rehabilitation is a treatment course that involves complex systems, no single measure is sufficient to evaluate progress adequately. For this reason, an OMB is recommended to assess sequentially (1) the physiological system, (2) the communication system, and (3) the psychological system (**Table 6–1**).

The physiological system is comprised of the auditory pathways that convert acoustical waveforms into meaningful neurologic events. This is the realm of diagnostic audiology, where frequency-specific and amplitude-controlled stimuli are used to measure the sensitivity of the auditory system. Significant loss of auditory sensitivity will negatively impact the communication system since understanding is impacted by hearing loss.

Performance of the communication system is one of the principle sources of complaints by patients when seeking medical attention because of the heavy reliance by most people on auditory input to convey information. Conversational speech is easily understood in most common listening environments by those with normal hearing. With hearing loss, particularly sensorineural loss, speech recognition is degraded, especially in the presence of background noise. Significant loss of speech recognition ability can negatively impact social interactions. The ability to communicate and interact is a major component of one's quality of life (QoL), and any degradation in the ability to communicate very often leads to isolation and/or depression. (For additional information on health-related quality of life [HRQoL] and improvements resulting from amplification, see National Council on Aging, 1999, and Abrams et al, 2005.)

The psychological system involves the set of behaviors associated with interpersonal communication. In the case of acquired hearing loss, otherwise normal behavior may change to the psychology of the hearing impaired. This may result in a loss in HRQoL, including miscommunications, frustration, social withdrawal, and depression. Patients often do not associate these behavioral changes with the hearing loss and do not realize how their QoL is being impacted.

A battery approach is a grouping of test instruments in which each test assesses a portion of the whole system. A typical diagnostic test battery includes observation of the external ear through otoscopy, evaluation of the middle ear through immittance audiometry, measurement of the function of the inner ear through air- and bone-conduction audiometry, and integrity of the auditory pathways using measurements of evoked potentials. For audiological rehabilitation, it is recommended that audiologists use an OMB approach that evaluates performance not only with these physiological tests but also with communication and psychological systems.

◆ The "How" of Outcome Measures

Using the World Health Organization (WHO) guidelines (2001), impairments are problems in bodily function or structure, such as a significant deviation or loss, where body functions are the physiological functions of the body systems (including psychological functions) and body structures are

Table 6–1 Overview of Outcome Measures Showing the Interdependent Relationships of What, How, When, Where, Who, and Why for Hearing Aid Fittings

What	How	When	Where	Who and Why
Processing Systems	**Identification (Pretreatment)**	**Assessment (Posttreatment)**	**Environment**	**Evaluator**
Physiological	Impairment	Amplification targets	Clinic	Audiologist (verification)
Communication	Activity limitation	Recognition improvement	Objective	Audiologist (verification)
Psychological	Participation restriction	Benefit/satisfaction	Home/work (subjective)	Patient (validation)

anatomical parts of the body, such as organs, limbs, and their components. Activity is the execution of a task or action by an individual, and activity limitations are thus difficulties an individual may have in executing activities. Participation is the involvement in a life situation and participation restrictions are problems an individual may have in involvement in life situations. (For additional discussion on the WHO guidelines with regard to audiology, see Abrams et al, 2005).

Assessment of hearing loss in the physiological system involves quantification of the impairment through identification of the location and degree of pathology. The result is a map of auditory sensitivity called the audiogram. From this map, amplification prescriptive targets may be constructed to restore audibility appropriately. Hearing aid performance measurements used to evaluate compliance to targets include electroacoustic tests, probe microphone measures, and sound-field measures.

The primary activity limitation resulting from a significant hearing loss is decreased communication. In fact, the primary symptom resulting in an assessment of hearing loss is a complaint of reduction in speech recognition, particularly in background noise. Based on the audiogram, reliable predictions may be made on the degree of speech recognition loss; based on the amplification prescriptive target, predictions may also be made as to the restoration of speech recognition. Outcome measurement instruments that quantify whether or not speech recognition has been adequately achieved include speech-based tests in quiet and in noise with measurements obtained at the phoneme, syllable, word, and sentence levels.

The participation restrictions that may result from a hearing loss are the behavioral changes resulting from decreased communication abilities. Although the audiologist is typically focused on identifying impairment in the physiological system and activity limitation in the communication system, the ultimate goal of any audiologic intervention is to reduce the participation restriction, as measured by favorable changes in behavior. Self-assessment questionnaires are commonly used to quantify behavior in the psychological system. These include scales of handicap, of benefit (or reduction in handicap), and of satisfaction (of which benefit is a major component).

Controversial Point

- The ultimate goal of audiologic intervention is to reduce the participation restriction, as measured by favorable changes in behavior.

♦ The "When" of Outcome Measures

Identification measurements of impairment, activity limitation, and participation restriction should be made prior to treatment and may all be made at the initial diagnostic session. The assessment of compliance to amplification prescriptive targets, improvement in speech recognition, and

benefit or satisfaction must be time sequenced as provision of amplification produces changes in recognition that, over time, can result in changes in behavior. The greater the complexity of the system being sampled (physiological, communication, then psychological), the more intervention time must be allowed to pass before post-treatment assessment begins. This requirement is necessary to provide ample time for adaptation to occur and multiple listening situations to be encountered (**Table 6–1**).

Assessment of the match between hearing aid performance and prescriptive amplification targets should occur at the beginning of the rehabilitation process. Reasons for measurement at the onset of treatment are that assurance of the proper implementation of the prescription sets the foundation for improvements in communication and benefit, and no adaptation time is needed for electroacoustic performance in the coupler or in the real ear, or for sound-field measures of threshold or comfort.

Assessment of improvement in the communication system should not occur until there is documentation that the physiological system is receiving proper amplification. This requires time for the patient to use the amplification system in a variety of listening environments and report back to the audiologist any situations that are unsatisfactory. Once electroacoustic modifications are complete and the patient has had time to adapt to the amplified signals presented to the impaired auditory system, speech recognition measures may be made to assess whether or not there has been an increase in recognition and a concomitant decrease in activity limitation.

Self-assessment questionnaires of participation restriction typically query the patient about his or her day-to-day performance in a variety of environmental situations, with an emphasis on any possible impact of hearing loss. Self-assessment measures of benefit look for a reduction in disability and handicap, and typically ask the patient about the amplified sound quality, the impact of amplification on speech recognition ability, and the effect of amplification on personal behavior in a variety of environmental situations. Self-assessment of satisfaction not only evaluates benefit but also looks at the patient's perception of the services provided, including satisfaction with the audiologist, the clinic, and the cost-effectiveness of the amplification solution provided. Because these questionnaires are global assessments of treatment efficacy, they should be administered toward the end of the intervention process.

Most outcome measures involve comparative data obtained before and after the administration of the services. First, a baseline is established, then performance is compared after the treatment to determine how the measure has changed. Some measures require that the baseline be measured before treatment, whereas others allow the baseline to be obtained at the same session that the treatment data are obtained because the treatment can be removed (e.g., comparison of unaided and aided performance). Other measures are made after treatment with the patient comparing conditions while expressing his or her opinions.

Baseline measures may be assessments of the physiological system. They may also be assessments of the communication system to evaluate what physical performance decrements are cognizant to the patient and to verify such complaints with a performance measure. These measures are also assessments of the psychological system to gain understanding of the impact of the hearing loss on the individual, to understand the areas of significance that can be improved from treatment, and to set realistic expectations of the potential improvement once treatment begins.

Interim measures can demonstrate that amplification provides a good fit to the physiological disability and that clinical goals are being met regarding change in auditory sensitivity with respect to frequency. Following this, there may be assessment of the communication system to evaluate speech recognition in quiet and in noise. For both physiological and communication assessments, change in performance from the baseline yields the indication of benefit. Some adaptation to the amplification system, however, may be needed before the optimal aided performance is obtained for speech recognition measures.

Postrehabilitation measures provide assessment of the whole person and substantiate that the physiological and communication benefit measured in the clinic have translated into psychological benefit in the real world. Because these are subjective measures using self-assessment questionnaires, the patient must have adaptation time to evaluate real-world performance across many listening environments.

The question of when postrehabilitation assessments should occur is a source of considerable investigation. Gatehouse (1993) reported that the benefit from amplification changed over time, whereas Surr et al (1998) reported no significant change in benefit with long-term hearing aid use. Although assessment of small-scale, long-term changes in group benefit is of high importance in research studies, the majority of hearing aid benefit in clinical applications has been obtained within the first 6 to 10 weeks of intervention (Horwitz and Turner, 1997).

♦ The "Where" of Outcome Measures

Hearing aid systems must operate successfully in a variety of environments that are of importance to the patient and that are often unavailable to the audiologist. In contrast, the audiologist performs hearing aid evaluations in the clinic, an environment that is of limited direct value to the patient. A balanced OMB must sample performance in both clinical and real-world environments (**Table 6–1**).

Audiologists work in a highly controlled world. Performance measurements are typically made in an audiometric test room, or other sound-controlled environment, where measurements of compliance to amplification targets and improvements to speech recognition can be made without interference from extraneous auditory stimuli. In the clinic, procedures are based on objective measures that are not biased by social or psychological factors. This level of control is necessary to maximize the sensitivity and reliability of the test. Comparisons to norms or other baselines are possible only if the measures are made in the same environment. Such control is not possible in the infinite variations encountered in the real world.

Patients, however, must successfully use hearing aids in the real world. Although environmental simulations can be constructed in the clinic, these are only an approximation for a few of the actual situations patients will encounter, such as in the car, at home, in the office, and in public. In the uncontrolled real world, clinical measures cannot be made reliably, but self-report surveys can be used to assess performance. These self-assessment questionnaires are considered subjective measures as they are records of an individual patient's psychological reactions to the treatment and may be influenced by day-to-day variations in feelings, moods, and opinions.

♦ The "Who" and "Why" of Outcome Measures

Outcome measures are needed to ensure that quality work processes are in place and to document that satisfactory results have been achieved. In the case of audiological rehabilitation, this is accomplished by simultaneous verification and validation using both the audiologist's and individual patient's perspectives (**Table 6–1**). Verification is generally understood to involve objective measurements made by the audiologist to improve hearing functions, whereas validation involves self-assessment measurements for improvement in activity limitation and participation restriction (Valente et al, 2006).

Outcome measures help the audiologist establish, and then meet, clinical goals and expectations, and they require communication between both parties. Outcome measures help the patient express his or her opinions and guide the patient's evaluation across a range of parameters that must be evaluated in terms of real-world performance. They help define appropriate expectations, as well as limits (with respect to performance and abilities). They also help conclude the process and define what has been accomplished.

For the audiologist, the diagnosis of hearing loss involves the verification of the impairment (in the physiological system) and the activity limitation (in the communication system) to determine if amplification should be recommended as treatment. These quantities are compared with norms or previous measures to verify a diagnosis or progression of hearing loss. If rehabilitation is recommended, the audiologist may apply treatment and measure the outcomes to verify appropriate amplification (physiological system) and improvement in speech recognition (communication system). The impact on social interactions, however, and overall behavior must be validated using questionnaires to understand the treatment effects as perceived by the patient.

The verification process confirms or substantiates—using reliable materials with repeatable methods—that the amplification chosen has met the electroacoustic performance goals that the audiologist intended. Verification involves performance measures that do not include the patient's opinion. The ability to detect, repeat, tolerate, interpret, or respond are all objective measures. This is not to say that objective measures cannot be biased (from attentiveness, effort, scoring, etc.), but these measures do not involve opinions.

Pearl

- Verification involves measures that do not include the patient's opinion.

If the goal of a hearing aid fitting is to improve speech recognition, a measure of speech recognition before and after the fitting would verify if a change has occurred. The amount of change may be statistically or quantitatively significant in that it can be reliably measured (the amount of change is within the sensitivity of the test in use), but it may not be clinically significant if it does not meet the patient's expectations about how much his or her performance should change. This is where the subjective measures come in.

For the audiologist, validation is support for expectations or beliefs that the rehabilitation process accomplished the right thing. Validation asks if the patient is aware of a change (specifically with hearing aids in auditory-related experiences). It is possible to verify a performance change and not validate that the patient believes there is a change. Conversely, subjective validation does not require a significant change in performance on a verification measure. Instead, validation measures require the patient to express the opinion that he or she is performing differently.

Pitfall

- Validation asks if the patient is aware of a change. It is possible to have verified a performance change but not have the patient validate the change.

There are many factors that contribute to a patient's self-evaluation. These do not express or verify performance improvements, but measure a patient's willingness to express that his or her lifestyle or personal interactions are different than before. Measures can be strongly biased by factors such as age (older patients' expectations are different), education, and income. Subjective measures validate patients' beliefs that they have received value, that services and products have met their expectations, or that their QoL has improved.

Separate from audiologists and patients, there are many third parties who have interests in the rehabilitation outcome as well. These may include individuals, such as family and friends; organizations, such as the clinic, an insurer, and an employer; government agencies, such as the Department of Veterans Affairs (VA) and the Food and Drug Administration (FDA; 1994); and self-regulating bodies, such as the Hearing Industries Association (HIA; 2002). Each entity has a different motivation for being interested in the patient's treatment. The audience for the OMB determines the level of detail and the organization of the battery.

In addition, many third-party payers are beginning to require proof of the value of services rendered, and therefore require outcome measures. Institutions under managed care, such as health maintenance organizations (HMOs) and the VA, negotiate large contracts for products and services for their patients and use outcome measures to optimize value. The proper use of outcome measures ensures that patients are experiencing a positive effect from the audiological rehabilitation for the money spent. Unless outcome measures are administered correctly and appropriately, audiologists may not be recognized for valuable services, or patients may be charged unnecessarily for unsatisfying or unbeneficial services.

◆ An Outcome Measures Battery Approach

Successful audiological rehabilitation requires a comprehensive OMB approach. Identification and measurement of impairment in the physiological system produces amplification prescriptive targets for assessment during treatment. Measurement of activity limitation in the communication system establishes guidelines for improvement in speech recognition. Quantification of the participation restriction establishes a baseline for treatment benefit and satisfaction (**Table 6–1**).

An OMB uses objective data collection from the audiologist's controlled world combined with subjective data from the patient's real world. The audiologist's task is to develop an OMB specific to each clinical setting that meets the needs of the audiologist, the patients, and the organization that supports the clinic. The battery of tests should combine clinical measures (objective) of the physiological and communication systems with self-assessments (subjective) of patients' behavior in different environments.

In planning an OMB, the audiologist must be aware that each test instrument evaluates at a certain level within a system (physiological, communication, or psychological) and has an individual degree of resolution within that level. There is also a system-level trade-off that becomes important in choosing from among different test instruments. As the audiologist evaluates at a higher level within the system, measurement resolution may be lost, but the evaluation may have greater relevance or applicability to the real world. For example, when evaluating speech recognition, a confusion matrix of consonant misunderstandings, using a consonant-vowel (CV) or vowel-consonant (VC) test, has high resolution, whereas a percent-understanding score of key words in sentences has high communicative value.

Special Consideration

- As the audiologist evaluates higher system levels, measurement resolution may weaken, but applicability to the real world may strengthen.

Table 6–2 Comparison of Test Methods to Assess Implementation of Amplification Targets in the Physiological System

	Coupler	Probe Microphone	Sound Field
Frequency response assessment	50 dB SPL gain curve	Real ear aided response (aided response − unaided response = insertion response)	Aided thresholds (aided threshold − unaided threshold = functional gain)
Maximum output assessment	90 dB SPL output curve	Real ear saturation response (real ear aided response at 90 dB SPL)	Aided maximum (aided maximum − unaided threshold = dynamic range)
Components of physical system assessed	Hearing aid in absentia; no real-ear complications	Hearing aid in situ: real-ear effects on microphone, vent, and receiver	Hearing aid in situ: real-ear effects, low-level auditory performance
Comparative strengths	High measurement resolution	High measurement resolution	Good real-world prediction
Comparative weaknesses	Poor real-world prediction	Accurate results technique-dependent	Low measurement resolution

SPL, sound pressure level.

Another key concept in planning an OMB is the comparative value of the various test instruments. To assess value, audiologists must know if a test instrument has performance guidelines, or targets for acceptable performance. Depending on the outcome measure of interest, the reference should be different. Therefore, the more benchmarks that are available, such as the normal-hearing population, the hearing-impaired population, and the hearing-impaired individual, the more outcomes that can be evaluated. This benchmarking may take the form of absolute ability (re normal) or improvement (re unaided or another hearing device).

In assessing the comparative value of outcome measures, each instrument has a specific utility resulting from its applicability to the real world, including the purpose of the instrument and generality of measure, the similarity of materials to the situation of interest, and the trade-off between sensitivity or statistical power and reality. In terms of statistical significance, each instrument has different levels of sensitivity when used to objectively verify clinical protocols. Clinical significance (a change in performance large enough to be recognized by the patient and impact satisfaction), as opposed to statistical significance, tends to require some measure of the psychological system and comes from changes in patient benefit. It is achieved by generating improved consumer satisfaction and can be documented with subjective measures.

Special Consideration

- Construct and use an OMB that demonstrates benefit, both clinically and in the real world, with the goal of significantly improving the HRQoL for patients.

◆ Outcome Measures for Evaluation of the Physiological System

A successful OMB approach begins with objective verification of the hearing loss and its etiology, followed by verification that the hearing aids are delivering proper amplification for the hearing loss under treatment. The three major methods for measuring hearing aid performance are coupler measures, which measure the electroacoustic response of the aids in a controlled environment of general characteristics; probe microphone measures, which measure the electroacoustic response of the aids in an uncontrolled environment specific to the characteristics of an individual's real ear; and sound-field measures with nonspeech stimuli, whereby minimal performance capabilities are documented.

For any of the three approaches used, performance prescriptive targets, such as National Acoustic Laboratories' nonlinear fitting procedure, version 1 (NAL-NL1; Byrne et al, 2001) and desired sensation level input/output (DSL [i/o]; Scollie et al, 2005), are available for a prescriptive approach. These three methods are all ways to implement and verify the frequency-specific and amplitude-dependent characteristics of the hearing aid fitting in accordance with a specified hearing loss. **Table 6–2** summarizes the key concepts that will be discussed in this section. (Refer to Chapters 4 and 5 in this volume for additional information on physical assessment of hearing aid performance with prescriptions.)

Electroacoustic Measures

Electroacoustic measures of hearing aid performance in a coupler provide a highly consistent and reliable method to evaluate performance (American National Standards Institute [ANSI] 1992, 2003) but have a low relevance to real-world performance. The value in these measurements comes from the stability of the hearing aid plus coupler system and allows the audiologist to easily perform comparisons among devices, styles, and manufacturers' products. A major component of the performance stability is that the measurements are made with the patient in absentia. This is also why the measurements have limited real-world value, as the patient's physical ear structures are not well represented by the 2 cc coupler. (Refer to Chapter 1 in this volume for additional information on electroacoustic measures of hearing aid performance.)

Based on the audiogram, 2 cc coupler amplification targets for gain and output are established. The gain target is most often specified for measurement with a 50 dB sound pressure level (SPL) pure-tone signal; the output target is

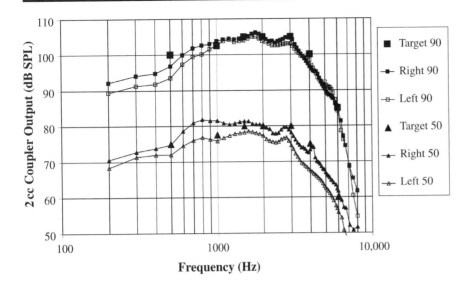

Figure 6–1 Display of 2 cc coupler responses to assess right and left device performance with respect to target. Coupler response targets are for a 50 dB sound pressure level (SPL) signal (*large closed triangles*) and a 90 dB SPL signal (*large closed squares*).

specified using a 90 dB SPL pure-tone signal. The gain target is an optimal frequency response configuration for low-intensity signals that is designed to restore audibility of conversational speech. The output target is a separate frequency response that limits maximum SPL from the hearing aid such that the amplification does not create pain or discomfort when used in the presence of high sound levels. **Figure 6–1** shows gain and output targets, with actual hearing aid settings, for a moderate sensorineural hearing loss.

Probe Microphone Measures

Probe microphone measures of hearing aid performance in the real ear provide a reliable method to evaluate performance (ANSI, 1997), with relevance to real-world performance. The value in these measurements comes from direct in situ measurement of the SPL of the hearing aid near the tympanic membrane. The measurement procedure uses the same high-resolution signals as coupler measurements, yet also incorporates external ear effects on the microphone input, vent effects on the frequency response, and residual ear canal volume effects on receiver efficiency. The major limitations to the measure are that accurate results are dependent on good technique, and, whereas the measure is in situ, it does not incorporate any documentation of actual auditory processing by the patient. (See Chapter 3 in this volume for additional information on physical assessment of hearing aid performance with probe microphones.)

Pitfall

• The major limitation to probe microphone measures is that results are highly dependent on technique.

As with coupler measures, probe microphone amplification targets for gain and output are based on the audiogram. Targets may be specified for pure-tone or broadband signals, and in the case of single-channel hearing aids,

either works satisfactorily. With the new digital, multichannel compression aids, however, pure-tone targets may overprescribe gain and output, unless the prescriptions have been adjusted for the specific multichannel architecture of the hearing aid. For this reason, broadband targets, which are generally insensitive to multichannel architecture, are recommended when measuring advanced technology devices.

Prescriptive targets for probe microphone measures may be specified in dB gain or dB SPL. Compliance to gain targets is typically evaluated with the real ear insertion response (REIR), which is the difference between the real ear aided response (REAR) and the real ear unaided response (REUR). Loudness discomfort to the output target is typically obtained with the REAR using a 90 dB input, which is also known as the real ear saturation response (RESR). **Figure 6–2** shows gain and output targets, with actual hearing aid settings, for a moderate sensorineural hearing loss.

Sound-Field Measures

Sound-field measures of hearing aid performance with nonspeech stimuli have a high relevance to real-world performance but are obtained with a lower resolution measurement scale than coupler or probe microphone measures. When assessing hearing aids at the physical system level, this is the only measure of the three techniques that involves the auditory pathways and requires patient responses. The major consequence is that measurement resolution is no longer 1 dB increments at 100 Hz intervals (as with coupler and probe microphones), but instead is 5 dB increments at half-octave intervals.

Nonspeech amplification targets for gain and output in a sound field are also audiogram-based. The functional gain target is specified as the difference between the aided threshold and the unaided threshold using frequency-modulated tones presented in a sound field. The aided dynamic range (in dB) is the difference between the aided maximum with frequency-modulated tones presented at high intensities and the aided threshold. The unaided dynamic range

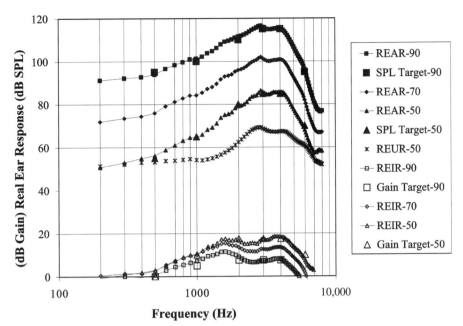

Figure 6–2 Display of probe microphone responses to assess real-ear performance with respect to targets. For a 50 dB SPL signal, real ear aided response (REAR) targets (*large closed triangle*) are plotted in dB SPL and real ear insertion response (REIR) targets (*large open triangle*) in dB gain. For a 90 dB SPL signal, REAR targets (*large closed square*) are plotted in dB SPL, and REIR targets (*large open square*) are plotted in dB gain. Real-ear measurements with 50, 70, and 90 dB SPL input are also plotted: REAR and real ear unaided response (REUR) in dB SPL and REIR in dB gain.

(in dB) is the difference between the unaided maximum and the unaided threshold (see **Table 6–2** and **Fig. 6–3**).

In evaluating the effectiveness of amplification performance using sound-field measures, 20 years of clinical experience and 10 years of algorithm development dictate that the aided thresholds should approach 20 dB hearing level (HL) values or should reduce the amount of threshold loss by at least 50%. To achieve this, greater amounts of functional gain must be achieved for greater amounts of hearing loss. Regardless of the amount of functional gain achieved, the aided maximum should be no lower than the unaided maximum; that is, the patient should not lose maximum tolerance for high input sounds in the aided condition. Functional gain at any frequency should never be negative, and the aided dynamic range should always be greater than the unaided dynamic range.

Pearl

- With functional gain measures, aided thresholds should approach 20 dB HL values. When this is not possible, threshold loss should be reduced by 50% or more.

It is important to note that the presence of sensorineural hearing loss results in a narrowing of the unaided dynamic range. Successful hearing aid fittings will produce an expanded dynamic range in the aided conditions through a combination of improved audibility for low-intensity inputs without changing the tolerance levels for high-intensity inputs. **Figure 6–3** shows the relationship of various sound-field measures obtained with nonspeech stimuli.

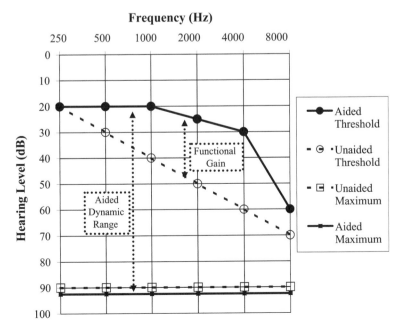

Figure 6–3 Display of unaided and aided values to assess sound-field performance. The difference between the aided thresholds and the unaided thresholds is functional gain. The difference between aided thresholds and aided maximum is the aided dynamic range.

Prescriptive Amplification Targets

Prescriptive amplification targets can be evaluated with couplers, probe microphones, or sound-field measures. All prescriptive methods produce a frequency-specific target that can be verified with any of these approaches. More sophisticated prescriptions, which incorporate nonlinear algorithms for wide dynamic range compression (WDRC) hearing aids, call for frequency-specific targets that are also level-dependent. As knowledge of the interactions among speech acoustics, hearing loss, and auditory processing for speech continues to grow, prescriptive approaches of the future will be designed specifically to improve speech intelligibility in noise (Byrne et al, 2001; Scollie et al, 2005).

With coupler measurement techniques, the best way to evaluate multilevel response curves on nonlinear hearing aids is by using the ANSI S3.42 guidelines (ANSI, 1992) for measurement with a family of broadband signals. For probe microphone measurement protocols, the best technique is to measure the REAR using a broadband stimulus with a range of input levels, such as 50, 65, and 80 dB SPL. For sound-field measures of nonlinear targets, loudness scaling must be used, incorporating aided judgments of soft, comfortable, and loud levels. Many current hearing aids incorporate dynamic signal processing features, such as multichannel compression, digital noise reduction, and feedback cancellation, to enhance speech communication. As such, speech or speechlike signals should be used whenever possible for these electroacoustic measurements (Valente et al, 2006).

◆ Outcome Measures for Verification of the Communication System

Once proper prescriptive amplification is in place, the OMB continues with objective verification that the hearing aids are providing improvement in speech recognition. These measures are made in the sound field with communicatively relevant materials, with the evaluation occurring at the phoneme, syllable, word, or sentence level (**Table 6–3**). Unaided measures are obtained to establish the activity limitation baseline; aided measures then determine change in ability, whether positive or negative. It is important to note that, although almost all hearing aid fittings successfully provide some degree of amplification, this does not necessarily translate into a guarantee of improved speech recognition, especially in noise.

Table 6–3 Comparison of Test Instruments to Assess Speech Recognition in the Communication System

Test	Signal	Masker	Procedure	Items	Test	Results
NST	Male, CVs or VCs with carrier phrase	Edited cafeteria noise	Fixed level; closed set	91 items organized into 11 subsets of 7 to 9 syllables	1 set unaided and aided (182 syllables)	Percent correct; auditory feature matrix
NU-6 and CID W-22	CVCs with carrier phrase	Optional, not standardized	Fixed level; open set	50 items, phonemically balanced word lists	1 list unaided and 1 list aided (100 words)	Percent correct
SPIN	Male, last word in sentence	12-talker babble	Fixed level; can vary SNR	50 sentences per list; both low- and high-probability lists	1 list unaided and aided (100 key words)	Percent correct
SSI	Male, synthetic sentences	Male, single talker	Fixed level varying SNR; closed set	10 sentences per list	3 lists unaided and four lists aided (70 sentences)	PI functions in noise
SIN	Female, IEEE sentences	4-talker babble	4 SNR (0, +5, +10, +15)	5 sentences with 5 key words per test condition	1 set unaided and aided (200 key words)	PI functions in noise
QuickSIN	Female, IEEE sentences	4-talker babble	6 SNR (0, +5, +10, +15, +20, +25)	1 sentence with 5 key words per test condition	1 set unaided and aided (60 key words)	SNR loss (re normal hearing)
HINT	Male, revised Bamford-Kowel-Bench sentences	Noise matched to Long-Term Average Spectrum of signal	Adaptive for Reception Threshold for Sentences with masker fixed at 65 dBA	10 phonemically balanced sentences per list; SNR	2 lists unaided and aided (40 sentences)	SNR for 50% correct in noise
CST	Female, continuous speech	6-talker babble	Fixed-level presentation	25 key words in 10 sentences per passage;	2 passages unaided and aided (100 key words)	Percent correct (RAU)

CID, Central Institute for the Deaf; CST, Connected Speech Test; CV, consonant-vowel; CVC, consonant-vowel-consonant (CVC); HINT, Hearing in Noise Test; IEEE, Institute of Electrical and Electronics Engineers; NST, nonsense syllable test; NU, Northwestern University; PI, performance intensity; QuickSIN, quick speech-in-noise test; RAU, rationalized arcsine unit; SIN, speech-in-noise test; SNR, signal-to-noise ratio; SPIN, Speech Perception in Noise; SSI, Synthetic Sentence Identification; VC, vowel-consonant.

Pitfall

- Although almost all hearing aid fittings successfully provide amplification, this does not guarantee improved speech recognition, especially in noise.

Controversial Point

- The ultimate goal of amplification and rehabilitation is to work toward the performance of normal-hearing listeners.

Phoneme and syllable identification tasks, such as with a CV or VC pairing, measure the basic ability to detect the components of speech. The physical characteristics of these stimuli are well characterized, and correct perception of the stimuli can be directly related back to audibility as measured frequency by intensity in the coupler, probe microphone, or sound field. CV and VC recognition also can be analyzed in the domain of speech features, such as voicing, manner, and place of articulation, yielding patterns of correct and incorrect perception. An example of this is the nonsense syllable test (NST; Levitt and Resnick, 1978).

Word identification tasks evaluate the ability to integrate speech components into semantic units carrying information. These tasks can be influenced by knowledge and experience with the semantic units typically used in language. Examples of word identification tasks are the Central Institute for the Deaf (CID) W-22 word lists (Hirsh et al, 1952), the Northwestern University NU-6 word lists (Tillman and Carhart, 1966), and the Speech Perception in Noise (SPIN) test (Bilger et al, 1984).

Sentence identification tasks determine the ability of the patient to combine units into meaningful structures. These tasks can be scored focusing on key words in a sentence or on the complete sentence. Sentence identification is influenced by word context, entropy, and familiarity with the speaker's voice and language. Examples of sentence identification tasks are the Synthetic Sentence Identification (SSI) test (Speaks and Jerger, 1965), the Connected Speech Test (CST; Cox et al, 1988), the Hearing in Noise Test (HINT; Nilsson et al, 1994), the speech-in-noise (SIN) test (Killion, 1997a), and the quick speech-in-noise (QuickSIN) test (Killion et al, 2004).

Prescriptive speech recognition targets provide guidance to assess the acceptability of aided communication. Like prescriptive targets of frequency by intensity for the physiological system, speech recognition targets provide guidance for the audiologist in determining acceptable aided performance for the patient. The targets can be established using (1) the performance level for the normal-hearing population, (2) the performance level of the hearing-impaired population, or (3) the performance level of the hearing-impaired patient.

Comparison of an individual's performance to the normal-hearing population tells the audiologist how well the individual is able to take advantage of all of the innate abilities of the auditory system. These targets are best-case values; unaided or aided hearing cannot be expected to be better than this. The ultimate goal of amplification is to work toward the performance of normal-hearing listeners, and this comparison will determine how closely performance matches this goal.

Comparison of an individual's performance to the hearing-impaired population determines whether the amount of difficulty the patient is experiencing is predicted by the amount of hearing loss measured. In other words, this comparison is used to help diagnose whether speech recognition deficits are solely peripheral or whether there may be other factors that the audiogram does not take into account (language experience, attention deficits, retrocochlear pathology, and central auditory processing disorder).

Comparison of an individual's performance to themselves, such as comparing aided to unaided or hearing aid A to hearing aid B, determines whether performance, as measured by multiple tests with the same person, is changing over time or with intervention. The ability of amplification to help with a hearing loss is initially calculated by comparing performance before and after the hearing aid fitting. The comparison can also determine if there are differences among various signal-processing algorithms, or even among various amplification targets. The analysis typically involves changes in performance, but it is not a gauge of absolute performance (which would involve the previous comparisons to normal-hearing or other hearing-impaired listeners).

Speech recognition in noise is the key performance measure of interest. Pure-tone thresholds have a strong predictive relationship to speech recognition measures in quiet; therefore, additional measures are of limited value. Speech measures in noise, however, are suprathreshold, involving complex auditory processing, and therefore are not well predicted by tonal thresholds or speech thresholds in quiet (Killion, 1997b; Plomp, 1978).

Clinical Implementation

Audiologists involved in fitting and dispensing hearing aids should establish expected performance levels for speech recognition test results. These performance targets should be based on measurements of both the normal-hearing population and the hearing-impaired population. Once these levels are established, hearing-impaired patients can be counseled regarding their unaided and aided ability, with respect to normal-hearing and hearing-impaired persons (Killion, 1997b; Taylor, 2003).

The first step in creating performance levels specific to a clinic is to select and repeatedly administer a set of test materials. Next, the test presentation must be standardized with respect to the intensity levels of the speech and noise, the loudspeaker configuration (single or multiple speakers), and the testing environment. Finally, the test must be administered to persons with a range of hearing abilities to establish expected performance levels. The example used

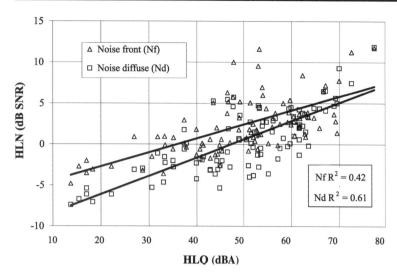

Figure 6–4 Unaided sound-field Hearing in Noise Test (HINT) measures from 101 normal-hearing or hearing-impaired subjects obtained in a clinical environment. The hearing level in quiet, measured in A-weighted decibels (HLQ, dBA) is plotted on the abscissa, and the hearing level in noise (HLN, dB signal-to-noise ratio [SNR]) is plotted on the ordinate. Performance for normal-hearing persons is in the lower left corner (< 20 dBA HLQ and < 0 dB SNR HLN). The two lines are the regression lines for best fit to the data, with the top line representing the "noise front" condition and the bottom line representing the "noise diffuse" condition.

will be with the HINT (Nilsson et al, 1994), using 20 sentence lists, administered with the masker fixed at 65 dBA and a loudspeaker array with each loudspeaker 1 m from the listener. In the "noise front" condition, the speech and the masker are administered simultaneously from 0 degrees azimuth and incidence. In the "noise diffuse" condition, the speech is as in the "noise front" condition, but the uncorrelated masker is administered simultaneously from four loudspeakers, respectively, at 45, 135, 225, and 315 degrees azimuth and 0 degree incidence (Nilsson et al, 2005).

Figure 6–4 plots performance data for the hearing level (for speech) in quiet (HLQ on the abscissa) and the hearing level in noise (HLN on the ordinate) for 101 subjects in the unaided condition. Each subject was tested three times: once without a masker, once in the "noise front" condition, and once in the "noise diffuse" condition. The two solid lines through the scatter plot are linear regression lines for best fit to the data for both "noise front" and "noise diffuse." The "noise diffuse" condition yields HLN values, on average, ~2 dB lower in signal-to-noise ratio (SNR) than the "noise front" condition.

In the lower left corner of the plot is a cluster of data points with HLQ thresholds < 20 dBA and HLN thresholds from −5 to −8 dB SNR for the "noise diffuse" condition and −2 to −4 dB SNR for the "noise front" conditions. These define the expected performance level for the normal-hearing population for this particular test environment.

The hearing-impaired population is characterized by the other data points where HLQ is > 30 dBA. It is important to realize that as HLQ increases from 30 to 70 dBA, the mean HLN SNR increases from −4 to +5 dB SNR for the "noise diffuse" condition and from −2 to +6 dB SNR for the "noise front" condition. This establishes that, using this particular test configuration, the expected increase in HLN is ~1 to 2 dB SNR per decade of HLQ for mild through severe sensorineural losses.

Once the normative data for a clinic have been established, individual data plotted on the graph can be used as a counseling tool, as shown in **Fig. 6–5**. For example, points 1U, 2U, and 3U represent similar unaided HLQ thresholds, at

~50 dBA, but markedly different unaided HLN thresholds, ranging from −4 to +3 dB SNR. In the unaided condition, patient 1 has an HLN of −4 dB SNR, which is ~4 dB better than expected for this degree of HLQ, but still 2 dB worse than the normal-hearing group. Patient 2 has an HLN that is in the expected range for his or her degree of HLQ but is 6 dB worse than the normal group. In contrast, patient 3 has an HLN of +3 dB SNR, which is 3 dB worse than expected for a moderate HLQ and 9 dB worse than the normal-hearing group.

In recommending hearing aid technology, it is possible that patient 1 could satisfactorily use a simple amplification system that overcomes the hearing loss for quiet, whereas patient 3 requires not only amplification in quiet but also extra assistance to improve hearing in noise. Because hearing aids incorporating multichannel compression, directional microphones, and/or digital noise reduction provide more advantageous benefit for those with greater SNR loss (Bray and Nilsson, 2001), patient 3 is clearly a candidate requiring an advanced technology system.

Following the hearing aid fitting and the necessary fine-tuning to ensure that the amplification prescription has been met, testing of speech recognition with the hearing aids is conducted. The aided score can be plotted on the graph alongside the unaided score. In **Fig. 6–5**, comparison of the unaided and aided scores shows a 20 dB shift to the left, representing a 20 dB gain in speech threshold for HLQ. For HLN, patient 1 has no change in performance, patient 2 has performance degraded by 2 dB SNR, and patient 3 has performance improved by 4 dB SNR. Hearing aid fittings that make HLN worse are unacceptable (see patient 2); fittings that do not make HLN worse are acceptable (patient 1); fittings that dramatically improve HLN are desirable (patient 3).

Controversial Point

- Hearing aid fittings that do not improve recognition of speech in noise are unacceptable. It is the professional responsibility of the audiologist to improve, not degrade, the patient's performance in noise.

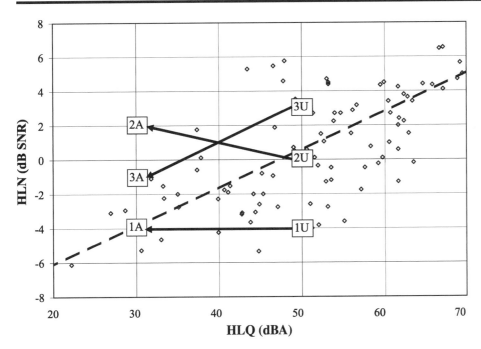

Figure 6–5 Unaided and aided sound-field Hearing in Noise Test (HINT) measures, for three hypothetical patients in the "noise diffuse" condition, plotted with respect to normative performance levels for the clinic, as shown in **Fig. 6–4.** Unaided (U) and aided (A) scores are plotted for patients 1, 2, and 3. In the unaided condition, all subjects have equal hearing loss in quiet (50 dBA) and different amounts of hearing loss in noise (–4 to +2 dB SNR). In the aided condition in quiet, all three patients move to 30 dBA thresholds, receiving an improvement of 20 dB. Also in the aided condition, patient 1 has unchanged performance in noise (acceptable results), patient 2 has degraded performance in noise (unacceptable results), and patient 3 has improved performance in noise (desired results). HLN, hearing level in noise; HLQ, hearing level in quiet.

In summary, the movement on the graph from right to left (change in HLQ) results from application of gain to increase thresholds in quiet. Movement on the graph from top to bottom (change in HLN) most often results from applications of advanced technology, such as excellent frequency shaping, multichannel compression, directional microphones, and digital noise reduction. In comparing the unaided to aided results for any patient, the aided value should always plot to the left of the unaided value (i.e., hearing in quiet is better) and should not be above the unaided value (i.e., hearing in noise is no worse). Hearing aid fittings that do not meet these criteria are to be considered unsatisfactory with regards to expected performance targets for speech recognition.

Figure 6–6 uses the HLQ/HLN format to display the result of a recent multisite field trial (Bray et al, 2005; Levitt et al, 2006). The subjects were adults with bilateral, symmetrical, sensorineural hearing loss of moderate degree. These subjects were fit with binaural behind-the ear (BTE) digital signal processing (DSP) hearing aids, including multichannel compression, directionality, and noise reduction. Subjects were measured in quiet and in noise, in the unaided condition and two aided conditions. The data are plotted as the mean value with the standard errors on both the HLQ and HLN scales.

In the unaided condition, the group performance was ~50 dBA for HLQ and 0 dB SNR for HLN. When aided with program 1, which was omnidirectional with noise reduction, performance improved to ~40 dBA for HLQ and –2 dB SNR for HLN. When aided with program 2, which was directional with noise reduction, performance improved to ~40 dBA for HLQ and –4 dB SNR for HLN.

Figure 6–7 shows the combined results of 195 DSP hearing aid fittings evaluated over the course of several years of clinical trials using a standardized test system for measurement

of speech recognition in diffuse noise using the modified HINT (Nilsson et al, 2005). The pooled subject data were divided into 5 decades of HLQ values from <30 dBA increasing to 60 to 70 dBA. For each of the five groups, SNR loss values, with respect to normal performance of –6 dB SNR, were plotted for three measurement conditions: unaided, aided in program 1 (omnidirectional microphone with digital noise reduction), and aided in program 2 (directional microphone with digital noise reduction). Each subgroup is plotted with the box defining the 25 to 75% quartile range and the

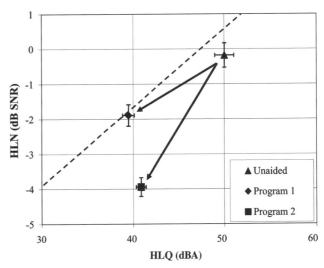

Figure 6–6 Clinical trial results for unaided and aided sound-field Hearing in Noise Test (HINT) measures for 84 subjects with moderate, bilateral, sensorineural hearing loss. Hearing level in quiet (HLQ) and hearing level in noise (HLN) values plotted are the means and standard errors for the unaided and two aided conditions (program 1 and program 2).

extended bars defining ± 2 standard deviations (SDs) from the mean.

The unaided data show an increase in SNR loss of ~1 to 2 dB for every decade of HLQ that is consistent with the scatter plot in **Fig. 6–5,** showing a similar change in HLN with respect to HLQ. The aided data for program 1, with respect to the unaided condition, show minimal benefit for milder HLQ values, growing to 3 dB SNR improvement for moderate to severe HLQ values. The aided data for program 2 show ~2 dB SNR improvement, with respect to program 1, for most of the HLQ groups.

In contrast to **Fig. 6–6,** which shows the mean and standard errors, **Fig. 6–8** shows the interquartile ranges along with 2 SDs. Although **Fig. 6–7** shows that significant group effects can be realized in speech recognition testing with hearing aids, **Fig. 6–8** shows there can also be a wide variation in performance in noise, even for individuals with similar amounts of HLQ. The key message from **Fig. 6–6** and **Fig. 6–7** is that hearing aids have well-documented group effects, which may be used for establishing appropriate expectations as part of the rehabilitation process, but that there is wide variation in individual results, meaning the process always requires verification for each individual patient.

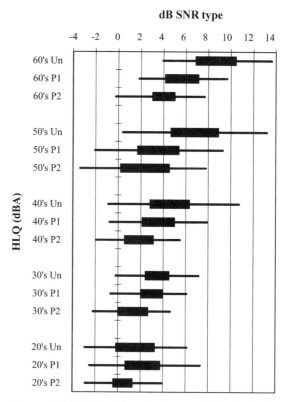

Figure 6–7 Clinical trial results for unaided and aided sound-field Hearing in Noise Test (HINT) measures for 195 subjects with bilateral, sensorineural hearing loss. The 195 subjects are grouped by degrees of hearing level in quiet (HLQ), from mild (< 30 dBA) to severe (60–70 dBA). HLQ and signal-to-noise ratio (SNR) loss values are the 25 to 75% interquartile ranges (boxes) ± 2 standard deviations for the unaided and two aided conditions (program 1 and program 2), where SNR loss is hearing level in noise (HLN) with respect to normal performance in the "noise diffuse" condition. Un, unaided; P1, aided in program 1; P2, aided in program 2.

Special Consideration

- Hearing aids have well-documented group effects, but wide variation in individual results will occur. Good clinical practice requires verification of each individual patient's performance.

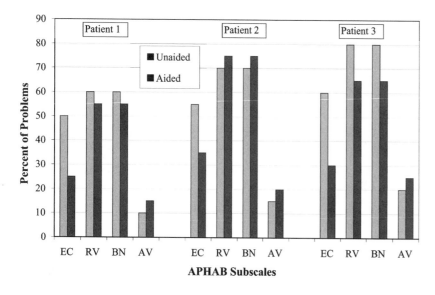

Figure 6–8 Abbreviated Profile of Hearing Aid Benefit (APHAB) graph of unaided and aided problems for the three hypothetical patients discussed in **Fig. 6–5.** APHAB subscales are ease of communication (EC), reverberation (RV), background noise (BN), and aversiveness (AV) of sounds.

◆ Outcome Measures for Evaluation of the Psychological System

The impact of hearing loss on the patient's behavior is multidimensional. Not only do behaviors change in response to physical stimuli (the patient cannot react to what he or she does not hear), but some behaviors and situations can be avoided altogether to alleviate the embarrassment or concern of others (social withdrawal). Therefore, most assessments of the psychological system attempt to evaluate the impact of the hearing loss on behavior with respect to multiple levels, such as expectations from hearing aids, unaided and aided performance in the real world, the impact of intervention on social interactions and personal image, and the patient's overall satisfaction with the rehabilitation process. It is also necessary to obtain subjective measures, as they appear to be largely independent of speech intelligibility in noise as assessed in the clinic (Beamer et al, 2000; Cord et al, 2000).

The self-assessment questionnaires are useful because they guide the patient in contemplating the global effect of the loss. Typically, a patient comes in for evaluation based on a single dimension whose participation restriction has become a dominant factor (e.g., "I can't understand my spouse"). A simple question assessing the patient's potential improvement in this one area will not produce evaluations of other behaviors that the patient has grown accustomed to as a result of the hearing loss (e.g., "I don't play bridge anymore; I can't follow the conversation"). The standardized questionnaires that are currently available sample a wide range of behaviors to more accurately assess the full impact of the disability on participation restriction across multiple dimensions (**Table 6–4**).

Participation Restriction

Participation restriction is the psychosocial disadvantage to the individual resulting from the physiological impairment and the communicative activity limitation. In the

Table 6–4 Comparison of Self-Report Questionnaires to Assess Domains in the Psychological System*

Test	Items	Ratings	Sections	H	P	B	E	S
APHAB	24 statements	7-point scale (always–never)	4 subscales	✓	✓	✓		
COSI	Patient picks up to 5 listening situations	5-point scale (degree of change)	16 categories	✓	✓	✓		
CPHI	145 items	5-point scale (agree–disagree)	4 subscales	✓				
ECHO	15 items	7-point scale (not at all–tremendously)	4 subscales				✓	
GHABP	24 questions (minimum)	5-point scale	6 subscales	✓	✓	✓		✓
HANA	11 questions	3-point scale	4 subscales	✓			✓	
HAPI	64 statements	5-point scale (helps–hinders)	4 subscales		✓			
HASS	34 items	5-point scale						✓
HAUQ	11 questions with subquestions	4-point scale						✓
HHIA	25 items	3-point scale (yes–no)	2 subscales	✓	✓	✓		
HHIA-S	10 items	3-point scale (yes–no)	2 subscales	✓	✓	✓		
HHIE	25 items	3-point scale (yes–no)	2 subscales	✓	✓	✓		
HHIE-S	10 items	3-point scale (yes–no)	2 subscales	✓	✓	✓		
HPI	158 situations	5-point scale (always–never)	6 subscales	✓				
HPI-R	90 situations	5-point scale (always–never)	6 subscales	✓				
IOI-HA	7 items	5-point scale						✓
PHAB	66 statements	7-point scale (always–never)	7 subscales	✓	✓	✓		
PHAP	66 statements	7-point scale	7 subscales		✓			
PIPSL	74 questions	7-point scale (always–never)	6 subscales	✓				
SADL	15 items	7-point scale (not at all–tremendously)	4 subscales + 1 global					✓
SHAPI	38 items	5-point scale (helps–hinders)	4 subscales		✓			

* Check marks indicate if the questionnaire evaluates handicap (H), aided performance (P), aided benefit (B), expectations (E), and/or satisfaction (S).

APHAB, Abbreviated Profile of Hearing Aid Benefit; COSI, Client Oriented Scale of Improvement; CPHI, Communication Profile for the Hearing Impaired; ECHO, Expected Consequences of Hearing Aid Ownership; GHABP, Glasgow Hearing Aid Benefit Profile; HANA, Hearing Aid Needs Assessment; HAPI, Hearing Aid Performance Inventory; HASS, Hearing Aid Satisfaction Survey; HAUQ, Hearing Aid User's Questionnaire; HHIA, Hearing Handicap Inventory for Adults; HHIA-S, Hearing Handicap Inventory for Adults–Screener; HHIE, Hearing Handicap Inventory for the Elderly; HHIE-S, Hearing Handicap Inventory for the Elderly–Screener; HPI, Hearing Performance Inventory; HPI-R, Hearing Performance Inventory–Revised; IOI-HA, International Outcome Inventory for Hearing Aids (IOI-HA); PHAB, Profile of Hearing Aid Benefit; PHAP, Profile of Hearing Aid Performance; PIPSL, Performance Inventory for Profound and Severe Loss; SADL, Satisfaction with Amplification in Daily Life; SHAPI, Shortened Hearing Aid Performance Inventory.

identification stage of the evaluation of the psychological system, measures of participation restriction serve as the unaided baseline for needed changes in the ensuing assessment of benefit. Self-assessment of participation restriction quantifies the disadvantage from the patient's perspective, and may or may not be consistent with the audiologist's expectations based on the hearing loss and communication deficit.

Measures of handicap include the Communication Profile for the Hearing Impaired (CPHI; Garstecki and Erler, 1996), the Hearing Handicap Inventory for Adults (HHIA; Newman et al, 1999), the Hearing Handicap Inventory for the Elderly (HHIE; Newman and Weinstein, 1988), the Hearing Handicap Scale (HHS; Tannahill, 1979), the Hearing Measurement Scale (HMS; Noble and Atherley, 1970), the Hearing Performance Inventory (HPI; Owens and Fujikawa, 1980), and the Performance Inventory for Profound and Severe Loss (PIPSL; Owens and Raggio, 1988).

Shortened measures of handicap include the Hearing Handicap Inventory for Adults–Screener (HHIA-S; Newman, Jacobson, et al, 1991), the Hearing Handicap Inventory for the Elderly–Screener (HHIE-S; Newman, Weinstein, et al, 1991), and the Hearing Performance Inventory–Revised (HPI-R; Lamb et al, 1983).

Handicap scales vary in their clinical feasibility and relevance. Shortened versions have been created to address concerns about test completion time, but the sensitivity and ability to interpret results vary. A good choice for measuring participation restriction should include no more than 25 items and provide normative data from a population similar to the patient, as well as guidelines as to significance.

Aided Performance or Aided Benefit

Both can be assessed following hearing aid intervention. Aided performance measures evaluate the aided participation restriction level without reference to the unaided condition (i.e., no unaided baseline), whereas the aided benefit measures determine a change in performance, or benefit, by establishing the difference in participation restriction between the unaided and aided conditions.

Measures of aided performance include the Hearing Aid Performance Inventory (HAPI; Walden et al, 1984) and the Profile of Hearing Aid Performance (PHAP; Cox and Gilmore, 1990).

Shortened measures of aided performance include the Abbreviated Profile of Hearing Aid Performance (APHAP; Purdy and Jerram, 1998), the Shortened Hearing Aid Performance Inventory (SHAPI; Jerram and Purdy, 1997), and the Shortened Hearing Aid Performance Inventory for the Elderly (SHAPIE; Dillon, 1994).

Measures of aided benefit include the Client Oriented Scale of Improvement (COSI; Dillon et al, 1999), the Glasgow Hearing Aid Benefit Profile (GHABP; Gatehouse, 1999), and the Profile of Hearing Aid Benefit (PHAB; Cox and Rivera, 1992).

Shortened measures of benefit include the Abbreviated Profile of Hearing Aid Benefit (APHAB; Cox and Alexander, 1995) and the International Outcome Inventory for Hearing Aids (IOI-HA; Cox et al, 2003).

Similar to participation restriction measures, aided performance or benefit measures also vary in their clinical feasibility and relevance. The same guidelines should be used when selecting a measure.

Satisfaction

Satisfaction measures go beyond assessing aided performance or benefit to include factors such as the patient's perspective of the rehabilitation process and the impact of the audiologist, facilities, and fees. Because satisfaction measures are quite global, they may be influenced by the patient's psychological mind-set prior to beginning the rehabilitation process. This preexisting mind-set, or baseline for satisfaction, can be assessed with expectations measures.

Measures of satisfaction include the Hearing Aid User's Questionnaire (HAUQ; Dillon et al, 1999), the MarkeTrak Hearing Aid Satisfaction Survey (HASS; Kochkin, 2005), and the Satisfaction with Amplification in Daily Life (SADL; Cox and Alexander, 2001).

Assessments of expectations include the Expected Consequences of Hearing Aid Ownership (ECHO; Cox and Alexander, 2000) and the Hearing Aid Needs Assessment (HANA; Schum, 1999). The ECHO is designed as a companion scale to the SADL; the HANA is a companion scale to the HAPI and the SHAPI.

Clinical Implementation

With so many self-report measures available, how does the audiologist choose which tool to use as part of the clinical battery? A 5-step guideline should be followed (see Cox, 2005, for details). Step 1 is to prioritize the clinical goals by determining what the data will be used for. For example, does the clinician need to provide a benefit measure to a third party? Step 2 is to understand the fundamentals of the questionnaires under consideration. How difficult is the measure to learn, administer, and score? Step 3 is to specify the essential features needed for clinical application. Considerations could include possible needs for computer administration and automated scoring. Step 4 is to narrow the field to a few choices that look appropriate, followed by a "report card" analysis to assess strengths and weaknesses of the final candidates. Finally, in step 5, select the best questionnaire.

A commonly used self-report measure in clinical and clinical research applications is the APHAB. In administering the APHAB, benefit is derived as the difference in ratings between the unaided and aided conditions. Ratings are categorized into four subscales: ease of communication in favorable conditions (EC); communication in reverberant rooms, such as classrooms (RV); communication in settings with high background noise (BN); and the aversiveness of environmental sounds (AV). The unaided conditions have been normalized to see how much participation restriction is perceived by the individual and whether or not there are any predictors for level of benefit with amplification.

An individual who expresses problems in the three communication subscales while unaided (EC, RV, and BN), is describing difficulty in almost all communication situations. If

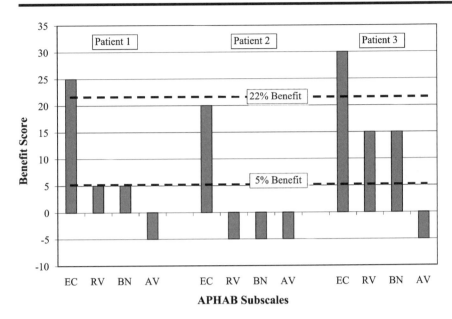

Figure 6–9 Abbreviated Profile of Hearing Aid Benefit (APHAB) graph of aided benefit for the patients profiled in **Figs. 6–5** and **6–8.** The benefit score is obtained by subtracting the aided percent of problems score from the unaided percent of problems score. Negative benefit scores on a subscale indicate the patient is having increased problems in the associated listening conditions as a result of wearing hearing aids. EC, case of communication; RV, reverberation; BN, background noise; AV aversiveness of sounds.

a patient's AV score is low, the patient has few problems tolerating environmental sounds and should have little difficulty adapting to amplification. If the AV score is high, some form of dynamic range compression or compression limiting will be necessary to control the harshness of typical environmental sounds (e.g., toilets flushing). An individual who expresses problems in only a single condition (e.g., BN) may or may not become a successful amplification user, as the limitations of amplification may outweigh the benefits. This user is more likely to require advanced-technology hearing aids to provide benefit in difficult listening conditions, without sacrificing performance in other listening conditions.

In measuring benefit, the change in perceived participation restriction between unaided and aided conditions is of great importance. The benefit is not an indication of the absolute number of problems encountered, but whether amplification has significantly reduced the number of problems experienced. Cox (1997) describes in detail several methods of interpreting APHAB scores with respect to a normal-hearing reference (which would quantify absolute performance level) and a hearing-impaired reference (which describes the individual's success relative to other, similar users of amplification), as well as comparisons between unaided and aided conditions or between two hearing aids on an individual (required differences between scores for significance are described).

In **Figs. 6–8** and **6–9,** the same patients are profiled with the APHAB as with the HINT speech recognition test results in **Fig. 6–5,** and similar interpretations are possible. Using the Cox guidelines (Cox, 1997), patient 1 obtains significant overall benefit from the > 22% improvement in the EC subscale; patient 2 does not obtain significant overall benefit; and patient 3 obtains significant overall benefit from both the > 22% improvement in the EC condition and the > 5% benefit on the EC, RV, and BN subscales.

It is important to remember that perceived benefit as indicated by a subjective measure is not guaranteed by improvements in measured physiological or communicative performance. For this reason, as part of a complete OMB, self-assessment questionnaires provide the needed additional level of detail characterizing patient performance, thereby verifying benefit and/or satisfaction from the patient's perspective.

Figure 6–10 displays the result of the recent multisite field trial discussed earlier in this chapter. **Figure 6–7** plotted the results of 84 subjects, of which 83 completed the APHAB for the unaided and aided conditions for program 2 (directional microphone plus digital noise reduction). Typical of groups with moderate hearing loss, they reported the most problems in RV and BN conditions, followed by EC, and the least with AV. The differences between the unaided and aided values are the benefit scores. Mean benefit for the group was ~30 points for EC, RV, and BN, with a negligible detriment for AV.

♦ Examples of the Outcome Measures Battery Approach

The OMB approach specifies premeasures and postmeasures across multiple auditory processing systems to identify and assess impairment, activity limitation, and participation restriction. Only with combined identification and assessment measures can benefit be calculated, which is an important evaluation of outcome. OMB approaches have been described in several proposals for standardized protocols (Arlinger, 1998; Humes, 1999; HIA, 2002; Valente et al, 1997, 2006; Walden, 1997), all of which measure across processing systems, as well as before and after treatment.

Valente et al (1997) describe a clinical OMB with the objective of improving patient satisfaction. The protocol includes evaluation of the hearing loss and disability during a prefitting session (using pure-tone and speech audiometry, immittance audiometry, real-ear measures, and the unaided

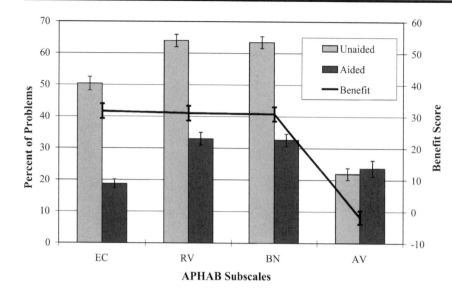

Figure 6–10 Clinical trial results for Abbreviated Profile of Hearing Aid Benefit (APHAB) measures for 83 subjects with moderate, bilateral, sensorineural hearing loss. Values plotted are the means and standard errors for unaided (white bars), aided in program 2 (black bars), and benefit score (black line, referenced to second y-axis). EC, case of communication; RV, reverberation; BN, background noise; AV aversiveness of sounds.

APHAB), followed by coupler measures of devices and real-ear comparison to fitting targets during the fitting. The second half of the APHAB is administered during a follow-up visit. This protocol depends more heavily on the benefit shown in the psychological system than evaluation of benefit in the communication system.

Walden (1997) recommends a research OMB with evaluation of the communication system in multiple environments (speech in quiet, speech in reduced cues, and speech in background noise) using the CST materials, followed by subjective measures of benefit using the PHAB. In this protocol, the subscales of the PHAB have been grouped according to their correspondence to four prototype listening situations (the three listed above as well as listening to environmental sounds) and can be used to determine the relationship between self-perceived benefit and the laboratory measures.

Arlinger (1998) describes a minimum OMB for clinical assessment of modern hearing aids and states that "[a]ssessment should contain at least the three dimensions: perceived hearing aid benefit (preferably including perceived sound quality and preference between test and reference aids), speech recognition in noise, and electroacoustic verification by means of real-ear measurements" (p. 50). Evaluation of the physiological system is performed using real-ear measures, evaluation of the communication system is performed with speech in noise (with no specific speech test recommended), and evaluation of the psychological system is performed again with the APHAB.

Another example of a proposal for an OMB comes from Humes (1999), who states,

> The most complete description of hearing aid outcome will be obtained when including at least one measure of aided speech recognition performance, one or more measures of objective benefit in speech recognition, one or two subjective measures of sound quality or listening effort, and one measure of either subjective benefit, satisfaction, or use. (p. 26)

Identification and assessment of the communication and psychological systems are suggested, with emphasis on benefit and satisfaction measures, and no stated evaluation of the physiological system. This OMB is not trying to focus on where the problem exists (as is done with a physical/diagnostic test battery), but is quantifying if treatment has been effective across multiple levels/systems.

Audiologists who conduct clinical trials as a part of industry-sponsored research should be aware that the OMB concept is included in the HIA (2002) guidelines to manufacturers, following up on an earlier FDA (1994) guidance document. The HIA guidelines outline a suggested protocol that clinical researchers should follow to obtain scientific data to substantiate hearing aid advertising claims. Specifically, the guidance recommends that

> . . . both objective (e.g., speech recognition or speech reception threshold in noise measures, such as NU-6, SPIN, SIN, or HINT) and subjective (e.g., self-assessment scales of benefit, satisfaction, or sound quality, including the APHAB, COSI, SADL, or IOI-HA) standard measurements may be included as substantiation. (p. 2)

♦ Summary

As part of his ongoing MarkeTrak analysis of consumer satisfaction with hearing aids, Kochkin (2000) intensively investigated the "in the drawer" (ITD) phenomenon exhibited by the 16.2% of hearing aid patients in the United States who no longer use their hearing aids. The top two reasons reported for not wearing hearing aids was "poor benefit" from the hearing aids (29.6% of respondents) and "background noise" (25.3% of respondents).

The biggest area of dissatisfaction that hearing aid consumers identified to Kochkin (2000) was poor benefit.

Benefit, from the patient's perspective, can be easily measured with a standardized questionnaire, such as the 24-item APHAB, or an individualized form, such as the 5-item COSI. Using on OMB approach, if the objective measures verify that the prescriptive target is appropriate and speech recognition in noise is improved, but the patient does not report satisfactory benefit, further investigation is indicated. Guidance as to where to look for the lack of perceived benefit can come from evaluation of the subscales in a questionnaire (such as EC, BN, RV, and AV of the APHAB) or in more global measures such as expectations and satisfaction from amplification.

The second largest dissatisfaction area reported is performance in noisy situations. This encompasses multiple aspects of aided performance, including poor speech recognition in noise and uncomfortably loud amplification of sounds. Both of these situations should be evaluated as part of the OMB. Acceptable tolerance to amplified sounds is the RESR (REAR-90) portion of the probe microphone battery or the aided tolerance measurement in the sound-field evaluation of the physiological system. Improved, and certainly nondegraded, speech recognition in background noise is the key performance measure in assessment of the communication system.

Audiologists who follow a three-step OMB, as recommended in this chapter, will not produce patients who have ITD hearing aids. The rationale for this argument is that satisfactory performance on outcome measures assures the audiologist that these two causes creating > 50% of patient dissatisfaction, and other "top 10" reported problems, such as "fit and comfort," "negative side effects," and "sound quality," have been overcome. In summary, it is hard to imagine that patients cannot successfully use hearing aids that (1) have gain, output, and frequency response appropriately set to improve audibility without increasing discomfort; (2) improve speech recognition in both quiet and in noise; and (3) produce significant benefit on a self-assessment scale comparing unaided to aided performance.

References

Abrams, H. B., Chisolm, T. H., & McArdle, R. (2005). Health-related quality of life and hearing aids: A tutorial. Trends in Amplification, 9, 99–109.

American National Standards Institute. (1992). Testing hearing aids with a broad-band noise signal (S3.42–1992). New York: Author.

American National Standards Institute. (1997). Methods of measurement of real-ear performance characteristics of hearing aids (S3.46–1997). New York: Author.

American National Standards Institute. (2003). Specification of hearing aid characteristics (S3.22–2003). New York: Author.

Arlinger, S. D. (1998). Clinical assessment of modern hearing aids. Scandinavian Audiology, 27(Suppl.), 49–53.

Beamer, S. L., Grant, K., & Walden, B. (2000). Hearing aid benefit in patients with high-frequency hearing loss. Journal of the American Academy of Audiology, 11, 429–437.

Bilger, R. C., Nuetzel, J., Rabinowitz, W., & Rzeczkowski, C. (1984). Standardization of a test of speech perception in noise. Journal of Speech and Hearing Research, 27, 32–48.

Bray, V. (1997, November). Outcome measures: Who, what, where, when, why and how. Presentation at the West Coast Conference of the American Academy of Audiology, San Diego, CA.

Bray, V., Ghent, R., Nilsson, M., & Murphy, P. (2005). Clinical study of a new directional system: Initial behavioral results. Hearing Review, 12(10), 54–55.

Bray, V., & Nilsson, M. (2001). Additive SNR benefits of signal processing features in a directional DSP aid. Hearing Review, 8(12), 48–51.

Byrne, D., Dillon, H., Ching, T., Katsch, R., & Keidser, G. (2001). NAL-NL1 procedure for fitting nonlinear hearing aids: Characteristics and comparisons with other procedures. Journal of the American Academy of Audiology, 12, 37–51.

Cord, M. T., Leek, M., & Walden, B. (2000). Speech recognition ability in noise and its relationship to perceived hearing aid benefit. Journal of the American Academy of Audiology, 11, 475–483.

Cox, R. M. (1997). Administration and application of the APHAB. Hearing Journal, 50(4), 32–48.

Cox, R. M. (2005). Choosing a self-report measure for hearing aid fitting outcomes. Seminars in Hearing, 26, 149–156.

Cox, R. M., & Alexander, G. (1995). The Abbreviated Profile of Hearing Aid Benefit (APHAB). Ear and Hearing, 16, 176–186.

Cox, R. M., & Alexander, G. (2000). Expectations about hearing aids and their relationship to fitting outcome. Journal of the American Academy of Audiology, 11, 368–382.

Cox, R., & Alexander, G. (2001). Validation of the SADL questionnaire. Ear and Hearing, 22, 151–160.

Cox, R. M., Alexander, G., & Beyer, C. (2003). Norms for the International Outcome Inventory for Hearing Aids. Journal of the American Academy of Audiology, 14, 403–413.

Cox, R. M., Alexander, G., Gilmore, C., & Pusakulich, K. (1988). Use of the connected speech test (CST) with hearing-impaired listeners. Ear and Hearing, 9, 198–207.

Cox, R. M., & Gilmore, C. (1990). Development of the Profile of Hearing Aid Performance (PHAP). Journal of Speech and Hearing Research 1990;33:343–357

Cox, R. M., & Rivera, I. (1992). Predictability and reliability of hearing aid benefit measured using the PHAB. Journal of the American Academy of Audiology, 3, 242–254.

Dillon, H. (1994). Shortened Hearing Aid Performance Inventory for the Elderly (SHAPIE): A statistical approach. Australian Journal of Audiology, 16, 37–48.

Dillon, H., Birtles, G., & Lovegrove, R. (1999). Measuring the outcomes of a national rehabilitation program: Normative data for the Client Oriented Scale of Improvement (COSI) and the Hearing Aid User's Questionnaire (HAUQ). Journal of the American Academy of Audiology, 10, 67–99.

Food and Drug Administration. (1994). Guidance to hearing aid manufacturers for substantiation of claims. Washington, DC: Author.

Garstecki, D. C., & Erler, S. (1996). Older adult performance on the Communication Profile for the Hearing Impaired. Journal of Speech and Hearing Research, 39, 28–42.

Gatehouse, S. (1993). Role of perceptual acclimatization in the selection of frequency responses for hearing aids. Journal of the American Academy of Audiology, 4, 296–306.

Gatehouse, S. (1999). Glasgow hearing aid benefit profile: Derivation and validation of a client-centered outcome measure for hearing aid services. Journal of the American Academy of Audiology, 10, 80–103.

Hearing Industries Association. (2002). Guidance for hearing aid manufacturers for substantiation of performance claims. Arlington, VA: Author.

Hirsh, I. J., Davis, H., Silverman, S., Reynolds, E., Eldert, E., & Benson, R. (1952). Development of materials for speech audiometry. Journal of Speech and Hearing Disorders, 17, 321–337.

Horwitz, A. R., & Turner, C. (1997). The time course of hearing aid benefit. Ear and Hearing, 18, 1–11.

Humes, L. E. (1999). Dimensions of hearing aid outcome. Journal of the American Academy of Audiology, 10, 26–39.

Jerram, J. C., & Purdy, S. (1997). Evaluation of hearing aid benefit using the Shortened Hearing Aid Performance Inventory. Journal of the American Academy of Audiology, 8, 18–26.

Killion, M. (1997a). SIN test: A speech in noise test. Elkgrove, IL: Etymotic Research.

Killion, M. (1997b). SNR loss: I can hear what people say, but I can't understand them. Hearing Review, 4(12), 8–14.

Killion, M. C., Niquette, P., Gudmundsen, G., Revit, L., & Banerjee, S. (2004). Development of a quick speech-in-noise test for measuring signal-to-noise ratio loss in normal-hearing and hearing-impaired listeners. Journal of the Acoustical Society of America, 116, 2395–2405.

Kochkin, S. (2000). MarkeTrak V: "Why my hearing aids are in the drawer." The consumer's perspective. Hearing Journal, 53(2), 34–42.

Kochkin, S. (2005). MarkeTrak VII: Hearing loss population tops 31 million people. Hearing Review, 12(7), 16–29.

Lamb, S. H., Owens, E., & Schubert, E. (1983). The revised form of the hearing performance inventory. Ear and Hearing, 4, 152–157.

Levitt, H., & Resnick, S. (1978). Speech reception by the hearing impaired: Methods of testing and the development of new tests. Scandinavian Audiology, 6, 107–130.

Levitt, H., Sandridge, S., Alvord, L., Kornhass, S., & Porcello, K. (2006, April). Interaction of noise reduction and directionality in aids. Presentation at the annual meeting of the American Academy of Audiology, Minneapolis.

National Council on the Aging. (1999). The consequences of untreated hearing loss in older persons. Washington, DC: Author.

Newman, C. W., Jacobson, G., Hug, G., Weinstein, B., & Malinoff, R. (1991). Practical method for quantifying hearing aid benefit in older adults. Journal of the American Academy of Audiology, 2, 70–75.

Newman, C. W., & Weinstein, B. (1988). The Hearing Handicap Inventory for the Elderly. Ear and Hearing, 9, 81–85.

Newman, C. W., Weinstein, B., Jacobson, G., & Hug, G. (1991). Test–retest reliability of the Hearing Handicap Inventory for Adults. Ear and Hearing, 12, 355–357.

Newman, C. W., Weinstein, B., Jacobson, G., & Hug, G. (1999). The Hearing Handicap Inventory for Adults: Psychometric adequacy and audiometric correlates. Ear and Hearing, 11, 430–433.

Nilsson, M., Ghent, R., Bray, V., & Harris, R. (2005). Development of a test environment to evaluate performance of modern hearing aid features. Journal of the American Academy of Audiology, 16, 27–41.

Nilsson, M., Soli, S., & Sullivan, J. (1994). Development of the Hearing in Noise Test for the measurement of speech reception thresholds in quiet and in noise. Journal of the Acoustical Society of America, 95, 1085–1099.

Noble, W., & Atherley, G. (1970). The Hearing Measure Scale: A questionnaire for the assessment of auditory disability. Journal of Auditory Research, 10, 229–250.

Owens, E., & Fujikawa, S. (1980). The Hearing Performance Inventory and hearing aid use in profound hearing loss. Journal of Speech and Hearing Research, 23, 470–479.

Owens, E., & Raggio, M. (1988). Performance Inventory for Profound and Severe Loss (PIPSL). Journal of Speech and Hearing Disorders, 53, 42–56.

Plomp, R. (1978). Auditory handicap of hearing impairment and the limited benefit of hearing aids. Journal of the Acoustical Society of America, 63, 533–549.

Purdy, S. C., & Jerram, J. (1998). Investigation of the Profile of Hearing Aid Performance in experienced hearing aid users. Ear and Hearing, 19, 473–480.

Schum, D. J. (1999). Perceived hearing aid benefit in relation to perceived needs. Journal of the American Academy of Audiology, 10, 40–45.

Scollie, S., Seewald, R., Cornelisse, L., et al. (2005). The desired sensation level multistage input/output algorithm. Trends in Amplification, 9, 159–197.

Speaks, C., & Jerger, J. (1965). Method for measurement of speech identification. Journal of Speech and Hearing Research, 8, 185–194.

Surr, R. K., Cord, M., & Walden, B. (1998). Long-term versus short-term hearing aid benefit. Journal of the American Academy of Audiology, 9, 165–171.

Tannahill, J. C. (1979). The Hearing Handicap Scale as a measure of hearing aid benefit. Journal of Speech and Hearing Disorders, 44, 91–99.

Taylor, B. (2003). Speech-in-noise tests: How and why to include them in your basic test battery. Hearing Journal, 56(1), 40–46.

Tillman, T., & Carhart, R. (1966). An expanded test for speech discrimination utilizing CNC monosyllabic words (Northwestern University Auditory Test no. 6, SAM-TR-66–55). Technical Report SAM-TR, 1, 1–12.

Valente, M., Abrams, H., Benson, D., et al. (2006). Guidelines for the audiological management of adult hearing impairment. Reston, VA: American Academy of Audiology.

Valente, M., Potts, L., & Valente, M. (1997). Development of a clinical protocol in an attempt to improve user satisfaction with hearing aids. Seminars in Hearing, 18, 19–28.

Walden, B. (1997). Toward a model clinical-trials protocol for substantiating hearing aid user-benefit claims. American Journal of Audiology, 6(2), 13–24.

Walden, B. E., Demorest, M., & Hepler, E. (1984). Self report approach to assessing benefit derived from amplification. Journal of Speech and Hearing Research, 27, 49–56.

World Health Organization. (2001). International Classification of Functioning, Disability, and Health. Geneva: World Health Organization.

Chapter 7

Fitting Approaches for Hearing Aids with Linear and Nonlinear Signal Processing

Francis K. Kuk

The transition of hearing aid signal processing from linear to nonlinear has been slow. It was not until the early 2000s that the majority of hearing aids (87%) dispensed in the United States were nonlinear (Strom, 2005). Along with the greater acceptance of this type of signal processing is a better understanding of how these devices should be fit and verified. This is evidenced by the introduction of several prescriptive formulas specifically for fitting hearing aids with nonlinear signal processing. This chapter will review the differences between linear and nonlinear signal processing and consider the factors that are important in selecting a prescriptive formula to fit hearing aids using these signal-processing types. Finally, the major prescriptive formulas that are used today will be examined for a better understanding of their rationale and applications.

♦ Purposes of Linear and Nonlinear Signal Processing

Differences between Linear and Nonlinear

Linear hearing aids maintain the same amount of gain at all input levels until saturation occurs. This is in contrast to nonlinear hearing aids, in which gain changes as the input level changes. **Figure 7–1A** illustrates the input/output (I/O) curve of three different hearing aids. Hearing aid A is linear until an input of 90 dB sound pressure level (SPL). Thereafter, the output is limited to ~120 dB SPL. Hearing aid B has kneepoints at 50 and 90 dB SPL. In this aid, the signal processing is linear below 50 dB SPL, nonlinear between 50 and

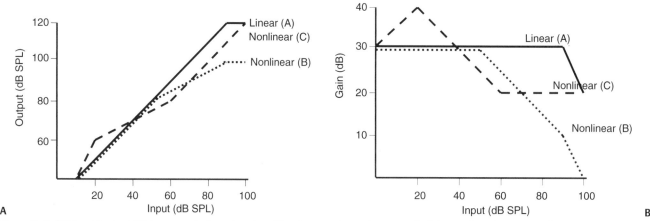

Figure 7–1 (A) Input/output (I/O) curves of a linear hearing aid and two nonlinear hearing aids. **(B)** Input/gain (I/G) curves for the same linear and nonlinear hearing aids. SPL, sound pressure level.

90 dB SPL, and with a constant output above 90 dB SPL. Hearing aid C has kneepoints at 20 and 60 dB SPL. Below 20 dB SPL, the signal processing is linear; between 20 and 60 dB SPL, the function is nonlinear; and between 60 and 90 dB SPL, it is linear once again. In all cases, output always increases (or stays the same) as input increases.

The type of processing (linear or nonlinear) becomes clearer if one replots the I/O curves as input/gain (I/G) curves **(Fig. 7–1B)**. An I/G curve is valuable because it directly reveals the gain and the type of signal processing at any input range. Linear processing is reflected by a flat line (indicating a constant 30 dB gain). Using the definition that linear processing provides the same gain at the inclusive input levels, one must agree that the region beyond 90 dB SPL is nonlinear because gain decreases as input increases. This suggests that even linear hearing aids can behave in a nonlinear manner at high input levels. Obviously, this nonlinearity is saturation distortion (i.e., peak clipping [PC]) and does not reflect the processing of the hearing aid at typical input levels.

In contrast to the flat line seen for the linear hearing aid (A), the I/G curve for nonlinear hearing aid B shows a flat line below an input level of 50 dB SPL. Above 50 dB SPL, gain decreases at a rate of 5 dB gain per 10 dB increase in input level until 90 dB SPL (i.e., a compression ratio [CR] of 2:1). From that input level on, gain decreases at a rate of 9 dB per 10 dB increase in input (i.e., a CR of 10:1). One would describe the hearing aid processing to be linear below 50 dB SPL, then nonlinear for input levels > 50 dB SPL. Specifically, gain reduction is seen as input increases. This type of nonlinear processing is called compression.

Nonlinearity does not always involve gain reduction. The I/O and I/G curves of nonlinear hearing aid C in **Fig. 7–1A** and **B** show gain increases as the input level increases from 0 to 20 dB SPL. This region is called expansion and is another form of nonlinear processing used in current digital hearing aids. Expansion is used for the purpose of reaching the desired gain at a particular input level without providing the same amount of amplification to sounds below that input level (so they remain inaudible). Only gain reduction nonlinearity (i.e., compression) will be elaborated in this chapter.

Pearl

• Linear hearing aids maintain the same gain at all input levels. Compression reduces gain as input increases. Expansion increases gain as input level increases.

Why Linear?

It is important to distinguish between linear signal processing and linear hearing aids. As explained in the previous section, linear processing is the type of signal processing whereby a constant amount of gain is applied regardless of input levels. As illustrated in the previous section, a linear hearing aid does not always stay linear. It becomes nonlinear at a high input level (> 90 dB SPL) because of the occurrence of saturation distortion. By the same token, linear processing is not restrictive to linear hearing aids only. Nonlinear hearing aids may have I/O characteristics that use linear processing for certain input levels, or they may use long time constants (longer than 2–3 seconds) to effectively achieve linear processing in the short term but nonlinear processing in the long term (Kuk, 1998). Thus, one must be clear on whether it is linear processing or linear hearing aid that is being evaluated.

The advantage of linear processing is that it preserves the intensity relationship of the input sounds. This would retain the suprasegmental cues within the speech signal (Kuk, 1998). Thus, linear processing is desirable.

Preserving the linearity or intensity relationship of the input signals cannot be the only objective in a hearing aid fitting. It is commonly acknowledged that the objectives in a hearing aid fitting are to ensure that (1) meaningful soft sounds are audible (above the wearer's thresholds) in as wide a frequency range as possible, (2) conversational level sounds are comfortable and provide the best speech recognition, and (3) loud sounds are below the wearer's loudness discomfort level (LDL). A properly fitted linear hearing aid can achieve the second and third objective easily by limiting the output to below the wearer's LDL. Furthermore, it can preserve the temporal structures of the input signal until saturation. However, to achieve the audibility of soft sounds, the wearer will need to regulate gain on the hearing aid through the use of a volume control. Consequently, using a linear hearing aid may not achieve all the objectives of a good hearing aid fitting unless the wearer actively participates in the use of the hearing aids (i.e., by adjusting the volume control). Thus, a linear hearing aid may not always be desirable.

Why Nonlinear?

Byrne (1996), Dillon (1996), and Souza (2002) provided excellent summaries of how compression is used in modern hearing aids. Simply, all nonlinear signal-processing methods minimize the need for a volume control by providing automatic gain change in accordance with the rationale to which nonlinearity is applied. Currently, there are at least three general uses for nonlinear signal processing.

Special Consideration

- Gain reduction and enhanced audibility appear to be paradoxical. In reality, when compression is applied for improved audibility, one purposely assigns more gain to the hearing aid first and then gradually decreases gain as the input level increases so the range of change in output narrows.

Minimize Saturation Distortion

Compression can be used to prevent the distortion caused by saturation (i.e., PC) as the output of a hearing aid exceeds a criterion level. The signal processing (linear or nonlinear) for input levels below the criterion remains constant. Beyond that input level, gain reduction (or further gain reduction) occurs as the input level increases. The result is that output remains minimally increased as the input level increases. This use of compression is referred to as compression limiting (CL) or output CL and has been known to provide better sound quality than PC when the input level is > 80 dB SPL (see, e.g., Hawkins and Naidoo, 1993).

Compression limiting should be desirable for all degrees of hearing loss. Because CL is associated with a loss of output above a conversational level input, there were concerns on its use for patients with a profound hearing loss. However, recent studies have shown that patients with a profound hearing loss also preferred CL and compression processing (e.g., Kuk et al, 2003).

The fitting considerations for a CL circuit are straightforward. Byrne (1996) recommended a compression threshold (CT) to be set to below the LDL of the hearing-impaired person if the CT is specified in output level (i.e., for automatic gain control—output [AGC-O]). Compression ratios used in CL hearing aids are generally greater than 5:1, with a typical value at 10:1 (i.e., every 10 dB increase in input level results in only 1 dB increase in output level).

Ensuring Audibility and Comfort without Volume Control

Alteration of Short-term Intensity Fluctuation   Compression has been used to compensate for the rapid growth of loudness perception that is often associated with sensorineural hearing loss. In order that the hearing-impaired person perceives changes in loudness at the same rate as a normal-hearing person, the hearing aid needs to use short attack and release time so the gain variation on the hearing aid can follow the intensity variation seen in the syllabic structures of the input signal. An attack time of < 5 msec and a release time of < 30 to 50 msec typically satisfy such a requirement. Such a hearing aid has been called a fast-acting wide dynamic range compression (WDRC) hearing aid.

Achieving the objective of a fast-acting WDRC results in a reduction of the output dynamic range (DR), a reduction of the intensity differences between low- and high-intensity sounds, and an increase in the proportion of consonantal syllables that are audible at a low input level (< 50 dB SPL). This could improve speech recognition at input levels < 60 dB SPL (re linear hearing aid). Some experts suggest, however, that reducing the short-term intensity relationship among speech segments reduces recognition, especially for those who are dependent on the temporal waveform. Souza (2002) provided a review of the literature in this area.

Preservation of Short-term Intensity Fluctuation (or Slow-acting WDRC)   To achieve long-term audibility (recognition) while preserving the short-term intensity contrasts among speech segments, one may use a WDRC hearing aid with a longer attack (e.g., several hundred milliseconds) and release time (e.g., several seconds). Compression hearing aids used in this manner are called slow-acting WDRC hearing aids. This approach is justified because the range of input variations (30–40 dB) in any typical listening environment is smaller than the residual dynamic range of hearing-impaired individuals with <80 dB hearing level (HL) thresholds (Kuk, 1998). Thus, the choice of attack and release time of a WDRC hearing aid could affect the appropriateness of its output and how it meets its stated objective.

Currently, all the fitting methods are targeted at WDRC hearing aids that attempt to ensure audibility and comfort (by preventing discomfort). The considerations behind these fitting methods will be the focus of this chapter.

Pearl

- It should be clear that CL and WDRC are independent of each other. CL is a method to limit output and eliminate or reduce distortion. Gain reduction occurs only at a high input level. The signal processing at conversational input levels can be either linear or nonlinear. WDRC is a form of signal processing. Gain reduction can occur at any input levels. WDRC can use either CL or PC for output control.

Noise Reduction

Whereas the previous sections described compression as an automatic gain change in response to stimulus levels, such a gain change can occur in response to the nature of the stimulus (e.g., speech or noise) in current multichannel hearing aids. These digital signal processing (DSP) hearing aids use complex statistical methods (e.g., percentile distribution) to estimate the nature of the input signal to differentiate between speech and noise. When a noise signal is identified, additional gain reduction beyond what typically occurs for a level change (i.e., compression) results. Depending on the spectrum of the noise signal, this action may change the frequency response of the hearing aid significantly. Hearing aids providing such changes in frequency response have been marketed as noise reduction hearing aids. In general, hearing aids using this technology improve the listening comfort of the wearers in noisy environments. However, their effectiveness in improving speech recognition in noise remains questionable.

Because using WDRC hearing aids for the purpose of noise reduction is a relatively recent development, there are no fitting methods that specifically describe or recommend how such a hearing aid should be fit. The important issues of its activation threshold, the speed of noise reduction, how much reduction, and so on, have not been formally evaluated. This will be an important topic in the coming years.

Pearl

- Compression and noise reduction share the same end result: gain of the hearing aid is reduced. The difference between the two features is that compression is triggered by the intensity level of the input signal, whereas noise reduction is triggered by the nature (i.e., speech or noise) of the input signal.

◆ Considerations behind Fitting Methods for Hearing Aids

The general objective of hearing aid fitting is to select the best settings on the wearer's hearing aids (e.g., frequency response and I/O), or to select the best hearing aids to provide such settings so that (1) soft sounds are audible; (2) conversational sounds are natural, meaningful, and comfortable; and (3) loud sounds are not uncomfortable. How closely a fitting method can achieve this objective depends on the design considerations taken by the developers of the fitting method. The following are some of these considerations.

Optimal Frequency Characteristics: Loudness Normalization versus Loudness Equalization

The rationale for loudness normalization is to provide sufficient amplification to all frequencies so the full range of sounds is perceived at the same loudness as a person with normal hearing. The assumption is that loudness perception of normal-hearing listeners is a reasonable target and should be important in providing hearing aid satisfaction and benefit. Typically, loudness growth functions, either by direct measurement or prescriptions, are determined to generate the frequency response and I/O characteristics of the WDRC hearing aid (Allen et al, 1990).

In fittings that use a loudness equalization rationale, each frequency is differentially amplified so they are equally loud. The rationale is to maximize speech recognition at a conversational (60–70 dB SPL) listening level (Byrne, 1996). Typically, empirical data are used to generate a statistical model that can be used to prescribe gain–frequency characteristics based on threshold information. Because lower frequencies contribute more to loudness than mid and high frequencies, low-frequency gain provided by an equalization approach is typically less than that prescribed by a normalization approach. This could have implications on the sound quality and speech recognition provided by hearing aids using these two different rationales.

Gain at Varying Input Levels

A linear hearing aid provides the same gain–frequency response for all input levels; thus, only gain for a conversational input (i.e., 60–70 dB SPL) is typically prescribed. A nonlinear hearing aid, in contrast, provides varying gain for different input levels. Consequently, fitting approaches for a nonlinear hearing aid would need frequency/gain/output recommendations for multiple input levels (e.g., soft, normal, and loud, or 50, 65, and 80 dB SPL input levels). Such recommendations can be made by considering the appropriate gain/output at each input level separately, or they may be estimated after specifying the optimal compression characteristics, such as CT, CR, and attack and release times.

Is There an Optimal Compression Threshold?

The CT is the point (input level) of maximum gain on the I/O curve (Kuk, 1999). Thus, gain decreases beyond the CT, and its theoretical value should be 0 dB HL with a gain value equal to the person's hearing loss (Dillon, 1996). This is especially the case if the objective of fitting is to restore normal loudness perception to the impaired ear. For example, a wearer with 80 dB HL will be assigned 80 dB of gain in order for a 0 dB HL input to be audible. Indeed, version 4.1 of the desired sensation level input/output (DSL [i/o]; Cornelisse et al, 1995) prescribed such a low CT. Because the typical CT occurs at a low (< 50 dB SPL) input level, the gain value at the CT often reflects the gain for soft sounds provided by the nonlinear hearing aid.

A low CT, assuming optimal gain/output at a conversational level, would result in more gain for soft sounds than a higher CT. Increased audibility of soft sounds, more consistent audibility of speech across listening environments, and partially overcoming the audibility limitation of a fixed directional microphone are some of the stated advantages of a low CT (Kuk, 1999). In practice, a CT at 0 dB HL may not be possible (because of feedback) or practical (because of circuit noise). Barker and Dillon (1999) adjusted the CT of a single-channel fast-acting WDRC hearing aid and reported that adults preferred a higher CT setting at 60 dB SPL. The decreased sound quality and the increase in the ambient noise level were cited as the major reasons for the preference for the higher CT (thus lower gain for soft sounds). Consequently, the final CT would depend on the maximum available gain of the hearing aid and the input level where one desires audibility. If hearing soft sounds (i.e., input level <50 or 60 dB SPL) is critical, then a low CT with high gain may be warranted.

The magnitude of the low CT may be different for a single-channel compression system than for a multichannel compression system. In a single-channel compression system, the effect of gain reduction (i.e., compression) is seen across all frequencies once the overall level of the input signal exceeds the CT. This means any intense sounds with a limited bandwidth, or a broadband sound at a moderate level, could trigger gain reduction across all frequencies. In a multichannel compression system, the effect of gain reduction may be experienced only at discrete frequency regions because each compression channel has its own CT, which specifies the overall intensity level of sounds for that channel to activate compression. A CT of 40 dB SPL (overall level) is low for a single-channel compression hearing aid because this level is lower than the typical level of soft speech. A multichannel nonlinear hearing aid, in contrast, "splits" the input into its component frequencies so that the effective input in each channel is lower than the overall input level. Thus, a CT of 40 dB SPL is relatively "high" in a multichannel nonlinear hearing aid. Indeed, one would expect a much lower CT than 40 dB SPL in a multichannel nonlinear hearing aid. Furthermore, one would expect a lower CT for the higher frequency channels than the lower frequency channels because the spectral level in the lower frequencies is higher than in the higher frequencies. One would also expect a lower CT in devices with more channels than ones with fewer channels because the overall level in each channel is lower from the increasing number of channels and narrowing of bandwidth. Obviously, the CT should be higher than the microphone noise of the hearing aid, which is typically between 15 and 20 dB SPL.

How Is the Compression Ratio Determined?

The CR used on a WDRC device may affect the acceptability of the hearing aids to the wearer. Because a higher CR (> 3:1) would inevitably lead to a greater reduction in intensity fluctuation of the output signals, most commercial WDRC hearing aids have CRs that are limited to < 3:1. Too much compression (high CR) could compromise speech perception for those who depend on the temporal envelope for speech recognition (Souza, 2002).

Knowledge of the gain values at multiple input levels allows one to estimate the CR. When the CR of a hearing aid is known, the output at multiple input levels can also be calculated. Direct loudness growth measurements and prescriptive approaches using normative data have been advocated to program the compression parameters of a nonlinear hearing aid. Differences between the two approaches reflect the

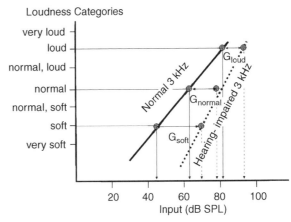

Figure 7–2 Hypothetical loudness growth function for a normal-hearing and hearing-impaired listener at 3000 Hz.

attention paid to individual variation in loudness perception. A brief description of these approaches follows.

Direct Loudness Measurement   During direct loudness measurement, the individual's loudness categories for signals at different frequencies and intensities are measured to either directly calculate the amount of necessary gain or compare with the loudness growth functions of normal-hearing individuals to derive the optimal compression settings. For example, **Fig. 7–2** illustrates that the normal ear (solid line) required 43, 62, and 82 dB SPL at 3000 Hz to reach the "soft," "normal," and "loud" loudness categories, respectively. The hearing-impaired ear (dotted line), on the other hand, required 69, 78, and 91 dB SPL to reach the same loudness categories. The difference between the solid (normal) line and the dotted (hearing-impaired) line represents the amount of gain at each input level (to the normal ear) to bring the impaired ear to the same loudness perception as the normal ear. In this case, 26 dB (69–43) of gain (G_{soft}) is required for soft sounds (input level of 43 dB SPL), 16 dB (78–62) of gain (G_{normal}) is required for conversational sounds (input level of 62 dB SPL), and 9 dB (91–82) of gain (G_{1oud}) is required for loud sounds (input level of 82 dB SPL) to reach normal loudness perception.

Figure 7–3 transforms the information from **Fig. 7–2** into an I/O curve. For example, one reads from **Fig. 7–2** that it requires 43 dB SPL for the normal ear and 69 dB SPL for the impaired ear to reach a "soft" loudness category at 3000 Hz. Consequently, the (x,y) coordinate on the I/O plane in **Fig. 7–3** is (43, 69). This point is identified as "soft." At the "normal" level, 62 dB SPL is required for the normal ear and 78 dB SPL for the impaired ear to reach the "normal" loudness category. Consequently, the (x,y) coordinate on the I/O plane to reach "normal" loudness is (62, 78). This process is repeated for the "loud" loudness category. These three coordinates are connected to create an I/O curve at 3000 Hz. In other words, this is the output at 3000 Hz the hearing aid must provide so the hearing-impaired person has the same loudness perception as the average normal-hearing person across intensity levels at 3000 Hz. Because the CR is defined as the change in input to the change in output

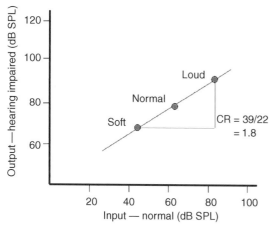

Figure 7–3 Desired I/O characteristics of a compression hearing aid to normalize loudness at 3000 Hz for the hypothetical listener in **Fig. 7-2.** CR, compression ratio.

(i.e., CR = input change/output change), one can easily calculate the CR at 3000 Hz to be 39/22, or 1.8:1.

Ratio of Dynamic Ranges   The CR may also be estimated by comparing the individual wearer's residual DR to that of normal-hearing individuals. For example, if a hearing-impaired person's DR (difference between threshold and upper limit of comfort) is 50 dB (from a threshold of 60 dB and an LDL of 110 dB) and a normal hearing listener is 100 dB (from LDL of 110 dB and threshold of 10 dB), the CR is

$$DR_n/DR_{hi} = (UL_n-TH_n)/(UL_{hi}-TH_{hi})$$
$$CR = (110-10)/(110-60)$$
$$= 2.0,$$

where DR_n is dynamic range in normal ear, DR_{hi} is dynamic range in hearing-impaired ear, UL_n is uncomfortable listening level in normal ear, TH_n is threshold in normal ear, UL_{hi} is uncomfortable listening level in hearing-impaired ear, and TH_{hi} is threshold in hearing-impaired ear.

Modified Linear Prescription   In this approach, the wearer's hearing thresholds are first specified so that the desired output may be estimated for a conversational input (i.e., 60–70 dB SPL) using either a loudness equalization or normalization philosophy. Once that information is available, the CR can be calculated based on output information at one or two input levels. For example, if one has determined the desired hearing aid output (87 dB SPL) for a conversational level input (67 dB SPL) and that the maximum output of the hearing aid must not exceed the wearer's LDL (110 dB SPL) for sounds > 90 dB SPL, these two points can be joined to form a straight line whose slope can be estimated to determine the CR **(Fig. 7–4)**. In this case, the slope between the conversational level (67 dB SPL) and the LDL (110 dB SPL) is 1 or linear. If an additional point such as the lowest input level (40 dB SPL) that audibility is desired (e.g., threshold is 75 dB SPL) is known, one can calculate more accurately the desired CR below the conversational level as well. In this case, the CR below the conversational level is 2:1. This

approach may even be useful to estimate the desired I/O curves with curvilinear characteristics.

> **Pitfall**
>
> - Although the prescriptive method using DR information is convenient, the calculated CR may be too high for patients with a severe to profound hearing loss. These individuals typically prefer a CR lower than 3:1.

The previous measurements determined the growth of loudness using narrowband signals. Real-life signals are typically broadband in nature. Because the loudness of a broadband signal is the sum of the loudness of all its component frequencies, loudness growth functions measured with narrow bands of signals must be corrected for the bandwidth effect to ensure that real-life broadband signals are not unacceptably loud.

In addition, Moore and Glasberg (1998) reported that the auditory bandwidth of hearing-impaired individuals may be wider than that of normal-hearing individuals. The difference in bandwidth increases as hearing loss increases and could be twice as wide on average. That means the growth of loudness to a broadband signal in a hearing-impaired person may be different from that of a normal-hearing person. Thus, the bandwidth correction must be made in reference to hearing-impaired ears and not to normal-hearing ears. Otherwise, the loudness growth information measured/predicted with narrowband stimuli would be unacceptable for real-life broadband stimuli.

Although the static CR can be estimated easily, the dynamic or effective CR (the actual CR in real life) is affected by other variables, such as vent diameter and the attack and release times. The impact of such factors will be discussed in a later section.

Direct Loudness Measurements versus Predicted Loudness
The choice between using a threshold-based prescription, such as DSL (i/o) or National Acoustic Laboratories' nonlinear fitting procedure, version 1 (NAL-NL1), and a suprathreshold-based approach, such as loudness growth

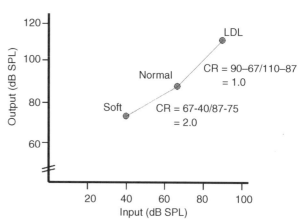

Figure 7–4 Desired I/O curve generated using the modified linear prescription (MLP) method. LDL, loudness discomfort level.

in octave bands (LGOB; Allen et al, 1990), to set the compression parameters on a nonlinear hearing aid has been controversial. One of the major goals for a WDRC hearing aid is to restore normal loudness perception. The implicit expectation is that wearers will receive maximum benefit from amplification when the processing is matched to the loudness growth functions of normal-hearing listeners across frequencies. Because loudness function varies for individuals with the same audiogram, direct measurement of this function could help program the precise compression parameters that could logically lead to improved audibility and speech recognition.

This need for direct loudness measurement has been questioned by several researchers and clinicians (Byrne, 1996; Dillon, 2001). First, there are no validation studies to support the efficacy of the approach. Second, there is a lack of uniformity for the definition of loudness perception. Third, loudness can be predicted fairly well in a majority of hearing aid wearers. Fourth, the real-life compression characteristics (e.g., the CR) are affected by the release time and vent diameter of the hearing aids. This means the prescribed setting based on the measured data will be different from real-life use of the hearing aids. Fifth, the loudness growth of broadband signals in real life is different from the loudness growth of narrowband signals used to measure loudness growth in the clinic. In addition, because loudness growth of a broadband signal is different between normal and impaired ears, the reference to normal ears may lead to a suboptimal recommendation. Sixth, Byrne (1996) questioned the importance of precise loudness judgment by noting that the long- and short-term spectra of speech vary considerably among talkers and acoustic conditions. Yet both normal-hearing and hearing-impaired listeners have little difficulty understanding speech as long as it is audible and comfortably loud. In addition, Byrne (1996) indicated that normal loudness perception may not always be the best for speech recognition and that restoring normalcy to some aspects of audition (e.g., recruitment compensation) could be counterproductive if other aspects (e.g., frequency resolution) remain abnormal. At least conservatively, there is no reason why a hearing aid cannot be fit using a prescriptive approach (or predicted loudness) as a starting point for the average wearer until additional evidence suggests otherwise.

Maximum Output or OSPL90 Setting

A critical factor in fitting hearing aids is the prescription of the output sound pressure level at 90 dB input (OSPL90) of the hearing aid so that its maximum output does not exceed the expected LDL of the hearing-impaired person to cause discomfort and/or to result in additional hearing loss. This information can be directly measured or predicted on the basis of available normative data (e.g., Pascoe, 1988). Although a direct measurement of LDL may have high face validity, this author prefers a predicted approach because of the difficulty and variability in instructions, the nontransference of LDL data measured using signals with narrow bandwidth to real-world broadband sounds, and the fact that data from the use of predicted LDLs appear to be favorable.

Whether the LDL is measured or predicted, the OSPL setting is typically adjusted to below the wearer's LDL.

Because the OSPL90 setting on a hearing aid affects the maximum output of the hearing aid, one should select an output level below the LDL of the wearer as the OSPL90 setting for both linear and nonlinear hearing aids. The issue of an "accurate" OSPL90 setting may be less critical in a nonlinear hearing aid than in a linear one, however, because of the decreasing gain characteristics as input level increases. With proper gain adjustment for the three different input levels (for soft, normal, and loud), it is less likely that the output of a nonlinear hearing aid reaches the maximum output of the hearing aid. Thus, many nonlinear hearing aids do not allow a separate adjustment of the OSPL90 setting; rather, a gain parameter for loud sounds is available instead to ensure that the maximum output of the hearing aid is acceptable.

There are additional concerns when it comes to programming the OSPL90 or insertion gain parameter for loud sounds for a multichannel nonlinear hearing aid. Because of power summation (i.e., output from each channel adding together to yield a higher output than from each individual channel), the loudness of the overall output may exceed the prescribed OSPL90 that is determined using narrowband stimuli. Thus, the final OSPL90 setting must be decreased by $\sim 10 \log (n)$, where n is the number of channels available on the nonlinear hearing aid (Dillon, 2001).

Changes in Frequency Response with Varying Input Levels

The typical WDRC hearing aid changes its output level while keeping its bandwidth as input level changes. The assumption is the frequency response that is optimal for a conversational level is also optimal for input levels above and below this level. There are compression hearing aids that are classified as bass increase at low levels (BILL) and treble increase at low levels (TILL) (Killion et al, 1990), in which the frequency response of the hearing aid changes as the input level changes. In the BILL circuit, low-frequency gain decreases as input increases; in the TILL circuit, the high-frequency gain decreases as input increases.

The BILL circuit was marketed as a noise reduction hearing aid when first introduced. A difference between the previous BILL circuit and current digital hearing aids with noise reduction is that the BILL circuit changes the frequency response (more specifically, the low-frequency gain) as a function of input level only. Current digital hearing aids change the overall output level as a function of input level but provide additional gain changes in specific frequency regions only when the input signals meet the criteria of "noise" defined by the algorithms of the hearing aids. Consequently, current digital hearing aids with noise reduction can yield a completely different frequency-output characteristic depending on the nature of the input signal. From a clinical perspective, clinicians will need to ensure not only the hearing aid provides an optimal level-dependent frequency output in a quiet listening condition but also a stimulus-dependent frequency response in noisy situations. This

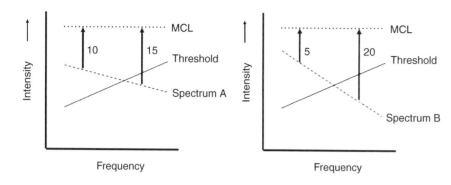

Figure 7–5 Desired gain to reach the most comfortable level (MCL) of a wearer using two stimuli (A and B) with different spectra.

means that for hearing aids with a noise reduction algorithm, it will be desirable that the fitting method provides two recommendations, one for "speech" listening and one for "noise" listening.

It is not a trivial matter to have a fitting method recommend a "noise" listening setting. In addition to the difficulty in agreeing on what is a typical noise signal and the criteria for acceptability (i.e., comfort or speech recognition), there is the variability in which different manufacturers implement their own noise reduction algorithms. The amount of noise reduction, the activation time for the noise reduction, the criteria used to identify noise, as well as the criteria for an optimal noise performance, vary greatly among manufacturers. This topic will need to be researched further in the years ahead.

Stimulus Used to Define a Target

Traditionally, a prescriptive fitting formula generates its target by measuring the required amount of gain to amplify a defined speech spectrum to a desirable level (e.g., most comfortable level [MCL] of the wearer). Let us assume that a hearing-impaired person has hearing thresholds and MCL levels indicated in **Fig. 7–5.** Let us also assume that two different signals with spectra indicated as A and B are used as the stimuli to generate the gain target. With stimulus A, 10 dB of gain is needed in the low-frequency region and 15 dB is needed in the high-frequency region to amplify spectrum A to the wearer's MCL. For spectrum B, 5 dB of gain in the low frequency and 20 dB of gain in the high frequency are needed to amplify spectrum B to the wearer's MCL.

If the gain settings on a linear hearing aid are adjusted to the gain target based on stimulus A (10 dB in the low frequency and 15 dB in the high frequency), the same gain curve will be evident if an alternate stimulus B is used to examine the gain on the hearing aid. Indeed, any stimuli (speech, sinusoids, etc.) can be used to verify that the target gain (of 10 dB in the low frequency and 15 dB in the high frequency) is achieved in the linear hearing aid. This is because gain is a characteristic of the linear hearing aid that is not changed by the choice of stimulus. This can be seen in **Fig. 7–6,** which shows the gain of a linear hearing aid to three stimuli—a pure-tone sweep at 50 dB, an American National Standards Institute (ANSI) S-3.22 speech-shaped noise, and an International Collegium of Rehabilitative Audiology (ICRA) speech-shaped noise (Dreschler et al, 2001).

Despite the difference in the spectral contents of these stimuli (see inset), gain of the linear hearing aid remains the same.

> **Pearl**
>
> • Specifying a gain target (instead of output) for linear hearing aids simplifies verification in that any stimuli (sinusoid, broadband noise) may be used for verification to yield the same results. The same is not true if an output target is used or when nonlinear hearing aids are considered.

The same is not true for a multichannel nonlinear hearing aid. **Figure 7–7** shows the gain of a 15-channel nonlinear hearing aid to the same stimuli. In contrast to the case of the linear hearing aid, one sees that the ICRA signal has the highest gain in the high frequencies, whereas the sweep sinusoid has the least high-frequency gain (**Fig. 7–7A**). The output of the hearing aid, however, showed the most high-frequency output with the ANSI speech-shaped noise and least with the ICRA speech-shaped noise (**Fig. 7–7B**). Such an observation can be explained by the spectrum of the input signal and the characteristics of a nonlinear hearing aid.

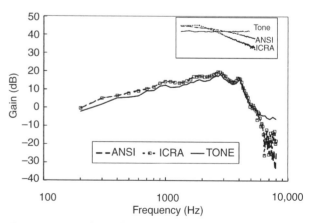

Figure 7–6 Equal gain from a linear hearing aid to three different stimuli (sinusoid, American National Standards Institute [ANSI], and International Collegium of Rehabilitative Audiology [ICRA] speech-shaped noise) despite the different spectra (see inset).

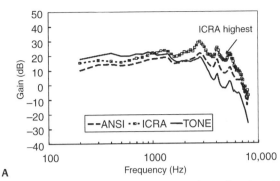

A

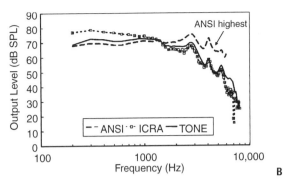

B

Figure 7–7 (A) Different gain from a nonlinear hearing aid to three different stimuli (sinusoid, ANSI, and ICRA speech-shaped noise). Note that the ICRA signal shows the greatest gain in the high frequencies.

(B) Different output from the same nonlinear hearing aid to the same stimuli. Note that the ANSI signal has the highest output.

Because a nonlinear hearing aid provides more gain for a lower input than a higher input, and the ICRA noise has less energy in the high frequency than the ANSI speech-shaped noise, the ICRA noise receives higher gain in the high frequencies. Despite the higher gain, the low input spectral level in the high frequency of the ICRA noise still yielded a lower high-frequency output than the ANSI speech noise.

This example has several implications. A fitting formula that uses the ANSI speech-shaped noise as a reference (e.g., NAL) will likely yield a different target than another one that uses the ICRA speech spectrum as the reference. This means that the choice of stimulus for verification is important for a nonlinear hearing aid when it comes to target matching. During gain verification of a nonlinear hearing aid, one must use the same stimulus in which the target was based. For example, if spectrum B **(Fig. 7–5)** is used to verify a fitting using a gain target that is based on spectrum A, one may find the high-frequency gain of the hearing aid to be higher than the prescribed target. If one lowers the high-frequency gain, one may have reduced the gain unnecessarily. One must know the characteristics of the stimulus that was used to define the prescriptive target so the identical stimulus is chosen during verification. Alternatively, one may adjust the target by making appropriate corrections. Not realizing the need for appropriate corrections to the target has been a source of confusion and frustration for many clinicians who try to verify. For the same reason, even though "real" speech may have high validity for verification, it is not appropriate for use in specifying prescriptive targets, nor should it be used for target-matching purposes because of the large variability in spectra across individuals.

Multichannel Summation

Whereas a linear hearing aid is single channel, current nonlinear hearing aids have varying numbers of channels (from 1 to as many as 20 channels). Furthermore, they vary considerably by their crossover frequencies as well as the steepness of the filter slope (i.e., specificity). This has significant implications on the target gain values as well as verification.

Figure 7–8 shows the output of four hearing aids to the ANSI (S-3.22) speech-shaped noise after they were closely

matched to the revised version of NAL (NAL-R; Byrne and Dillon, 1986) target frequency response with a sweep tone stimulus (see inset of figure). These hearing aids were produced by the same manufacturer and differed in the number of processing channels. They include a single-channel linear hearing aid (Logo), a 2-channel WDRC (Bravo), a 3-channel WDRC (SensoC8+), and a 15-channel WDRC device (Diva). The output of the hearing aids differed significantly among each other when presented with the broadband noise (ANSI speech-shaped noise). The 15-channel device yielded 8 to 10 dB greater output than the single-channel and the 2-channel devices.

The observations can be easily explained. When a sinusoid was used to adjust gain of the hearing aid, the output of the hearing aid was based on one frequency at a time. Any potential interactions among frequencies, which will be present in the real world when broadband signals are encountered, would not be evaluated or evident. However, if a broadband stimulus such as speech is presented, the output of each frequency channel would add and result in a higher output as the final output of the hearing aid. Indeed, the higher the CR, the more channels there are, and the shallower the filter slopes, the greater will be the output difference between a single-channel device and a multichannel

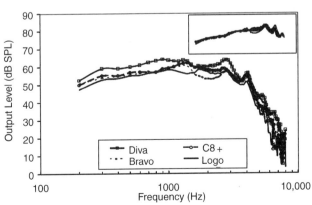

Figure 7–8 Output of four hearing aids (15-channel Diva, 3-channel SensoC8+, 2-channel Bravo, and single-channel Logo) when presented with an ANSI speech-shaped noise after equated in gain to a sinusoidal stimulus (see inset).

device. Similar considerations are also applicable in the OSPL90 prescription described earlier.

Clinically, this suggests any nonlinear fitting formulas that recommend a gain (or OSPL90) target must consider the number of channels in the nonlinear device and the appropriate stimulus to be used for target matching. If the target is to be verified with a sinusoidal stimulus, then knowledge of the number of channels as well as the crossover frequencies must be specified. This is required so the target can be compensated for a multichannel device by subtracting an amount of gain equal to the impact of the channel summation. An alternative is to examine the aided output (instead of gain) of the multichannel hearing aid with a broadband stimulus. In this case, the result of potential channel summation will be reflected in the overall aided output. This is another reason for using a broadband signal and examining the aided output instead of the aided gain or insertion gain during verification.

Target Candidates

Children versus Adults

To recommend a suitable gain–frequency/output setting, fitting methods designed for pediatric use often include considerations of the developmental differences between adults and children in their target formulation. From the physiological standpoint, it is well known that children under 5 years of age have ear canals that are substantially smaller than adults'. This results in a higher resonance frequency and SPL at the ear canal. In addition, it makes the use of an insertion gain target (difference between the real ear unaided response [REUR] and the real ear aided response [REAR]) problematic because such a gain target assumes adult REUR. Use of an aided output target or an aided gain target will bypass such a bias. Alternatively, one may modify the insertion gain targets based on the age-appropriate REUR information. Obviously, one would have to assume that the child is an "average" of the specific age group with normal external and middle ear characteristics.

Because most children may not be able to remain cooperative during the evaluation, the fitting method must require minimal information that can be obtained quickly and yet accurately. The determination and use of real ear-to-coupler difference (RECD) corrections to predict real-ear output from hearing aid coupler results has been advocated (Moodie et al, 1994). This simplifies the fitting, selection, and verification because one can derive the desired coupler response given any real ear aided gain (REAG) target or estimate the real-ear aided output given the coupler response of a hearing aid. This is especially beneficial when several hearing aids are considered as potential candidates.

Another consideration that may be necessary for pediatric fitting is the optimal gain. Currently, the only model that allows one to calculate speech recognition is based on adult considerations. Although there is no evidence to suggest that such a model is not appropriate for pediatric use, several researchers (e.g., Nozza et al, 1991) have shown that at least in normal-hearing children, young children required a higher sensation level to perform like adults on speech

discrimination and recognition tasks. If this observation can be extrapolated to hearing-impaired children and adults, this suggests an adult and a child with the same degree of hearing loss should be prescribed different amounts of gain for optimal performance. Unfortunately, there is no consensus on how much more gain is needed and which gain parameter (for soft, medium, and loud sounds) should be adjusted. On a theoretical level, such adjustments should be made in the gain for soft sounds (either through the gain parameter or the CT to ensure more consistent audibility) and normal conversational sounds, so that such sounds are also more easily and loudly heard for better speech discrimination and identification. Such gain increase will not be necessary for loud sounds to ensure comfort and prevent the likelihood of additional hearing loss. It is important that a fitting method explain what considerations have been taken when it is earmarked for pediatric use.

Severity of Hearing Loss

Another consideration in examining a prescriptive method is its appropriateness for different severity of hearing loss. There are two main reasons for this consideration. First, Byrne and his colleagues (1991) reported that the preferred gain used by patients with more than a moderately severe hearing loss (> 60 dB HL) is higher than what is typically recommended for patients with a lesser degree of hearing loss. Indeed, the original NAL-R fitting formula (Byrne and Dillon, 1986) found that for hearing loss to 60 dB HL, a gain factor that was ~0.46 times the degree of hearing loss provides appropriate gain recommendation. As the degree of hearing loss increases, this gain factor is increased to 0.6 times to provide adequate gain, especially for the lower frequencies.

A second reason is that spectral resolution becomes poorer as hearing loss increases. Moore and Glasberg (1998) have shown that the width of the auditory filter increases as hearing loss increases (i.e., poorer spectral resolution). This widening means that individuals with a severe hearing loss will be less likely to discriminate spectral differences and be more dependent on temporal cues for discrimination. Any disruptions in temporal intensity fluctuations may lead to a reduction in speech recognition ability (e.g., Souza, 2002). Unfortunately, a potential drawback of compression is the reduction of intensity contrasts. This raises the question of the appropriateness of nonlinear processing for such patients. Indeed, the higher the CR, or the faster the attack/release time, the more reduction in the temporal intensity contrast one may expect. Thus, it is reasonable to expect that hearing-impaired patients with more than a mild degree of hearing loss (> 40–50 dB HL) will more likely experience difficulty with fast-acting WDRC because of its potential alteration of the temporal-intensity contrasts. Thus, they may not be good candidates for such hearing aid processing. Especially for fitting methods targeted at fast-acting WDRC hearing aids, it will be necessary to indicate the fitting range of the specific method. Souza (2002) provided summaries of studies to show that subjects with a mild to moderate degree of hearing loss showed more benefit with WDRC on sentence recognition than did subjects with more severe losses.

"Dead" Region?

The concept of a "dead" region is considered by some fitting methods (e.g., Byrne et al, 2001; Moore and Glasberg, 1998). Moore (2001) provided a detailed description of the clinical picture of individuals with a dead region. Specifically, a dead region is an area within the cochlea with no surviving inner hair cells. Individuals typically would have a precipitous (defined as hearing loss in excess of 50 dB/octave) hearing loss that can be either rising or sloping, severe to profound, and leads to poor word recognition scores that are not commensurate with the degree of hearing loss. From an amplification standpoint, it has been reported that providing amplification or audibility in the dead region may result in poorer speech recognition than not amplifying the region (Ching et al, 1998; Moore, 2001). To avoid such an occurrence, a fitting method that considers the implication of a dead region will recommend less gain in the high-frequency region if it assumes that the inner hair cells in a precipitous high-frequency hearing loss are dead. This is implemented in the NAL-NL1 nonlinear fitting formula where a hearing loss desensitization factor is added to lower the high-frequency gain as the degree of hearing loss increases. Because a severe degree of high-frequency hearing loss may not always mean the presence of a dead region, fitting formulas may refine their recommendations by providing a different gain target to patients with the same degree of hearing loss but different hair cell survival (presence or absence of dead region). In this case, suprathreshold information such as tuning curves or masking functions that reflect the tuning of the cochlea would be required.

The issue becomes more complicated when the concept of a dead region is applied to fittings of children with a precipitously sloping high-frequency hearing loss. This is because the same severity and hearing loss configuration in an adult that is suggestive of a dead region may still benefit from amplification in children. Mackersie et al (2004) reported the speech scores on two groups of listeners who had the same degree of hearing loss. One group was identified on the Threshold Equalizing Noise (TEN; Moore, 2001) test to have a dead region, and the other group did not have a dead region. Mackersie et al (2004) found that as the bandwidth of amplification increased, speech recognition scores in quiet improved for both groups of listeners. In a noisy environment, the authors found that the group without a dead region still improved their speech scores when the bandwidth of amplification was increased. However, the group of subjects with a dead region did not show any improvement in speech scores with an increase in bandwidth. However, their speech scores did not decrease with increasing bandwidth. This suggests that amplification of a dead region may not always lead to deleterious results. Clearly, the issue of dead region and its implication on the fitting target is unsettled at best. It would be meaningful to understand if the fitting method has considered the issue to interpret how the recommended target may be different from other fitting methods.

Conductive and Mixed Hearing Loss

Although the majority of hearing losses that a clinician encounters are sensorineural in nature, there are patients with a conductive or mixed hearing loss who present themselves for amplification. Typically, a conductive hearing loss introduces an attenuation component in the hearing loss that can best be overcome with linear processing. In the case of a nonlinear hearing aid, changing the processing from nonlinear to linear would require an increase in the gain for loud sounds (e.g., IG loud). This will effectively overcome the intended design of a nonlinear hearing aid of decreasing gain with increasing input to result in more linear processing. However, how much gain increase varies from one fitting method to another, from one quarter the magnitude of the air–bone gap to three quarters this magnitude.

Binaural versus Monaural Amplification

It is well established that binaural hearing has several advantages over monaural hearing. One of the advantages is that the overall loudness perception is increased by 6 to 8 dB over the monaural case. It is also recognized that this advantage (and others) are evident when using binaural hearing aids. Thus, if a monaural hearing aid yields a comfortably loud perception, the use of binaural hearing aids could result in a loudness percept that is "too loud." A prescriptive formula needs to have different targets for monaural and binaural fits. Indeed, for the same degree of hearing loss, a gain recommendation that is 3 to 5 dB less is often used in a binaural fit than in a monaural fit. Clinicians who normally use a fitting approach that is intended for a binaural fit will have to increase the gain setting on the hearing aid if a particular fit is for a monaural hearing aid. Likewise, clinicians who normally use a fitting method that is intended for monaural use will have to lower the recommended gain when the fitting target is for a binaural instrument.

Is Experience with Hearing Aids Important?

A clinical observation that many dispensing professionals frequently encounter is that the prescribed gain for a new hearing aid wearer is "too loud." This has led to the implementation of "adaptation managers" used in several commercial hearing aid fitting systems. In essence, less overall gain is prescribed for a first-time wearer. Gain is gradually increased over time as the wearer becomes acclimatized to the hearing aid.

Convery et al (2005) reviewed 14 studies on the issue of changes in preferred gain over time. Of these studies, only one (Marriage et al, 2004) found that new wearers preferred 3 dB less gain than experienced wearers on a prescriptive target. All the other studies showed no preferred gain difference between experienced and new wearers or with new wearers over time.

Convery et al's (2005) review is in stark contrast to the current clinical observation and practice. There are several important implications. If the effect of adaptation were real, then the current fitting methods should include considerations of such an effect in their formulation. That is, rather than just optimizing on a theoretical construct such as the maximum Speech Intelligibility Index (SII; ANSI, 1997) or speech recognition, one may need to include a new set of criteria that consider hearing aid experience and make corrections in the target gain/output recommendation. Suffice to say, using this criterion (or corrections) would affect how well the fitting meets the original criteria of maximum speech recognition. An ensuing question is, when can one increase the gain setting to match the original target? Also, will the wearer likely accept the new settings at that time after he or she has adapted to the current settings? This is a complex question that is important to consider.

Accounting for Hearing Aid Effect

Venting

The effects of vent diameter on hearing aid performance and wearer satisfaction have been well documented. From a physical standpoint, an increase in vent diameter increases the loss of low-frequency output of the hearing aid, reduces the occlusion effect, and limits the amount of usable gain on the hearing aid (Dillon, 2001). However, Kuk (1991) reported that when two hearing aid fittings were matched in insertion gain characteristics but differed in the use of a vent, subjects preferred the vented hearing aid over the unvented hearing aid. This observation raised several interesting questions.

First, should a vented fitting always be recommended over an unvented fitting? If so, what would be an optimal vent diameter for a specific degree and configuration of hearing loss? Such a consideration would involve understanding the trade-offs between a "relief" from the occlusion effect with venting and the "sacrifice" in audibility from increases in vent diameter. A second question is, should the gain/output target for a vented hearing aid be different from that for an unvented hearing aid? One may argue that the recommended gain/output is based on audibility considerations. Consequently, how one reaches the target is less important than that one indeed reaches the target (i.e., vented and unvented hearing aids should have the same target). In that case, a fitting method would recommend the same REAR, although the coupler response to reach the same REAR may be different between the vented and unvented hearing aid conditions.

A consequence of increasing the vent diameter is the limitation of the maximum available gain before feedback from the hearing aid. For example, Dillon (2001) reported that

the maximum available gain at 3000 Hz for a behind-the-ear hearing aid was 41 dB with an occluding earmold. That decreased to 23 dB when a tube fitting was attempted. In other words, the maximum aided gain from an open fitting will be limited to 23 dB. If the average ear canal resonance of an adult is ~15 to 20 dB at ~2700 to 3000 Hz, and if one were to use an insertion gain target (REAR–REUR), one may only receive a maximum of 3 to 8 dB of insertion gain at 3000 Hz regardless of the wearer's hearing loss at that frequency. One may conclude that an open fitting does not meet an insertion gain target at 3000 Hz. Despite this inability, wearers of open-fitting hearing aids report high satisfaction with their devices. Clearly, hearing aid wearers use a different criterion other than speech recognition ability in judging their hearing aid satisfaction. The prescribed target in such a case will need to be modified to reflect the potential change in criteria with venting (e.g., more comfort than speech recognition) as well as the gain limitation with venting (i.e., less available gain as vent diameter increases). That is, prescriptive targets may include vent effects in their recommendations. For example, a method that considers open fitting may alter its gain target such that the maximum recommended insertion gain does not need to exceed 10 to 15 dB (from previous discussions) to be considered acceptable. This will be a paradigm shift in how one considers an acceptable fitting.

Controversial Point

- The success of open fitting raises an important question: should one maximize comfort (as in minimizing occlusion effect but compromising speech intelligibility) or maximize speech intelligibility (as in minimizing vent diameter to prevent loss of gain) in a hearing aid fitting?

Attack and Release Times

A critical element on a nonlinear hearing aid is its attack and release times. Commercial nonlinear hearing aids vary greatly in their attack and release times depending on their design rationale. The impact of the difference in release time is that the static CR of the nonlinear hearing aid would be reduced. Ellison et al (2003) reported significant waveform change in the speech signals as they were processed by hearing aids fitted with generic fitting formulas like the NAL-NL1 and DSL [i/o] when release times of 40 and 640 msec were compared. The amplified dynamic range was less compressed (or wider) with the longer release time. To achieve the static I/O characteristics, very short attack and release times must be used. On the other hand, several perceptual studies showed that hearing-impaired listeners preferred a longer release time (seconds instead of fractions of a second) because it resulted in a more natural sound quality (e.g., Hansen, 2002).

Consequently, two hearing aids fitted with the same generic prescriptive target could likely lead to different perceptions if they differ in their attack and/or release times. A fitting target designed for nonlinear hearing aids with long attack and release times may not be as appropriate for use in hearing aids with short attack and release times. Unfortunately, it is not clear how a fitting method should adapt to different attack and release times used in commercial hearing aids. Would the increased loudness from the longer release time enhance sound quality while keeping the percept comfortably loud? If it is louder, should one decrease the output of a slow-acting WDRC hearing aid from the target for it to be equally loud as a fast-acting WDRC hearing aid? These and many others questions await more research for clarification.

Curvilinear Input-Output

Advances in modern digital technology have resulted in digital nonlinear hearing aids that are more sophisticated in their intensity processing than those with a traditional I/O curve with uniform characteristics. Today, many premier digital hearing aids have multisegment I/O curves that deviate from the recommended compression characteristics with conventional I/O characteristics. For example, it is not uncommon to find on the I/O curve a region of expansion below the CT, followed by several segments of compression processing each with its own CR and CT. The implication of this development is that it becomes more difficult to apply a generic prescription directly to a specific nonlinear hearing aid. A generic approach that has considered the diversity in real-world I/O characteristics may have a better chance of yielding a more satisfactory fitting than one that assumes uniform compression characteristics. Another view is that a given target or fitting method will need to be integrated into the manufacturer's fitting software to ensure appropriate performance of the specific hearing aids. This is seen in the higher incidence of generic formulas being integrated into a manufacturer's fitting software.

◆ Fitting Approaches

This section describes the common fitting methods that are used for linear and nonlinear hearing aids. From a historic perspective, fitting methods were originated for linear hearing aids first. As technology evolved, nonlinear versions of the fitting methods became available. A commonality of these methods is that they are prescriptive approaches requiring primarily the wearer's audiometric thresholds to begin the fitting process. Suprathreshold measures such as the individual's LDL and RECD are also accepted in some methods (e.g., DSL). In addition, these methods have included age-appropriate transfer functions and transducer corrections to increase the accuracy of the fitting.

Linear Hearing Aids

Desired Sensation Level: Linear Version

The DSL (Seewald et al, 1985) method is a prescriptive approach that is specifically earmarked for fitting linear amplification to infants and children. To use this method, the

child's hearing loss, his or her age, and the transducers used to measure thresholds are entered into the fitting software to generate the prescription. The goal of this method is to amplify conversational sounds so they are at a desirable intensity level above the child's in situ hearing thresholds (i.e., sensation level). In addition, a prediction of the maximum real ear saturation response (RESR) is available as a function of hearing loss and frequency.

The DSL fitting method has explicitly considered many physiological and behavioral differences between adults and children noted in the earlier sections. One major difference between the DSL and other fitting approaches is that it advocates an REAG target (difference between REAR and sound-field input) instead of real ear insertion gain (REIG) target to bypass the bias introduced by the adult ear canal resonance.

The DSL method requires using the eardrum as the reference during verification. Thus, the use of probe microphone measurement is highly recommended. To simplify fitting, the DSL advocates the use of RECD correction factors that convert a coupler output to the individual's real-ear output. This simplifies the fitting, selection, and verification in that one can adjust for the target coupler output given any REAG target or estimate the REAR given the coupler output of a hearing aid. When applied to the coupler OSPL90 setting, it can also predict the RESR of the hearing aid.

The characteristics of the speech spectrum used to calculate gain in the original DSL differed substantially from other prescriptions. This is because DSL placed high importance on the child's ability to monitor his or her own voice. Thus, the speech spectrum that was used in the DSL was a composite of the average speech levels recorded at a reference distance of 30 cm of adult male and female and children's speech (averaged) and the children's own speech production measured at the ear level of the children. This could have a significant implication in two ways. First, the recommended target frequency gain characteristic will be different from others that use a typical speech spectrum (Byrne et al, 1994). Second, during verification, one must use a signal with the same spectral characteristics; otherwise, one may risk not matching the target without further unnecessary adjustment. This could be especially important in verifying nonlinear multichannel hearing aids. In recent years, the DSL fitting software has included targets for other speech spectra.

NAL

The NAL fitting formula was first proposed in 1976 based on the empirical observations that the preferred gain at 1000 Hz equaled 0.46 times its thresholds. Gain at frequencies below and above 1000 Hz was computed by mirroring the long-term speech spectrum such that less gain was applied to frequencies that were more intense, and more gain was applied to frequencies that were less intense. The overall gain was then adjusted to the MCL level of the average wearer with the same degree of hearing loss.

Later, Byrne and Dillon (1986) revised the original NAL prescription to reflect the shape of the audiogram. Specifically, while gain still changed at 0.46 times the three-frequency (500, 1000, and 2000 Hz) average threshold, the shape of the frequency response curve was modified to be 0.31 times the shape of the audiogram. This is commonly known as the NAL-R formula.

The latest revision to the NAL-R formula was motivated by a change in the prescribed gain for individuals with a severe to profound loss. Specifically, for individuals with a three-frequency average greater than 60 dB HL, the required gain increased to 66% of the hearing loss instead of 46% of the hearing loss for the milder loss. In addition, less high-frequency amplification was prescribed. This is known as the NAL-RP formula (Byrne et al, 1991). Despite all the revisions, the goal of the NAL fitting formula is to amplify conversational speech so that all frequencies within the speech bands are equally loud (i.e., loudness equalization). The rationale is that maximum speech intelligibility results when all amplified frequencies are equally loud.

The NAL's recommendation on the OSPL90 settings is different from other fitting methods. Instead of setting the OSPL90 to be just below the LDL, the NAL-SSPL (saturation sound pressure level) procedure derived its recommendation by considering the saturation level of the hearing aid as well (Dillon, 2001). Thus, it first determined a minimum acceptable output level that is below the saturation limit of the hearing aid when loud speech (root-mean-square level of 75 dB SPL) is added to the gain of the hearing aid. This criterion minimizes the possibility of an OSPL90 setting that is too low, which could affect the amount of usable gain. The second factor NAL-SSPL considered was the predicted LDL of the wearer. The average of these two levels became the prescribed OSPL90 of the hearing aid for the wearer.

As with other linear prescriptive formulas, one may use either sinusoids or any broadband signals to verify if the gain target is achieved. Compensation for mixed or conductive losses is also considered by adding 25% of the air–bone gap to the prescribed gain for the sensorineural hearing loss. This formula has been used for both adults and children internationally.

Pearl

- There is no reason why a linear target cannot be applied to a single-channel nonlinear hearing aid for a conversational input level (65–70 dB SPL). It may require modification only when it is applied to a multichannel nonlinear hearing aid.

Cambridge

The Cambridge formula developed by Moore and Glasberg (1998) is based on their loudness model generated empirically from psychoacoustic research. There are one linear and two nonlinear versions of the fitting formula. This formula has not been specifically earmarked for pediatric use, although there is no reason why it can only be used with adults.

The linear version of the Cambridge formula aims to provide an amplified output that is equally loud across frequencies to a speech input (long-term spectrum defined by Byrne

et al, 1994) presented in the free field at 65 dB SPL with binaural listening. Audiometric thresholds are required, and REIG targets can be verified using any stimuli (sinusoids and broadband stimuli). The target REIG is calculated approximately at 0.48 times the degree of hearing loss and subtracting almost 10 dB below 500 Hz. No specific mention was made on the prescription of the OSPL90 setting.

Moore and Glasberg (1998) compared the calculated articulation index (AI) and loudness level (in sones) for speech at a 65 dB SPL input level fitted with the NAL-R, DSL, and Cambridge-linear formulas. For a mild-to-moderate sloping high-frequency hearing loss, the loudness pattern formed by the Cambridge formula was flat between 500 and 4000 Hz (i.e., equal loudness). Equal loudness was seen below 1600 Hz with the NAL. The modeled loudness resulting from the DSL was significantly higher than the Cambridge equation (42 sones vs 23 sones), especially between 3500 and 5300 Hz. For a moderately flat hearing loss, the Cambridge-linear formula provided the highest calculated AI and the most comfortable loudness when 1.2 dB was subtracted from the prescription. It prescribed a higher loudness level and a higher AI than NAL but a lower loudness level and a lower AI than DSL.

Pitfall

- Prescriptive formulas for linear hearing aids were designed for gain recommendation so that optimal perception of conversational speech may result. These formulas assume that the wearers will use the volume control under the right listening condition. Unfortunately, this assumption is not always followed by adults and is almost unrealistic for infants and young children.

Nonlinear Hearing Aids

The following description is intended for nonlinear WDRC hearing aids. Although the earlier approaches such as the LGOB aimed at restoring "normal loudness perception" in the hearing-impaired ear (i.e., normalization philosophy), the more recent ones such as the NAL-NL1 and Cambridge formula are designed with the "equalization" principle.

Loudness Growth by Octave Band

The LGOB method was proposed by Allen et al (1990) to compare the loudness growth functions (LGFs) of the hearing-impaired person to patients with normal hearing to determine the optimal compression characteristics for a WDRC hearing aid. In this method, one-half octave bands of noise centered at octave intervals from 500 to 4000 Hz are presented randomly through calibrated insert earphones. The subject responds to the loudness of these stimuli by pressing the appropriate buttons on a pad, which are labeled "too loud," "very loud," "loud," "comfortable," "soft," "very soft," and "did not hear." An LGF is formed when one plots the loudness category on the y-axis and the SPL (re calibrated 2 cc coupler) required for that loudness category on the x-axis

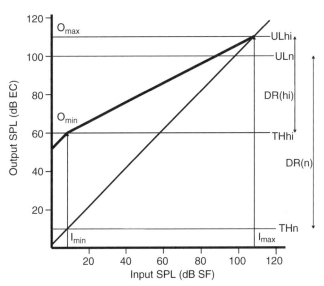

Figure 7–9 Hypothetical I/O function for a 60 dB hearing level (HL) using the desired sensation level input/output (DSL [i/o]) formula. EC, ear canal, compression threshold; SF, sound field-to-eardrum transforms. (From Cornelisse, L. E., Seewald, R. C., & Jamieson, D. G. (1995). The input/ output formula: A theoretical approach to the fitting of personal amplification devices. Journal of the Acoustical Society of America, 97, 1854–1864, with permission.)

(see **Fig. 7–2**). The manner in which the desirable insertion gain is estimated or how the CR is determined has been described in the previous section.

DSL [i/o]

The nonlinear version of the DSL formula, the DSL [i/o], is an extension of the original DSL formula for nonlinear hearing aids (Cornelisse et al, 1995) based on theoretical considerations. It has all the critical ingredients of the DSL-linear approach described previously. The difference between the linear and the nonlinear versions is that gain recommendations are made at several input levels in the nonlinear version.

The theoretical concept behind the DSL [i/o] can be best illustrated in **Fig. 7–9**. This figure shows all the necessary indices in formulating the recommended compression settings with a hypothetical hearing loss of 60 dB SPL (measured at the eardrum) at 1000 Hz. Other than the obvious inclusion of the wearer's threshold and measured LDL information, this I/O curve is similar to the typical I/O curves of WDRC hearing aids with a linear region below the CT, a compression region, and a limiting region that is bounded by the upper limit of comfort of the listener.

Pearl

• The derivation of the DSL [i/o] formula appears complex and confusing. This is because of the introduction of the sound field-to-eardrum transforms (SF). To simplify its appearance, pretend that SF does not exist (i.e., set the SF$_t$ to 0), and the equations will appear more straightforward.

The DSL [i/o] recommends a theoretical CT at 0 dB HL and a CR equal to the ratio of the DR of a normal-hearing person to the DR of a hearing-impaired person. In this example, the hearing-impaired person's DR is the difference between threshold (Th$_{hi}$, e.g., 60 dB) and the upper limit of comfort (UL$_{hi}$, e.g., 110 dB) or a DR of 50 dB. The DR of a normal-hearing listener should be the same as the aided DR of the wearer. In this case, the softest level that any wearer (normal or hearing impaired) should hear will be I$_{min}$ (10 dB). The maximum input level for discomfort should still be 110 dB SPL. Thus, the aided DR of the wearer should be similar to that of a normal-hearing listener, or 100 dB. A CR of 2:1 can thus be calculated. Despite the simplicity in the DSL [i/o] formulation, Cornelisse et al (1995) indicated that the target defined by the DSL [i/o] for conversational speech is similar to that recommended by the original DSL (linear) formula.

The DSL fitting method has been widely used for fitting hearing aids, both linear and nonlinear, to children with good success. Scollie et al (2000) compared the preferred listening levels (PLLs) of children fit with the DSL target to targets recommended by the NAL-RP and NAL-NL1. The authors reported that the PLLs were similar to the DSL targets, and that the NAL-RP and NAL-NL1 targets prescribed less gain than PLLs.

The DSL fitting method has been refined and improved over the years. In addition to its unique emphasis on pediatric fitting, the most recent version of the DSL [i/o] fitting software, version 5.0 (Scollie et al, 2005), has updated the following features:

1. RECD predictions that include normative data for using foam tips and earmolds obtained in 1-month intervals. This increases the accuracy of the prediction when individual RECDs cannot be obtained.

2. Tone-evoked auditory brainstem response (ABR) thresholds are reported in normalized hearing level (nHL) and are transformed into dB SPL by adding the appropriate RECD and reference equivalent threshold SPLs for inserts (RETSPLs) for ABR measurement. This permits the use of electrophysiological thresholds to estimate optimal gain settings on hearing aids.

3. Conductive hearing losses are compensated by increasing the output level (O$_{max}$) by 25%. This results in an I/O curve that is more linear than the nonconductive hearing loss.

4. In contrast to the original uniform I/O curve shown in **Fig. 7–9,** the revised desired sensation level multistage input/output (DSL m[i/o]) algorithm considers more complex I/O curves (i.e., multistage I/O) by providing thresholds for regions of expansion, linear, WDRC, and compression-limiting functions.

5. Targets for a wider range of stimuli are provided, including different speech spectra, speech at different vocal efforts, and broadband and narrowband signals. This is desirable because by adjusting the target values accordingly for different stimuli, one is ensured a more accurate interpretation during hearing aid verification. Considerations for the effect of vent diameter and mode of amplification (binaural vs monaural) are also included.

6. An alternative gain/output target for listening in noise is included by modifying the original DSL targets with the frequency-importance weightings used in the speech intelligibility index (SII).

7. The DSL target is modified to be age dependent so younger children receive a higher sensation level than older children and adults. Thus, the I/O curve for adults will have a higher CT and a lower CR than children (i.e., less gain for soft to loud sounds).

NAL-NL1

The NAL-NL1 target is derived by examining how much amplification is needed to amplify the long-term speech spectrum (Byrne et al, 1994, similar to ANSI-92 speech-shaped noise) to maximize the SII (ANSI, 1997) for a particular hearing loss. The SII is a mathematical model that predicts speech intelligibility based on the amount of audible information (signal above the masked or unmasked thresholds) at each frequency channel and the speech importance of each channel. The sum of these products (importance by audibility) across channels provides an estimate of speech intelligibility.

In addition to maximizing the SII, the NAL-NL1 method included a second criterion in that the loudness of the amplified speech should not be louder than that perceived by someone with normal hearing. This was calculated using Moore and Glasberg's loudness model (Moore and Glasberg, 1998), which has accounted for the difference in loudness perception between normal-hearing and hearing-impaired listeners. If a lower loudness level results in a higher SII, gain on the hearing aid will be reduced to achieve the higher SII. Thus, the NAL-NL1 method does not attempt to maximize audibility for soft sounds; rather, it attempts to maximize speech recognition.

Another unique consideration taken by NAL-NL1 is its management of "dead" regions. Ching et al's data (1998) reported decreases in speech recognition with increasing input levels and increasing hearing loss (i.e., hearing loss desensitization). A correction factor is entered into the SII model to reduce the prescribed gain for a precipitously sloping hearing loss. Thus, the prescribed frequency response would result in less high-frequency emphasis than a fitting method that does not consider hearing loss desensitization and/or level distortion. Despite the different approach taken by NAL-NL1 in its formulation, Byrne et al (2001) reported that the NAL-NL1 recommendation for an average speech level (65–70 dB SPL) closely agrees with the NAL-RP prescription (i.e., equal loudness). The final NAL-NL1 prescription averages the differences between the two prescriptions (NAL-RP and NAL-NL1) as the final gain recommendation for conversational input levels. This method provides less amplification of the low-frequency region than other formulas that "normalize" loudness. Consequently, tasks that maximize listening comfort and those that depend on the availability of low-frequency amplification, such as localization, detection, and sound quality judgment, may not be optimized using NAL-NL1.

The NAL-NL1 also prescribes CT and CR based on the hearing loss of the wearer. The default CT is set so that soft speech at 52 dB SPL will activate the compression circuit (the channel-specific CT will be lower in a multichannel device). The CR is calculated from the I/O curve above the CT based on the ratio of input change to output change. In addition, the NAL-NL1 formula allows for channel summation correction (up to four channels) when pure tones are used for verification of hearing aid output. Finally, the NAL-NL1 formula assumes binaural fittings (i.e., lower gain is prescribed than for a monaural fitting).

Byrne et al (2001) compared the insertion gain recommended by the NAL-NL1 formula to those by the NAL-RP and DSL [i/o] for different configurations and degrees of hearing loss. For a flat 60 dB HL, the authors found that the NAL-NL1 formula offered significantly less low-frequency gain than DSL [i/o]. For a reverse slope audiogram, the DSL [i/o] formula recommended more low-frequency gain than the NAL formulas. For a moderately sloping hearing loss, both formulas prescribed similar gain in the midfrequencies, but DSL [i/o] prescribed more low-frequency gain than the NAL-NL1 formula. DSL [i/o] also prescribed more gain above 4000 Hz than the NAL-NL1. For a precipitously sloping hearing loss, the NAL-NL1 formula prescribed similar gain as DSL [i/o] along the slope of the audiogram, but much less gain in the higher frequencies (> 2500 Hz) than DSL [i/o].

The noted differences may be due to two factors. First, NAL-NL1 is based on maximizing speech intelligibility while ensuring "normal" loudness perception. To that end, the prescription in the low frequencies for a moderate loss is much less than at other frequencies because of their relative input level as well as their contribution to speech recognition. Another distinctive feature of the NAL-NL1 is that it does not prescribe significant amounts of gain at the most extreme frequencies, especially in the high frequencies, because of potential hearing loss desensitization. That is why it prescribes less gain in the low frequency for a flat loss and less gain in the high frequency for a sloping loss than DSL [i/o].

The second reason for the difference is the slope rule used by NAL-NL1 and DSL [i/o]. Many of the linear formulas use a half-gain to two-thirds-gain rule, whereas NAL-NL1 (as well as the NAL-R) uses a one-third-gain rule. The reason is that the effects of hearing loss desensitization and level distortion were included in the NAL-NL1 formula but not in the DSL [i/o].

At the time of this writing, NAL is planning to introduce a revised version of its nonlinear fitting software. The new software, NAL-NL2, has additional considerations in the following areas (Dillon, 2003). First, the extent to which hearing loss desensitization contributes to speech recognition will be updated. The gain targets for frequency regions that are "dead" will not be amplified to the same extent as regions with the same degree of hearing loss that are not "dead." This would require clinicians to enter suprathreshold information (tuning curve, results on the TEN test, etc.) that would indicate the survival status of the remaining inner hair cells. The gain targets will automatically be modified to accommodate the individual differences in psychophysical abilities. Furthermore, an improved optimization procedure is used to ensure sufficient gain for the "dead" regions so they can maximize their use of the available audible information.

Second, the target gain is less than the NAL-NL1 target. This is because the authors observed that the preferred loudness by hearing-impaired (and normal-hearing) individuals is less than normal loudness (which is what NAL-NL1 attempted to achieve). Third, an independent gain target for children is available to account for the observation that some children preferred higher than NAL-NL1 prescribed gain. The impetus for that consideration originated from the cooperative study between the NAL and the University of Western Ontario that compared the efficacy of the NAL-NL1 and DSL [i/o] prescriptive targets in children (Dillon, 2002/2003). Their results showed that Australian children in the study preferred each target almost equally, whereas Canadian children in the study preferred the DSL [i/o] prescribed gain (which tended to be higher than the NAL-NL1 prescribed gain). This conflicted with the persistent findings that adults typically prefer even less gain than the NAL-NL1 target. Finally, the effect of acclimatization and the choice for a lower CT were made available in the new prescription.

Cambridge: CAMEQ and CAMREST

There are two nonlinear fitting options that can be selected from the Cambridge formula: CAMEQ and CAMREST. The CAMEQ is designed to achieve equal loudness of speech (equalization) presented in a free-field level at 65 dB SPL (i.e., the same for linear hearing aids) and audibility of soft speech presented in the free-field at 45 dB SPL. The special emphasis placed on the audibility for soft speech distinguishes this procedure from its linear version and from NAL formulas (NAL-RP and NAL-NL1). A key consideration for this formula is its correction for the difference in frequency tuning between normal and hearing-impaired individuals by assuming auditory information is integrated over a 2 ERB (equivalent rectangular bandwidth) instead of the normal 1 ERB. This formula is appropriate only for hearing loss to 80 dB HL. Similar to the DSL method, this approach advocates the use of real-ear measurements and reports gain as REAG as well as REIG with sinusoids. Adjustment to the target gain from multichannel processing will be automatic once the number of channels and crossover frequencies on the nonlinear hearing aid are specified.

The CAMEQ calculates the CR as the ratio of the input change to the output change from an overall level of soft speech (45 dB SPL) to normal speech (65 dB SPL) at each channel. If the calculated CR is > 3, it is automatically set to 2.92. The calculated CT is the lowest input level at which gain reduction occurs (from linear). To avoid "overamplification" of the microphone noise level, the calculated CT below 15 dB SPL is set to 15 dB SPL. To facilitate fitting with sinusoids, the authors provide REIG targets for sinusoidal inputs at free-field levels of 50, 65, and 80 dB SPL.

Both the NAL-NL1 formula and the Cambridge formula are based on the loudness model of Moore and Glasberg (1998). The Cambridge formula has a goal to equalize loudness, which will maximize the AI. The NAL-NL1 aims to maximize the SII, which tends to equalize loudness. Because of the inclusion of the level distortion factor and hearing loss desensitization factor in the NAL-NL1 formula, a one-third slope rule is seen in NAL-NL1, whereas a one-

half slope rule is used in the Cambridge formula. Thus, the CAMEQ will prescribe more gain in the high frequencies than NAL-NL1.

The CAMREST procedure determines the gain needed to restore normal loudness perception for speechlike stimuli over a wide range of input levels. The REIG recommended by this procedure is derived by considering the gain level needed for a speech-shaped noise (same spectrum as Byrne et al, 1994) at overall levels of 65 and 85 dB SPL (normal and shouted speech, respectively) to be equally loud to normal-hearing listeners. Both the CAMEQ and CAMREST formulas allow clinicians to specify the number of channels (up to 20) and crossover frequencies so gain correction for loudness summation can be applied if pure-tone signals are used for verification and gain measurement.

With the CAMREST targets, it was shown that the loudness patterns calculated for the 65 and 85 dB SPL speech noise were similar between a normal-hearing listener and hearing-impaired listeners with a flat 50 and 70 dB HL, a sloping loss, and a reverse slope audiogram. When the REIG recommended by the CAMREST was compared with the CAMEQ recommendations with several hearing loss configurations (flat, sloping, and reverse slope) at 50, 65, and 80 dB SPL sinusoidal inputs on a five-channel system, both systems recommended similar insertion gain for the 80 dB SPL input level. However, at lower input levels (50 and 65 dB SPL), CAMREST prescribed less gain than CAMEQ for frequencies above 1000 Hz and more gain than CAMEQ in the lower frequencies.

Marriage et al (2004) compared the CAMEQ and CAMREST with DSL [i/o] using a commercial 14-channel fast-acting compression hearing aid on 20 experienced and inexperienced subjects with a mild to moderately severe sloping hearing loss. The gain prescribed by the CAMEQ and CAMREST was significantly lower than that prescribed by the DSL [i/o] formula, especially in the high frequencies. Also, the amount of adjustment made after the initial fitting with the CAMEQ and CAMREST formulas was less than the DSL [i/o] formula for real-world use. Performance on the subjective questionnaire was not significantly different among the three formulas after fine-tuning adjustment. The authors concluded that the Cambridge formulas were effective for the initial setting of a compression hearing aid with as many as 20 channels.

◆ Summary

It is not surprising to note differences in the prescribed frequency gain characteristics of nonlinear hearing aids from different prescriptive targets. These differences arose as a consequence of the reported differences in the rationale behind these approaches (e.g., loudness normalization vs loudness equalization), the use of different speech spectra (e.g., DSL's speech spectrum vs NAL's speech spectrum), or additional assumptions or constraints placed on the fitting formula (e.g., NAL vs Cambridge view of the importance of soft sounds).

One may summarize the comparison studies this way. When the comparisons were made among fitting formulas that advocate a loudness normalization approach (LGOB, DSL, and DSL [i/o]) to those that advocate a loudness equalization approach (NAL-RP, NAL-NL1, CAMEQ, and Cambridge-linear), those advocating a normalization principle tend to recommend higher overall loudness (and gain) as well as a broader frequency response (i.e., more gain in the high frequency and in the low frequency) than those with an equalization principle. There could be several implications. First, for a first-time adult hearing aid wearer, it is more likely that he or she will prefer less than the recommended gain if one starts with a formula that advocates normalization. A possible exception is that the target is modified by device-specific factors or corrected for acclimatization. Second, for a pediatric fitting, the child will likely receive higher gain if the fitting formula advocates normalization than equalization. Third, regardless of the philosophy or subjective preference, there are no validation studies to document a significant difference in speech recognition scores between hearing aids fitted with normalization and equalization principles.

When the comparison was made between the linear version and the nonlinear version of a particular fitting, such as NAL-RP with NAL-NL1, DSL with DSL [i/o], and Cambridge-linear with CAMEQ/CAMREST, the authors reported that the resulting settings recommended by the linear version of the fitting approach were similar to those recommended by the nonlinear approach for conversational input levels. This is reasonable because the difference in recommendations between a linear and a nonlinear fitting should not be at the conversational level, but rather at input levels that are lower and higher than the conversational level. This is also encouraging because many of these approaches have extensive validation studies for the linear version, whereas the nonlinear version has only become popular in the last few years.

Which prescriptive formula (or approach) should one use to fit a nonlinear hearing aid? Hopefully, it is clear to the readers that none of the formulas have considered all the variables for every hearing-impaired person. Every formula emphasizes what it feels to be the most important for the wearer—normal loudness, maximum intelligibility (at normal level of all input levels), comfortable hearing, perception of other sounds, and so on. It is thus important that clinicians fully understand the considerations made by each approach and adopt those that agree with their own philosophy and patient needs. Regardless of the approach, it is important to recognize that the recommendation is only the first step in the hearing aid fitting process. Additional follow-up and fine-tuning will be necessary to ensure wearer satisfaction and benefit.

References

Allen, J. B., Hall, J. L., & Jeng, P. (1990). Loudness growth in 1/2 octave bands (LGOB): A procedure for the assessment of loudness. Journal of the Acoustical Society of America, 88, 745–753.

American National Standards Institute. (1997). Methods for the calculation of the Speech Intelligibility Index (ANSI S3.5–1997). New York: Author.

Barker, C., & Dillon, H. (1999). Client preferences for compression threshold in single-channel wide dynamic range compression hearing aids. Ear and Hearing, 20, 127–139.

Byrne, D. (1996). Hearing aid selection for the 1990s: Where to? Journal of the American Academy of Audiology, 7, 377–395.

Byrne, D., & Dillon, H. (1986). The National Acoustic Laboratories' (NAL) new procedure for selecting the gain and frequency response of a hearing aid. Ear and Hearing, 7, 257–265.

Byrne, D., Dillon, H., Ching, T., Katsch, R., & Keidser, G. (2001). NAL-NL1 procedure for fitting nonlinear hearing aids: Characteristics and comparisons with other procedures. Journal of the American Academy of Audiology, 12, 37–51.

Byrne, D., Dillon, H., Tran, K., et al. (1994). An international comparison of long-term average speech spectra. Journal of the Acoustical Society of America, 96, 2108–2120.

Byrne, D., Parkinson, A., & Newall, P. (1991). Modified hearing aid selection procedures for severe/profound hearing losses. In G. Studebaker, F. Bess, & L. Beck (Eds.), The Vanderbilt Hearing Aid Report II (pp. 295–300). Parkton, MD: York Press.

Ching, T. Y., Dillon, H., & Byrne, D. (1998). Speech recognition of hearing-impaired listeners: Predictions from audibility and the limited role of high-frequency amplification. Journal of the Acoustical Society of America, 103, 1128–1140.

Convery, E., Keidser, G., & Dillon, H. (2005). A review and analysis: Does amplification experience have an effect on preferred gain over time? Australian and New Zealand Journal of Audiology, 27, 18–32.

Cornelisse, L. E., Seewald, R. C., & Jamieson, D. G. (1995). The input/output formula: A theoretical approach to the fitting of personal amplification devices. Journal of the Acoustical Society of America, 97, 1854–1864.

Dillon, H. (1996). Compression? Yes, but for low or high frequencies, for low or high intensities, and with what response times? Ear and Hearing, 17, 287–307.

Dillon, H. (2001). Hearing Aids. New York: Thieme Medical Publishers.

Dillon, H. (2002/2003). Basis of NAL-NL2. National Acoustic Laboratories Research and Development Annual Report, 48–49.

Dreschler, W. A., Verschuure, H., Ludvigsen, C., & Westermann, S. (2001). ICRA noises: Artificial noise signals with speech-like spectral and temporal properties for hearing instrument assessment. International Collegium for Rehabilitative Audiology. Audiology, 40(3), 148–157.

Ellison, J. C., Harris, F. P., & Muller, T. (2003). Interactions of hearing aid compression release time and fitting formula: Effects on speech acoustics. Journal of the American Academy of Audiology, 14, 59–71.

Hansen, M. (2002). Effects of multi-channel compression time constants on subjectively perceived sound quality and speech intelligibility. Ear and Hearing, 23, 369–380.

Hawkins, D. B., & Naidoo, S. (1993). Comparison of sound quality and clarity with asymmetrical peak clipping and output limiting compression. Journal of the American Academy of Audiology, 4, 221–228.

Killion, M. C., Staab, W. J., & Preves, D. A. (1990). Classifying automatic signal processors. Hearing Instruments, 41(8), 24–26.

Kuk, F. K. (1991). Perceptual consequences of venting in hearing aids. British Journal of Audiology, 25, 163–169.

Kuk, F. K. (1998). Rationale and requirements for a slow acting compression hearing aid. Hearing Journal, 51(6), 41–53.

Kuk, F. (1999). Optimizing compression: The advantages of a low compression threshold. Hearing Review Supplement (High Performance Hearing Solutions III: Marketing and Technology), 44–47.

Kuk, F. K., Potts, L., Valente, M., Lee, L., & Picirrili, J. (2003). Evidence of acclimatization in persons with severe-to-profound hearing loss. Journal of the American Academy of Audiology, 14(2), 84–99.

Mackersie, C. L., Crocker, T. L., & Davis, R. A. (2004). Limiting high-frequency hearing aid gain in listeners with and without suspected cochlear dead regions. Journal of the American Academy of Audiology, 15, 498–507.

Marriage, J., Moore, B., & Alcantara, J. (2004). Comparison of three procedures for initial fitting of compression hearing aids: 3. Inexperienced versus experienced users. International Journal of Audiology, 43, 198–210.

Moodie, K. S., Seewald, R. C., & Sinclair, S. T. (1994). Procedure for predicting real-ear hearing instrument performance in young children. American Journal of Audiology, 3, 23–31.

Moore, B. C. (2001). Dead regions in the cochlea: Diagnosis, perceptual consequences, and implications for the fitting of hearing aids. Trends in Amplification, 5, 1–34.

Moore, B. C., & Glasberg, B. R. (1998). Use of a loudness model for hearing-aid fitting: 1. Linear hearing aids. British Journal of Audiology, 32, 317–335.

Nozza, R. J., Rossman, R. N., & Bond, L. C. (1991). Infant-adult differences in unmasked thresholds for the discrimination of consonant-vowel syllable pairs. Audiology, 30, 102–112.

Pascoe, D. P. (1988). Clinical measurements of the auditory dynamic range and their relation to formulas for hearing aid gain in presbyacousis and other age related aspects. In J. H. Jensen (Ed.), Proceedings of the 13th Danavox Symposium (pp. 129–147). Copenhagen.

Scollie, S. D., Seewald, R. C., Moodie, K. S., & Dekok, K. (2000). Preferred listening levels of children who use hearing aids: Comparison to prescriptive targets. Journal of the American Academy of Audiology, 11, 230–238.

Scollie, S., Seewald, R., Sinclair-Moodie, S., Cornelisse, L., Bagatto, M., & Beaulac, S. (2005). The desired sensation level (DSL) method in 2004: DSL m[i/o] version 5.0.

Seewald, R. C., Ross, M., & Spiro, M. (1985). Selecting amplification characteristics for young hearing-impaired children. Ear and Hearing, 6, 48–53.

Souza, P. E. (2002). Effects of compression on speech acoustics, intelligibility, and sound quality. Trends in Amplification, 6(4), 131–165.

Strom, K. E. (2005). The HR 2005 dispenser survey. Hearing Review, 12(6), 18–36.

Chapter 8

Counseling for Diagnosis and Management of Auditory Disorders

Kristina M. English

Give sorrow words: the grief that does not speak
Whispers the o'er-fraught heart, and bids it break.

(*Macbeth*, Act 4, Scene 3)

In this scene from *Macbeth*, a nobleman has just been informed that his wife and children had been killed. A prince advises him to verbalize his reactions, to put his grief into words. Notice he does not say that the sorrow will "break the heart," but that the unexpressed grief will. Shakespeare knew 400 years ago that grief is manageable, but those who experience it need others to listen while they express that grief.

On a daily basis, audiologists work with patients who carry different kinds of grief. Sometimes patients do "give sorrow words" by telling us directly, "I am so frustrated" or "This hearing problem is a miserable thing." Sometimes their expressions of grief are indirect and may not be well understood even by the patients themselves. Whether clearly expressed or not, patients are expecting audiologists not only to understand the problems of living with hearing loss but also to care about and provide support for those problems. This may sound like an odd statement, because, of course, audiologists care; it's why they chose this profession. But as Glass and Elliot (1992) indicate, when our communication focuses only on information, patients leave the appointment feeling "that's not enough." This chapter will consider how our counseling efforts also need to provide the psychological and emotional support our patients are seeking.

◆ Two Types of Audiologic Counseling

Audiologic counseling is a term that covers two types of counseling. One is informational counseling, in which the audiologist answers questions and describes test results, anatomy, amplification use, communication repair strategies, and so on. Informational counseling is teaching and is a skill that requires practice and feedback (Margolis, 2004). Patients typically understand only 50% of what a health care provider says and accurately remember only 50% of that content. That represents a 75% communication failure rate.

Developing effective informational counseling skills has yet to be addressed in the audiologic literature. This chapter will focus on the second type of audiologic counseling, termed *personal adjustment counseling*. As the name suggests, this type of counseling is used to help patients express, understand, and accept their emotional and psychological reactions to their hearing loss.

Personal adjustment counseling has three components: (1) understanding the effects of hearing loss on our patients' lives, (2) listening carefully to patients as they attempt to describe those effects, and (3) responding carefully and appropriately in ways that convey empathy, hope, and trust in the individual patient's ability to handle the problem. These components are ordered not only chronologically during the development of the audiologist–patient relationship but also in terms of difficulty.

The easiest of the three components of personal adjustment counseling is understanding, or "knowing about" how hearing loss affects patients' lives. Reading this chapter, the references cited within, and other materials will provide some of that information. The second component, listening carefully, or hearing what patients really mean when they speak to us, is one of the great challenges of being human. Bookshelves overflow with advice on this topic, indicating the continual need to improve our listening skills.

But when we do improve our ability to "listen between the lines," what do we say in reply? This third component of audiologic counseling is the most difficult: if we are not careful, we are likely to provide solutions and "fix" the problems but not provide patients with the opportunity to "own" both the problems and the solutions. What can we say to let patients know we are heeding them carefully, and also help patients accept and transcend the problems?

The last component reflects an approach found in other rehabilitative and health care fields. Although the professional can provide information and recommendations, the patient is the one who "owns" the problem. Only the patient can do the "ditch-digging hard work" (Kennedy and Charles, 2001, p. 379) of accepting the diagnosis, following the recommendations, and committing to that decision over time. In other health care fields, professionals are reminded to ask themselves, Who owns the problem? In audiology, we must ask ourselves, Who owns the hearing loss? This question keeps us patient-centered, a concept that will be described in more depth in a subsequent section.

The second and third components of audiologic counseling, then, take audiologists beyond "knowing about" patients' reactions to hearing loss, to "knowing how" to counsel. All three components will be used as headings for this chapter—but first, a caveat.

Counseling Is an Integrated Skill

If it were possible to ask the reader to identify the influential people in his or her life, there would be no shortage of names. The reader will have had parents, other family members, teachers, coaches, scout leaders, and others who provided care and support during childhood and the adult years. When considering the characteristics of these supporters, it becomes apparent that they do not somehow "add" care to their interactions; rather, care has been fully integrated into these interactions.

Why make this rather obvious point? Because there is a risk that audiologic counseling will be perceived as yet another skill readers must add to their repertoire ("First, I will learn how to test patients, then how to provide a range of treatments, then—eventually—how to be an effective counselor"). Additionally, they may begin to wonder how to "add" counseling to appointments, when there is already precious little time for testing and treatment.

This chapter will encourage readers to think about how to integrate, not add on, audiologic counseling into patient care. As audiologists greet new patients or welcome returning ones, as we listen to their experiences, as we convey test results, as we make recommendations, do we actively attend and respond to patients' psychological and emotional reactions to hearing loss? Or do these interactions resemble business transactions?

And does it matter? Research indicates it does. Health problems are personal, and a business-type or other impersonal approach is not compatible with patient expectations. The medical literature provides very compelling data indicating that when practitioners attentively listen to their patients' stories, actively acknowledge their emotional and psychological state, and respect their abilities to handle their problems (fundamental counseling strategies), patients are more likely to adhere to their recommendations. For example, Golin and colleagues (1996) found that when physicians employed these counseling strategies, patients were far more likely to adhere to the recommendations made for diabetes management. Stewart and colleagues (1999) reported similar results with cancer patients. In fact, dozens of studies have associated higher levels of patient adherence with the clinician's counseling skills. (See Stewart et al, 2003, for a meta-analysis of these studies.)

Providing Patient-Centered Care

The studies mentioned above were conducted because it was apparent that the traditional clinical method did not result in the kind of patient adherence that practitioners were hoping for. The clinical method, which bases treatment on observation and data collection, sees disease as an entity located in the body, unrelated to the sick person. By definition, this model of care does not address the human aspects of disease or disability: emotional reactions, life events, relationships, or environmental challenges. Not surprisingly, patients have not been satisfied with this approach.

In 1964, Balint described an alternative to the clinical method, which he termed "patient-centered." He proposed that two perspectives should be considered: not only does the clinician interpret the health problem in terms of symptoms, but the patient also has a perspective in terms of experience (i.e., what it is like to live with the health problem). Exchanging perceptions should result in the development of mutual understanding, of common ground. In the patient-centered model, clinicians are not detached observers and dispassionate dispensers of information and treatment. Being patient-centered means attending carefully to "problems of living" and providing help to reduce those problems. The patient-centered approach views patients not as machines with broken parts but rather as organisms who can grow, heal, learn, and transcend problems.

In the counseling field, Rogers (1961) had already adopted this approach. A review of other counseling approaches is provided by Clark and English (2004), including behaviorism, which emphasizes positive and negative reinforcement (Skinner, 1953). In contrast, the rational emotive behavioral approach (Ellis, 1996) strives to change patients' thinking about a problem, to change how they feel and act about the problem. The reader is encouraged to become familiar with as many approaches as possible. As "nonprofessional counselors" (Kennedy and Charles, 2001), audiologists are usually most comfortable with the patient-centered approach.

Pearl

- Patient-centered care requires the audiologist to use test results and patients' self-defined goals to address the problems of living with hearing loss.

Most of us, as students, entered the profession of audiology with the desire to help others, but it would be naive to assume that patients will passively accept our help and obey our recommendations. Patients resist hearing help for a variety of reasons. We will now examine these reasons, then consider how audiologists can help patients help themselves.

◆ Understanding the Effects of Hearing Loss on Patients' Lives

When the audiologist confirms to an adult patient that he or she does indeed have a hearing loss as suspected, the audiologist has dealt that patient a "verbal blow" (Martin, 1994). Even when expecting this diagnosis, the patient's self-concept is now being challenged ("I have always been a person with good hearing, and now I am not"). This challenge should not be overlooked, because it likely accounts for many patients' reactions to the diagnosis and their reluctance to seek hearing help. The next section will describe how individuals develop and maintain their self-concepts,

and how acquiring hearing loss can affect patients' sense of well-being.

What Is Self-Concept?

Self-concept is defined as the way one describes oneself: perceptions of one's traits, attitudes, abilities, and social natures. (The term *self-esteem* is often used as a synonym, but that more accurately means the value, positive or negative, one puts on these traits, abilities, etc.).

Developmental psychologists have determined that self-concept is learned from infancy, and only as a result of social interactions with significant others. Caregivers' attitudes and verbal messages toward infants convey a child's value by the amount of acceptance and concern provided. Children gradually internalize the attitudes and messages given by significant others and accept these messages as valid appraisals of self. In other words, "I see myself the way you tell me you see me" (English, 2002, p. 18).

An individual's self-concept is not immutable. During childhood, adolescence, and many times in adulthood, each person is challenged with the decision to accept those early inputs or reject them. One's self-concept is altered not only by the acceptance/rejection of earlier input from significant others but also by the events of one's life. The onset of hearing loss is one such event that may significantly alter one's self-concept. Changing our perception of "who we are" may be one of the hardest challenges faced in life. Shames (2000) reminds us that "[l]etting go of who we are or the way we were can be fraught with both fears and pain: pain over the past and fears about the future" (p. 14). Although there are inherent difficulties in changing one's self-concept, at the same time we all have resources to manage these changes. The process of modifying one's self-concept will be unique to each individual.

Hearing Loss, Hearing Aids, and Self-Concept

The diagnosis of hearing impairment is just the first attack on a patient's self-concept. An audiologist's best recommendation to improve the hearing problem involves visible prosthetic devices. For many patients, the prospect of changing their body image with hearing aids is more than they can accept. Hearing aids have a long-observed social stigma, first described as "the hearing aid effect" by Blood et al (1977). These researchers found that when they showed images of individuals with and without hearing aids, persons with hearing aids were rated significantly lower in the areas of intelligence, achievement, personality, and appearance.

Patients frequently worry about being the subject of these negative impressions. Doggett et al (1998) showed that these worries may actually affect how one projects oneself to others. Women in this study who wore hearing aids were perceived to be significantly less confident, friendly, and intelligent than women without hearing aids; however, the raters did not report even noticing any hearing aids. Because the raters did not make a direct association between hearing aids and personal attributes, the researchers concluded that the negative ratings likely originated from the self-images projected by the hearing aid users.

Many patients take challenges and change in stride and have a history of coping effectively with adversity. In other words, they approach problems rather than avoid them. However, when working with patients who find the adjustment to the changes in their hearing a challenge, audiologists should not be surprised and should be ready to help patients through these reactions.

Loss and Grief

This chapter opened with a quote about responding to grief, a concept that may seem overstated when applied to hearing loss. Tanner (1980), however, points out that any loss in one's life stimulates a grief response to some degree, and hearing loss is not exempt. Following is a summary of Tanner's discussion of the classic "grief cycle" as first presented by Kübler-Ross (1969), integrated with Smart's (2001) inclusion of shock as the first stage.

Shock

In this stage, the individual feels overwhelmed and confused because of the unexpectedness of the event. For a short time, it is difficult to think or feel anything. Even adults with gradually acquired hearing loss report experiencing a sense of shock upon diagnosis. Whether because it "officially" defines the situation, or it describes a loss worse than they anticipated, or it is not treatable as they had hoped, the shock is still real, and the inability to make immediate decisions can explain initial patient behaviors. Feelings associated with shock are bewilderment, panic, and uncertainty.

Denial

After the initial shock has worn off, individuals are quite likely to deny the event even occurred ("Your tests have got to be wrong; I hear fine most of the time"). Audiologists often perceive denial as worrisome, but this reaction is a vitally necessary buffer or defensive mechanism. Denial allows patients to maintain their self-identity temporarily, protects them from overwhelming pain and confusion, and gives them time to assimilate the implications of the situation. It is an effort to hold on to the preferred past. Individuals will often "stay in denial" longer when they are feeling rushed, threatened, coerced, or belittled. Feelings associated with the stage of denial include alienation, tension, impatience, and frustration.

Anger

As reality begins to sink in, individuals start to resent, resist, and fight back against it. In the case of hearing loss, patients may ask why this disability is happening to them. They may become focused on finding out how it could have been avoided and possibly look for sources to blame. The answer to questions such as What caused this? Is there something I could have done to prevent it? may appear to be I should have known better. This conclusion can result in feelings of guilt, especially if it seems as if the hearing loss is a burden to others. Feelings associated with the anger stage include a sense of betrayal and bitterness.

Bargaining

During this stage, individuals are "grasping at straws," making promises to God or professionals or even themselves as a way to substitute a preferred scenario for reality. This stage provides additional time to prepare for a "new normalcy" (Atkins, 1994), but because it is not effective, it is generally short-lived. Adults with sudden hearing loss are more likely to bargain compared with those who have gradually acquired hearing loss. Bargaining seems to be a private stage, not demonstrated openly and therefore not likely to be observed by the audiologist. Feelings associated with bargaining include panic, desperation, shame, and loneliness.

Depression

Whereas denial, anger, and bargaining stages attempt to "stop the clock" and hold on to the past, individuals in this stage gradually realize that in fact the present will be different, resulting in a sense of sorrow or mourning and deep sadness or (usually nonclinical) depression. Individuals in this stage may have trouble sleeping, concentrating, or caring about appearances and things that normally interest them. They generally have little energy to take on the challenges of rehabilitation. Tanner (1980) cautions that attempts to "cheer up" the patient should not be overly aggressive, because the patient needs to feel the full extent of this loss. This suggestion can make the audiologist feel uncomfortable, because he or she may feel obligated to make people feel better. This inclination needs to be countered by an understanding of who "owns" the hearing loss. It is a mark of psychological maturity on the part of the audiologist to acknowledge that this "emotional work" is the patient's.

Integration and Growth

Kübler-Ross (1969) described the last stage of grief as acceptance, meaning only that individuals at this point are no longer angry, bargaining, or depressed. Smart (2001) also includes in this stage efforts to establish new goals and using one's strengths and abilities to contribute to the quality of one's life, or "transcend the loss." Associated feelings include resignation and even an enthusiasm for a chance to improve a difficult situation.

It is important to remember that grief in all its forms is a normal experience and that the resolution of each stage contributes to overall emotional maturity. It is also essential to realize that we cannot possibly predict how a person will manage grief, nor is our judgment regarding grief management warranted.

Stress and Hearing Loss

While adults with acquired hearing loss come to terms with a change in their self-concepts, another psychological response is simultaneously occurring, and that is dealing with the stress of living with a chronically challenging condition. Unless an audiologist has a hearing loss, it is difficult to appreciate fully the chronic stress that patients experience. Selye (1956) provided the classic definition of stress as "the state of wear and tear" (p. 55) on an individual in response to either an acute crisis or to a chronic stressor. Hearing loss is a chronic stressor because it is a persistent life difficulty concomitant with social strain and the potential to threaten or alter one's self-concept. The strain of ongoing hearing problems could explain a great deal of the frustration, anger, and even despair expressed by patients.

Patients with hearing loss actually experience three kinds of stress. First is the daily effort of living with an impaired system, that is, not being able to hear well and struggling to understand communication. Second is the stress of adjusting to a new self-concept, addressed above. Third, individuals must deal with the stress of living with how society reacts to those with a disability, also discussed above. Opinions, attitudes, and reactions from others are powerful influences. As social beings, all persons care, worry about, and are affected by the positive or negative reactions we receive from those around us. The social environment can modify the impact of chronic stressors such as hearing loss by mitigating or exacerbating people's responses to them. Developmental psychologists report that as most people enter their 50s, they become less concerned about others' opinions, but that seems hard to believe when audiologists see so many 50+-year-old patients insisting, "I want the hearing aids you can't see!"

Special Consideration

- In addition to the strain of listening with an impaired auditory system, patients have two other stressors: they must work through their own emotional reactions to hearing loss and decide how much importance should be placed on social approval and acceptance.

Withdrawal

The stress of living with hearing loss can cause an individual to seek relief by partially or fully withdrawing from family and friends, creating an even more adverse condition of social isolation. Isolation can be both physical and emotional (Crow, 1997). Occasional physical isolation will provide necessary respite, but emotional isolation is not a preferred state for human beings. Individuals with hearing loss frequently report this kind of emotional isolation even while sitting in a room with friends and family: because they are unable to follow the conversations swirling around them, they might as well be alone. The patient may not be fully cognizant of the dynamics of this situation, and the family members are even less likely to understand it. Therefore, withdrawal may need to be a topic of conversation as audiologists talk to patients about the impact of hearing loss.

Summary

This section reviewed some of the psychological and emotional reactions adults tend to experience as they develop and live with hearing loss. A threat to a hard-fought-for self-concept will lead to reactions of grief, stress, and withdrawal. By no means should this section be considered an exhaustive list. Clark (1990a) described more subtle psychoemotional responses to ponder: for example, why might patients be more inclined to please the audiologist rather than satisfy their own needs? Why might patients seem unable to make a decision? Might patients be hostile not only because they have a hearing loss but also because the audiologist represents authority? For all these reactions and more, how do we help these patients advance toward hearing help? Some suggestions will be provided in a subsequent section.

♦ Listening Carefully

At this point, we can say that we "know about" just a few of the psychological and emotional difficulties adult patients may experience. However, "knowing about" these reactions is not enough; to genuinely help patients, our responses must convey to each patient that we are actively attending to his or her unique story, and we are working hard to understand it. If our responses do not convey this effort and interest, the patient will not be able to see that we do care and we do want to help. Whether the disclosures have been spontaneous or elicited, direct or indirect, we have an obligation to acknowledge and respond to them in ways that let patients know they can trust us and work with us.

The Risk of Communication Mismatch

The first step in careful listening is to recognize the risk of "missing the real point" to a patient's comments. Audiology is steeped in science, research data, and technical manuals, and therefore clinicians' mind-set may only be on the information or content associated with audiology. However, as was presented, the patient's conversation may be focused on stress, loss, and other emotions associated with hearing problems. If we are not careful, we will answer all comments or questions with information, even though information was not requested.

For example, a patient may say, "I feel so self-conscious when I wear these hearing aids." We could respond with facts ("The hearing aids are so small, no one can see them" or "The main thing is they improve your hearing") or with a comment that is audiologist-centric (seeing the situation only from our point of view), such as, "You should feel even more self-conscious when you can't hear people." However, the patient is not asking for facts or an editorial, but instead is asking that we attend to and acknowledge a psychological reaction. Remember, this patient said, "I feel self-conscious," and did not ask, "Do these hearing aids improve my hearing?" When we reply instead with information, we have caused a communication mismatch. It appears that, if careful listening is not actively practiced and routinely considered, audiologists do not perceive requests for personal support, and instead provide information although it was not requested (English et al, 2000).

Requests for Information or for Personal Support

How does the listener know what the speaker is asking? How does the listener become aware that the question asks for more than information? The mindful listener will want to develop a skill called differentiation (Cormier and Hackney, 1999), which requires a second or two of consideration and observation. That is, we stop and ask ourselves the following:

♦ Is a parent literally asking about when the school bus will arrive to take her child to a special education program, or is there something more?

♦ Is an older patient casually mentioning that his only son is moving his family to another state to make conversation, or is there something more?

♦ When a child tells his parents he left his hearing aids at school, and tells his teachers he left them at home, is he becoming absentminded? Or is there something more?

Even a comment as seemingly innocuous as "What size batteries do I need to buy?" can be more than just a request for information. A patient was observed asking this, and the audiologist understood that there was "something more" to this question. After all, that information had been provided verbally and had been highlighted on the written material. More telling was how the question was asked: with tension, almost panic. The audiologist answered the question, then asked an intentionally vague question: "Is there something about the batteries?"

The patient nodded: "So much to remember! And I don't even know where to buy them, much less know how much they cost or how long they last. Hearing aids are more complicated than I expected; it feels like, if I have to remember one more detail, I will forget everything altogether. I feel totally overwhelmed."

The audiologist differentiated correctly: this question was much more than just a request for information. It has been shown that audiologists can acquire the skill of differentiation (English et al, 2000), but it is safe to say one never truly masters it—patients will invariably catch us off guard, and

we will miss an occasional cue. When we realize it later, though, we need to address it.

The Problem with Assumptions

One of the author's professional joys is teaching a counseling course via distance education on the Internet. In the first week of every semester, the following case is presented:

After canceling three appointments, Ms. B arrives at the audiology clinic with her 4-year-old daughter, Margie. She says, Margie just refuses to wear those hearing aids. I guess it's been 3 weeks since she used them last.

The assignment is to post an answer to the question What do you hear? Enrollees are audiologists with a master's degree, averaging 15 years' experience. At this early point in the semester, the students have read more than 30 pages on listening, stress, grief, and related topics. Even with these readings, though, it seems that, in every term, over 90% of the audiologists "hear" a mother in denial, a mother who has lost control of the situation, or a mother who is not convinced of the value of amplification.

The students are then provided additional information: when Ms. B. is asked (nonjudgmentally) for more of the story, they learn that Ms. B's own mother is very ill and perhaps has only a few more weeks to live. Ms. B spends every possible moment at the hospice with her mother, and Margie is left with a babysitter for 12 hours a day. She does not even know what Margie is eating for dinner these days, much less how consistent the child's hearing aid use is. Ms. B is devastated about losing her mother and, except for the babysitter, has no help with home responsibilities.

Of course, this additional information changes everything. But why would audiologists assume so much when so little is known about the situation? We now feel chagrined about judging this mother in any light except as a parent who is doing the best she can at the moment, even when we lack the "deep background."

Empathy

When patients indicate how their hearing loss is affecting the quality of their interpersonal relationships and their own self-concept, as nonprofessional/personal counselors, we are not asked to feel sorry for them (sympathy) but instead to put ourselves in their position and understand what they are feeling (empathy). Josselman (1992) says that to be empathic, we must "put aside our own experience, at least momentarily, and reverberate to the feelings of another" (p. 203).

Pearl

♦ The metaphor of the sounding board found in pianos and violins is helpful: a sounding board provides no music on its own; it simply reverberates with the notes played near it.

Interestingly, Sigmund Freud observed that talking out a problem somehow made that problem easier for the patient to manage and solve. He called this process the "talking cure," although he did not know how to explain it. Recent research now shows that as individuals talk about their difficulties, neurons in the brain reorganize their connections, leading to improvements in processing, integrating, and understanding both information and emotions (Vaughn, 1997). Audiologists' role as a "sounding board" has legitimate clinical validity.

As essential as empathizing is, it is not easy, because people are, by nature, egocentric, and empathy is the antithesis of egocentricity. In addition, empathic responses are not normally used in everyday conversations. Note, however, that when we talk to patients about the psychological and emotional challenges they face, by definition we are not involved in everyday conversations. Empathic responses can be drawn upon to mark the importance of the moment as we try to understand.

Natural egocentrism is the ultimate barrier to empathizing with another, but more specific barriers have been delineated to help counselors analyze their own behaviors. A leading obstacle to responding with empathy is habituation, a reduction in response as a result of repeated exposure to a stimulus. In this situation, audiologists become numb to patients' remarks and perceived complaints, thinking that they have "heard this all before" (Kennedy and Charles, 2001). Just a few years in practice can lead audiologists to feel exactly that way: that all patients say the same things, so there is no longer any need to attend to their individual stories.

Habituation is related to another barrier, generalization, whereby we hold preconceived notions (or assume that we can predict from an audiogram and past experiences with patients) of how a specific patient will respond to hearing loss. Because research proves the contrary (e.g., Garstecki and Erler, 2001), the audiologist has an ongoing challenge to set aside assumptions and respond only to what the patient is disclosing. Empathy requires us to hold back on planning and solving, for the moment, and to focus only on the "here and now" experiences as reported by the patient.

Empathy has a cost. It requires energy and an ability to be temporarily selfless. On days when audiologists' own energy is low, worries are piling up, and distractions are beyond control, empathy is hard to sustain. It is important for audiologists to realize their own limitations and not be overly critical of themselves if they are not models of empathy every day of the week.

Audiologists have reason to be concerned about the degree to which they successfully convey empathy. Patients have registered strong complaints about audiologists as a group, finding them indifferent, brusque, or pessimistic, even occasionally shouting at patients (Martin et al, 1989). Glass and Elliot (1992) summarized a patient survey stating that not only do audiologists not seem to know about living with hearing loss, "they don't seem to want to know—or to care" (p. 27). This perception does not have to be perpetuated; in fact, audiology students enrolled in doctoral programs have identified their interest in improving patient interactions (English and Zoladkiewicz, 2005). There is always room for improvement in developing and conveying empathy for patients' emotional and psychological experiences.

Controversial Point

- In the study by English and Zoladkiewicz (2005) mentioned earlier, one student made this request: "I would like input from supervisors about our interactions with patients, how I 'read' the patient's nonverbal cues, etc. I get input about the way I conduct the testing, deliver the hearing aids, etc., but not really if I 'matched' my help to the way the patient was acting." Supervisors do tend to overlook evaluating students' counseling skills, but they must assume this responsibility to help students translate course content to direct patient care.

Summary

This section described some ways to improve listening skills. Differentiation is the cognitive act of determining the nature of a patient's comment (asking for information or personal support) and is needed to avoid communication mismatches. Avoiding assumptions will help us keep an open mind (and therefore an "open ear") to patients' situations and needs, and empathy will help us see those situations and needs from patients' point of view. The next section will provide some guidance on how to respond.

◆ Responding Carefully

We now find ourselves listening carefully and recognizing that a comment or question could be far more complicated than it seems to be. We open our mouths and, in response, say . . . what? Should we say that everything will be OK? Or that other people have problems far worse than the patient's? Or perhaps that bad things can happen to good people?

We were cautioned at the beginning of the chapter that responding carefully is by far the most difficult component of audiologic counseling. The first response that comes to mind may not be the most helpful thing to say. Before we consider helpful responses, it might be helpful to review one approach we should try to avoid. It is inappropriate reassurance, or the "Don't Worry—Be Happy" response.

Inappropriate Reassurance

Clark (1990b) was the first to note that audiologists are likely to try to make patients "feel better" by telling them not to worry, or that their worries are unfounded. Even with good intentions, the outcome of these reassurances is problematic: patients in fact do not feel better, but instead feel dismissed or admonished for not trusting the professional. For example:

Patient: I just am not making as much progress as I was expecting with these new hearing aids. Every day is a struggle.

Audiologist: You've made more progress than a lot of my patients. You just need to give this some time.

The reader is reminded of the discussion earlier in the chapter about the idea of ownership of the hearing loss. The easy reassurance in this sample dialogue conveys the impression that the audiologist owns the hearing loss: (1) the audiologist is the expert and should not be questioned, (2) the patient's experiences are neither important nor interesting, and (3) there is nothing more to say about this issue.

What is the patient's reaction to this exchange? Most likely, it is along these lines: (1) the audiologist is not interested in my situation, (2) the audiologist is not someone I can trust with my struggles, (3) that's easy for others to say when they have normal hearing.

Consider the outcome when the audiologist actively acknowledges the patient's stress and the patient as "owner" of the problem:

Patient: I just am not making as much progress as I was expecting with these new hearing aids. Every day is a struggle.

Audiologist: You're disappointed, it sounds like. Or tired—maybe both?

Patient: A little disappointed, yes, but also discouraged and definitely tired. I had no idea the adjustment process would wear me out like this.

Audiologist: Until you go through it, it's not something you can expect.

Patient: That's for sure; it's a real process. Not impossible, mind you, just hard.

Audiologist: Hard work, and yet you are sticking with it.

Patient: Well, it's important to me. I'm willing to give it time, and I'll figure out how to make the most of it.

The conversation in this example kept moving forward because the patient was given the opportunity to express her thoughts and feelings, instead of having those feelings brushed aside. Notice, too, that the audiologist refrained from saying, "We talked about this 2 weeks ago, when you first received your hearing aids, about how the new input could tire you out." Clearly, the first time this information was given, it did not make an impression; there is no need to chastise the patient for not processing it at the time.

This concept of inappropriate reassurance is complicated, and the reader is therefore encouraged to study it further. Lundburg and Lundburg (1995) have written an excellent layperson's guide on the topic.

Empathic Responses

Earlier we considered empathy, the act of temporarily stepping away from our own perceptions so that we can share our patients' outlooks. Consider again the second dialogue above. Let us examine each comment made by the audiologist. Essentially, the audiologist is acknowledging, "This is what it's like for you—am I getting it right?"

♦ *You're disappointed, it sounds like. Or tired—maybe both?*   This statement tried to summarize the emotions expressed by the patient. If we are correct, the patient will confirm it; if we are wrong, the patient will correct it. Either way, we are verbally trying to understand.

♦ *Until you go through it, it's not something you can expect.*   This statement attempts to reflect the unexpected degree of work involved with the adjustment process. Important: No information is added; the comment is a "verbal mirror."

♦ *Hard work, and yet you are sticking with it.*   This statement acknowledges the commitment and the persistence as described by the patient. The patient is not being showered with compliments, but instead is being acknowledged as being capable of meeting this challenge.

This exchange took a little longer, perhaps another minute, but the patient is far more likely now to persist in the hard work of adjustment, and also to begin to reevaluate expectations. Is less than perfect acceptable? This position may now be tolerated. As Stone and colleagues (1999) put it, "People almost never change without feeling understood" (p. 29).

There is no "empathy script" or other secrets to learn to be an empathic responder. However, here are some sample responses we can use to convey that we are trying to understand:

"Helping cues" when we do understand the response:

♦ *It sounds like you feel. . . .*

♦ *You seem to be feeling. . . .*

♦ *My impression is. . . . Am I understanding you correctly?*

♦ *The part that I understand is. . . .*

"Helping cues" when we do not understand the response:

♦ *The part that isn't clear to me is. . . .*

♦ *Could you tell me . . . ?*

♦ *Can you say more about . . . ?*

♦ *How is that for you?*

♦ *What does that mean to you?*

♦ *Is this what you're saying?*

"The Readiness Is All"

Patients may or may not be ready to make any changes in their status quo. For change to occur, the psychological state of readiness is essential, or, as Hamlet put it, "The readiness is all" (Act V, Scene 4). We would be gravely mistaken to assume that every patient is fully ready for change, to obtain hearing aids, and to work through the adjustment process. Informal queries of colleagues indicate that on some days, up to 80% of their patients make appointments at the behest of loved ones, not because the patients themselves are interested in improving their hearing status.

Rather than trying to guess, or to read from body language, whether a patient is ready, audiologists can use a simple counseling strategy to find out. We can ask the patient to consider a readiness scale from 1 to 10, where 1 is "no way" and 10 is "absolutely ready." With this scale, we can ask a patient the following:

Audiologist: We've been discussing your hearing challenges, and my best recommendation is to make sounds louder for you with amplification. But before we talk about hearing aids, I need you to tell me: on a scale from 1 to 10, how ready are you for this next step in your treatment plan?

We can try to predict what the patient will say, but what matters most is the patient's reply:

Patient X: I'm a 1! I have no interest in hearing aids; I just made this appointment to appease my spouse.

Patient Y: "Hmm, maybe a 4 . . . but I have a lot of questions first.

Patient Z: Although I'm not thrilled about it, I'd say 9. Things are just getting too bad to let it stay that way.

Early on, information was presented about providing patient-centered care; this strategy directly demonstrates that approach, by giving the patient the opportunity to define the starting point and to discuss the barriers created.

Give It Words: Two Coping Strategies

In her memoir, writer Amy Tan (2003) describes growing up in a bilingual home and her experiences with language. She was a young adult when she first learned the word *mauve* and the color that word described. Once she learned the word, she saw mauve everywhere. Of course, the color had always existed, but until she learned the word, she did not truly see it.

This chapter began by considering how to "give sorrow words"; in this section, we also want to try to "give help words." When people are consistently challenged to live with a disability, they tend to use one of two modes of coping: vigilance or respite. Living with a hearing loss requires a patient to maintain a high level of mental and physical alertness and effort (vigilance) to detect, process, and respond rapidly to unpredictable or hard-to-hear input. Because this heightened state of attention depletes physical and psychological energy, patients will also employ different strategies to conserve and regain that energy (i.e., seeking respite), including social or physical withdrawal or even sleeping. This kind of temporary withdrawal will recharge the individual's "batteries," but if it is not understood, family members will perceive this strategy as rudeness or lack of interest. Naming these behaviors as expected coping strategies (by way of patient-friendly handouts, for instance) can help both the patient and his or her family "see" the stress associated with hearing loss, and reduce the tendency to blame the patient as unmotivated or self-absorbed.

Summary

This section provides a few strategies on how to respond when patients express their emotional and psychological reactions to hearing loss and hearing aid use. Understanding the pitfalls of inappropriate reassurance will help us avoid cutting off conversation or conveying undue expertise. Empathic responses are needed when we hear patients describing their psychoemotional state. As the counseling conversation progresses (remembering it is integrated into every step of the appointment), we may see the need to check for readiness or to provide a working vocabulary (vigilance, respite) to help patients give words to their coping strategies. In audiology settings, readers are encouraged to consult regularly with colleagues to evaluate the effectiveness of their responses. Invariably, we all miss important cues sometimes, but we still need to hold to a commitment to improve these counseling skills, and it helps when we have a supportive work environment that nurtures and supports this development.

♦ Family-Centered Audiology: When a Child Has Hearing Loss

Statistically, most patients with impaired hearing are adults. However, several million children in the United States alone also have hearing loss, and their unique concerns are embedded within the context of their family. In this section, we will briefly consider two aspects of audiologic counseling related to children and their families: how we tell parents that their child has a hearing loss and how to capitalize on the contributions of family support groups.

Breaking the News: Informing Parents of Their Child's Hearing Loss

Informing parents of their child's hearing loss may be an audiologist's greatest challenge. Even if a parent has suspected a hearing loss for some time, the news will be upsetting. This process must be carefully considered and must be managed with as much sensitivity as can be mustered.

Guidelines for "breaking the news" to parents are described in Clark and English (2004) and are summarized here: ensure privacy and adequate time; assess parents' understanding of the situation; encourage parents to express feelings; respond with empathy and warmth; give a broad time line; briefly discuss treatment options.

This process will sound familiar to the reader, who has been encouraged to develop patient-centered audiologic counseling practices. When we serve children, we expand our approach to be family centered. Family-centered practices acknowledge the parent's role as collaborator and decision maker, and the family as a system with a range of resources and goals (Sass-Lehrer, 2004). Family-centered practices strive to develop a partnership, rather than an expert-based relationship, between family and audiologist. In other words, the family is our patient, and our responsibility is to help the family manage the hearing loss. The person with the hearing loss (the child) will not really be an independent patient for many years to come.

This approach, by definition, requires our best listening abilities: we must listen carefully, with empathy, to differentiate the nature of families' questions, to hear and respond to their grief and stress, and to support them as they redefine their self-concept as a family (English, 2002). Additionally, we must practice extra restraint from "solving" families' situations, so as not to undermine their growth process. It is tempting to admonish parents to follow our directions, to trust us as we start making earmolds and phone calls to early intervention programs, but the reader can see that this approach is the opposite of family centered. Although we feel much urgency for parents to make decisions quickly, we once again must ask ourselves, Who owns this hearing loss? When a child has a hearing loss, the answer is, the parents (or caregivers). These adults "own" the loss just as they own the responsibility for their child's overall health, safety, and development. Audiologists must strive to team with families, acknowledging the leading role of the parents and other family members.

Family Support Groups

When asked what helps them most, parents invariably put "contact with other parents" at the top of their list of answers. Regular meeting times (with child care) or regular telephone contacts provide parents an opportunity to confide with seasoned parents dealing with similar problems. Parents who have "been there" will be deeply sensitive to other parents' struggles, and their suggestions will be more readily considered. Support groups can also be designed for children with hearing loss, especially when they interact with few other children with hearing loss and even more especially when they enter the teen years (Oliva, 2004). Audiologists must remember that support groups "belong" to the members, not the professionals. As soon as professionals try to control meeting times or guest speakers, members will lose interest, and the group will disband.

Summary

Clearly, this section cannot possibly do justice to the complex topic of childhood hearing loss and family adjustment. Readers interested in this topic are directed to cited readings for more in-depth coverage.

♦ Referring to a Professional Counselor

We have been considering our role as nonprofessional counselors, which requires us to stay within the audiologic scope of practice. That is to say, if a patient's reactions are related to hearing loss, and we perceive no other stressor,

we are within our scope of practice to help patients through the help-seeking process.

However, on occasion we are likely to have patients who are experiencing problems that involve more than living with hearing loss. Just like individuals with normal hearing, our patients may be contending with very serious life problems: clinical depression, unmanageable anger, eating disorders, marital discord, financial worries, dysfunctional relationships, to name a few. If we perceive an encroachment on our professional boundaries, we must refer to professional counselors (Stone and Olswang, 1989). A referral procedure should be in place before a crisis presents itself, and we are not to feel that somehow we have failed a patient when we make the referral. In fact, the opposite is true: we have best served the patient by directing him or her to someone qualified to help with problems other than hearing loss.

♦ Summary

Audiologic counseling is expressed in many ways and throughout our interactions with patients and their families. By our choice of words and body language, and in other ways, we communicate the following:

- ♦ We care about patients' struggles and suffering.
- ♦ We understand that they face barriers to accepting hearing help.
- ♦ We honor the courage needed to face those barriers.
- ♦ We respect patients' ability to improve their situation.

At the beginning of the chapter, we considered how counseling skills need to be regularly considered and integrated into every stage of our preprofessional and professional experiences. To support the development of these personal adjustment counseling skills, a checklist is given in Appendix 8–1 (from Clark and English, 2004). This checklist is designed for students and practitioners alike; input from others can help audiologists as they grow as nonprofessional counselors. Readers can safely assume that developing effective listening and responding skills will take years, if not a lifetime, to master, but the effort is well worth it.

Acknowledgments   The chapter "Counseling for Diagnosis and Management of Auditory Disorders in Infants, Children, and Adults," by Jane R. Madell, Ph.D., director, Hearing and Learning Center, Beth Israel Medical Center, New York, served as a guide for this chapter. Dr. Madell's work appeared in the first edition of this volume.

Appendix 8–1

Audiology Counseling Growth Checklist

The Audiology Counseling Growth Checklist (ACGC) may be used as a self-assessment measure for those wishing to increase their awareness of effective audiologist–patient dynamics or as a means to appraise the effectiveness of others whose service delivery approach may serve as a springboard toward growth in counseling. While observing another, or upon reflection of a concluding patient visit that you have conducted, simply circle the most appropriate response to the statements presented. All items are worded so that a yes response signifies a positive behavior on the part of the audiologist. The word *patient* refers to the individual seeking services during the session, whether this is the individual with the hearing loss or that individual's parent, guardian, or spouse. If you are working with a supervisor, comparison of your self-assessment on the ACGC with that of the supervisor can be beneficial in developing a constructive dialogue toward growth. Notation of examples of observed behaviors or responses, or examples of lost opportunities to present a behavior or response, can further discussion and facilitate the development of counseling skills.

Greeting and Opening

1. The audiologist introduced himself/herself by name (or greeted the patient if formerly met) with a handshake and direct eye contact.

    Yes   No   Not applicable

2. The audiologist seated himself/herself at eye level with the patient.

    Yes   No   Not applicable

3. The audiologist began with an appropriate opening that invited the patient to express his/her immediate concern and actively acknowledged and addressed this concern.

    Yes   Example: _____

    No   Example: _____

    Not applicable

Demeanor and Delivery

4. The audiologist maintained eye contact with the patient.

    Yes   Example: _____

    No   Example: _____

    Not applicable

5. The audiologist's facial expressions were appropriate to the context at hand.

    Yes   Example: _____

    No   Example: _____

    Not applicable

6. The audiologist maintained an attentive yet relaxed posture conveying a responsiveness of an undivided attention.

    Yes   Example: _____

    No   Example: _____

    Not applicable

7. The audiologist's nonverbal expressions were appropriate to the dialogue and not distracting.

    Yes   Example: _____

    No   Example: _____

    Not applicable

8. The audiologist's voice was easily heard by the patient and maintained a tone of interest.

    Yes   Example: _____

    No   Example: _____

    Not applicable

9. The audiologist spoke at an appropriate rate to enhance understanding.

    Yes   Example: _____

    No   Example: _____

    Not applicable

10. The audiologist avoided jargon within his/her comments, making every effort to ensure that meaning was understood.

    Yes Example: _____

    No   Example: _____

    Not applicable

11. The audiologist avoided both verbal statements and nonverbal expressions that might appear judgmental.

    Yes Example: _____

    No   Example: _____

    Not applicable

12. The audiologist seemed aware of potential conflicts between his/her social style and that of the patient.

    Yes Example: _____

    No   Example: _____

    Not applicable

Patient Affirmation

13. The audiologist appeared conscious of multicultural issues that might influence the dynamics of the interaction.

    Yes Example: _____

    No   Example: _____

    Not applicable

14. The audiologist employed reflective listening responses to ensure patient's meanings were understood correctly and to display a desire to attain that understanding.

    Yes Example: _____

    No   Example: _____

    Not applicable

15. The audiologist made affirmative statements regarding perceived patient strengths.

    Yes Example: _____

    No   Example: _____

    Not applicable

16. The audiologist seemed aware of and responded to the feelings underlying the patient's statements.

    Yes Example: _____

    No   Example: _____

    Not applicable

17. The audiologist used statements that affirmed something expressed by the patient.

    Yes Example: _____

    No   Example: _____

    Not applicable

Patient Encouragement

18. The audiologist avoided closed questions that might elicit simple yes/no responses.

    Yes Example: _____

    No   Example: _____

    Not applicable

19. The audiologist made appropriate use of silence to encourage further comment from the patient on a current topic before changing the direction of discussion.

    Yes Example: _____

    No   Example: _____

    Not applicable

20. The audiologist's nonverbal expressions were encouraging to the continuation of dialogue.

 Yes   Example: _____

 No   Example: _____

 Not applicable

21. The audiologist interjected positive affirmations (yes, hmm, etc.) to encourage continuation or expansion of the patient's comments.

 Yes   Example: _____

 No   Example: _____

 Not applicable

22. The audiologist encouraged the patient to express his/her feelings.

 Yes   Example: _____

 No   Example: _____

 Not applicable

23. The audiologist avoided signs of defensiveness or expressed feelings or anger, frustration, and so on, that may have appeared directed at the audiologist.

 Yes   Example: _____

 No   Example: _____

 Not applicable

Exploration

24. The audiologist appropriately challenged statements made by the patient that might impede the positive actions taken by the patient and helped him/her to identify more positive views.

 Yes   Example: _____

 No   Example: _____

 Not applicable

25. If exploring solutions for specific communication breakdowns, the audiologist asked the patient to identify at least one action that might be taken to address the problem.

 Yes   Example: _____

 No   Example: _____

 Not applicable

26. The audiologist suggested alternative actions that might be useful.

 Yes   Example: _____

 No   Example: _____

 Not applicable

27. The audiologist helped the patient to develop actions that might facilitate an identified goal.

 Yes   Example: _____

 No   Example: _____

 Not applicable

28. The audiologist provided an opportunity to practice identified actions.

 Yes   Example: _____

 No   Example: _____

 Not applicable

29. The audiologist encouraged the patient to critique the effectiveness of actions taken to address the identified goal when attempted at home, work, or during social activities.

 Yes   Example: _____

 No   Example: _____

 Not applicable

30. The audiologist recognized when a topic could not be fully explored during current time constraints and offered an opportunity to return for further exploration.

Yes Example: _____

No   Example: _____

Not applicable

From Clark, J. G., & English, K. E. (2004). Counseling in audiologic practice: Helping patients and families adjust to hearing loss. Boston: Allyn & Bacon, with permission.

References

Atkins, D. (1994). Counseling children with hearing loss and their families. In J. G. Clark & F. Martin (Eds.), Effective counseling for audiologists: Perspectives and practice (pp. 116–146). Englewood Cliffs, NJ: Prentice Hall.

Balint, M. (1964). The doctor, his patient, and the illness (2nd ed.). New York: International Universities Press.

Blood, G. W., Blood, I. M., & Danhauer, J. (1977). The hearing aid effect. Hearing Instruments, 28, 12–16.

Clark, J. G. (1990a). Emotional response transformations: Redirections and projections. ASHA, 32(6), 67–68.

Clark, J. G. (1990b). The "Don't Worry—Be Happy" professional response. Hearing Journal, 4(4), 21–23.

Clark, J. G., & English, K. (2004). Counseling in audiologic practice: Helping patients and their families adjust to hearing loss. Boston: Allyn & Bacon.

Cormier, S., & Hackney, H. (1999). Counseling strategies and interventions (5th ed.). Boston: Allyn & Bacon.

Crow, T. A. (1997). Emotional aspects of communicative disorders. In T. A. Crow (Ed.), Applications of counseling in speech-pathology and audiology (pp. 30–47). Baltimore: Williams & Wilkins.

Doggett, S., Stein, R., & Gans, R. (1998). Hearing aid effect in older women. Journal of the American Academy of Audiology, 9(5), 361–366.

Ellis, A. (1996). Better, deeper, and more enduring brief therapy: The rational emotive behavioral approach. New York: Brunner/Mazel.

English, K. (2002). Counseling children with hearing impairment and their families. Boston: Allyn & Bacon.

English, K., Rojeski, T., & Branham, K. (2000). Acquiring counseling skills in mid-career: Outcomes of a distance education course for practicing audiologists. Journal of the American Academy of Audiology, 11, 84–90.

English, K., & Zoladkiewicz, L. (2005). AuD students' concerns about interacting with patients and families. Audiology Today, 17(5), 22–25.

Garstecki, D. C., & Erler, S. F. (2001). Personal and social conditions potentially influencing women's hearing loss management. American Journal of Audiology, 10(2), 78–90.

Glass, L., & Elliot, H. (1992). The professionals told me what it is, but that's not enough. SHHH Journal, 13(1), 26–29.

Golin, C. E., DiMatteo, M. R., & Gelberg, L. (1996). The role of patient participation in the doctor visit: Implications for adherence to diabetes care. Diabetes Care, 19(10), 1153–1164.

Josselman, R. (1992). The space between us: Exploring the dimensions of human relationships. San Francisco: Jossey-Bass.

Kennedy, E., & Charles, S. (2001). On becoming a counselor: A basic guide for nonprofessional counselors and other helpers (3rd ed.). New York: Crossroad.

Kübler-Ross, E. (1969). On death and dying. New York: Macmillan.

Lundburg, G., & Lundburg, J. (1995). "I don't have to make it all better": Six practical principles that empower others to solve their own problems while enriching your relationship. New York: Penguin.

Margolis, R. (2004). What do your patients remember? Hearing Journal, 57(6), 10–17.

Martin, F. (1994). Conveying diagnostic information. In J. G. Clark & F. Martin (Eds.), Effective counseling in audiology (pp. 38–67). Boston: Allyn & Bacon.

Martin, F., Krall, L., & O'Neal, J. (1989). The diagnosis of acquired hearing loss. ASHA, 31(11), 47–50.

Oliva, G. (2004). Alone in the mainstream: A deaf woman remembers public school. Washington, DC: Gallaudet University Press.

Rogers, C. (1961). On becoming a person. Boston: Houghton Mifflin.

Sass-Lehrer, M. (2004). Early detection of hearing loss: Maintaining a family-centered perspective. Seminars in Hearing, 25(4), 295–307.

Selye, H. (1956). The stress of life. New York: McGraw-Hill.

Shames, G. (2000). Counseling the communicatively disabled and their families. Boston: Allyn & Bacon.

Skinner, B. F. (1953). Science and human behavior. New York: Free Press.

Smart, J. (2001). Disability, society, and the individual. Gaithersburg, MD: Aspen.

Stewart, M., Brown, J. B., Boon, H., Galadja, J., Meredith, L., & Sangster, M. (1999). Evidence on patient–doctor communication. Cancer Prevention and Control, 3(10), 25–30.

Stewart, M., Brown, J. B., & Freeman, T. (Eds.). (2003). Patient-centered medicine: Transforming the clinical method (2nd ed.). Abington, UK: Radcliffe Medical Press.

Stone, D., Patton, B., & Heen, S. (1999). Difficult conversations: How to discuss what matters most. New York: Viking Press.

Stone, J. R., & Olswang, L. B. (1989). The hidden challenge in counseling. ASHA, 31, 27–31.

Tan, A. (2003). The opposite of fate: A book of musings. New York: Putnam.

Tanner, D. C. (1980). Loss and grief: Implications for the speech-language pathologist and audiologist. ASHA, 22, 916–928.

Vaughn SC. (1997). The talking cure: The science behind psychotherapy. New York: Grosset-Putnam.

Section II

Applications

Chapter 9

Medical and Surgical Treatment of Middle Ear Disease

Elizabeth A. Dinces and Richard J. Wiet

This chapter is not intended to fully discuss all treatments of disease occurring in the middle ear. Instead, the authors present the more common pathological conditions and some current standard treatments. The surgical treatments outlined here are intended to provide the audiologist with an example of how the middle ear is altered during the most common surgical procedures. The authors do not mean to imply that they are the only surgical techniques to be used. Understanding the anatomy of the middle ear is critical to understanding how middle ear disease occurs, how middle ear disease becomes chronic or resolves, and how the anatomy of the middle ear is related to the varied pathological conditions.

♦ Anatomy

The anatomy of the middle ear determines the response of the middle ear to disease. The developments of the middle ear structures are linked together. This helps the reader understand how middle ear disease arises, progresses, and responds to treatment (**Fig. 9–1** and **Fig. 9–2**).

External Auditory Canal

The external auditory canal (EAC) derives from the first branchial groove. Initially, this area is solid. At the seventh month, the epithelial core begins to absorb at the medial end, leaving a layer of cells to form the tympanic membrane

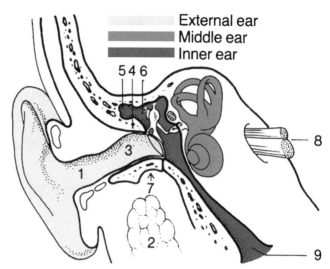

Figure 9–2 Relationship of the external auditory canal (EAC) and middle ear: 1, cartilaginous EAC; 2, parotid gland; 3, bony EAC; 4, lateral wall of the attic; 5, entrance to the mastoid; 6, attic; 7, temporomandibular joint; 8, internal auditory canal; 9, eustachian tube.

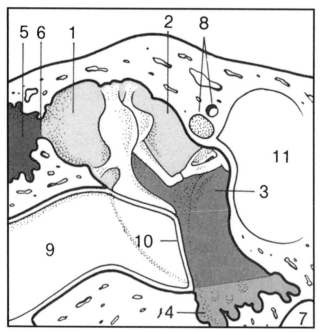

Figure 9–1 Anatomy of the middle ear: 1 and 2, epitympanum or attic; 3, mesotympanum; 4, hypotympanum; 5, mastoid antrum; 6, entrance to the antrum; 7, internal jugular vein; 8, facial nerve narrowing the lower part of the attic (2); 9, external auditory canal; 10, tympanic membrane; 11, labyrinthine vestibule.

(TM). The medial aspect of the external canal is formed by the tympanic ring. Malformation of this tympanic ring can lead to a bony atretic plate at the level of the TM (Bellucci, 1981). In the infant, the TM is found just at the medial edge of the cartilaginous EAC. As the mastoid bone develops and is pneumatized, it grows around and lateral to the tympanic ring, thus extending the bony canal and effectively moving the TM medially. Because the external ear and canal form at a different time in fetal development from both the middle ear and the inner ear, an abnormality may exist in one, with normal structures and function in the other two. Frequently, however, abnormalities of the first branchial pouch (external ear and canal) are accompanied by abnormalities of the first and second branchial arches (ossicles) (Bellucci, 1981). Because the stapes footplate develops from the otic capsule, it is usually present and normal in ears with congenital atresia.

Abnormalities of the stapes footplate may be seen in conjunction with aberrant facial nerves. In the human, facial nerves that develop between the embryonic stapes superstructure and the otic capsule can prevent contact between the otic capsule and the stapes superstructure, causing discontinuity of the ossicular chain. This can also lead to failure of development of the oval window (Lambert, 1990).

Tympanic Cavity

The middle ear consists of the tympanic cavity and the eustachian tube (ET). The tympanic cavity is bordered by the TM laterally and the bony labyrinth medially. Superiorly, the tegmen separates the tympanic cavity from the dura of the middle fossa. The inferior boundary is the skull base with a thin layer of bone over the jugular foramen and a variable system of air cells, which may track underneath the bony labyrinth toward the petrous apex. The tympanic portion of the facial nerve and the chorda tympani (both arising from cranial nerve 7 [CN VII]) run through the tympanic cavity, along with a network of small blood vessels and nerves.

Two muscles act within the tympanic cavity. The tensor tympani muscle arises from the superior edge of the ET orifice (in the anterosuperior portion of the tympanic cavity). It then courses within its bony semicanal to turn at the cochleariform process and attach to the neck of the malleus. The stapedius muscle enters the tympanic cavity at its posterior edge through a triangular piece of bone called the pyramidal process, and its tendon then extends from this pyramidal process to the head of the stapes.

The chorda tympani enters the tympanic cavity just lateral to the pyramidal process and courses under the malleus to its canal in the anterior wall of the cavity. The facial nerve enters the middle ear just lateral to the cochleariform process and courses laterally within the bony facial canal superior to the oval window toward the mastoid **(Fig. 9–3)**. Any course of the facial nerve over the oval window or through the stapes crura is aberrant and can be seen in atretic ears and in otherwise normal ears. Dehiscences in the tympanic portion of the facial canal have been reported in up to 50% of temporal bones (Moreano et al, 1994). The facial recess is located between the chorda tympani and the pyramidal process. This area is important because disease can be difficult to eradicate from this deep and narrow recess. The scutum is that portion of bone that forms the lateral wall of the epitympanum or attic. The epitympanum is the space above the tympanic cavity. It is separated from the

cavity by malleolar and incudal ligaments and contains the head of the malleus and the body of the incus. Both the attic and the scutum can become involved with cholesteatoma, and changes on computed tomographic (CT) scanning in these areas can indicate the presence of cholesteatoma.

Vascular Supply

The blood supply to the middle ear consists of branches of the anterior tympanic and deep auricular arteries, each of which arises from the internal maxillary artery. The anterior tympanic artery supplies the mucosa of the middle ear and has a branch that is the main supply to the incus and malleus. The deep auricular artery supplies the TM. The middle meningeal artery supplies the superficial petrosal artery that sends branches to the geniculate ganglion and facial nerve. From here separate branches are sent to the stapedial tendon, the incudostapedial joint, and the posterior crura of the stapes. The superior tympanic artery supplies the tensor tympani and some of the middle ear mucosa, and joins with the inferior tympanic artery to form a plexus to the anterior stapes. Caroticotympanic arteries arise from the carotid and anastomose with this plexus along with a branch from the ascending pharyngeal artery.

Tympanic Membrane

The TM is conical shaped and is ~9 to 10 mm wide and 8 to 9 mm high. The TM sits at an oblique angle at the medial end of the external canal, with the posterior edge being the most lateral edge. The normal TM is ~0.1 mm thick and has three layers: an outer layer consisting of squamous epithelium, a middle fibrous layer, and an inner layer of mucosa that is in continuity with the middle ear mucosa. Landmarks seen through a normal TM can include the short process and handle (long process) of the malleus, the lenticular process of the incus, the incudostapedial joint, the round window niche, the ET orifice, and the chorda tympani nerve. The umbo is the end of the handle of the malleus and is the point from which the radial fibers of the middle layer of the TM emanate. The umbo also defines the deepest or most medial portion of the TM. The TM has been described as a canterary lever, which is thought to enhance sound transmission.

The TM consists of the pars tensa, which makes up most of the TM, and the pars flaccida. The pars flaccida begins at the short process of the malleus and extends superiorly to the uppermost portion of the tympanic ring. This portion of the TM is also known as Shrapnell's membrane and is thought to be more compliant because of a difference in the arrangement of the fibrous layer at this portion of the TM. It is from retractions or perforations of the pars flaccida that attic cholesteatomas form.

Middle Ear Mucosa

The mucosa of the middle ear and ET consists largely of ciliated respiratory epithelium and mucus-secreting cells. It also contains some B cells that secrete immunoglobulins to

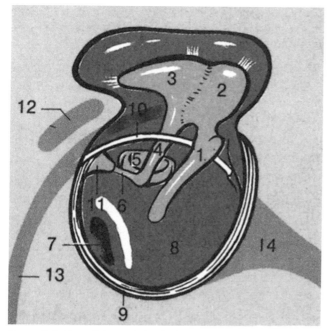

Figure 9–3 View of the medial wall of the middle ear. The facial nerve (13) enters the middle ear behind the head of the malleus (2) and body of the incus (3) superior to the stapes (5) and turns into the mastoid at the lateral semicircular canal (12). It then sends off the chorda tympani (10), which traverses the middle ear lateral to the pyramidal eminence between the long processes of the incus (4) and malleus (1) to exit near the eustachian tube (14).

assist in the body's defense against invading organisms. The cilia beat selectively toward the nasopharynx. They form the "motor" for a mucociliary blanket that is produced by the secretory cells. This blanket of mucus and immune system proteins sits on top of the ciliary layer; as the cilia beat, they act to sweep secretions from the middle ear and antrum toward the nasopharynx by way of the ET. A healthy oxygenated environment is needed to maintain the function of the cilia.

Ossicles

The incus and the malleus develop from the cartilages of the first and second branchial arches in the embryo before the 16th week of development. These arches develop cartilaginous connections during development. It is from these connections in the roof of the tympanic recess (which will become the tympanic cavity) that the body of the incus and the head of the malleus develop (Hanson et al, 1962). The forming ossicles then develop inferiorly, extending processes, which form the long process of the incus and the handle of the malleus. Failure of any of these processes to develop or ossify will result in ossicular abnormalities. The ossicular chain is normally attached directly to the TM along the handle of the malleus. The incus is attached to the malleus and to the stapes by means of joints that are susceptible to the same pathological processes as other similar bony joints in the body. In addition, the ossicles themselves can be affected by systemic and local disease.

The stapes is the third bone in the ossicular chain, and its superstructure is thought to develop from the second branchial arch cartilage. The footplate of the stapes develops and ossifies in conjunction with the otic capsule and thus takes its origin from the otic placode in the embryo. An absent or anomalous superstructure does not rule out a normal and mobile stapes footplate within the oval window. The stapes is shaped like a stirrup, with the arch developing as a result of the stapedial artery coursing through the cartilage as it ossifies. Eventually this artery regresses and may leave a small remnant behind. The head or capitulum of the stapes articulates with the long process of the incus, and its articulating surface is covered by cartilage. The tendon of the stapedial muscle extends from the pyramidal process to the posterior crus of the stapes, which usually is thicker and more curved than the anterior crura. Contraction of this muscle helps to dampen loud sounds to help protect the cochlea from noise trauma. The footplate of the stapes sits in the oval window and transmits sounds through this window to the inner ear (**Fig. 9–4**).

An annular ligament attaches the footplate to the margins of the oval window and enables the stapes to move in a complex fashion within the window. Five other ligaments are found within the tympanic space and act to suspend the ossicular chain within the tympanic space. Three ligaments suspend the malleus: the anterior, lateral, and superior malleolar ligaments. Two other ligaments suspend the incus, the superior incudal ligament, and the ligament of the short process, which is found within the fossa incudis.

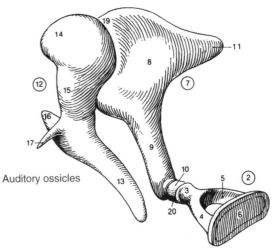

Figure 9–4 The ossicles: view of the articulation and positions of the ossicles from the middle ear looking out. The stapes (2), anterior crus (5), posterior crus (4), footplate (6), capitulum (3). The stapes articulates with the long process of the incus (9) at the incudostapedial joint (10). The incus also has a short process (11), and its body (8) articulates with the head of the malleus (14) at the incudomalleolar joint (19). The malleus (12) has a neck (15), a lateral process (16) (or short process), and an anterior process (17), which usually regresses.

Middle Ear Transformer Function

The TM normally acts as a physical barrier between the EAC and the middle ear space. The TM and ossicular chain also act as a transformer to enable sound waves traveling through the air to act within the fluid of the inner ear and stimulate the organ of hearing (the organ of Corti within the cochlea). In addition, the middle ear acts as an impedance-matching device, increasing the transmission of sound from air to the higher impedance fluids of the inner ear. Without the middle ear, most sound energy in our environment would not be of sufficient magnitude to vibrate the surface of the cochlear fluid. The transformer function of the middle ear is accomplished through three factors. First, because of the difference in surface area between the TM and the footplate of the stapes, the gain in sound pressure at the stapes footplate has been shown to be ~18:1 (Wever and Lawrence, 1954). Second, the sizes and connections of the ossicles within the ossicular chain enable the chain to act as a lever. The malleus head moves a greater distance than the long process of the incus in response to TM motion; thus, the incus will exert a greater pressure over the shorter distance in the transmission of that force. The gain based on the ossicular chain lever is ~3:1 (Békésy, 1960). The third factor is the cone shape of the TM (canterary lever), which enables some areas of the membrane to vibrate at greater amplitude than others do, adding force to the vibrating ossicular chain. Applying these factors, the middle ear transformer adds 25 to 30 dB of sound pressure to the signal that reaches the inner ear. The TM also transmits changes in ambient pressure through its motion and thus can change the effective size of the middle ear space. It is most compliant when the pressure is equal on both sides, and its stiffness increases with positive or negative pressure. Diseases of the TM change its compliance and thus influence the effectiveness of sound transmission. At low frequencies, the entire TM transmits sound as it acts to displace the ossicles. At high frequencies (> 1500 Hz), it acts as a baffle, directing the sound to the handle of the malleus, which is displaced directly by the sound wave (Tonndorf and Khanna, 1970).

Eustachian Tube

The middle ear is part of a system whose function depends on the anatomy and health of its surroundings. The ET is the corridor by which nasopharynx and middle ear/mastoid systems communicate. Normally the ET is closed, preventing the flow of secretions or infections into the middle ear from the nasopharynx. This also protects the middle ear from the dramatic changes in nasopharyngeal pressure seen commonly with coughing, sniffing, sneezing, and nose blowing. In the infant, the ET lies in a horizontal plane, and its opening into the nasopharynx is a slit parallel to the skull base at rest. This opening is controlled by the tensor veli palatine muscle, which, when contracted, pulls on the lateral edge of the ET cartilage in the nasopharynx to open the ET. The levator veli palatine muscle inserts onto the medial portion of this cartilage and aids the tensor in the opening of the ET in the adult. The entrance of the ET into the middle ear is in the anterosuperior portion of the middle ear and can often be seen through a translucent and intact TM. The ET has three functions: (1) to aid in the removal of secretions from the middle ear space, (2) to aerate the middle ear and to equalize pressure between the nasopharynx and the middle ear, and (3) to prevent nasopharyngeal secretions from entering the middle ear space. The ET achieves these three functions by being passively closed and actively opened. Because the muscles of the nasopharynx and palate control the opening of the ET, diseases or anatomical malformations of the nasopharynx or palate can lead to dysfunction of the ET. The distal two thirds of the ET consists of an incomplete cartilaginous tube, which is flexible enough to collapse and close when the attached muscles are relaxed. Because the mucosa of the ET is in continuity with both the mucosa of the middle ear and the mucosa of the nasopharynx, the pathological processes that may be occurring in either of these two locations affect it. Changes in the mucosal lining of the ET affect how well it performs each of its three functions. The success of the ET in performing its functions can be impacted by any pathological condition affecting its neighboring spaces. Because the system is closed at rest, resorption of the gases of the middle ear and mastoid results in negative pressure within the middle ear and mastoid. Swallowing opens the ET, and air is pulled into the middle ear space from the nasopharynx because of this negative pressure. The proper functioning of the ET depends on the integrity of the middle ear system, the ET itself, and the nasopharynx. Any change in the anatomy or function of these spaces will affect the ET's ability to perform any or all of its three functions.

Special Consideration

- Because of its course through the temporal bone, the facial nerve is at risk for injury during any otologic procedure.
- A stenotic or atretic EAC can be associated with normal middle ear structures.
- The otoscopic examination can be normal in the presence of middle ear pathology.
- A limited blood supply to the long process of the incus puts it at risk for necrosis when middle ear disease is present.
- ET function depends on the anatomy and physiology of the middle ear, the nasopharynx, and the skull.

♦ Pathological Conditions of the External Auditory Canal

The EAC links the middle ear with the external environment. It directs sound to the middle ear but can also act as a conduit for obstruction of that sound. The canal is lined with skin containing cerumen glands. The canal skin is directly attached to cartilage in the lateral two thirds of the ear canal and bone in the medial one third.

General dermatological diseases can affect the skin of the EAC. The most commonly seen dermatological diseases are local inflammatory reactions, infections (both fungal and bacterial), squamous cell carcinoma, basal cell carcinoma, and melanoma. Autoimmune diseases of the skin affect the EAC, and psoriasis, lupus erythematosus, and scleroderma can all cause lesions within the external canal. The cartilaginous portion of the external canal is susceptible to perichondritis from local infection and systemic causes. Edema and obstruction of the EAC occur with the progression of cartilaginous and dermatological diseases and can cause hearing loss, dysfunction, and discomfort of hearing aids. Cutaneous reactions to shampoos, medications, and foreign material in the ear canal can be severe and require rapid attention to prevent scarring and stenosis of the soft tissues of the EAC.

Some common diseases affect the bony portion of the external canal. Osteomas and exostoses of the bone can cause complete obstruction of the canal and a significant conductive hearing loss. Osteomas are singular benign bony tumors, often with no identifiable cause. Exostoses of the EAC are rounded multiple bony outgrowths that occur because of chronic irritation of the canal. The most common cause of exostoses of the EAC is cold-water swimming in childhood. These lesions are usually bilateral and can continue to grow for many years, even after the patient is no longer swimming. Tumors and obstructing lesions of the EAC require surgical excision with some type of canal reconstruction (called canaloplasty). Diagnosis of lesions of the EAC is made based on a careful history and cultures or biopsy when appropriate.

Otitis Externa

Otitis externa is an infection of the EAC. It commonly occurs as "swimmer's ear" and often results from contaminated water retained in the canal after swimming or bathing. Otitis externa can also occur in patients wearing poorly vented hearing aids that prevent the evaporation of perspiration from the canal. The retained water macerates the skin and allows organisms to enter and infect the skin. It can also occur after trauma to the canal skin and can be worsened by retained cerumen or other debris within the canal. Fungal infections are often seen in the setting of chronic antibiotic use, both topical and systemic. The most common fungal pathogen found in ear canal infections is *Aspergillus* (Singer et al, 1952).

Initially, the patient experiences mild edema and itching. When infection progresses, there is increased edema, and the TM becomes thickened and less compliant. The canal can narrow as a result of edema, preventing medications from entering and allowing the accumulation of sloughed skin and debris. The patient can experience conductive hearing loss because of canal occlusion and TM thickening. If the infection progresses or spreads, it can involve the cartilage of the EAC, the soft tissue overlying the mastoid, and/or the parotid and produces severe pain, local swelling, and erythema. Fungal and bacterial pathogens may coexist. Some patients develop a chronic inflammatory otitis in this situation.

In chronic otitis externa, the skin can be chronically irritated by scratching, chemical irritation, recurrent low-grade infections, or other causes, such as dermatologic manifestations of systemic disease. Thickening of the canal skin with decreased or absent production of cerumen is present. Occasionally, the patient may have a serous effusion in the middle ear space or an associated thickening of the TM with scarring, which contributes to the hearing loss. Treatment consists of frequent cleaning of the canal and ear wicks to help carry topical medications to the medial portion of the canal and to help reduce edema. Acetic acid drops can help to acidify the canal skin and aid in reestablishing a normal microbial-resistant environment. Antibiotic drops applied topically will help to remove bacteria from the skin crevices, and often a steroid is included in the drops to reduce inflammation, itching, or pain. Occasionally, systemic antibiotics are required when cellulitis, adenopathy, severe pain, or fever accompanies the infection. Of utmost importance is the instruction of the patient to avoid placing fingers or foreign bodies (e.g., cotton-tipped applicators or bobby pins) into the canal and maintenance of water precautions to prevent additional infections and/or spread of the current infection.

In uncomplicated otitis externa, the above treatments will usually normalize the canal within 2 weeks. Avoidance of occluding plugs or hearing aids, as well as keeping the ear canal dry, is necessary. If infection persists despite vigilant care, cultures of the canal skin and occasionally biopsies of any lesions may be warranted. With prolonged infection, irreversible changes in the skin of the EAC may render it susceptible to recurrent or chronic otitis externa. Consequently, the canal skin becomes thickened and does not produce adequate cerumen. Treatment may require skin excision and grafting in severe cases.

Necrotizing otitis externa (also called malignant otitis externa) is a potentially fatal form of otitis externa. This disease is most often seen in diabetic patients, but it can also be seen in patients with other immunodeficiencies. This disease originates as an otitis externa in the skin of the EAC but quickly becomes invasive with infection of surrounding soft tissue cartilage, vascular channels, and eventually bone. The hallmark of malignant otitis externa is granulation tissue in the floor of the EAC with pain out of proportion to the visible disease. Infection can involve the TM and middle ear structures, with destruction of the bony canal and ossicles. Infection often extends into the parotid gland and glenoid fossa with local tissue destruction. The facial nerve is at risk in the parotid gland and mastoid process and at the skull base. Once the bone and soft tissues of the skull base become involved, the patient is at risk for cranial nerve palsies, meningitis, intracranial thrombosis, and brain abscess. The disease progresses rapidly if not treated because of inadequate or tenuous blood supply. Tissue ischemia and inability of the patient's immune system to mount an effective response enable unchecked bacterial invasion. The presence of cranial nerve involvement is associated with a mortality of up to 20% despite treatment (Singh et al, 2005). Treatment involves antibiotics and strict control of blood glucose. Hyperbaric oxygen and surgical debridement are used for resistant cases as necessary. The antibiotics chosen should be effective against *Pseudomonas* infection because this is the most common pathogen in malignant otitis externa.

◆ Tympanic Membrane Diseases

Although the TM often remains unaffected by disease in the EAC, the skin of the canal is in continuity with the external epithelial layer of the TM. External disease can impinge on the TM's ability to move normally or can invade the TM itself.

Dermatitis of the Canal Skin and Tympanic Membrane

Exfoliative dermatitis can cause sloughing of the skin of the EAC and outer layer of the TM with secondary infection. Both middle ear and external infections can cause thickening of the TM with calcified deposits or scarring that is visible years later and that can potentially affect the sound transmission properties of the TM. A chronically thickened and stiff TM that causes hearing loss may require tympanoplasty (replacement or reconstruction of the middle ear structures) to restore the compliant properties of the TM and improve hearing. Replacement of all or part of the TM with grafted material often results in improvement of the air–bone gap and can be undertaken in conjunction with a reconstruction of the ossicular chain when indicated.

Patients with seborrheic dermatitis of the scalp or other cutaneous areas can also have this condition develop in the skin of the EAC and external surface of the TM. Otitis externa that does not respond to the usual cleansing and topical treatments and that presents as dry, scaly skin with itching may be the result of seborrheic dermatitis. Eczema and fungal infections cause significant pruritus but are also associated with other signs. Weeping of the skin with crusting is seen in eczematous dermatitis, and a grayish membrane and fungal hyphae are seen with fungal infections. The treatment of seborrheic dermatitis of the EAC is similar to that for the scalp or any other skin involvement. Topical medications and shampoos are tried first. Tar preparations can be applied to a wick placed in the canal. All wicks placed in the EAC should be removed or changed every 7 to 10 days to avoid superinfection of the canal. Frequent cleanings under microscopic view may be necessary in refractory cases.

Myringitis

Infections of the EAC can involve the TM, causing a myringitis in the absence of otitis media (OM). Acute myringitis can also be the result of middle ear infections because the medial or innermost layer of the TM consists of mucosa in continuity with the middle ear mucosa. Acute myringitis is characterized by thickening of the TM with edema of the involved layer and increased vascularity. An inflammatory reaction with invasion of the layers of the TM by white blood cells is common in the presence of infection. Focal cell death by the pressure of a middle ear effusion or by local invasion of the TM itself by infecting organisms usually leads to TM perforation.

Treatment of myringitis is usually symptomatic, with analgesics and topical drops containing steroids to reduce the inflammation and associated pain. In the presence of middle ear disease and an intact TM, a systemic antibiotic taken orally is usually also prescribed.

Viral Myringitis

Bullae or blisters on the external surface of the TM are the result of acute inflammation often caused by viral disease like that seen with influenza virus. Serum and blood collect between the fibrous and squamous epithelial layers and are often, but not always, painful. The associated viral infection can lead to hearing loss by damaging the inner ear without causing lasting middle ear pathology. Treatment of viral myringitis is similar to that of bacterial myringitis in that topical medications are often required to make the patient more comfortable. In addition, opening the blisters and relieving pressure can speed recovery. When this is necessary, water precautions and topical antibiotic drops are prescribed until the TM reepithelializes to help prevent concurrent bacterial infection.

Tympanic Membrane Retractions and Middle Ear Atelectasis

Pathological processes affecting the TM most commonly arise from associated middle ear disease. They can lead to healing with scar or chronic perforations. A diseased TM usually causes some degree of hearing loss. Treatment of any underlying problems improves the success of treatment of the TM pathology.

Obstruction of the ET in the setting of chronic otitis media (COM) or otitis media with effusion (OME) leads to negative pressure in the middle ear and mastoid as gases and fluid are reabsorbed by the middle ear mucosa. This negative pressure pulls the TM inward. In some patients, as the TM is pulled back toward the ET, it slowly yields to this negative pressure, causing retraction pockets in areas of increased compliance within the TM. In severe cases, complete obliteration of the middle ear space can occur.

In middle ear atelectasis, the TM is pulled back onto the ossicles and exerts pressure on them, initially transmitting sound directly, but eventually increasing the stiffness of the ossicular chain and causing a conductive loss. Over time, the pressure of the TM on the ossicles compromises the blood supply to the long processes of the incus and malleus, resulting in erosion and, eventually, ossicular discontinuity. Thinning of the TM, from recurrent episodes of acute otitis media (AOM), causes it to become more susceptible to retraction and atelectasis. The TM goes through stages of retraction and atelectasis before it eventually becomes adherent to the bone of the promontory and ossicles with the absence of intervening middle ear mucosa. Once the TM adheres to the bone with no intervening mucosal surfaces, the condition is called adhesive otitis. Treatment of middle ear atelectasis before the adhesive stage is often initiated with myringotomy and tube insertion.

When the negative pressure acts only on areas of increased compliance within the TM (e.g., the pars flaccida or dimeric areas resulting from healed perforations), retraction pockets result. If the negative pressure is allowed to continue acting on these areas, the retractions will be pulled backward toward the mastoid antrum or into anatomical niches like the sinus tympani or ET orifice. Retraction of the TM into tight anatomical spaces leads to the formation of closed cystic spaces where the epithelium of the TM is trapped as it desquamates and eventually develops into a cholesteatoma.

Placement of a ventilating tube has been shown to reverse or arrest the progression of retractions of the TM (Sade et al, 1989). When a ventilating tube is unsuccessful, erosion of the ossicular chain or adhesive otitis is present; tympanoplasty is an option to re-create an aerated middle ear space with healthy mucosa. In situations in which the mastoid process has become sclerotic or contracted from COM, a mastoidectomy may be indicated to help aerate the middle ear and prevent recurrence of retraction and adhesion.

Tympanostomy Tubes

The placement of tympanostomy tubes has become a frequent therapy for chronic or recurrent OM and OME. These tubes act to hold open a surgically created opening in the TM and can sometimes lead to TM and middle ear disease, as well as help to eradicate them. The most common complications of tympanostomy tubes include failure of the TM to close after the tube falls out (or is removed) and chronic drainage from the tubes while they are in place. Drainage occurs either because the middle ear disease is persistent or because the tubes themselves are a source of irritation to the middle ear mucosa.

The choice of tympanostomy tube depends on the disease and the surgeon's preference. Tubes placed for chronic middle ear effusion should have a wide bore to allow drainage and are usually short. They drain fluid well but can easily become plugged by cerumen. Tubes placed for retractions and middle ear ventilation are fairly long and are less susceptible to plugging from cerumen but do not drain effusions as well. Typically, tubes last from 6 months to 1 year and are extruded from the TM. Tubes designed to last longer than 1 year have extended flanges that help to prevent extrusion. Occasionally, a tube will remain in place longer than the surgeon intended, and it will then be removed to allow the TM to heal the perforation. Tubes are removed when they are deemed no longer necessary or when they are causing problems such as chronic drainage in the absence of infection (**Fig. 9–5**).

Tympanic Membrane Perforation

Most TM perforations heal spontaneously regardless of their cause. Infection and trauma are by far the most common causes of TM perforation. Loss of a large portion of the TM or a prolonged or recurrent infection can lead to permanent TM perforations. Perforations are classified as (1) central perforations, which occur in the pars tensa and leave at least a rim of TM by the annulus intact; (2) marginal perforations, which also occur in the pars tensa and go up to or involve the annulus; and (3) attic perforations, which involve the pars flaccida at the superior aspect of the TM. Complications of TM perforations occur when the squamous epithelium of the external layer of the TM grows to cover the edge of the perforation, preventing its closure.

The degree of conductive hearing loss from a small TM perforation (in the presence of an otherwise normal middle ear) depends on the location of the perforation and on an individual's specific anatomy. Despite little conductive loss, small chronic dry perforations can cause other symptoms that lead a patient to choose surgical repair. A sensation of

fullness in an ear with a TM perforation is common and is uncomfortable for some patients. This can be due to a lack of TM mobility or changes in the middle ear mucosa from exposure to the external environment (e.g., changes in temperature and low humidity). Occasionally, patients may complain of intermittent ear pain associated with a chronic dry perforation. Discomfort with temperature extremes, especially cold air, is also reported by our patients. Patients will rarely complain of vertigo when cold air hits the exposed middle ear.

Small anterior perforations and perforations of the pars flaccida often cause little if any conductive loss if they do not interfere significantly with the middle ear transformer mechanism. Small dry perforations in the posterior quadrant can enable sound waves to bypass the middle ear transformer and act directly on the incudostapedial joint or the stapes footplate, with a resultant conductive hearing loss. Perforations that allow sound waves to access the round window directly can also cause a significant conductive hearing loss.

Medium and large central perforations of the TM usually cause hearing loss. The cause of the perforation will often determine the condition of the ossicular chain and middle ear mucosa. Dry medium or large perforations will usually permit visual inspection of the remainder of the middle ear, including the ossicles, under microscopic view. The symptoms of fullness, tinnitus, ear pain, and sensitivity to environmental changes are common with medium to large central perforations. In the absence of infection or ingrowth of squamous epithelium, these perforations should be watched carefully for the development of complications. The most immediate health concern in a patient with a chronic perforation of the TM is repeated or prolonged infection of the middle ear, associated drainage from the perforation, and chronic changes to the remaining TM and middle ear mucosa. Chronic or repeated infections of the middle ear cause damage to the blood supply and tissues of the TM, ossicles, and middle ear mucosa. This can result in an enlarging perforation, ossicular erosion, scarring, and tympanosclerosis, as well as the complications associated with AOM (e.g., meningitis). Patients with chronic TM perforation must be extremely careful to avoid moisture in the EAC and to treat the onset of infection aggressively. The second most immediate health concern is the growth of squamous epithelium around the edges of a perforation and into the middle ear. The presence of squamous epithelium in the middle ear invariably leads to the formation of cholesteatoma, either the creeping, spreading type or the formation of keratin pearls and cysts. Careful and frequent follow-up of chronic dry central perforations to monitor the middle ear space for the development of cholesteatoma is necessary.

Medical Management of Perforations

The medical management of draining perforations begins with cleaning under the microscope and topical antibiotic drops. Occasionally, acute purulent drainage or pain associated with drainage or water exposure is treated with oral antibiotics. Coverage for *Staphylococcus*, *Streptococcus*, and

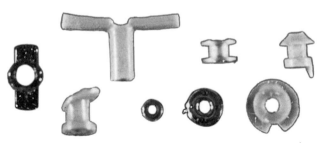

Figure 9–5 Examples of short- and long-acting tympanostomy tubes.

Pseudomonas, when appropriate, is required in these situations. Dilute acetic acid preparations and sterile irrigations can also be effective in curing an acute infection in the presence of a perforation.

Dry TM perforations can be managed with watchful waiting, depending on the individual circumstances. In the absence of infection, a perforation may require very little care to avoid complications. Avoidance of water or other substances that may potentially carry infection is critical. Swimming with earplugs in chlorinated or other disinfected water is allowed by some practitioners, but the patient must be prepared to treat any discomfort or drainage immediately to avoid a serious infection. The conductive hearing loss that often accompanies perforation of the TM can be treated with hearing aids if the patient chooses that option. Discomfort in an ear with a TM perforation exposing middle ear mucosa can be treated with plugging of the meatus to prevent temperature or humidity fluctuations from affecting the middle ear. Tinnitus can often be successfully treated with a hearing aid or other masking device. Long-term observation of perforations is necessary to evaluate for the development of cholesteatoma. Cholesteatoma can develop even in ears with long-standing stable perforations. The development of cholesteatoma requires surgery to avoid serious complications.

Surgical Management of Perforations

Once the patient decides on surgical closure of a chronic TM perforation, the surgeon must decide on the type of procedure and the approach. Options include TM grafting with and without ossicular reconstruction, cartilage grafting, and tympanomastoidectomy with or without ossicular reconstruction.

In a cooperative patient, myringoplasty or patching of a small (< 10%) chronic perforation can be attempted in the office setting. The TM is anesthetized with topical medication (phenol or topical anesthetic) or, alternatively, by canal injections of 2% lidocaine with 1:100,000 epinephrine. The edges of the perforation are freshened. A cigarette paper patch, piece of moist gelatin sponge, or fat from the earlobe is applied to the perforation. The patient is instructed to avoid Valsalva's maneuvers and to adhere to strict water precautions. The TM is followed at regular intervals to assess healing. If this method fails, or the situation is not amenable to patching, tympanoplasty is considered.

The principle behind tympanoplasty is a reconstruction of the sound-transmitting mechanism of the middle ear. Tympanoplasty involves re-creation of (1) an air-containing middle ear space; (2) a properly placed, intact, and vibratory TM; (3) an intact connection between the oval window and the TM; and, sometimes, (4) reconstruction of the EAC.

At present, the material of choice for tympanoplasty is temporalis fascia. This material provides a strong fibrous framework for epithelialization, is resistant to infection, will not be rejected by the patient's immune system, and results in a repair of nearly equal thickness to the original TM. Temporalis fascia can be easily manipulated into position and can be precisely shaped. Perichondrium is an excellent second choice when a cartilage graft will be used or if temporalis fascia is unavailable. Alternatively, vein grafts have been used with similar success rates to temporalis fascia. The main disadvantage of vein grafts is that a separate surgical field must be prepared.

Tympanoplasty can be performed through the EAC or through a postauricular approach. The choice of surgical approach for a small central TM perforation depends on the condition of the ossicles and on the location of the perforation. Perforations in the posterior half of the TM in the absence of mucosal disease can be approached through the canal (transcanal) provided the middle ear mucosa is normal and the ossicular chain is intact and mobile. Often the middle ear mucosa can be inspected under a high-power microscope through the existing perforation.

One way to determine the condition of the ossicular chain is by placing a temporary paper patch over the perforation. If the hearing is normal when the hole is patched, and the patient experiences no discomfort, tinnitus, or fullness, a normal middle ear beyond the known perforation is assumed. With a normal middle ear, repair of the perforation alone can successfully restore hearing to its premorbid state. Alternatively, the remainder of the middle ear can be evaluated by the placement of a thin, angled endoscope through the perforation to inspect the ossicular chain, middle ear mucosa, and ET orifice. CT scanning may also be used to evaluate aeration of the mastoid cavity and middle ear space.

Very anterior central perforations and situations in which the integrity of the ossicular chain and middle ear mucosa is in question require the postauricular approach. This type of approach provides a better angle of view for visualizing the anterior aspect of the middle ear space and enables the surgeon to evaluate and repair any ossicular pathology that may be present.

Once the approach and type of repair have been determined, preoperative audiograms are obtained, and the risks and benefits of surgery are discussed in detail with the patient. The risks of surgery include sensorineural hearing loss, tinnitus that may appear or worsen after surgery, failure of the TM graft, injury to the facial nerve, infection, bleeding, and reaction to the anesthetic.

Whether the TM repair is performed through the canal or through the postauricular approach, the principles of tympanoplasty remain the same. These principles include the creation of a framework that bridges the perforation and is stable. This framework acts to allow the migration of healthy epithelium along with an adequate vascular supply that will restore the middle ear transformer in a sterile environment. The achievement of these principles depends on (1) the freshening of the edges of the perforation to stimulate new blood supply and epithelial growth, (2) a framework that is resistant itself to infection and that will survive until a local blood supply is established, (3) adequate coverage of the perforation without slippage of the graft, and (4) the creation of an aerated middle ear space free of infection with healthy middle ear mucosa. Given the best-case scenario, ~90% of perforations will be successfully closed on the first surgical attempt.

For successful tympanoplasty, the surgery should be performed in a sterile environment, usually in an operating room. Injections of epinephrine solution are made within the canal skin to help prevent excessive bleeding. The perforation is visualized with a microscope, and the edges of the perforation are freshened or removed. The middle ear mucosa on the underside of the TM is roughened to encourage adhesion of the graft and epithelial growth of the mucosa along the underside of the graft. Incisions in the canal skin are made to allow elevation of the TM and annulus from the bony tympanic ring while preserving a strip of canal skin attached laterally. If the middle ear is accessed through the postauricular approach, the incision behind the ear is carried to the edge of the bony EAC. The skin of the posterior EAC is then elevated to the level of the canal incisions. The remaining canal skin and annulus are then elevated to the level of the malleus handle and turned forward to provide adequate visualization of the middle ear space and ossicular chain. Key to the procedure is visualization of the underside of the TM anterior to the perforation to ensure placement of the graft well beyond the margins of the perforation.

The middle ear is packed with a dissolvable gelatin sponge to hold the graft in place while it adheres to the TM remnant. The ET orifice is often packed with the gelatin sponge as well to prevent negative pressure on the graft during the healing and epithelialization process. The gelatin sponge will take 2 to 4 weeks to dissolve, and its presence contributes to an initial conductive hearing loss.

For an underlay technique, the graft material is then cut to the appropriate size, placed on top of the gelatin sponge, and tucked underneath the remaining TM. The graft is shaped to extend along the posterior bony canal wall beyond the original canal incision. The reflected TM with the annulus still attached is then unfolded on top of the graft. The posterior canal skin (created during the initial incisions) is placed on top of the new TM graft, helping to secure it in place and providing a blood supply and source of squamous epithelium. Care is taken to unravel all the edges of the TM remnants and the canal skin. The canal is then packed to hold all the elements in place. Choices for packing include dissolvable gelatin sponge, antibiotic ointment, expanding cellulose sponges, and gauze strips. If a postauricular incision has been used, it is closed at this time, and the ear is dressed with a mastoid dressing. For the transcanal approach, packing of the canal is adequate to control any bleeding, and the donor site is covered with a sterile dressing.

Large central perforations, such as those resulting from long-standing chronic infection, tuberculosis (TB), or slag burns to the TM, may be repaired with a similar underlay technique, provided there remains an anterior remnant of TM to anchor the graft. More frequently, larger perforations will leave little viable TM remnant and will require an overlay graft technique. In skilled hands, the overlay and underlay techniques have equal failure and complication rates, and the choice of technique is entirely based on the anatomy of the remaining TM and the surgeon's preference. Overlay grafting requires the presence of at least some of the malleus handle to keep the graft from lateralizing in the canal.

The overlay technique requires a postauricular approach and drilling of the bony anterior canal wall bulge to completely visualize the anterior annulus. Removal of the anterior canal wall skin and its later replacement as a free skin graft allow drilling of the anterior canal wall while maintaining its epithelial covering. All squamous epithelium must be denuded from the TM remnant to prevent trapping of epithelium and subsequent intratympanic cholesteatoma from forming.

Temporalis fascia is used as the grafting material and must be cut to fit the edges of the annulus in the anterior canal exactly. The fascia graft is tucked underneath the handle of the malleus and then pulled up on top of the denuded annulus. Gelfoam within the middle ear space holds the graft lateral to the promontory, and the canal is packed to hold the graft in its placed position. Overlay graft techniques are also used for anterior perforations with too little anterior remnant to support an underlay graft.

Tympanoplasty with ossicular reconstruction is performed when damage has occurred to the ossicular chain and to the TM. Regardless of the cause, erosions of the ossicular processes can occur without affecting the overall function of the ossicular chain or causing hearing loss. When the mobility or continuity of the ossicular chain is compromised, however, ossicular reconstruction becomes an important option. Adequate exposure of the middle ear is necessary to evaluate and reconstruct the middle ear. Therefore, tympanoplasty with ossicular reconstruction is usually performed through a postauricular incision.

The lenticular process of the incus has a tenuous blood supply that is easily compromised by chronic infection; therefore, the incus is the most common ossicle to require replacement. The choice of which ossicular reconstruction device is used is made based on the repair needed and the surgeon's preference **(Fig. 9–6)**. Often the damage to the ossicles cannot be fully assessed before surgery, and the choice of prosthetic cannot be made until the surgeon has explored the middle ear.

Pearl

- Repair of a perforated TM does not ensure improvement of a conductive hearing loss.
- Pathology within the middle ear does not always cause hearing loss.
- Because of poorer ET function, young children have a lower expected rate of success for tympanoplasty than adults do.
- Surgery may be recommended to prevent future pathology, even in the presence of normal hearing.

◆ Pathological Conditions of the Eustachian Tube

The most common type of ET dysfunction is obstruction. Because the ET is actively opened, disease affecting the ET tends to prevent the opening of the ET and frequently leads to disease of the middle ear and mastoid.

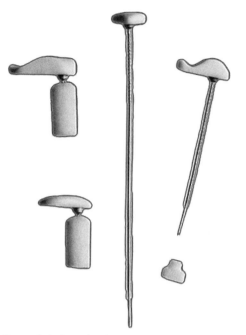

Figure 9–6 Ossicular chain prostheses. (*Right top and center*) Total ossicular replacement prostheses (from stapes footplate to tympanic membrane [TM] or malleus). (*Right bottom*) Incudostapedial joint prosthesis. (*Left top and bottom*) Partial ossicular replacement prostheses (from head of stapes to TM or malleus handle).

Patulous Eustachian Tube

In abnormal patency of the ET, the ET is open at rest or, to a lesser extreme, has a lower opening pressure than normal. This can lead to a higher incidence of OM because nasal secretions have easier access to the middle ear than with normal ET function. Nose blowing, sniffing, sneezing, and crying all create pressure at the ET opening, which may be greater than the opening pressures of a patulous ET, resulting in the forced entry of nasal secretions into the middle ear space.

Symptoms of a patulous ET consist of hearing respiratory noises in the ear, tinnitus, and paradoxical stuffiness in the affected ear. Autophony (hearing one's own voice echoing in the ear) is the most common complaint with patulous ET. Exercise, loss of weight, and fatigue aggravate the symptoms. They improve with nasal stuffiness, as seen with allergy or upper respiratory infection. TM movements in synchrony with respirations can be seen on physical examination. In some patients, the autophony is so loud that it interferes with normal hearing (Falk and Magnuson, 1984). A careful history will distinguish dysacusis (distorted hearing) from true autophony.

Weight loss is the most common cause of a patulous ET. As little as 6 pounds of weight loss can cause a loss of tissue mass in the peritubal area, potentially leading to patulous ET (Pulec, 1967). Pregnancy has been found to be associated with patulous ET (the cause of this association is unclear at this time). Scarring of the nasopharynx (as seen in radiation treatments), atrophy of nasopharyngeal muscles (as seen in multiple sclerosis and cerebral palsy), and dysfunction of

the tensor veli palatine are also thought to be contributors to the cause of patulous ET.

Tympanograms can document mobility of the TM during respiration, indicating that the ET is not closing passively, as is seen with normal physiology. Treatment of a patulous ET is offered in severe cases only. Such treatment includes placement of irritating substances into the ET orifice at the nasopharynx to cause scarring within the tube and to decrease its patency (Virtanen and Palva, 1982). Injection of space-occupying tissues, such as fat, into the wall of the cartilaginous ET through the nasopharynx has also been tried (Doherty and Slattery, 2003) Obliteration of the ET orifice within the middle ear can be a permanent solution if the condition is severely disturbing the patient's ability to function (Dyer and McElveen, 1991). ET obliteration requires concomitant placement of a permanent tympanostomy tube to avoid chronic effusion and to avoid barotrauma to the middle ear.

Palatal Myoclonus

Because of the anatomical connections between the ET and the palatal muscles, a condition known as palatal myoclonus, or chronic spasm of the palate, can lead to opening and closing of the ET. This causes a sensation of clicking or a pulsating tinnitus. Treatment of the palatal muscles leads to resolution of the symptoms. This may involve partial paralysis of these muscles with botulinum toxin injections or use of antispasmodic, antiseizure, or muscle-relaxing medications.

Eustachian Tube Obstruction

Anatomical ET obstruction occurs with pathology in the nasopharynx that obstructs the nasopharyngeal opening of the ET. Tumors of the nasopharynx and other tumors extending into the nasopharynx can obstruct the ET. Hypertrophy of the lymphoid tissue, normally present at the nasopharyngeal orifice of the ET, and hypertrophy of the adenoid bed can occur with chronic infections, diseases that cause lymphoid hypertrophy, lymphoma, leukemia, and immunodeficiency syndromes.

The ET can also be obstructed in the nasopharynx by scarring of the orifice due to radiation treatments, inadvertent injury during adenoidectomy, or other nasopharyngeal surgeries. Chronic infections such as sinusitis can cause hypertrophy and polyp formation within the mucosa of the nasopharynx, creating obstruction as well.

Anomalies of the muscles that would normally open the ET orifice in the nasopharynx can also effectively act as an anatomical obstruction to the ET opening. Such anomalies are seen with craniofacial syndromes, clefting of the palate, musculoskeletal syndromes, and neurological syndromes.

Treatment of ET obstruction usually involves treatment of the associated middle ear disease that invariably accompanies such obstruction. Placement of tympanostomy tubes is the most common otologic treatment. Treatment of the diseases of the nasopharynx causing obstruction of the nasopharyngeal orifice of the ET can lead to resolution of the obstruction and normal ET function. Improvement of ET function after cleft palate repair is an example of this. Adenoidectomy is frequently recommended when the adenoids obstruct the nasopharynx.

Special Consideration

- Patulous ET syndrome is treated only in severe cases.
- ET dysfunction can be caused by nasopharyngeal disease. More commonly, it results from recurrent middle ear infection.
- Medical treatment of ET dysfunction seeks to normalize the respiratory tract mucosa.
- Surgical treatment of ET dysfunction usually includes tympanostomy tubes.
- Tympanostomy tubes relieve the symptoms of ET dysfunction but only rarely improve long-term ET function.

♦ Mucosal Disease

Mucosal diseases can affect the ability of the middle ear to clear infection or effusions. These diseases can cause disruption of the normal transformer function of the middle ear, resulting in conductive hearing loss and chronic symptoms for the patient. They can also lead to serious complications and pathology beyond the middle ear.

Otitis Media and Effusions

Otitis media with effusion is defined as persistent fluid in the middle ear space after an episode of AOM. OME can also be seen in the setting of recurrent or frequent infections, ET obstruction, or mucosal disease in the absence of prior infection. Middle ear effusion is identified by pneumotoscopic examination and can cause a conductive hearing loss in some patients. Up to 90% of children will clear a middle ear effusion within 3 months of an OM, with most clearing their effusions within 1 month (Teele et al, 1980).

Evaluation of the circumstances contributing to the presence and persistence of fluid in the middle ear is essential when deciding on the treatment options. ET dysfunction, either from a stable anatomical abnormality or from local mucosal changes caused by a particular disease process, is the most common cause for effusion in the middle ear. The fluid can be serous (thin and transparent), mucoid (thick and transparent), or mucopurulent (thick and opaque that indicates infected or infected secretions). OME is more frequent in the winter months when upper respiratory infections occur more often. The presence of virus in the upper respiratory tract causes inflammation in the middle ear, ET and nasal mucosa. This can cause dysfunction of the ET and help prevent clearance of fluid from the middle ear space. Viral infections can present in the middle ear as AOM in the absence of other upper respiratory symptoms. Alternatively, OME can occur in association with an upper respiratory viral infection in the absence of any otologic symptoms of infection.

The effusion resulting from a single episode of AOM or acute upper respiratory illness is initially treated with watchful waiting. Because 90% of children with an acute effusion will clear it within 3 months (Teele et al, 1980), effusions that persist longer should be considered for treatment. Children with symptoms associated with their effusions (unsteadiness, vertigo, discomfort, and hearing loss are the most commonly reported symptoms) are often treated more aggressively, with earlier use of medical or surgical management to help clear the effusion.

Clinical practice guidelines on OME in children have been published by the U.S. Department of Health and Human Services (Rosenfeld et al, 2004). The specific management depends on the patient's medical history and the type of effusion present.

With moderate to severe symptoms, children are offered myringotomy with or without tube placement, depending on their prior otologic history and the presence of other confounding factors. Children may have frequent AOM develop in the presence or absence of middle ear effusion. Frequent infections with clearing of any fluid in the intervals between infections define recurrent AOM. Recurrent AOM has also been implicated in language delay and decreased quality of life for children. Recurrent AOM or OME in the presence of adenoid hypertrophy warrants consideration of adenoidectomy (removal of the lymphoid tissue pad from the posterior wall of the nasopharynx) in addition to myringotomy and the placement of tubes. Chronic adenoiditis can be a source of both viral and bacterial middle ear pathogens. The performance of adenoidectomy in conjunction with myringotomy and tubes has become common. Recent randomized trials have shown minimal benefit in children younger than 4 years old (Hammaren-Malmi et al, 2005) and benefit only in patients in whom the adenoidal tissue actually abuts the opening of the ET in the nasopharynx (Nguyen et al, 2004).

Effusions of the mucoid or mucopurulent type are thicker and can be more difficult to clear. Mucoid and mucopurulent effusions may be a sign of underlying mucosal or systemic disease. Mucosal disease and anatomical obstructions should be treated when possible.

Clinical Guidelines for Otitis Media with Effusion in Children

The most recent clinical guidelines as of this volume's publication date advocate distinguishing children at risk for speech or learning problems from low-risk individuals. Low-risk children can be treated with watchful waiting for 3 months. Moderate- to high-risk children with OME and those with OME that persists past 3 months need audiometric evaluation and follow-up evaluations with an otolaryngologist. Abnormalities of the TM or middle ear on otoscopy and any hearing loss that is clinically significant should prompt consideration of surgical intervention with myringotomy and tube placement. Tympanostomy tubes have definitively been shown to be more effective than antibiotic prophylaxis. Antihistamines and decongestants have been shown to be ineffective as a treatment for OME. Antibiotics and steroids are not recommended (Rosenfeld et al, 2004).

Controversial Point

- At least one study has shown no benefit of adenoidectomy in children under 4 years old who required tubes for OME (Hammaren-Malmi et al, 2005).
- Despite the above guidelines, steroids continue to be used by many practitioners.

Pitfall

- Chronic OME has not been shown to respond significantly to antibiotics.
- OME can cause language delay in young children and should be aggressively managed.
- OME can exist in the absence of a history of AOM.
- Antibiotics for OME in children should be considered short term, and only in patients with signs and symptoms of bacterial infection.
- The overuse of antibiotics for OM is believed to contribute significantly to the increasing prevalence of antibiotic-resistant bacteria in OM.
- Because large clinical trials have not shown consistent benefit, steroid use for OME should be based on individual patient considerations only.

Acute Bacterial Otitis Media and Mastoiditis

Bacterial invasion of the middle ear space can occur by way of the ET, through a perforation, or by direct invasion of the TM. The development of an infection, after such an invasion has occurred, depends on several factors. These include the degree of the immune response of the host to the invasion, the virulence of the invading organism, and the effectiveness of the treatment given. The range of acute infection extends from mild inflammation (e.g., OME) with few symptoms to severe suppuration with necrosis of tissues and possible inner ear and intracranial complications that can threaten the patient's hearing and even the patient's life.

The most common bacteria causing AOM are *Streptococcus, Staphylococcus,* and *Moraxella* infections. Even more frequent are viral infections of the middle ear space. Purulent bacterial AOM is often treated with antibiotics. In cases where infection is not responsive to first-line therapy, tympanocentesis (drawing out of fluid from the middle ear with a needle) can help relieve pressure buildup behind the TM and provide a means of identifying the responsible microbial agent. Frequent infections are often treated more

aggressively with newer antibiotics; failure of resolution of pain, erythema, or fever warrants a change in medications or a switch to intravenous therapy to prevent complications. Despite the high incidence of AOM, true emergencies arising from complications of AOM have become rare. Most patients with OM will resolve their infections without sequelae. Because the overuse of antibiotics in the community has resulted in the increasing development of antibiotic-resistant strains, the use of prophylactic antibiotics should be limited (Poole, 1998). Children who are still acquiring language and who also have frequent or severe infections should be referred to an otolaryngologist for workup and treatment. Tympanostomy tubes are strongly recommended in such patients (Bergus and Lofgren, 1998). It is believed that avoidance of exposing children to unnecessary courses of multiple drugs can help to reduce the rate of antibiotic-resistant bacterial strains in the community.

Patient-related factors associated with an increased incidence of AOM include unrepaired cleft palate, craniofacial abnormalities, immune deficiency syndromes, ciliary dysfunction, nasotracheal or nasogastric intubation, and nasal obstruction. Cleft palate is a congenital deformity in which the two shelves of the palate do not fuse during development, resulting in improper alignment of the muscles involved in palatal function. Some of the muscles of the palate (tensor and levator veli palatine) insert on the nasal end of the ET, resulting in opening of the ET during elevation of the palate, as in swallowing. When the palatal muscles are misaligned, as in cleft palate, they cannot act effectively on the ET and result in ET dysfunction. Surgical correction of palatal clefts often results in improved ET function. Pathological conditions that may have developed before a surgical correction for cleft palate are not always reversible, and OM or chronic problems related to ET dysfunction may persist. Craniofacial abnormalities are also associated with increased incidence of AOM. They often are associated with cleft palate but also contribute separately to AOM by altering the anatomical relationships of the middle ear, ET, and nasopharynx.

Edema, acute inflammatory cell invasion, and engorgement of the vascular structures of the middle ear mucosa cause thickening of the TM and local obstruction of the ET orifice in the middle ear. The cilia of the middle ear and ET are often damaged by these changes in the mucosa, and this destruction of cilia further hampers the clearance of secretions and debris from the middle ear space. Intubation of the nasopharynx obstructs the normal clearance of secretions from the nasopharynx and allows backflow of infected secretions, increasing the likelihood of infection of the middle ear space.

Complications of Otitis Media

Most acute infections will resolve without any permanent changes to the middle ear structures or mucosa. If, however, infections become recurrent or chronic, irreversible pathological changes can occur. These changes can involve the TM, middle ear mucosa, or ossicles. Severe complications of acute bacterial infections include bacterial invasion of the inner ear through the round window membrane, facial nerve infection with facial weakness, thrombosis of the sigmoid sinus, extradural abscess, and brain abscess.

Prolonged, inadequately treated, or severe infection can lead to resorption of bone and facial paralysis after osteitic invasion with mastoiditis, ossicular destruction, and exposure of the dura to bacterial invasion. Evidence of destruction of the mastoid's trabeculated bone on radiographic studies is an indication for surgical intervention. Patients may present with destruction of the mastoid cortex by an infective focus with edema, pain, and inflammation of the overlying skin, and subperiosteal abscess formation. Infection that breaks through the mastoid cortex and tracks down into the neck forms Bezold's abscess.

Treatment of these serious complications involves complete eradication of the infecting organisms. Intravenous antibiotics, surgical removal of infected bone and tissue (debridement), wide-field myringotomy, drainage of abscesses, and removal of infected clot are all part of the treatment armamentarium of these life-threatening complications. Bacterial or suppurative labyrinthitis can lead to encephalitis or meningitis and is frequently treated aggressively with emergency labyrinthectomy (surgical exenteration of the labyrinth). This procedure, although it causes unilateral deafness, can be lifesaving. Patients with acute coalescent mastoiditis may also require surgical treatment if intravenous antibiotics fail to provide a rapid eradication of the infection. Severe complications of OM occur in < 3% of children with AOM (Culpepper, 1997).

Special Consideration

- Normal ciliary function is necessary for mucosal and middle ear health.
- Craniofacial anomalies are associated with an increased incidence of OM.
- The most common bacteria causing AOM are *Streptococcus, Staphylococcus,* and *Moraxella.*
- Resistant strains of *Streptococcus* in the community limit the effectiveness of many commonly used antibiotics for OM.
- Despite a vast array of antibiotics, complications of OM continue to occur.
- Complications from bacterial OM can be life threatening and may require emergency surgery.

Chronic Otitis Media and Cholesteatoma

Infections that persist longer than 6 weeks are, by definition, chronic infections. COM can cause changes to the TM. Often chronic infections result in perforations to the TM, either with or without chronic drainage. The perforation can range from pinpoint to a total loss of the membrane. The severity of the infection is not necessarily related to the perforation size. Changes to the membrane, other than perforation, can be evident on otoscopic examination, with thickening, hypervascularity, scarring, retractions, and loss of the normal landmarks.

Chronic infections involve the mastoid cavity and are often characterized by drainage from a perforated TM. When they organize within the middle ear or mastoid, such infections may develop into what is called a cholesterol granuloma—a locally destructive process. Foul-smelling drainage is a sign of anaerobic infection or *Pseudomonas* infection. Granulation tissue, polypoid mucosal changes, and local edema are all frequently seen in the setting of chronic infection. Granulations forming on dura through dehiscences of the tegmen indicate infection of the epidural space. Aggressive treatment with intravenous antibiotics, mastoid debridement, and close follow-up is needed.

Cholesteatoma formation is commonly associated with COM. Cholesteatoma arises from trapped squamous epithelium within the temporal bone. Congenital cholesteatomas are thought to arise in the absence of infection. They originate in epithelial rests sequestered within the temporal bone during embryonic development. Most cholesteatomas are acquired (secondary), with squamous epithelium implanted or extending into the temporal bone through a perforation. Deep retraction pockets in the TM, as a result of ET obstruction, can also lead to entrapment of squamous epithelium into the recesses of the middle ear or through the attic into the mastoid, resulting in cholesteatoma. As the top layers of the trapped epithelium shed or desquamate, the accumulated keratin debris collects to form a cyst. This cholesteatoma cyst continues to expand as long as the epithelial lining is viable. Expansion of the cyst leads to pressure and destruction on the surrounding bone.

Infection of cholesteatoma either through a TM perforation or in conjunction with an acquired OM cannot be adequately treated with antibiotics and topical medications, primarily because no blood flows to the center of a cholesteatoma. Collagenases and other substances produced at the edge of the cyst prevent local scarring from impeding its growth. Cholesteatoma, left without treatment, will erode through the mastoid cortex, destroy the ossicles, and invade the oval and round windows and the otic capsule, causing sensorineural hearing loss and vertigo. Chronic ear drainage that does not clear up with medical therapy should initiate a search for a hidden cholesteatoma within the mastoid or attic space.

Cholesteatoma has also been shown to erode through the tegmen, invade the dura, and eventually the brain. Fistulas of the semicircular canals, uncovering of the bone of the facial nerve, and invasion into the facial nerve are commonly found in patients with extensive or long-standing cholesteatomas. These patients rarely have facial nerve symptoms but have intermittent vertigo and sensorineural hearing loss. Further sensorineural hearing loss and injury to the facial nerve can occur during removal of cholesteatoma.

Cholesteatoma originating in the middle ear space can erode through the attic and tympanic ring and present within the EAC or at the level of the TM. Often the drainage and discomfort associated with an infected cholesteatoma are the first clues to its presence. COM and cholesteatoma are frequently seen together. Untreated cholesteatoma can lead to significant morbidity and mortality. Currently, no medical therapy is available for cholesteatoma.

Surgical Treatment of Chronic Otitis Media and Cholesteatoma

Mastoidectomy or surgical exenteration of the mastoid air cells and opening of the antrum is the basic operation offered for complicated OM, COM, and cholesteatoma. In the case of complications from OM, the goal of surgery is to remove areas of infection and provide aeration to the mastoid and middle ear space with a minimum of morbidity for the patient. For cholesteatoma, surgical goals include complete eradication of squamous debris or exteriorization of the epithelium to prevent accumulation or formation of future cholesteatoma cysts, eradication of infection, and, when possible, repair or reconstruction of the middle ear mechanism.

An operating drill is used to open the mastoid cortex just behind the auricle and to carefully and systematically clean out any areas of trapped infected secretions. Landmarks for this dissection include the bony posterior canal wall, the thin layer of bone over the dura of the temporal lobe, and the sigmoid sinus. Once all these landmarks have been identified and fully defined, the dissection is continued through Körner's septum to expose the antrum.

Within the antrum of the mastoid, the horizontal semicircular canal can usually be found protruding laterally at the level of the vertical facial nerve. As the antrum is opened widely, the short process of the incus can be seen within the fossa incudis. In the case of serious infection or suspected extensive cholesteatoma, the facial recess is often carefully opened to further help aerate the middle ear and to visualize the tympanic recess. This is the area where infection and cholesteatoma can hide, causing recurrence or failure to eradicate disease, but it is also the area where the facial nerve is at most risk for injury during mastoid surgery. Often, in acute disease and during the first surgery for moderate cholesteatoma or COM, the canal wall is left intact. If all the disease can be removed, a canal wall intact procedure will leave the patient with the potential for normal middle ear function.

Tympanoplasty to reconstruct a damaged ossicular chain is commonly deferred in the case of acute infection or extensive cholesteatoma. It can be attempted concurrently in an ear with COM if minimal infection is present and the surgeon believes there has been complete removal of all cholesteatoma. (See the section on tympanoplasty.)

In ears that have failed previous surgical attempts at cure and in ears with extensive cholesteatoma invading critical structures (facial nerve, oval window, the labyrinth, or involving the dura), the canal wall is taken down to exteriorize the mastoid bowl and any remaining cholesteatoma matrix. Complete removal of the contents of the middle ear and closure of the ET orifice along with a canal wall down mastoidectomy constitutes a radical mastoidectomy. Middle ear reconstruction is rarely successful when a radical mastoidectomy had been performed.

When preservation or reconstruction of a middle ear space and ossicular chain with canal wall down mastoidectomy can be accomplished, the operation is termed a modified radical tympanomastoidectomy, and the ET is left open. The extent of the surgical procedure is determined by the balance of preservation of the hearing mechanism and the risk of a recurrence or serious complication of the disease process.

Special Consideration

- Cholesteatoma is an invasion of squamous epithelium into the temporal bone structures where it is normally not present.
- The optimal treatment for cholesteatoma and COM is tympanomastoidectomy.
- Attempts are made, where possible, to reconstruct the middle ear.
- Cholesteatoma, causing facial nerve, dural, or labyrinthine dehiscence, or that involves the oval or round windows, or the ET, necessitates surgery that is more radical.
- Cholesteatoma within the facial recess can be treated with a modified radical tympanomastoidectomy or with a facial recess approach, leaving the canal wall intact.
- A radical mastoidectomy does not leave any middle ear space and usually results in a maximal conductive hearing loss.

Tympanosclerosis

Chronic infections or other chronic inflammatory conditions of the TM and middle ear mucosa cause submucosal and subepithelial fibrosis and thickening. Deposits of hyalin and calcium called tympanosclerosis appear on the TM and within the middle ear mucosa as white patches and can lead to a change in compliance of the TM and middle ear transformer. Occasionally, new bony formations can occur within the TM in association with this process. Coalescent tympanosclerosis involving a significant portion of the pars tensa or extending to the ossicular chain can be a major cause for conductive hearing loss in affected individuals.

Tympanosclerotic patches of the TM are avascular and will not be able to provide a blood supply to a graft. If tympanoplasty is contemplated for a perforation in the presence of significant tympanosclerosis of the TM remnant, that involved remnant will need to be replaced. The placement of a larger graft and the presence of well-vascularized epithelial strips are required in this situation to avoid postoperative failure of the repair. If most of the TM is involved with tympanosclerosis, a lateral graft technique with complete replacement of the diseased TM is usually required for successful repair.

For successful hearing restoration, tympanosclerosis within the middle ear mucosa must be removed when it immobilizes the ossicular chain or obstructs the oval or round windows. No specific medical management exists for the prevention or treatment of tympanosclerosis of the TM or middle ear mucosa. Timely treatment of AOM with systemic antibiotics may be effective in reducing the amount of TM scarring resulting from recurrent infection and thus in the resultant amount of tympanosclerosis. Ossicular replacement prostheses are used when tympanosclerosis fixes the ossicular chain, necessitating removal of the involved ossicles for hearing restoration.

◆ Ossicular Disease

Ossicular disease can present in the setting of OM, as an isolated event or as part of a systemic disease. The TM is commonly normal, and clues to the presence of the disease are based on the patient's history and on audiometric examinations coupled with the physical examination.

Otosclerosis

Otosclerosis (OS) is a disease of the stapes footplate and bony labyrinth. It usually presents in the second or third decade of life. This disease is often noted only when stapes involvement causes hearing loss. A familial association has been shown in some cases (Larsson, 1960). OS is bilateral in more than 80% of affected individuals, with slight female predominance (Cawthorne, 1955). It can progress more rapidly during pregnancy (Gristwood and Venables, 1983). Disease involving the oval window will commonly cause fixation of the footplate with an associated conductive hearing loss. Early in OS, fibrous connections develop between the oval window niche and the bony footplate, causing a mild conductive hearing loss. As bony ankylosis of the stapes footplate occurs, a conductive hearing loss of up to 40 dB is seen. Fixation of the anterior portion of the footplate is the most common lesion seen at surgery. Because OS can involve the bony labyrinth, sensorineural losses and vestibular disturbances are also seen in some patients with OS.

On microscopic examination of otosclerotic lesions, the initial process involves resorption of bone around vessels replaced by abnormal, immature, collagen-poor bone. This remodeling of bone progresses irregularly, creating foci of OS within the normal bone. The resorption of bone with increased perivascular spaces is the "active" or spongiotic phase of the disease. These increased perivascular spaces form connections with the submucosal vessels, resulting in increased blood flow and an increase in the capillary vessels within the submucosa. It is this increase in capillary vessels that is responsible for Schwartze's sign, a reddish hue on the promontory seen through the TM indicating active disease. The increase in blood flow over the promontory also can cause tinnitus. As the new collagen-deficient bone matures, the bone becomes sclerotic.

Within a single portion of the labyrinth, both active and mature regions of OS may exist. In some patients, bone within the cochlea becomes involved, causing sensorineural hearing loss by encroaching on the nerve fibers (Richter and Schuknecht, 1982; Sando et al, 1974). Sensorineural hearing loss is also thought to occur through inner ear damage by inflammatory mediators released by otosclerotic foci within the labyrinth. Seven percent of temporal bones examined by Schuknecht and Barber (1985) had involvement of the round window niche by otosclerotic lesions. Such lesions

can lead to greater air–bone gaps than expected from ossicular fixation alone. Once a patient notices significant handicap from progressive hearing loss caused by OS, he or she comes to the attention of the audiologist and otolaryngologist. The range of disease that can cause conductive pathological conditions includes isolated foci of OS at the anterior or posterior edge of the oval window, bipolar involvement at both ends of the footplate, narrowing of the oval window niche, and complete obliteration of the round window niche by otosclerotic bone.

The actual diagnosis of OS fixing the stapes can be confirmed only at surgery. Once the stapes is fixed, a round window reflex (seen on palpation of a mobile and intact ossicular chain) is absent. Surgical options for mature disease have ranged from lateral semicircular canal fenestration and stapes mobilization procedures in the first half of the 20th century to the stapedectomy and small fenestra stapedotomy procedures that are commonly practiced today. Whenever possible, small fenestra stapedotomy is performed because it provides the best result with the smallest surgical risk. The stapedotomy technique can be performed with the patient under local or general anesthesia, depending on the surgeon's and patient's preference. Incisions are made, and a tympanomeatal flap of canal wall skin in continuity with the TM is elevated. The fibrous annulus is then elevated from the tympanic ring, and the entire flap with the posterior portion of the TM is reflected anteriorly. This opens the middle ear space just over the incudostapedial joint in the posterosuperior quadrant. If an overhang of the bony tympanic ring obscures the view of the oval window, it must be drilled or curetted away.

Successful placement of the fenestra of the footplate and of the stapes prosthesis depends on direct visualization of the incudostapedial joint and the oval window niche. Once the stapedial tendon is in view, the surgeon will have an adequate view of the posterior footplate. The ossicular chain is then palpated to determine whether the ossicles are mobile. Lack of footplate mobility and lack of a round window reflex together confirm a fixed footplate.

Once the diagnosis has been established, the operation proceeds to a stapedotomy. If the OS has completely obliterated the oval window niche, and its location (along with the location of the facial nerve running above the oval window) cannot be precisely determined, the surgeon may close without proceeding with the stapedotomy. If the round window niche is completely obliterated by otosclerotic disease, the surgery will also be aborted. Such situations often prevent correction of the hearing loss despite otherwise excellent technique, and the risk/reward ratio for the surgery becomes unacceptable. An aberrant facial nerve that crosses the footplate or courses between the crura of the stapes will also cause the surgeon to consider terminating the surgery. This situation puts the facial nerve at risk for injury during placement of the prosthesis.

Once the surgeon chooses to proceed with stapedotomy, the next step is to remove the stapes superstructure. This is accomplished by cutting the stapedial tendon, separating the incudostapedial joint, and fracturing the stapes suprastructure. A laser is often used for these procedures because it is precise, hemostatic, and does not create pressure on the

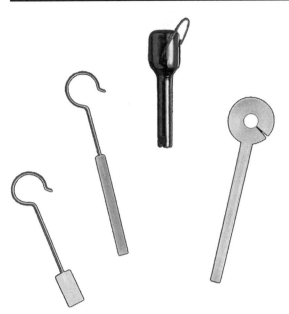

Figure 9–7 Examples of different stapes prostheses.

footplate. These elements help to prevent complications during surgery.

The distance from the footplate to the long process of the incus is measured, and a hole is then made with a laser, or a small drill, in the posterior portion of the footplate. Care is taken to use the laser just to vaporize the bone over the vestibule and to avoid penetration of the perilymph by the laser light. The stapedotomy is then enlarged with a rasp or with picks to ~0.8 mm. A stapes prosthesis is then placed into the stapedotomy hole and crimped around the long process of the incus. This re-creates a connection between the TM and the vestibule. Proper sizing of the prosthesis is critical to a good result, and each manufacturer's prosthesis is sized differently. Finally, a soft tissue seal is created around the base of the prosthesis (see **Fig. 9–7** for different types of prosthetics). As with all conductive pathological conditions, the patient may forgo surgery and purchase hearing aids.

Pearl

- OS can be inherited.
- Progression of disease is frequently associated with progressive hearing loss.
- Small fenestra stapedectomy is currently the surgical treatment of choice.
- OS involving the round window or obliterating the oval window niche is usually nonoperative.

Ossicular Erosion

Air–bone gaps of 50 dB or more are a sign of ossicular discontinuity or immobility, especially in the presence of abnormal TM. Ossicular discontinuity can be the result of trauma or loss of the blood supply to bone caused by infection, cholesteatoma, or tympanosclerosis. Occasionally, a retraction of the TM onto the head of the stapes will bypass an ossicular discontinuity, resulting in near normal hearing despite significant middle ear pathology.

COM commonly leads to erosion or resorption of parts of the ossicles. Pathologically, the inflammatory reaction of the mucosa to chronic infection can extend to involve the ossicles, causing an osteitis (or direct inflammatory reaction within the bone). The lenticular process of the incus is at greatest risk for resorption once osteitis occurs because of its relatively poor blood supply. Once a significant amount of bone is lost from the long process of the incus, the result is ossicular discontinuity. Occasionally, ossicular discontinuity exists in the absence of infection. A severe blow to the head can dislocate the ossicles as a result of transmitted force alone or associated with a temporal bone fracture. The incus is most often dislocated during trauma. Fractures of the stapes superstructure or of the malleus neck can occur with more severe head traumas.

Ossicular discontinuity is also seen in congenital malformations of the middle ear. Abnormal development of the ossicles often leads to discontinuity of the ossicular chain. Because the embryological origins of each ossicle are from more than one branchial arch, abnormalities of the branchial arches (also called branchial arch syndromes) can lead to ossicular abnormalities and conductive hearing loss. Absence of one of the ossicles or part of an ossicle can be seen without other noted congenital abnormalities.

Abnormalities of the ossicles are commonly seen in atretic and microtic ears. They can be found (rarely) in an otherwise normal individual. Treatment of ossicular discontinuities and malformations is with surgical repair or replacement of the ossicles (ossiculoplasty), often in conjunction with surgery for canal anomalies or with assistive listening devices.

◆ Systemic Disease Affecting the Middle Ear

Systemic disease can present for the first time with otologic symptoms. Many systemic diseases can affect the middle ear. The most common ones are presented here.

Osteogenesis Imperfecta

Osteogenesis imperfecta is also known as van der Hoeve's syndrome. This genetically transmitted disorder of collagen formation is inherited as an autosomal dominant disease with variable severity. The most severe form results in multiple fractures occurring during fetal development and is incompatible with life. The spectrum has been divided into four types. Type I is the only form in which hearing loss is frequent, with close to 100% of patients experiencing significant air–bone gaps by middle age (Kosoy and Maddox, 1971).

Although these patients have been described as having stapes fixation consistent with OS, the disease of osteogenesis imperfecta is microscopically different from OS (Brosnan et al, 1977). The bony structure of ossicles in osteogenesis imperfecta is immature with osteoid that is disordered and less dense than normal, providing a weak underlying structural framework. The ossicles can exhibit areas of thinning with increased fragility (Nager, 1988). They then become susceptible to pathological fractures and erosion and can be so delicate as to be ineffective in the transmission of sound energy. When this fragility is noted, the conductive hearing loss can be due to incudostapedial joint separation.

In osteogenesis imperfecta, an involved stapes footplate is thick, chalklike, and frequently immobile in the oval window (Brosnan et al, 1977). Occasionally, true otosclerotic foci are found to be fixing the stapes (Armstrong, 1984). When OS exists in the setting of osteogenesis imperfecta, it has been shown to be more aggressive (Nager, 1988). Despite the presence or absence of OS, a careful stapedectomy is the treatment for the fixed footplate. In these patients, the success rate for closure of the air–bone gap is lower than for patients with stapes fixation due to isolated OS. As with OS, these patients can choose hearing aids or other alternative listening devices for treatment of their conductive hearing loss.

Arthritis

The ossicles are susceptible to arthritic conditions because they have joints that contain cartilage, and therefore are susceptible to the degeneration associated with aging, autoimmune processes, accumulation of deposits, and inflammation. Autoimmune reactions and changes diagnostic for rheumatoid arthritis have been found to involve the cartilage of the ossicular joints (Belal and Stewart, 1974). Treatment of the ensuing pain and conductive hearing loss from joint fixation can include ossiculoplasty and nonsteroidal anti-inflammatory medications. The patient's candidacy for surgery depends on the severity of the disease.

Wegener's Granulomatosis

Wegener's granulomatosis is a systemic disease of the connective tissue characterized by inflammatory reactions around blood vessels. Involved tissue shows necrotizing granulomas on microscopic pathological examination. In the middle ear, Wegener's granulomatosis can manifest as OM, either of the serous or suppurative type, or as chronic mastoiditis. Suppurative OM is often associated with thickening or perforation of the TM and granulations within the middle ear and mastoid. Unilateral serous OM can be an early manifestation of this disease. Often the middle ear effusion will not respond to the usual medical therapy or to placement of ventilating tubes, and this may be a clue that a systemic process is responsible for the effusions. Surgery of the mastoid (used in severe cases with recurrent bacterial infections) can help to maintain an aerated middle ear space but is not indicated in most cases. Management is for the systemic disease and involves immune suppressants such as cyclophosphamide and steroids as needed.

Other systemic granulomatous diseases, such as sarcoid, polyarteritis nodosa, systemic lupus, TB, and syphilis, can lead to granulomatous lesions of the middle ear. Such lesions can interfere with hearing by obstructing the ET, blocking normal mucociliary flow within the middle ear, physically preventing motion of the ossicular chain or TM, and acting as a nidus for infection with associated effusion.

Tuberculosis

Tuberculosis is caused by a mycobacterial infection that is transmitted by airborne particles and can be ingested through the unpasteurized milk of cows. TB infections of the middle ear can be the result of the ET's admitting infected secretions, hematogenous spread, or lymphatic spread. TB OM is typically painless. A purulent middle ear effusion develops early in the course of the disease, causing a conductive hearing loss. The TM may appear thickened or red. If the infection progresses, inflammation, fibrosis, and granuloma formations occur as the body's defenses respond to the mycobacteria and its irritative capsule.

A profuse immune response to the TB organism can cause erosion of the ossicular chain and multiple perforations of the TM. Coalescence of the TM perforations can leave a large central perforation or complete loss of the TM. Extension of this infection into the mastoid cavity with the accompanying mucosal response frequently occurs. Diagnosis of mycobacterial infection is made on culture or stain of acid-fast bacilli from infected material. Clinically, the disease may mimic other granulomatous disorders such as Wegener's disease, and histological examination with acid-fast staining is required to make the diagnosis. Mastoidectomy performed in the absence of systemic treatment will often lead to a chronically draining infected cavity, with the disease progressing to adjacent sites. Once the patient has been diagnosed and is taking appropriate antituberculous medication, tympanomastoidectomy may become necessary to remove necrotic sequestered bone, to aid in healing, and to reconstruct the middle ear.

Syphilis

Syphilis is caused by a microorganism called *Treponema pallidum,* a spirochete. Infection reaches the otologic structures through the bloodstream.

Congenital syphilis is transmitted from mother to fetus in utero. It can be present at birth or can first manifest in early adulthood. The otologic manifestations are not distinguishable from acquired syphilis. Syphilitic infection of the ear is termed otosyphilis and can involve the middle ear, mastoid, and the inner ear. Early otosyphilis is characterized by inflammatory tissue accumulating around the site of infection. As scarring and fibrosis of the tissues occur, the characteristic gumma of syphilis forms with a necrotic center surrounded by a raised fibrotic area. Spirochetes can be demonstrated under dark-field microscopy in scrapings from accessible lesions (including perilymph), and serologic testing is positive for antibodies to the organism. Typically, areas of bony involvement are scattered throughout the temporal bone. Both the inner and middle ear can be involved, and infection of CN VIII is frequently seen (Martinez and Mooney, 1982). Within the middle ear, fibrosis in the submucosa, involvement of the ossicles with deformities, and fusions of the joints can be found. Infection of the TM causes perforation and scarring and can be accompanied by cholesteatoma. Middle ear involvement in syphilis often results in conductive hearing loss. When the inner ear is involved, patients can present with Meniere's-type symptoms, low-frequency hearing loss, sudden sensorineural hearing loss, and vestibular symptoms.

A diagnosis of otosyphilis is made with serologic tests. These tests are typically positive in early congenital syphilis and in the secondary stage of acquired syphilis but can become nonreactive in the later stages of the disease. Two reagin tests, the Venereal Disease Research Laboratory (VDRL) test and the rapid protein reagin (RPR) test, are not specific for syphilis, and false-positive results occur in up to 40% (Hughes and Rutherford, 1986). When the suspicion for syphilis is high, antibody levels to specific treponemal antigens can be measured by the fluorescent treponemal antibody absorption test and the microhemagglutination assay for *Treponema pallidum*. These antibody titers are positive in 100% of cases of secondary and tertiary syphilis.

For all stages of both congenital and acquired syphilis, the treatment of choice is intramuscular injection of penicillin G. For patients with penicillin sensitivity, other antibiotics, such as erythromycin, tetracycline, and cephalosporins, can be used. The dose and time course of treatment vary with the stage of disease (Dobbin and Perkins, 1983). Concomitant steroids are also given for associated sensorineural hearing loss because the prognosis for hearing recovery has been shown to improve with steroid treatment (Balkany and Dabs, 1978).

Immotile Cilia Syndromes

Immotile cilia syndromes are genetic diseases that result in a microscopic defect in the cell structures normally responsible for ciliary beating. Immotile cilia can be seen with Kartagener's syndrome and in diseases such as cystic fibrosis. In the upper respiratory tract, ciliated cells help to clear secretions from the middle ear and ET, from the sinuses, and from the nasal cavity and nasopharynx. When these specialized cell structures are not functioning normally, the mucus produced in the upper respiratory tract is stationary. Without the normal clearance mechanisms, water is absorbed from the mucous blanket, and the mucus becomes viscous. It then can act as a medium for bacteria to grow and can physically block normally open spaces, such as the ET orifice in the middle ear. In the middle ear, immotile cilia syndromes are manifest as chronic mucoid OM. Associated middle ear atelectasis is common and can result in cholesteatoma if severe retractions occur.

With immotile cilia, effusions are difficult to clear from the middle ear space even when the ET is patent and opening normally. Treatment involves active removal of the effusion through myringotomy, placement of wide-bore tympanostomy tubes, and instillation of antibiotic and steroid drops to reduce the viscosity of the effusion and the inflammation of the mucosa. Some patients may require steroids

to improve the conductive hearing loss, but effusions with associated hearing loss tend to recur in these patients once the steroids are discontinued. Perforations resulting from previous infections are often left open, with aural hygiene, observation, and water precautions as the basic treatment. Many patients will also require frequent suctioning of the gluelike effusions to minimize their hearing loss.

Immunoglobulin Deficiency

Immunoglobulins are essential components of the immune system that act to protect and defend the body against foreign invading organisms. Specific deficiencies in the production and secretion of immunoglobulins can be present in the first decade of life and significantly affect the body's ability to fight off infection. Immunoglobulin A (IgA) and G (IgG) are found in high concentrations in the normal middle ear. All the major classes of immunoglobulins can be found in chronic middle ear effusions. IgA is normally produced by lymphoid tissues in the upper respiratory tract mucosa. It is the main immunoglobulin found in middle ear effusions. These molecules are produced with a specific affinity for certain antigens (or portions of infecting microbials). IgA has been shown to interfere with a microbial's ability to adhere to the mucous membranes and can help stop viral invasion of local cells. IgG is the most common immunoglobulin found in the blood. In the middle ear, IgG is found in effusions of patients with COM and AOM. The lymphoid tissues of the middle ear are thought to produce IgG locally.

Most children and adults with recurrent episodes of OM have normal concentrations of immunoglobulins and have no apparent defects in their immune systems either locally within the middle ear or systemically. Usually some other reason can be identified to explain the recurrent infections (often ET dysfunction). However, a few patients have an otherwise undiagnosed immunodeficiency syndrome. IgA and IgG deficiencies will predispose an individual to recurrent sinus, pulmonary, and middle ear infections. Occasionally, no other signs or infections are present except recurrent OM to suggest an underlying immunodeficiency, and diagnosis in many of these patients can be delayed. Once a deficiency of IgA or IgG has been identified, adjunctive treatment with replacement of immunoglobulins in conjunction with the usual OM treatment options helps to clear the infection. For patients with chronic or recurrent severe infections, prophylactic replacement of immunoglobulins can be given at regular intervals.

Infection with Human Immunodeficiency Virus

Human immunodeficiency virus (HIV) infection affects the T-cell and B-cell components of the immune system, the complement system, and the ability of immune system cells to phagocytose and kill invading microorganisms. Most middle ear infections in HIV-infected individuals are caused by the common pathogens of OM. In addition, HIV-infected individuals are at risk for infection with unusual, opportunistic, or particularly virulent microbials. For all these reasons, these patients should be treated aggressively with intravenous antibiotics if they fail an initial course of oral medications. An essential component in the treatment of resistant OM in an HIV-infected patient is aspiration of the middle ear contents for culture. Because of the risk for recurrent infections in the setting of immunocompromise, the placement of tympanostomy tubes in patients with poorly controlled HIV should be considered with caution. A chronic effusion with mild hearing loss can be inadvertently converted into a chronically draining ear with a perforation that is resistant to healing. Perforation of the TM in an immunocompromised individual puts that person at an increased risk for chronic mastoiditis and its associated complications. HIV-infected individuals who are responding well to antiretroviral therapy do not have an increased risk of OM or of complications of OM and do well with usual treatment.

Pearl

- The failure to search for systemic disease in patients with persistent and progressive COM can lead to permanent changes in hearing and more severe otologic disease.
- Wegener's disease of the middle ear causes suppurative OM with chronic effusions and middle ear granulomas that are difficult to treat locally.
- Otosyphilis (both congenital and acquired) can lead to middle ear fibrosis and effusions.
- TB OM, usually painless with large or multiple TM perforations and thin grayish discharge, fails to improve with conventional treatments.
- Patients with immotile cilia syndromes will have recurrence of their symptoms despite tubes and frequent aural hygiene measures.
- The pathogens commonly causing OM in HIV-infected individuals are generally the same as those pathogens commonly causing OM in non-HIV-infected individuals.

◆ Tumors of the Middle Ear

Tumors of the middle ear are rare. When present, they cause hearing loss and middle ear disease through mechanical obstruction of normal structures or through displacement or destruction of those structures. Often obstruction of the ET will lead to chronic effusions.

Leukemia

Leukemic infiltrates are found in the submucosa of the middle ear in patients with chronic leukemic syndromes (Zechner and Altmann, 1969). They cause thickening of the TM with chronic, often suppurative effusions and recurrent bleeding into the middle ear and mastoid process. Conductive hearing loss is a common complaint in these patients. The effusions are treated with methods to improve ET function, such as Valsalva's maneuvers and decongestants. Tympanostomy tubes may be placed to relieve pressure and conductive hearing loss, but the risk of recurrent infections and chronically draining ears is high in these immunocompromised individuals. Radiation and chemotherapy are the mainstays of treatment for leukemia.

Paragangliomas

Also referred to as glomus tumors, paragangliomas in the middle ear arise from paraganglioma cells of (1) the jugular bulb to invade the middle ear or from (2) the middle ear portions of CN X (Arnold's nerve) or (3) CN IX (Jacobson's nerve) (Ogura et al, 1978). Ten percent of these tumors are familial, and ~10% of paragangliomas have been found to be bilateral (Spector et al, 1975). Paragangliomas are the most common tumors of the middle ear. They present with a history of aural pulsation, pain, fullness, tinnitus, hemorrhage, and/or symptoms of cranial neuropathy. When these tumors arise from the jugular bulb (as ~85% do), they can cause lower cranial nerve palsies and destruction of the skull base. All can extend to the intracranial space and erode into the otic capsule.

Treatment options for glomus tumors include surgical removal, embolization (placement of blocking substances into blood vessels feeding the tumor), and radiation treatment. Occasionally, glomus tumors can cause unstable and difficult-to-treat hypertension. Radiation treatment can slow or stop growth of paragangliomas. It is offered as primary therapy to patients who are not good surgical candidates or who refuse surgery (Konefal et al, 1987) and as an option for other selected patients. Radiation is also used in patients with recurrent disease that cannot be completely resected. Embolization can be offered in conjunction with other treatments, such as surgery and radiation. Surgery is preceded by angiogram with embolization of major feeding vessels to reduce blood loss and to aid in preserving vital structures of the skull base and reducing surgical time.

Surgery for glomus tumors is based on the degree of involvement of the skull base and any intracranial involvement (Jackson et al, 1982). This surgery is usually a team effort. The surgical team consists of a neurotologist, a head and neck surgeon, and a neurosurgeon. Because these tumors arise in the skull base and neck, they frequently involve cranial nerves and the carotid artery. Attempts to preserve these vital structures through new microsurgical techniques and computer-assisted navigation make surgery lengthy but have significantly improved outcomes. Control of the major vessels is achieved in the neck, and the involved structures (usually those of the jugular foramen and the facial nerve) are followed up to the skull base. An extensive mastoidectomy with skeletonization of the carotid artery within the temporal bone is frequently needed. This portion of the surgery involves careful dissection of the facial nerve, which often must be transposed (moved out of its bony canal) to access the medial aspect of the tumor. Transposition of the facial nerve always results in postoperative weakness. The lower cranial nerves must all be identified in the neck and/or at the brainstem and traced through tumor whenever possible. Injury to these nerves, by tumor invasion, compression, or during surgical resection, often results in permanent deficits in speech, swallowing, and shoulder motion.

When the tumor extends intracranially, a craniotomy with careful dissection from above the skull base may be necessary but adds to the risk and difficulty of the procedure. Injury or involvement of the carotid artery puts the patient at risk for stroke. Preoperative temporary occlusion of the carotid artery with a balloon catheter on the involved side can help to determine whether the patient can tolerate an attempt at total tumor removal when the carotid is involved. If necessary, a layer of tumor cells may be left behind to avoid unacceptable morbidity from surgery. A second surgery, or radiation therapy, is often necessary if any residual tumor grows. Patients with large glomus tumors of the skull base may receive a tracheotomy during surgery to protect the airway in anticipation of swallowing and vocal cord dysfunction after surgery. Because complete tumor removal can be difficult to determine in extensive tumors, close follow-up with CT or magnetic resonance imaging (MRI) and physical examinations is maintained in all these patients.

Adenomas of the Middle Ear

Primary adenomas of the middle ear are rare. They are benign tumors that arise from the glands found naturally in the middle ear mucosa and are usually slow growing. Despite their benign pathology, they can be life threatening when they extend intracranially. They are often discovered during the workup for conductive hearing loss or OME. Most adenomas of the middle ear do not respond well to radiation or chemotherapy; therefore, treatment of these tumors is surgical. Mastoidectomy and tympanoplasty are the most common surgical procedures performed for these tumors. Although extremely rare, primary adenomas can be aggressive, destroying bone and recurring when the resection is incomplete. Postoperative CT scans should be obtained to follow any potential recurrences.

Basal Cell Carcinoma

Basal cell carcinoma is a common slow-growing, locally invasive neoplasm of the basal cells of the skin. It is most often seen in men older than 60 and usually results from sun exposure. When it arises in the EAC, it often extends into the subcutaneous tissues and middle ear before the tumor is discovered. This tumor is a malignancy with a tendency to invade soft tissues and bone if left untreated. Resection with wide margins and postoperative radiation treatments may be needed to prevent recurrence.

Other tumors found in the middle ear include rhabdomyosarcoma, melanoma, and benign neuromas. Discussion of these tumors has been left out here because they are rare.

◆ Trauma

Trauma can cause TM pathology, with tears in the membrane related to temporal bone fractures. Temporal bone fractures can also cause hemotympanum when the TM remains intact. Other types of perforations can be seen with external trauma from foreign bodies being forced through the TM through the external canal. Slag burns (such as seen in welders) and small batteries (usually placed by children in their ears) cause a necrosis of the TM and middle ear mucosa. Pressure trauma from blasts, sound, or a closed blow to the ear all can cause large or total perforations.

Temporal Bone Fractures

Transverse fractures of the temporal bone are often the result of a blow to the occiput. The fracture can run across the labyrinth or through the middle ear. The hearing loss is usually sensorineural and total; facial paralysis or weakness occurs about half of the time, and hemotympanum is common. These fractures tend to occur in conjunction with serious head trauma, and the hearing impairment and facial nerve injuries can go unrecognized and untreated for extended periods.

In longitudinal fractures, the external canal is often lacerated, the TM may be torn, and the ossicles are often injured. Only 25% of these patients will have facial nerve weakness. With either of these fractures or with mixed fractures, the ossicles may be damaged or dislocated. A CT scan will help determine the extent of middle ear injury. Treatment of ossicular injury or dislocation with or without TM injury is nonurgent middle ear exploration with tympanoplasty and ossiculoplasty as needed (**Fig. 9–8** and

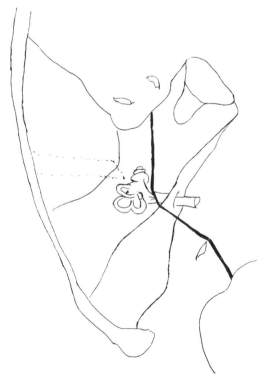

Figure 9–8 Schematic drawing of a longitudinal temporal bone fracture. The fracture line usually extends from the petrous apex, lateral to and around the bony labyrinth, and along the external auditory canal. These fractures frequently cross the facial nerve and ossicular chain and can tear the tympanic membrane.

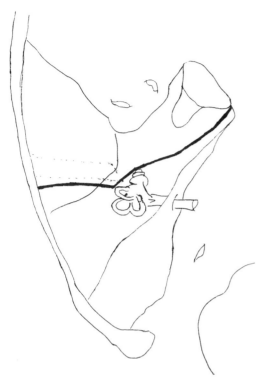

Figure 9–9 Schematic drawing of a transverse temporal bone fracture. The fracture line usually extends from the foramen magnum across the internal auditory canal, medial to the bony labyrinth, and only rarely involves the middle ear.

Fig. 9–9). Paralysis of the facial nerve resulting from temporal bone trauma requires rapid intervention, especially when it occurs immediately. Facial paralysis from temporal bone trauma can be delayed for up to several weeks. This usually is indicative of a better prognosis for recovery than immediate paralysis. When the facial nerve has been disrupted at a fracture line or contused severely, the patient experiences immediate paralysis. Decompression of the injured segment (removal of the surrounding bony canal) and anastomosis (reattachment of severed ends) or grafting (placement of a connecting nerve between severed ends) can improve the final outcome.

Temporal bone fractures can result in cerebrospinal fluid (CSF) leak either from the EAC or from the nasal cavity through the ET. Acutely, bleeding associated with the head injury can obscure a CSF leak. CSF leaks are of concern because they indicate possible intracranial injury and can lead to meningitis. Isolated CSF leaks, in an otherwise stable patient, are initially managed conservatively with bed rest, head elevation, and avoidance of straining. Two weeks of such treatment will determine whether the leak will close spontaneously. If conservative measures fail, lumbar drainage of the CSF or surgical repairs of the leak at the skull base are indicated. Once a CSF leak is recognized or suspected, nothing that is not sterile should be placed in the ear. Unsterile cotton, eardrops, wicks, unsterile ear swabs, irrigations, or ear probe tips all can introduce bacteria into the ear. These bacteria can travel through the leakage path and cause meningitis.

Perilymphatic Fistulas

Perilymphatic fistulas can occur spontaneously and are a more common cause of sudden hearing loss in children than in adults. These patients present with a sudden decrease in hearing, tinnitus, and/or vertigo. Leakage of perilymph into the middle ear can be a sequela of barotrauma in susceptible individuals. Spontaneous perilymph fistulas can be associated with inner ear malformations.

A search for associated malformations should be undertaken in children with sudden hearing losses attributed to fistulas. Bed rest will frequently lead to resealing of the fistula with resolution of the vertigo. Hearing can be stabilized with fistula closure (spontaneous or surgical) but often does not recover completely. If recovery does not occur after 1 week of bed rest, the patient can opt for exploratory tympanotomy with fat, vein, or fascia placed as a patch over the fistula. Patients with proven fistulas may need reoperation if recurrent or progression of symptoms develops after patching.

Barotrauma to the Middle Ear

Usually, barotrauma results in inflammation of the middle ear and mastoid mucosa because of the rapid development of negative pressure within the middle ear/mastoid system. Such pressure causes edema of the mucosa and TM retraction (Farmer, 1985). The negative pressure can draw transudate into the middle ear space from the tissues, creating an effusion. Bleeding into the middle ear can result from the rapid development of very negative pressure. Often middle ear barotrauma causes pain, hearing loss, tinnitus, and sometimes vertigo. During diving, the TM can rupture from rapid pressure differentials of as little as 100 mm Hg (Farmer, 1982). Patients with ET dysfunction are at increased risk for barotrauma of the middle ear with only mild to moderate stress, such as gradual airplane descent or when diving.

Barotrauma can occur rapidly in susceptible individuals during elevator rides from high floors or when traveling over mountains. Mechanical obstruction of the ET by nasal edema from upper respiratory infection or allergy can contribute to or worsen ET dysfunction and lead to barotrauma during flight. Restoration of normal middle ear pressure with Valsalva's maneuvers, decongestants, or myringotomy will usually correct the problem.

Prevention of barotrauma during air travel in individuals with known ET dysfunction can be facilitated with the use of Valsalva's maneuvers during airplane descent, special baffled earplugs, or the placement of tympanostomy tubes (in selected individuals) to equalize the pressure on both sides of the TM. Diving should be avoided in individuals with ET dysfunction, history of perilymphatic fistula, or chronic ear disease.

♦ Complications of Surgery

Because of the complex anatomy of the temporal bone, surgery in this area can sometimes be complicated and risky. Often diseases of the middle ear and mastoid process obscure or eliminate the usual landmarks, putting the patient at increased risk for intraoperative and postoperative complications. Occasionally, the disease process results in involvement of the structures of the middle ear that necessitates changing the surgical plan to ensure the patient's best possible outcome.

Facial Nerve Complications

Extensive cholesteatoma can be a particularly damaging disease. The facial nerve in its tympanic course in the middle ear can be uncovered, displaced, or invaded by this disease (which often acts like a malignancy of the temporal bone). This puts the facial nerve at high risk for injury from infection, local compression, and cholesteatoma removal.

Immediate recognition of a facial nerve injury gives the patient the best chance for recovery of acceptable facial function. If the facial nerve has been transected and can be primarily anastomosed, this is done immediately. Any need to transpose the facial nerve out of its bony canal for repair changes its orientation. When the neuronal fibers regrow, they rarely all find their original paths. This leads to synkinesis and incomplete recovery of facial function. In the worst case, the nerve is injured such that a portion of the nerve is absent and length is insufficient for a primary anastomosis. In such a case, an interposition graft, usually taken from the greater auricular nerve, is anastomosed between the cut edges of the facial nerve. The result is asymmetric facial motion in the best of circumstances. Delays in repairing a transected facial nerve can lead to scarring and neuroma formation at the transection site, with a worse prognosis for the eventual outcome.

Incomplete Removal of Cholesteatoma

If cholesteatoma intimately involves the facial nerve or causes a hole to form into the cochlea or labyrinth, it becomes necessary to leave cholesteatoma matrix (a layer of epithelial cells) over the involved structure to avoid a more serious complication. Enclosure of this remaining matrix behind a canal wall or reconstructed TM will invariably lead to a recurrence of the complications of cholesteatoma, with the potential for further damage of the involved structures.

The solution is often exteriorizing the matrix of cholesteatoma that is purposely left behind so that it can be cleared or decompressed through the EAC. This canal wall down procedure sometimes includes sacrifice of the middle ear structures in a radical mastoidectomy procedure and a permanent, surgically created conductive hearing loss. Only rarely can a radical mastoid cavity be revised, with an attempt to re-create an air-containing middle ear space and ossicular reconstruction. For most patients who are not able to have the middle ear reconstructed after surgery, hearing aids are a good option for hearing rehabilitation.

Open middle ear cavities with remaining tight corners or mucosa left within the mastoid tip can become infected. Trapping of moisture, cerumen, and squamous debris within a deep or creviced space or behind a high facial ridge can create optimal conditions for bacterial growth. Such infections that persist cause chronic drainage, can progress to invade intracranially, and usually require a surgical revision. Persistent infections can be an early sign of recurrence of cholesteatoma, which also requires surgical revision.

Postoperative Dizziness and Hearing Loss

Surgery of the middle ear often involves manipulation of the ossicular chain. Occasionally, a fistula of the lateral semicircular canal or the oval window is present. Manipulations of the ossicular chain and of tissues on or near a lateral canal fistula can result in disturbance of the perilymph of the labyrinth and result in postoperative dizziness that can be disabling if it does not resolve.

Manipulation of the stapes footplate, as occurs during stapedectomy, can disturb the perilymph of the vestibule and result in postoperative dizziness. The treatment for such postoperative dizziness is bed rest and head elevation for 2 to 5 days. In the case of stapedectomy when the vestibule has been opened, a noninfectious serous labyrinthitis (inflammatory reaction within the inner ear) can develop and cause delayed postoperative dizziness. In these cases, a short course of oral steroids is added to the postoperative regimen and helps to resolve the dizziness. Dizziness immediately after stapedectomy can result if the prosthesis, placed during the procedure, is too long. This dizziness will persist beyond the first postoperative week and often requires reoperation for resolution. Careful measurements before placement of the prosthesis are essential in preventing this complication.

Failure in the development of an adequate seal around the stapes prosthesis can result in a persistent postoperative perilymph fistula, with intermittent vertigo and, possibly, a decline in hearing. Usually, additional bed rest and head elevation will be enough to allow a soft tissue seal to develop, closing the leak. Infections of the middle ear space shortly after stapedectomy are of particular concern because any opening in the footplate puts the patient at risk for both labyrinthitis and meningitis until an adequate seal at the oval window has occurred. Perioperative antibiotics, careful timing of surgery in children, and the placement of oval window tissue seals can help prevent these very serious complications.

Any time surgery is performed on the structures of the ear, there is the potential for a permanent sensorineural hearing loss. Surgery on the oval and round windows carries the highest risk because this surgery occurs at the middle ear–inner ear interface. Surgery for extensive or aggressive cholesteatoma also carries a high risk of hearing loss if a labyrinthine or an oval window fistula is present. Once an opening into the perilymphatic space is made or discovered during surgery, care must be taken to avoid aggressive suctioning of the perilymph. If the vestibule is kept clean of bone dust and cholesteatoma debris, and the pressure within the perilymphatic space is not significantly reduced by suctioning, there is often no residual effect on the function of the inner ear. Children with inner ear malformations who undergo manipulation of the stapes can often have perilymph gushers from the direct effect of CSF pressure on the perilymph. Opening the vestibule in this situation can lead to rapid drops in perilymph pressure, severe dizziness, and permanent profound hearing loss. Obtaining a preoperative CT scan that adequately evaluates the inner ear structures and vestibular aqueduct will help the surgeon predict a potential complication. Surgery should be undertaken with extreme caution in these children.

Conductive Hearing Loss

Removal of mucosa from the surface of the ossicles can lead to scar, causing devascularization of these structures and loss of bone mass. The long processes of the incus and the incudostapedial joint are at particular risk for this process. Over time, such devascularization will create bone loss with ossicular discontinuity and an associated conductive hearing loss. Postoperative scarring of the middle ear mucosa and fixation of portions of the TM and ossicles can occur in some individuals. This can be minimized by removing a minimum of diseased middle ear mucosa and by placing material as a barrier to scar, such as absorbable gelatin film or silicone elastomer, between the promontory and the undersurface of the TM. Scarring around the ossicles can be very difficult to prevent in susceptible individuals. Scarring can also occur in the EAC, causing stenosis. Stenosis can prevent adequate visualization of the middle ear and mastoid cavity, cause accumulation of debris and cerumen in the EAC, and contribute to a conductive hearing loss. We have found the laser particularly useful in removing scars from the external canal safely, while helping to prevent recurrence of the stenosis. Stenosis of the EAC can be prevented by removing conchal cartilage during a meatoplasty (always performed in conjunction with a canal wall down mastoid procedure), by the application of permanent sutures to hold the meatal skin open, and by minimizing trauma to the EAC skin during middle ear surgery.

Drainage after Tympanostomy Tube Insertion

Chronic drainage from a tympanostomy tube occurs because of infection of the middle ear mucosa, foreign body reaction to the material of the implant, systemic mucosal disease, or unrecognized cholesteatoma. Drainage that fails to respond to topical antibiotic/anti-inflammatory combinations can be due to any of these causes. Up to 40% of ears with tympanostomy tubes will drain (Gates et al, 1986). Occasionally, the tympanostomy tube will become colonized with unusual bacteria that do not respond to topical therapy. Culture of the drainage will usually identify any persistent microbials, and removal of the existing tympanostomy tube will be necessary to stop the drainage. When reintubation is necessary after tube removal for drainage, specially treated tubes are often used. Occult cholesteatoma can be ruled out with CT scanning. In addition, care should be taken when considering placing a tympanostomy tube for effusion or conductive hearing loss in the presence of systemic disease. Unless the systemic disease is well controlled, the middle ear mucosa will continue to discharge, and the patient will just be trading one problem for another. (See section on mucosal disease.)

Persistent Perforation after Tympanostomy Tubes

Failure of closure of the perforation resulting from tympanostomy tubes is treated like a perforation from any other cause. With observation and water precautions, the perforation can be managed indefinitely, barring other complications (e.g., the development of cholesteatoma). Once surgery is considered (as in chronic or recurrent infections, or a clinically significant conductive hearing loss), the size and location of the perforation determine the optimal treatment.

Lateralization of the Tympanic Membrane

A conductive hearing loss can also occur if the TM lateralizes and separates from the ossicular chain, or prosthesis, as it heals from tympanoplasty. Lateralization of the TM can occur when a large perforation is repaired. Failure to place the graft under the malleus handle during lateral grafting and lack of an appropriate length of the malleus handle remnant lead to lateralized grafts. Grafting of the anterior TM without re-creation of the anterior sulcus will also lead to anterior blunting, with an associated air–bone gap. Lateralization can also occur when the total replacement prosthesis used is too short or if the prosthesis tips over. Ossicular reconstruction can be redone with a longer prosthesis.

Reoperation

Postoperative infections can be particularly troublesome, resulting in new or recurrent perforation (failed tympanoplasty). Development of ET or attic obstruction also contributes to infection or additional TM pathologies. Extrusion of the prosthesis, scarring, or thickening and lateralization of the TM all contribute to a persistent conductive hearing loss after surgery with failure of the tympanoplasty. Reoperation or use of a hearing aid is often recommended in such situations.

If the dura of the middle or posterior fossa is injured during mastoid or middle ear surgery, a rare complication of CSF leakage or brain herniation can occur. These rare complications often require corrective surgery. Herniated nonviable brain tissue must be carefully amputated and any openings in the dura repaired. Neurosurgical consultation and involvement in the treatment of such complications are critical to proper handling.

Bleeding

Any dehiscence of the vascular structures of the skull base into the middle ear, or thinning of the overlying bone, puts these structures at risk during middle ear and mastoid surgery. The carotid canal forms the medial portion of the bony ET. Openings of this bone (surgically created, congenitally present, or due to trauma) can expose the carotid artery to injury at the middle ear orifice of the ET or in the hypotympanum. Injury to the carotid artery wall puts the patient at risk for stroke, future bleeding, and possibly death.

The jugular bulb sits in the hypotympanum and is usually covered by bone. Congenital dehiscence; erosion of the covering bone by infection, cholesteatoma, or tumor; and aggressive drilling in the hypotympanum during middle ear surgery can injure the jugular bulb. Myringotomy in the inferior quadrant of the TM can inadvertently lead to a hole in an unrecognized dehiscent jugular bulb. Jugular injuries can cause severe bleeding, clot formation into the lateral sinus with brain edema, and lower cranial neuropathies.

Bleeding is controlled, for both the jugular bulb and the carotid artery, with packing material such as surgical cellulose or thrombin-soaked gelatin foam. This material assists in clot formation along the opening in the vessel. Often further exposure of the carotid artery is needed to maintain control of the bleeding. In severe cases, ligation of the vessels may be necessary to control bleeding.

♦ Summary

This chapter has provided the reader with the most common medical and surgical managements of diseases affecting the middle ear. Some of these diseases are poorly understood, and research is ongoing to improve the treatment options and aid in prevention. Overuse of antibiotics remains a source of altered strains of pathogens, which are becoming more difficult to treat medically. Surgical treatments are currently the mainstay for most middle ear diseases. Future management will involve improved surgical techniques and newer medical and therapeutic regimens to increase our success in treating these pathological conditions.

References

Armstrong, B. W. (1984). Stapes surgery in patients with osteogenesis imperfecta. Annals of Otology, Rhinology and Laryngology, 93, 634–635.

Balkany, T. J., & Dabs, P. E. (1978). Reversible sudden deafness in early acquired syphilis. Archives of Otolaryngology, 104, 66–68.

Békésy, G. von. (1960). Experiments in hearing. New York: McGraw-Hill.

Belal, A., & Stewart, T. J. (1974). Pathological changes in the middle ear joints. Annals of Otology, Rhinology and Laryngology, 83, 159–167.

Bellucci, R J. (1981). Congenital aural malformations: Diagnosis and treatment. Otolaryngologic Clinics of North America, 14, 95–124.

Bergus, G. R., & Lofgren, M. M. (1998). Tubes, antibiotic prophylaxis, or watchful waiting: A decision analysis for managing recurrent acute otitis media. Journal of Family Practice, 46(4), 304–310.

Brosnan, M., Burns, H., Jahn, A. F., & Hawke, M. (1977). Surgery and histopathology of the stapes in osteogenesis imperfecta tarda. Archives of Otolaryngology, 103, 294–298.

Cawthorne, T. (1955). Otosclerosis. Journal of Laryngology and Otology, 69, 437–456.

Culpepper, L. (1997). Routine antibiotic therapy of acute otitis media: Is it necessary? Journal of the American Medical Association, 278, 1643–1645.

Dobbin, J. M., & Perkins, J. H. (1983). Otosyphilis and hearing loss: Response to penicillin and steroid therapy. Laryngoscope, 93, 1540–1543.

Doherty, J. K., & Slattery, W. H. III. (2003). Autologous fat grafting for the refractory patulous eustachian tube. Otolaryngology–Head and Neck Surgery, 128(1), 88–91.

Dyer, R. K. Jr., & McElveen, J. T., Jr. (1991). The patulous eustachian tube: Management options. Otolaryngology–Head and Neck Surgery, 105, 832–835.

Falk, B., & Magnuson, B. (1984). Eustachian tube closing failure. Archives of Otolaryngology, 110, 10–14.

Farmer, J. C. (1982). Otologic and paranasal sinus problems in diving. In P. B. Bennet & D. H. Elliott (Eds.), The physiology and medicine of diving (3rd ed., pp. 507–536). London: Bailliere Tindall.

Farmer, J. C. (1985). Eustachian tube function and otologic barotrauma in eustachian tube function: Physiology and role in otitis media. Annals of Otology, Rhinology and Laryngology, 94, 45–47.

Gates, G. A., Avery, C., Prihoda, T. J., & Holt, G. R. (1986). Post-tympanostomy otorrhea. Laryngoscope, 96, 630–634.

Gristwood, R. E., & Venables, W. N. (1983). Pregnancy and otosclerosis. Clinical Otolaryngology, 8(3), 205–210.

Hammaren-Malmi, S., Saxen, H., Tarkkanen, J., & Mattila, P. S. (2005). Adenoidectomy does not significantly reduce the incidence of otitis media in conjunction with the insertion of tympanostomy tubes in children who are younger than 4 years: A randomized trial. Pediatrics, 116(1), 185–189.

Hanson, J. R., Anson, B. J., & Strickland, E. M. (1962). Branchial sources of the auditory ossicles in man. Archives of Otolaryngology, 76, 200–215.

Hughes, G. B., & Rutherford, I. (1986). Predictive value of serologic tests for syphilis in otology. Annals of Otology, Rhinology and Laryngology, 95, 250–259.

Jackson, C. G., Glasscock, M. E., & Harris, P. F. (1982). Glomus tumors: Diagnosis, classification, and management of large lesions. Archives of Otolaryngology, 108(7), 401–410.

Konefal, J. B., Pilepich, M. V., Spector, G. J., & Perez, C. A. (1987). Radiation therapy in the treatment of chemodectomas. Laryngoscope, 97(11), 1331–1335.

Kosoy, J., & Maddox, H. E. (1971). Surgical findings in van der Hoeve's syndrome. Archives of Otolaryngology, 93, 115–122.

Lambert, P. R. (1990). Congenital absence of the oval window. Laryngoscope, 100(1), 37–40.

Larsson, A. (1960). Otosclerosis: A genetic and clinical study. Acta Otolaryngologica Supplementum, 154, 1–86.

Martinez, S. A., & Mooney, D. F. (1982). Treponemal infections of the head and neck. Otolaryngologic Clinics of North America, 15, 613–620.

Moreano, E. H., Paparella, M. M., Zelterman, D., & Goycoolea, M. V. (1994). Prevalence of facial canal dehiscence and of persistent stapedial artery in the human middle ear: A report of 1000 temporal bones. Laryngoscope, 104(3, part 1), 309–320.

Nager, G. T. (1988). Osteogenesis imperfecta of the temporal bone and its relation to otosclerosis. Annals of Otology, Rhinology and Laryngology, 97, 585–593.

Nguyen, L. H., Manoukian, J. J., Yokovitch, A., & Al-Sebeih, K. H. (2004). Adenoidectomy: Selection criteria for surgical cases of otitis media. Laryngoscope, 114(5), 863–866.

Ogura, J. H., Spector, G. J., & Gado, M. (1978). Glomus jugularae and vagale. Annals of Otology, Rhinology and Laryngology, 87, 622–629.

Poole, M. D. (1998). Declining antibiotic effectiveness in otitis media—A convergence of data. Ear, Nose, and Throat Journal, 77, 444–447.

Pulec, J. L. (1967). Abnormally patent eustachian tubes: Treatment with injection of polytetrafluoroethylene (Teflon) paste. Laryngoscope, 77, 1543–1554.

Richter, E. (1980). Quantitative study of human Scarpa's ganglion and vestibular sensory epithelia. Acta Otolaryngologica, 90, 199–208.

Richter, E., & Schuknecht, H. F. (1982). Loss of vestibular neurons in clinical otosclerosis. Archives of Otorhinolaryngology, 234(1), 1–9.

Rosenfeld, R. M., Culpepper, L., Doyle, K. J., et al. (2004). Clinical practice guideline: Otitis media with effusion. Otolaryngology–Head and Neck Surgery, 130(Suppl. 5), S95–S118.

Sade, J., Luntz, M., & Pitashny, R. (1989). Diagnosis and treatment of secretory otitis media. Otolaryngologic Clinics of North America, 22(1), 1–14.

Sando, I., Hemenway, W. G., Miller, D. R., & Black, F. O. (1974). Vestibular pathology in otosclerotic temporal bones: Histopathological report. Laryngoscope, 84(4), 593–605.

Schuknecht, H. F., & Barber, W. (1985). Histologic variants in otosclerosis. Laryngoscope, 95, 1307–1317.

Singer, D. E., Freeman, E., Hoffert, W. R., et al. (1952). Otitis externa: Bacterial and mycological studies. Annals of Otology, Rhinology and Laryngology, 61, 317–330.

Singh, A., Al-Khabori, M., & Hyder, M. J. (2005). Skull base osteomyelitis: Diagnostic and therapeutic challenges in atypical presentation. Otolaryngology–Head and Neck Surgery, 133(1), 121–125.

Spector, G. J., Ciralsky, R., & Maisel, R. H. (1975). Multiple glomus tumors in the head and neck. Laryngoscope, 85, 1066–1075.

Teele, D. W., Klein, J. O., & Rossner, B. (1980). Epidemiology of otitis media in children. Annals of Otology, Rhinology and Laryngology Supplement, 89, 5–6.

Tonndorf, J., & Khanna, S. M. (1970). The role of the tympanic membrane in middle ear transmission. Annals of Otology, Rhinology and Laryngology, 79, 743–753.

Virtanen, H., & Palva, T. (1982). Surgical treatment of patulous eustachian tube. Archives of Otolaryngology, 108, 735–739.

Wever, E. G., & Lawrence, M. (1954). Physiological acoustics. Princeton, NJ: Princeton University Press.

Zechner, G., & Altmann, F. (1969). The temporal bone in leukemia: Histological studies. Annals of Otology, Rhinology and Laryngology, 78, 375–387.

Chapter 10

Medical and Surgical Treatment of Sensorineural Hearing Loss

John Gail Neely

- ♦ **Surgical Anatomy of the Temporal Bone**
- ♦ **Role of the Clinical Audiologist**
- ♦ **Diagnostic Tools**
- ♦ **Red Flags in a Busy Office Practice**
- ♦ **Specific Diseases Causing Sensorineural Hearing Losses**

  General Considerations

- ♦ **Causes of Sensory Hearing Losses**

  Mechanical

  Medicinal/Toxic

  Metabolic

  Congenital/Genetic/Developmental

  Collagen Diseases/Immunologic/Allergic

  Neoplastic/Growth

  Infectious

  Degenerative/Idiopathic

- ♦ **Causes of Neural Hearing Losses**

  Lesions Detectable by Imaging

  Lesions Not Detectable by Imaging

- ♦ **Summary**

Sensory hearing loss is defined in this chapter as a lesion in the inner ear causing hearing loss, and *neural hearing loss* is a lesion referable to the eighth cranial nerve (CN VIII) or lower brainstem. The term *lesion* refers to any anatomical or physiological deviation from the norm. Because the potential impact on the care of a patient is so great, false-positive results suggesting a neural hearing loss are more tolerated than false-negative results. Also, because neural lesions are not often purely neural and may be concomitant with conductive or sensory losses, even the slightest hint of a neural lesion must be carefully evaluated.

♦ Surgical Anatomy of the Temporal Bone

Viewing the anatomy as a surgeon would in planning an approach to a lesion, we can see the ghosted outline of the labyrinth and the facial nerve anterior to the sigmoid sinus, with the posterior aspect of the jaw joint acting as the anterior wall of the external auditory canal (EAC). The floor of the middle cranial fossa forms the roof of the jaw joint, middle ear, and mastoid. Surgical approaches may go anterior to the sigmoid sinus, through the mastoid, and around

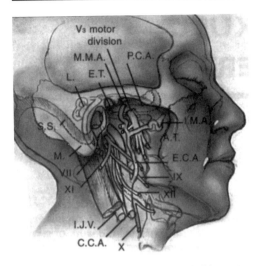

P.C.A. - Petrous Cartoid a.
M.M.A. - Middle Meningeal a.
I.M.A. - Internal Maxillary a.
A.T. - Auriculo-temporal n.
E.C.A. - External Cartoid a.
XI - Accessory n.
IX - Glossopharyngeal
X - Vagus n.
C.C.A. - Common Cartoid a.
I.J.V. - Int. Jugular v.
VII - Facial n.
M. Mastoid
S.S - Sigmoid sinus
L. - Labyrinth
E.T. - Eustacian tube
XII Hypoglossal n.

Figure 10–1 Illustration of the lateral skull base view with surface landmarks and ghosted deep anatomy. (From Pensak, M. L. (1997). Revision skull base surgery. In V. N. Carrasco & H. C. I. Pillsbury (Eds.), Revision otologic surgery (pp. 143–159). New York: Thieme Medical Publishers, with permission.)

the labyrinth into the posterior fossa, a retrolabyrinthine approach. Alternatively, an approach may go above the labyrinth into the middle fossa and subsequently into the posterior fossa by means of the middle fossa. The posterior fossa may also be reached by going through the labyrinth and, at times, the cochlea, in a translabyrinthine or transcochlear approach, respectively. The posterior fossa may be approached posterior to the sigmoid sinus in a retrosigmoid or suboccipital approach (**Fig. 10–1**).

Looking at the skull base with the calvarium (top of the skull) and the brain removed, CN V to XII are seen to course through or about the temporal bones, which form most of the lateral walls of the posterior fossa and much of the middle fossa (**Fig. 10–2**).

A posterolateral view with the temporal bone removed shows the intimate relationship of the cochlea, vestibular labyrinth, CN VIII, facial nerve (CN VII), other nerves, cerebellum, pons, and medulla oblongata (**Fig. 10–3**).

Figure 10–4 illustrates how the facial nerve is intimately related to all parts of the ear, the posterior fossa internal auditory canal (IAC), the labyrinth, the middle ear by the stapes, and the mastoid. In **Fig. 10–5**, a facial recess approach from the mastoid to the middle ear and from the middle fossa to the middle ear along the facial nerve are illustrated; the facial nerve is a surgical landmark in most surgical approaches to the temporal bone. A closer view of the relationship of the facial nerve to the stapes is seen in **Fig. 10–6**.

◆ Role of the Clinical Audiologist

The primary focus of audiology in a medical setting is to determine the site and the degree of each independent lesion affecting the auditory system and to monitor those lesions

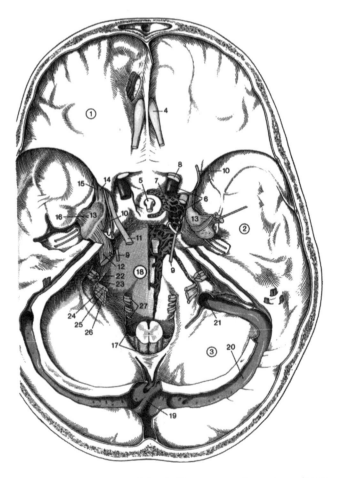

Figure 10–2 Illustration of the skull base as seen from above. (From Roeser, R. J. (1996). Roeser's audiology desk reference: A guide to the practice of audiology. New York: Thieme Medical Publishers, with permission.)

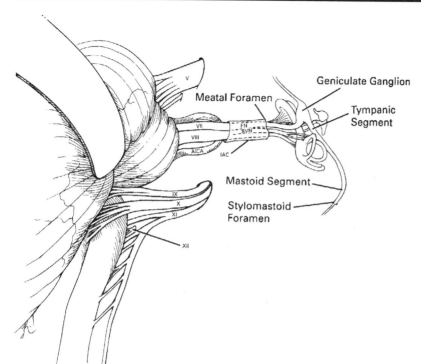

Figure 10–3 Illustration of the posterolateral view of the posterior fossa showing the 5th to 12th cranial nerves (CN V–XII). OW, TK; RW, TK. (From Rubinstein, J. T., & Gantz, B. J. (1997). Facial nerve disorders. In G. B. Hughes & M. L. Pensak (Eds.), Clinical otology (2nd ed., pp. 367–380). New York: Thieme Medical Publishers, with permission.)

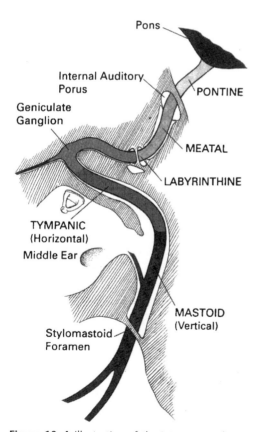

Figure 10–4 Illustration of the intratemporal course of the facial nerve. (From Gulya, A. J. (1997). Anatomy and embryology of the ear. In G. B. Hughes & M. L. Pensak (Eds.), Clinical otology (2nd ed., pp. 3–34). New York: Thieme Medical Publishers, with permission.)

throughout the course of the disease, which may extend for the life of the patient. For example, conductive or long-standing sensory hearing loss does not immunize the patient from a host of serious illnesses, some of which may be reversible or, conversely, deadly.

Patients with neural lesions may have minimal to profound auditory, vestibular, or facial motor complaints. Patients may, and often do, present with conductive hearing loss with or without middle ear effusion. For example, a patient may demonstrate normal pure-tone thresholds and word recognition scores but reveal reflex decay or elevated reflex thresholds at 500 and/or 1000 Hz along the afferent limb of the reflex arc. Other patients might reveal normal pure-tone thresholds and speech and immittance audiometry but a delay of wave V on auditory brainstem response (ABR) ipsilateral to a patient's report of subjective tinnitus. These two examples are actual patient presentations of the author. Each patient had large solitary vestibular schwannomas with brainstem compression. Another patient may have middle ear effusion and a mild neural hearing loss and have a large petroclival meningioma. Or a patient might have bilateral moderate to severe noise-induced hearing loss for which he or she has regularly been followed and fitted with hearing aids for 20 years. Later, a mild progressive difference in the word recognition score may be discovered in one ear without any change in pure-tone thresholds. In this last example, the patient was found to have a 2 cm solitary vestibular schwannoma on that side.

Repeated measurements of all audiometric parameters, obviously important in the initial diagnosis, are always required to be repeated to assess the clinical course of the

Facial Recess Approach

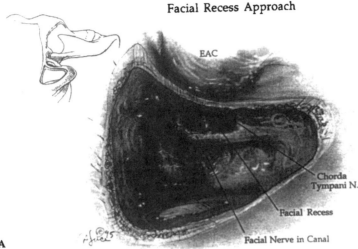

A

Middle Fossa Approach

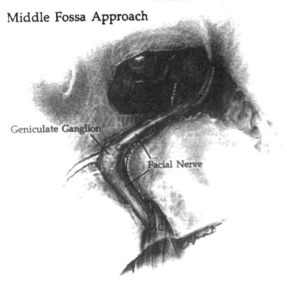

B

Figure 10–5 (A) Diagram of the facial recess approach from the mastoid to the middle ear. **(B)** Middle fossa exposure of the facial nerve in the labyrinthine and tympanic segments. (From Huang, M. Y., & Lambert, P. R. (1997). Temporal bone trauma. In G. B. Hughes & M. L. Pensak (Eds.), Clinical otology (2nd ed., pp. 251–267). New York: Thieme Medical Publishers, with permission.)

disease for diagnostic confirmation, management planning, disease, and therapeutic monitoring. In the management of complex otological and neurotological cases, it is a serious error in clinical judgment to fail to obtain a comprehensive audiogram, covering speech reception thresholds, word recognition scores, and immittance audiometry, including reflex measures in contralateral and ipsilateral conditions for both ears and reflex decay throughout the clinical course. Any results of any one of these tests may change independently and can have major implications for the progressive or retrogressive pathophysiology of the disease.

Skilled audiologists are crucial partners with medical specialists. They must be knowledgeable about ear diseases for diagnosis and monitoring the medical, surgical, and rehabilitative management of the patient. Every patient with a hearing loss is, or may become, a medically or surgically treatable candidate.

Pearl

- The primary objective of an audiological assessment is to determine the site of lesions within the auditory system and the degree to which they are involved. To do this, a comprehensive audiogram, including speech and immittance audiometry, is required initially and every time audiological assessment is clinically necessary.

◆ Diagnostic Tools

Diagnostic tests are either anatomically based, meaning they are designed to evaluate distortions of anatomy, or physiologically based, meaning they are designed to evaluate the

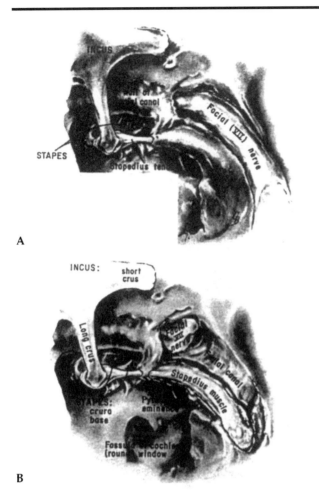

A

B

Figure 10–6 **(A)** Illustration of the facial nerve in relation to the stapes and stapedial tendon and **(B)** muscle. (From Arts, H. A. (1997). Anatomy of the ear. In P. S. Roland, B. F. Marple, & W. L. Meyerhoff (Eds.), Hearing loss (pp. 1–25). New York: Thieme Medical Publishers, with permission.)

physiology of a system or region. It often takes both types of tests to fully identify a disease and characterize its extent.

The case history, taken by a physician and audiologist with a depth of knowledge of the systems involved, remains the most important single tool for diagnosis. The audiologist is a crucial partner in this venture because of his or her expertise in accurately defining the site and degree of specific independent lesions within the auditory system. The first question in diagnosis is, Where is the lesion?

Each symptom or sign is viewed by the author as a three-dimensional object in space on its separate timeline; the duration of each episode and frequency of occurrence are graphed on the x-axis, the intensity of each episode is graphed on the y-axis, and the quality of each episode is graphed on the z-axis. For example, a patient with Meniere's disease may present with episodic vertigo on one timeline, which has a sudden onset, last minutes to hours, is severely intense, and has the quality of spinning. Fluctuating

hearing loss on a separate timeline may slowly progress prior to vertigo, peak during the vertigo, have low-frequency distortion, and slowly recover over days. Patterns of aggregates of signs and symptoms are then compared with known patterns of specific disease. When there is a match, a new diagnostic menu is generated to explore the specific diseases that can match that exact scenario. For example, if the aggregate of signs and symptoms suggests Meniere's disease, syphilitic labyrinthitis, Cogan's syndrome, delayed endolymphatic hydrops, perilymphatic fistula, and other diseases may exactly match the clinical scenario of Meniere's disease. Ultimately, by the use of this technique and by filtering it with an in-depth knowledge of the anatomy and physiology of the systems involved, a diagnostic impression is formulated, which contains a differential diagnostic list in which each disease may be confirmed or rejected. Confirmation or rejection of a candidate disease may require the use of imaging techniques and/or laboratory tests.

The imaging studies most often used are computed tomography (CT), magnetic resonance imaging (MRI), magnetic resonance angiography (MRA), conventional angiography, and conventional radiography of the skull or chest. CT is used when looking at bone is the primary concern, for example, for bone-destructive lesions of the petrous apex. MRI is predominantly useful to look at the nerves and brain without bone obscuring the view, for example, to examine the IAC and posterior fossa in search of a solitary vestibular schwannoma. MRA is used to look at large arteries and venous sinuses, for example, when concerned about a dural venous thrombosis or vascular malformation. Conventional angiography is required when a detailed look at the vessels is needed. Standard radiographs are still useful to look at the skull and the chest; several diseases, for example, tuberculosis, sarcoidosis, and Wegener's granulomatosis, may affect the lungs and the auditory system.

Special laboratory tests often used are noninvasive. These may include (1) electrophysiological tests of cardiac and vascular function; (2) cultures or serological tests for viral, spirochetal, rickettsial, bacterial, or deep fungal infections; (3) blood tests for function of the immune systems, metabolic systems, and hematopoietic system; and (4) toxicological tests. Physiological tests of other systems are sometimes required, such as the vestibular, visual, and renal systems.

The clinical course during treatment is also a vital part of the process of confirmation and surveillance to ensure resolution of the disease and that no new diseases arise without detection.

◆ Red Flags in a Busy Office Practice

The following are a few "red flags" that may occur in a busy practice that may alert the audiologist to a serious problem. Some of the more common warning signs are given in **Table 10–1.** The best way to understand and evaluate

Table 10–1 "Red Flags" Indicating a Potentially Serious Problem

"Red Flag"	Explanation
An audiometric retrocochlear finding that seems to have spontaneously resolved	Serious problems can get better without disappearing.
A chronically draining ear with fever or pain	Such ears rarely present this way unless a complication or cancer is present.
A nose that runs unilaterally	Unilateral rhinorrhea may indicate a foreign body, severe infection, cancer, or a cerebrospinal leak.
Reduced ability to attend or inconsistent results	Serious developmental, psychiatric, cardiovascular, pulmonary, renal, CNS disease, drug or alcohol abuse, or dangerously excessive medication can present this way.
Minimal or no hearing loss with subtle retrocochlear signs	There is very little correlation between tumor size and hearing loss; any retrocochlear sign is too much.
Long-duration, circumstantially "explained" hearing loss that has not been medically evaluated	It is not unusual for large benign tumors to exist and slowly and progressively enlarge without changing the pure-tone thresholds in moderate to profoundly affected ears; this has been observed to occur in long-persistent, nonprogressive mild losses as well.
Asymmetric pure-tone thresholds, unilateral tinnitus, and/or asymmetric word intelligibility scores	Very subtle asymmetries may be the only presentation of serious disease; ABR or imaging is usually necessary to resolve the issue. The size of the lesion does not have to correlate with the audiometric dysfunction. There is increasing evidence that ABRs may give false-negative results in some of these lesions.
Facial paralysis or twitching	All facial paralysis is not Bell's palsy; tumors, infections, and trauma may present this way with few other signs or symptoms. Bell's palsy, per se, is treatable for better outcome if seen very early.
A child who complains of dizziness	Children are not often dizzy, especially when they lie down. Brainstem gliomas may initially present with only this symptom. Children may have other treatable, or dangerous, causes of dizziness similar to adults.
Hoarseness persisting for 2 weeks, or which frequently recurs	Base of skull or other discrete or systemic lesions capable of causing neural hearing loss may initially present with hoarseness; a good example is the glomus jugulare tumor extending along CN X into the posterior fossa.
Retro-orbital pain behind one eye	Such pain tends to come from deep orbital or petroclival infections or tumors that may or may not be associated with neural hearing loss but that are urgently serious.
Double vision, or diplopia	A host of petrous apex, neural, or brainstem lesions may present this way.
Anyone under age 40 presenting with the slightest CN VIII finding	Young people may have huge bilateral acoustic tumors and many other neurofibromas and meningiomas intracranially and within their spine, characteristic of NF2, and present only with the slightest hearing loss.
Persistent or frequent headaches, especially severe ones and those that awaken the patient	Headaches that awaken a patient are associated with a high incidence of intracranial pathology.
An unusually dark hue to the middle ear	A high-lying jugular fossa, dehiscent of bone, or blood behind the eardrum from a base of skull fracture present this way.
Unilateral ear infections or unilateral serous otitis media	Acute recurrent otitis media or chronic serous otitis media are usually bilateral; when these occur unilaterally, it is imperative to investigate the nasopharynx and petrous apex for the presence of nasopharyngeal cancer, petrous apex tumors, or occult cholesteatomas. These will often not be otherwise apparent.
Unsteady gait, ataxia	Ataxia is not caused by inner ear disease; instead, the brain or spinal cord is implicated. Even when the patient is severely vertiginous, off balance, and deviating to the involved side, this passes, and persistent ataxia does not occur.
Rapidly progressive hearing losses over weeks, months, or 2 years	Such losses are dangerous if proven to be neural and often reversible if proven to be sensory.
Vague symptoms of dizziness or an off-balance feeling	Most of the time these symptoms are not associated with serious disease; however, these symptoms associated with a neural hearing loss are often from dangerous disease.
Falling down or passing out (becoming unconscious), with or without dizziness	Inner ear problems do not make people fall down, with the rare exception of the otolithic crisis of Tumarkin, or pass out. These signs are usually from cardiovascular or CNS disease.

ABR, auditory brainstem response; CN VIII, eighth cranial nerve; CN X, 10th cranial nerve; CNS, central nervous system; NF2, neurofibromatosis type 2.

patients is to have a thorough knowledge of the anatomy and physiology of these integrated systems and be ever vigilant to identify the slightest deviation from the norm. Also, it is necessary to triangulate all the signs and symptoms to one site of lesion capable of explaining the clinical signs.

Confirmation of the disease process requires special tests to verify the existence of the lesion. Slight deviations from the expected clinical course of a simple, uncomplicated, common disease are often the only clue that a serious problem exists or has arisen.

Table 10–2 Initial Diagnostic Matrix for Investigation of Hearing Loss

	EE	ME	IE	CN VIII	LBS	HBS	TL	O
Mechanical								
Medicinal/toxic								
Metabolic								
Congenital/genetic/developmental								
Collagen diseases/immunologic/allergic								
Neoplastic/growth								
Infectious								
Degenerative/idioplastic								
Psychogenic								

Sites of lesion: EE, external ear; ME, middle ear; IE, inner ear; CN VIII, eighth cranial nerve; LBS, low brainstem; HBS, high brainstem; TL, temporal lobe; O, other sites (e.g., heart, cervical, or cerebral vasculature).

Sites germane to this chapter: IE, sensory hearing losses; CN VIII and LBS, neural hearing losses.

Pitfall

- On repeat testing during the clinical course of the disease, it is a serious error to obtain only pure-tone thresholds. Each audiometric variable can change independent of the others; this can have important medical implications.

Pearl

- Minimal, subtle, or transient signs and symptoms with recovery do not mean the lesion is resolved or that the disease process is not serious.

◆ Specific Diseases Causing Sensorineural Hearing Losses

General Considerations

Etiology is the cause of a disease. Nosology is the classification of diseases, grouped by common etiologies. For each anatomical point in the body, a full nosological array of diseases may apply. One nosological array that this author has used successfully since senior year in medical school is (1) mechanical (e.g., trauma), (2) medicinal/toxic, (3) metabolic, (4) congenital/genetic/developmental, (5) collagen diseases/immunologic/allergic, (6) neoplastic/growth, (7) infectious, (8) degenerative/idiopathic, and (9) psychogenic. Within each nosological category, there may be many specific diseases.

When investigating the cause of hearing loss in a patient, it is useful to create a mental multiple column by row (C × R) table as the first diagnostic matrix to guide the investigation. The columns are the sites of possible lesions, and the rows are the nosological categories (**Table 10–2**). As the history, physical examination, and subsequent audiometry, imaging, and/or laboratory tests are performed, columns and rows may be eliminated. Eventually, remaining cells may be exploded, and the discrete diseases within each cell may be considered.

◆ Causes of Sensory Hearing Losses

Mechanical

Head injury (temporal bone fracture and concussion), noise trauma, and barotrauma may cause cochlear hearing loss. The sensorineural hearing loss may be transient or permanent. Hearing loss is the most common sequela of head injury. Twenty to 40% of patients with head injury have hearing loss. Ten to 24% of patients with head injury have high-frequency sensorineural hearing loss. Nearly 15% of patients with brain concussion, without skull fracture, have hearing loss.

Temporal Bone Fractures

Temporal bone fractures are generally classified as longitudinal or transverse. Longitudinal fractures occur through the EAC, often tear the tympanic membrane (TM), and fracture longitudinally through the shock-absorbing pneumatized spaces of the middle ear and mastoid lateral to the otic capsule. Transverse fractures, however, fail to take advantage of the shock-absorbing characteristics of the EAC, TM, and lateral pneumatized spaces and fracture through the hardest bone in the body, the otic capsule, and petrous bone from foramen to foramen through the vestibule, often right through the facial nerve, and transmit trauma directly to the intracranial contents (**Figs. 10–7** and **10–8**).

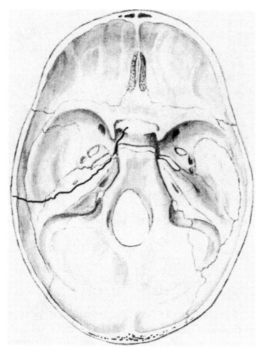
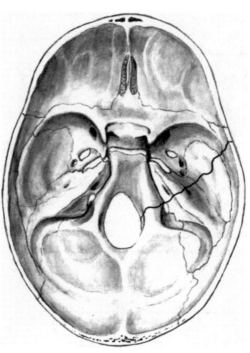

A

B

Figure 10–7 Drawings of **(A)** a longitudinal temporal bone fracture and **(B)** a transverse temporal bone fracture. (From Jahrsdoerfer, R. A., & Ghorayeb, B. Y. (1996). Temporal bone trauma. In H. H. Naumann, J. Helms, C. Herberhold, et al (Eds.), Head and neck surgery (2nd ed., Vol. 2, pp. 131–157). New York: Georg Thieme Verlag, with permission.)

Either fracture can create a cerebrospinal fluid (CSF) leak that externalizes through the torn TM as CSF otorrhea and/or down the eustachian tube as CSF rhinorrhea. Often CSF leaks are obvious if looked for; however, they may be occult. Meningitis, although not extremely common, can occur immediately following trauma or be delayed for months or years.

Immediate treatment is usually confined to caring for any brain, facial nerve, or other associated injuries. Later, care may be directed at any persistent CSF leaks, perilymph

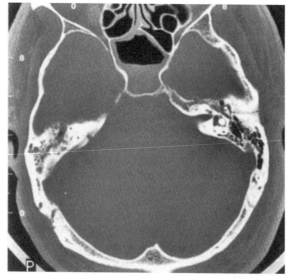
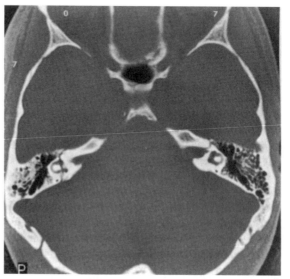

A

B

Figure 10–8 (A) Computed tomography (CT) scan showing a left longitudinal fracture through the superior wall of the external canal, right side of the left image. **(B)** CT scan showing a right transverse fracture through the horizontal semicircular canal, left side of the right image. (From Huang, M. Y., & Lambert, P. R. (1997). Temporal bone trauma. In G. B. Hughes & M. L. Pensak (Eds.), Clinical otology (2nd ed., pp. 251–267). New York: Thieme Medical Publishers, with permission.)

fistulas (PLFs) with fluctuating or progressive sensory hearing loss with or without constant instability, persistent positional or episodic vertigo, ossicular discontinuity, entrapment cholesteatomas, or EAC stenoses.

It is wise to inform the patient of and be personally diligent for delayed meningitis, especially during the onset of an acute ear infection months or years later. The earlier meningitis can be identified, the better the chances of survival. Early signs of meningitis are headache, with or without confusion, and a generalized feeling of illness, with or without diaphoresis (profuse sweating). Classic later signs are fever and stiff neck. Rapid deterioration to coma and death may follow.

Pearl

- Transverse fractures are potentially much more serious and injurious to the brain than longitudinal fractures.

Sensorineural hearing loss (cochlear or retrocochlear) occurs more commonly with transverse temporal bone fractures. Cochlear hearing loss occurring with temporal bone fractures may be due to a direct fracture through the otic capsule, as in transverse fractures, a perilymphatic fistula from disruption of the stapes in the oval window, or by labyrinthine concussion. Head injury causing labyrinthine concussion may occur with or without associated skull fracture. Labyrinthine concussion describes a nonfracture injury to the labyrinthine capsule that results in vertigo, disequilibrium, with or without hearing loss, aural fullness, and tinnitus.

Treatment of hearing loss from head trauma is usually directed at restoration of middle ear function if the ossicles are fixed or separated and the repair of perilymphatic fistulas is suspected and ultimately found at surgery. Vestibular rehabilitation may be useful in hastening recovery. Surgical exploration for perilymph fistula (PLF) should be considered in patients with head trauma who continue to have fluctuating hearing loss and vertigo (Roland and Marple, 1997). After head trauma, some patients have typical attacks of what appears to be Meniere's syndrome (post-traumatic endolymphatic hydrops): vertigo, aural fullness, and hearing loss that may last hours. The treatment of post-traumatic endolymphatic hydrops is the same as the treatment for Meniere's disease.

Perilymph Fistula

Perilymph fistula is an abnormal communication between the labyrinth and the middle ear spaces that can allow passage of perilymph into the middle ear spaces, air into the labyrinth, or a mixture of perilymph and endolymph if a tear is present in the membranous labyrinth. The most common site for PLF is the oval window, followed by the round window; however, cholesteatomas or fractures may produce fistulas directly into the cochlea or, more commonly, into the horizontal semicircular canal. PLFs may also be congenital and can occur bilaterally. The congenital form is associated with craniofacial malformation, birth trauma, and inner ear malformations such as large vestibular aqueduct syndrome and common cavity deformity, as in Mondini's dysplasia. Acquired PLFs are associated with head trauma, noise trauma, barotrauma (swimming/diving, nonpressurized airline travel, scuba diving, skydiving, forceful nose blowing, and sneezing), recent ear surgery, cholesteatoma, tumors of the middle ear and mastoid, and vigorous physical activity.

PLF symptoms include fluctuating or progressive sensorineural hearing loss and fluctuating or progressive vertigo or disequilibrium. Symptoms seem to be improved in the morning or after periods of rest and worsen in the evening or after prolonged periods of activity (Brookhouser, 1996). The "gold standard" for diagnosis is visualization, during exploratory tympanotomy, of clear fluid leaking from a definite opening in the inner ear. However, even during surgery, the differentiation between accumulation of perilymph, transudate, CSF, irrigation, or anesthetic solutions in the middle ear space is difficult. Western blot assays for β_2-transferrin (a marker believed to be unique to perilymph and CSF) have been advocated to help with this problem; however, no widely available rapid analysis technique has been developed (Brookhouser, 1996; Roland and Marple, 1997).

A relatively new type of fistula of unknown etiology is dehiscent superior semicircular canal (Minor et al, 2003). This defect in the middle fossa convexity of the superior semicircular canal creates a widely varied complex of hearing and vestibular symptoms. These symptoms include, but are not limited to, fluctuating sensory hearing loss and episodic vertigo associated with pressure or sound, unusually good hearing levels, or conductive hearing loss suggesting otosclerosis but not responding to stapes surgery.

Noise Trauma

Sound, ranging from high-intensity, short-duration, to lower intensity, long-duration exposure, may result in cochlear (sensory) hearing loss that is either transient or permanent. Tinnitus and threshold shifts after noise exposure are indications of cochlear injury that may contribute to permanent threshold shifts (Brookhouser, 1996).

Sudden, extremely intense sounds can tear the membranous labyrinth; this is termed *noise trauma*. More commonly, less intense sound over longer durations resulting in hearing loss is termed *noise-induced hearing loss*.

Permanent cochlear hearing loss from intense sound may be ameliorated with amplification. However, prevention is the principal focus in this disorder.

Pearl

- Noise trauma is distinctly different than noise-induced hearing loss.

The reader may refer to Chapter 20 in this volume for use of hearing protection to reduce effects of noise exposure. Genetic predisposition for noise-induced hearing loss seems to be very important. Thus, individuals who seem to have a more rapid or greater hearing loss for the amount of noise exposure should be informed of this predisposition and warned of the consequences for themselves specifically.

Barotrauma

Barotrauma occurs when the ear is subjected to sudden changes in pressure or more gradual changes in pressure that cannot be equalized by the eustachian tube. Activities such as scuba diving, skydiving, airline travel, severe sneezing, lifting, straining at the stool, and vigorous sexual activity may be associated with cochlear hearing loss. Barotrauma causing cochlear hearing loss is much less common than the conductive hearing loss from barotrauma-induced middle ear effusion. The resulting sensorineural hearing loss from barotrauma may be partial or complete. Causes include perilymphatic fistulas, rupture of the membranous labyrinth, and intralabyrinthine hemorrhage. Initial treatment is directed at avoidance of activities associated with sudden changes in external or internal pressure across the middle or inner ear, such as the Valsalva's maneuver, coughing, sneezing, and airline travel. Patients with symptoms that persist after conservative treatment may require surgical exploration.

Medicinal/Toxic

Numerous medications are known to cause hearing loss. Most clinical ototoxic hearing loss, however, is caused by aminoglycoside antibiotics, loop diuretics, and antineoplastic agents. Hearing loss, tinnitus, and balance instability are symptoms of ototoxicity. Hearing loss from ototoxic antibiotics is sensorineural and initially seen in the high frequencies. Hearing loss with loop diuretics usually produces a flat or gradually sloping hearing loss (Brookhouser, 1996). Although most ototoxic drugs have both cochleotoxic and vestibulotoxic properties, some are predominantly cochleotoxic, whereas others are predominantly vestibulotoxic.

Aminoglycoside Antibiotics

Aminoglycosides are a group of antibiotics that are used to treat many gram-negative bacterial, staphylococcal, and mycobacterial infections. Hearing loss may be seen in the first few days of treatment or several months after the completion of therapy. The outer hair cells of the basal turn are most vulnerable to injury, corresponding to the high-frequency hearing loss often seen with aminoglycoside treatment. The magnitude of hearing loss is related to dose, rate of infusion, serum peak and trough levels (i.e., serum high and low levels measured at various times after dosing), and duration of treatment. Toxic effects, however, can be idiosyncratic, meaning the effects may occur in a given individual even when no clear reasons exist why such toxicity should occur. In addition, these events may prove to be genetic, meaning the patient is genetically predisposed to the toxic effects of a specific compound.

These antibiotics are excreted in the urine and can also be nephrotoxic (i.e., toxic to the kidney). In addition, any renal impairment may allow increased circulating levels of the drug and increase the risk of ototoxicity. Streptomycin, neomycin, cactinomycin, kanamycin, gentamicin, tobramycin, amikacin, netilmycin, and sisomycin are examples of aminoglycoside antibiotics.

If ototoxicity is identified, the medication must be discontinued, unless no alternative treatment exists for a serious disease. Unfortunately, little can be done to reverse or arrest ototoxicity from aminoglycoside antibiotics once it has begun. It is possible for hearing loss to progress after the discontinuation of the medication; however, ototoxicity often spontaneously stops at some level.

Ideally, monitoring audiometry (i.e., complete audiologic evaluation, including speech, tympanogram, acoustic reflexes, reflex thresholds, and high-frequency audiometry) would be completed before potentially ototoxic drugs were administered and repeated periodically during treatment. In addition, complaints of dizziness or tinnitus should be reported to the physician. The physician uses this information to evaluate antibiotic selection and dosing.

Although no reliable method exists to avoid aminoglycoside ototoxicity, measurement of serum peak and trough levels remains important to avoid potentially ototoxic levels. Antioxidants, however, may play a role in protecting against ototoxicity (Rybak and Whitworth, 2005).

Pearl

- The best way to "treat" ototoxicity is to identify the decrease in hearing early and take steps to prevent further hearing loss (i.e., change medicine, dose, and dose frequency).

Interestingly, the concomitant use of iron-chelating agents with aminoglycoside administration has been shown to prevent ototoxicity in laboratory animals. Clinical trials will be needed to see whether this will be of benefit to humans; a search of www.clinicaltrials.gov did not reveal any trials to date.

Nonaminoglycoside medications that have potentially ototoxic or vestibulotoxic side effects are erythromycin, vancomycin, loop diuretics, antineoplastic agents, anti-inflammatory agents, and antimalarial agents.

Metabolic

Diabetes Mellitus

Diabetes is a disorder of carbohydrate metabolism resulting in difficulties controlling blood glucose. An association exists between sensorineural hearing loss and diabetes. In addition, an association exists between the interaction of diabetes and hypertension (a common problem in the diabetic patient) in the pathogenesis of sensorineural hearing loss. The mechanism by which diabetes may participate in producing hearing loss is unclear. There is a rare hereditary neurodegenerative disease known as Wolfram syndrome, which results in diabetes insipidus, diabetes mellitus, optic atrophy, and deafness. Some reports correlate diabetic hearing loss with general vascular disease and the severity of diabetes. No correlation exists between hearing loss and the duration of diabetes, insulin dosage, and family history of diabetes. No treatment reverses or prevents diabetic cochlear hearing loss except, perhaps, adequate diabetic control (Monsell et al, 1997).

Renal Disease

As with diabetes, the mechanism of sensorineural hearing loss commonly seen in patients with renal disease is unclear. Metabolic abnormalities, such as accumulation of uremic toxins, electrolyte imbalance, osmotic shifts during dialysis, or endocrine abnormalities, are believed to contribute to the sensorineural hearing loss. Fluctuation in low-frequency hearing is occasionally observed after dialysis; however, hearing loss is not proportional to elevated blood urea nitrogen or serum creatinine levels. Other possible explanations for hearing loss seen in patients with renal failure may be associated with the use of ototoxic diuretics/antibiotics, anemia, presence of infection, coexisting diabetes, hypertension, small vessel disease, and hemodynamic changes associated with dialysis and kidney transplantation. No treatment reverses or prevents cochlear hearing loss associated with renal disease except, perhaps, appropriate control of the renal disease and correction of associated diseases (Monsell et al, 1997).

Hypothyroidism

The mechanism causing sensorineural hearing loss associated with low levels of thyroid hormone (hypothyroidism) is also poorly understood. Endemic cretinism is a congenital form of hypothyroidism caused by a lack of iodine. Affected children have goiter, mental retardation, and mixed hearing loss. Thyroid hormone supplementation may improve the mental retardation but not the hearing loss. Athyroid cretinism results from abnormal lack of development of the thyroid gland. During development, the fetal metabolism is supported by maternal thyroid hormone crossing the placenta. Shortly after birth, however, the infant becomes hypothyroid. Adult forms of hypothyroidism may occur after infections, radiation, surgery, or drug treatment. Occasionally, the sensorineural hearing loss associated with hypothyroidism is improved with thyroid hormone supplementation (Monsell et al, 1997). There is some evidence that some cases of Meniere's disease is associated with hypothyroidism. Patients with thyroid disease, even hereditary conditions like Pendred's syndrome, should be followed carefully because thyroid carcinoma can arise.

Pitfall

- In patients with early hearing loss, failure to identify and treat hypothyroidism may result in deafness.

Other Metabolic Disorders

Other metabolic disorders, such as vitamin D deficiency, hypophosphatemia/hyperphosphatemia, and abnormalities in bilirubin metabolism, are known to be associated with sensorineural hearing loss. Some patients with adrenocortical insufficiency have symptoms of Meniere's disease, and this is thought to be due to a defect in regulation of sodium.

Congenital/Genetic/Developmental

A general fact sheet from the American Academy of Otolaryngology–Head and Neck Surgery summarizes the epidemiology of genetic hearing loss as follows: approximately 3 of every 1000 babies born have birth defects resulting in hearing loss; 60% of these are inherited. Seventy percent (70%) of the inherited causes are nonsyndromic (80% of these are recessive, 20% are dominant, and 2% are X-linked or mitochondrial), and 15 to 30% are syndromic, meaning other parts of the body are abnormal. More than 400 syndromes associated with hearing loss have now been discovered.

Hearing loss may be inherited in the following ways:

Autosomal dominant A single parent with the gene may transmit the defect to 50% of his or her offspring.

Autosomal recessive Two unaffected parents (heterozygous) carrying the gene may transmit the defect to 25% of their offspring. The fact that 70% of inherited deafness is nonsyndromic and that 80% of nonsyndromic deafness is recessive emphasizes the importance of finding rapid methods of genetic screening.

X-linked recessive The defect is transmitted from the mother in the X chromosome and usually affects male offspring (XY chromosomes); female offspring will have one X chromosome from the mother and one from the father. The normal X chromosome usually predominates, but if the father is affected, and the mother also carries the abnormal X chromosome, a female offspring may inherit the disorder.

Mitochondrial The intracellular mitochondria have their own deoxyribonucleic acid (DNA), separate from the nucleus, and that abnormal mitochondrial DNA comes from the mother's egg, because sperm has no mitochondria; thus, only affected mothers may transmit the disease, not affected fathers. All offspring, male or female, from an affected mother will have the disease; none of the offspring from the affected father will inherit the disease. Some defective mitochondria cause the offspring to be abnormally sensitive to aminoglycoside antibiotics, which can cause deafness even when the dose is not excessive.

Congenital Syndromes with Hereditary Hearing Loss

When evaluating an adult or child with hearing loss, it is prudent to look carefully at the patient's overall appearance, especially his or her face, eyes, skin, hair, ears, and skeletal structure, and evaluate basic functions of the thyroid, kidneys, heart, and nervous system. If something is abnormal with one or more of these areas, it is probable that the individual has a syndromic type of hereditary hearing loss.

Medical treatment consists of searching for and addressing dangerous, correctable, or controllable associated conditions. Some of these associated conditions are Meniere-type symptoms, proteinuria (proteins in the urine), uremia (excess urea in the bloodstream) or renal failure, and potential for hyperthermia. Progressive neural foramina stenosis amenable to decompression, stapedial fixation amenable to stapedotomy, potential for CSF gusher after stapes surgery or trauma, susceptibility for long bone fractures, cataracts, and glaucoma are other associated problems. Additional associated diseases are diabetes mellitus, exudative retinitis, epilepsy, potential for excessive sunburning, sudden death from cardiac dysrhythmia, skin ulceration or infection, dental deterioration, kyphoscoliosis, indifference to pain leading to severe injury, severe inner ear dysplasia with abnormal dehiscences into the intracranial cavity potentially leading to recurrent meningitis, and diabetes insipidus (Grundfast and Toriello, 1998). Medical treatment may eventually extend to cochlear or brainstem implantation.

Common syndromes (Brookhouser, 1996; Grundfast and Toriello, 1998) include the following:

- Waardenburg's syndrome is an autosomal dominant inherited disorder that may present with sensorineural hearing loss and abnormalities of pigmentation, such as white forelock, premature graying of hair, or two eyes of different color (heterochromia iridis). In addition, craniofacial abnormalities, such as high, broad nasal root, confluent eyebrows, and lateral displacement of the medial canthi of the eyes (dystopia canthorum), may be evident.

- Pendred's syndrome presents with a congenital hearing loss with an enlarged thyroid gland (goiter). On further investigation, the patient may actually have hypothyroidism.

- Branchio-otorenal syndrome may present with hearing loss, malformed pinna, preauricular pits, and/or branchial cleft cysts or fistulas. Identification of this disorder is important because many patients also have renal anomalies.

- Goldenhar's syndrome patients have varying degrees of hemifacial asymmetry or mandibular hypoplasia, with mixed hearing loss. On further examination, these patients may possess abnormalities of the ocular, renal, skeletal, and central nervous system (CNS).

- Treacher Collins syndrome (mandibulofacial dysostosis) presents with symmetric malar hypoplasia with underdeveloped zygomatic arches (small cheekbones), mandibular hypoplasia (small mandible), downward sloping eyelids, microtia (small ears), and aural meatal atresia (narrow ear canals) with mixed or sensorineural hearing loss.

- A patient with sensorineural hearing loss and a family history of renal failure or hematuria (blood in the urine) might have Alport's syndrome. This includes hereditary progressive glomerulonephritis and sensorineural hearing loss. Interestingly, this syndrome affects women more commonly and men more severely. Fifty to 75% of affected males have end-stage renal failure develop by 20 to 40 years of age and require extensive treatment for the renal disease.

- Usher's syndrome presents as young congenitally hearing-impaired children who are slow to sit, stand, or walk and may be experiencing an additional vestibular disorder and difficulty with vision. This syndrome may accompany a constellation of symptoms, ranging from poor night vision to blindness, mild sensorineural hearing loss to deafness, and normal balance to complete loss of vestibular function. Diagnosis may be assisted by a complete ophthalmologic examination and electroretinography.

- An obese patient who has progressive sensorineural hearing loss may have undiagnosed Alström syndrome, an autosomal recessive disorder that may eventually lead to diabetes, retinal degeneration, and blindness.

- A child being evaluated for congenital bilateral profound deafness with a history of syncopal attacks (complete loss of consciousness) and sudden lapses of consciousness or family history of a sibling with sudden unexplained death in childhood may have the autosomal recessively inherited Jervell and Lange-Nielsen syndrome. Electrocardiograms (ECGs) of these patients will have an abnormally prolonged QT interval (the interval between the Q wave and T wave of the ECG). Syncopal attacks begin at age 3 to 5 years; before the development of appropriate cardiac medication, most affected individuals died by age 15.

Pearl

- It is important to recognize syndromic hearing loss to identify coexisting potentially treatable medical conditions and provide information for possible genetic counseling and identification of family members with undiagnosed genetically related medical problems.

Nonsyndromic Hereditary Hearing Losses

All sensorineural hearing losses in adults and children should be considered to derive from a definable disease, some of these dangerous to life. Many of those deemed unexplained, or idiopathic, after thorough investigation are, indeed, genetic and often hereditary. Khetarpal and Lalwani (1998) suggested a diagnostic algorithm that includes the following:

1. A thorough case history and physical examination

2. Complete diagnostic audiometry

3. A more detailed medical examination of the unexplained cases, including

   a. History of pregnancy

   b. Postnatal history

c. Family history

d. Otological examination

e. Eye examination

f. Laboratory tests for renal and thyroid function, diabetes, anemia, infection, syphilis, immunological and autoimmune disease, specific viral disease such as cytomegalovirus (CMV), and rubella

4. ECG

5. High-resolution CT of the temporal bones

Nonsyndromic hereditary hearing losses are identified and further classified by inheritance pattern, audiometric characteristic, vestibular signs/symptoms, and radiographic findings.

The specific identification of the type of hereditary hearing loss may lead to therapeutically important implications, beyond managing the hearing loss with amplification, special education, and cochlear implantation in profound cases. For example, a small proportion of Meniere's disease cases that can respond to medical or surgical treatment may present with an autosomal dominant inheritance pattern for sensorineural hearing loss. Mondini's dysplasias, which can be seen in some cases of syndromic or nonsyndromic hereditary sensorineural hearing losses, can be severe enough to create a defect in the otic capsule medially through the vestibule into the IAC and laterally through the stapedial footplate into the middle ear; this can predispose the patient to have a delayed onset of recurrent meningitis with middle ear infections. Unusual sensitivity to aminoglycoside antibiotics or diabetes mellitus can result from mitochondrial genetic defects, causing sensorineural hearing loss.

Otosclerosis, familial conductive hearing loss, and X-linked progressive mixed hearing loss can all be associated with genetic defects capable of causing sensorineural hearing loss, and the conductive loss is potentially treatable with surgery; however, in the X-linked cases, the probability of a CSF gusher through the stapedial surgical defect is increased and can have serious consequences for persistent CSF leak, recurrent meningitis, and damage to the membranous labyrinth, resulting in profound deafness on that side.

Hone and Smith (2003) published an excellent review of the genetics of hearing loss. Interested readers are encouraged to study this work.

Prenatal and Perinatal Noxious Events

Symptomatic, or usually asymptomatic, maternal infection during the first trimester with rubella, CMV, toxoplasmosis, or syphilis can result in a severe or progressively severe to profound sensorineural hearing loss. Infants often have congenital inner ear, eye, cardiac, and nervous system birth defects. Diagnosis is made by the characteristic array of defects, history of rash or infection of the mother in the first trimester, and early serological testing of the neonate.

No effective medical treatment exists against congenital rubella; however, surgery to correct the cataracts or heart defects can help in some cases. Immunizing against rubella,

even in adults, has proven an effective way to prevent congenital rubella. Congenital CMV is treatable with the antiviral foscarnet. Congenital toxoplasmosis may be treated with pyrimethamine and sulfadiazine, spiramycin combined with pyrimethamine and sulfadiazine, or spiramycin alone for approximately 1 year beginning the first months of life. Congenital syphilis is treated with high doses of penicillin.

Perinatal trauma, infection, or anoxia may cause sensorineural hearing loss. A seriously ill neonate may receive ototoxic aminoglycosides or diuretics for survival. This neonate may become hypoxic, or high levels of unconjugated bilirubin may develop, which stains the basal ganglia in the brain in a condition known as kernicterus. Aggressive pulmonary ventilation, antibiotics, blood exchange transfusions, and careful monitoring of drug levels are all ways of keeping the infant alive and preventing hearing loss. Once the hearing loss occurs, however, very little more can be done to improve hearing (Irving and Ruben, 1998).

Collagen Diseases/Immunologic/Allergic

Autoimmune Inner Ear Disease

Clinically, autoimmune inner ear disease (AIED) presents as bilateral, asymmetric progressive sensorineural hearing loss over a period of days to months. Although AIED may occur at any age, it is more frequently seen in the middle-aged female. It may occur in association with other systemic autoimmune diseases, such as Wegener's granulomatosis, Cogan's syndrome, polyarteritis nodosa, rheumatoid arthritis, ulcerative colitis, Crohn's disease, systemic lupus erythematosus, ankylosing spondylitis, multiple sclerosis, relapsing polychondritis, and postvaccination serum sickness. The hearing loss may be fluctuant, but progressive and not sudden (<72 hours). In addition, half the patients may have vestibular symptoms, making the initial diagnosis difficult to separate from Meniere's disease. In fact, many patients with classic Meniere's disease have been shown to have serologic testing suggestive of AIED (Roland and Marple, 1997).

AIED is thought to occur when the patient has antibodies, autoantibodies, or a cell-mediated immune response develop against the patient's own cochlear and/or vestibular antigens, which then causes an inflammatory response damaging the inner ear.

Excluding retrocochlear causes of the hearing loss with ABR testing and/or MRI is important to avoid missing the diagnosis of multiple sclerosis or acoustic neuroma before initiation of treatment of AIED. Blood tests that may be useful include complete blood count, erythrocyte sedimentation rate, antinuclear antibody titer, rheumatoid factor, syphilis serology, thyroid function testing, C-reactive protein, C3 and C4 complement levels, Raji cell assay for circulating immune complexes, and immunoglobulin levels. Western blot assays for the patient's own antibodies against 68-kDa inner ear protein antigen is becoming one of the standards to confirm this disease.

Initial therapy for patients whose hearing loss is suspected to be autoimmune mediated consists of a therapeutic trial of high-dose anti-inflammatory steroid (prednisone

40–60 mg daily) for 3 to 4 weeks. Audiograms are performed at patient presentation and again in 3 weeks. The objective is to determine the maximum hearing improvement possible before beginning to reduce the medication significantly. Subsequently, the steroid dose is gradually decreased. The patient's hearing is monitored with serial audiograms. The objective in this titration phase is to maintain the improved hearing and reduce the medication to reduce complications. Occasionally, hearing improvement is not demonstrated, but hearing stabilization is seen; therefore, the same technique is used in these cases. The ultimate goal is to arrest the disease and stop prednisone treatment. If the hearing loss begins to recur during dose reduction, the dose must be increased, and additional treatments may be considered, such as plasmapheresis or cytotoxic agents.

Special Consideration

- It is crucial to determine whether immunological inner ear disease is associated with a systemic collagen disease. The latter can be devastating to vital structures for life.

Cogan's Syndrome

Cogan's syndrome is a disorder generally affecting young adults characterized by a sudden onset of interstitial keratitis and vestibuloauditory symptoms. Interstitial keratitis presents with eye pain, blurred vision, and lacrimation. Associated vestibuloauditory symptoms include vertigo, tinnitus, and sensorineural hearing loss occurring concomitantly. These symptoms usually occur with a sudden onset with waxing and waning and progressive hearing loss.

The cause of this disease is believed to be of cell-mediated autoimmune origin, with the autoimmune response being directed at the eye and ear. Cogan's syndrome may be associated with polyarteritis nodosa, which is discussed later.

Treatment is directed at suppressing the immune response with steroids, methotrexate, cyclophosphamide, and, rarely, plasmapheresis. Cochlear implantation in patients with Cogan's syndrome and sensorineural hearing loss is being studied.

Pitfall

- Failure to identify and treat Cogan's syndrome can result in blindness and deafness.

Polyarteritis Nodosa

Polyarteritis nodosa is a systemic necrotizing vasculitis of small and medium-sized arteries thought to be of immune complex deposition in origin. It most commonly affects middle-aged individuals, with a male/female ratio of ~2:1. Vessels of the kidneys, heart, liver, gastrointestinal tract,

peripheral nerves, mesentery, testes, and skeletal muscles are commonly involved. Symptoms include fever, weight loss, fatigue, abdominal pain, skin lesions, and joint pain. In addition, symptoms of renal failure, myocardial infarction, heart failure, and cardiac dysrhythmia may develop. Hearing loss, although not always present, may be mixed, conductive, or sensorineural, depending on vessel involvement.

Diagnosis by arteriography may demonstrate segmental narrowing of small and medium-sized vessels in the gastrointestinal tract. Biopsy of involved tissue may demonstrate necrosis, polymorphic infiltrate, thrombosis, and small vessel aneurysm formation. Treatment options consist of corticosteroids, cytotoxic agents, and/or plasmapheresis.

Vogt-Koyanagi-Harada Syndrome

Vogt-Koyanagi-Harada syndrome is believed to be an autoimmune-mediated response against melanocytes contained in the eye, skin meninges, and the inner ear. Symptoms include sensorineural hearing loss, vertigo, depigmentation of the hair and skin with uveitis, and nonbacterial meningitis. Treatment options are similar to that of polyarteritis nodosa.

Wegener's Granulomatosis

Classic Wegener's granulomatosis consists of necrotizing granulomas with systemic vasculitis affecting the upper and lower respiratory tracts and kidneys. Common problems associated with this illness are sinusitis, epistaxis (nosebleeds), otalgia, and hearing loss. Eighty-seven percent of patients with Wegener's granulomatosis have pulmonary disease. Left untreated, the illness is rapidly fatal, with renal involvement being the most frequent cause of death. Hearing loss is the presenting feature in 6 to 15% of the cases.

Early diagnosis and treatment are important in improving the long-term prognosis. Unfortunately, no single laboratory test is diagnostic for Wegener's granulomatosis. Complete blood count, erythrocyte sedimentation rate, urinalysis antinuclear antibodies, rheumatoid factor, creatinine level, sinus CT scan, and chest x-ray films are useful during the initial diagnostic process. Cytoplasmic staining anticytoplasmic antibodies have been found to be elevated in patients with active disease, and changing levels may correlate with activity of disease. Intranasal or lung biopsy specimens may show the pathological features of granulomatous changes, small and medium vessel vasculitis, and necrosis.

Treatment is often directed by a rheumatologist. Combinations of anti-inflammatory steroids, cyclophosphamide, methotrexate, and trimethoprim-sulfamethoxazole have been used to induce remission. Surgery, other than diagnosis by biopsy, is only useful in controlling occurrences of complications: sinusitis, otitis media, dacrocystorhinitis, proptosis, subglottic stenosis, and renal failure.

Sarcoidosis

Sarcoidosis is an inflammatory disease of unknown cause affecting multiple organ systems, particularly the lower respiratory tract. Noncaseating granulomas and Langhans' giant cells may be identified in any organ system. Respiratory failure, lymphadenopathy, splenomegaly, hepatic dysfunction, and cutaneous lesions may be seen in patients affected by this disease. Perivascular lymphocytic infiltrate, demyelinization, and axonal degeneration of CN VII and VIII have been identified in temporal bone sections of a patient with sarcoidosis. Patients with Heerfordt's disease, a variant of sarcoidosis, have uveitis, parotid enlargement, and bilateral facial paralysis. CNS involvement is seen in nearly 10% of patients with sarcoidosis. Treatment primarily consists of corticosteroids; however, the ultimate outcome may not change.

Poststapedectomy Granuloma

A noninfectious process that may occur 2 to 6 weeks after stapedectomy is foreign body granuloma formation at the site of the stapes implant. Typically, patients experience sensory and conductive hearing loss with significant reduction in word recognition scores. They may experience vertigo and tinnitus. A gray or erythematous mass in the posterosuperior quadrant of the middle ear space noted on otoscopy combined with the appropriate history is helpful in making the early diagnosis. With modern nonferromagnetic prostheses, MRI may be valuable in differentiating causes of sensorineural hearing loss following stapedectomy/stapedotomy.

Pearl

- Early and complete surgical excision may stabilize or reverse permanent sensorineural hearing loss in cases with poststapedectomy granuloma.

Neoplastic/Growth

Malignancies invading the temporal bone may be classified into those originating in the temporal bone (primary) or metastasizing to the temporal bone from other sites (secondary or metastasis). They are uncommon and rarely cause a sensorineural hearing loss until the labyrinth is involved. Squamous cell carcinoma is the most common malignancy involving the temporal bone in adults (85%). The remaining 15% of adult temporal bone malignancies are due to basal cell carcinomas, glandular tumors, regionally invasive cancers, and metastases. In the pediatric population, rhabdomyosarcoma is by far the most common temporal bone malignancy, followed by leukemia, fibrosarcoma, Ewing's sarcoma, and aggressive papillary adenoma.

Metastatic tumors to the temporal bone may originate from carcinomas of the breast, kidney, thyroid, lung, bone, and gastrointestinal tract. Metastases from melanoma, leukemia, and lymphomas occur occasionally.

Pain is the most common and noteworthy symptom of temporal bone malignancy, followed by hearing loss, pruritus, bleeding, headache, tinnitus, and vertigo. Typical signs of temporal bone malignancy are ear canal ulcerated mass, aural drainage, periauricular swelling, facial paralysis, and cervical adenopathy. Diagnosis is usually made by biopsy with additional information from CT and MRI scanning.

Treatment for most temporal bone malignancies usually consists of local measures (i.e., wound care and control of infection) and options of surgical resection, radiation therapy, and chemotherapy. It should be remembered that many antineoplastic agents are capable of causing ototoxicity.

Hematopoietic malignancies such as lymphoma and leukemia may involve the temporal bone and have a granular friable mass in the ear canal or middle ear space, thickened TM, otitis media, hearing loss, mastoiditis, and facial nerve paralysis. Acute lymphocytic leukemia produces more otologic symptoms than the other leukemias. Involvement of the temporal bone occurs in 20% of patients with leukemia. The temporal bone is affected by leukemic infiltrates, hemorrhage, and infection. Leukemic infiltrate of the labyrinth is rare.

Treatment is directed at controlling the leukemia and any secondary infection. Chemotherapy, culture, antibiotics, myringotomy and tube placement, and mastoidectomy may become necessary. Aural complications usually improve with treatment of the underlying leukemia.

Special Consideration

- Lytic bone lesions are malignant until proven otherwise.

Infectious

Cytomegalovirus

Infection with CMV, a herpes-type virus, is the most common congenital infection occurring in 1 to 2% of live newborns in the United States. It is the most common cause of early acquired sensorineural hearing loss in infants and children. Most infections in adults and children with intact immune systems are asymptomatic. Ninety to 95% of CMV neonatal infections are asymptomatic. However, 1 to 5% have CMV inclusion disease and may have multiorgan disease, causing dysfunction of the brain, liver, spleen, eye, and inner ear. One in 1000 congenitally infected asymptomatic patients have sensorineural hearing loss beyond the first year of life. Five to 15% of these patients eventually have mild to moderate bilateral hearing loss. Hearing loss is poorer at the high frequencies. Fowler and others (Fowler et al, 1997) found that asymptomatic congenital CMV infection is likely a leading cause of sensorineural hearing loss in young children. Furthermore, among CMV-infected children with an earlier hearing loss, further deterioration in hearing occurred in 50%.

CMV infections acquired after birth in nonimmunocompromised patients rarely progress to sensorineural hearing loss. In immunocompromised patients, such infections may lead to more serious complications associated with multiorgan system involvement. CMV may be passed transplacentally during an acute infection or during reactivation of a latent infection in mothers who previously demonstrated immunity. A 20-fold increase is found in parental infection in families with a child actively excreting virus and a 10-fold increase in parental infection in day care workers.

Diagnosis of CMV in the newborn may be made by (1) isolation of virus in urine, saliva, or umbilical cord blood; or (2) detection of CMV DNA by polymerase chain reaction. Detection of neonatal immunoglobulins to CMV may be helpful if performed in the first weeks of life. Active infection is treated with acyclovir, gancyclovir, or foscarnet sodium (Pass, 2005).

Toxoplasmosis

Toxoplasma gondii is an obligate intracellular protozoan parasite that can infect humans or other warm-blooded species. It is commonly acquired after ingestion of material contaminated with feces from infected cats, which are a reservoir for the oocyst-containing parasites. Nonimmunocompromised adults and children may experience a flulike illness. The fetus of a first-time infected mother may have congenital toxoplasmosis develop. Ninety to 95% of subclinically infected infants may eventually have symptoms of infection develop up to 16 years of age, predominantly retinal and choroid problems. Hearing loss occurs in 25% of these patients if not treated. In these untreated cases, the progressive hearing loss is due to the continued inflammatory response within the cochlea caused by the presence of the organism. Five to 10% of congenitally infected neonates are born with severe complications of toxoplasmosis with involvement of the CNS and eye. Diagnosis is made on clinical suspicion, serologic testing of the mother and infant, and occasionally CT scan of the neonate brain.

Spiramicin is used to treat mothers until definitive diagnosis. If infection is confirmed, a regimen of pyrimethamine-sulfonamide is initiated. Pyrimethamine-sulfonamide is alternated with spiramicin and continued for 1 year in the infected neonate. Patients with acquired immunodeficiency syndrome (AIDS) with toxoplasmosis are treated with pyrimethamine, trisulfapyrimadines, prednisone, and clindamycin. Risk of infection may be reduced by immunizing kittens with antitoxoplasma vaccine and heating food to at least 70 °F for 10 minutes.

Congenital Rubella

Rubella virus infection during pregnancy may lead to a wide variety of congenital problems, ranging from delayed sensorineural hearing loss to congenital heart defects, ocular defects, hepatosplenomegaly, thrombocytopenia, microcephaly, mental or motor retardation, long bone radiolucencies, interstitial pneumonitis, encephalitis, and low birth weight. The severity of complications is associated with duration of infection during pregnancy. First trimester infections are associated with poorer outcomes than third trimester infections.

The classic triad of the congenitally infected infant is congenital hearing loss, cataracts, and cardiac defects. The sensorineural hearing loss is usually flat in configuration and severe or profound. Fifty percent of infants born with symptomatic congenital rubella have hearing loss. Infants born with infection later in the pregnancy may be asymptomatic at birth. Ten to 20% of these asymptomatic children have hearing loss that may be progressive.

Clinical suspicion should be elevated in the patient with congenital hearing loss with a mother having a history of a skin rash during pregnancy. Diagnosis of congenital rubella may be made by (1) isolation of rubella virus or detecting rubella ribonucleic acid (RNA) from urine or throat cultures; (2) detection of neonatal immunoglobulin M (IgM) antibodies in the first weeks of life; (3) detection of increasing antirubella antibody titer in the first few months of life; and (4) ophthalmologic examination, which may reveal pigment abnormalities diagnostic of rubella embryopathy.

Unfortunately, no treatment for preventing the sequelae of congenital rubella infection exists after infection occurs. However, prevention of rubella infection with the introduction of the rubella vaccine has significantly reduced the incidence of congenital rubella in the United States.

Mumps (Epidemic Parotitis)

The mumps virus causes a flulike illness with sore throat, chills, fever, malaise, and parotid gland swelling in children and young adults. Deafness occurring with mumps usually occurs at the end of the first week of parotitis. It is unilateral in 80% of the cases and is usually profound and permanent. Tinnitus and fullness in the affected ear are common.

Mumps may be diagnosed by viral isolation from throat cultures, CSF, or detection of a rise in mumps antibody titers between acute and convalescent titers. At present, no treatment exists for mumps infection; however, mumps vaccine given at an early age prevents infection in later life.

Measles

Measles is a highly communicable viral disease causing fever, sore throat, cough, and rash in the pediatric to young adult age group. It is caused by the rubeola virus. Deafness occurs in 0.1% of patients with measles. The bilateral and usually abrupt onset of hearing loss occurs at the time of the rash. Usually a greater degree of hearing loss is seen in the higher frequencies. No specific treatment for measles or its associated hearing loss exists. Measles and deafness caused by measles are now rare because of the widespread use of the rubeola vaccine.

Varicella zoster Virus

The *Varicella zoster* virus is a herpesvirus that is identical to the virus that causes chickenpox (varicella) and shingles (zoster). Infections by this virus (herpes zoster oticus or Ramsay Hunt syndrome) cause painful vesicular eruptions of the ear canal and external ear, facial paralysis, and occasionally sensorineural hearing loss and vertigo. Sensorineural hearing loss occurs in 6% of these patients.

The diagnosis is based on a high level of clinical suspicion. The isolation of virus from vesicles, detection of virus DNA in vesicle fluid or CSF, and demonstration of multinucleated giant cells in vesicle scrapings can confirm herpes zoster oticus. Treatment consists of local care of the vesicles, acyclovir, and anti-inflammatory steroids.

Human Immunodeficiency Virus

AIDS is caused by the human immunodeficiency virus (HIV). Sensorineural hearing loss is seen in 49% of HIV-infected patients. Worsening cochlear and vestibular dysfunction is correlated with longer durations of infection. Causes of sensorineural hearing loss in HIV-infected patients are (1) use of potentially ototoxic medication; (2) opportunistic infection; (3) neoplastic processes affecting the temporal bone, IAC, and CNS; (4) idiopathic causes; and (5) CNS infections or demyelination. Potentially ototoxic medications used to treat HIV complications are aminoglycosides, amphotericin B, azydothymidine, pentamidine, and azythromycin. HIV-infected patients are predisposed to syphilis and cryptococcal meningitis, which can cause sensorineural hearing loss. Occult meningitis may be the cause of hearing loss in these patients.

Otosyphilis should be considered in any HIV-infected patient complaining of hearing loss or vertigo. Patients may complain of sudden, progressive, or fluctuating hearing loss with or without tinnitus, aural fullness, or disequilibrium. Diagnosis may be made with fluorescent treponemal antibody absorption test (FTA-ABS) and Venereal Disease Research Laboratory (VDRL) test.

Treatment of otosyphilis in the HIV-infected patient should consist of high-dose penicillin given over several weeks. Corticosteroids, normally used in treating non-HIV otosyphilis, should be used with caution in the HIV population because they may worsen the preexisting immunocompromised condition. In addition, previously treated HIV-syphilis patients may have reactivation of latent syphilis; therefore, recurrent otosyphilis should be suspected in any treated patient with cochleovestibular complaints.

Sensorineural hearing loss caused by cryptococcal meningitis may have headache, nausea/vomiting, disorientation, and cranial nerve abnormalities. Hearing loss is the most common cranial nerve abnormality and may be the initial presenting symptom. Cryptococcal meningitis causes a predominantly retrocochlear hearing loss. Diagnosis can be made by serum cryptococcal antigen and evaluation of CSF by lumbar puncture. Cryptococcal meningitis is treated with amphotericin B and 5-fluorocytosine followed by lifelong suppression with fluconazole.

Central auditory dysfunction unrelated to cryptococcal meningitis is a common cause of sensorineural hearing loss in the patient with HIV and is related to demyelination of the central auditory tract. Evaluation of sensorineural hearing loss in the HIV-infected patient should include a thorough history, head and neck examination, pure-tone audiometry with evaluation of stapedial reflex, and word recognition scores. In addition, electronystagmography (ENG) may be useful in the evaluation of patients with disequilibrium. VDRL test, FTA test, serum cryptococcal antigen, antinuclear antibodies, erythrocyte sedimentation rate, and rheumatoid factor may be useful. MRI or CT scan should precede lumbar puncture in patients with neurologic signs or symptoms.

Treatment of HIV-infected patients with hearing loss should concentrate on the underlying cause of hearing loss.

Caution should be exercised with the use of anti-inflammatory steroids because of their inherent risk of increasing immunosuppression (Monsell et al, 1997).

Other Viruses and Mycoplasma

Adenovirus, influenza virus, and *Mycoplasma* (a nonviral cause of pneumonia) have been associated with sensorineural hearing loss. In addition, sudden sensorineural hearing loss occurs in the presence of an upper respiratory tract infection in 25% of patients. Epidemiologic clusters of upper respiratory tract infections associated with sensorineural hearing loss have been observed (Roland and Marple, 1997).

Meningitis

Meningitis is caused by inflammation of the brain or spinal cord and may be caused by bacteria, viruses, or, more rarely, disseminated fungal infections, disseminated malignancies, and chemicals or toxins. Symptoms of meningitis are fever, headache, stiff neck, and vomiting. This may progress to disorientation, coma, or death. One third of all noncongenital hearing loss is due to complications of bacterial meningitis. Persistent sensorineural loss occurs in 10% from bacteria or their toxin invading the inner ears from the CSF. Deafness may occur at any point during the course of meningitis; however, it commonly occurs early. Bacteria most commonly associated with sensorineural hearing loss after meningitis are *Streptococcus pneumoniae, Neisseria meningitides,* and *Haemophilus influenzae.*

Diagnosis is made by case history, physical examination, and CSF cellular, electrolyte, and protein evaluation and culture from lumbar puncture.

Treatment is aimed at appropriate antibiotic therapy and corticosteroids. Corticosteroids reduce the inflammatory process in the labyrinth, thereby lessening the chances or intensity of hearing loss.

Labyrinthitis

Labyrinthitis is due to an inflammatory process within the labyrinth. It may be secondary to direct invasion by bacteria, viruses, spirochetes, protozoa, or fungi or their toxic effects. The types of labyrinthitis are stratified into perilabyrinthitis and endolabyrinthitis. Perilabyrinthitis is caused by substances entering the perilymph and defined by what enters the fluid. In serous labyrinthitis, toxins enter; in suppurative labyrinthitis, bacteria enter; and in chronic labyrinthitis, soft tissue enters, like the matrix of a cholesteatoma. Endolabyrinthitis is from hematogenous dissemination of viruses to the membranous labyrinth. End-stage obliteration of the labyrinth with fibrous tissue is called fibrous labyrinthitis, and obliteration with new bone is known as labyrinthine ossificans. Serous labyrinthitis is one of the most common complications of otitis media. It is caused by bacterial toxins entering the labyrinth from an adjacent acute otitis media. These toxins may enter the inner ear from the CSF in cases of meningitis.

Clinically, the patient experiences vertigo, tinnitus, and sensorineural hearing loss associated with otitis media or meningitis. The accompanying irritative nystagmus beats toward the affected ear until it rapidly becomes paralytic to the labyrinth and reverses direction. The cochleovestibular symptoms can be reversible. Treatment for serous labyrinthitis includes supportive care, appropriate antibiotic coverage, and myringotomy in patients with bacterial otitis media. It can rapidly progress to bacterial labyrinthitis and meningitis.

Pearl

- Sudden onset of severe vertigo, tinnitus, nausea, and vomiting with sudden hearing loss in the setting of an acute or chronic otitis media indicates that labyrinthitis has developed. Within a very short time, this can progress to meningitis.

Suppurative labyrinthitis occurs with direct bacterial invasion of the labyrinth. Signs and symptoms are the same as serous labyrinthitis; however, recovery does not occur, and meningitis can rapidly result. Therefore, patients with these signs and symptoms and an ear infection should be considered a medical emergency. The ultimate recovery profile will determine whether it is suppurative or serous.

Treatment for suppurative labyrinthitis consists of hospitalization, hydration, vestibular suppressants, and appropriate antibiotic therapy. Antibiotic selection depends on the results of culture obtained from the patient and the specific antibiotic sensitivities of the cultured organism. When acute otitis media is the source of infection, myringotomy for drainage and bacterial identification is necessary. Mastoidectomy may be required to resolve a subacute or chronic infection.

Chronic labyrinthitis is a complication of chronic middle ear disease, characteristically with cholesteatoma, resulting in fistula through the otic capsule, usually over the horizontal semicircular canal. Other causes of fistula are granulation tissue, cholesterol granuloma, and tumors of the middle ear. A patient with a history of chronic ear disease presenting with fluctuating mild vertigo or hearing loss that is worsened by the Valsalva's maneuver or pressure on the ear should be suspected of having a labyrinthine fistula. A positive fistula test is found by creating positive or negative pressure in the EAC that causes vertigo with nystagmus. Patients with this problem are predisposed to suppurative labyrinthitis. Mastoidectomy is usually required to resolve this problem.

Pitfall

- Failure to make the diagnosis of labyrinthine fistula may result in permanent loss of cochleovestibular function.

Labyrinthine fibrosis and ossification are common sequelae to suppurative labyrinthitis. This process begins within months of a suppurative labyrinthitis and is caused by fibrous replacement of the inner ear structures. This fibrous process is followed by bony replacement of the labyrinth. Clinically, deafness is complete, the incapacitating vertigo has disappeared, and the patient may continue to have mild disequilibrium.

Although little can be done to stop ossification, it is important to recognize its early development in potential cochlear implant patients. Insertion of the complete electrode array is difficult once labyrinthine ossification begins. In addition, performance of patients implanted after the ossification process is poorer than those implanted before ossification. Temporal bone CT and/or MRI confirms labyrinthine fibrosis and/or ossification.

Fungal Infections

Fungal infections of the labyrinth are rare. Species associated with fungal labyrinthitis are *Candida, Mucor, Cryptococcus,* and *Blastomyces.* Infections of this nature usually occur in patients with immunocompromise (i.e., AIDS and transplant patients), diabetes, leukemia, or terminal illness. The source of infection may be middle ear, meninges, or blood borne. When possible, treatment is directed at correcting the underlying cause and administration of intravenous amphotericin B (Haruna et al, 1994).

Syphilis

Otitic syphilis is caused by the spirochete *Treponema pallidum.* Often the presenting symptoms are similar to those of Meniere's disease: fluctuating progressive sensorineural hearing loss, aural fullness, tinnitus, and vertigo. Otitic syphilis, however, has a higher incidence of bilateral disease. Syphilis as a cause of sensorineural hearing loss occurs during the late congenital and tertiary acquired stage of syphilis.

Symptoms are due to a resorptive osteitis of the labyrinth that can destroy the inner ear, cause hydrops, or cause fistulization of the bony labyrinthine wall. A positive Hennebert's sign (vertigo and nystagmus with pressure applied to the ear canal) and Tullio's phenomenon (vertigo seen with high-intensity sound) can be associated with otosyphilis.

Diagnosis is suspected if there is a positive FTA-ABS or VDRL test result in a patient with these symptoms. Neurosyphilis must be excluded or confirmed by evaluating the CSF for organisms and/or positive CSF, FTA-ABS, and VDRL test findings.

Treatment consists of high-dose, long-term penicillin and anti-inflammatory corticosteroids (Roland and Marple, 1997).

Pearl

- In patients with fluctuating hearing loss with or without vertigo, it is important to consider syphilis, a treatable disease.

Degenerative/Idiopathic

Presbycusis

Presbycusis is the loss of hearing associated with the aging process. Schuknecht (1993a) defined four histopathologic types: sensory, neural, strial, and cochlear conductive. Sensory presbycusis is due to flattening and atrophy of the basal turn of the organ of Corti because of loss of hair cells and supporting cells. It produces a progressive bilateral, sharply sloping high-frequency sensorineural hearing loss that begins in middle age. Neural presbycusis is initially due to atrophy of the spiral ganglion and nerves of the osseous spiral lamina in the basal turn of the cochlea. Neural presbycusis produces a moderate-sloping high-frequency hearing loss that is bilateral and gradual in progression. The organ of Corti is usually intact compared with sensory presbycusis. Word recognition scores are disproportionately poorer than pure-tone thresholds, making the benefit from amplification more difficult. Strial presbycusis is due to atrophy of the stria vascularis producing a flat sensorineural hearing loss with preservation of word recognition scores. Word recognition scores are usually preserved until pure-tone averages exceed 50 dB hearing level (HL). Cochlear conductive presbycusis is believed to be due to excessive stiffness of the basilar membrane; however, histopathological findings are absent. It produces an elevation of pure-tone thresholds and decrease in word recognition scores. Audiometric evaluation demonstrates a bilateral symmetrical gradually sloping sensorineural hearing loss.

At present, little can be done to prevent or slow the progression of presbycusis. However, moderately severe hearing loss, or poorer, is usually not because of aging alone. After the occurrence of significant hearing loss, amplification, hearing assistive technology (HAT), or cochlear implantation may be the only treatment options available.

Sudden Idiopathic Sensorineural Hearing Loss

Sudden sensorineural hearing loss is defined by a sensorineural hearing loss of 30 dB HL or greater over at least three audiometric frequencies occurring within 3 days or less. With the exception of presbycusis, most of the previously discussed causes of sensorineural hearing loss (infections, neoplasms, trauma, ototoxicity, immunologic, metabolic, and developmental) may have what initially appears to be idiopathic sudden sensorineural hearing loss. It is the obligation of the practitioner to attempt to identify the source of any hearing loss by thorough case history, physical examination, appropriate audiometric evaluation, laboratory examination, and diagnostic imaging. A careful patient history will identify a cause in 10 to 15% of these sudden cases. The "diagnosis" of sudden idiopathic hearing loss can only be made when other identifiable causes of hearing loss are ruled out.

Sudden sensorineural hearing loss occurs in approximately 1 patient per 5000 population per year. It is likely that more cases actually occur than present clinically because of possible spontaneous resolution before obtaining medical advice. No predilection for either ear or gender exists. No apparent occupational predisposition exists. The degree of hearing loss is variable and usually unilateral. Ten percent are bilateral. Seventy percent of patients with sudden deafness present with tinnitus, and 40% have some form of vertigo or disequilibrium. Two thirds of patients improve without treatment within 2 weeks. Fifteen percent of patients with hearing loss progress. A poorer prognosis for recovery is associated with severity and duration of hearing loss, presence of vertigo, advanced age, and reduced word recognition scores. In addition, the shape of the audiogram appears to have some relationship to prognosis. Rising and trough configurations have a better prognosis for recovery than sloping or flat configurations.

When identifiable, treatment of sudden sensorineural hearing loss is based on the cause. Treatments of sudden idiopathic sensorineural hearing loss, however, are numerous, based on suspected cause. Viral infection, labyrinthine hypoxia, and autoimmune disease have been suggested as potential factors. In the past, treatment regimens have aimed at (1) improving blood flow or oxygenation to the inner ear, (2) fighting possible viral infection, (3) reducing inflammation or autoimmune response, (4) preventing further injury (rest), and (5) reducing the potential causes of hydrops. The current, generally accepted approach includes an initial trial of bed rest, anti-inflammatory corticosteroids, low-salt diet, and a diuretic. Others would consider the addition of oral antiviral medication and the vasodilating properties of carbogen, an inhaled mixture of oxygen and carbon dioxide. When medical therapy fails and there is suspicion of PLF, surgical exploration may be warranted.

Meniere's Disease

Meniere's disease, in its classical form, describes an aggregate of signs and symptoms in which the patient has recurrent episodes of vertigo lasting minutes to hours, with associated fluctuating roaring tinnitus, aural fullness, and sensory hearing loss. These episodes may be accompanied by nausea and vomiting. Meniere's disease typically is unilateral and presents with a rising audiometric configuration. Early in the disease, the patient's hearing is usually preserved between attacks. The course of this illness is highly variable. Some patients may have a few mild episodes, whereas others may endure numerous debilitating episodes and gradually lose hearing over time. In some cases, the illness is said to "burn out" over time with fewer, less intense occurrences as the patient's hearing decreases. Twenty percent of patients will have a family history of Meniere's disease. Forty percent of patients will develop bilateral involvement. Meniere's disease may occur at any age; however, its onset is most common in the third to sixth decade of life (Roland and Marple, 1997).

Meniere's disease is not curable; however, 75 to 85% of patients respond to medical treatment. The goals of treatment are to alleviate symptoms during the acute attack and to reduce the frequency of recurrence. Labyrinthine suppressants such as antihistamines (meclizine), benzodiazepines (Valium), anticholinergics (scopolamine), and antiemetics (perchlorperazine maleate [Compazine] and promethazine [Phenergan]) are used to control acute symptoms of vertigo, nausea, and vomiting. Low-salt diet and avoidance of caffeine and alcohol may be useful in reducing recurrences. In addition, triamterene with hydrochlorothiazide (Dyazide), a diuretic used to treat mild hypertension, has been found to reduce recurrences in some patients (Roland and Marple, 1997).

For those patients who fail conservative medical therapy, surgical options may be considered. It should be remembered that 20 to 40% of patients with Meniere's disease will have bilateral involvement. Therefore, any surgical procedure potentially compromising hearing must be carefully considered. A thoughtful and progressive approach to interventions is advisable, stopping at the level of satisfactory efficacy. The following is the author's progressive interventional protocol to date, following medical treatment.

An old, but effective, intervention is the insertion of a tympanostomy tube in the eardrum on the affected side. This intervention has been proven experimentally to reduce endolymphatic hydrops (Kimura and Hutta, 1997).

A new treatment, which first requires the insertion of a tympanostomy tube, is the low-pressure pulse generator (Meniett device). The low-pressure pulsing is thought to reduce hydrops and alleviate episodic vertigo in Meniere's disease (Gates, 2005).

If these efforts fail, office intratympanic gentamicin titration using a fine needle on a tuberculin syringe to inject through the intact anesthetized eardrum or tympanostomy tube at intervals no closer than 3 to 4 weeks is effective and has a low incidence of inducing hearing loss (Chia et al, 2004).

Complete ablation of the inner ear or vestibular nerve, such as with a vestibular nerve section or labyrinthectomy, is rarely required. Endolymphatic sac surgery is uncommon today.

Pearl

- The initial treatment for Meniere's disease is aimed at medical control of symptoms. Generally, invasive techniques with lower surgical risk and risk of hearing loss may be considered for those patients who initially have medical therapy fail. Invasive techniques associated with a higher risk of hearing loss or associated complications may be considered in patients who have a permanent severe loss or those in whom more conservative therapy has failed.

Each patient should be evaluated individually, with therapy directed to the highest benefit/risk ratio for that patient.

Cochlear Otosclerosis

Otosclerosis is usually associated with conductive hearing loss presenting with progressive hearing loss. Lesions of this disease of otic capsule bone usually cause fixation of the stapes footplate. These lesions, however, may spread extensively within the otic capsule and cause both sensory and conductive hearing loss. If cochlear hearing loss occurs without the conductive component, it is known as cochlear

otosclerosis; otherwise, it may be described as oval window and labyrinthine otosclerosis. Rarely does otosclerosis cause a sensorineural loss without conductive hearing loss.

Oral sodium fluoride may be given in an attempt to stabilize hearing. Serial audiograms are used to monitor hearing during sodium fluoride therapy. Because of similarities between osteoporosis and otosclerosis and growing evidence supporting an association between the two diseases (Clayton et al, 2004), interest is growing in the potential use of diphosphonates (alendronate [Fosamax], etidronate [Didrocal], and risedronate [Actonel]) to attempt to reverse or stall the progression of otosclerosis, especially those with sensorineural losses. Two reports, however, suggest these compounds may be associated with deterioration in hearing. A recent class-action suit against one of these drugs further dampens enthusiasm. Cochlear hearing loss may be due to a multitude of factors. It is the responsibility of the practitioner to identify the cause of hearing loss and to evaluate the other potential associated medical ramifications to treat the patient as a whole. Complete audiologic assessments are crucial in the initial evaluation and subsequent therapeutic monitoring of sensorineural hearing losses.

◆ Causes of Neural Hearing Losses

Neural lesions may or may not create a mass or anatomical distortion detectable by imaging techniques. Because of this, it is helpful to consider neural lesions detectable by imaging and those that are not. Cellular, or subcellular, dysfunctions of the primary auditory neurons and pathways manifest as neural auditory defects. Cellular dysfunctions in other systems may be genetically or physiologically related to the auditory neuronal function. Leads to these disorders come from a careful and professionally performed case history; confirmation requires specific tests determined by this medical sleuthing.

These patients may have profound auditory, vestibular, or facial motor complaints, or none at all. They may also present with conductive hearing loss with or without middle ear effusion. Therefore, it is imperative to evaluate each type of hearing loss independently.

Lesions Detectable by Imaging

Congenital/Genetic/Developmental

Paget's Disease   Paget's disease is an autosomal dominant polyostotic (meaning more than one separate bone) bone disease of laminar bone of the neurocranium, sacrum, spine, pelvis, femur, and tibia. It deforms the local architecture by progressive osteoclastic osteolytic (meaning bone destruction by special cells adjacent to bone called osteoclasts) bone resorption and replacement with fibrous and vascular tissue, followed by osteoblastic (special cells adjacent to bone that build bone) new bone formation, which creates a mosaic pattern of an excess, but weak, bony mass.

Conductive and sensory hearing losses are more common than neural hearing loss. The cause of these losses is not clear; obliteration of the round window niche with fibrous tissue or with a markedly enlarged jugular bulb and sigmoid sinus may be implicated. Bony distortions of the skull base can result in basilar impressions, resulting in vertebrobasilar ischemia (underperfusion of tissues), compression of cranial nerves, or cerebral or cerebellar dysfunction.

Treatment is predominantly medical by calcitonin, sodium etidronate, or the combination of both. The objective of treatment is to arrest progression of the disease and symptoms. Surgery can be hazardous and ineffective, except in few select cases.

Osteosarcoma, fibrosarcoma, or giant cell tumor transformation can arise from a Paget's lesion. A rapid or unusual change in symptoms causing pain, pathological fractures, or bone enlargement should alert the caregiver to this possibility.

Osteopetroses   Osteopetroses are a group of hereditary metabolic bone diseases generally classified, by time of clinical onset and clinical course, into a congenital (early onset), or lethal, form and a tarda (delayed onset), or adult, form; the former is transmitted in an autosomal recessive fashion, and the latter is autosomal dominant, except Albers-Schönberg disease, which is autosomal recessive. The tarda form may involve all the skull, type I, such as Englemann's disease, or only the skull base, type II. The disease obliterates spaces and foramina (anatomical holes or passages in bone), resulting in compression neuropathies and conductive and neural hearing losses.

Medical treatment is ineffective; surgical intervention can be helpful. Reconstruction of the external ear canal, middle ear space, and ossicular reconstruction can be useful. Facial nerve decompression can be effective to avoid progressive or recurrent paralysis; decompression of the IAC may be effective in stabilizing neural hearing losses but remains to be proven.

Neoplastic/Growth

Solitary Vestibular Schwannomas (Acoustic Neuromas)
Schwannomas, also known as neurinomas and neurilemmomas, originate from Schwann's cells comprising the neurilemmal, rather than the glial portion of cranial and peripheral nerves. Common usage, albeit erroneous, has led to the terms *acoustic neuromas* and *acoustic tumors*. Eighth nerve schwannomas arise within the vestibular nerve and expand within the trunk of CN VIII and its branches in all directions. These tumors destroy some fibers, infiltrate between others, encasing some fibers in the peripheral substance of the tumor mass, and dispersing and displacing other fibers on the surface of the tumor in large or very small aggregates. Because of this pathobiology, hearing preservation surgery with total tumor removal, though possible, is very difficult (Lin et al, 2005). **Figures 10–9** and **10–10** demonstrate small and large solitary vestibular schwannomas and the value of gadolinium-enhanced MRI to detect these tumors.

Treatment options are (1) expectant observation to determine if and when enlargement occurs, (2) stereotactic radiotherapy to retard growth, and (3) surgical removal. Each case is special and should be considered in detail with the patient by an experienced neurotologist/neurosurgical team.

Three surgical approaches are appropriate for tumors of any size. The approach primarily depends on the surgical objective and the experience of the surgeon. Middle fossa approaches and retrosigmoid, retrolabyrinthine approaches are usually used for hearing conservation. Translabyrinthine or the extended transcochlear approaches are used when hearing conservation is not a feasible objective.

Controversial Point

- Hearing conservation surgery may increase the risk of incomplete tumor removal. If incomplete removal does happen, it may or may not result in recurrence.

Neurofibromatosis Type 2   Neurofibromatosis type 2 (NF2) is an autosomal dominant genetic condition phenotypically presenting with bilateral vestibular schwannomas, schwannomas of other cranial nerves, meningiomas, and other low-grade brain malignancies throughout the intracranial cavity and spine. The NF2 gene is on chromosome 22q12. Because of the bilateral and multicentric presentations of these tumors, MRIs of the head and complete spine are necessary. Audiometric and genetic screening of at-risk family members during infancy is appropriate. MRI screening may be appropriate at 10 to 12 years of age (Evans et al, 2005).

Very conservative management by centers with considerable experience with these cases is the central focus of these progressively difficult cases (Evans et al, 2005). If some cochlear nerve can be spared with tumor removal, cochlear implantation can result in serviceable hearing, but at the risk of tumor recurrence (Aristegui and Denia, 2005). Brainstem auditory stimulating implants may be required to give some awareness of sound; unfortunately, open set speech may be difficult in these cases. Chapter 13 in this volume addresses brainstem auditory stimulating implants in detail.

Controversial Point

- Bilateral neurofibromas of CN VIII almost invariably lead to bilateral profound sensorineural hearing loss, either from the disease or its treatment. However, because of a few isolated cases of successful tumor removal or stabilization with irradiation with hearing conservation, the issue of when and how to intervene in NF2 remains challenging and controversial.

Other neoplastic Schwann's cell lesions that may mimic acoustic neuromas are facial nerve (CN VII) trigeminal nerve (CNV), and jugular, foramen schwannomas.

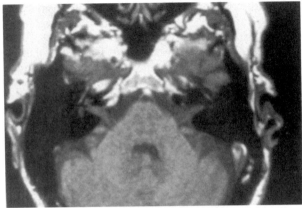

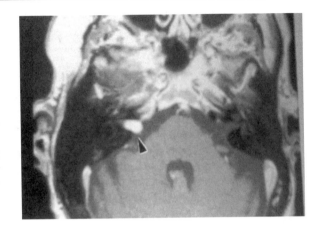

A

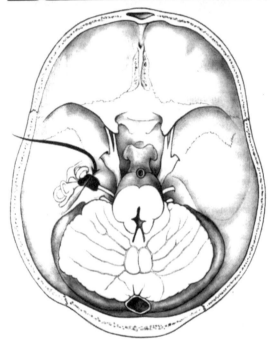

B

Figure 10–9 (A) Magnetic resonance imaging (MRI) without and with contrast gadolinium, showing a small right intracanalicular solitary vestibular schwannoma (*arrow*). **(B)** Illustration showing the tumor (*arrow*) drawn on the left for easy comparison with the MRI, which, by convention, shows the patient's right side on the examiner's left. (From Lustig, L. R., & Jackler, R. K. (1997). Benign tumors of the temporal bone. In G. B. Hughes & M. L. Pensak (Eds.), Clinical otology (2nd ed., pp. 313–334). New York: Thieme Medical Publishers, with permission.)

Treatment may be surgical or stereotaxic radiotherapeutic. Manipulation of a facial neuroma alone may result in facial paralysis; however, occasionally, the facial nerve may be spared and the tumor removed. If preoperatively involved by a jugular foramen tumor, CN IX, X, and/or XI cannot be saved; however, return of function of CN VIII can occur with resection of the compressing jugular foramen tumor.

Controversial Point

• Even the slightest manipulations of facial neuromas can result in total facial paralysis and a poor outcome. Conversely, the longer a partial paralysis progresses, the poorer the outcome, even with grafting. These two points power the controversy of when and how to intervene in a facial nerve schwannoma.

Meningiomas   Meningiomas arise from arachnoid meningothelial cells in a variety of intracranial locations and are usually benign. Four characteristic locations from which meningiomas arise relative to the temporal bone are IAC, jugular foramen, geniculate ganglion, and greater and lesser petrosal nerves (Nager, 1993; **Fig. 10–11** and **Fig. 10–12**). Meningiomas are usually globular, encapsulated tumors tightly adherent and invasive of dura but not of brain, and often highly vascular from the adjacent dural vascular supply.

Posterior fossa, or infratentorial, meningiomas may be subdivided into six groups according to location: petroclival, cerebellopontine angle, cerebellar convexity, fourth ventricle, foramen magnum, and jugular foramen. Any of these meningiomas may mimic vestibular schwannomas by direct impingement on or by distortion of CN VIII, or they may occur simultaneously with NF2 bilateral CN VIII schwannomas.

Treatment is surgical resection; the approach depends on the site and extent of the lesion and the residual function of

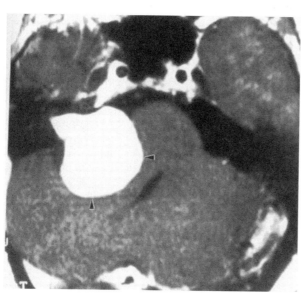

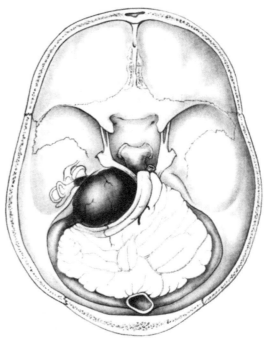

Figure 10–10 (A) MRI with contrast gadolinium, showing a large right solitary vestibular schwannoma. **(B)** Illustration showing the tumor drawn on the right for easy comparison with the MRI, which by convention, shows the patient's right side on the examiner's left. (From Lustig, L. R., & Jackler, R. K. (1997). Benign tumors of the temporal bone. In G. B. Hughes & M. L. Pensak (Eds.), Clinical otology (2nd ed., pp. 313–334). New York: Thieme Medical Publishers, with permission.)

the involved nerves. Treatment for recurrent or incompletely resected tumors may include radiotherapy.

Pitfall

- Meningiomas can get quite large and have slight symptoms. They are easily missed or underestimated.

Cholesteatomas (Epidermoids) of the Deep Petrous Bone or Meninges Congenital epidermoids, or congenital cholesteatomas, may be divided into four groups: mesotympanic, perigeniculate, petrous apex (extradural, cranial,

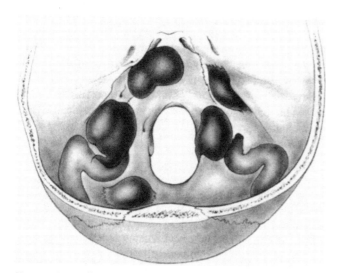

Figure 10–11 Illustration showing the common location of meningiomas that are associated with the temporal bone. (From Lustig, L. R., & Jackler, R. K. (1997). Benign tumors of the temporal bone. In G. B. Hughes & M. L. Pensak (Eds.), Clinical otology (2nd ed., pp. 313–334). New York: Thieme Medical Publishers, with permission.)

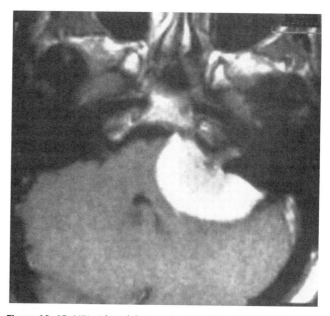

Figure 10–12 MRI with gadolinium, showing a large left cerebellopontine angle meningioma, characteristically sessile and broad based adjacent to the temporal bone, but not extending into the internal auditory canal. (From Roland, P. S., & Marple, B. F. (1997). Disorders of inner ear, eighth nerve, and CNS. In P. S. Roland, B. F. Marple, & W. L. Meyerhoff (Eds.), Hearing loss (pp. 195–256). New York: Thieme Medical Publishers, with permission.)

or diploic), and cerebellopontine angle (intradural, intracranial). By far the most common are those that arise in the mesotympanum of the middle ear, which rarely cause neural hearing loss. Those arising in the perigeniculate (more lateral to the otic capsule) and petrous apex (more medial to the otic capsule) locations erode bone to impinge on the facial nerve, inner ear, and CN VIII but usually remain extradural even if they expand into the posterior or middle fossae. Those arising in the cerebellopontine angle may become quite large before presenting like vestibular schwannomas. Facial twitching is unusual, but more common in the latter three.

Because of the proximity to the eustachian tube, like many other mass lesions in the petrous apex or protympanum, mesotympanic, perigeniculate, and petrous apex, cholesteatomas may present as a unilateral serous middle ear effusion, with or without sensorineural loss. This emphasizes the need to evaluate unilateral effusions or mixed hearing losses very carefully relative to each component of the anatomy and hearing loss.

Treatment is surgical and is designed to remove the mass or to marsupialize it (marsupialize means to remove the lateral wall of the cyst and all tissues lateral, or external, to the cyst so that the contents of the cyst are exposed to the outside). The surgical approach is designed to accommodate the remaining function and the exact site and extent of the lesion. A transtympanic, transmastoid approach, with extradural middle fossa or posterior fossa perilabyrinthine extensions, may be used to resect or marsupialize the lesions limited to the osseous and extradural areas, which have function and in which the anatomy makes this appropriate. Otherwise, a translabyrinthine or transcochlear approach may be necessary. For intradural lesions, approaches for vestibular schwannomas are used. Marsupialization is not an option; however, incomplete resection occasionally is necessary.

Special Consideration

- Petrous apex lesions can obstruct the eustachian tube and present only as unilateral serous otitis media.

Petrous Cholesterol Granulomas Petrous apex cholesterol granulomas are slowly expanding bone-erosive lesions in the petrous apex formed by foreign body tissue reaction about cholesterol crystals as a consequence of red cells, the source of the cholesterol, in the presence of a relative vacuum. As these painless, occult lesions expand, they may compress CN VIII or nerves adjacent to the apex, such as CN VI or VI.

Complete resection of these lesions is not usually possible or necessary. Surgical drainage with aeration into the middle ear or mastoid is effective. Infracochlear or infralabyrinthine approaches through an enlarged EAC or mastoidectomy with stenting the opening is usually sufficient. Careful and perpetual surveillance is necessary.

Chondromas and Chondrosarcomas Chondromas are rare benign tumors of hyaline cartilage arising from areas of synchondroses (where embryonic cartilage origin bones join) within the base of skull. They may arise from or extend into the cerebellopontine angle from primary sites as distant as the parasellar region and compress CN VIII, mimicking signs and symptoms of solitary vestibular schwannomas. As they expand within the petrous bone, they create a radiographically lytic (bone-destructive) lesion with irregular margins. Rarely, they may become malignant and metastasize.

Chondrosarcomas are rare malignant tumors of cartilage arising from areas of endochondral ossification within the base of the skull. The degree of malignancy tends to correlate with the histological findings. These tumors are difficult to distinguish from benign chondromas; histological examination of the surgical specimen is crucial in this differentiation.

Treatment is surgical resection using one or more of the extradural or intradural approaches to the skull base. Preservation of neural function is expected if the anatomy of the lesion allows. Unresected, these lesions can become quite large.

Treatment of chondrosarcomas with total removal was once considered impractical or impossible; however, with infratemporal fossa or transcochlear approaches, these can sometimes be totally resected. Preservation of neural function is not the primary concern in these tumors. These are relatively radioresistant (not susceptible to irradiation); however, some response is seen with high doses of irradiation.

Chordomas Chordomas are uncommon but less rare than chondromas and derive from aberrant remnants of the notochord; these tend to arise in children and young adults. The embryonic notochord is predominantly midline; however, these tumors may originate or extend to lateral locations. They occur in the vertebrae, the sacrococcygeal area (the pelvic bone), and the spheno-occipital region of the skull. In the skull base, they may involve the sella (sella turcica, wherein sits the pituitary gland), clivus, or petrous apex and become quite large, compressing cranial nerves. They may involve CN VII or VIII within the petrous bone or with the cerebellopontine angle. They may present like a vestibular schwannoma; however, imaging shows a large destructive lesion in the petrous bone. These lesions are clinically difficult, if not impossible, to differentiate from chondromas, except chordomas are more common. Rarely, they may become malignant and metastasize.

Treatment is surgical resection using one or more of the extradural or intradural approaches to the skull base. Preservation of neural function is expected if the anatomy of the lesion allows. Often, these lesions are soft and can be evacuated almost totally with suction; recurrences can occur. Unresected, these lesions can become quite large.

Jugulotympanic Paragangliomas (Glomus Tumors) Paragangliomas are tumors arising from one or more of the small aggregates of branchiomeric (taking origin from the embryonic branchial arches), extra-adrenal (not within the adrenal glands) paraganglia (small aggregates of these special cells, also called glomus bodies in the ear) along the glossopharyngeal and vagus nerves, from the temporal bones to the aortic arch. The tumors may arise and remain limited to the middle ear over the promontory, hypotympanum external to the jugular bulb, or in the adventitia (fibrous tissue on the external surface of a vessel) of the jugular bulb. They may extend from these sites of origin to involve the other sites, the mastoid, the internal carotid artery, the infralabyrinthine and petrous apex regions, and extend intracranially into the posterior fossa, extradurally or intradurally. The usual presentation of these tumors is pulsatile tinnitus and conductive hearing loss. However, if the tumor mass invades the pars nervosa (the portion of the foramen associated with CN IX, X, and XI and the origin of the cochlear aqueduct) of the jugular foramen, it can compress, invade, and paralyze CN IX, X, and XI (**Fig. 10–13**).

These tumors may be differentiated as sporadic (without current evidence of hereditary transmission; these are most common) or hereditary; the hereditary group is much more commonly multicentric. Hereditary tumors may be associated with the multiple endocrine neoplasia type II (MEN II), which includes pheochromocytomas, medullary thyroid carcinoma, and parathyroid hyperplasia; patients with a paraganglioma should be evaluated for multicentricity and, if found, should be evaluated for these other lesions. Recently, it was discovered that, even in sporadic cases, the genetic characteristics suggest multicentric or malignant possibilities (Schiavi et al, 2005).

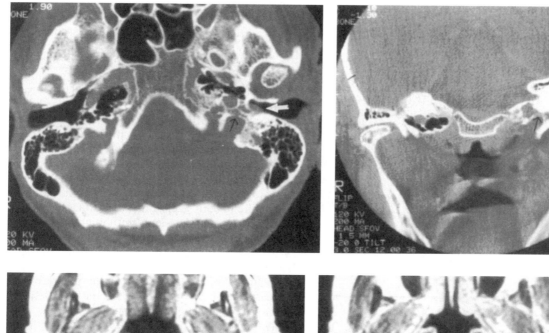

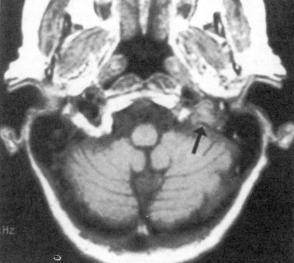

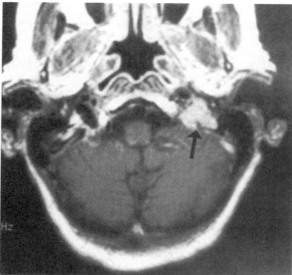

Figure 10–13 Jugulotympanic paragangliomas, left side. **(A)** Axial and **(B)** coronal views of a left middle ear mass (*white arrow*) and erosion of the superolateral bony wall of the jugular foramen (*black arrow*). **(C)** T1-weighted image without contrast and **(D)** T1-weighted image with contrast gadolinium demonstrate that the CT findings are due to a highly vascular jugular foramen mass (*arrows*) that fills the jugular bulb and extends into the middle ear.

Treatment for paragangliomas is predominantly surgical; however, in special circumstances, their growth can be arrested with irradiation. Salvage and restoration of CN VIII function is often possible; however, if the lower cranial nerves (IX, X, XI) are preoperatively involved by tumor invasion, return of function is not possible. Additional procedures, on a temporary or permanent basis, may be required for voice and deglutition (swallowing) restoration.

Pearl

- Multiple or bilateral glomus tumors or carotid body tumors suggest a probable hereditary origin or the possibility of MEN II.

Brainstem Gliomas   Intrinsic (originating within the brain, in contrast to extra-axial lesions like vestibular schwannomas or meningiomas) brain tumors, such as brainstem gliomas, can occasionally involve the audiologist in the evaluation for "dizziness," which, in fact may be vomiting, with or without ataxia. It is important to be ever vigilant in the search for a diagnosis in children presumed to have inner ear dizziness or vertigo. Intraoperative monitoring and post-treatment surveillance in these cases may also involve the audiologist (Jerger et al, 1980).

Brainstem gliomas are classified as diffuse intrinsic infiltrating tumors and focal, exophytic (bulging outward) tumors. The diffuse variety tend to be malignant astrocytomas or glioblastoma multiforme. These have a very poor prognosis and are treated with chemotherapy and radiotherapy. The focal, exophytic variety are low-grade astrocytomas or gangliogliomas and tend to be cystic or solid. These have a much better prognosis and are treated surgically by resection and cyst evacuation.

Pitfall

- Brainstem gliomas can be very subtle and present only as minor dizziness.

Degenerative/Idiopathic

Vascular Lesions Vascular Loop Compression   Little doubt exists that vascular compression of cranial nerves by aneurysms, ectatic vessels, and vascular loops does occur, giving rise to symptoms specific to those nerves. The difficulty is to differentiate these causes from other causes presenting the same symptoms. In the posterior fossa tic douloureux (trigeminal neuralgia), hemifacial spasm, and glossopharyngeal neuralgia are, perhaps, more generally recognized as originating from this mechanism. There is some consideration that tinnitus, fluctuating hearing loss, episodic or positional vertigo, or constant imbalance may arise from vascular compression of portions of CN VIII. Differentiating this cause from a host of other causes convincingly, however, awaits improved diagnostic techniques.

Treatment is by microvascular decompression of the nerve involved by moving the offending vessel(s) and wedging pieces of soft Teflon felt (Dow Co., Midland, MI) between the nerve and the vessel(s). This requires surgical entry into the posterior fossa (Jannetta, 1996).

Aneurysms   Seventh and eighth nerve signs and symptoms are rare, even in aneurysms of the posterior fossa circulation; however, headache, dizziness, diplopia (double vision), and transient cerebral ischemic attacks are not rare symptoms of aneurysms, with or without sentinel bleeding (small amount of bleeding signaling much more severe bleeding to come). These same symptoms can be present in patients being evaluated for hearing loss or dizziness and should be taken seriously and evaluated. An aneurysm rupture can have a mild headache and stiff neck or can be quite dramatic with the sudden onset of severe headache and rapid onset of coma.

Treatment of aneurysms is predominantly surgical by microvascular hemostatic clip application.

Stroke   Stroke is defined as a "sudden, nonconvulsive, focal neurological deficit" (Adams et al, 1997b). The principal underlying cause is cerebrovascular arteriosclerotic disease, although aneurysms and arteriovenous malformations may participate. Strokes are classified clinically as thrombotic (blood clot originating within the vessel), embolic (clot originating somewhere else and moving to the affected vessel), or hemorrhagic (rupture in the blood vessel). It is important to remember that transient ischemic attacks (TIAs) are warnings of generalized arteriosclerosis and indicate not only a higher probability of a full-blown stroke but also a myocardial infarct. Chronic hypertension increases the probability of both stroke and heart attacks; smoking and birth control pills in patients with migraine also increase the chances of stroke. The audiologist may encounter a patient being evaluated for dizziness, tinnitus, transient unilateral blindness, or speech and language problems who may, in fact, be having these symptoms as a result of TIAs.

Treatment of TIAs is focused on reducing risk factors, such as smoking, hypertension, birth control pills, and diets high in cholesterol, and the prophylactic (preventive) use of aspirin. Definite ischemia may require thrombolytic agents, anticoagulants, and occasionally surgical remedies for occluded cervical vessels. Treatment of embolic strokes must look closely at the usual origin of the embolic thrombus, the heart. Atrial fibrillation, previous infarctions, and valve disease are common cardiogenic causes of occult thrombi capable of embolizing. Hemorrhagic strokes require extensive monitoring and care of the comatose patient, control of the hypertension, and occasionally surgical evacuation of cerebral or cerebellar hematoma or clipping an offending aneurysm or intraluminally occluding an arteriovenous malformation.

Special Consideration

- Transient ischemic attacks can be a warning not only of an impending stroke but also of a heart attack.

Monostotic Fibrous Dysplasia   Fibrous dysplasia is a progressive bone disease of uncertain cause in which marrow and bony septae are replaced by fibro-osseous proliferation in which osteoblastic and osteoclastic activity abound. Fibrous dysplasia may be classified as polyostotic or monostotic (affecting only one bone); the monostotic form may involve the temporal bone. These lesions must be differentiated from bone lesions resulting from hyperparathyroidism by blood chemistry tests showing normal serum levels of calcium, phosphorus, and alkaline phosphatase.

Conductive hearing loss from stenosis of the EAC, with or without an entrapped canal cholesteatoma, and cosmetic deformity from a laterally expanding temporal bone are the predominant symptoms and signs of monostotic fibrous dysplasia. Sensorineural hearing loss is unusual.

No medical treatment exists for this disease; surgery is the only effective intervention, when necessary to open the EAC or to resculpture the lateral temporal bone for cosmesis. Surgical decompression of the IAC has been successful in reversing sensorineural hearing loss (Morrissey et al, 1997).

Special Consideration

- Some bone diseases can, on rare occasions, undergo malignant transformation. If the reader is following a case of a defined bone disease, and the patient tells of an area of bone that seems to be expanding or has become painful, immediate investigation, which may require biopsy, is indicated.

Lesions Not Detectable by Imaging

Infectious

Intracranial Complications of Suppurative Otitis Media
Imaging does play a role in the characterization and diagnosis of some of these complications; however, most are detectable clinically. Acute or chronic middle ear infections can spread intracranially and can be fatal. Aural (mastoiditis, subperiosteal abscess, petrositis, labyrinthitis, and facial paralysis) or intracranial complications of suppurative ear disease may be suspected when an acute ear infection lasts more than 1 week, an acute infection recurs within 2 weeks of treatment, or a chronic ear infection gets worse. Aural or intracranial complications may occur at any time, especially if there is a foul discharge that persists even with treatment. The intracranial complications are extradural granulations or abscess, sigmoid sinus thrombophlebitis (inflammation of the wall of the vessel, with or without partial or complete occlusion), brain abscess, subdural abscess, meningitis, and otitic hydrocephalus (increased intracranial pressure without meningitis or brain abscess). Any of these can result in a neural hearing loss as a result of active infection, associated intracranial pressure, or early or late sequelae, from the infection.

Treatment is surgical drainage and exenteration of the ear disease, intravenous antibiotics, and surgical drainage of intracranial abscesses. An exception to this rule is that some brain abscesses respond to antibiotics alone. Neural dysfunctions resulting from pressure or toxicity often recover, whereas dysfunctions resulting from direct infection of the specific conducting tissue usually do not (Neely, 2005).

Pitfall

- Failure to suspect an impending complication can result in serious morbidity or mortality.

Bacterial Meningitis   Bacterial meningitis usually occurs as a result of hematogenous dissemination from the respiratory system. Devastating effects from the bacteria can occur throughout the CNS, the cranial nerves, and the inner ear.

Treatment is predominantly life support and specific intravenous antibiotics given in sufficient doses and for an appropriate duration. Systemic steroids have been shown to reduce sequelae, such as deafness (McIntyre, 2005).

***Mycoplasma* and Viral Infections**   *Mycoplasma* organisms, influenza viruses, mumps, measles (rubeola), rubella, herpes zoster virus, herpes simplex virus, cytomegalovirus, and Epstein-Barr virus (mononucleosis) can have systemic influenza symptoms, a skin eruption, hemorrhagic painful blebs on the TM or face, swollen salivary glands, or many other symptoms suggesting a systemic illness with generalized or localized manifestations. Any of these can also cause single or multiple cranial nerve deficits or meningoencephalitis, which can be sudden and stable or progressive.

Treatment is generally supportive; however, antiviral medications are being developed very rapidly, and medications such as acyclovir may have some use in some of the viral infections. Steroids can, at times, reduce inflammation and sequelae. *Mycoplasma,* somewhat between bacteria and viruses, are responsive to the macrolides (erythromycin, azithromycin, clarithromycin) or, alternatively, doxycycline or respiratory quinolones (levofloxacin, gatifloxacin, moxifloxacin).

Fungal Infections   Fungi can cause brain or cranial nerve infection. The patient is often immunocompromised, either from disease, such as AIDS, or from medications to suppress organ rejection, and becomes infected by opportunistic fungi. *Cryptococcus* sp. (cryptococcosis), *Aspergillus* sp. (aspergillosis), and *Phycomycetes* sp. (mucormycosis) are some of the fungal species that can penetrate deeply and infect tissues. Commonly, these originate in the lungs or nose and paranasal sinuses and spread hematogenously or by direct extension to the intracranial cavity. Rapidly progressive CNS or cranial nerve destruction by the organisms and by invasive vasculitis can be fatal.

Treatment is predominantly by systemic use of rather toxic antifungal medications, such as amphotericin B, and, occasionally, by extensive local debridement, as in cases of mucormycosis.

Syphilis A spirochete (a special family of bacteria named for their long-flowing hairlike architecture), *T. pallidum,* causes syphilis. This organism reproduces in the early stages only every 30 to 33 hours; in later stages, it may lay dormant for years and rarely reproduce. It is only during reproduction that penicillin can kill this organism; therefore, once infected, if any organisms were missed in the initial treatment, the patient may have delayed disease develop. The two types of transmission stratify syphilis into acquired syphilis (acquired after birth) and congenital syphilis (transmitted to the fetus by the mother).

In both strata, clinical stages of the disease are characterized by time from exposure and clinical signs. Clinical stages in acquired syphilis are (1) primary (initial local chancre, or ulcerated sore, at entry site [e.g., the labia or penis]), (2) secondary (several weeks later a rash, lymphadenopathy, and systemic fever and illness), (3) latent (recurrence of symptoms years later; early latent is within 2 years, and late latent is < 2 years later), and (4) tertiary (3–10 years after onset, specific target organ destruction: "benign" tertiary syphilis of bone, skin, and viscera; cardiovascular syphilis; and neurosyphilis). Clinical stages in congenital syphilis are (1) early (infantile), with skin rash, blisters, and liver and spleen enlargement) and (2) late (tardive), occurring in late childhood or adulthood with specific target organ destruction, such as "saddle nose," "saber shins," interstitial keratitis, Hutchinson's notched teeth, and sudden deafness. Sensorineural hearing loss from infection of CN VIII or the inner ear may occur in any of the clinical stages of both congenital and acquired strata.

Treatment for syphilis is large doses of penicillin. Hearing loss is treated with long-duration steroids. Steroids are begun at high levels and titrated so that the maximal hearing improvement or stabilization is first achieved. Then, the dose is slowly decreased over many weeks to months to define the optimum lowest dose to maintain effect and minimize the serious side effects and possible complications from long-duration steroids. If the medication can be discontinued, any sudden loss or progressive loss is considered a medical emergency, and high, or higher, doses are reinstituted.

Lyme Disease Lyme disease, named after Lyme, Connecticut, a town in which the first recognized cases were identified, is a systemic disease caused by a spirochete, *Borrelia burgdorferi,* transmitted by a common deer tick vector. Initially, a rash and influenza-type symptoms occur. Weeks or months later, this neurotropic organism may cause dysfunction of cranial nerves and can cause a chronic meningitis. Sudden deafness may result from Lyme disease, even without the stigmata of the disease. This disease is treatable; however, prognosis for hearing recovery may be poorer in elderly patients (Peltomaa et al, 2000). Treatment is by ceftriaxone, cefuroxime, doxycycline, or amoxicillin or, alternatively, cefotaxime, penicillin G (high dose), erythromycin, clarithromycin, or azithromycin.

Degenerative/Idiopathic

Most of the diagnoses believed to be idiopathic (having an unknown cause), which have been given a clinical name, associated with sensorineural hearing loss affect the inner ear, not CN VIII or the brainstem. In the experience of the author, however, instances can occur in which a CN VIII lesion is demonstrated without a clear cause; most of these cases have not been given a clinical name. This is graphically illustrated in the review of articles assessing the false-positive and false-negative rates of the ABR in comparison to an MRI in identifying solitary schwannomas of the vestibular nerve. The focus is usually on how the result of the ABR poorly compares with the finding of the MRI in identifying these tumors. An alternative way to investigate these data is to determine how poorly the MRI may be in identifying a demonstrated CN VIII lesion as defined by an ABR. This comparison would seem to be a fruitful area of future research.

Controversial Point

- Most retrocochlear lesions defined by audiometry remain idiopathic. This is a fruitful area for further research.

Neural Presbycusis Schuknecht (1993b) classified presbycusis as sensory, neural, strial, and cochlear conductive. Neural presbycusis is defined by a progressive loss of word recognition in the presence of stable pure-tone thresholds (i.e., phonemic regression).

Currently, no medical or surgical treatment exists for this disorder; however, it should be emphasized that this is a clinical diagnosis of exclusion, requiring that no other identifiable lesion exists in the inner ear, nerve, or low brainstem causing the progressive loss.

Pearl

- Four types of presbycusis exist, one of which results in neural hearing loss. However, other causes of neural hearing losses must be excluded, even in the elderly.

Cranial Neuropathies Acute cochlear neuritis and acute vestibular neuritis have sudden, spontaneous onset of neural-type lesion and are the result of a direct viral attack on the cochlear nerve or one of the vestibular nerves. Acute cochlear neuritis presents as a sudden idiopathic sensorineural hearing loss. Vestibular neuritis presents as a sudden onset of constant severe vertigo without auditory symptoms. The vertigo can remain severe for days before gradually reducing to intermittent positional vertigo, and ultimately resolving over weeks to months. Diabetic cranial neuropathies, conversely, are the result of microangiopathies usually affecting CN III, IV, or VI. In these cases, however, the vestibular nerve may be involved and may have the same symptoms of vestibular neuritis (Schuknecht, 1993b).

Multiple cranial neuropathies must be assessed carefully with the location of the lesions and associated dysfunctions defined precisely relative to temporal and spatial characteristics. Primary neuropathies must be differentiated by clinical pattern and exclusion of other diseases mentioned in this chapter. In addition, the site of neuropathy must be identified as extra-axial or intra-axial. Secondary lesions on the surface of the brainstem involve adjacent cranial nerves, often unilaterally and sometimes painfully, and involve long sensorimotor tracks much later. Lesions occurring within the brain may rapidly involve the long sensorimotor tracks and cranial nerves bilaterally.

Steroids or antiviral agents have been used for the presumed viral-induced illnesses; however, steroids may be contraindicated in the diabetic patient. Good diabetic control is the principal treatment for diabetic neuropathies.

Pitfall

- Multiple cranial neuropathies must be evaluated carefully to ensure they are primary rather than a result of other diseases.

Primary Auditory Neuropathy   Primary auditory neuropathy is characterized by abnormal ABR and normal outer hair cell functions as measured by otoacoustic emissions (OAE) and cochlear microphonics (CM). This type of neuropathy appears to be inherited in an autosomal dominant pattern and tends to progress over 10 to 20 years. Marked improvement of auditory functions may occur after cochlear implantation (Starr et al, 2004).

Secondary Cochlear Neuron Degeneration   Secondary (retrograde) cochlear neuron degeneration occurs as a function of multiple inner ear disease processes. Modern imaging techniques may be able to detect some degrees of nerve survival. Currently, no medical or surgical treatment halts or prevents secondary degeneration; however, cochlear prosthesis or brainstem auditory prosthesis implantation seem to be effective (Nadol, 1997).

Leukodystrophies   Leukodystrophies are almost always fatal in early infancy or early childhood; however, unusual cases may survive into the third decade of life. These diseases are congenital or early onset, postnatal rapidly progressive demyelinating diseases of the white matter of the CNS and may be transmitted in an autosomal recessive fashion. Cochlear agenesis may be present; however, cochlear neurons may still be fairly abundant. At present, no treatment, except supportive, for this tragic group of diseases exists. Theoretically, cochlear implantation may or may not be effective; however, there are no data to support either contention.

Multiple Sclerosis   Multiple sclerosis is one of a group of demyelinating diseases that meet the following criteria for inclusion: destruction of myelin sheaths of nerve fibers, relative sparing of other neural cellular components, perivascular inflammatory infiltration, specific distribution of lesions to perivenous white matter, and relative lack of wallerian neural degeneration. The cause may be a delayed, viral-reactivated autoimmune reaction to a previous viral insult years before. Although MRI can often detect larger lesions suggesting multiple sclerosis, diagnosis is principally made on the basis of clinical presentation, clinical course, and CSF analysis. Audiometrically, this disease may present with a fluctuating neural hearing loss, which may improve with treatment, making a complete diagnostic audiologic evaluation looking for CN VIII signs important with each visit.

The pathology of these scattered lesions, from a millimeter to several centimeters in size, with a periventricular predilection, is initially myelin destruction with astrocytic reaction and infiltration of mononuclear cells and lymphocytes. Later these "plaques" become a matted fibroglial scar. Fluctuating and recurring symptoms arise from surrounding waxing and waning edema and conduction blockade. Ultimately, the demyelination areas create more permanent dysfunction. Some sporadic remyelination does occur.

Weakness, fatigue, numbness, tingling, diplopia, evidence of internuclear ophthalmoplegia, dizziness, and ataxia are common presenting symptoms; scanning speech, nystagmus, and intention tremor (Charcot's triad) is a classic, but late, presentation. Sudden or fluctuating neural hearing loss may rarely be the only, but more commonly an associated, symptom.

Treatment of acute exacerbations for more rapid resolution of symptoms is by adrenocorticotropic hormone (ACTH), methylprednisolone, prednisone, cyclophosphamide, or interferon-β. However, long-duration, continued use of these agents has not yet proved to change the ultimate course of the disease or prevent recurrences. Much therapeutic research is ongoing in this potentially debilitating disease (Frohman et al, 2005).

◆ Summary

Audiologic assessments are crucial in the initial evaluation and subsequent therapeutic monitoring of sensorineural hearing losses. Because the primary purpose is to determine which components of the auditory system are changing and to what degree, a full diagnostic audiometric evaluation, including immittance audiometry with ipsilateral and contralateral acoustic reflexes and speech audiometry, is mandatory at each evaluative session. Shortcuts are not acceptable, even in hearing aid follow-up visits. The wearing of hearing aids does not immunize a patient from subsequent disease, sometimes initially only detectable audiometrically.

The specific diagnosis of the cause of the hearing loss has important medical ramifications relative to the cause of the hearing loss, per se, and other potentially associated medical conditions that can result in increased morbidity and, in some cases, mortality.

References

Adams, R. D., Victor, M., & Ropper, A. H. (1997a). Deafness, dizziness, and disorders of equilibrium. In R. D. Adams, M. Victor, & A. H. Ropper (Eds.), Principles of neurology (6th ed., pp. 284–310). St. Louis: McGraw-Hill.

Adams, R. D., Victor, M., & Ropper, A. H. (1977b). Principles of neurology (6th ed., pp. 777–873). St. Louis: McGraw-Hill.

American Academy of Otolaryngology - Head Neck Surgery. (2003). Fact sheet: your genes and hearing loss. Retrieved July 31, 2007, from http://www.entnet.org/healthinfo/hearing/Genetic_Hearing_Loss.cfm

Aristegui, M. , & Denia, A . (2005). Simultaneous cochlear implantation and translabyrinthine removal of vestibular schwannoma in an only hearing ear: Report of two cases (neurofibromatosis type 2 and unilateral vestibular schwannoma). Otology and Neurotology, 26(2), 205–210.

Brookhouser, P. E. (1996). Diseases of the inner ear and sensorineural hearing loss. In C. D. Bluestone, S. E. Stool, & M. A. Kenna (Eds.), Pediatric otolaryngology (3rd ed., Vol. 1, pp. 649–670). Philadelphia: W. B. Saunders.

Chia, S. H. , Gamst, A. C. , Anderson, J. P. , & Harris, J. P . (2004). Intratympanic gentamicin therapy for Meniere's disease: A meta-analysis. Otology and Neurotology, 25(4), 544–552.

Clayton, A. E. , Mikulec, A. , Mikulec, K. , Merchant, S. , & McKenna, M. (2004). Association between osteoporosis and otosclerosis in women. Journal of Laryngology and Otology, 118(8), 617–621.

Evans, D. G. , Baser, M. , O'Reilly, B. , et al. (2005). Management of the patient and family with neurofibromatosis 2: A consensus conference statement. British Journal of Neurosurgery, 19(1), 5–12.

Fowler, K. B. , McCollister, F. , Dahle, A. , et al. (1997). Progressive and fluctuating sensorineural hearing loss in children with asymptomatic congenital cytomegalovirus infection. Journal of Pediatrics, 130(4), 624–630.

Frohman, E. M. , Stuve, O. , Havrdova, E. , et al. (2005). Therapeutic considerations for disease progression in multiple sclerosis: Evidence, experience, and future expectations. Archives of Neurology, 62(10), 1519–1530.

Gates, G. A . (2005). Treatment of Meniere's disease with the low-pressure pulse generator (Meniett device). Expert Review of Medical Devices, 2(5), 533–537.

Grundfast, K. M., & Toriello, H. (1998). Syndromic hereditary hearing impairment. In A. K. Lalwani & K. M. Grundfast (Eds.), Pediatric otology and neurotology (pp. 341–363). Philadelphia: Lippincott-Raven.

Haruna, S. , Haruna, Y. , Schachern, P. , Morizono, T. , & Paparella, M. (1994). Histopathology update: Otomycosis. American Journal of Otolaryngology, 15(1), 74–78.

Hone, S. W. , & Smith, R. J . (2003). Genetic screening for hearing loss. Clinics in Otolaryngology, 28, 285–290.

Irving, R. M., & Ruben, R. J. (1998). The acquired hearing losses of childhood. In A. K. Lalwani & K. M. Grundfast (Eds.), Pediatric otology and neurotology (pp. 375–385). Philadelphia: Lippincott-Raven.

Jannetta, P. J. (1996). Posterior fossa neurovascular compression syndromes other than neuralgia. In R. H. Wilkins & S. S. Rengachary (Eds.), Neurosurgery (Vol. III, pp. 3227–3233). St. Louis: McGraw-Hill.

Jerger, J., Neely, J. G., & Jerger, S. (1980). Speech, impedance, and auditory brainstem response audiometry in brainstem tumors: Importance of a multiple test strategy. Archives of Otolaryngology, 106, 218–223.

Khetarpal, U., & Lalwani, A. K. (1998). Nonsyndromic hereditary hearing impairment. In A. K. Lalwani & K. M. Grundfast (Eds.), Pediatric otology and neurotology (pp. 313–340). Philadelphia: Lippincott-Raven.

Kimura, R. S. , & Hutta, J . (1997). Inhibition of experimentally induced endolymphatic hydrops by middle ear ventilation. European Archives of Oto-rhino-laryngology, 254(5), 213–218.

Lin, V. Y. , Stewart, C. , Grebenyuk, J. , et al. (2005). Unilateral acoustic neuromas: Long-term hearing results in patients managed with fractionated stereotactic radiotherapy, hearing preservation surgery, and expectantly. Laryngoscope, 115(2), 292–296.

McIntyre, P . (2005). Should dexamethasone be part of routine therapy of bacterial meningitis in industrialised countries? Advances in Experimental Medicine and Biology, 568, 189–197.

Minor, L. B. , Carey, J. , Cremer, P. , et al. (2003). Dehiscence of bone overlying the superior canal as a cause of apparent conductive hearing loss. Otology and Neurotology, 24(2), 270–278.

Monsell, E. M., Teixido, M. T., Wilson, M. D., & Hughes, G. B. (1997). Nonhereditary hearing loss. In G. B. Hughes & M. L. Pensak (Eds.), Clinical otology (2nd ed., pp. 289–312). New York: Thieme Medical Publishers.

Morrissey, D. D. , Talbot, J. M. , & Schleuning, A. J. II. (1997). Fibrous dysplasia of the temporal bone: Reversal of sensorineural hearing loss after decompression of the internal auditory canal. Laryngoscope, 107(10), 1336–1340.

Nadol, J. B. , Jr. (1997). Patterns of neural degeneration in the human cochlea and auditory nerve: Implications for cochlear implantation. Otolaryngology–Head and Neck Surgery, 117(3, Pt 1), 220–228.

Nager, G. T. (1993). Meningiomas. In G. T. Nager (Ed.), Pathology of the ear and temporal bone (pp. 620–670). Philadelphia: Williams & Wilkins.

Neely, J. (2005). Facial nerve and intracranial complications of otitis media. In R. Jackler & D. Brackmann (Eds.), Neurotology (2nd ed., pp. 912–925). Philadelphia: Elsevier Mosby.

Pass, R. F . (2005). Congenital cytomegalovirus infection and hearing loss. Herpes, 12(2), 50–55.

Peltomaa, M. , Pyykko, I. , Sappala, I. , Viitanen, L. , & Viljanen, M . (2000). Lyme borreliosis, an etiological factor in sensorineural hearing loss? European Archives of Oto-rhino-laryngology, 257(6), 317–322.

Roland, P. S., & Marple, B. F. (1997). Disorders of inner ear, eighth nerve, and CNS. In P. S. Roland, B. F. Marple & W. L. Meyerhoff (Eds.), Hearing loss (pp. 195–256). New York: Thieme Medical Publishers.

Rybak, L. P. , & Whitworth, C . (2005). Ototoxicity: Therapeutic opportunities. Drug Discovery Today, 10(19), 1313–1321.

Schiavi, F. , Boedeker, C. , Bausch, B. , et al. (2005). Predictors and prevalence of paraganglioma syndrome associated with mutations of the SDHC gene. Journal of the American Medical Association, 294(16), 2057–2063.

Schuknecht, H. F. (1993a). Disorders of aging. In H. F. Schuknecht (Ed.), Pathology of the ear (2nd ed., pp. 415–446). Philadelphia: Lea & Febiger.

Schuknecht, H. F. (1993b). Neural disorders. In H. F. Schuknecht (Ed.), Pathology of the ear (2nd ed., pp. 319–344). Philadelphia: Lea & Febiger.

Starr, A. , Isaacson, B. , Michalewski, H. , et al. (2004). A dominantly inherited progressive deafness affecting distal auditory nerve and hair cells. Journal of the Association for Research in Otolaryngology, 5(4), 411–426.

Chapter 11

Treatment of (Central) Auditory Processing Disorders

Teri James Bellis

Intervention for auditory disorders is a key component of the audiologist's scope of practice. Indeed, it might be argued that the diagnosis of any auditory deficit, including (central) auditory processing disorder ((C)APD), is of questionable value unless it can be used to develop a plan of intervention for the presenting disorder.

This chapter will discuss treatment and management approaches that may be employed for individuals with (C)APD. Key components of a comprehensive intervention program will be delineated, and several specific examples of activities or strategies within each component category will be described. In accordance with current consensus regarding (C)APD (American Speech-Language-Hearing Association [ASHA], 2005a,b), this chapter will focus on a multidisciplinary approach to (C)APD intervention.

Several key concepts will be emphasized throughout this chapter. Most importantly, readers must be aware that there is no one intervention approach that is appropriate for all individuals with (C)APD. Therefore, although several methods of treating and managing (C)APD will be described, the applicability of each will depend entirely on the nature of the individual's specific auditory deficit(s), as well as several higher order, cognitive, language, and related factors. Therefore, as with any disorder, the key to effective treatment is accurate and comprehensive diagnosis. Furthermore, to design a deficit-specific, individualized intervention plan for children or adults with (C)APD, one must have a strong foundation of knowledge in the current science relative to central auditory processing and its disorders. Thus, this chapter will begin with an overview of the current definition and nature of (C)APD.

♦ Current Conceptualizations of (Central) Auditory Processing and Its Disorders

The definition of any disorder will inform directly how it is both diagnosed and treated. Additionally, any definition of a disorder must be consistent with the current scientific knowledge regarding how the system in question works. As such, it is important for clinicians to understand the nature of (C)APD. For additional information on processing disorders in children and adults, see Chapters 16 and 17 in *Audiology: Diagnosis*, second edition. A vast body of literature in the general and auditory neurosciences, cognitive sciences, neuropsychology, and related disciplines illuminates the manner in which information, including auditory information, is processed in the central nervous system (CNS). This literature forms the basis for our current conceptualization and definition of (C)APD. See Chapter 3 in *Audiology: Diagnosis*, second edition, for additional information on the anatomy and physiology of the central auditory nervous system (CANS).

As our knowledge base has evolved over the past several years, so too have our definitions of (C)APD and our recommendations regarding diagnosing and treating it. Historically, definitions of (C)APD have ranged from the rather amorphous (e.g., "what we do with what we hear") to the very restrictive (e.g., "an auditory-specific deficit that is not attributable to peripheral hearing loss" [Jerger and Musiek, 2000, p.1]). More recently, however, clinicians have begun to recognize that, because of the inherent complexity of the CNS and its myriad functions, combined with the heterogeneity of various types and combinations of central auditory deficits, no simple definition can capture accurately its true essence. Instead, recent definitions of (C)APD have striven to provide a detailed, operational construct that can guide clinicians through the often-confusing labyrinth of differential diagnosis and intervention. Moreover, it is likely that, as our knowledge base regarding CNS function continues to evolve, our definitions of disorders of that system, including (C)APD, likewise will be modified.

ASHA (2005a) defines central auditory processing ((C)AP) as "the perceptual processing of auditory information in the CNS and the neurobiologic activity that underlies those processes and gives rise to the electrophysiologic auditory potentials" (p. 2). Operationally, (C)AP involves the mechanisms and processes that underlie a variety of auditory behaviors, including sound localization and lateralization, performance with competing and/or degraded acoustic signals, discrimination of both speech and nonspeech auditory stimuli, and auditory temporal processing and pattern recognition. These auditory behaviors, in turn, are presumed to play a role in more complex auditory-verbal learning and communication tasks, including comprehension of verbally presented information, perception of prosodic elements of speech, phonological awareness abilities, and following verbal directions and instructions. It is recognized further that, as is the case with auditory deficits in general, central auditory dysfunction may coexist with and/or contribute to language and learning difficulties, including disorders of reading and spelling, deficits in language processing, and problems in other academic, social, and vocational areas. Although the importance of the auditory system should not be underestimated, it is important to realize that (C)AP is but one, small component of these and related higher order, more global functions and that ultimate listening, learning, and communicative success is dependent on a host of interlocking factors, many of them unrelated to the auditory system. Thus, although the comorbidity of (C)APD and various cognitive (including attention), language, and learning deficits is well recognized, it is very difficult if not impossible to draw a simple, direct one-to-one correlation between specific, circumscribed central auditory skills and higher order language/learning/communication outcomes in large groups of individuals (ASHA, 2005a; Bellis, 2003). The existence of considerable overlap between symptoms of (C)APD and those of other higher order deficits further confounds the issue. As such, although the audiologist is identified as the professional qualified to diagnose (C)APD (ASHA, 2005a,b), an individualized and multidisciplinary approach to (C)APD differential diagnosis and treatment is critical.

Special Consideration

- The terms *diagnosis* and *assessment* are not synonymous. *Diagnosis* refers to the identification of a disorder, whereas *assessment* refers to the overall data-gathering process to identify areas of strengths and weaknesses. Because (C)APD is an auditory disorder, the audiologist is the professional qualified to diagnose (C)APD. Speech-language pathologists are uniquely qualified to delineate the cognitive-communicative and related speech-language sequelae that may be associated with (C)APD and to diagnose language-processing disorders (ASHA, 2005b,c). Nonetheless, (C)APD should not be diagnosed in a vacuum. Because of the complexity and heterogeneity of central auditory processing and its disorders, a multidisciplinary approach involving audiologists, speech-language pathologists, and other professionals is critical to overall assessment, differential diagnosis, and treatment of individuals with (C)APD.

Notwithstanding its inherent complexity and heterogeneity, it should be emphasized that (C)APD is conceptualized as an auditory disorder. That is, it should manifest itself primarily, if not solely, in the auditory modality. There has been a great deal of controversy in recent years regarding the modality specificity of (C)APD. Some contend that, in order for (C)APD to be a useful diagnostic construct, one must be able to demonstrate that the disorder is present in the auditory modality to the exclusion of other modalities (e.g., McFarland and Cacace, 1995). Others have suggested that, because of the significant amount of cross-modal and multimodal interaction within the human brain, combined with the finding of relatively few if any entirely circumscribed CNS regions dedicated to a single modality, the expectation of complete modality specificity as a diagnostic criterion for (C)APD is neurophysiologically untenable (e.g., ASHA, 2005a,b; Bellis, 2003; Musiek et al, 2005).

Controversial Point

- Does (C)APD even exist as a valid diagnostic construct? It seems to depend on how the disorder is defined. There is a paucity of evidence supporting the existence of a completely auditory modality-specific disorder that directly correlates with reading and related academic outcomes. If (C)APD is defined as a modality-specific disorder that is limited to the auditory system, then one might argue that such a disorder does not exist, and, therefore, to use the "label" of (C)APD would be of limited clinical utility (e.g., McFarland and Cacace, 1995). However, current consensus definitions of (C)APD (e.g., ASHA, 2005a) recognize both the interactive and multimodal nature of information processing and the heterogeneity of auditory, learning, and related disorders. Thus, these definitions reject the notion of complete modality specificity as a diagnostic criterion for (C)APD as neurophysiologically untenable and emphasize that the relationship between auditory processing and ultimate listening, communication, and learning outcomes will depend on a host of interlocking factors. Under this construct, a diagnosis of (C)APD provides direction for deficit-specific treatment of the identified auditory deficit(s) while, at the same time, not attributing all learning and related difficulties to an underlying auditory disorder.

These positions are not necessarily mutually exclusive. That is, although complete modality specificity of (C)APD may not be a reasonable expectation based on what is known about CANS function, it is reasonable to expect that individuals with (C)APD have as their primary complaint auditory difficulties. Furthermore, it is critical that, to enable a diagnosis of (C)APD, a central auditory deficit that cannot be accounted for by peripheral auditory, cognitive, language, or other factors must be demonstrated conclusively using tests that have been shown to be sensitive and specific to disorders of the CANS (ASHA, 2005a,b; Bellis, 2003; Chermak and Musiek, 1997; Musiek et al, 2005). To differentiate (C)APD from other disorders that may manifest similar symptoms, including language processing and other speech/language disorders, attention deficits, and cognitive disorders, multidisciplinary exploration of function in other modalities and at other CNS processing levels and regions is critical. This multidisciplinary approach to differential diagnosis of (C)APD also serves to ensure that our treatment and management of the disorder is both consistent with fundamental neurobiological principles and highly individualized to address the person's unique confluence of auditory and higher order difficulties.

Our current conceptualization of (C)APD is influenced further by theories of information processing and resource allocation. Information-processing theory demonstrates that processing occurs in both a bottom-up and top-down manner (Massaro, 1975). Message comprehension relies on the extraction of information at various stages, and complex interactions between sensory and higher order cognitive, language, and related factors occur. Bottom-up factors are those that occur before higher level cognitive, language, and related operations. These are "data-driven," and they rely on the acoustic parameters of the incoming signal and the integrity of the central auditory pathways. Neurobiology demonstrates that there is a great deal of redundancy in the CANS, and bottom-up processing is not merely a hierarchical relay from one ascending structure to the next. Rather, there are patterns of convergence and divergence as well as parallel processing, in addition to hierarchical processing. At various stages throughout the CANS, specific features of the acoustic signal are enhanced, and a great many regions subserve overlapping functions (see Musiek et al, 2005, and Chapter 3 in *Audiology: Diagnosis*, second edition, for reviews).

In addition, top-down factors such as cognition, attention, language, and related factors also come into play when processing auditorily presented information. Although adequate (C)AP is necessary for successful listening and comprehension, it is not sufficient. Instead, effective listening is subserved by multiple knowledge bases and skills, and even the most deceptively simple of auditory tasks is influenced by higher order functions, such as attention, motivation, cognition, memory, and executive function. For example, listening in backgrounds of noise recruits additional, higher level and multimodal brain circuitry than those employed when listening in quiet (Salvi et al, 2002). Similarly, familiarity with the language and vocabulary of a message facilitates spoken word recognition even when fine-grained auditory discriminations are required (Bradlow and Pisoni, 1999). Additional contextual and language cues have a significant effect on what is ultimately perceived, even when the acoustic signal itself is held constant (e.g., Elliott, 1995). Furthermore, the relative reliance on bottom-up versus top-down factors changes with the demands of the listening situation, so that more reliance on top-down factors is to be expected when the bottom-up acoustic signal is degraded, distorted, or presented in a noisy environment, or when a disorder exists that affects the integrity of that signal, including hearing loss and (C)APD.

Recent research, however, has suggested that, when a greater expenditure of effort is required to process the incoming auditory signal, either due to a perceptual deficit or to environmental factors such as reverberation or noise, fewer cognitive and related resources may be available "upstream" to comprehend and retain the message (e.g., McCoy et al, 2005). Thus, this resource allocation, or "effortfulness," theory (McCoy et al, 2005) holds significant implications for the treatment of (C)APD in children and adults and may help to explain why these individuals also often exhibit apparent "auditory memory" and related deficits.

◆ General Principles of Treatment and Management

The scientific bases of (C)AP discussed in the previous section provide the framework for treatment and management of (C)APD. That is, the neurobiology of the system should inform both the specific components of any treatment/management program and the manner in which such intervention is implemented. Based on this underlying science, several general principles of (C)APD treatment and management can be identified.

First, because information processing occurs in both a bottom-up and top-down direction, intervention for (C)APD likewise should include targeted activities and strategies that address both bottom-up and top-down processing. Thus, intervention should focus on addressing those factors that are critical for accessing and processing the acoustic features of the incoming signal while, at the same time, recruiting and strengthening higher order cognitive, language, multimodal, and related central resources to assist in compensating for deficiencies in the auditory system.

Second, intervention for (C)APD should be both intensive and extensive. Specifically, intervention should include deficit-specific auditory stimulation activities that are challenging, intense, and frequent so as to maximize

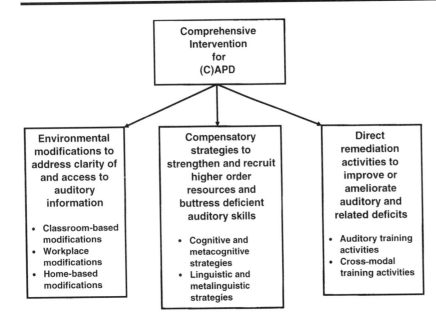

Figure 11–1 Components of a comprehensive treatment and management program for children and adults with (central) auditory processing disorders (C)APD.

plasticity of the CANS and effect improvement in those specific auditory deficit areas identified during the diagnostic process. In addition, intervention should be extensive, including activities that facilitate generalization to real-world situations and that address daily functional listening and related deficits. Throughout all intervention activities, whether intensive or extensive, inclusion of salient reinforcement will optimize learning and result in maximum benefit. Thus, intervention for (C)APD must be multidisciplinary in nature so that both specific auditory deficits and daily functioning in the classroom, workplace, or other communicative environments may be addressed. Intervention also must be individualized to target the specific difficulties present in a given child or adult. There is no "one size fits all" intervention approach that is appropriate for all individuals with (C)APD.

Finally, any comprehensive intervention plan for (C)APD should include three primary components **(Fig. 11–1)**: (1) modifications that address the learning, work, and communicative environment; (2) compensatory strategies that focus on recruitment of higher order central resources to buttress deficient auditory skills; and (3) direct remediation activities that target, in a deficit-specific manner, the auditory deficiencies identified (ASHA, 2005a). Following is a detailed discussion of each of these three components.

Environmental Modifications

The primary purpose of environmental modifications is to improve access to, and thereby facilitate acquisition and comprehension of, the intended message. Intervention plans for (C)APD should address the communicative environment from both a bottom-up and top-down perspective. Bottom-up modifications are those that address the clarity of the acoustic signal itself. Top-down modifications are those that focus on the manner in which information is

imparted so that opportunities for comprehension are maximized. Whether the individual with (C)APD is a child or an adult, both types of modifications are critical to facilitate success in day-to-day communicative situations.

It is important once again to emphasize that there are few, if any, environmental recommendations that are appropriate for all children or adults with (C)APD. The selection and implementation of classroom, workplace, and home modifications should be based on the unique needs of the individual. Moreover, rather than producing an exhaustive list of any and all suggestions that may be appropriate for a given person, focus should be placed on those modifications that are most likely to have a significant impact on daily functioning for the patient in question. By selecting "high-impact" modifications, the likelihood of compliance will be maximized.

> **Pearl**
>
> - Clinicians should avoid the temptation to use generic and lengthy lists of recommendations for children and adults with (C)APD. Instead, they should analyze carefully the individual's learning and communicative environment and practice the "80/20 rule" by identifying those 20% of the possible solutions that have a maximum likelihood of addressing 80% of the individual's unique functional difficulties.

Following is a brief discussion of several environmental modifications that may be appropriate for individuals with (C)APD. Again, it is important to note that this list is not exhaustive, and other modifications may be indicated depending on a particular individual's presenting difficulties.

Furthermore, the selection of which of the following recommendations are indicated in a given situation should be made carefully, as few of them are appropriate for all persons with (C)APD, and, indeed, several actually may be contraindicated in certain circumstances.

Pitfall

- Some classroom-based suggestions that seem at first glance to be appropriate for any child with an auditory deficit actually may make the situation worse for some children with (C)APD. For example, the addition of visual or multimodality cues, although a good suggestion for many, may result in confusion for children with (C)APD arising from inefficient interhemispheric communication and for whom multimodal integration skills are compromised. Similarly, the use of repetition may be an efficacious clarification strategy for some, whereas rephrasing key information may confuse rather than clarify. Thus, all individuals with (C)APD should be carefully monitored to ensure that the recommendations implemented do, indeed, yield the desired outcome.

Table 11–1 Selected Environmental Modifications

Classroom-Based Modifications
- Analyze the acoustic environment.
- Consider use of personal frequency modulation (FM) system.
- Augment with visual or multimodality cues.
- Ensure preferential seating.
- Practice principles of clear speech.
- Provide a note taker.
- Preteach new information and vocabulary.
- Repeat or rephrase information.
- Employ methods of gaining attention.
- Make frequent checks for comprehension.
- Schedule auditory breaks throughout the day.

Workplace-Based Modifications
- Provide directives in written form (e.g., e-mails, memos).
- Conduct communications in quiet backgrounds.
- Paraphrase and clarify.
- Consider use of hearing assistive technology.

Home-Based Modifications
- Write down and post key instructions and chores.
- Turn off television or other noise sources during critical communications.
- Schedule family conference time.
- Make frequent checks for understanding.
- Allow for "down time."
- Blame the disorder, not the person.

Note: This is not an exhaustive list of environmental modifications for (C)APD. The relative appropriateness of each of these modifications will depend on the nature of the auditory deficit identified in a given individual, and some modifications may be contraindicated for certain types of auditory deficits.

Classroom-Based Modifications

It should be remembered that a school-aged child is in the classroom on a daily basis to learn science, mathematics, language, social studies, and other specific topic areas. Therefore, classroom-based modifications should assist in ensuring that the student has access to the information he or she is supposed to be learning, and the focus should be on the message itself, rather than on specific auditory or related skills, per se. In general, classroom modifications can be separated into two primary categories: those that focus on the acoustic environment and signal (bottom-up) and those that focus on methods of imparting information, including instructional strategies (top-down). These modifications are discussed below and are summarized in **Table 11–1**.

Acoustic Signal Enhancement

It is well established that a hostile acoustic environment will impede listening and learning and that learning is best facilitated when the signal-to-noise ratio (SNR) is optimal. This is true even for individuals with no disorder whatsoever, but it is particularly important for very young children and those with auditory disorders such as (C)APD and for whom listening in noise is often a primary complaint. It is incumbent upon all clinicians to be familiar with the current standards for classroom acoustics and to assist in ensuring that schools comply with these guidelines. Certainly, relatively low-cost acoustic enhancements will benefit everyone in a given classroom, including installation of carpeting, acoustic tiles, mitigation of other reverberant

surfaces, and removal of sources of excess noise. It would be most desirable if every classroom in the country were fitted with sound-field amplification so as to maximize listening and learning for all students. However, that goal, though admirable, may be overly idealistic at present given the current fiscal situation in our schools. Therefore, the acoustic conditions of classrooms of children with (C)APD should be given particular attention and should be one of the first considerations when a (C)APD is identified. Attention also should be paid to the acoustic characteristics of other environments in which learning and listening occur, including assembly areas, auditoriums, learning laboratories, and libraries. Methods of evaluating and documenting both the acoustic conditions of specific classrooms and the efficacy of acoustic interventions have been described, and readers are referred to Chapter 18 in this volume for additional information.

Historically, the use of personal frequency modulation (FM) systems or other hearing assistive technologies (HATs) were recommended in a blanket fashion for most, if not all, children with (C)APD. More recently, however, the appropriateness of this recommendation has been called into question (e.g., Bellis, 2003; Rosenberg, 2002). Although personal FM systems or other HATs may well be indicated for many school-aged children with (C)APD, as with any intervention recommendation, a HAT should be recommended only after careful ascertainment of the need for and efficacy of such a device. Rosenberg (2002) points out that, whereas the benefit of sound-field amplification for all children has been well documented, there is a paucity of empirical data supporting the efficacy of personal FM use for children with (C)APD in the literature. She advocates for a four-step approach to determining need for personal HATs for children with (C)APD: (1) analysis of the specific nature and functional deficit profile of the child, including indicators that support or contraindicate the use of a personal HAT; (2) evaluation and, when needed, modification of the classroom acoustical environment; (3) selection and fitting of the personal HAT if deemed appropriate; and (4) in-service training and careful monitoring of the efficacy of HAT use. For further information on HAT, refer to Chapter 17 in this volume.

Most, but not all, children with (C)APD have some degree of difficulty listening in noisy or competing backgrounds. Certainly, the presence of such a complaint should be a primary factor in the determination of appropriateness of personal HAT use, as should be an estimation of degree of benefit the individual child should expect to enjoy from the device. For some types of (C)APD, message clarity is not the primary concern, and therefore the need for personal HATs may be questionable. Consideration also should be given to the specific acoustic characteristics of the child's learning environment(s), as even children with speech-in-noise difficulties nonetheless may report little or no problem in their primary classrooms, or may have difficulty isolated to specific rooms or specific teachers. The subject matter and instructional methods employed also may be factors affecting the degree of benefit that can be expected from HAT use. For example, a course that consists primarily of group discussion and interaction or one that employs small-group, center-based activities and instruction may not lend itself easily to use of a personal HAT. Indeed, in certain situations, personal HAT use actually may interfere with a student's ability to participate fully in the class experience, and this potential impact should be assessed carefully and thoughtfully.

Another consideration that should be given careful thought is that of the age of the child or adolescent and the importance of socialization to the growth and well-being of the individual. It should always be remembered that children learn many things in the school setting, not all of which fall under the umbrella of academics. A large portion of a student's school life is devoted to developing appropriate social communication skills, self-esteem, and self-identity. Indeed, it may be argued that these lifelong issues carry more importance overall than do the myriad details of algebra, biology, or other topic-specific information, much of which likely will be forgotten once examinations are completed. In addition, conformity in appearance and dress and the ability to fit in often are of primary import for school-aged children, particularly those in the middle-school years or higher. For some of these children, forced use of personal FM systems may lead to a feeling of isolation and thus hinder socioemotional growth. It is important to respect these concerns and not underestimate their impact. The whole child must always be taken into account, and, if the ultimate goal of our interventions is to facilitate communication, we likewise must recognize when an otherwise logical intervention works in opposition to that goal.

Special Consideration

- Clinicians should not underestimate the importance of social interaction in children and adolescents. All too often, attention is placed solely on facilitating academic achievement, and social concerns are considered secondarily, if at all. However, some of the most important skills learned during the school-age years are acquired outside the classroom. The ability to develop and maintain interpersonal relationships is integral to an individual's self-esteem and socioemotional well-being. Children with (C)APD, as with any disorder, should be afforded the same opportunities to be accepted, to participate in extracurricular activities, and to pursue personal goals as any other child. When making recommendations regarding accommodations, therapy schedules, or other interventions specific to a child's disorder, clinicians should make every attempt to ensure that the recommendations do not interfere with these other, equally important, considerations.

Finally, even when all indications suggest that a personal HAT will be of benefit to a particular child, actual benefit of the device should be monitored and documented regularly through the use of both functional evaluations of speech recognition in noise and related skills and subjective questionnaires. In addition, opportunities to engage in daily listening activities without the use of the HAT should be provided on a regular basis. It has been this author's clinical experience that ongoing and continuous use of personal HATs without concomitant opportunities for and training of listening in noise skills can lead to an overreliance on the HAT and an actual worsening of speech-in-noise difficulties when the HAT is not available. This may well represent an incidence of plasticity in which those networks necessary for speech-in-noise abilities simply are not employed regularly and thus fall into disuse. As a result, these children may find themselves at an even greater disadvantage in environments in which a HAT is not available, such as in social situations or upon leaving the K–12 educational environment for either postsecondary education or the workplace. In these cases, it could be argued that regular use of a personal HAT, while facilitating acquisition of information presented during the school years, may have done a disservice to the student overall. Therefore, this author advocates for withdrawing the HAT during daily activities or courses in which acoustic access to verbal instruction is less critical (e.g., music, art class, and physical education) so as to provide opportunities for children to practice real-world listening-in-noise skills on an ongoing, daily basis.

- The use of personal FM or other assistive listening devices may be the most commonly recommended accommodation for children with (C)APD. But are they truly appropriate for all children? And, if deemed appropriate for a given child, should the device be used regularly? There is no agreement on these points. Certainly, all listeners benefit from improvement in the SNR. However, given the funding limitations of most school districts, combined with several other factors, determining whether a specific child actually needs a personal FM system to receive educational benefit is of primary importance, and some types of (C)APD may not affect acoustic signal clarity. Moreover, it is possible that constant use of HAT, even when indicated for a specific child, may decrease opportunities to practice real-world listening-in-noise skills and exacerbate speech-in-noise difficulties over time. The obvious solution appears to be the placement of sound-field amplification and implementation of appropriate acoustic standards in all classrooms everywhere, which is an ideal that, unfortunately, will be very difficult to attain in the foreseeable future without significant public support and funding.

In summary, this author does not support the blanket recommendation of personal HATs for all children with (C)APD. Instead, such a recommendation should occur only when the nature of a child's auditory deficits indicates the need for such a device and when the benefits clearly outweigh the possible disadvantages. When used, efficacy of the device should be monitored carefully.

Visual and Other Signal Augmentations

For many children with (C)APD, as with most listeners, it is particularly important that the auditory signal be augmented with other forms of information to facilitate access to—and, ultimately, comprehension and retention of—the verbal message. Recommendations for preferential seating, addition of visual and multimodal cues, provision of a note taker, and similar suggestions are commonplace for these children. However, as with any intervention recommendation, these suggestions also should be analyzed carefully for their applicability to the particular child in question. Even more important, the individual child's presenting auditory deficits and functional complaints should be examined along with the learning environment to determine the best means of carrying out these suggestions in an optimal manner.

For example, the term *preferential seating* often has been associated automatically with a "front and center" placement approach. However, given the unique physical arrangement of many classrooms, especially those in lower elementary grades, this approach may not be the most efficacious for children with listening difficulties. Instead, focus should be on placement in the classroom in which the best visual access to the speaker is afforded while, at the same time, keeping auditory, visual, and other distractions to a minimum. Likewise, attention should be given to nonauditory factors that influence optimal placement, including lighting conditions, location of windows and doors, presence of "busy" backgrounds that may interfere with visual figure–ground skills, and similar factors. It also should be recognized that, for some children, the addition of visual and multimodal augmentations actually may confuse rather than clarify the message. In these cases, it may be most beneficial to place the child where he or she can attend fully to the auditory signal alone. For many classrooms, the determination of optimal seating may differ depending on the activity being undertaken at a given point in time. Therefore, flexibility in seating will be required, and clinicians are encouraged to analyze each learning environment for purposes of determining the meaning of "preferential" or "optimal" placement on a room-by-room basis.

- Clinicians should not assume that "preferential seating" always means a front-and-center approach. Instead, careful observation of the classroom environment, combined with an analysis of the student's listening needs, should guide placement recommendations. Furthermore, it should be remembered that, for children with some types of (C)APD, placements that minimize visual input actually may facilitate listening skills by avoiding the need for division of attention and multimodal integration.

Children with auditory deficits, including (C)APD, often have great difficulty with the inherent division of attention needed for note taking, copying from the board, or other multimodal tasks. Previously in this chapter, the topic of resource allocation theory was discussed. If, as in the case of (C)APD, an inordinate amount of energy is being placed on accessing and decoding the incoming auditory signal, less energy may be left over for manipulating, comprehending, or remembering that signal. When further energy is diverted to the writing process (often a difficult task in and of itself for children with central auditory deficits and associated reading/spelling sequelae), both listening and note taking may be affected adversely. As a result, acquisition and retention of the target information may be impeded. In these cases, provision of a note taker should be considered. In some cases, this can be accomplished simply via copying notes from another student whose notes have been examined and determined to be sufficiently clear and accurate. More preferable, however, is the provision of teacher-generated notes, particularly in lecture-based classes. When these notes can be provided in advance of the lecture and reviewed by the student, familiarity with both the vocabulary and topic matter is enhanced, and auditory closure abilities are facilitated. Thus, preteaching of upcoming new vocabulary and information often is a very useful instructional strategy for many children with (C)APD, and the material from these topics also may be incorporated into therapy sessions so as to maximize generalization of skills learned from the therapy room to the classroom and beyond.

Another suggestion that this author has encountered frequently in clinical reports is that of allowing the student to tape-record class sessions or lectures for playback later. Although this strategy appears, on the surface, to have some merit, as it allows the student additional exposure to the subject matter and verbal messages, it has been my experience that it is rarely beneficial for children with (C)APD. Because most individuals with (C)APD experience particular difficulty with degraded auditory signals and fare more poorly when in the absence of visual or other contextual cues, listening to typically low-fidelity taped lectures often represents an activity that is more challenging than clarifying. Nonetheless, it is possible that such a strategy may be useful for select students, which underscores the need for highly individualized recommendations that are accompanied by careful monitoring of the efficacy of the interventions implemented.

Finally, a word should be said about employing methods of sensory deprivation to ease listening in the classroom. Because so many children with (C)APD exhibit some difficulty with binaural hearing skills, it may seem useful to plug one ear (usually the left) so that information is presented primarily to the "better" ear; this is a recommendation that has been made not infrequently in the past. However, this author cautions against any recommendation that essentially represents a form of sensory deprivation and that, via neuroplasticity, can result in undesirable organizational changes within the CANS. As has been illustrated in the animal literature (Gold and Knudsen, 2000), monaural occlusion for extended periods of time and other alterations in auditory experiences lead to significant structural reorganization of bilateral pathways within the CANS and concomitant functional changes in binaural skills, frequency tuning, and other auditory abilities. It is possible, perhaps even likely, that plugging one ear may result in the same undesirable reorganizations in children with (C)APD and lead, over time, to exacerbation of binaural listening and related auditory difficulties. For this reason, this author does not advocate such approaches for any child with (C)APD. Clinicians always should weigh both the seemingly apparent short-term benefits and the potential long-term effects of any intervention recommendation and avoid any strategy that holds even the possibility of long-term harm.

Controversial Point

- Many children with (C)APD exhibit exaggerated ear (usually right ear) advantages under dichotic listening conditions. These children also may report that listening is easier when sound is directed to the right ear only. This has led some to recommend use of a left earplug in the classroom to facilitate classroom listening skills. However, when one considers the literature regarding monaural occlusion or other forms of sensory deprivation and undesirable central auditory reorganization, one must seriously question the advisability of such a recommendation. Nonetheless, there is no clear-cut evidence at present specifically documenting harm resulting from the use of monaural occlusion in children as an aid to classroom listening, and this recommendation still is supported by some clinicians and educators.

Instructional and Related Modifications

Instructional modifications may be thought of as methods of enhancing access to the message itself, rather than focusing solely on the auditory signal. As such, these typically address linguistic, conceptual, and other higher order factors and, therefore, tend to be top-down in nature. Most of the following suggestions can be implemented with little or no additional time required on the part of the teacher and in such a manner as to be relatively unobtrusive so as not to draw undue attention to the child with (C)APD. One of the most beneficial instructional modifications for many children with (C)APD is that of preteaching new vocabulary and information. As previously discussed, the relative importance of bottom-up versus top-down processing shifts with changing listening demands. In often-noisy classrooms and other real-world environments, familiarity with vocabulary and topic matter assists in the ability to achieve auditory closure, or to fill in the missing elements of a message. For some children with (C)APD, auditory closure deficits are of primary concern.

Another common suggestion for classroom teachers of children with (C)APD or other auditory disorders is that of repetition or rephrasing of key information. However, it should be remembered that repetition and rephrasing are very different, and the appropriateness of each of these strategies will depend on the nature of the individual child's auditory deficit. For example, if a child does, indeed, have difficulty with auditory closure abilities, repetition may be a useful strategy, as he or she will have additional opportunity to "fill in" the pieces of the message that were missed on the first delivery. However, rephrasing may result in confusion for that same child, as he or she is likely, then, to encounter new missing elements and may even think that an entirely new message was delivered. For other auditory deficits, however, particularly those that are accompanied by language, memory, and/or other related difficulties, rephrasing using smaller linguistic units often is far more effective than repetition as a message clarification strategy. Therefore, the relative utility of repetition versus rephrasing will depend on the type of deficit that is present, as is the case with virtually all intervention recommendations for (C)APD.

Pearl

- Children for whom acoustic signal clarity and auditory closure are of primary concern likely will benefit most from repetition of the message as a clarification strategy. In contrast, for children with accompanying or secondary language, memory, or related difficulties, rephrasing the message using smaller linguistic units is likely to be more effective.

General Considerations

For most children with (C)APD, ensuring that attention is engaged prior to speaking, as well as making frequent checks for comprehension, is important. However, it is not sufficient merely to request that the child pay attention, nor is it advisable to draw repeated attention to a given child in this manner. Instead, it may be useful for the teacher to have some type of attention-getting strategy designed either for the entire class or only for the child in question. For example, the teacher may clap his or her hands in a familiar rhythm, and the class is to respond with the rest of the pattern. Or the teacher may have a "secret signal" that has been planned in advance with the individual child and that can be used to reengage attention without disrupting the entire class or drawing undue attention to the child.

Similarly, frequent checks for comprehension should be made; however, simply asking "Do you understand?" is unlikely to illuminate whether or not message comprehension was attained. Instead, teachers should observe performance for target behaviors or ask the child (again, in a manner that does not draw attention) to rephrase or paraphrase the instructions given.

Practicing principles of clear speech, that is, speaking slightly slower and slightly louder than normal, is a good communicative strategy in general, and is particularly effective for children with (C)APD. For other types of (C)APD, however, it may be more important to focus on ensuring that the child is placed with a teacher who makes good use of speech prosody—the rhythm, stress, and intonational contours of speech that allow us to identify key words in a message as well as intuit the underlying intent of a verbal communication—rather than focusing on signal clarity, per se.

Many children with (C)APD must expend a great deal of physical energy to listen successfully throughout a school day. This is particularly true of those children with (C)APD that affects speech-in-noise skills and for whom active listening and attention are critical. This effortful listening for hour after hour can be exhausting, regardless of the student's age. For those children for whom this seems to be a concern, effort should be made to arrange the course schedule so that auditory fatigue can be avoided to the greatest extent possible. For example, rather than scheduling all substantive lecture-based courses in the morning, they should be spread throughout the day. Breaks can be in the form of courses that represent fewer listening demands (e.g., art and physical education) or through scheduling of recesses and lunch. Again, the optimum schedule should be identified based on the needs of the individual child.

Finally, the efficacy of each classroom-based recommendation, as well as the teachers' compliance with such recommendations, should be monitored on a regular basis. It should be remembered that, despite best attempts, there may be situations in which classroom- or teacher-specific difficulties cannot be overcome for a particular child. When all options have been exhausted, consideration of an alternative placement, either with another teacher or even, perhaps, at a different facility, may be necessary.

Modifications for Postsecondary Educational and Workplace Settings

The fundamental listening needs of individuals with (C)APD in postsecondary educational settings (e.g., college) often are the same as those in the K–12 system, and the types of classroom modifications required, similarly, may be the same. However, the manner in which these modifications are implemented changes with increasing educational level. Thus, in college, the responsibility for informing central services (e.g., the Office of Disabilities), instructors, and others as to educational needs, ensuring that compliance occurs, and ultimate listening and learning success falls to the student, rather than to a designated educational team. Whereas the student may have received special education services afforded via federal law during the public school years and may have had an Individualized Education Plan (IEP) that delineated needs and goals and carried the weight of a legal contract, Individuals with Disabilities Act (IDEA) extends only through graduation from secondary education. College students with disabilities, including (C)APD, are protected under civil rights legislation that prevents discrimination against any individual with a disability from accessing education and other services that receive federal funding.

It is not uncommon for a previously undiagnosed (C)APD (or one that had been managed successfully) to create difficulties when a young adult arrives at college. This is due in part to the large class sizes of many freshman general education courses, as well as to the reliance on lectures in these courses and the increasing need for independent learning skills and self-monitoring in the college setting. Given all of the other changes that going to college brings, including expanded social activities, it is often difficult for students to identify an underlying cause for academic difficulties. Postsecondary educational facilities typically have some sort of mechanism in place to provide assistance to students having difficulty in the first year of college. It is important that, when appropriate, the possibility of (C)APD be considered and assessed so that modifications can be recommended.

Pearl

- Whether in K–12 or postsecondary educational settings, one of the most effective recommendations for students with (C)APD is to avoid auditory fatigue. Therefore, classes should be scheduled so that listening-intensive courses are divided regularly throughout the day by classes that are less verbal in nature, such as art, music, physical education, reading, and applied mathematics.

Similarly, adults with (C)APD may find it difficult to function in the workplace, particularly if their jobs involve communication in noisy backgrounds. Accommodations in the workplace may include carrying on conversations with supervisors and others in quiet settings, using memos and e-mails to provide instructions in writing, and developing a system of paraphrasing and/or clarifying instructions to ensure accurate task comprehension and facilitate task completion. In some cases, assistive technology, such as a personal FM system, may be indicated. The needs of the individual with (C)APD combined with the unique communicative challenges of the workplace setting will determine the types of accommodations needed. It is important that clinicians have a clear understanding both of the underlying auditory deficit(s) present in a given individual and of the characteristics of the workplace and the specific difficulties the individual is having for individualized accommodations to be designed. For specific suggestions regarding college and workplace modifications, readers are referred to Bellis (2002a).

Special Consideration

- At present, there is no agreed-upon method of rating the severity of (C)APD, nor may such an approach be appropriate. Because of the complex interaction of bottom-up and top-down factors in auditory processing, performance on measures of central auditory function may not reflect accurately the degree to which function is impaired in real-world listening situations. Furthermore, the listening demands of a specific environment will be a primary determining factor in the degree of difficulty an individual with (C)APD experiences, and an otherwise "mild" auditory deficit may be significantly disabling for an individual who is required to work in an exceptionally noisy setting.

Home Modifications

For many children and adults with (C)APD, some of the primary communicative frustrations occur not at school or in the workplace, but at home with parents, siblings, or spouses. In typical households, frustration often arises when a child fails to complete an assigned chore or a spouse "forgets" to pick up important items from the store. These frustrations often are compounded by the presence of a (C)APD that interferes with message acquisition. Several home-based modifications are available that may assist children and adults in the home setting. For example, key instructions or chores can be written down for clarification and retention; a write-on/wipe-off white board is particularly useful for this purpose. Similarly, if difficulties in competing acoustic conditions are identified, all attempts should be made to ensure a quiet listening environment when important conversations are occurring or critical information or instructions are being delivered, and carrying on a conversation while the television is on or the water is running should be avoided. Additionally, all attempts should be made to engage in conversation only when all participants are in the same room, rather than attempting to converse from different rooms. As in the school setting, making frequent checks for comprehension, asking the child or adult to paraphrase instructions, and other appropriate modifications may be helpful.

As in all settings, the key to effective communication at home is education and understanding on the part of all involved. Therefore, involving the entire family in developing and implementing home-based modification strategies can both ensure compliance with the recommendations and facilitate a supportive home environment. At all times, family members should attempt to avoid the temptation of exclaiming in exasperation, "You never listen to me!" or making other critical statements that assign blame to and undermine the listener. Effective family counseling can assist in helping family members learn to blame the disorder, not the person, for misinterpretations or miscommunications. Because of recent findings that suggest that adult males may exhibit auditory difficulties that differ from those of females and that occur earlier in the adult life span (Bellis and Wilber, 2001), cross-gender counseling of couples may be an important component of family counseling.

Finally, it should be remembered that everyone has a need for rest and relaxation at home. No one is a "good listener" all day, every day, least of all children or adults with (C)APD. All too often, especially with children, individuals with (C)APD are required to put forth great listening effort throughout the day, perhaps engage in after-school therapy (in addition to extracurricular activities), and still complete homework assignments each evening. By the end of the day, these individuals may be exhausted from the great effort put into listening throughout the day. It is important that "down time" be afforded them when in the home environment. To this end, it may be helpful to schedule family conferences during which important information can be imparted and then allow the child or adult time simply to rest and rejuvenate, or simply to engage in play or other enjoyable endeavors, without the need for continued vigilance and active listening. Bellis (2002a) provides additional discussion of home-based modifications that may be appropriate for individuals with (C)APD.

Compensatory Strategies

As the term implies, compensatory strategies assist an individual with (C)APD to compensate for residual auditory deficit(s). Specifically, these are activities that train the individual to strengthen higher order, top-down skills so that these central resources can be recruited to buttress deficient auditory skills. As discussed previously, resource allocation theory illustrates that available energy is allocated across sensory systems and higher order cognitive, language, and related functions. When a disproportionate amount of energy is spent on processing the incoming acoustic signal, less energy is left over for interpreting, comprehending, remembering, and acting upon the message. Thus, these higher order resources support auditory processing and are critical to overall listening, learning, and communicative success. Compensatory strategies training maximizes generalization of learned skills to the ever-changing demands of the day-to-day environment and teaches patients methods of taking responsibility for their own listening success. Several compensatory strategies that may be appropriate for individuals with (C)APD will be discussed in this section and are summarized in **Table 11–2**.

Because effective listening involves more than just peripheral and central auditory processes and functions, it is critical to address these higher order and pansensory central resources in any intervention program for (C)APD. Many of us automatically develop strategies to compensate for less than ideal listening situations and implement those strategies virtually subconsciously. However, individuals with auditory or related disorders may, over time, develop secondary motivational deficits due to repeated listening

Table 11–2 Selected Compensatory Strategies

Cognitive and Metacognitive Strategies
- Active listening techniques
- Attribution training
- Problem solving
- Self-instruction and reciprocal teaching
- Assertiveness training
- Metamemory techniques
  - Chunking
  - Elaboration
  - Transformation
  - Reauditorization
  - Use of external aids

Linguistic and Metalinguistic Strategies
- Contextual derivation
- Schema induction and discourse cohesion devices
- Prosody training and perception of body language cues
- Key word recognition and extraction

failures and, as such, become passive listeners and learners. These individuals, then, may not develop compensatory strategies, or may implement nonadaptive strategies. Therefore, for many children and adults with (C)APD, these skills need to be trained explicitly. Compensatory strategies fall into two general categories: cognitive and metacognitive strategies (including metamemory), and linguistic and metalinguistic strategies. Chermak (1998) and Chermak and Musiek (1997) have been credited with the application of many of these techniques to individuals with (C)APD, and readers are referred to these works as well as to Bellis (2002a, 2003) for further details regarding compensatory strategies.

Cognitive and Metacognitive Strategies

The overall purpose of cognitive and metacognitive strategies is to promote active self-regulation and monitoring of listening behaviors and to strengthen higher order attention, memory, and related cognitive resources (Chermak, 1998; Chermak and Musiek, 1997). These strategies require the listener to learn to pay attention to and take responsibility for his or her own listening and learning behaviors, and to develop problem-solving and self-monitoring techniques to overcome comprehension difficulties. As such, most of these techniques can be considered collectively as cognitive behavior modification techniques. Cognitive and metacognitive strategies that may be appropriate for individuals with (C)APD include but are not limited to the following.

Active Listening Techniques Although many children and adults with (C)APD are aware that they need to become "better listeners," the mechanisms by which to accomplish this goal may be less than clear. Furthermore, these individuals may not be aware of the behaviors that impede their ability to focus and listen, and may be unable to monitor and regulate their own attention and related internal cognitive skills. Therefore, telling an individual to "pay attention" or "listen more closely" often is ineffective. Active listening techniques, including "whole body listening" (Bellis, 2002a), may provide an easy-to-learn, yet effective, means of refocusing attention and aiding in listening success.

Active listening involves teaching the individual to make physical (rather than cognitive or attentional) adjustments in behavior. Specifically, he or she is taught to (1) sit up straight, (2) incline the head toward the speaker, (3) watch the speaker carefully, and (4) cease extraneous movement (e.g., foot jiggling or finger tapping). Because the mind follows where the body goes, the application of these four simple steps automatically ensures that the individual is actively involved in the listening process. The fifth step involves self-monitoring of one's own physical state so that, when focus is lost, the individual can reimplement the four physical steps immediately and reengage in the listening process. Because the focus in active listening is on self-regulation and self-monitoring of behavior, the individual with (C)APD is empowered to take responsibility for his or her listening success.

> **Pearl**
>
> - Individuals with (C)APD often develop secondary motivational difficulties and adopt a passive approach to listening and communication. Therefore, training that focuses on the provision of skills needed to allow them to participate actively in their own intervention, mitigates feelings of helplessness, and facilitates the development of self-empowerment is likely to enhance the success of all other accommodations and direct remediation activities implemented. In contrast, even a well-designed, deficit-specific, and appropriately implemented intervention plan may yield less than desirable results if the individual with (C)APD remains a passive listener and learner.

Attribution Training   In attribution training, the individual is taught to attribute failures to factors under his or her control (e.g., insufficient effort) rather than adopting an external locus of control (i.e., blaming the problems on the sensory problem, the speaker, or others). Here, again, the primary focus is on ensuring that the individual takes responsibility for listening and learning success. The role of the clinician is to provide opportunities for patients to confront listening situations in which they were less than successful and to identify ways in which increased effort may have assisted. Careful wording, support, salient feedback, and ensuring that the individual does indeed experience improved success with greater expenditure of effort are critical aspects of attribution training.

Problem Solving   Both of the above strategies may be thought of as forms of problem solving. Additional direct problem-solving skills training often is helpful, particularly in the areas of situational analysis and generation (and implementation) of possible solutions. This strategy also requires the individual to engage in self-monitoring to determine whether the solution generated was successful and, if not, to generate alternate solutions to the problem. For example, when faced with a challenging SNR, the individual might analyze the noise situation and determine the source of the noise, identify possible solutions (e.g., relocate to another spot in the room, turn off a noisy piece of equipment, or ask the speaker to move to another location), select a solution appropriate for the situation, implement the solution, determine whether the solution addressed the problem, and implement another solution if the first proves unsuccessful. Similarly, children or adults who frequently misinterpret instructions even when they think they have heard them correctly may analyze the situation (e.g., realize that what was heard may not be accurate), generate and implement a solution (e.g., paraphrase the instructions with the teacher or supervisor—"Let me see if I understand . . . you would like me to . . ."—to reveal any misunderstandings and provide opportunity for clarification), and evaluate the outcome (e.g., determine if task completion was accomplished successfully). Because it is impossible to prepare for all possible situations that may arise, problem-solving training empowers individuals with (C)APD to

self-identify methods of dealing with any contingency and can, therefore, increase self-esteem and self-confidence, as well as improve overall listening and learning success.

> **Pitfall**
>
> - Children and adults with (C)APD may not be aware when they have heard messages incorrectly. As a result, they may carry out instructions only to learn, after the fact, that their actions were in error. This can result in considerable frustration and embarrassment for the individual with (C)APD and his or her communicative partners, educators, supervisors, and others. Therefore, problem-solving skills and clarification strategies should not focus solely on repairing communication breakdowns. More general and automatic message clarification strategies and other means of ensuring that what was heard actually conformed to what was said should be a key component of the intervention program, as well.

Self-Instruction and Reciprocal Teaching   This technique involves instructing patients to "coach" themselves through challenging listening, learning, or communicative situations. In the beginning, the clinician talks out the steps of a particular problem or task as the child or adult carries them out. Then, the individual with (C)APD is taught to do the same, first aloud, then subvocally, and finally silently. Reciprocal teaching involves having the patient and clinician switch roles, so that the individual with (C)APD coaches the clinician through a particular task. This is useful to facilitate the transfer of responsibility for self-regulation and problem solving from clinician to patient, and can enhance self-esteem and accountability.

> **Pearl**
>
> - Individuals with (C)APD often find it very difficult to self-monitor and identify means of addressing communication or listening difficulties that they, themselves, are experiencing. When witnessing another person undergoing similar difficulties, in contrast, they may well be able to analyze the situation more objectively and arrive at an appropriate solution. For this reason, reciprocal teaching is a very effective strategy, especially for those individuals who exhibit difficulty in self-analysis and problem solving.

Assertiveness Training   It is critical that individuals with (C)APD, as well as those with other disorders, learn to advocate for their own needs, rather than relying on others to provide for them. Clinicians, educators, and parents often are so focused on ensuring that the needs of patients (especially children) with (C)APD are met that they forget that there will not always be someone looking out for the individual on a day-to-day basis. Teaching problem-solving and related skills is useless unless the child or adult is able to implement the solutions identified, which often requires the ability to assert himself or herself with others to make his or her needs known. As with all of these techniques, assertiveness training fosters self-empowerment and shifts the individual's cognitive framework from an external locus of control in which he or she is entirely reliant on others to an internal locus of control in which self-advocacy and self-responsibility are of primary focus.

Metamemory Techniques   Because individuals with auditory disorders expend a great deal of effort on decoding the incoming message, there may be few resources remaining "upstream" to remember and act upon the information (McCoy et al, 2005). Therefore, activities that target awareness and use of memory strategies to enhance comprehension and recall often are useful additions to the overall intervention program. A variety of metamemory techniques exist, and the decision regarding which to choose often depends on the individual patient as well as on the task demand or listening situation. Language-based memory strategies include mnemonic devices, which are contrived techniques that facilitate recall through the use of artificial aids to information organization. Examples of these include chunking, or grouping similar items together into categories; elaboration, or the use of acronyms or analogies to aid item recall (e.g., ROYGBIV for the colors of the rainbow, "On Old Olympus' Towering Top . . ." for the names of the cranial nerves); and transformation, in which complex information is stored in another form such as an equation ($E = mc^2$) or in pictorial form. These sketches then are referred to later to facilitate recall of the key information. Finally, re-auditorization, or repetition of the incoming message, when used selectively, also may enforce the auditory memory trace and thus enhance recall.

Additional methods of enhancing memory and recall include the use of external aids, such as notepads, organizers, electronic planners, and similar devices. Many of us use these devices daily to maintain organization and provide reminders of important information and events. Explicit training in their use can be a useful adjunct to the overall intervention plan even for very young children.

Linguistic and Metalinguistic Strategies

A primary functional implication of (C)APD is difficulty understanding spoken language. Therefore, language-based strategies that aid in comprehension of the intended message are critical to overall communicative success. Linguistic and metalinguistic strategies involve explicit training in the deployment of language-based knowledge and skills to assist message comprehension. Several language-based strategies are described below.

Contextual Derivation   An important skill for comprehension is the ability to use surrounding context to fill in missing pieces of a message or communication and achieve closure. Knowledge of the subject matter, combined with analysis of the surrounding words and information, combine to assist in achieving this goal. Contextual derivation activities focus on teaching the individual to rely on surrounding context and other knowledge to make educated hypotheses about the nature of missing information or gaps in the incoming message. Specific auditory closure activities may include (from least to most difficult) passages and sentences in which entire words are missing, missing syllable exercises, and missing phoneme exercises (Bellis, 2002a, 2003). Another activity that focuses specifically on use of context to derive meaning is vocabulary building (Chermak and Musiek, 1997). This technique uses written material to enhance closure and vocabulary skills. When an unfamiliar word is encountered, the reader is instructed to repeat the word aloud (reauditorization) and then to attempt a definition of the word based on surrounding context. At that point, the actual definition of the word is provided and is reinforced through having the reader reword the definition and/or use the word in a sentence or alternate context. The final result is that the reader is able to identify the new word both auditorily and visually, thus expanding his or her vocabulary, while at the same time enhancing the ability to use context to derive meaning and improving general closure skills.

Pearl

- Whenever possible, clinicians should attempt to incorporate vocabulary and other material that is likely to be encountered in the individual's daily life into therapy activities. For example, by using material culled from upcoming topics in coursework for intervention activities rather than those designed solely for the therapy setting, skills learned in the therapy setting will generalize more readily to the classroom environment, and the potential for academic success will be maximized.

Schema Induction and Discourse Cohesion Devices   For some individuals with (C)APD, particularly children, training in the rules of language may be indicated to facilitate improvement in and recruitment of higher order linguistic and related skills. For example, explicitly teaching recognition and use of linguistic markers that serve to connect components of complex messages, organize and integrate information, and signal relationships among elements can assist greatly in general auditory comprehension. These formal schemata and discourse cohesion devices include but are not limited to tag words that indicate order or sequence (e.g., *first, last, next, then*), adversative terms (*however, although*), referents (e.g., pronouns and proverbs), additives (e.g., *and*), and causal terms (e.g., *if/then, because, therefore*).

Prosody Training and Perception of Body Language Cues
Comprehension of a spoken message does not rely solely on perception of the phonological and linguistic elements of the signal. Instead, how something is said often is just as important as what is said. Therefore, the ability to recognize both linguistic and prosodic elements of speech and to link them together is critical to overall spoken language comprehension. This is especially important in the comprehension of forms such as sarcasm, which is typified by a mismatch between linguistic and prosodic elements; however, it comes into play in general communication situations, as well. Some individuals with (C)APD have particular difficulty with prosodic elements of speech, or those rhythm, stress, and intonation characteristics of running speech that convey what is meant in relation to what is said. For these individuals, activities that employ stimuli in which prosodic changes alter meaning may be indicated (Bellis, 2002a,b, 2003; Chermak and Musiek, 1997). These may include heteronyms (e.g., sub*ject* vs sub*ject*, con*vict* vs

con*vict*), sentences in which segmentation and rhythm alters meaning (e.g., "I saw the snow *drift* by the window" vs "I saw the *snowdrift* by the window"), and sentences in which relative stress alters meaning (e.g., "You can't go to the store with *me*" vs "You can't go to the *store* with me" vs "*You* can't go to the store with me"). In addition, activities that focus on both tone of voice and nonverbal, body language cues that signal emotion (e.g., happy, surprised, angry, and threatening), as well as communications employing sarcasm and punch line humor, may facilitate overall comprehension of communicative intent for those with prosodic difficulties. Reading aloud with exaggerated prosodic features is a final activity that may improve both perception and production of these intonational cues, particularly in children.

Special Consideration

- Not all forms of (C)APD affect speech-sound discrimination and related abilities. Instead, perception of the prosodic elements of speech and social communication skills may be the primary auditory concern in some types of (C)APD, particularly those that affect right hemisphere auditory skills. Therefore, prosody training and other activities that target specifically these right hemisphere communication functions may be the primary focus for the intervention efforts in these individuals.

Identification of important elements of a message relies on the ability to perceive relative stress, as it is the critical words that are typically given more emphasis in spoken communication. An inability to resolve differences in relative stress, such as occurs in some individuals with (C)APD, can significantly impede comprehension. In these cases, explicit training in key word recognition and extraction is indicated. These activities, which often are most appropriate for children but may be indicated for some adults as well, focus on anticipating and actively listening for specific elements, such as subject, verb, object, distinctive adjectives (e.g., "The *blue* book"), and key prepositions (e.g., "Put it *under* the table") while, at the same time, paying less attention to relatively unimportant words, such as articles and some conjunctions. It should be noted that key word recognition and extraction activities also can be instrumental in improving note-taking skills, as note taking involves listening for, identifying, and writing down the most important words in a message in outline form.

Direct Remediation Activities

The activities that have been discussed thus far in this chapter have addressed the individual's ability to access information that is being presented auditorily and to compensate for the auditory deficit(s) that is/are present. However, none of them have focused directly on improving or ameliorating the deficits themselves. As such, although the foregoing recommendations may be thought of as management approaches for (C)APD and are critical components of the overall comprehensive intervention program, they cannot, in truth, be considered to be treatment activities. In contrast, the primary goal of direct remediation activities is actually to improve, to the greatest extent possible, the child's or adult's auditory deficit(s) through the use of targeted auditory training (AT) activities. A significant body of literature substantiates both structural reorganization and functional improvement in auditory behaviors as well is in neurophysiologic representation of acoustic stimuli following AT (see Musiek et al, 2002, 2005 for reviews). Structural reorganization may take the form of either activation of previously inactive neuronal tissue or the development of new and/or more efficient synaptic connections within the brain. Of key importance is the accurate identification of the auditory deficit(s) present and the manner in which AT is administered.

Bellis (2002a,b, 2003) emphasizes that, first and foremost, the selection of which direct remediation activities to implement should arise logically from the diagnostic test results and should be deficit-specific in nature. Just as there are few, if any, management recommendations that are appropriate for all individuals with (C)APD, there is no "one size fits all" direct remediation approach or AT activity that will "cure" all central auditory deficits, no matter how badly such a program is desired nor how many anecdotal reports of such programs exist. Instead, the specific AT activities that are recommended must be based on the individual's presenting functional deficit profile, must be appropriate to his or her developmental level, and must be administered in such a manner that training is frequent, intense, and challenging (but not overly frustrating) by working near the patient's skill threshold (Chermak and Musiek, 2002). Finally, although some AT programs exist that purport to effect beneficial changes in auditory function while requiring nothing more than passive listening on the part of the individual, these approaches are inconsistent with what is known about the importance of active participation and engagement in maximizing CNS plasticity and perceptual learning. Therefore, AT activities must require that the child or adult respond actively to the auditory stimuli and should incorporate both immediate feedback and salient reinforcement so as to maintain motivation, induce plasticity, and maximize learning.

Based on their clinical experience, Chermak and Musiek (2002) suggest several additional guidelines for AT activities. These include employing varied stimuli and tasks, working at a level at which 30 to 70% accuracy is maintained, verifying attainment of 70% accuracy prior to moving on to more demanding tasks, ensuring that training is frequent (i.e., five to seven sessions per week), and presenting stimuli at comfortable listening levels or slightly louder. The authors note that the progression of AT activities should occur in accordance with normal development of auditory skills, so that detection and discrimination activities, if indicated, precede identification, recognition, and other, more advanced skills.

Direct remediation activities may include formal AT administered by an audiologist using appropriate audiometric equipment and acoustically controlled, usually nonverbal or very simple verbal stimuli. They also may be informal, implemented in the school or home setting by a speech-language pathologist, resource teacher, parent, or others and using more language-based stimuli. Ideally, formal and informal AT both should be employed to maximize generalization of specific learned auditory skills to real-world communicative experiences. Several issues, however, impede delivery of audiologist-implemented formal AT services to children and adults with (C)APD, including lack of third-party reimbursement for audiologists for aural rehabilitation, paucity of audiologists with the training and/or the time to design and deliver such services, and issues related to the patient's distance from the nearest audiometric equipment and need for daily travel to and from the clinical setting. Thus, most of the direct remediation for (C)APD currently is overseen by speech-language pathologists or others in the school and/or home setting. Nonetheless, with a bit of creativity and knowledge, combined with the recent advent of computer-assisted therapy programs and the promise on the horizon of additional, more acoustically controlled, commercially available compact disc (CD)—based AT activities that target fundamental auditory skills, direct remediation can and should be undertaken for anyone, child or adult, with (C)APD.

Several AT activities appropriate for specific central auditory deficits are described briefly in this section and are summarized in **Table 11–3**. Readers are referred to Bellis (2002a,b, 2003), Chermak and Musiek (1997, 2002), and Musiek et al (2002) for additional information on these procedures.

Verbal and Nonverbal Discrimination Activities

Auditory discrimination is a skill that is fundamental to almost all auditory tasks. Therefore, auditory discrimination

Table 11–3 Selected Formal and Informal Deficit-Specific Remediation Activities

Verbal and Nonverbal Auditory Discrimination Activities
- Phoneme discrimination
- Word discrimination
- Frequency, intensity, and duration discrimination

Temporal Processing Training Activities
- Gap detection/auditory fusion
- Temporal sequencing/ordering activities
  - Multitone ordering
  - Sequencing of rapid auditory events with varied interstimulus intervals
  - Imitation of nonverbal patterns
  - Following directions of increasing length and complexity

Distorted or Degraded Speech Recognition Activities
- Low-pass filtered words (in isolation and in context)
- Time-compressed words (in isolation and in context)
- Words in reverberation (in isolation and in context)
- Speech-in-noise training

Binaural Interaction and Localization/Lateralization Activities
- Sound source identification
- Interaural intensity differences
- Interaural temporal offsets

Dichotic Listening Training
- Binaural separation
- Binaural integration
- Interaural intensity and/or timing differences

Auditory Vigilance Activities

Cross-modality Activities

deficits identified during diagnostic testing should be addressed directly. These activities may focus on discrimination of phoneme cognate pairs (both vowels and consonants), as well as on words containing similar-sounding phonemes in various positions, including rhyming words. If testing reveals difficulty with discrimination of nonverbal stimuli and/or suprasegmental elements of speech (e.g., duration, intensity, and frequency), then difference-limen training should be implemented.

Computer-assisted programs and/or specialized audiologic equipment are particularly useful for formal discrimination training, as they provide the ability to vary systematically the difference between pairs to be discriminated. Thus, for example, the use of synthesized syllables allows for the systematic varying of the third formant transition in the /da/-to-/ga/ continuum, and the use of auditory signal delivery equipment permits tonal signals differing in frequency to be varied by a matter of only a few hertz. In addition, computer-controlled algorithms that automatically increase the difference between cognate pairs following an incorrect response and decrease the difference following a correct response can, when combined with salient reinforcement, induce rapid improvement in fundamental discrimination skills. Several commercially available computer-assisted programs include such auditory discrimination activities, including Fast ForWord (1998) and Earobics (1998). These and other computer-assisted programs will be discussed in a later section of this chapter.

Research in neuroplasticity has demonstrated that formal discrimination training results in both physiologic and behavioral changes in the central auditory system. Moreover, physi-

ologic changes typically precede behavioral improvement in discrimination skills, indicating that electrophysiologic techniques may play an important role in monitoring treatment efficacy (Tremblay et al, 1998). Finally, discrimination skills trained may generalize to other, untrained cognate pairs, perhaps reflecting an overall improvement in timing in the CANS (Tremblay et al, 1998).

Informal auditory discrimination training activities also may be implemented, and typically use phoneme stimuli either in syllables or in words. This activity, also a hallmark of AT for hearing-impaired children, typically is conducted in a live-voice manner, and also may be combined with speech-to-print skills training to facilitate improved reading and spelling abilities. Although live-voice stimuli cannot approximate the very precise acoustic control of computer-generated stimuli, informal phoneme discrimination training is important for generalization of learned fundamental discrimination skills to real-world listening and learning situations. Similarly, higher level phonological awareness activities involving phoneme analysis, synthesis, and segmentation also promotes generalization to daily listening tasks involving spoken language.

Special Consideration

- Although auditory synthesis, segmentation, and other phonological awareness abilities are reliant, in part, on adequate central auditory processing, these are considered higher order language-related functions and thus are not included in the definition of (C)APD (ASHA 2005a,b). It is important that clinicians recognize that, although informal auditory training activities may incorporate such activities to facilitate generalization of specific auditory skills trained, phonological awareness difficulties either may be absent in individuals with (C)APD or may arise from factors entirely unrelated to the auditory system. Therefore, tests of phonological awareness are not considered to be diagnostic of central auditory function, and not all individuals with (C)APD will benefit from treatment focused on phonological awareness skills.

Temporal Processing Training

Temporal processing, or timing-related aspects of processing, may be considered to be the foundation of all auditory processing. Indeed, a variety of temporal processing deficits have been associated with learning and related deficits in children (e.g., Tallal, 1980; Wright et al, 1997). It should be noted that there are many types of temporal processing, however, and timing plays a role in virtually every auditory activity and skill discussed in this chapter. The nature of an individual's temporal processing deficit will dictate the type of temporal processing training that is indicated. Thus, for example, children and adults who demonstrate deficit in temporal resolution, such as gap detection (i.e., the ability to detect a very short silent period in a signal) or auditory fusion (i.e., the ability to discriminate whether one or two short signals occur when separated by a short silent period), may require specific training to improve these thresholds prior to beginning higher level activities that rely on fine timing in the system, such as verbal and/or nonverbal discrimination. Alternatively, some patients demonstrate deficits in temporal sequencing or ordering, as evidenced by poor performance on pitch- or duration-patterns testing. In these cases, temporal sequencing activities (e.g., multitone ordering; sequencing of rapid auditory events with variable interstimulus intervals; and imitation of nonverbal patterns that incorporate changes in rhythm, intensity, and frequency) are indicated and, for some individuals, may be a necessary prerequisite before higher level patterning activities, such as prosody training, can be introduced. To facilitate generalization of sequencing skills, training in following directives of increasing length and complexity is a useful informal AT activity.

Distorted or Degraded Speech Recognition Training

In the previous discussion of compensatory strategies, the topic of contextual derivation to facilitate auditory closure skills was introduced. From a formal AT perspective, training in distorted or degraded speech recognition, incorporating words either in isolation or in context, also addresses auditory closure skills. Speech may be degraded by low-pass filtering, time compression, and/or via the addition of noise or reverberation. The ability to recognize distorted or degraded speech relies, in turn, on intact auditory discrimination and temporal resolution abilities. Therefore, these fundamental skill areas may need to be addressed before degraded speech recognition training can commence.

Binaural Interaction and Localization/Lateralization Training

A skill that is fundamental to hearing in noise and related abilities is localization of the sound source. Specific training in localization and lateralization may be indicated when deficits in binaural processing are identified. Typically, localization training is conducted in a sound field using speakers set at varying azimuths, whereas lateralization training is conducted under headphones and can be accomplished via varying the interaural intensity of the sound and/or the temporal offsets of a leading versus following signal so as to engage the precedence effect. The goal of binaural interaction training is to improve the listener's sound source identification acuity. Informal AT to improve localization skills can occur in virtually any daily listening environment that affords opportunities for sound source identification.

Dichotic Listening Training

Deficits in binaural separation and binaural integration, as evidenced by poor performance on dichotic speech tests, are particularly amenable to dichotic listening training. Dichotic listening involves the presentation of disparate signals to each ear simultaneously. During dichotic listening training, listeners are instructed to attend to a target ear while ignoring competing speech presented to the opposite ear (binaural separation). Alternatively, listeners may be instructed to monitor both ears for a target word or phrase,

and to respond when the target is presented in either ear (binaural integration). Typically, the interaural intensity difference is rendered more difficult by increasing the presentation level of the competition gradually while, at the same time, decreasing the level of the target over time. In addition, temporal offsets may be incorporated so that the competition lags in time relative to the target, which improves performance. As the temporal offset is reduced, the task becomes more challenging. These activities can be done formally under highly acoustically controlled conditions or more informally on an at-home basis using familiar sound equipment such as portable CD devices, televisions, or radios, and commercially available headphones or earbuds. Dichotic listening training involving interaural temporal offsets typically is formal in nature because of the need for acoustic control of signal timing.

Pearl

- Motivation and compliance are key factors in the success of home-based training activities, such as dichotic listening training. Therefore, materials that are inherently interesting to the individual with (C)APD should be used for this activity whenever possible. The local library or video rental store may offer an unexpected wealth of material for dichotic listening training, including books on tape and popular movies that can be selected with the individual child's or adult's interests and language level in mind.

Other Auditory Training and Related Activities

Additional training in auditory vigilance may be indicated, particularly for those individuals who have developed secondary motivational deficits and/or passive listening behaviors. The active listening techniques discussed in the section on compensatory strategies may be thought of as forms of auditory vigilance training, as may activities involving following instructions of increasing length and complexity. Another form of auditory vigilance training involves instructing the patient to listen for a predetermined target word in a sentence or passage, then to recall the word that immediately preceded the target. This task can be rendered more difficult by not revealing the target word until after the sentence is presented, thus requiring the listener to attend to and remember the entire sentence to successfully complete the task (e.g., Sweetow and Henderson-Sabes, 2004). In the latter condition, both auditory vigilance and working memory are challenged. Additional activities that train auditory vigilance include listening for specific prosodic elements (e.g., stressed words), linguistic markers (e.g., adjectives, adverbs), or other specific components of messages of increasing length.

Cross-modality training tasks can facilitate generalization of skills learned to other contexts and engage multimodal integration areas of the brain. Exercises that require rapid interhemispheric transfer via the corpus callosum may be indicated for many individuals with binaural separation and/or integration deficits, specifically those that are presumed to arise from inefficient interhemispheric interaction. These activities can involve virtually any skill that requires the two hemispheres of the brain to communicate and cooperate with one another, including verbal-to-motor (and reverse) transfers, verbal identification of objects held in the nondominant (usually left) hand, and video games and music lessons that require rapid and coordinated bimanual responses. Tasks involving communications that require the linking of prosodic and linguistic elements of speech (e.g., sarcasm and humor) or differential identification of the lyrics versus the melodies of songs are additional examples of interhemispheric integration activities.

In summary, there are several direct remediation activities that may be appropriate for individuals with (C)APD. As the purpose of these activities is to reduce or ameliorate the auditory deficit, it is critical that they be deficit-specific in nature. Thus, as with all aspects of intervention for (C)APD, the choice of which specific therapy activities to implement for a given individual is entirely dependent on accurate and comprehensive diagnosis of the underlying auditory deficit(s). In addition, because the ultimate goal of (C)APD intervention is to improve daily function, it is important that auditory deficits be related to the functional complaints, difficulties, and sequelae exhibited by the individual so that ecologically valid treatment plans may be developed. Methods of interpreting (C)APD diagnostic testing and relating the findings to multidisciplinary results and functional complaints for the purpose of developing comprehensive intervention plans have been discussed elsewhere, and readers are referred to Bellis (2002a,b, 2003) for a review.

◆ Computer-Assisted Therapies and Other Popular Programs

In recent years, there has been a dramatic increase in commercially available computer-assisted or similar therapy programs to address various types of disorders, including (C)APD and other auditory deficits. Many of these programs have the advantage of being able to engage the listener through the use of entertaining graphics and fun activities, ensuring that the listener is challenged by employing synthesized signals and computer-based algorithms that converge on skill threshold levels in a manner that is not possible using live-voice stimuli, and maintaining motivation via the provision of immediate and salient feedback to the listener. Several of these programs were developed for specific populations; however, their use has extended to those with (C)APD. For example, Fast ForWord (1998) originally was designed to address the temporal processing deficits observed in children with specific language impairment (SLI). Nonetheless, the activities in this program may be appropriate for those children with (C)APD who exhibit specific auditory deficits in temporal processing even if SLI is not diagnosed. Similarly, Earobics (1998) is a more general auditory skills training program that addresses a variety of areas, including phoneme discrimination and speech-to-print skills, rhythm, sequencing, speech

in noise, and rhyming words, among others. Depending on the individual's identified auditory deficit(s), one or more components of this program may be applicable.

Pitfall

- Clinicians should be cautious of and guard against becoming caught up in the "bandwagon" phenomenon when considering commercially available therapy programs for (C)APD. No matter how many anecdotal reports exist attesting to a given program's efficacy and no matter how successful the program may have been for others in a clinician's caseload, this does not mean that the program in question will be appropriate for every individual. Clinicians must remain objective and carefully analyze any program's task demands and scientific claims before recommending it for a child or adult with (C)APD.

Other programs have appeared in recent years, and many more are on the horizon, making it difficult to determine which may be appropriate for children and adults with (C)APD. This is particularly true given the paucity of specific treatment efficacy studies using well-defined populations with (C)APD. Therefore, it is important that readers keep in mind several general "rules" regarding these or, indeed, any programs that purport to address (C)APD.

First, clinicians should analyze the task demands and activities of any program and determine whether they target the identified auditory deficit(s) present. As emphasized previously, there is no "one size fits all" program appropriate for all individuals with (C)APD. Therefore, whereas many of these popular programs may be appropriate for some individuals with (C)APD, their applicability will depend entirely on accurate and specific diagnosis of the problem and careful analysis of the task demands of the AT program. One should never enter into the therapy arena using a "shotgun" approach, trying everything in the hopes that something will work. Instead, any direct remediation activity, whether computer-assisted or not, should be selected carefully and with a specific purpose and rationale in mind.

Second, clinicians always should keep in mind what is known about neuroplasticity and perceptual learning, as discussed previously in this chapter. Specifically, one should remember the importance of active participation and motivation on the part of the listener, as well as the need for salient reinforcement. In general, programs that purport to alter auditory function through mere passive listening violate these principles and are likely to be far less effective than programs that actively train specific auditory skills.

Third, the scientific bases of all programs should be examined carefully for consistency with the current peer-reviewed literature. Programs that purport to effect change through means that are anatomically and/or physiologically untenable or that are inconsistent with the science underlying audition and auditory processing should be viewed with extreme caution. Similarly, programs that claim to address a wide range of disorders, from autism to (C)APD to attention deficit and beyond, should raise some suspicion in the mind of the clinician, as these claims are highly suspect given the significant differences between and complexity of these types of disorders.

Finally, any program that carries a risk of harm of any kind should never be recommended for individuals with (C)APD or, indeed, any disorder. Thus, programs that include prolonged sensory deprivation, use potentially damaging sound presentation levels, or include caveats that normal function may in some way be altered following the program should be avoided at all costs. In addition, clinicians should resist the "bandwagon" phenomenon that often accompanies the introduction of any new program. Specifically, regardless of the plethora of anecdotal reports of treatment efficacy that may exist for a given program, clinicians always should approach any therapy critically and scientifically. Recommending one program in a "blanket" manner for all individuals in one's caseload goes against the principles of deficit-specific intervention and suggests a lack of objectivity on the part of the clinician.

With the exception of Fast ForWord and Earobics, this author has intentionally resisted listing specific names of various programs in this section. This is due, in part, to the large number of programs available at this time, as well as to the fact that new programs undoubtedly will be available by the time this chapter comes to print. Instead, the above general principles should provide a guide for clinicians to evaluate the appropriateness of any program, past, present, or future, for individuals with (C)APD. Nevertheless, two additional treatment paradigms do deserve specific mention: Auditory Integration Training (AIT; Stehli, 1994) and Listening and Auditory Communication and Enhancement (LACE; Sweetow and Henderson-Sabes, 2004).

AIT, developed by Dr. Guy Berard, an otolaryngologist in France, was first described as an intervention for autism by Stehli (1994). Since that time, several anecdotal reports have appeared to support the efficacy of AIT "sound therapy" approaches, including the Berard method and the Tomatis and Clark methods for a variety of disorders. As a result, popular demand for these programs has skyrocketed. However, systematic, peer-reviewed research documenting efficacy of these approaches for children with (C)APD is lacking. In addition, concerns have been raised regarding the significant and numerous inconsistencies between the scientific claims made by the developers and proponents of these programs and the basic science relative to auditory system structure and function. Additional concerns have been expressed regarding the potential for harm that may occur through the use of unregulated sound levels with these programs (see ASHA, 2004a, for a review). As a result, ASHA (2004b) recently took the position that AIT "has not met scientific standards for efficacy that would justify its practice by audiologists and speech-language pathologists" (p. 1), although well-designed research protocols to explore the efficacy of AIT are encouraged. In a study specifically addressing the use of AIT for children with (C)APD, Yencer (1998) found no evidence supporting its efficacy for this purpose. As a result of these findings and concerns, this author does not, at present, recommend AIT or related programs for children or adults with (C)APD, despite their current popularity.

Controversial Point

- Should AIT and other "sound therapy" programs be recommended for children with (C)APD? Despite a paucity of peer-reviewed evidence supporting the efficacy of such programs and the decision by ASHA (2004a,b) to consider such programs experimental in nature, there are many clinicians throughout the world who continue to implement these programs regularly. AIT also is used by professionals in other disciplines, including occupational therapy, often to the exclusion of other auditory interventions. Of further concern is the inaccuracy of the scientific claims made by the developers of such programs and the potential for harm that exists due to inadequate monitoring of sound levels. Nonetheless, proponents of AIT and AIT-like auditory therapies point out—and rightly so—that few, if any, auditory training programs for (C)APD have undergone the level of scientific validation that is required to demonstrate conclusively an intervention's efficacy. This controversy underscores the need for controlled, large-scale clinical trials and treatment efficacy studies in (C)APD, as in many other areas relating to auditory and communication disorders.

LACE is a home-based computer program designed to provide specific AT for hearing-impaired adults who have been fit with amplification. The aim of the program is to address the central auditory changes that occur secondary to peripheral hearing loss, as well as to train specific compensatory strategies and skills so that better listening is facilitated. An analysis of the components of this program suggests that it conforms to the key principles of neuroplasticity and perceptual learning, as well as to the basic tenets of information processing and resource allocation theory. Furthermore, it includes many of the activities appropriate for some individuals with (C)APD that have been discussed in this chapter, such as degraded and competing speech training, auditory vigilance, contextual derivation, and additional communication strategies training. As such, although research to date has addressed the use of LACE only with post-hearing-aid-fit adults (Sweetow and Henderson-Sabes, 2004), it is this author's opinion that this program may, with further research, prove to be beneficial for some individuals with (C)APD and normal peripheral hearing sensitivity, as well.

Pearl

- Many of the auditory training activities that have been in use for many years for individuals with peripheral hearing loss may be appropriate for those with central auditory disorders, as well. Depending on the needs of the individual patient, clinicians may uncover a wealth of appropriate and deficit-specific materials by perusing time-honored curricula and activities that address auditory skills in hearing-impaired children and adults.

In summary, computer-assisted therapies provide a valuable addition to the treatment armamentarium; however, they must be analyzed carefully for appropriateness to specific individuals with (C)APD. Even when deemed applicable for a given individual's auditory deficit, they should be used to complement, rather than to replace, other components of the overall intervention program.

◆ Intervention in Special Populations

Throughout this chapter, the need for accurate and comprehensive assessment and diagnosis of (C)APD as a prerequisite to developing an individualized intervention plan has been emphasized. However, the question often arises as to what can be done when an accurate diagnosis cannot be made due to young age, hearing loss, or presence of additional confounding or comorbid disorders that may impact the ability to perform diagnostic central auditory tests. For example, because of the inherent variability of CNS structure and function in very young children, diagnostic tests of (C)APD typically cannot be interpreted reliably in children younger than approximately 7 years of age. Similarly, it is now well recognized that elderly individuals may exhibit age-related changes in central auditory function that cannot be accounted for by peripheral hearing loss (e.g., Bellis et al, 2000; Bellis and Wilber, 2001; Chmiel and Jerger, 1996). Yet many elderly individuals do, indeed, exhibit peripheral hearing loss of varying degrees, rendering it difficult to disentangle the central auditory component from the hearing loss component via available psychophysical tests. The same is true for others of any age who exhibit concomitant peripheral hearing loss or comorbid disorders, such as attention deficit hyperactivity disorder (ADHD). Although the presence of intra- and intertest patterns on central auditory tests (e.g., ear differences on dichotic listening tasks given symmetrical hearing sensitivity; specific patterns across tests indicative of CANS dysfunction) may be identified in these latter two groups of individuals, testing may not be possible in young children or in those with significant comorbid hearing loss or attention deficit. Nonetheless, it is important that intervention be undertaken as soon as possible in these populations, even when a complete diagnostic profile cannot be ascertained.

To this end, it is critical that clinicians make use of all available information, including any multidisciplinary testing that may have been conducted and in-depth analyses of specific listening complaints, to attempt to identify those auditory processes and mechanisms that appear to be intact in a given individual versus those that may be compromised. Although a discussion of central auditory test interpretation and differential diagnosis is not within the scope of this chapter, readers may refer to Bellis (2003) for an in-depth view of how this may be accomplished. The goal of these analyses is to use all available data to make educated hypotheses as to the likelihood of the presence and nature of a specific (C)APD in these populations and, based on that information, develop individualized intervention plans that are as individualized as possible,

with the understanding that, in some cases, (C)APD cannot be diagnosed definitively.

Pearl

- Analysis of central auditory and multidisciplinary test results for patterns of auditory dysfunction based on well-established neuroaudiologic and neuropsychologic tenets provides a means of determining whether a central auditory deficit may be present in a hard-to-test individual and can direct treatment efforts even when a (C)APD cannot be diagnosed definitively.

Virtually all of the intervention techniques and strategies discussed in this chapter can be modified for very young or elderly individuals, as well as for those with peripheral hearing loss or other conditions. For example, the use of games such as Marco Polo and Duck-Duck-Goose (using minimal pair phoneme contrasts) can assist in training localization and phoneme discrimination skills, respectively. Several computer programs have lower extensions appropriate for young children, including Earobics and Fast ForWord, and other programs may be implemented even with elderly clients (e.g., LACE and the adolescent and adult version of Earobics). Dichotic listening training conducted at adequate listening levels and using engaging, age-appropriate materials can be implemented for individuals of all ages, as long as adequate listening levels are ensured. Games such as Simon (Milton Bradley) can assist in training cross-modality sequencing abilities. Compensatory strategies training, including attribution training and problem solving, is important even for very young children, as it can foster self-empowerment and mitigate the loss of self-esteem and the sense of helplessness that often develops when listening or related difficulties exist. In short, even when an accurate diagnosis of (C)APD cannot be made, it is incumbent upon the clinician to analyze carefully the presenting auditory difficulties in any individual and attempt to provide appropriate environmental modifications, compensatory strategies, and direct remediation activities as soon as possible once a central auditory deficit is suspected.

◆ Outcome Measures and Evidence-Based Practice

The primary goal of any intervention program is to ensure optimum outcomes for individuals and thereby improve quality of life and ability to undertake activities and participate in society. Outcomes may be measured objectively through the use of test paradigms that evaluate central auditory and related function or subjectively through the use of questionnaires, patient report, or other measures that rely on the patient's perception of his or her own functioning levels. Ideally, the efficacy of intervention for (C)APD will be reflected both in performance on specific auditory tests and in functional daily listening and related skills.

Evidence-based practice (EBP) allows for the maximization of opportunities for success in these arenas from the time of diagnosis by guiding selection and implementation of those intervention techniques that have the most likelihood of effecting positive change. This requires the integration of individual clinical experience and judgment skills with evidence gleaned from systematic research documenting treatment efficacy. The quality of treatment efficacy research can be described in terms of levels and grades of evidence that support specific intervention activities (e.g., large or small randomized clinical trials, nonrandomized controlled studies, historical controls and expert opinion, and case series or uncontrolled studies). This grading scheme can allow for clinical practice guidelines in which recommendations can be made with varying strength and conviction for specific disorders.

Most of our clinical recommendations for audiologic treatment and management paradigms, including amplification, aural rehabilitation, and intervention for (C)APD, are based on expert opinion and indirect evidence rather than on high-level, randomized controlled trials (Abrams et al, 2005). Numerous studies exist documenting the effects of specific AT in improving psychophysical performance, neurophysiologic representation of acoustic stimuli, and listening and related abilities in children and adults, as discussed previously. These studies, combined with relevant literature in the cognitive and general neurosciences, neuropsychology, and related disciplines, provide the foundation for the intervention approaches discussed in this chapter.

Special Consideration

- Because the ultimate goal of any intervention program is to improve daily functioning, outcome measures of treatment efficacy should not be limited solely to pre- and post-therapy central auditory test results. Instead, questionnaires and other measures of functional listening skills and perceived handicap in the classroom, workplace, and at home also should be used to document treatment efficacy. Electrophysiologic measures of auditory function may provide an early indicator of treatment efficacy, even before behavioral improvements are evident (Tremblay et al, 1998).

As with most disorders involving the auditory system, as well as those affecting learning, language, communication, and related function, future research is needed to document the validity and efficacy of specific treatment and management programs for various types of (C)APD, using controlled, high-level, randomized trials. Nonetheless, as ASHA (2005a,b) concluded, there is sufficient evidence at present to guide intervention for (C)APD using the combined approach delineated in this chapter when appropriate and accurate diagnosis of the disorder, along with multidisciplinary assessment of relative strengths and weaknesses across functional domains, has been obtained.

◆ Summary

This chapter has provided an overview of basic principles of treatment and management of (C)APD in children and adults. Consistent with the current scientific knowledge base regarding central auditory processing and its disorders, intervention for (C)APD should be both bottom-up and top-down in nature and should include three primary components: environmental modifications that address the clarity of the acoustic signal and other issues related to access to auditorily presented information, compensatory strategies that focus on harnessing higher level resources to assist in buttressing deficient auditory skills, and direct remediation activities to improve or ameliorate the auditory deficit(s). In all instances, intervention recommendations should arise logically from and be based on accurate and comprehensive diagnosis of (C)APD using testing paradigms that have been shown to be valid for the identification of CANS dysfunction. Finally, it has been emphasized throughout this chapter that treatment and management of (C)APD must be deficit-specific and individualized. As such, there is no "one size fits all" approach to (C)APD intervention that is appropriate for all individuals presenting with the disorder.

References

Abrams, H. B., McArdie, R., & Chisolm, T. H. (2005). From outcomes to evidence: Establishing best practices for audiologists. Seminars in Hearing, 26(3), 157–169.

American Speech-Language-Hearing Association. (2004a). Auditory integration training [technical report]. Retrieved from http://www.asha.org/members/deskref-journals/deskref/default

American Speech-Language-Hearing Association. (2004b). Auditory integration training [position statement]. Retrieved from http://www.asha.org/members/deskref-journals/deskref/default

American Speech-Language-Hearing Association. (2005a). (Central) auditory processing disorders [technical report]. Retrieved from http://www.asha.org/members/deskref-journals/deskref/default

American Speech-Language-Hearing Association. (2005b). (Central) auditory processing disorders—the role of the audiologist [position statement]. Retrieved from http://www.asha.org/members/deskref-journals/deskref/default

American Speech-Language-Hearing Association. (2005c). Speech-language pathology (SLP) preferred practice patterns. Retrieved from http://www.asha.org/members/deskref-journals/deskref/default

Bellis, T. J. (2002a). When the brain can't hear: Unraveling the mystery of auditory processing disorder. New York: Pocket Books.

Bellis, T. J. (2002b). Developing deficit-specific intervention plans for individuals with auditory processing disorders. Seminars in Hearing, 23(4), 287–295.

Bellis, T. J. (2003). Assessment and management of central auditory processing disorders in the educational setting: From science to practice (2nd ed.). Clifton Park, NY: Thomson Learning.

Bellis, T. J., Nicol, T., & Kraus, N. (2000). Aging affects hemispheric asymmetry in the neural representation of speech sounds. Journal of Neuroscience, 20, 791–797.

Bellis, T. J., & Wilber, L. A. (2001). Effects of aging and gender on interhemispheric function. Journal of Speech, Language, and Hearing Research, 44, 246–263.

Bradlow, A. R., & Pisoni, D. B. (1999). Recognition of spoken words by native and non-native listeners: Talker-, listener-, and item-related factors. Journal of the Acoustical Society of America, 106, 2074–2085.

Chermak, G. D. (1998). Managing central auditory processing disorders: Metalinguistic and metacognitive approaches. Seminars in Hearing, 19(4), 379–392.

Chermak, G. D., & Musiek, F. E. (1997). Central auditory processing disorders: Current perspectives. San Diego, CA: Singular Publishing Group.

Chermak, G. D., & Musiek, F. E. (2002). Auditory training: Principles and approaches for remediating and managing auditory processing disorders. Seminars in Hearing, 23(4), 297–308.

Chmiel, R., & Jerger, J. (1996). Hearing aid use, central auditory disorder, and hearing handicap in elderly persons. Journal of the American Academy of Audiology, 7, 190–202.

Earobics. (1998). Evanston, IL: Cognitive Concepts.

Elliott, L. L. (1995). Verbal auditory closure and the Speech Perception in Noise (SPIN) test. Journal of Speech and Hearing Research, 38, 1363–1376.

Fast ForWord. (1998). Berkeley, CA: Scientific Learning Corp.

Gold, J. I., & Knudsen, E. I. (2000). A site of auditory experience-dependent plasticity in the neural representation of auditory space in the barn owl's inferior colliculus. Journal of Neuroscience, 20, 3469–3486.

Jerger, J., & Musiek, F. (2000). Report of the consensus conference on the diagnosis of auditory processing disorders in school-aged children. Journal of the American Academy of Audiology, 11, 467–474.

Massaro, D. W. (1975). Understanding language: An information-processing analysis of speech perception, reading, and psycholinguistics. New York: Academic Press.

McCoy, S. L., Tun, P. A., Cox, L. C., et al. (2005). Hearing loss and perceptual effort: Downstream effects on older adults' memory for speech. Quarterly Journal of Experimental Psychology A, 58(1), 22–33.

McFarland, D. J., & Cacace, A. T. (1995). Modality specificity as a criterion for diagnosing central auditory processing disorders. American Journal of Audiology, 4, 32–44.

Musiek, F. E., Bellis, T. J., & Chermak, G. D. (2005). Nonmodularity of the CANS: Implications for (central) auditory processing disorders. American Journal of Audiology 14, 128–138.

Musiek, F. E., Shinn, J., & Hare, C. (2002). Plasticity, auditory training, and auditory processing disorders. Seminars in Hearing, 23(4), 263–275.

Roeser, R. J., Valente, M., & Hosford-Dunn, H., eds. (2007). Audiology: Diagnosis (2nd ed.). New York: Thieme Medical Publishers.

Rosenberg, G. G. (2002). Classroom acoustics and personal FM technology in management of auditory processing disorder. Seminars in Hearing, 23(4), 309–317.

Salvi, R. J., Lockwood, A. H., Frisina, R. D., et al. (2002). PET imaging of the normal human auditory system: Responses to speech in quiet and in background noise. Hearing Research, 170, 96–106.

Stehli, A. (1994). Auditory integration training: The use of a new listening therapy within our profession. American Journal of Speech-Language Pathology, 3(2), 12–15.

Sweetow, R., & Henderson-Sabes, J. (2004). The case for LACE: Listening and auditory communication enhancement training. Hearing Journal, 57(3), 32–40.

Tallal, P. (1980). Auditory temporal perception, phonics, and reading disabilities in children. Brain and Language, 9, 182–198.

Tremblay, K., Kraus, N., & McGee, T. (1998). The time course of auditory perceptual learning: Neurophysiological changes during speech-sound training. Neuroreport, 9, 3557–3560.

Wright, B. A., Lombardino, L. J., King, W. M., et al. (1997). Deficits in auditory temporal and spectral resolution in language-impaired children. Nature, 387, 176–178.

Yencer, K. A. (1998). Is auditory integration training an effective treatment for children with central auditory processing disorders? In M. G. Masters, N. A. Stecker, & J. Katz (Eds.), Central auditory processing disorders: Mostly management (pp. 151–173). Needham Heights, MA: Allyn & Bacon.

Chapter 12

Counseling and Orientation toward Amplification

David Citron III

- ♦ **Counseling Defined**

    Affect

    Theory of the Psychology of Hearing Loss

- ♦ **Counseling**

    Basic Helping Skills

    Helping Skills Model

    Initial Interview

    Postassessment Interview/Consultation

- ♦ **Consultation**

    Personality Typing

    Matching Hearing Technology to Patient Needs

- ♦ **Orientation**

    The Orientation Session

    Expectations and Suggestions for Adapting to Hearing Aid Use

- ♦ **Summary**
- ♦ **Appendix**

Counseling is perhaps the most overlooked aspect of the process of fitting amplification and at the same time is probably the most important professional service an audiologist can provide for patients and their families (Garstecki and Erler, 1997). Most audiologists perceive counseling as orientation in the care and use of amplification (Wilkinson, 1995). Certainly, this is a critical part of the audiologic rehabilitation process. However, it is clear that such a narrow focus on "product solutions" is only one small portion of a set of necessary components of audiologic rehabilitation. O'Neill (1988) raised the issue of why so many hearing instrument patients fail to accept and use amplification. Smedley and Schow (1990) investigated this problem by surveying adult hearing aid candidates and found that poor use patterns were secondary to certain aspects of the patient's hearing loss, the nature of the hearing aid technology, and unrealistic expectations from the use of amplification. Reports from unsuccessful users included "worthless in noisy settings, a damn nuisance, making them nervous, and feeling uncomfortable." It is evident that a large patient population requires counseling support during the amplification process, and it is critical that audiologists deliver these helping skills directly to their patients or provide an appropriate referral to a mental health professional.

Another problem lies in the fact that audiologists frequently feel uncomfortable in their counseling role, often expressing insecurity as to how far their counseling should extend (Clark and English, 2004). Also, master's and doctor of audiology (Au.D.) training programs do not provide sufficient training in basic helping skills (Crandell, 1997; Herzfeld and English, 2001), though distance-learning Au.D. training programs have developed effective coursework to teach counseling competencies (Crandell and Weiner, 2002). Four-year residential Au.D. programs have proliferated over the past few years, but at the time of this writing, there is no uniform national standard that provides inclusion of counseling in course curricula.

This chapter will provide an extensive overview of the counseling and orientation processes, along with the importance of differentiating these services. An additional goal of this chapter is to furnish the necessary tools for training audiologists in the use of basic helping skills. Audiologists will then be able to deliver hearing instrument fittings in which (1) psychological barriers to the use of amplification are identified, (2) appropriate strategies in managing those barriers are implemented, (3) a balanced picture of the advantages and limitations of amplification is presented to the patient, and (4) most management and resolution of psychological barriers occur prior to fitting. Patients must realize the importance of accepting their hearing loss and the aspects of adapting to hearing aid use before the actual fitting process.

Pearl

- Appropriate management of psychological barriers to the use of amplification should reduce hearing instrument returns and in-the-drawer (ITD) hearing aid nonuse.

◆ Counseling Defined

A common mistake made by audiologists is to define counseling as providing information as a part of the hearing aid orientation process. It is easy to see how this misconception occurs, because most dictionaries provide the same ambiguity in their definitions of counseling and orientation. For instance, *The American Heritage Dictionary of the English Language* (1992) and *Webster's New Twentieth Century Dictionary–Unabridged* (1966) define *counseling* as "advice or guidance, especially as solicited from a knowledgeable person." *Orientation* is defined as "an adjustment or adaptation to a new environment, situation, custom, or set of ideas; introductory instruction concerning a new situation." *Merriam-Webster's Collegiate Dictionary* (1993) defines *counseling* as "professional guidance of the individual by utilizing psychological methods, esp. in collecting case history data, using various techniques of the personal interview, and testing interests and aptitudes," whereas *orientation* is defined as "to set right by adjusting to facts or principles; to acquaint with existing situation or environment." If as audiologists we apply these principles to audiology and amplification, it appears that we will often ignore the psychological aspects of the counseling process, particularly affect and emotional phenomena. Clark and English (2004) divide counseling into content (information-based) and personal adjustment (affect-based) components. These components often overlap and constantly change during a patient visit, as the specifics of earmold insertion (content) and the underlying frustration of being unable to insert the earmolds (personal adjustment) can occur within seconds of each other.

Affect

One measure of separation between personal adjustment counseling and content counseling/orientation is the identification of patient affect. Most audiologists receive little or no training in managing patient affect. Affect can best be described as "feeling" states. Certainly, any of these can be present in our patients, and the keys in audiologic counseling are the recognition and management of affective behaviors. When these emotional reactions are unchecked, they can be increased to the point where they cause severe lifestyle and personality changes.

Rezen and Hausman (2000) state that anyone who undergoes a physical or emotional change goes through the same stages of denial, projection, anger, depression, and acceptance. These categories are similar to those described by Kübler-Ross (1969) as a cycle of grief for patients coping with death and dying. Not all patients will experience all of these stages, but all will experience at least one of the following before they come to grips with their hearing loss. These emotions will appear randomly, then may reappear at later times. It is also important to realize that grieving is a normal process, and the management and resolution of these components add to overall emotional maturity (Kennedy and Charles, 2001). Defining and understanding these emotional stages are critical in effective personal adjustment counseling.

Denial is an expected initial reaction if someone is faced with a threat to his or her physical or emotional health. Acceptance of hearing loss is certainly unpleasant, and denial creates a mechanism for the patient's emotions to "stall for time" to build up the necessary emotional energy to come to grips with the problem. The slow, progressive nature of hearing loss can make denial an easy alternative because the change in hearing sensitivity is often so gradual that it is frequently not discernible to the patient. Denial can often be carried to extreme lengths by patients to avoid dealing with their hearing loss. For instance, a spouse can bring to the attention of the patient that he or she did not understand most of the communication that occurred at the social function that they just attended. "Baloney," replies the patient. "The conversations were so boring that I did not care to listen to any of it. I can hear when I want to hear." It is clear that this will almost always cause emotional distress within the family, and it will not change until the patient realizes a problem exists and wishes to deal with it in an effective fashion. Often, patients are stuck in this stage for some time and practice the philosophy of Lucy Van Pelt from "Peanuts" who said, "No problem is so big or so complicated that it cannot be run away from." Denial is not a river in Egypt.

Projection is the next effective avoidance measure and involves shifting the blame for the hearing loss to another person. A common example of projection is the patient who responds, "I hear fine; people mumble. If everyone would stop their mumbling, I would hear just fine. Especially, my wife." The individual may also blame the acoustics of the room for not being able to hear the television unless it is turned to loud levels. This is a similar patient defense mechanism, but many elderly patients are convinced that the youth of today all mumble and do not produce speech in a clear fashion. Just as in the case of denial, erroneous lack of awareness of the slow, progressive nature of hearing loss can lead to projection. The underlying psychological behavior is that nothing is better than a good scapegoat to avoid solving a problem.

Anger typically follows projection and usually involves a general sense of anger at things in general or may be anger directed at a specific individual, most often the significant other in the patient's everyday life. No question exists that anger can cause a breakdown in the most solid family relationships. However, significant others must take care in managing patients who exhibit anger in that they can reinforce the lack of positive behavior in dealing with their hearing loss. For instance, the husband who tells his wife, "You did not hear anything at the Waxmans' last night and made me feel like a real idiot," can often serve to reinforce the patient's anger and defensiveness. Angry patients may also say, "If you are frustrated to be with me, why don't you go out by yourself?"

Depression develops once the anger is spent and is often accompanied by a sense of isolation and further withdrawal. A sense of lethargy grows, and some patients will be acutely aware that the birds no longer chirp, television seems distorted, and traffic noises once heard from the living room have faded. Patients may internalize their embarrassment of their lack of receptive communication and subsequently impose a long-term isolation. Depressed patients will state, "I know I can't hear well, but I don't mind having to ask my family to repeat things" or "I just don't think that I can face my friends again because I feel so ashamed of my hearing loss." In some patients, this sense of isolation can last for many years before they seek help for their hearing loss.

Acceptance occurs when depression fades, and patients finally realize that the problem lies not with themselves but with their hearing. This is the only stage in which patients can take action to seek treatment for their hearing loss. They come to the realization that they do not wish to be deprived of positive life experiences and understand that they cannot communicate effectively in certain situations. It is well documented in the mental health literature that elderly patients manifest denial, projection, anger, and depression as a result of other psychological problems within their lives (Novalis et al, 1993). This can be illustrated with the following case.

Case Vignette

- An 80-year-old woman arrived at our facility for amplification consultation accompanied by her daughter. She had recently undergone audiologic evaluation at a hospital in Boston, and test results demonstrated a bilateral mild to moderately severe sensorineural hearing loss. Although the patient's daughter was completing the necessary forms, the patient sat in the waiting room with her arms folded tightly across her chest, with a sad, waxen facial expression. She maintained both postures in the examination room. When asked by the audiologist to "tell me about your hearing loss," she replied, "I'm here because of her," and pointed to her daughter. When asked to elaborate, the patient stated that "I know that I can't hear well, but I have no problems having to ask people to repeat." Further case history information revealed recent vision deterioration that necessitated an end to driving, as well as a recent move into the daughter's residence. The patient clearly had no motivation to pursue amplification, and when it was discussed with her that she had to be self-motivated to seek help, she asked, "Aren't you going to try to talk me into it?" At the end of the session, the patient did ask if she could speak with two of the other patients who were successful users of amplification. After receiving permission from these two patients who were similar in age and lifestyle, their names and phone numbers were forwarded to the patient's daughter. Four months passed, and the two patients were never contacted; the patient did return subsequently for amplification consultation, and thanked the audiologist for not "pressuring" her to pursue amplification when she was not motivated.

Clearly, this patient had depression that was a result of a myriad of other issues in her life and not just hearing loss. If hearing aid use had been "pushed," nonuse or a return for credit was likely. In this case, the patient needed time to deal with the recent changes in her life and ultimately was able to accept her hearing loss. Despite the fact that this patient decided to move in a positive direction to accept her hearing loss and pursue amplification, the orientation session and follow-up visits illustrated some interesting behaviors.

During the amplification consultation session, the patient was questioned as to whether she was "ready" to pursue hearing aid use. Some degree of apprehension was displayed, and the patient stated that she was not certain that she would be able to physically operate the hearing aids. Practice with replica instruments was helpful to reassure the patient that she could change the battery and insert/remove the instruments with little or no difficulty. Also, she appeared to understand that an adjustment period was normal for all new users of amplification.

Throughout the course of the fitting session, the patient displayed an attitude of apprehension about the entire concept of hearing aid use. When informed that it would take a few weeks to adjust to hearing her voice differently and the audibility of new sounds, she displayed the same physical posture as in the first meeting, with her arms folded tightly across her chest. She stated, "This is all so complicated and overwhelming." In addition to constant reassurance to the patient that these were normal feelings of new users, she was placed on a wearing schedule that would permit a more gradual acclimatization to hearing aid use. Her daughter, who accompanied her to the fitting session, was motivated to provide positive support for her mother during the initial weeks of hearing aid use. Despite all the positive encouragement, the patient requested that she not wear the instruments home and begin a gradual introduction of amplification at home. A follow-up visit was scheduled for 2 weeks.

At the time of the follow-up visit, the patient and her daughter arrived ~15 minutes late. After waiting ~10 minutes and remarking to her daughter that "I haven't used these that much and don't know if I will keep them," they could not wait any longer and decided to leave the office.

The patient did return for further follow-up 3 weeks later. She reported that she has begun to adapt to hearing new sounds again and has experienced significant improvement in communication. Despite those positive interactions, she stated that it was still "an effort" to use the hearing aids consistently and that in many ways she was "happier without them."

Upon examination of this patient's history, it is apparent that she is depressed from all the other issues in her life and that any change from her depressed state is too large of an emotional jump for her to make. Certainly, her behavior during the fitting session could have been a predictor, but how much user apprehension is acceptable? How much "encouragement" can the audiologist provide before it is clear that the audiologist is pushing the patient into something that she does not want and may not use?

Often, patients will have other problems in their lives, such as the recent loss of a spouse, serious illness, or changes in lifestyle, that are not related to hearing loss. Many patients will be able to manage these issues successfully and accept their hearing loss, whereas others will be "stuck." During the course of the interview, patients will make it apparent how they cope with age-related changes in their health and lifestyle. Many will state, "They call it the golden years . . . it certainly has not been golden for me, but I'm ready to seek help." At the same time, audiologists have seen patients in rehabilitation facilities where relearning to walk, feed themselves, and fasten their clothes are far higher priorities than obtaining amplification. Most of these patients will seek help for their hearing loss when they are less burdened with more pressing medical and personal problems.

The above case vignette is quite common for audiologists who manage adults with hearing loss. Approximately 1 in 10 American adults suffer from depression (Narrow, 1998). Several studies have shown a larger than normal prevalence of depression in adults with hearing loss (Bridges and Bentler, 1998; Strawbridge et al, 2000). Carmen (2001) summarizes basic symptoms of depression in older adults and recommends using a checklist to recognize its primary signs. It is not necessary for audiologists to review this checklist with the patient on an item-by-item basis, but understanding the myriad of manifestations that accompany depression will enable audiologists to refer to appropriate mental health professionals when indicated. Approximately 80% of older adults with depression improve with proper treatment that includes psychotherapy, medication, or both (Little et al, 1998).

Theory of the Psychology of Hearing Loss

What are the sources of denial, projection, anger, and depression that we observe in many of our patients? A better understanding of these psychological states can provide valuable assistance for audiologists in learning to manage their patients and assist them in receiving help for their hearing loss.

One of the more popular theories of the bases of psychological disorders is described by Beck (1979) and is known as cognitive therapy. He stated that individuals manage to approach external forces around them much like a scientist in that they make observations, create hypotheses, check their validity, and eventually form generalizations that will subsequently serve as a guide for making quick judgments of situations. Throughout the course of their development, individuals use the basics of the experimental method without recognizing it. They acquire an array of techniques and generalizations that enable judgment as to whether they are reacting realistically to situations to resolve conflicts and to deal with rejection, disappointment, and danger. By virtue of personal experience and emulation of others, individuals learn to make use of the tools of common sense: forming and testing hunches, making discriminations, and reasoning. They also use these tools to fine-tune observations and reasoning over time.

A good example of this process is driving an automobile. We learn as student drivers that when the traffic signal turns yellow, we are supposed to slow down and get ready to stop. Of course, a red signal means stop. We also discover how to react quickly to various driving conditions, such as cars pulling out quickly in front of us, tailgaters, and operating the vehicle in snow and ice. This learning and reasoning

may have occurred initially in a small town in Ohio. A further need to test hypotheses and reason may be required on moving to Boston. Drivers in Boston believe that a yellow light means "speed up" and will always attempt to speed through the intersection before it turns red. Often, many drivers will accelerate when the light turns red before their vehicle enters the intersection. This is a part of the standard driving culture, so that there is virtually no enforcement of this phenomenon by the local police. Unaware of the culture, new residents will often slow down and stop at a yellow light, only to hear the honking of horns from the drivers behind them who fully intended to run the light. Wise reasoning will cause a change in new residents' driving habits; they will soon learn that survival dictates that they accelerate when the signal turns yellow.

Beck (1979) theorized that psychological disorders occur from ordinary problems, such as flawed learning, making incorrect inferences on the basis of insufficient or false information, with an inability to distinguish between imagination and reality. Our inner workings can suppress or twist around the signals from the outside, leaving our perceptions completely opposite what is going on around us. Emotional disturbances can be related to the types of misconceptions an individual has experienced throughout cognitive development. In other words, the deviant meanings create the cognitive distortions that form the essence of emotional disorders. This approach to the neuroses is known as cognitive therapy because reality testing, insight, learning, and introspection are all basically cognitive processes.

The cognitive therapy theory reported by Beck (1979) has interesting application to the emotional aspects of hearing loss. As hearing sensitivity deteriorates, the patient will apply hypothesis testing. Some awareness may be present, for example, that the television is more difficult to hear; raising the level of the sound solves the problem. The individual may have noticed that communication in restaurants has started to become more demanding and reasoned that it must due to the poor acoustics in the restaurant. The voices of the individual's spouse and grandchildren now seem faint and hard to discriminate; if so, they must be mumbling. The erroneous misinterpretation is that nothing is wrong with the individual; instead, there must be an external problem, whether the acoustics of the room or other people not speaking loudly and clearly. Thus, the individual's thinking is unrealistic because it is derived from misconceptions that he or she experiences numerous times a day.

Anger and depression occur as a further response to the fallacious thinking described by Beck (1979). Mistaken thoughts that constitute projection ("It's them—*they* mumble") lead to anger when the hearing-impaired individual is a recipient of "noxious verbal assault," which is an attack on his or her self-esteem. A significant other, such as a spouse, is the most common source of the verbal abuse. Typically, that other person will continually criticize the hearing-impaired individual for his or her inability to communicate. The behavior of the offender indirectly exposes the individual to self-devaluation. Anger may be the first reaction: "If you are so embarrassed to go to the Coopers' with me, I can just stay home."

According to Beck (1979), depression develops when the person becomes sensitized by particular varieties of life situations, such as chronic rejection by peers or spouse. It could also be a chain of experiences that the individual views as diminishing in some fashion. Included in these experiences may be those that relate to the hearing loss: frustration because he or she cannot always communicate in a consistent fashion; sadness caused by changed relationships with spouse, family, and friends; isolation from activities that the individual used to enjoy but are now difficult because of the hearing loss. Individuals may regard themselves as inadequate, unworthy, and deficient, and they are susceptible to attributing unpleasant events to their own deficiencies. They often become self-critical and blame themselves for their difficulties. Sadness, hopelessness, apathy, and subsequent loss of motivation can trigger depression.

Treatment of these emotional disorders through cognitive therapy can be integrated into the counseling process. Beck's (1979) protocol involves offering the patient productive procedures for conquering blurred perceptions, blind spots, and self-deceptions. It is called cognitive therapy because the main psychological problem and the psychological treatment are both concerned with the patient's thinking (or cognitions).

Many methods exist that can assist patients in making more realistic self-evaluations and linking them to their world. Beck (1979) described an "intellectual" approach that identifies misconceptions, tests their validity, and substitutes more appropriate concepts. The need for change often occurs when the patient recognizes that the rules he or she has relied on to guide thinking and behavior ("people mumble") have served to deceive and defeat. "The "experiential" approach exposes the patient to experiences that are in themselves strong enough to change misinterpretations. Specific application of cognitive therapy techniques for hearing-impaired patients will be described in later sections on interviewing and consultation.

♦ Counseling

Carl Rogers (1951), one of the pioneers of modern psychotherapy, stresses the importance of the counseling "relationship." Patients must possess a sense of "safety and freedom" to express their feelings and concerns and feel confident in the skills of their audiologist. The external environment is a critical component in providing comfort to the patient during the hearing aid counseling and selection process.

Comfort and emotional safety begin at the front desk of your facility. Are patients greeted in a timely and friendly fashion? Does the front office staff provide assistance in completing forms? Observe the telephone manners of your staff. How many times are patients placed on hold before they are appropriately served? How quickly can patients receive an appointment? Is there flexibility in scheduling appointments (early mornings, evenings, and weekends) to accommodate patient needs? How frequently do patients have to wait past their scheduled appointment times?

Office layout and structure are equally important in creating a "counseling-friendly" environment. Chairs need to be comfortable and have arms so patients can move about in an easy fashion, and soft lighting (incandescent) is preferred for waiting areas. Examination and waiting areas must possess adequate space to accommodate wheelchairs and patients and their families. Magazines and audiology brochures should be current, well organized, and within easy reach. Examination rooms must be neat and respect patient privacy. Sessions should only be interrupted in case of emergency. These issues may appear to be trivial, but successful counseling and hearing aid orientation can be limited if the professional environment does not create a sense of emotional safety and comfort.

Basic Helping Skills

Most audiologists possess little or no training in basic helping skills. Our knowledge base of understanding hearing loss, amplification, and follow-up aural rehabilitation is exceptional, but do audiologists know how to be good listeners and integrate patients' emotions and attitudes in the audiologic rehabilitation process? The intent is not for audiologists to become psychologists; rather, the goal is to improve patient care and minimize ITD hearing instruments and those returned for credit. In addition, training and understanding of basic helping skills will help audiologists to determine when patients need to seek further help from mental health professionals.

Helping Skills Model

Carkhuff (2000) has developed an excellent model for training basic helping skills. It is based on his theory that people are constantly undergoing intrapersonal processing, the basic process for human growth and development. Intrapersonal processing involves exploring, understanding, and acting. This is a personal process in which the helpee (patient) relates to personally relevant experiences and transforms them into human actions for human purposes. In a strict sense, intrapersonal processing is quite similar to Beck's (1979) underlying theory behind cognitive therapy. This model will be reviewed in a somewhat simplistic fashion; the goal is to provide specific strategies that audiologists can use to improve their counseling skills.

Interpersonal processing or helping skills facilitate the intrapersonal processing of others. The phases of interpersonal processing that compose Carkhuff's (2000) model are seen in **Fig. 12–1**. Attending skills involve the helpees in the helping process. Responding skills expedite understanding by the helpees. Personalizing skills facilitate understanding by helpees. Initiating skills encourage acting by the helpees. Feedback that occurs from the helpee's actions recycles the stages of intrapersonal and interpersonal processing.

Attending (Prehelping)

Attending involves communicating undivided attentiveness to the patient. It serves to direct the audiologist's listening and observing skills to the patient's verbal and behavioral

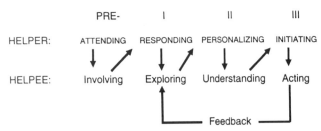

Figure 12–1 Phases of interpersonal processing. (From Carkhuff, R. R. (1993). The art of helping (4th ed.). Amherst, MA: HRD Press, with permission.)

description of his or her experiences. It also functions to express a strong concern in the experiences of the patient and encourage him or her to become engaged in the helping process.

Physical attending is another important ingredient of pre-helping. It is critical that the audiologist give complete and undivided attention to the patient. This involves making eye contact, fully facing the patient, and leaning forward at least 20 degrees so that the forearms can rest on the thighs. Consistency in attentive behaviors communicates interest in the patient and his or her problems. Egan (1977) suggests a helpful tool (SOLER) to employ proper attending behavior:

♦ *S*traight, face-to-face body orientation, with

♦ *O*penness in body posture and a slight, forward

♦ *L*ean, while maintaining

♦ *E*ye contact, and all done in a

♦ *R*elaxed manner.

Yogi Berra, a member of Major League Baseball's Hall of Fame and a premier philosopher, once said, "You can observe a lot by watching" (Berra, 1998). Observing consists of viewing the appearance and behavior of the patient. This can begin in the waiting room by observing the patient's body movements, posture, grooming, and facial expressions. For instance, poor grooming, a slouched appearance, slow body movements, a furrowed brow, and downcast eye movements all suggest low energy level and minimal readiness for helping, whereas fast body movements and fidgeting can indicate anxiety.

The ability of audiologists to listen and respond to the verbal expressions of patients is most critical in the helping process. Certainly, listening is hard work and necessitates deep concentration. Carkhuff (2000) describes numerous ways to sharpen listening skills, which include having a purpose for listening, suspending judgments or preexisting attitudes, focusing on the patient and the content, and recalling the patient's verbal and nonverbal expressions while listening for common themes. Just as hearing aids are often reprogrammed after listening to and processing a patient's descriptions of his or her amplification experiences, so too can the audiologist learn about a patient's emotional attitudes and readiness to seek help by listening and processing the patient's verbal and nonverbal expressions. Some

excellent case studies are presented by Carkhuff (2000) to provide practice in developing helping skills.

Stage I: Responding

Responding consists of reacting to the content, feelings, and meaning of the patient's expressions. Responding to content helps to clarify the patient's experiences, whereas responding to feelings identifies the affect that is a part of the experience. Clarification of the reason for the feeling occurs by responding to meaning.

The first step is to respond to the content of patient's expressions. This is accomplished by using Carkhuff's (2000) "5 W's": Who and what was involved? What did the patient do? Why and how did the patient do it? When and where did the patient do it? This will help the audiologist to organize the patient's thoughts. A good response does not parrot the statement but rephrases the expression in a fresh fashion. An appropriate response format is "You are saying that . . . " or "In other words. . . ."

Responding to feeling is perhaps the most critical helping skill because it mirrors the patient's emotional experience of himself or herself in relation to the patient's everyday world. Most audiologists are uncomfortable in relating to patients in the affective domain. A simple way to think during patient interchanges is, If I were the patient, how would I feel? Carkhuff (2000) organizes these different emotions into seven different categories: happy, sad, angry, scared, confused, strong, and weak. **Table 12–1** provides a division and classification of these feelings. This can provide valuable assistance in expanding a feeling vocabulary. Having a laminated copy of a "feelings table" within easy reach in an examination room can greatly assist the audiologist in the development of good helping skills. It is best to first choose the general feeling category (happy, sad, angry, scared, confused, strong, or weak) and the severity of the feeling (high, medium, or low). The statement is then selected that reflects the content and intensity of the feeling. This can be presented to the patient in the following format:

"You feel (*very sad*)."

With further practice, general feelings can be transferred into more specific feelings:

"When I feel (*depressed*),

I feel (*lost*)."

Because feelings represent the most basic quality of human experience, it becomes critical for the audiologist to understand and identify the affective forces that patients bring into the hearing rehabilitation process. Learning to respond to emotional issues can help to facilitate appropriate counseling.

Proper responses to the affect and content of the patient's statements are not adequate. According to Carkhuff (2000), feelings must be integrated with content to provide patients with emotional meaning to their expressions.

Table 12–1 Categories of Feelings Grouped According to Intensity and Affect State

Levels of Intensity	Categories of Feelings						
	Happy	Sad	Angry	Scared	Confused	Strong	Weak
High	Excited Elated Overjoyed	Hopeless Depressed Devastated	Furious Seething Enraged	Fearful Afraid Threatened	Bewildered Trapped Troubled	Potent Super Powerful	Overwhelmed Impotent Vulnerable
Medium	Cheerful Up Good	Upset Distressed Sorry	Agitated Frustrated Irritated	Edgy Insecure Uneasy	Disorganized Mixed up Awkward	Energetic Confident Capable	Incapable Helpless Insecure
Low	Glad Content Satisfied	Down Low Bad	Uptight Dismayed Annoyed	Timid Unsure Nervous	Bothered Uncomfortable Undecided	Sure Secure Solid	Shaky Unsure Bored

From Carkhuff, R. R. (1993). The art of helping (4th ed.). Amherst, MA: HRD Press. Reprinted with permission.

It is based on the principle of cause and effect, in that every feeling is precipitated by some particular reason or causes.

Pearl

- One of the most important objectives in counseling is to recognize the patient's reason for each true feeling.

It is easy to practice responding to feeling and content by using examples in our own lives, then extending them into typical patient expressions:

Feeling	Content
"I feel happy	because I was promoted."
"I feel sad	because my son moved away."
"I feel upset	about my sister's divorce."

Stage II: Personalizing Meaning

Stage II of Carkhuff's (2000) model involves personalizing the meaning of the patient's experiences and expressions. It is probably the most demanding helping skill to master and use during counseling. It tends to happen over a long time and may exceed the format of the typical hearing aid consultation session. However, it can provide the necessary information to assess the emotional stage of the patient and whether the patient is close to setting goals to resolve hearing problems. Personalization consists of introducing the patient's experiences into the responses by use of the format "You feel (*feeling*) because *you* (*meaning, problem, or goal*)." This can be applied to the patient with hearing loss by using the following examples:

Personalizing meaning   "You feel frustrated because you wish people would stop mumbling."

Personalizing problems   "You feel sad because you cannot understand your grandchildren."

Personalizing goals   "You feel upset because you cannot hear at Rotary meetings, and you want to stay active."

Ultimately, personalizing goals can shift into decision making and action to begin to take positive steps toward problem solving.

Stage III: Initiating to Facilitate Acting

During the final stage of Carkhuff's (2000) helping process, the audiologist assists the patient in a program for action (amplification). It is important for the audiologist to define and focus the patient's personalized goals in developing an action plan. Implementing the program will resolve the patient's problem and achieve his or her goals. Feedback is necessary throughout this stage. Often, a patient will cling to emotional barriers such as depression while initiating solving the hearing problem. This occurred in the case vignette that was described earlier. Feedback involves recycling into those emotions that can serve to block acting. For example, in the case vignette, even though the patient was willing to pursue amplification, her depression still served to make the process difficult; every step along the way felt "overwhelming." The plan was subsequently modified to "ease" her into the amplification experience. The acting stage requires hard work and high motivation on the part of the patient. Many will succeed with support and encouragement; others will border the emotional line so that any negative experience during the process (e.g., poor shell fit) will result in termination of the amplification process.

Initial Interview

Certainly, the importance of a thorough patient case history cannot be overstated. It is a starting point to use the basic helping skills that have been described previously. It is the natural place in the counseling process to identify a patient's attitude toward his or her hearing loss and the use of amplification.

After the medical portion of the case history, the audiologist can begin to inquire about the patient's perception of his or her hearing loss and those of significant others. It is critical to include items that will probe for affect-based attitudes. Pertinent questions include

- "Tell me about your hearing loss."

- "When is it most noticeable?"

- "How does your spouse/family feel about it?"

- "How does it affect watching television?"

- "How does it affect going to (church/synagogue/mosque, etc.)?"

- "How does it affect the movies/theater?"

- "How does it affect social gatherings with family and friends?"

- "Have there been any recent changes in your lifestyle over the past few years?"

- "What changes in your vision or general health have occurred over the past few years?"

- "Have you, any family members, or friends ever used hearing aids?"

- "What size and type of instruments were worn and for how long?"

- "Tell me about your/their experiences with amplification."

- "How do you feel about wearing amplification?"

This list is not designed to be all-inclusive but will furnish the necessary information concerning the patient's emotional attitude toward his or her hearing loss and the use of amplification. For instance, the practitioner can use it to identify which stage the individual may be in (denial, projection, anger, depression, or acceptance); appropriate helping strategies can subsequently be used to address the emotional barriers to amplification. The list can also be used to recognize preconceived beliefs the patient may possess about the advantages and limitations of hearing aid use.

Validation of affect can begin to take place during the initial interview. Use appropriate statements, such as "I understand how frustrating it is to feel as if people are mumbling all the time" or "I know how confined you feel since you have moved in with your daughter." These validation techniques improve the counseling relationship and provide the patient with the comforting notion that the audiologist understands what he or she is feeling. Management of these affect-based behaviors is best accomplished when the test results are reviewed or during a hearing aid consultation session. Inappropriate intervention early in the counseling process with a statement such as "People do not mumble; you have a hearing loss" can only serve to create a confrontational counseling relationship and can often be interpreted by the patient as being judgmental.

Postassessment Interview/Consultation

After the completion of the audiologic evaluation, it is customary to review the test results with the patient and any significant others. The importance of having the patient understand the audiogram and the effects of hearing loss on communication cannot be overstated. Explanation of the audiometric data needs to be detailed but understandable.

Involvement of the significant other is a critical part of the counseling process. Questionnaires such as the Significant Other Assessment of Communication (SOAC) and its companion Self Assessment of Communication (SAC; Schow and Nerbonne, 1992) can help to screen for primary communication problems and for secondary social and emotional consequences. The SOAC and SAC are short and easy to administer. Results can greatly assist the audiologist in evaluating discrepancies between a patient's assessment of communication and that of the significant other. Hoover-Steinwart and colleagues (2001) found a significantly positive impact of hearing aid benefit as a result of early involvement by significant others.

Several different strategies are effective in describing the patient's audiogram and its effects on communication. Harford and Curran (1997) use shading critical areas of the audiogram that affect communication, along with an overlay that contains vowels and critical consonants. This is illustrated in **Figs. 12–2** and **12–3**. **Figure 12–2** shows an audiogram with a typical high-frequency sensorineural hearing loss, with shading in the area of the hearing loss. **Figure 12–3** illustrates the critical consonants and vowels that can subsequently be placed over the patient's audiogram. The "Count the Dot" articulation function (Mueller and Killion, 1990) can also be used to show how much critical speech information is missing as a function of the patient's hearing loss. It is necessary for patients who exhibit word recognition scores that are poorer than 70% to understand the limitations of poor word recognition and its impact on hearing aid performance.

Computer-based hearing loss simulation is an additional tool to assist patients in understanding their hearing loss. GN Otometrics (Taastrup, Denmark), MedRx Inc. (Elk River, MN), Audioscan (Dorchester, Ontario), and others use a system called visible speech mapping (VSM), which displays the patient's audiogram on a computer monitor. Sound libraries selected from a menu include, but are not limited to, such sound snippets as male speech, female speech, music, a train approaching, and a soda can opening. The voice of the significant other can also be recorded and used in the simulation demonstration. Each sample is played first in the "normal" mode and switched into the "simulated" condition. The end result is that the patient and significant other can instantly hear the difference between "normal" and "simulated" using real-world stimuli to comprehend the impact of the patient's hearing loss on daily living. VSM also includes a module that incorporates the above-mentioned stimuli in real-ear measurements for fitting verification. In other words, the voice of the significant other or other speech stimulus can be used in the fitting process to verify optimum performance with amplification. A sample display of VSM data is shown in **Fig. 12–4**. Our center uses VSM simulation and/or a modified version of the method described by Harford and Curran (1997). The audiogram and its configuration are reviewed with the patient and significant other. A modified item from the California Consonant Test (Owens and Schubert, 1977) is selected: *cheek, chief, cheese, cheap, cheat.*

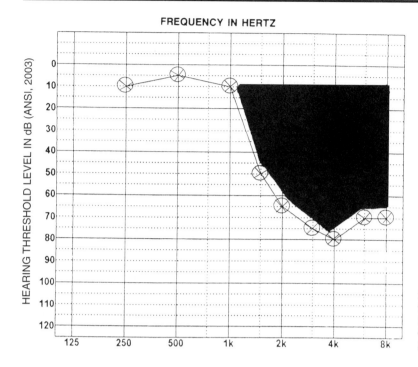

Figure 12–2 A typical high-frequency hearing loss, with the area of loss shaded. (From Harford, E. R., & Curran, J. R. (1997). Managing patients with precipitous high-frequency losses. Hearing Review Supplement, 1, 8–13, with permission.)

It is explained to the patient that the softer consonants in the English language—/k/, /t/, /z/, /p/, and /f/—supply the critical information in speech, whereas vowels are much louder and do not carry much information. It is easy for the patient to see that by changing one consonant sound, the meaning of the entire word changes, and the frequency range of the patient's hearing loss is such that he or she cannot hear those softer consonants, especially if the speaker is a woman or child. The author uses an analogy from the television show *Wheel of Fortune*. The vowels /a/, /e/, /i/, /o/, and /u/ have a lot of sound energy/loudness, but they do not help us "solve the puzzle." The critical consonants /s/, /f/, /t/, /h/, /p/, and /z/, in contrast, are very soft and give much needed information.

The author also uses an anatomical chart to explain how the hair cells are damaged much like a worn carpet and do not grow back once they are altered. Often, patients will have the erroneous notion that they have "nerve deafness" and that their "nerve" is just fine. They are often told by their physician that amplification will not help nerve deafness.

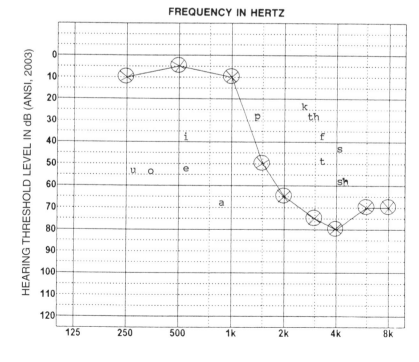

Figure 12–3 A typical high-frequency hearing loss. Critical high-frequency consonants and vowels can be laid over the audiogram in the form of a transparency. (From Harford, E. R., & Curran, J. R. (1997). Managing patients with precipitous high-frequency losses. Hearing Review Supplement, 1, 8-13, with permission.)

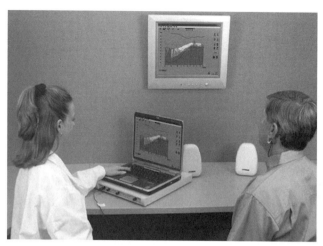

Figure 12–4 An example of visual speech mapping measurements. (Courtesy of MedRx Corp.)

The use of the chart and audiogram can act as tools to facilitate patient education and help to indicate to the patient that most successful hearing aid fittings are on individuals physicians refer to as having nerve deafness. Certainly, patients can then turn around and educate their family and friends about the erroneous concept of nerve deafness.

Pearl

- The use of visual aids and analogies to explain the effect of high-frequency hearing loss on communication will help in resolving the patient's erroneous assumption that "people are mumbling." Using the term *sensorineural hearing loss* is too technical for most patients. Our practice uses the preferred term *inner ear* or *hair cell damage*.

This is also the point in the counseling process in which the principles of Beck's (1979) "erroneous assumptions" can be implemented. Use of the VSM hearing loss simulator can be very helpful at this stage in counseling. It is critical to communicate simply and clearly to the patient that hearing loss is very slow in its progression, so much so that he or she may be unaware that it is changing; it is very common for others around the patient to be more conscious of the deterioration in his or her hearing sensitivity. In addition, it is the softer "information-loaded" consonants that patients cannot perceive, so that the false impression he or she receives is that "people are mumbling." It is also important to share with the patient that communication problems are often situational, and it is perfectly normal for the patient to experience an array of environments where he or she will communicate effectively. In the words of Dr. Mark Ross, "The biggest problem with hearing loss is that you don't know what you don't hear."

An appropriate follow-up to the effects of gradual hearing loss on the perception of softer consonant sounds is to provide a transition into hearing aid consultation. Patients

can be questioned about their feelings and attitudes concerning hearing aid use and provided with preliminary basic information about the improvements in hearing aid technology. They can be informed that the present technologies can now boost the softer sounds that they cannot hear so that they can understand speech in a much clearer fashion without overamplification of louder, annoying sounds, such as dish noises and paper rattling. As a result, they will not have to lower the volume or remove the instruments every time there is a louder sound in their listening environment. Many patients will feel overwhelmed by this process and will require time to digest the information, accept their hearing loss, and feel comfortable enough to move forward to using amplification. In the author's practice, patients are given brochures that describe general facts about hearing loss and hearing aids, as well as new technologies and how they differ from conventional instruments. Most are scheduled for a full hearing aid consultation within a week's time, which will review the various hearing aid technologies, sizes, and fee structure. Those individuals who are still in denial, projection, anger, or depression and are not ready to pursue amplification are also given information and encouraged to return for consultation once they are ready to receive help. Our experience with this population shows that most will return within a time frame that varies from 1 week up to 5 years; others return with instruments purchased elsewhere that have been sitting in a drawer. Another group of individuals will continue to search for a reason to avoid dealing with the problem. An audiologist with good helping skills may be able to isolate the patient's emotional barrier that prevents him or her from moving forward; a well-trained mental health professional may be necessary to facilitate positive change in the patient's emotional behavior.

♦ Consultation

A brief review of the audiogram is often necessary when a patient returns for hearing aid consultation. This is also an appropriate time to administer a questionnaire such as the SOAC, SAC, or Characteristics of Amplification Tool (COAT). It is critical that the patient's apprehensions be validated while at the same time creating an emotionally positive atmosphere for evaluating amplification.

Personality Typing

Van Vliet (1997) describes an assortment of patient personality types known as high-risk users, which audiologists will frequently encounter during the process of audiologic assessment and hearing instrument selection.

I'm not vain, but . . .   These are individuals who will take one look at a behind-the-ear (BTE) instrument and feel faint. Vanity may not be the only issue for these patients. They may present with feelings that others will perceive them as infirm or disabled if the hearing instruments are visible. Certainly, completely-in-the-canal (CIC) instruments can provide an alternative for these patients, but in many circumstances they may not be candidates for a CIC fitting because of dexterity issues, ear canal anatomical problems, audiometric constraints, or limitations resulting from above-average cerumen production.

So, I have a slight hearing problem . . . thank goodness it is not enough for me to use amplification   These patients are not unlike those in denial or projection. Many are not ready to accept their hearing loss and will often understate their handicap to avoid dealing with it.

Do I have to wear two?   It is quite common for patients to feel "twice as deaf" wearing two instruments. In many circumstances, patients have just accepted their hearing loss, so it is an emotional stretch just to use one hearing instrument. Frequently, patients will state, "Am I that bad?" Often, they will report that their best friends and relatives wear only one instrument and perform quite well, or they may mention that others remove one instrument in noise because everything is too loud. Financial issues may be a source of concern for patients, but more often it is the psychological "load" of two instruments. It is similar to the cane versus walker dilemma, in which individuals may feel much more handicapped and infirm with a walker than while using "just" a cane.

I could never spend that   Many patients are on fixed incomes that limit their ability to afford amplification. There are programs and foundations, however, that can provide assistance to those in need. On a local level, service organizations such as Lions, Rotary International, Kiwanis, Knights of Columbus, and Quota have provided various levels of support. Hear Now, Starkey Foundation, Sertoma, and Miracle-Ear Children's Foundation, among other organizations, furnish financial aid for amplification on a national level. Specific information concerning these national organizations is found in Appendix 12–1.

Patients, however, will often use financial limitations as an excuse to postpone or avoid dealing with their hearing loss. Dychtwald and Flower (1989) report that members of the 50+ population purchase 80% of all luxury travel, gamble more than any age group, spend more per capita in the supermarket than any other age group, own 77% of all the financial assets in the United States, and account for a whopping 40% of total consumer demand. Many individuals would much rather take that trip to Europe than invest both financially and psychologically in their hearing loss.

• *Same as 20 years ago:* Audiologists will encounter patients who enter their offices wearing a 20-year-old linear BTE instrument with the original earmold and tubing attached. The user will request that the same instrument style, circuit, and original earmold be fitted while they wait. Discussions about new technologies and the importance of comprehensive audiologic assessment are fruitless; these patients will reply, "My hearing hasn't changed in 20 years. If it ain't broke, don't fix it." A formal waiver may be an option for these patients; certainly, detailed documentation in their record is a necessity.

If everyone talked like you . . .   Most doctor–patient communication takes place in quiet rooms at distances that seldom exceed 4 feet, so patients are often unaware that hearing loss is not "black and white" and that their ability to communicate will depend on the listening environment. Projection will often serve as a convenient roadblock. Patients often will state, "You speak so clearly, but my husband and children mumble."

I understand that. I'm an engineer . . .   Some users have such extreme confidence in their ability to understand the technology that they will attempt to control the entire hearing rehabilitation process. These patients will request a screwdriver so they can operate the instrument's trimmers, or they will ask for a copy of the programmable software so they can perform their own programming alterations. Many of these users will have unrealistic expectations and feel that by adjusting the acoustic characteristics, they can solve all of their problems. A fact-based approach is useful in dealing with "engineers"; descriptions of hair cell physiology and of studies that show that sensorineural-impaired patients require a more favorable signal-to-noise ratio (SNR) for accurate communication can be very helpful in managing this group of users.

What did you do before computers?   Many patients can be phobic about computers; demonstrating programmable technologies in front of them can cause them to feel "overwhelmed" and think that amplification is "much too complicated." Sometimes a simple explanation may be helpful, such as "Before computers, we had to keep sending the hearing aids back to the factory for changes." For some individuals, the process needs to be made as simple as possible.

Traynor and Buckles (1997) report that identifying the user's personality style through a formal personality evaluation may provide helpful information regarding the patient's hearing rehabilitative needs. They analyzed the Myers-Briggs Type Indicator (MBTI; Myers et al, 1993), which is used on a large scale in many industries to furnish information concerning employees, and believed that it could be applied to gain knowledge about a patient's personality type, learning style, and coping mechanisms for incorporation into the individual's hearing rehabilitation program.

The MBTI was based on the theories of Jung (1974), who suggested that people are different in fundamental ways in that they possess different motivations, purposes, urges, aims, values, needs, impulses, and drives. None of these instincts is ranked as better or more important than another, but their value is in how they influence functional personal choices. Individual preferences for a specific function are indicative of how a person interacts with his or her instincts. The end result is that an individual can be "typed" according to his or her choices.

The MBTI is composed of 126 questions about individual preferences, diverse situations, and reactions to different word pairs. The scores are plotted using a point system that is adjusted according to gender and are presented as a tendency toward one end or the other of four scales, or continuums.

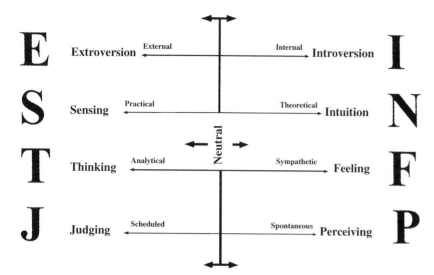

Figure 12–5 Myers-Briggs Type Indicator (MBTI) preference continuums. (From Traynor, R. M., & Buckles, K. M. (1997). Personality typing: Audiology's new crystal ball. Hearing Review Supplement, 128, 31, with permission.)

Figure 12–5 shows the preference continuums for the MBTI: extroversion (E)/introversion (I), sensing (S)/intuition (N), thinking (T)/feeling (F), and judging (J)/perceiving (P). The MBTI scores on these four continuums compose 16 different personality types. The scores start at zero from the neutral position and become higher as one moves toward each end of the four different continuums. For example, if the individual scores toward the "I" side of the first continuum and the "S" side of the second, the "F" side of the third and the "P" side of the fourth, the individual's personality type will be scored as ISFP.

Traynor and Buckles (1997) discuss the MBTI personality types in detail and their possible role in the aural rehabilitation process. In a study of 30 patients, they found that 80% of those identified by the MBTI as possessing extroverted personalities were satisfied with their first choice of amplification. These patients were often excited about the amplification process and very good communicators with the audiologist about the hearing aid selection process. Introverts, in contrast, were more interested in receiving a highly detailed explanation of hearing aid technology as opposed to accepting the audiologist's rationale for hearing aid use. They need to be convinced of the benefit of the amplification before they use it. If introverts are comfortable enough in the counseling environment, they may be good candidates for in-office demonstration of the different hearing aid technologies.

Knowing and understanding these personality types is certainly important to serve our patients in a more thorough fashion; the time necessary to administer, score, and interpret a 126-item test, however, can be excessive for most practice settings. Traynor and Buckles (1997) state that a retrospective study is necessary with at least 1600 patients to correlate audiologic complaint to personality. Future research in personality assessment may assist in providing an amended or abridged version of the MBTI for use by audiologists.

The Keirsey Temperament Sorter (KTS; Keirsey and Bates, 1984) reduces the MBTI evaluation, making it a more useful clinical tool. It delineates four personality temperament groupings: Sensing-Perceiving (SP), Sensing-Judging (SJ), Intuitive-Feeling (NF), and Intuitive-Thinking (NT). The assessment can be accessed online at www.Keirsey.com, offering audiologists and patients the opportunity for evaluation and scoring at no charge.

Traynor (2003) provides a summary of the four different Keirsey categories, with detailed considerations for audiology practitioners in managing each personality style. Additionally, the audiologist's personality styles are analyzed, with recommendations and concerns for patient management.

Dawson (1985) describes four different personality styles as they relate to decision making and buying behavior. What follows is a description of these personality types and their application to the processes of counseling and orientation toward amplification.

The Pragmatic

Dawson (1985) describes the pragmatic individual as being fact-driven, bottom-line-focused. The pragmatic will always try to get to the point of a topic and is very conscious of time management. As a result, he or she will often use time-efficiency gadgets, such as personal organizers. The pragmatic will write daily reports or read the newspaper while waiting in the audiologist's office; that behavior will continue during the wait for the ear impressions to harden. As an active individual, the pragmatic has difficulty sitting and watching anything; he or she is a doer, not a listener or observer. You will not often see the pragmatic sitting in the bleachers at a baseball game; instead, he or she will either be on the tennis court or listening to the game on the radio while writing a memo. In a hearing aid consultation session, the pragmatic will not desire folksy detailed explanations of every hearing aid technology; a quick synopsis of advantages and limitations will be more than sufficient. The pragmatic will often state his or her preferences at the beginning of a consultation and will try to control the session. The pragmatic is strictly business and will often base any decision, including amplification, on facts. He or she will want fee quotations, warranty information, loss damage protection, and service visit policies to be spelled out in very precise terms. Programmable technology may appeal to the pragmatic in that no volume controls need to be adjusted, and such an individual will like the "gadget" concept of multiple memories and remote controls.

The Extrovert

Dawson's (1985) second category is the extrovert, who is motivated, emotional, very friendly, and easily impressed. Unlike the pragmatic, the extrovert enjoys an animated, folksy, humorous approach. He or she loves to share in the emotions of a crowd, such as at a sporting event, and will get very excited over big issues but may not always think things through completely. The extrovert is willing to take risks and has a good sense of the ins and outs of business. He or she makes decisions quickly but is also quite emotional; this individual will see something he or she likes and take to it almost immediately. The extrovert is not afraid to say no, but will almost always do it in a friendly manner. Much like the pragmatic, the extrovert does not like detailed explanations but may need tempering of his or her often emotional responses.

The Amiable

The third type of personality described by Dawson (1985) tends to be a creature of habit who frequently creates obstacles around himself or herself. The amiable may have an unpublished phone number and a "No Soliciting" sign on their home or business. He or she often makes lifetime bonds to people and attachments to homes, automobiles, and surroundings. The ambience of an environment and middle-of-the road personality are appealing. The amiable will have a difficult time buying a new automobile, for instance, because of his or her bond to the old car and a fear of being pressured by salespeople. The amiable tends to be very nice, warm, friendly, and observant, someone who will remember the names of your children and identify the mood of a crowd. During a hearing aid consultation session, the amiable may want to have a 10-year-old hearing aid repaired because he or she does not wish to part with an old friend, or when it finally dies, the amiable will want exactly the same replacement instrument.

The Analytical

The fourth personality style described by Dawson (1985) is best recognized by his or her profession: accountant, engineer, mathematician, actuary, or some other analytical job. The analytical thrives on detail and loves gadgetry, desiring to be the first on the block to acquire a combination TV remote/garage door opener/digital cellular phone. Unlike the pragmatic, who seeks results, the analytical searches for causes of a problem. He or she will pursue every morsel of critical information that even remotely relates to an issue before attacking it. The analytical is methodical and curious, wishing to digest every aspect of a question before venturing a solution. He or she will devour detailed instrumentation manuals with gusto and will often phone toll-free help lines

with further requests. Because the analytical is obsessed with facts and detail, he or she is punctual and likes to have fees and contracts quoted to the penny. Such an individual tends to be withdrawn and prefers gadgets and details to relationships, but once the analytical makes a decision, it will typically hold up in the most challenging of situations.

Most audiology practitioners have interesting stories to share about analytical patients. Even the detailed digital hearing instrument brochures that are written from an engineering slant are insufficient for some of these patients; they will check out the manufacturer's Web site and annual report, and wish to communicate with the company's director of research and development. Analyticals will also request schematics of the instrument's directional microphones and may ask for a copy of the programming software so they can make their own modifications. Remote controls and multiple memory instruments/microphone arrays can be their best friends. Before the development of programmable technology, analyticals would tend to carry a screwdriver with them to change their trimmer settings. It can be a frustrating experience to work with these patients; referring to anatomy and hair cell physiology can be helpful in managing analyticals.

These personality styles are not necessarily distinct categories. No patient will have all of the attributes of one style of personality without possessing some of the characteristics of the others. Analyzing our own personality and how it fits into Dawson's (1985) scheme can be quite valuable.

Figure 12–6 illustrates how the four personality styles can be graphed according to degree of assertiveness and organizational level. It is divided into quadrants, with the analytical in the upper left-hand corner, the pragmatic in the upper right-hand corner, the amiable in the bottom left corner, and the extrovert in the bottom right corner.

The vertical line on the graph represents the organizational and emotional levels of the various personalities. Dawson (1985) suggests that pragmatics and analyticals are very organized people who have an excellent sense of time management and completing projects, with very neat work spaces. Decisions are usually made in advance with a fair amount of insight and virtually no emotion.

Amiables and extroverts occupy the opposite side of the organizational scale. They tend to make decisions and plan activities in a more spontaneous fashion, usually on the basis of emotion. Their working and home environments are unstructured, cluttered, and disorganized.

On the horizontal line are the levels of assertiveness and attention span of the four personality styles. High levels of assertiveness are on the right side of the graph. Extroverts and pragmatics possess strong degrees of assertiveness; they will volunteer in group activities because they want to lead. Both are aggressive types and will desire to take charge of situations. Amiables and analyticals, on the other hand, would rather do many other things than lead an activity.

Analyticals and amiables possess longer attention spans. Most analyticals will sit through an hour-long hearing aid consultation loaded with information about digital technology and leave feeling as if they had just started the session. Amiables have very long-lasting relationships with everything around them, taking a long time to reach a decision

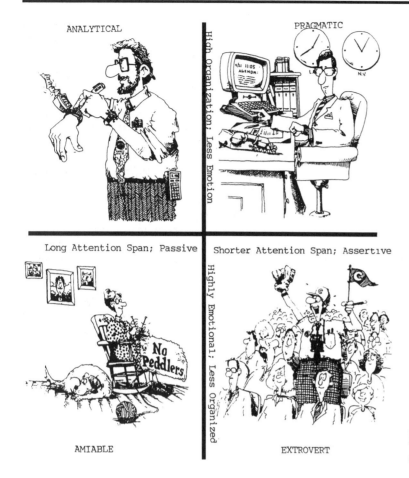

ANALYTICAL

PRAGMATIC

High Organization; Less Emotion

Long Attention Span; Passive

Shorter Attention Span; Assertive

No Peddlers

Highly Emotional; Less Organized

AMIABLE

EXTROVERT

Figure 12–6 Personality styles. (From Dawson. R. (1985). You can get anything you want, but have to do more than ask. New York: Fireside Books, with permission.)

on most issues, but will not analyze things as thoroughly as an analytical.

On the right-hand side of the graph are the extroverts and the pragmatics. They will have a lot of trouble sitting through a play or a board meeting and will always feel distracted by other matters that they must accomplish immediately. Pragmatics and extroverts become very unsettled when they have to sit and watch things for extended periods; they are ready to move on to the next life issue. These individuals will look at a proposal and reach a decision quickly, without requiring much time to mull things over.

According to Dawson (1985), conflicts arise when individuals of different personalities attempt to negotiate or communicate with each other. The maximum conflict occurs when personality styles in opposite quadrants on the graph interact. If you are a pragmatic or extrovert who practices fast decision making, and you are in the middle of a hearing aid consultation with an analytical or amiable personality, his or her slow, methodical decision process will drive you crazy. On the other hand, amiables and analyticals may feel pressured by the fast decisions of pragmatics and extroverts and may abandon or withdraw from seeking further help for their hearing loss. If you are interacting with a pragmatic, spend less time with small talk and anecdotes.

It is apparent that slow decision makers feel threatened by rapid decision makers, and that fast decision makers are irritated by methodical decision makers. Sessions can flow

more smoothly if you can discover the personality style of the individual patient. A self-assessment is valuable; once you have analyzed your own personality style, you may find that sources of conflict are easier to perceive.

Clark and English (2004) describe four different social styles—driver, expressive, amiable, and analytical—based on the work of Wilson Learning Corp. (1978). These are similar to the pragmatic, extrovert, amiable, and analytical categories reported by Dawson (1985). Clark and English's (2004) questionnaire can be used to identify the social style of the audiologist and practitioner. The authors also offer recommendations on how to modify the counseling style of the practitioner to accommodate the social style of each patient.

Matching Hearing Technology to Patient Needs

Bevan (1997) stresses that the hearing aid fitting system should take into account the needs of the real patient. Most patients will state, "I want to hear better," but the specific lifestyle and communication needs of the individual patient will determine which specific technology is appropriate. Ask the patient to provide information regarding specific situations in which hearing instruments must solve his or her communication problems. These may include church, TV, club meetings, sporting activities, movies, family gatherings, and the like. In this counseling method, the audiologist is an advocate and empowers the patient to make an informed choice.

One of the most successful retail chains selling discount designer apparel is Syms, whose radio and television advertisements feature the tag line "An educated consumer is our best customer." This philosophy should be stressed to the patient and his or her significant other or family member; they should be briefed on the advancements in hearing aid technology, describing the changes from basic linear instruments into digital instruments that do not require the use of a volume control and are programmed with a computer, including the innovation of noise reduction and adaptive directional microphone technology. It is important that the explanations avoid the use of technical terms and be brief; the sole purpose is to make the patient aware of the problems of the past and how hearing aid technologies have improved. Many patients will enter the consultation session reporting a negative experience with amplification; being sensitive to those experiences and explaining the differences among technologies will help to improve the patient's confidence in pursuing amplification. It should be emphasized that multiple strategies are available and that the specific amplification solution will depend on the nature of each person's lifestyle and needs, as well as budget.

Pearl

- Determination of patient goals for amplification should take place before reviewing specific technology solutions.

Setting Realistic Expectations and Goals of Hearing Aid Use

Selection of hearing instrument technology will be made on the basis of the patient's communication needs and lifestyle. An assessment can be conducted using the Client Oriented Scale of Improvement (COSI; Dillon et al, 1997), Abbreviated Profile of Hearing Aid Benefit (APHAB; Cox and Alexander, 1995), or other self-assessment measure. The COSI **(Fig. 12–7)** provides important information in helping to set patient-specific goals for amplification. Up to five specific user needs are listed in order of significance at the time of the initial hearing aid consultation. It is critical that the listening needs are stated in a specific condition (e.g., "To communicate better with my spouse in a restaurant" as opposed to "To hear better in noise"). These individual requirements can also assist in selecting a particular type of hearing aid technology for each patient. For instance, if the most

COSI

The NAL Client Oriented Scale of Improvement

Name: ____________________

Audiologist: ____________________

Date: 1. Needs established ____________________

2. Outcome assessed ____________________

Degree of Change — "Because of the new hearing instrument, I now hear . . ."

Final Ability (with hearing instrument) — "I can hear satisfactorily . . ."

SPECIFIC NEEDS	Indicate Order of Significance	Worse	No Difference	Slightly Better	Better	Much Better	Hardly Ever 10%	Occasionally 25%	Half the Time 50%	Most of Time 75%	Almost Always 95%
	☐										
	☐										
	☐										
	☐										
	☐										

901 76 311 07/01.96

Figure 12–7 The National Acoustic Laboratory (NAL) Client Oriented Scale of Improvement (COSI). (From Dillon, H. James, A., & Ginis, S. (1997). Client Oriented Scale of Improvement (COSI) and its relationship to several other measures of benefit and satisfaction provided by hearing aids. Journal of the American Academy of Audiology, 8, 27–43, with permission.)

critical patient need is to communicate effectively while working in a large exhibit hall, a binaural digital system incorporating optional dual microphones with multiple memories may be the optimum choice.

At the time of the patient's initial 3- to 4-week postfitting checkup, the COSI is completed. It is possible to measure how well the instruments performed relative to the patient's user requirements. The results can be used to pinpoint problem areas that may require further orientation or in-depth counseling if the patient has unrealistic expectations of hearing aid performance. At the time of the postfitting checkup, the patient should reflect on his or her performance with amplification, followed by discussion of a specific degree of change for each particular user need. Final ability with the hearing instruments can also be quantified by having the patient summarize how often he or she can communicate successfully in each of the specific situations.

Sandridge and Newman (2006) have developed the Characteristics of Amplification Tool (COAT; **Fig. 12–8**). It has patients list the top three situations where they would like to

Characteristics of Amplification Tool (COAT)

Name: _____ Date: _____

Audiologist: _____

Our goal is to maximize your ability to hear so that you can more easily communicate with others. In order to reach this goal, it is important that we understand your communication needs, your personal preferences, and your expectations. By having a better understanding of your needs, we can use our expertise to recommend the hearing aids that are most appropriate for **you**. By working together **we** will find the best solution for you.

Please complete the following questions. Be as honest as possible. Be as precise as possible. Thank you.

1.   Please list the top three situations where you would most like to hear better. Be as specific as possible.

   _____

   _____

   _____

2.   How important is it for you to hear better? Mark an X on the line.

   Not Very Important   --   *Very Important*

3.   How motivated are you to wear and use hearing aids? Mark an X on the line.

   Not Very Motivated   --   *Very Motivated*

4.   How well do you think hearing aids will improve your hearing? Mark an X on the line.

   I expect them to:

   Not be helpful   --   *Greatly improve my*
   at all   *hearing*

5.   What is your most important consideration regarding hearing aids? Rank order the following factors with **1** as the most important and **4** as the least important. Place an **X** on the line if the item has no importance to you at all.

   ____   Hearing aid size and the ability of others not to see the hearing aids

   ____   Improved ability to hear and understand speech

   ____   Improved ability to understand speech in noisy situations (e.g., restaurants, parties)

   ____   Cost of the hearing aids

Figure 12–8 The Characteristics of Amplification Tool (COAT). (From Sandrige, S. A., & Newman, C. W. (2006). Improving the efficiency and accountability of the hearing aid selection process. Retrieved March 2006 from http://www.audiologyonline.com, with permission.)

6.   Do you prefer hearing aids that: (check one)

_____   are totally automatic so that you do not have to make any adjustments to them.
_____   allow you to adjust the volume and change the listening programs as you see fit.
_____   no preference

7.   Look at the pictures of the hearing aids. Please place an X on the picture or pictures of the style you would **NOT** be willing to use. Your audiologist will discuss with you if your choices are appropriate for you – given your hearing loss and physical shape of your ear.

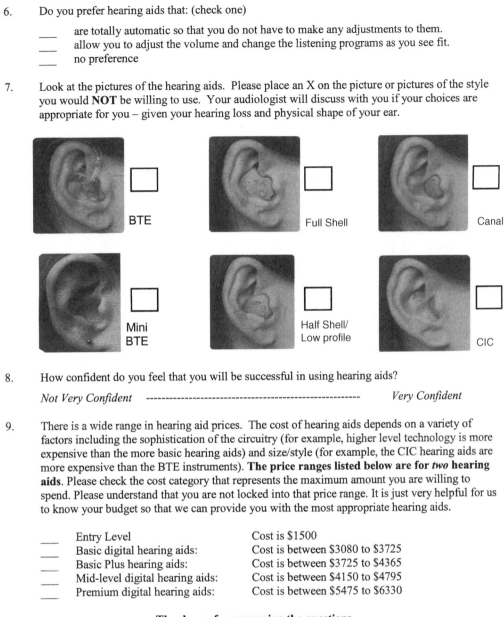

8.   How confident do you feel that you will be successful in using hearing aids?

   Not Very Confident   ---   *Very Confident*

9.   There is a wide range in hearing aid prices. The cost of hearing aids depends on a variety of factors including the sophistication of the circuitry (for example, higher level technology is more expensive than the more basic hearing aids) and size/style (for example, the CIC hearing aids are more expensive than the BTE instruments). **The price ranges listed below are for *two* hearing aids**. Please check the cost category that represents the maximum amount you are willing to spend. Please understand that you are not locked into that price range. It is just very helpful for us to know your budget so that we can provide you with the most appropriate hearing aids.

_____	Entry Level	Cost is $1500
_____	Basic digital hearing aids:	Cost is between $3080 to $3725
_____	Basic Plus hearing aids:	Cost is between $3725 to $4365
_____	Mid-level digital hearing aids:	Cost is between $4150 to $4795
_____	Premium digital hearing aids:	Cost is between $5475 to $6330

Thank you for answering the questions.
Your responses will assist us in providing you with the best hearing healthcare.

Figure 12–8 *(Continued)*

communicate more effectively. They also have to rank their attitudes concerning how important it is to communicate more effectively, how motivated they are to wear and use amplification, and how well they think that hearing aids will improve their hearing, as well as their confidence in successfully using amplification. Patients are also required to rank the importance of the size of the instruments, the improved ability to hear and understand speech in quiet and noisy environments, and the cost of the hearing aid system. The COAT also lists photos for patients to choose any of the different sizes of hearing aids that they would not be willing to use. Five different "tiers" of technology are also listed, along with a cost range for each tier. Patients then select which of the cost categories would represent the maximum amount they would be willing to spend.

The COAT is an excellent instrument to facilitate the hearing aid selection process, as it identifies patient communication needs, personal preferences, expectations, and financial considerations. A detailed summary and analysis of outcome measures can be found in Chapter 6 in this volume.

It is important to include the discussion of hearing aid limitations as a part of setting realistic goals for hearing instrument performance. **Figure 12–9** describes expected benefits from amplification for both new and experienced

EXPECTED BENEFITS FROM AMPLIFICATION

INEXPERIENCED USERS

IN QUIET, AIDED PERFORMANCE WILL BE SIGNIFICANTLY BETTER THAN UNAIDED PERFORMANCE

IN NOISE, AIDED PERFORMANCE WILL BE SIGNIFICANTLY BETTER THAN UNAIDED PERFORMANCE HOWEVER, AIDED PERFORMANCE **IN NOISE** WILL NOT BE AS GOOD AS AIDED PERFORMANCE **IN QUIET**!

SOFT SOUNDS WILL BE SOFT, BUT AUDIBLE; **LOUD SOUNDS** WILL BE LOUD, BUT NOT UNCOMFORTABLE!

• EXPERIENCED USERS

• **IN QUIET**, AIDED PERFORMANCE WILL BE SIGNIFICANTLY BETTER THAN AIDED PERFORMANCE WITH THE PREVIOUS HEARING AID

• **IN NOISE**, AIDED PERFORMANCE WILL BE SIGNIFICANTLY BETTER THAN AIDED PERFORMANCE WITH THE PREVIOUS HEARING AID

• HOWEVER, AIDED PERFORMANCE **IN NOISE** WILL NOT BE AS GOOD AS AIDED PERFORMANCE **IN QUIET**!

• **SOFT SOUNDS** WILL BE SOFT, BUT AUDIBLE; **LOUD SOUNDS** WILL BE LOUD, BUT NOT UNCOMFORTABLE!

Figure 12–9 Expected benefits from amplification. (Courtesy of Washington University School of Medicine, Adult Audiology Division.)

users used by Valente and his colleagues at the Washington University School of Medicine's Adult Audiology Division. Copies can be given to users to help ensure realistic expectations from hearing aid use. Often patients will perceive that the hearing aids will "eliminate noise," based in part on some of the early consumer advertising on radio and television. Perhaps the most significant statement in reviewing expected benefits is that the instruments will perform better in noise than without amplification but not as well as in a quiet environment. A frank discussion of the concept of SNR should contain some basic facts that sensorineural-impaired individuals require a more favorable SNR than normal listeners for effective communication, even with advanced technology instruments (Killion, 1997). Patients with poorer word recognition will require education on how to use their vision appropriately and manipulate their listening environment to supplement their communication skills.

Pearl

• Making the patient aware that hearing instruments are only one component of hearing rehabilitation will help to prevent unrealistic expectations of hearing aid performance.

Many patients fully comprehend the importance of binaural amplification, particularly in helping to optimize communication in the presence of noise. Others will react negatively ("You mean I have to wear *two*?"). The benefits of binaural amplification are stressed, particularly if their primary goal is improved communication in groups. Audiologists should also attempt to create a risk-free environment, assuring patients that they can return the second instrument if there is no significant improvement from binaural use. Although some patients will fully understand the benefits of binaural amplification and the fact that they have a

risk-free environment for evaluation, others will feel "twice as deaf" and are not yet ready to consider binaural amplification. Many of them have just reluctantly accepted their hearing loss and feel that monaural amplification is a major emotional step. A large proportion of these individuals will ultimately upgrade from monaural to binaural amplification at a later date, which can vary from 1 month to many years.

In some practices where the patient desires a monaural fitting but a binaural fitting is recommended by the audiologist, patients are required to sign a legal release that states that "binaural amplification results in better long-term performance than one instrument." Typically, the primary basis behind a patient's preference for monaural amplification is the "psychological load" of two instruments. In our practice, staff audiologists believe that presentation of such a form can serve to place a psychological barrier between the audiologist and the patient. After discussion of the benefits of binaural amplification, detailed notes are entered into the patient record that show that binaural amplification was discussed and the reason(s) why monaural amplification was chosen.

Digital Signal Processing

Because of the higher sampling rates and processing speeds that are inherent in digital signal processing, these instruments are reported to provide cleaner and clearer sound quality with the intent of maximizing speech recognition, particularly in the presence of noise. Many of these systems feature multiple channels and frequency bands that can serve to provide even greater precision in matching the amplification characteristics to the user's audiometric profile and dynamic range, particularly in those patients who have irregular audiometric configurations that require multiple channels for signal processing. Advantages of all-digital instruments may lie in their ability to maximize audibility and dynamic range rather than to produce large improvements in enhancing SNR (Killion, 1997). Adding dual microphones, multiple microphone arrays, and adaptive microphone technology in coordination with digital programming can provide significant improvement in SNR (Valente, 1998).

Additional information regarding the various hearing instrument technologies is found in Chapters 4, 5, 6 and 13 in this volume.

All these technology "tiers" are available in our practice for patient demonstration using BTE demonstration units coupled to stock earmolds. VSM is employed to evaluate and verify performance of the various technologies, including performance with directional microphones. Other demonstrations can involve taking the user to the cafeteria of the facility or outside on a busy street. Although not perfect, these mini-demonstrations can provide positive listening experiences under different listening conditions for patients before fitting, particularly for analytical personality types who require a lot of specific detail before making a decision. These demonstrations can be structured to match the individual's unique communication needs. An additional advantage of the demonstration is that it can help patients to realize that they can indeed understand softer voices; this can correct their erroneous assumptions that "people mumble."

Size Preferences

Samuel Lybarger, in his timeless definition of a hearing aid, states, "It is an ultra-miniature electroacoustical device [that] is always too large." Certainly, it is well known that patients are preoccupied as to how they will appear to others while wearing their hearing instruments. This stigma is referred to as the "hearing aid effect." Johnson and Danhauer (1997) summarize these attitudes as (1) an excuse or form of denial for rejecting amplification, (2) negative experiences from dissatisfied hearing aid users, (3) an excuse used by patients who have financial limitations to purchase amplification, (4) marketing forces that stress the cosmetics and size of the hearing aids, and/or (5) patients who feel possible adverse reactions to the visual appearance of hearing instruments.

No question exists that counseling patients who are cosmetically sensitive presents a major challenge to practitioners. Certainly, these individuals bring their fear and apprehension into the hearing selection process. Often, many cosmetically sensitive patients are just over the brink of denial and depression. For many, it is a big emotional step just to sit in the audiologist's office. As a result, they may be driven by the fear of stigma so that they have yet to accept their hearing loss. Others who work in the business world may feel additional apprehension or shame that they will appear weak or infirm if their clients or friends "see" the instruments.

Counseling strategies should focus on validating the cosmetically sensitive patient's emotional attitudes. Beck's (1979) theory of "erroneous thinking" may be the source of the apprehension; the patient fears that he or she will be viewed as disabled and rejected by peers if the instruments are noticeable. In some cases, patients can be reassured that most individuals they encounter would view them as a "total person" and would ultimately feel that the patient's hearing loss may be more conspicuous than the physical visibility of the instruments, though some patients may interpret this as a judgmental response from the audiologist. Many of these patients can accept this idea and will pursue amplification; others will continue to rank size as their major priority. The COAT is an effective tool for patients to indicate which style of instrument they would not be willing to use and can be employed prior to hearing aid consultation.

In our practice, the audiology staff treat instrument size as a patient-choice option. All sizes can be demonstrated, regardless of the degree of hearing loss, along with a discussion of the fact that not all sizes are appropriate for all hearing losses. Audiologists will gently recommend against the choice of a smaller instrument if it is outside the patient's fitting range. Audiologists should keep individual replicas of custom instruments and earmolds so patients can have a real perception of how they appear in an individual's ear. Patients are also encouraged to interact with the replicas so that they can realize the dexterity necessary to change the battery and operate smaller in-the-canal (ITC) and CIC instruments. They are also informed of the effects of cerumen on the performance of smaller instruments. Stocks of earmolds that blend with the user's skin tone are also demonstrated, along with smaller sized BTE hearing aids, which are less conspicuous. The effect of these mini-demonstrations can help patients to realize they may not be able to physically operate smaller instruments; new smaller BTEs and mini open-fit instruments may be more appealing, especially when they can obtain a loaner instrument if repairs are necessary.

Some prospective users will readily understand that not all instrument sizes are appropriate for their hearing loss; others will continue to be "emotionally stuck." A confrontation that "it must be this size or no instrument" will tend to cause some patients to "shop" for someone who will dispense what they desire, often with limited benefit. The end result is that audiologists will frequently see these patients at a later date when they arrive in our offices complaining that they were "ripped off."

The use of the 30-day satisfaction guarantee (60 days in the author's practice) can serve as a security blanket to provide a low-risk evaluation of hearing aid performance for cosmetically sensitive patients. For some individuals, the experience of inadequate performance may be necessary to provide the evidence that performance is more important than instrument size. Others may be happily satisfied but find themselves at the upper end of the fitting range of programmable CICs, with no capacity to increase the instruments' gain or output. Many of these patients place a low priority on further programming; they tend to live in the present but fully understand that they may need to replace the instruments if any changes are present in their hearing sensitivity. These experiences may be one of the factors that contribute to a higher return rate for CIC instruments; it may be of interest to investigate the percentage of the returns that were ultimately fitted with larger hearing aids. As well, circumstances exist in which experienced ITC or CIC users will reject standard in-the-ear (ITE) fittings because of insertion difficulties or physical discomfort. Mini-BTEs with slim-tube open fits have created another option for cosmetically sensitive patients who are candidates for this new technology.

The "hearing aid effect" continues to be an important concern in counseling prospective users. It is certainly critical that audiologists prioritize performance, satisfaction, and the importance of the outcome of "better hearing" as opposed to the "hearing aid." However, it is most critical that audiologists validate patients' emotional apprehensions concerning size preferences. Recent improvements in CIC technology have helped to bridge some of the gaps between cosmetic preference and instrument effectiveness.

◆ Orientation

The primary goal of hearing aid orientation is to furnish the hearing aid user with the necessary information concerning the operation and use of the instruments so that optimum benefit is derived. Extensive amounts of information are presented to the patient, including adapting to hearing aid use, operation of the components and batteries, troubleshooting techniques, warranty, loss/damage protection, telephone use, limitations, cleaning, wax guard system, and insertion and removal instructions.

In a survey conducted by Eggen and Stanford (1988), they found that the median time to accomplish hearing aid orientation is 30 minutes. Critical variables such as manual dexterity, memory, vision, and aging can certainly have an impact on the success or orientation and subsequent satisfaction in hearing aid use.

Tirone and Stanford (1992) examined the specific amount and type of information that a new user is exposed to during hearing aid orientation. Eighteen new users of ITE amplification were videotaped throughout a hearing aid orientation session. Tapes were reviewed, and bits of information presented to the user were counted. "Bits of information" was defined as any new information presented with respect to the patient's amplification device and any demonstration of an adjustable technique. These bits of information could be a single word or phrase. The topic areas discussed included batteries, wax guard, physical adjustment, Dri-Aid (Hal-Hen Co., Inc., New Hyde Park, NY) kit, warranty/product information, hearing aid adjustment, hearing aid description, troubleshooting, precautions, cleaning, trial period, accessing facility/fees, and hearing assistance technology (HAT). Results revealed that the mean number of information bits was 93, with a range of 61 to 136. In some cases, five information bits were presented to the patient in < 1 minute.

It is apparent from this study that many new users are literally overloaded with much new information that must be integrated and retained to ensure successful hearing aid use. Many elderly patients do not possess sufficient memory to retain all the necessary critical facts concerning hearing aid use. Time management is crucial; information concerning warranty, accessing facilities, fees, and troubleshooting can be provided in written form. Tirone and Stanford (1992) recommend the use of a programmed videotape on maintenance, cleaning, and physical manipulation of the instruments in addition to one-to-one interaction. Paraprofessionals can also be used to provide assistance for patients who require additional training in basic skills.

Ranking the importance of all the necessary information that must be covered during an orientation session is indeed a challenge for the audiologist. Virtually all patients need to practice insertion/removal and operation of the instruments unless a caregiver is present on a consistent basis to provide that function. It is paramount that patients understand the limitations of amplification and the process of relearning to adapt to new sounds. This does not limit the importance of all the other information; it will be based on the unique needs and characteristics of the specific user.

Special Consideration

- Some patients do not have the memory capacity and/or attention span to absorb all of the new bits of information presented during initial hearing aid orientation and performance verification. A second orientation visit may be necessary.

The Orientation Session

Pearl

- Just as airline pilots are required to use a checklist for items to be confirmed before takeoff, audiologists need a checklist to specify what information is to be covered during a hearing aid orientation/fitting session.

Uniformity of patient care is important not only for audiologists but also for all health care practitioners. Many managed care organizations require practice guidelines before issuing contracts to their providers. A comprehensive checklist of items covered during hearing aid orientation and fitting helps to ensure a consistent quality and uniformity of care. This is exceptionally important in practice settings where multiple audiologists are providing hearing aid dispensing services. Just as the pilot has a list of safety and airplane function items that need to be confirmed before takeoff, the audiologist needs a similar item inventory so all critical aspects are addressed during a fitting session.

Figure 12–10 is a sample dispensing check-off sheet. Although it is quite specific, no weighting is given to any of the items. This permits some space for individual interpretation while at the same time defining specific areas to be addressed during the fitting process. Not every item on the list will be reviewed in this chapter, but those factors that involve interaction between the use environment and the patient will be discussed.

Performance Verification

Other chapters in this text provide detailed discussion of performance verification with tools such as real-ear measures

SOUTH SHORE HEARING CENTER
Hearing Aid Fitting Checklist

Patient: _____ Fitting Date: _____

Audiologist: _____

Right Aid: _____ Serial #: _____

Left Aid: _____ Serial #: _____

Warranty Repair Exp Date: _____ Loss and Damage Exp Date: _____

Discuss: Extended Manufacturer Warranty / ESCO / Replacement Fee / Return Policy (see contract)

*Fitting Verification: Real Ear: _____   VSM: _____

Functional Gain: _____   Other: _____

*Fit Modifications: Make: _____   Venting: _____

Model: _____   Tubing Type: _____

Material: _____   Wax Guard: _____

* Reasonable Expectations:
        Own voice, male/female voices
        Wearing hearing aids in quiet, noisy or group settings
        Importance of lip reading and structuring environment
        Effects of monaural vs. binaural listening; localization
        Hearing aid use in theaters, auditoriums and houses of worship
        Use of FMs and ALDs

*Identification and Use of Controls

*Feedback: Causes and Prevention

*Cleaning and Maintenance:
        Cerumen management
        Turning it off when not in use
        Tips for avoiding loss
        Avoiding water, hairspray, humidity Dri-Aid Kit 25$, Air Blower 10$
        Tubing replacement

*Battery: Size _____
        Toxicity
        Low battery signal/when to change/tracking battery life
        How to change
        Where to purchase
        Tamper lock: _____ Tool needed? _____

* Insertion and Removal

* Telephone: T-coil   Amplified telephone   Acoustic coupling

* Follow-up Issues/Listening needs: _____

_____

_____

PLEASE NOTE CHANGES TO ORIGINAL FIT ON BACK

Figure 12–10 Hearing aid fitting checklist.

(Chapter 3), functional gain (Chapter 4), and loudness scales (Chapter 6). Certainly, verification of optimum acoustical performance is an absolute necessity during the initial fitting session. Hawkins and Cook (2003) showed that relying on manufacturers' simulated predictive fitting formulas for programming resulted in gain reduction errors in the high frequencies by as much as 10 to 15 dB. It was recommended that real-ear measurements should be employed for verification to resolve these errors. Cunningham et al (2002) reported a 48% reduction in the total number of follow-up visits when verification was accomplished with VSM.

Pearl

- Verification of benefit from amplification using real-ear measurements during the initial fitting will reduce follow-up visits and optimize patient performance.

Expectations and Suggestions for Adapting to Hearing Aid Use

The Occlusion Effect

The effect of hearing aid or earmold placement on the user's voice quality is a well-known process, and its management is discussed in detail in Chapter 2 in this volume. Certainly, the "hollow, barrel over the head" feeling created by the occlusion effect needs to be minimized, but new users must understand that all hearing aid microphones will pick up and amplify their own voice and that it is a normal process, regardless of the instrument's size or type of signal processing. As well, a realistic time frame of patient adaptation to his or her own voice should be discussed. For some patients, it may take up to 8 weeks before they are completely comfortable with the manner in which they perceive their own voice while using amplification.

Audibility of New Sounds

Another amplification interaction effect is the almost instant audibility of new sounds that the patient may not have perceived for quite some time. This effect is particularly common in wide dynamic range compression (WDRC) technologies, which have low-threshold kneepoints (40–50 dB sound pressure level [SPL]) that provide greater amplification for low-input signals. Patients will typically report that "the hearing aids are making noise," when what the listeners actually hear is a soft sound in the environment that may include the computer fan/hard drive, room ventilator, or footsteps in the hallway. In most circumstances, these are sounds that are not audible to the hearing aid user when the instruments are removed but are perceptible to individuals with normal hearing sensitivity.

Gatehouse and Killion (1993) suggest that listeners with hearing loss require a significant period of time to learn to make optimum use of the new set of speech cues to receive maximum performance from their amplification. They theorize that as a high-frequency sensorineural hearing loss

slowly progresses, the neural representation in the cortex of the low-input, high-frequency sounds will no longer receive stimulation. As a result, the brain will begin to "fill in" those gaps with surrounding frequencies and intensities to those areas that are unstimulated. In view of the fact that most sensorineural hearing losses are slowly progressive, the process may take years to run its course.

When the patient is fitted with appropriate amplification, the sounds that were previously inaudible to the user are now perceived and presented to the cortex. If those auditory areas were "filled in" by surrounding frequencies and intensities, it may take a significant amount of time for the rewiring/unmapping of the brain to take place. Gatehouse and Killion (1993) suggest that the time frame for the relearning process can take weeks or even months and may be correlated to how much of the high-frequency information was absent—and for how long.

This pattern is also present in the visual system. Ophthalmologists and optometrists (Calnan, 1997; personal communication, C. A. Gustafson, 2006) report that patients who manifest moderate to severe vision deficits that are uncorrected will often require gradual refraction changes for optimum vision improvement. They report that a single change in refraction from severe vision deficit to normal will often produce headaches and rejection of the eyeglass/contact lens fitting because the change in visual acuity is too large for the brain to handle in an effective fashion. In addition, it is a well-known fact that bifocals require a period of acclimatization for the visual system to process the changes in visual image that occur when the user looks down. Calnan (1997) and Gustafson also point out that much variability exists among patients with similar visual acuity in the amount of time that is necessary for their visual systems to adapt fully to bifocal use.

Pearl

- The nature of the brain rewiring/adaptation process for amplification, with parallels in the visual system, need to be stressed to the patient during all stages of hearing aid counseling/orientation.

The phenomenon of relearning has been confirmed by Cox and Alexander (1992), who showed increases in both measured and perceived benefits from amplification over a 3-month period. Gatehouse (1992) measured speech identification scores in noise for both narrowband and wider band hearing instruments and found that no changes in speech identification abilities occurred over a 16-week period for the narrowband instruments, but performance increased gradually using a wider band condition.

Whether one supports the idea that the brain is rewiring itself or adapting to new stimuli, this new audibility of both speech and nonspeech signals has critical application to the hearing aid orientation process. An individual interaction between the user and the hearing instruments will be unique. It is also important to demonstrate to the patient the difference between "audibility" and "annoyance." *Audibility* can be defined as the identification of new sounds that have been absent for some time, whereas *annoyance* refers to overamplification of louder sounds, such as crackling paper, dishes rattling, and traffic noises.

It is clearly evident that the large "jump" in audibility that is experienced by new users of amplification, particularly WDRC instruments, requires significant time of the brain to learn to use and categorize new sounds. Some listeners may need to be introduced gradually to this style of amplification. Where users start will vary significantly, but the audiologist can begin by raising the compression kneepoint by 5 to 10 dB or lowering the amplification for low-input sounds to minimize the effect of too many soft sounds in the initial stage of amplification. Some programmable hearing aid systems are equipped with software called adaptation managers, which allows listeners to be introduced to new amplification in small steps, similar to small changes in refraction for eyeglass or contact lens users.

Wearing Schedules/User Diaries

Although many users will perform well by using their hearing instruments on a full-time basis each day, others may require a more gradual, steady period of acclimatization. Selected hearing aid manufacturers have developed wearing schedules and user diaries to assist selected patients to "ease in" to the process of adjusting to the use of amplification. Palmer and Mormer (1997) use a specific wearing schedule as part of their hearing aid orientation process. It is a 9-day schedule that consists of 1 hour of use the first day, followed by a 1-hour "rest period" that is followed by another hour of use. For the second and third days, use time increases in 1-hour intervals, with the same 1-hour "time-out." Listening activities during the first 3 days are limited to activities inside the home, such as listening to household sounds (e.g., a fan, water running, doorbell ringing, and toilet flushing). Television and radio use and quiet conversation with low background noise are also integrated in the first 3 days of use.

Days 4 and 5 increase the time to 4 to 5 hours of use, followed by an hour of rest, with another 4 to 5 hours of use. Listening activities are increased to include quiet indoor work activities at home or in the work environment. Days 6 and 7 provide the same 1-hour increment in use time and 1 hour time-out, with an increase in listening activities to include quiet outdoor activities. By the end of the ninth day, the user is engaged in full-time use with the same 1-hour break period.

It is often difficult to predict which patients will adapt readily to new amplification. Even those who fully understand the process of relearning to hear and integrate new sounds may require gradual increments in use time to accomplish both success and satisfaction with hearing aid use. Others will require a more regimented approach of using the hearing aids consistently each day while fully understanding that the brain will never "rewire" itself if the patient uses the instruments only 1 hour per day. Part-time use can be a facade for denial in that many patients will say, "You mean, I have to use them all the time? . . . My hearing isn't that bad!" Many new users will wish to remove the

hearing aids in the office right after a thorough and successful fitting/orientation session, not wanting to wear them home. Audiologists will constantly be challenged to identify the difference between psychological acceptance of the hearing loss in the form of use of amplification and the process of the auditory system physically adjusting to hearing aid use. In the author's experience, audiologists should encourage patients to use their instruments full time, with a brief rest period each day, while stressing that if they do not use the hearing aids consistently, the brain will never accept the change. A wearing schedule similar to that reported by Palmer and Mormer (1997) is subsequently used in situations in which patients require a more gradual introduction to amplification and will not use the schedule as a tool to avoid hearing aid use.

A user diary can help new hearing aid patients to provide a structured summary of their experiences with amplification. This can greatly assist the audiologist in providing necessary reprogramming and quantifying benefits from hearing aid use and realistic expectations. Oticon (Smørum, Denmark) and GN ReSound (Bloomington, MN) are among the companies who have structured user diaries.

Hearing Instrument Use in Various Listening Environments

A brief discussion of hearing aid use in different listening environments is a meaningful part of a hearing aid orientation session. Specific situations can be taken from the list of individual patient goals. For example, reassurance to the patient that, with amplification, he or she will be able to hear the television now without "blasting" his or her spouse out of the living room can boost the user's self-confidence. The deleterious effects of poor acoustics and distance should be described to help the patient cope with communicating in churches, auditoriums, and theaters. The role of infrared and frequency modulation (FM) systems for improved communication in large-area listening environments can be briefly mentioned. More detailed information on HAT can be found in this volume in Chapter 17. Communication in noise should also be reviewed, with discussion of why individuals with inner ear damage require a more favorable SNR than normal listeners and the importance of binaural amplification in group listening situations. Discussion of performance limitations in everyday environments can help users to form realistic expectations of hearing aid performance. This can go a long way to dispel the myth that newer digital technologies "eliminate noise."

Feedback

Demonstration of the causes and prevention of feedback is critical during hearing aid orientation. Feedback should not interfere with satisfactory hearing instrument performance; this places an additional burden on hearing instrument manufacturers and earmold laboratories to furnish a good-fitting shell and on practitioners to provide good ear impressions. Multiple remakes are not uncommon, particularly in advanced technology instruments. Telephone use must be accomplished without having to remove the instrument because of instrument feedback. Many new technologies are now available with feedback managers that can greatly assist in reducing feedback without deleterious effects on hearing instrument performance. Specific strategies in managing feedback are provided in this volume in Chapter 1.

Battery Issues

At present, zinc-air button cells are the preferred choice for most hearing instruments. Certain programmable systems use silver oxide or alkaline batteries for remote controls. Zinc-air cells tend to "dry out" in ~60 days once the tab is removed, so that silver oxide cells will provide significantly longer life for long-term, low-drain applications such as remote controls. Some power instruments demonstrate more consistent operation with silver oxide cells or "high-performance" zinc-air batteries. It is important that patients understand the shelf life of a zinc-air cell once the tab is removed; some users will try multiple batteries in an instrument as a means of troubleshooting and reduce the shelf life on an entire package of batteries to 60 days.

Controversial Point

- Variability in performance/reliability of zinc-air cells can exist among manufacturers. Audiologists should consult with hearing aid manufacturer product managers with specific questions concerning battery performance.

Calculation of the relative battery life of a hearing instrument is rather simple. American National Standards Institute (ANSI; 2003) hearing instrument specifications include a battery drain figure that can then be used to insert into a chart, which is available from most battery manufacturers. This chart is shown in **Fig. 12–11** and displays battery life in hours or days as a function of cell size and current drain. Specification sheets typically will publish cell drain with the instrument run at full-on gain. Many of the newer hearing instrument test chambers include the ability to calculate specific battery drain.

During a hearing aid orientation session, users can be trained to track the battery life of their instruments. In our practice, audiologists instruct patients to place the battery tab onto a calendar when a new cell is inserted so that they can count the number of days before it loses its power. They are also provided with a miniature plastic case to store a spare cell for quick access. The shelf life of unopened cells often exceeds 2 years; unopened packages do not require refrigeration. Storage should be in a cool, dry location, such as a desk or dresser, and cells should not be carried loose with other metal objects, which may cause the battery to discharge.

Most circuits provide an internal warning system: an audible tone or hum occurs when battery voltage begins to deteriorate. It is the recommendation of audiologists that all instruments use some sort of battery warning feature.

Unless it is certain that a caregiver will provide battery insertion/removal, all patients should receive ample practice in changing the battery in their instruments during initial orientation or as a part of preliminary consultation. Many wax loops come with magnets attached to the opposite end; these can provide assistance in battery insertion/removal for patients with more limited dexterity.

Directions concerning battery toxicity are provided to all new users. Virtually all hearing instrument instruction booklets contain the necessary required information. Tamper-resistant battery doors should be used in pediatric fittings, and battery toxicity is a required topic in a dispensing check-off sheet. Some practices use a signed waiver, which describes the hazards of accidental battery ingestion.

Care of Instruments

Certainly, it is essential that all users be educated concerning the effects of water, humidity, perspiration, and heat on hearing instrument performance. In a practice, nearly all users of BTE instruments should be provided with Dri-Aid kits (seen in **Fig. 12–12**), as well as individuals who are exposed to high humidity or moisture on a consistent basis.

GN ReSound has recently introduced ReStore, a small, extremely portable heat-based hearing aid drying case. Two power BTE instruments with earmolds can fit in the case, and the system functions with the case lid either open or closed. It quickly and gently dries instruments in 3 hours. ReStore can be seen in **Fig. 12–13**.

More extensive control of moisture and humidity has occurred with the introduction of Dry & Store, from Ear Technology Corp. (Johnson City, TN), an electronic desiccant/sanitizing agent that can be seen in **Fig. 12–14**. The instrument operates with a fan, which causes the air inside the chamber to circulate and increase in temperature. The heat and moving air cause the water molecules to move out of the instruments and into the charged desiccant. A germicidal ultraviolet lamp, which is activated electronically for the last 30 seconds of each hour, also functions to help disinfect the instruments. The total drying/sanitizing cycle takes approximately 6 hours.

Earhooks on BTE instruments should be changed on a regular basis; dirt and moisture can clog the dampers in the ear hook, resulting in a deleterious effect on the instrument's frequency response. Super Seals (shown in **Fig. 12–15**), from Hal-Hen, are disposable latex sheaths that are mounted onto the case of a BTE instrument to reduce perspiration.

The Hearing Aid Sweat Band, from VanB Enterprises (West Valley, NY), is a soft fabric sleeve that helps to protect BTE instruments from the damaging effects of moisture. It is shown in **Fig. 12–16**. Unlike latex sleeves, it can be installed without a tool and is easily removed, with easy access to instrument controls. Made from a specially designed fabric, it sheds water instead of holding or trapping moisture. It has the ability to be reused multiple times, and can be hand washed a few times without losing its effectiveness. Six sizes and six colors are available. The Sweat Band is acoustically transparent for sound; tests have shown sound dampening effects of only 2 dB.

Earmold air blowers from Hal-Hen can be seen in **Fig. 12–17** and are another important accessory to remove obstructions in earmold tubing for BTE users; earmold tubing that

Hearing Aid Battery Life Chart

Life/hrs. = $\frac{mAh}{mA}$ (16 hours of use per day)

Battery Drain Current (mA) per ANSI (S3.22 1976)	PRO LINE PREMIUM ZINC AIR*								MERCURY					
	312A 130mAh		13A 255mAh		675A 600mAh		10A 70mAh		R312 60mAh		R13 60mAh		HR675 270mAh	
	Hours	Days	Hours	Days	Hours	Days	Hours	Days	Hours	Days	Hours	Days	Hours	Days
.1mA	1300	81	2550	159	6000	375	700	44	600	37	1000	63	2700	169
.2mA	650	41	1275	80	3000	188	350	22	300	19	500	31	1350	84
.3mA	433	27	850	53	2000	125	233	15	200	13	333	21	900	56
.4mA	325	20	638	40	1500	94	175	11	150	9	250	16	675	42
.5mA	260	16	510	32	1200	75	140	9	120	8	200	13	540	34
.6mA	217	14	425	27	1000	63	117	7	100	6	167	10	450	28
.7mA	186	12	364	23	857	54	100	6	86	5	143	9	386	25
.8mA	163	10	319	20	750	47	88	5	75	5	125	8	338	21
.9mA	144	9	283	18	667	42	78	5	67	4	111	7	300	18
1.0mA	130	8	255	16	600	38	70	4	60	4	100	6	270	16
1.1mA	118	7	232	15	545	34	64	4	55	3	91	6	245	16
1.2mA	108	7	213	13	500	31	58	4	50	3	83	5	225	15
1.3mA	100	6	196	12	462	29	54	3	46	3	77	5	208	13
1.4mA	93	6	182	11	429	27	50	3	43	3	71	5	188	12
1.5mA	87	5	170	11	400	25	47	3	40	3	67	4	180	11
1.6mA	81	5	159	10	375	23	44	3	37	2	63	4	169	11
1.7mA	76	5	150	9	353	22	41	2	35	2	59	4	159	10
1.8mA	72	5	141	9	333	21	39	2	33	2	56	4	150	9

*IMPORTANT NOTE: Maximum battery life with any zinc-air battery will not typically exceed 60 days regardless of what is indicated by the chart. The battery will dry out and no longer be effective.

Figure 12–11 Hearing aid battery life chart. (Courtesy of Rayovac Corp.)

is pretreated with desiccant to reduce moisture that can build up in the tubing is also available from laboratories. Windscreens are also helpful to help prevent dirt and cerumen particles from entering the microphone, particularly on custom products. GN ReSound has recently developed microphone filters that can be easily replaced in the office to prevent debris from clogging microphones on ITEs, half-shells, ITCs, and CICs. Phonak (Stäfa, Switzerland) and Unitron

Hearing have office-replaceable microphone filters for BTE products.

Cerumen Control

Controlling cerumen buildup in the receiver of custom hearing instruments is one of the most common problems faced by dispensing audiologists. On the basis of the high

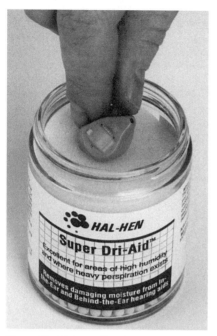

Figure 12–12 Dri-Aid kit. (Courtesy of Hal-Hen Co., Inc.)

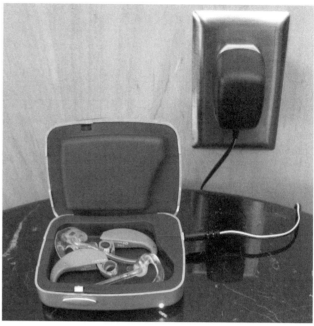

Figure 12–13 ReStore heat-based portable hearing aid dryer. (Courtesy of GN ReSound Corp.)

cost of replacing hearing instrument receivers as a result of cerumen contamination, manufacturers have designed an array of wax guard options. These include spring dampers, wax baskets, wax plungers, and element dampers, which are mounted inside the receiver tubing to prevent the cerumen from clogging the receiver.

Certainly, patients need to be instructed in detail concerning the effects of cerumen and proper cleaning techniques. Experience has shown that no single strategy is effective in controlling cerumen buildup in receiver tubes. Extending receiver tubes can cause discomfort in the ear canals of some

users; wax springs and baskets can easily become obstructed and can require biweekly replacement in some patients. Oticon has developed a "wax buster" cerumen cleaning system (shown in **Fig. 12–18**). The system incorporates a spring-loaded plunger; the user pushes the tip of the instrument down on a paper towel, and the piston pushes cerumen debris out of the sound bore. **Figure 12–19** shows the HF-3 wax guard system developed by GN ReSound. The small green filter has a screen, acts as a wax barrier, and can be changed by the user at weekly or monthly intervals. The

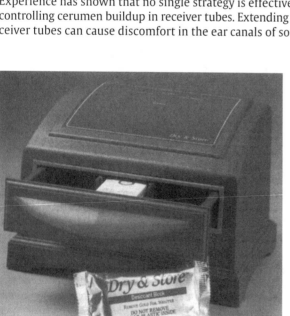

Figure 12–14 Dry & Store electronic hearing instrument desiccant/germicide system. (Courtesy of Ear Technology Corp.)

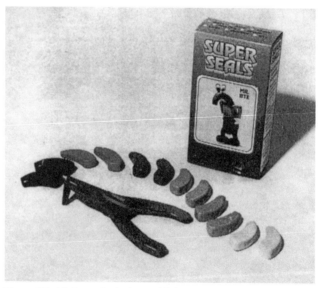

Figure 12–15 Super Seals disposable latex hearing aid covers. (Courtesy of Hal-Hen Co., Inc.)

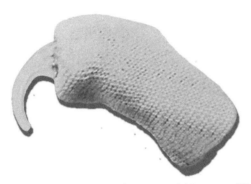

Figure 12–16 Hearing Aid Sweat Band. (Courtesy of VanB Enterprises.)

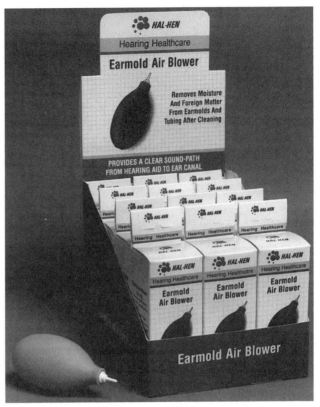

Figure 12–17 Earmold air blower. (Courtesy of Hal-Hen Co., Inc.)

Widex CeruStop system (Widex Hearing Aid Co.), also used by Unitron and Phonak, is shown in **Fig. 12–20** and is similar to the GN ReSound HF-3. It has an additional advantage in that it can be used in smaller ear canals. Kochkin (2001) reported on the use of a wax filter system, the Wax Buster. The data showed that those companies that had high usage rates for the wax filter system were nearly 8 times less likely to return the receivers for replacement.

Some manufacturers insert small removable coils into the instrument's receiver tube to help prevent cerumen from spreading into the receiver. Experiences with these coils have indicated that they clog easily; one new hearing aid user had the instrument coil become completely obstructed with cerumen within 48 hours after his initial fitting. Patients have also pushed the coil with their wax tool or cleaning brush down into the instrument's receiver. In our facility, a variety of techniques are used; audiologists often use the first year of use to help select the most effective wax control option for a particular patient, but we prefer systems like Wax Buster, HF-3, and CeruStop that can easily be replaced by the patient.

Many patients use a facial tissue to wipe the earmold or shell after removal or before insertion. Although this can be an effective method of removing pieces of cerumen or dirt from the instrument, many facial tissues (e.g., Puffs) contain perfumes or other additives that can result in dermatitis of the external ear if the instrument is placed into the ear immediately after it is wiped (personal communication, E. S. Cole, 1996). The symptoms can be the same as if the external ear had an allergic reaction to the plastic composition of the shell. Antibacterial wipes are available from supply houses that can be used to clean shells on instruments for

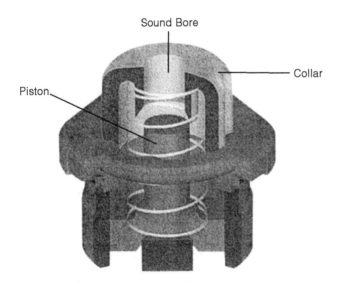

Figure 12–18 Wax Buster system. (Courtesy of Oticon, Inc.)

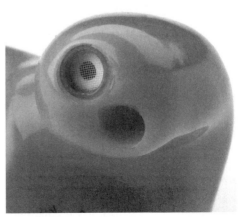

Figure 12–19 HF-3 wax guard system. (Courtesy of GN ReSound Corp.)

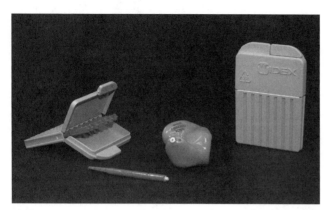

Figure 12–20 CeruStop wax protection system. (Courtesy of Widex Hearing Aid Co., Inc.)

patients with draining ears or for infection control. Those wipes can introduce moisture into the hearing aid. The Dry & Store can be helpful for those patients who require routine germicidal treatment. Some patients will also use their instruments while they sleep; lack of ventilation can often cause severe otitis externa and excessive cerumen problems. Instruments can also be lost or damaged if worn in bed. Alerting devices are a much better alternative for patients who express concerns for monitoring their listening environment during sleep.

Instrument Insertion/Removal

All patients must receive sufficient time to practice instrument insertion and removal. Caregivers and significant others can help provide support for patients with limited motor skills and dementia, but under most circumstances, the patient is the responsible individual.

Instrument removal is a preferred place to begin. Most patients perform this task with little or no difficulty; most will push up from the bottom of the external ear, between the lobe and the antitragus. This typically causes the instrument to slide out of the ear gently, with minimal discomfort. For individuals with firm ear texture or dexterity problems, earmolds and custom shells can be equipped with optional handles and notches to facilitate removal.

For many users, instrument insertion is an extremely demanding task; some patients who live alone use personal listening devices strictly because they are unable to insert and operate any type of traditional hearing aid. Proper hearing aid insertion is a challenge for many patients.

Some users with limited vision will require color coding or a notch to differentiate the left and right instruments, particularly half-shell, ITC, and CIC models. Despite some limited practice during initial hearing aid consultation to screen for dexterity issues, many patients will struggle with insertion. Although some individuals will recognize poor insertion from instrument feedback or tactile awareness, others will have no idea that the hearing aids are inserted incorrectly, leading to sore spots on the external ear, poor acoustic performance, and/or loss. No one size of instrument is immune: ITE hearing aids will protrude because the helix is not

inserted; canal instruments will not be fully seated or will be inserted sideways; BTE earmold tubing will be twisted, or the helix will protrude.

Audiologists should always have patients use a mirror as a validator following their best attempt at insertion. This will reinforce correct insertion technique and will also serve to provide visual feedback to users to show where they have made a mistake; most will be able to see if the instrument is protruding. The use of a portable plastic ear is also helpful for patients to visualize the insertion process. Individuals who experience insertion problems during initial fitting are contacted within 48 hours after orientation and can be scheduled for follow-up before their routine 2-week postfitting visit.

Telephone Use

Proper use of the telephone with hearing instruments is another significant part of the hearing aid orientation process. Unless it is an open fitting incorporating a large vent with large amounts of high-frequency gain, it should not be necessary for users to remove the hearing instrument to use the telephone successfully. Choices of various telephone accessories are described in Chapter 17 in this volume.

Choosing between acoustic and inductive coupling for telephone use presents a challenge to the audiology practitioner. Lowe and Goldstein (1982) evaluated speech recognition using the Speech Perception in Noise (SPIN) test for both acoustic and inductive coupling and found no significant differences between the two methods of telephone use, with some users performing better with acoustic coupling, and others demonstrating improved speech recognition with inductive coupling. Both coupling methods have advantages and limitation that can affect practical use. Users should be educated concerning compatibility problems with inductive coupling and the use of instruments with certain cellular phones.

Many users require a significant amount of time to activate the telecoil in a BTE instrument and hold the receiver in the correct position for effective communication; some report that the phone stops ringing before they can make the necessary adjustments. Others report that sitting near a computer monitor causes a significant hum when the telecoil is active. Some telephones are not compatible for use with inductive coupling, but there has been a large increase in the choice of compatible cellular and land telephones. Also, most digital instruments feature the ability to program a separate frequency response for either telecoil or acoustic coupling. Many manufacturers incorporate a feature called Easy Phone, which allows the hearing aid to shift automatically into the telecoil mode when an inductive telephone handset is placed near the instrument. It is clear that there is no preferred method of coupling for telephone use, but it is recommended that the hearing aid system have both coupling options available.

Acoustic coupling is also successful for many users. It can be limited from feedback that takes place when the handset is positioned on the ear; angling the phone or positioning the receiver a bit higher so it is directly on the hearing aid microphone can be effective in reducing feedback. Patients are also instructed in lowering the volume control on conventional instruments that may accomplish easy telephone use without annoying feedback. Circular pads are available that mount onto the telephone receiver and create a larger cavity volume, subsequently reducing feedback. Their limitation is that they can interfere with the ability to hang the telephone up properly and cannot be used easily with coin-operated phones.

Pitfall

- Feedback should not limit appropriate telephone use; users should be able to use either acoustic or inductive coupling without having to remove their hearing instruments.

Proper determination of the patient's telephone use patterns will identify whether acoustic or inductive coupling is more beneficial; many patients will use both systems. Some patients will use acoustic coupling for quick telephone use, while using inductive coupling for noisy environments or assistive device application. Detailed instruction during fitting is important: most patients do not position the phone correctly for effective use. Even with extensive practice during initial orientation, many users will require reinstruction during follow-up. Some states have subsidized programs for patients to acquire amplified handsets or special phones at no charge or for a reduced cost. Erber (1985) provides a comprehensive overview of telephone communication and hearing aid use.

Service Policy

During initial orientation, all users receive written information regarding instrument warranty, loss/damage protection, and follow-up visits. The differences between warranty and accidental loss/damage are reviewed in detail; many users think that their loss/damage plan will cover routine repairs. They are also instructed as to the length of time given to cover follow-up services and instrument reprogramming. Many patients who spend the winter months in other locations are given materials so they can ship the instruments to the clinic for repairs if needed. In addition, patients are provided with the names of practitioners in their area, with instructions that they may be charged for shipping or office

visits if the instrument needs servicing or reprogramming, even if the warranty is in effect.

Follow-up visits are extremely important in hearing aid orientation. Typically, they are scheduled for 2 to 3 weeks after initial fitting. Their general purposes are to evaluate patient satisfaction and make certain that the goals of the user are met. The scope of a follow-up visit varies and can include any of the following: reprogramming the instrument; managing user apprehension, denial, and projection; shell remake or modification; environmental manipulation strategies; discussing realistic expectations; real-ear measurements; functional gain measurements; evaluation of performance in noise; practice with insertion/removal; cleaning instructions; orientation on telephone use; assistive listening devices; outcome measures; and discussion of performance in restaurants and elsewhere. Certainly, if the prestated realistic goals of patients are met, and they decide to use and keep the instruments, they will achieve satisfaction. Long-term success may entail more than just keeping the instruments past the 60-day satisfaction guarantee period. It is best defined by Palmer and Mormer (1997), who describe successful use as when the patient's prestated communication needs are met, combined with the use of hearing instruments, assistive listening devices, counseling, communication strategies, and environment manipulation.

◆ Summary

There is little doubt that counseling and orientation toward amplification are complex processes. Greater knowledge and management of the psychological aspects of hearing loss will not only reduce the number of instruments that sit in the drawer but will also improve the proportional number of successful hearing aid users. Audiologists are not expected to become mental health professionals; rather, it is hoped that the information contained in this chapter will provide dispensing audiologists with some of the tools that are essential to improve their helping skills and fitting proficiencies.

Acknowledgments I thank Robert Beckhardt, M.D., and Herbert Goldberg, Ph.D., for their valuable input in the area of the psychology of hearing loss.

Appendix 12–1

Sources of Financial Assistance for Amplification

Audient: An Alliance for Accessible Hearing Care
Northwest Lions Foundation for Sight and Hearing
901 Boren Avenue, Suite 810
Seattle, WA 98104–3534
Phone: (877) AUDIENT (283–4368)
Fax: (206) 838–7195
Web site: www.audientalliance.org

Miracle Ear Children's Foundation
P.O Box 59261
Minneapolis, MN 55459–0261
Phone: (800) 234–5422
Web site: http://www.miracle-ear.com

Sertoma International
1912 East Meyer Boulevard
Kansas City, MO 64132
Phone: (816) 333–8300
Fax: (816) 333–4320
E-mail: infosertoma@sertoma.org
Web site: http://www.sertoma.org

Starkey Hearing Foundation
HEAR NOW Program
6700 Washington Avenue South
Eden Prairie, MN 55344
Phone: (800) 648–4327
Fax: (952) 947–4997
E-mail: nonprofit@starkey.com

References

American Heritage dictionary of the English language. (1992). New York: Houghton Mifflin.

American National Standards Institute. (2003). Specifications of hearing aid characteristics (ANSI S3.22–2003). New York: Author.

Beck, A. T. (1979). Cognitive therapy and the emotional disorders. New York: Meridian Books.

Berra, Y. (1998). The Yogi book. New York: Workman Publishing.

Bevan, M. A. (1997). Matching hearing technology to hearing *needs*. Hearing Review, 1(Suppl.), 32–36.

Bridges, J. A., & Bentler, R. A. (1998). Relating hearing aid use to well-being among older adults. Hearing Journal, 51(7), 39–44.

Carkhuff, R. R. (2000). The art of helping in the 21st century. Amherst, MA: Human Resource Development Press.

Carmen, R. E. (2001). Hearing loss and depression in adults. Hearing Review, 8(3), 74–79.

Clark, J. G., & English, K. M. (2004). Counseling in audiologic practice. Boston: Allyn & Bacon.

Cox, R. M., & Alexander, G. C. (1992). Maturation of hearing aid benefit: Objective and subjective measurements. Ear and Hearing, 13(3), 131–141.

Cox, R. M., & Alexander, G. C. (1995). The abbreviated profile of hearing aid benefit. Ear and Hearing, 16(2), 176–183.

Crandell, C. C. (1997). An update on counseling instruction within audiology programs. Journal of the Academy of Rehabilitative Audiology, 6, 77–84.

Crandell, C. C., & Weiner, A. (2002). Counseling competencies in audiologists: Efficacy of a distance-learning course. Hearing Journal, 55(9), 42–47.

Cunningham, D. R., Lao-Davila, R. G., Eisenmenger, B. A., & Lazich, R. W. (2002). Study finds use of live speech mapping reduces follow-up visits and saves money. Hearing Journal, 55(2), 43–46.

Dawson, R. (1985). You can get anything you want, but have to do more than ask. New York: Fireside Books.

Dillon, H., James, A., & Ginis, S. (1997). Client Oriented Scale of Improvement (COSI) and its relationship to several other measures of benefit and satisfaction provided by hearing aids. Journal of the American Academy of Audiology, 8(1), 27–43.

Dychtwald, K., & Flower, J. (1989). Age wave. Los Angeles: Jeremy P. Tarcher.

Egan, G. (1977). You and me: The skills of communicating and relating to others. Pacific Grove, CA: Brooks/Cole.

Eggen, S., & Stanford, L. S. (1988). A survey of hearing aid orientation procedures in Michigan audiologists. Mt. Pleasant, MI: Central Michigan University.

Erber, N. P. (1985). Telephone communication and hearing impairment. San Diego, CA: College Hill Press.

Garstecki, D. C., & Erler, S. F. (1997). Counseling older adult hearing instrument candidates. Hearing Review. 1(Suppl.),14–18.

Gatehouse, S. (1992). The time course and magnitude of peripheral acclimatization to frequency responses: Evidence from monaural fitting of hearing aids. Journal of the Acoustical Society of America, 92, 1256–1268.

Gatehouse, S., & Killion, M. C. (1993). HABRAT: Hearing aid brain rewiring accommodation time. Hearing Instruments, 44(10), 29–32.

Harford, E. R., & Curran, J. R. (1997). Managing patients with precipitous high-frequency losses. Hearing Review, 1(Suppl.), 8–13.

Hawkins, D. B., & Cook, J. A. (2003). Hearing aid software predictive gain values: How accurate are they? Hearing Journal, 56(7), 26–34.

Herzfeld, M., & English, K. M. (2001). Survey of AuD students confirms need for counseling as part of audiologist's training. Hearing Journal, 54(5), 50–54.

Hoover-Steinwart, L. M., English, K. M., & Hanley, J. E. (2001). Study probes impact on hearing aid benefit of earlier involvement by significant other. Hearing Journal, 54(11), 56–59.

Johnson, C. E., & Danhauer, J. L. (1997). The "hearing aid effect" revisited: Can we achieve hearing solutions for cosmetically sensitive patients? Hearing Review, 1(Suppl.), 37–44.

Jung, C. (1974). Psychological types. Princeton, NJ: Princeton University Press.

Keirsey, D., & Bates, M. (1984). Please understand me. Del Mar, CA: Prometheus Nemesis Books.

Kennedy, E., & Charles, S. (2001). On becoming a counselor: A basic guide for nonprofessional counselors and other helpers (3rd ed.). New York: Crossroad.

Killion. M. C. (1993). The K-Amp hearing aid: An attempt to present high fidelity for persons with impaired hearing. American Journal of Audiology, 2(2), 52–74.

Killion, M. C. (1997). The SIN report: Circuits haven't solved the hearing-in-noise problem. Hearing Journal, 50(10), 28–32.

Kochkin, S. (2001). The effectiveness of a wax protection system in reducing receiver replacements. Hearing Review, 8(9), 40–41.

Kubler-Ross, E. (1969). On death and dying. New York: Macmillan.

Little, J. T., Reynolds, C. F., Dew, M. A., et al. (1998). How common is resistance to treatment in recurrent, nonpsychotic geriatric depression? American Journal of Psychiatry, 155(8), 1035–1038.

Lowe, R. G., & Goldstein, D. P. (1982). Acoustic versus inductive coupling of hearing aids to telephones. Ear and Hearing, 3(4), 227–234.

Merriam Webster's collegiate dictionary. (1993). Springfield, MA: Merriam-Webster.

Mueller, H. G., & Killion, M. C. (1990). An easy method for calculating the articulation index. Hearing Journal, 43(9), 14–17.

Myers, I., Kirby, L. K., & Briggs, K. D. (1993). Introduction to type (5th ed.). Palo Alto, CA: Consulting Psychologists Press.

Narrow, W. E. (1998). One-year prevalence of depressive disorders among adults 18 and over in the U.S.: NIMC ECA prospective data. Population estimates based on the U.S. census estimated residential population age 18 and over on July 1, 1998 (NIH Pub. No. 99–4584). Bethesda, MD: National Institutes of Health.

Novalis, P. N., Rojcewicz, S. J., Jr., & Peele, R. (1993). Clinical manual of supportive psychotherapy. Washington, DC: American Psychiatric Press.

O'Neill, J. (1988). Are we marketing the right product? Hearing Journal, 4(11), 21–22.

Owens, E., & Schubert, E. D. (1977). Development of the California consonant test. Journal of Speech and Hearing Research, 20, 463–474.

Palmer, C., & Mormer, E. (1997). A systematic program for hearing instrument orientation and adjustment. Hearing Review, 1(Suppl.), 45–52.

Rezen, S. V., & Hausman, C. (2000). Coping with hearing loss. New York: Barricade Books.

Rogers, C. R. (1951). Client centered therapy: Its current practice, implications and theory. Boston: Houghton Mifflin.

Sandridge, S. A., & Newman, C. W. (2006). Improving the efficiency and accountability of the hearing aid selection process. Retrieved March 2006 from http://:www.audiologyonline.com

Schow, R. L., & Nerbonne, M. A. (1982). Communication screening profile: Use with elderly clients. Ear and Hearing, 3(2), 135–147.

Smedley, T., & Schow, R. L. (1990). Frustrations with hearing aid use: Candid observations from the elderly. Hearing Journal, 43, 21–27.

Strawbridge, W. J., Wallhagen, M. I., Shema, S. J., & Kaplan, G. A. (2000). Negative consequences of hearing impairment in old age: A longitudinal analysis. Gerontologist, 40(3), 320–326.

Tirone, M., & Stanford, L. S. (1992). Analysis of the hearing aid orientation process. Paper presented at the annual meeting of the American Speech-Language-Hearing Association, San Antonio, TX.

Traynor, R. M. (2003). Personal style and hearing aid fitting. Hearing Review, 10(9), 16–22.

Traynor, R. M., & Buckles, K. M. (1997). Personality typing: Audiology's new crystal ball. Hearing Review Supplement, 128, 31.

Valente, M. (1998). The bright promise of microphone technology. Hearing Journal, 51(7), 10–16.

Van Vliet, D. (1997). Personality types. Paper presented at the annual meeting of the Academy of Dispensing Audiologists, Orlando, FL.

Webster's new twentieth century dictionary—Unabridged. (1966). Cleveland, OH: World Publishing.

Wilkinson, D. (1995). Counseling: Every patient is different. Hearing Journal, 48(7), 63–66.

Chapter 13

Middle Ear Implantable Hearing Devices

Douglas A. Miller and Carol A. Sammeth

Over the past decade, audiologists have heard increasingly more about the topic of middle ear implantable hearing devices (MEIHDs), which in this chapter will be referred to simply as middle ear implants (MEIs). According to Spindel (2002), more than 1500 MEIs had been implanted worldwide as of a few years ago, and presumably that number has continued to increase. In the United States, there is currently limited MEI availability on the commercial market. However, research, development, and clinical trials on several devices continue, with the expectation of market introduction of more devices in the future.

The goal of this chapter is to introduce this relatively new and growing area of amplification technology, but also to provide an update to earlier published reviews on the topic (e.g., Hüttenbrink, 1999; Miller and Fredrickson, 2000; Spindel, 2002). The information presented herein was accurate, to the best of the authors' knowledge, at the time this book chapter was submitted for publication. Given the rapid pace at which the field has developed and the scarcity of published information, however, it is possible that there may be changes even by the time this material reaches its readers.

So why has there been such an interest in MEIs? The primary reason is that these devices potentially offer some advantages not found with conventional hearing aids. Most patients with nonmedically correctible conductive hearing loss, and those with mild to moderate sensorineural hearing loss, demonstrate excellent performance with the use of conventional (acoustic) hearing aids, especially given recent advancements in digital signal processing and newer options such as multimicrophones. However, patients with greater degrees of sensorineural hearing loss often experience limitations with conventional high-power hearing aids, including the occlusion effect (e.g., patients report that their own voice is too loud or that it sounds as if they are speaking "in a barrel"), discomfort from wearing tight and fully occluding earmolds, problems with acoustic feedback, poor perceptual sound quality, and high levels of distortion at the hearing aid output. Theoretically, MEIs may be able to provide these patients with higher levels of undistorted amplified sound and with better sound quality. Furthermore, because there is nothing placed in the ear canal with most types of MEIs, there is no occlusion effect or other problems associated with the use of an earmold. Although feedback is still possible with most MEIs, the potential for a significant feedback problem may be reduced with some of these devices relative to acoustic high-power amplifiers.

For these reasons, the majority of MEIs currently under development are intended for patients whose hearing loss is considered to be too severe for satisfactory performance with conventional hearing aids, but that is not severe enough to meet the criteria for a cochlear implant (see Chapters 14 and 15 for more information on cochlear implants in children and adults). Patients with recurrent otitis media are not good candidates for implantation in the middle ear, but MEIs may also be a reasonable option for patients who should not have their ear canal occluded with an earmold, for example, as a result of allergies or sensitivities to earmold materials, or because of chronic otitis externa. (There are alternatives that may be appropriate for some patients whose ear canals should not be occluded, including bone-conduction hearing aids, a bone-anchored hearing device [Baha, formerly BAHA, Cochlear Ltd, Sydney, Australia], and open contralateral routing of signals [CROS] earmolds. None of these options will work very well, however, for patients who require high levels of high-frequency gain.). In addition, a few MEIs have been developed specifically to assist patients with conductive or mixed hearing loss. At this time, MEIs are available only for adult patients and are not intended for children.

The most notable MEI advancement in recent years has been the advent of fully implantable, rather than just semi-implantable, models. Many companies working in the MEI field state that they have in development a fully implantable model, in addition to or instead of an earlier semi-implantable version, and one fully implantable model was briefly on the market in Europe. In fully implantable MEIs, all components, including the microphone, are placed under the skin, creating a "bionic ear" of sorts.

Special Consideration

- Beyond MEIs, there are also other types of implantable hearing devices currently available, including cochlear implants (see Chapters 14 and 15). Another implantable device is the Baha, an alternative to conventional bone-conduction hearing aids for patients with conductive hearing loss or to a CROS aid for patients with single-sided deafness. An auditory brainstem implant (ABI) has also now received approval from the U.S. Food and Drug Administration (FDA) for patients who have had their auditory nerve severed or damaged. Although these are also interesting topics, those devices are intended for different patient populations and will not be presented in this chapter.

◆ What Are Middle Ear Implants?

Like conventional hearing aids, MEIs pick up sound with a microphone and have circuitry for signal processing. Unlike the output speaker (or receiver) of a conventional hearing aid that delivers amplified sound through the external auditory canal, however, an MEI delivers sound directly to an implanted portion that stimulates some structure of the middle ear. Thus, there is no electric-to-acoustic transduction as provided by the output speaker of a conventional hearing aid, but rather transduction from electric to mechanical vibratory energy. In most MEIs, the ossicles are the structure receiving the vibrational stimulation; these MEIs are sometimes referred to as ossicular stimulators. Stimulation can also be to a different structure, such as the tympanic membrane itself, or even to the round window to the cochlea.

Types of Middle Ear Implants

In general, MEIs can be divided into three types based on the transduction mode used: piezoelectric, electromagnetic, and electromechanical. Devices of each type have advantages and disadvantages to be considered in terms of such factors as power and efficiency, frequency response, and reliability. The method of delivery of the transduced energy also varies across devices of each type, as described later in this chapter.

Piezoelectric

In the first type of MEI, piezoelectric materials are used for the transducer. These materials have the property that when a voltage is applied, there is a resulting deformation of the material that can be used as the mechanical energy to stimulate the middle ear ossicles or other structure. Piezoelectric devices are typically found in two basic configurations: the monomorph, which utilizes expansion and contraction of the material directly to provide displacement, and the bimorph, which uses two pieces of piezoelectric materials bonded together with opposite polarities to cause bending of the structure. This is illustrated schematically in **Fig. 13–1**. There are many piezoelectric materials available, but lead titanate zirconate is a material often chosen due to its high efficiency (Dumon et al, 1995; Yanagihara et al, 1983).

The major disadvantage with piezoelectric devices is that there appears to be an inherent limitation in output and frequency response capability. At least with current piezoelectric materials, gain does not appear to be as high as that achieved with other types of MEIs, and there is controversy about whether adequate high-frequency response energy can be achieved for as broad a bandwidth. This may prevent production of high enough levels of amplification for the patient with moderate to severe hearing loss who is currently the primary target for candidacy of most MEIs, because these are the patients believed most likely to receive insufficient benefit from conventional hearing aids. The development of new piezoelectric materials in the future may result in higher power/gain devices of this type.

Electromagnetic

In the electromagnetic type of MEI, the transducer consists of a magnet and an energizing coil. The magnet, which is usually of the "rare earth" type (either samarium cobalt or neodymium iron boron), is attached to either the ossicular chain or the round window membrane. A fluctuating magnetic field is generated when the coil is energized by a signal corresponding to the acoustic input, and the magnetic field causes the magnet to vibrate. This in turn causes movement of either the ossicular chain or the cochlear fluids directly, depending on where the magnet is placed. This concept is illustrated in **Fig. 13–2**.

Coils in the electromagnetic devices are generally "air core," which means the wire is not wound around a ferrous metal core. Although it is true that a ferrous core coil will increase power output, there are some disadvantages to this

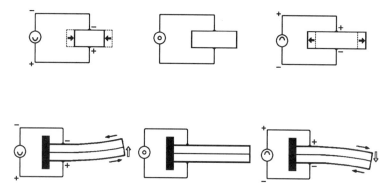

Figure 13–1 (A) Piezoelectric transducers work on the principle that when a voltage is applied across the material, it will contract or expand, depending on the direction of current flow. **(B)** If two piezoelectric materials are bonded together with opposing polarities, then as a voltage is applied across this bimorphic material, one will expand, while the other will contract. It is this "push-pull" action that causes the bimorph to bend. (From Yanagihara, N., Gyo, K., Suzuki, K., & Araki, H. (1983). Perception of sound through direct oscillation of the stapes using a piezoelectric ceramic bimorph. Annals of Otology, Rhinology, and Laryngology, 92(3, Pt. 1), 223–227, with permission.)

configuration. There is a tendency for the magnet to be attracted to the ferrous core, and this can cause a bias of the magnet toward the core when it is inactive, potentially dislodging it. For the same reason, only a "push force" is generated by the coil, causing the magnet to only be pushed toward the ossicle, not pulled away from it. Also, magnet weight must be kept at 50 mg or less (Goode, 1989) so that a substantial "mass effect" is not produced, altering the frequency response characteristics of the ossicular chain and thus reducing the higher frequency response.

In all electromagnetic devices, another common problem is that the magnet and coil must be close to one another to provide an efficient transmission system. The force generated is inversely proportional to the square of the distance between the components, so that, for example, a doubling of the distance between the magnet and coil results in an output force of only one fourth of that produced at the original distance. If the relationship between the components varies, for instance, due to displacement of the coil with jaw movement, there may be variations in the frequency response and fluctuations in the output level.

Electromechanical

The third type of MEI was partly designed as a response to the problem of varying magnet and coil distance, and can be considered a subtype of the electromagnetic devices. With electromechanical MEIs, the energizing coil and magnet are housed together within a single assembly so optimized spatial and geometric relationships are maintained. The mechanical energy produced is transmitted by a direct connection of the electromechanical transducer to (usually) the ossicular chain, as illustrated schematically in **Fig. 13–3**.

An advantage of this type of device is that it can be designed as a closed magnetic circuit, which is more efficient and can have a more flexible frequency response. A disadvantage of this technique is that it is generally a more complex device and therefore more susceptible to fatigue factors. The greater the number of components comprising the transducer, the greater the possibility of a device failure due to component wear or defect. Also, the design process is longer, and it is more difficult to produce a reliable device than for the other transduction methods.

Hardware and Software

The hardware and software of most MEIs are based on conventional air-conduction hearing aid components and signal-processing algorithms. In some MEIs, a conventional air-conduction hearing aid has simply been modified to transcutaneously transmit the signal to the implant via a radio-frequency (RF) link. Other implantable devices have developed special-purpose hardware and software, but without deviating significantly from the types of signal processing used in conventional hearing aids. Signal processing in MEIs has ranged from simple analog linear

— Coil leads connected to signal source

— Electromagnetic coil

Magnet attached to middle ear structure
(ossicle, round window, etc.)

Figure 13–2 Schematic of electromagnetic theory. Electromagnetic devices send the processed audio signal through leads to an electromagnetic coil. The magnetic field generated by this coil causes the magnet to vibrate in synchrony with the signal, thus causing the ossicle to also be vibrated.

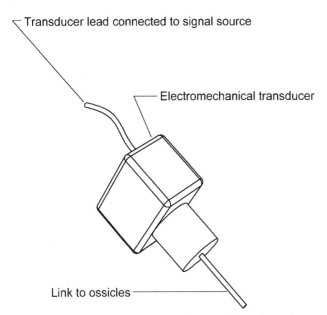

Transducer lead connected to signal source

Electromechanical transducer

Link to ossicles

Figure 13–3 Schematic illustration of electromechanical stimulation theory, used in a subcategory of electromagnetic devices. Electromagnetic transducers generate vibratory motion in synchrony with the signal but within an enclosure. This mechanical stimulus is then transmitted to the ossicular chain via a physical link to the ossicles (as opposed to a magnetic field link).

amplification to state-of-the-art digital signal processors incorporating multiband filtering and multichannel compression, depending on the stage of development of the device.

After implantation by an ear, nose, and throat (ENT) surgeon and a sufficient healing period, the fitting and adjustment of an MEI are accomplished by an audiologist, as with conventional hearing aids and cochlear implants. Fitting algorithms for MEIs at this time are also essentially based on current knowledge of fitting conventional hearing aids, including use of common prescriptive formulas (see Chapters 4 and 5 for information on prescriptive formulas for use in children and adults). As more knowledge is gained regarding differences between direct vibratory middle ear stimulation and conventional stimulation via air conduction hearing aids, both signal processing and fitting techniques will likely need to be adjusted to take into account different characteristics of stimulation with the implanted device.

Pearl

- Because the goals of fitting for conventional hearing aids and MEIs are essentially the same, similar approaches can be used to verify the fittings. Aided thresholds can be used to verify the adequacy of gain for low-level inputs, and for those devices incorporating compression, loudness measurements, and speech recognition at soft, conversational, and loud input levels can be used to assess suprathreshold performance.

Pitfall

- Because many MEIs place internal components in a recess in the mastoid bone, when a bone vibrator is placed on the mastoid postsurgery for measurement of bone-conduction thresholds, it can sometimes set an MEI into vibration and result in thresholds that actually appear improved relative to preoperative measures. This, of course, is not a true reflection of cochlear function in the implanted ear, but merely a measurement artifact. If this occurs, forehead bone vibrator placement can be used instead of mastoid placement (with appropriate calibration or correction factors applied, and masking of the non–test ear as needed).

Materials and Biocompatibility

Materials used in the design and construction of any implantable device must take several factors into consideration. The electrical conductors chosen must have good conductivity (i.e., low resistance), be accepted by the body (be biocompatible), and be capable of withstanding the hostile corrosive environment of bodily fluids. Gold is a good choice because it is nearly as good a conductor as copper and is highly resistant to corrosion. In addition, gold has been used for decades in other medical devices and instruments. A less conductive but stronger material is an alloy of 90% platinum and 10% iridium. Both platinum and iridium are very resistant to corrosion, and a platinum iridium alloy is well accepted by the body.

In some applications, electrical conductors require insulation. If the conductor is to be subjected to bending, the insulator must be flexible. Often, polytetrafluoroethylene, more commonly known as Teflon, is used for this purpose. A ceramic material is chosen instead if the insulator can be rigid or if it is necessary that it be bonded to a metal, such as an electrical feedthrough in an enclosure. One such ceramic is aluminum oxide, which has a long history of use in ossicular replacement prostheses. Both Teflon and aluminum oxide ceramics are nonreactive and well tolerated when placed in the body. Aluminum oxide and hydroxyapatite are also commonly used where osseointegration of the component is required.

Components constructed of materials that are not biocompatible also must frequently be used in an MEI device, but they must then be hermetically encased in a material that is biocompatible. Titanium and ceramics have both been used for this purpose because they are well tolerated, perform well, and have a long history of success in implantations. Of the two, titanium enclosures are easier to manufacture, because they are sealed by welding after the contents are in place, and not as prone to hermeticity breach from impacts. Titanium is also used for structural components of implanted devices, such as mounting platforms and anchors. Finally, sometimes components of an implant need to be encapsulated in a flexible shell to maintain their positional relationships and to provide a soft surface for overlying tissue. Silicone elastomers, in a cured, solid form, are often used in this role and have been shown to be inert and well tolerated.

Potential Advantages of Middle Ear Implants

As previously mentioned, there are several potential advantages of MEIs. Some advantages result from the fact that MEIs offer better impedance matching with the middle ear than do conventional hearing aids. In a normal ear, the ossicular chain acts to improve the impedance mismatch between the air in the external auditory canal and the cochlear perilymph, so that more sound is transmitted through, rather than reflected from, the auditory pathway. Still, there is a large amount of acoustic energy reflected from the tympanic membrane and, in a hearing aid user, it can leak past the earmold, be picked up by the microphone of a hearing aid, and cause feedback. Furthermore, the output speaker (receiver) of a conventional hearing aid is the "weak link" in that it often introduces significant amounts of distortion in the electric-to-acoustic transduction. Because the outer ear is bypassed with MEIs, the impedance mismatch between the air in the external auditory canal and the fluid of the cochlea is eliminated, thus resulting in the possibility for more energy to be transferred to the cochlea and less energy to be lost due to reflection back out of the external auditory canal. Also, the electric-to-mechanical transduction used in MEIs is expected to create less distortion than acoustic output speakers.

It has been proposed that the more efficient energy transmission in MEIs compared with conventional acoustic amplifiers might provide lower levels of distortion, higher fidelity sound quality, higher levels of usable gain, and a reduced potential for feedback problems. All these things could conceivably result in improved speech recognition scores in difficult listening situations, which would be of great importance to the targeted population.

Because there is nothing worn in the ear canal with most MEIs—for example, the Esteem (formerly Envoy) Hearing Implant (Envoy Medical Corp., St. Paul, MN), the MET Ossicular Stimulator and the Carina (Otologics LLC, Boulder, CO), and the Vibrant Soundbridge (Vibrant Med-El Hearing Technologies GmbH, Innsbruck, Austria)—a clear advantage is that the often significant discomfort of wearing an earmold or hearing aid shell is avoided. Furthermore, patients who have difficulty due to allergies to earmold materials, who have persistent problems with cerumen blockage in an in-the-ear (ITE) hearing aid receiver, or who are predisposed to recurrent bouts of otitis externa when moisture accumulates in the occluded canal could potentially benefit from an MEI. The occlusion effect will not occur in the majority of MEIs, but these benefits may not fully accrue with those models of MEIs that place an energizing coil in the external ear canal, for example, the Direct System from Soundtec Inc. (Oklahoma City).

An additional advantage is cosmetic. Although the authors believe cosmesis should not be a primary reason for invasive implant surgery, some of the semi-implantable MEIs can be unobtrusive if the patient's hair covers the external piece (which is usually placed superior and posterior to the pinna), and there is no unattractive earmold and

tubing, or ITE casing, as with conventional hearing aids. When consideration is made of the fully implantable devices—for example, the Esteem and Carina—the cosmetic advantage is obvious.

Beyond the cosmetic consideration, there are other potential advantages of a fully implantable device. In these devices, all components are placed under the skin and/or in the mastoid bone, including placing the microphone under a thin layer of skin or cartilage. Thus, the patient can actually walk in the rain, take a shower, and even swim while using his or her amplifying device without fear of moisture causing microphone and electronics breakdown. If feedback does not prove to be a problem, these devices may also allow patients to sleep with amplification turned on, thus being able to hear a baby cry or a telephone ring during the night. If the microphone is not placed under the skin in the ear canal, cerumen buildup will also not be a performance issue.

Controversial Point

- Clearly, the fully implantable MEI is the culmination of the search for an "invisible" hearing aid, which also resulted in the development of completely-in-the-canal (CIC) models of conventional hearing aids. Some argue that the additional benefits of fully implantable devices would make them appropriate even for patients with milder degrees of hearing loss who do well with conventional hearing aids. This controversial idea is likely to be hotly debated in the future, particularly because some fully implantable MEIs require disarticulation of a normal ossicular chain.

Finally, one of the potential advantages of some models of MEIs (e.g., Direct System and Vibrant Soundbridge) is that, unlike cochlear implant surgery, MEI surgery may be "reversible." That is, it may be possible that the MEI could later be explanted and the ear more or less returned to its preimplant state, should performance prove less than satisfactory. This will not be possible for those models of MEIs that disarticulate the ossicles for placement of the MEI (e.g., Esteem).

Potential Disadvantages

One must also consider that there are potential disadvantages of MEIs. An obvious one is that invasive surgery is required for placement of the devices, and this comes with its attendant potential complications. Benefits from the device must therefore outweigh the need for surgery; that is, the level of performance and satisfaction must exceed that offered by nonimplantable technology.

The majority of MEIs developed to date have used a surgical approach that includes a postauricular incision and drilling of the mastoid bone, and thus are done under general anesthesia at a hospital as a same-day surgery. Although otologists have been entering the middle ear for many decades through the mastoid approach, MEI surgeries are moderately complex because the surgeon must identify and preserve important anatomical structures as the middle ear is exposed. Surgical risks vary with the type of implant and its method of implementation. There are the common risks associated with any surgery, including infection and wound complications, and the potential for anesthesia reactions. In some procedures, the surgeon is required to work closely enough to the facial nerve to pose a risk of facial paralysis, although this risk is extremely small. Another remote, but possible, risk is trauma to the inner ear caused by excessive manipulation of the ossicular chain. In some MEIs (e.g., Esteem), the ossicular chain is intentionally disarticulated as part of the procedure for placing the MEI, which makes the surgical implantation a nonreversible procedure (i.e., if the device is later explanted, presurgical hearing sensitivity and middle ear status are not restored), and in other devices, there is a risk of accidental disarticulation.

One model of MEI, Direct System, uses a simpler surgical approach, through the external auditory canal. Thus, an advantage unique to this MEI is that the implantation can be accomplished under local anesthesia as an in-office procedure. There are also fewer surgical risks with the procedure and a shorter recovery time.

Surgery time varies across devices, but 1 to 2 hours is typical for most MEIs. Healing time prior to activation of the implant and fitting of the signal processor also vary by device, but ranges from ~8 to 10 weeks, during which time the patient cannot use a hearing aid on the implanted ear. For surgeries in which the middle ear is opened, there must be adequate time for fluid to clear from the middle ear space, as well as wound healing. It is also important to note that, like cochlear implants, persons implanted with an MEI must not undergo magnetic resonance imaging (MRI) after implantation without removal of either the magnet or the entire device.

Although in the early days of development, it was believed that MEIs would "eliminate" the possibility of feedback, this has not been found to be true (except for those devices that disarticulate the ossicles). In fact, although it is not expected to occur as frequently or at as high a level as with a conventional high-power amplifier, feedback has been reported with several MEIs. The mechanism is as follows: the ossicular vibration produced by the MEI transducer actually transmits energy back to the tympanic membrane (as well as onto the cochlea), causing it to act as a speaker diaphragm, producing sound in the external auditory canal that can be picked up by the microphone of the device.

At this point in development, most MEIs are still in semi-implantable form, requiring an external unit and thus being subject to some of the same maintenance and breakdown issues seen with conventional air-conduction hearing aids. The exception to this is that the lack of an output speaker placed in the ear canal precludes some common problems, such as cerumen impaction and breakdown due to canal moisture. The transcutaneous RF transmission used in many semi-implantable devices could have susceptibility to interference, or if the internal RF coil is placed too deeply, to less robust transmission and inadequate magnetism to hold the external coil.

Pearl

- When a feedback problem occurs with an MEI, it can be difficult to resolve. Initial efforts can involve the same types of signal-processing changes used with conventional hearing aids. This may include reduction of gain in the channel in which feedback is occurring, an increased compression ratio, or a lower compression threshold. In intractable cases, an earmold or earplug may need to be used, which will, unfortunately, take away the MEI benefit of an open ear canal.

With fully implantable MEIs, these potential problems are precluded. Currently, however, implantable microphone technology has not been perfected, and there is likely to be at least some loss of sensitivity for a microphone placed under the skin. Finally, if there are reliability problems for implanted components (for semi- or fully implantable models), or if they fail after a period of time, another surgical intervention is needed to repair or replace them. Although some devices allow transcutaneous software upgrades for future technology improvements, an additional surgery will be needed to replace outdated hardware components.

There has also been some notable variability in individual performances with nearly all MEIs developed to date, in that even patients with similar audiometric profiles may perform differently with the device in place. This is probably related to anatomical and physiological differences among ears, and to the fact that placement of the MEI impacts the normal biomechanics of the ossicular chain (e.g., Hüttenbrink, 2001). Ossicular mechanics are complex, and placement of many MEI transducers results in ossicular loading and/or stiffening that changes the resonance of the ossicular chain and reduces efficiency of energy transmission. It also can produce postsurgical air–bone gaps (an iatrogenic conductive hearing loss component) in some patients, for which higher levels of device gain are needed to compensate.

Finally, the cost of implantation with an MEI is high. The cost of the MEI itself may eventually be only a little more than a top-of-the-line digital hearing aid, but there is the additional cost of the surgical procedure to consider.

Special Consideration

- Third-party reimbursement through insurance and U.S. government Medicare/Medicaid programs has been an issue for all types of implantable hearing devices. Cochlear implants were the first to be reimbursed, and the first MEI to be placed on the U.S. commercial market, the Vibrant Soundbridge, also made significant strides in insurance coverage. More recently, the surgery and processor for the Baha bone-anchored hearing aid were approved for coverage by Medicare. It remains to be seen, however, if third-party reimbursement will be available for all MEIs entering the U.S. market.

◆ History of Middle Ear Implants Development

Probably the earliest work on direct stimulation of the middle ear was done by Alvar Wilska more than 70 years ago (Wilska, 1935). Wilska placed iron particles on the tympanic membrane and vibrated them with an electromagnetic field to demonstrate that pure tones could be heard by a subject via mechanical stimulation of the ossicles. In the late 1950s, Rutschmann also successfully stimulated the ossicles by gluing 10 mg magnets onto the umbo of the tympanic membrane and causing it to vibrate via application of a modulated magnetic field by an electromagnetic coil (Rutschmann, 1959). The University of Pittsburgh's Department of Electrical Engineering described the design of an implantable hearing aid in 1967, but a device based on the patent was apparently never fabricated and tested (Goode, 1970).

Although the placement of devices into the middle ear was suggested earlier, the concept was not well developed until the late 1970s (e.g., Fredrickson et al, 1973, Nunley et al, 1976). Early benchtop and animal experimentation during this period paved the way for development of MEIs intended for trial in human subjects. The first evaluations of an MEI in human subjects occurred in Japan in the 1980s (e.g., Suzuki et al, 1985; Yanagihara et al, 1983, 1987). Preclinical research in the field (i.e., work done prior to human implantation) has been conducted for many years by several different groups using a variety of techniques. Laboratory experiments using models and temporal bones have helped researchers to better understand how the middle ear reacts to direct vibrational stimulation. In addition, many animal studies have been performed to evaluate in vivo performance of these devices compared with measurements obtained with acoustic stimulation via earphones (e.g., Dumon et al, 1995; Maniglia et al, 1995; Park et al, 1995; Spindel et al, 1995; Welling and Barnes, 1995). Auditory brainstem responses (ABRs) have been the most common tool for acquiring information about the performance of MEIs in animal studies, but laser Doppler vibrometry (LDV) and other approaches have also been used (e.g., Gan et al, 1997; Javel et al, 2003; Needham et al, 2005).

Special Consideration

- Laser Doppler vibrometry techniques, which have a linear phase response and high accuracy, can be quite useful in assessing small vibratory movement of the ossicular chain (in cadavers or intraoperatively) when an MEI transducer is in place. The technique is based on the Doppler principle, whereby, for example, the acoustical tone of a moving vehicle changes as it passes you by on a highway. The same principles can be applied to light propagation from a laser. When a light wave is reflected by the moving object and detected by the measurement system, the frequency shift can be calculated. For a known wavelength, the velocity of movement or displacement can then be determined from the induced frequency shift.

After preclinical laboratory research, if a device appears promising, it is then taken to clinical (human) trials. In the United States, the FDA regulates clinical trials of medical devices, including middle ear implants. In 2003, the FDA developed recommended guidelines specifically for research on MEIs (http://www.fda.gov/cdrh/ode/guidance/1406.pdf), which, like cochlear implants, are class III medical devices. Typically, a phase I clinical trial is first conducted using a small number of subjects to illustrate general safety of the device and its implantation, as well as the potential for efficacy relative to other available remediation approaches. Upon successful completion, a larger phase II clinical trial is run with the goal of obtaining approval for U.S. commercial release and to support marketing claims. Sometimes a phase III clinical trial is also done, when further information on the device is requested. In other countries, the process for market introduction of a product differs and is sometimes less rigorous. In Europe, a product can be commercially released when it has obtained certification known as the CE mark (officially CE marking). There are several MEIs worldwide that are now in, or have completed, clinical trials, and some devices have been marketed.

Devices Developed to Date

The following section reviews known device development by transducer type, and any known preclinical research, clinical trials, or marketing of the devices as of January 2006. Some MEIs have not moved beyond bench study, whereas others have been commercially released. This review is based on published information in English-language journals and personal communications, but newer work may have been done on some of the devices, as presentation of results has tended to lag behind product development in this field. To date, MEIs have been introduced only for an adult population, not for pediatric patients.

Piezoelectric-based Devices

Rion RDE (Yanagihara and Suzuki; Ehime and Teikyo Universities, Japan) One of the first piezoelectric MEIs was developed as a result of work done since 1978 by Yanagihara and colleagues at Ehime University, in collaboration with Suzuki and colleagues at Teikyo University, both in Japan, and in association with Rion and Sanyo Electric companies (e.g., Suzuki et al, 1985, 1994; Yanagihara et al, 1983, 1987, 1995, 2001). This semi-implantable ossicular stimulator is illustrated in **Fig. 13–4**. It was originally called the PIHA (Partially Implantable Hearing Aid) but was renamed the Rion Device E-type, or RDE. In Japan, the device has been implanted in humans in clinical trials.

Candidates for the Rion RDE are bilaterally hearing impaired and with a mixed loss that is not believed to be well remediated with surgical means or a conventional hearing aid (e.g., due to chronic adhesive otitis media, fibrosis of the tympanic cavity, or tympanosclerosis, with no active middle ear infection at implantation). The pure-tone average (PTA) bone-conduction hearing threshold should not exceed 50 dB hearing level (HL), speech recognition should be > 70%, and the poorer ear should be implanted (Yanagihara et al,

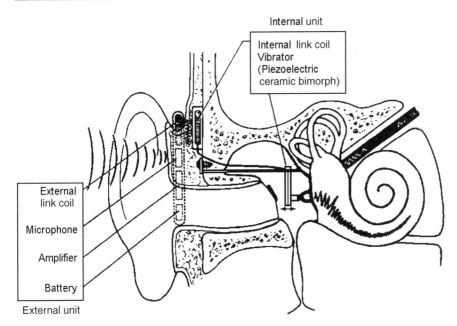

Internal unit

Internal link coil
Vibrator
(Piezoelectric
ceramic bimorph)

External
link coil

Microphone

Amplifier

Battery

External unit

Figure 13–4 The Rion Device E-type (RDE) uses a piezoelectric transducer to provide vibratory stimulus to the ossicles. A subcutaneously placed electronic circuit receives signals from a modified behind-the-ear hearing aid, which holds the processor, microphone, and battery. (From Yanagihara, N., Aritomo, H., Yamanaka, E., & Gyo. K. (1987). Implantable hearing aid: Report of the first human applications. Archives of Otolaryngology–Head and Neck Surgery, 113(8), 869–872, with permission.)

2001). The fact that the surgical procedure requires removal of a portion of the ossicular chain makes this device undesirable for patients with a normal middle ear. One of the techniques used to evaluate the efficacy of this approach and to determine candidacy is intraoperative vibratory testing done during reconstructive middle ear surgeries (Yanagihara et al, 2001).

The Yanagihara and Suzuki device has had some of the longest-term clinical studies of any of the MEIs. In general, patients using the RDE have expressed an appreciation for the good perceptual quality of the sound. In 2001, data were reported for 39 patients fitted with this MEI (Yanagihara et al, 2001). None reported feedback problems with the device, and satisfaction levels were high. For those nine patients who had worn their device for more than 10 years, the mean preoperative PTA air-conduction threshold was 58.1 dB HL (standard deviation [SD] = 8.2), and the mean preoperative PTA bone-conduction threshold was 35.2 HL (SD = 6.8). Three months postoperatively with the MEI, the mean PTA sound-field threshold for these patients was 22.4 dB HL (SD = 6.7). After 10 or more years of usage, the mean PTA sound-field threshold was poorer, at 38.8 dB HL (SD = 6.8), which the researchers attributed to decreased ossicular vibrator sensitivity caused by aging of the mechanism and tissue reaction impeding its vibratory function.

Dumon (University of Bordeaux, France)   Another early device was investigated at the University of Bordeaux, in France (Dumon et al, 1995). This device was used to stimulate the cochlear fluids more directly, in 12 guinea pigs. The device consisted of a small piezoelectric bimorph with a tiny platinum ball extending from the end that was placed in contact with the round window membrane. The other end of the bimorph was anchored in the mastoid bulla. Auditory evoked potentials obtained over a 7-month period illustrated stable and reproducible responses that were similar

to those obtained with acoustic stimulation. This group also developed a method for placing a piezoelectric device in contact with the ossicular chain in human temporal bones. It was reported, however, that there was not always sufficient space in the middle ear for the approach.

Welling and Barnes (Ohio State University)   Welling and Barnes at Ohio State University in Columbus developed a piezoelectric device that was not dissimilar to that developed by Yanagihara and Suzuki (Welling and Barnes, 1995). In several cats, and one volunteer human patient (who was undergoing a posterior semicircular canal occlusion for intractable benign paroxysmal positional vertigo), the ossicular chain and a fenestrated semicircular canal were stimulated intraoperatively for measurement of cochlear microphonics. Results demonstrated good correlation in frequency response and coherence functions between responses obtained with mechanical stimulation with the MEI and with acoustic stimulation. To our knowledge, however, no further development work has been done on this device.

Implex Totally Implantable Cochlear Amplifier (Leysieffer and Zenner; University of Tübingen, Germany)   A piezoelectric-based MEI that was marketed for a time in Europe is the Implex TICA (Totally Implantable Cochlear Amplifier, model LZ-3001). This was the first fully implantable device, developed by Leysieffer, Zenner, and colleagues at the University of Tübingen in Germany (e.g., Zenner and Leysieffer, 1998, 2001; Zenner et al, 2004). The device, shown in **Fig. 13–5,** incorporates a microphone implanted beneath the skin inside the external auditory canal, which provides the signal to a processor placed subcutaneously in a bony recess created in the squamosal portion of the temporal bone. The ossicles are then stimulated by connection to a piezoceramic disk that is controlled by a digitally programmable

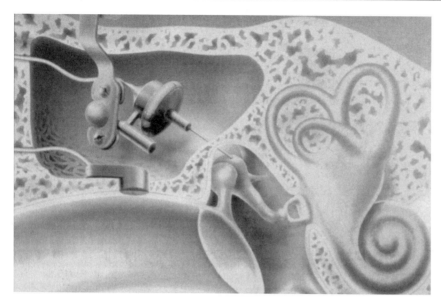

Figure 13–5 The Implex TICA uses a microphone placed beneath the skin of the external auditory canal to pick up the sound in the canal (shown here just above the canal). The signal from the microphone is sent to a processor placed subcutaneously behind the ear (not shown). The processed signal is then sent to a piezoelectric transducer (the cylindrical object with the pin attached to the incus). (From the front cover of the German language journal HNO (Hals-Nasen-Ohren-Heilkunde), 45(10), 1997, with permission.)

three-channel audio processor. The processor battery is recharged via a transcutaneous inductive link, with ~50 hours' usage with 2 hours of recharging time. The patient uses a wireless, inductive remote control that allows selection among four programs, volume adjustment, and an on/off switch.

The TICA is intended for persons with bilateral moderate to severe degrees of high-frequency sensorineural hearing loss (Zenner and Leysieffer, 2001). Specifically, candidates have hearing loss at 500 Hz ≤ 30 dB HL, with a slope of the hearing loss between 500 and 2000 Hz of ≥ 30 dB, leading to a maximum hearing loss at ≥ 3000 Hz of 90 dB HL. Maassen et al (2001) suggested that, with modifications, it might also be useful for patients with conductive or mixed hearing loss resulting from ossicular chain interruption.

In a retrospective study, Zenner et al (2004) reported results from 20 subjects who had been fitted with the TICA. Only 19 finished the study, when 1 subject withdrew due to complaints of inadequate gain. At 6 months postsurgery, 17 of the 19 subjects were reported to have significantly improved phonetically balanced (PB) word recognition with the TICA relative to the preoperative unaided condition (no comparisons were done relative to a conventional hearing aid), and 16 of the 19 felt they received benefit from the TICA relative to unaided listening. Three subjects did not benefit from the implant, and it was noted that many had postoperative air–bone gaps.

Implex's TICA obtained the CE mark and was made commercially available in 1999 in Europe, and there was talk of impending clinical trials in the United States. However, Implex subsequently went out of business. According to Spindel (2002), reasons for the company's demise included device performance problems—insufficient output, negative impact of the device on residual hearing, and feedback. As reported by European surgeons, there was the need for ossicular dislocation in some TICA patients due to unresolvable feedback problems. This was because the microphone

in this device was placed in the ear canal, so that it readily picked up energy reflected outward by the tympanic membrane when the ossicular chain was set into motion by the device. Although the TICA technology was later purchased by Cochlear Ltd. (Lane Cove, Australia), a cochlear implant manufacturer, the device has not been reintroduced to the market.

Hüttenbrink (Technical University, Dresden, Germany) Hüttenbrink and colleagues at the Technical University Dresden, Germany, have proposed a transmission mode based on "hydroacoustic" principles for piezoelectric-transduced sound (Hüttenbrink, 2001; Hüttenbrink et al, 2001). Specifically, in their device, a liquid-filled flexible tube is attached to one end of a piezoceramic transducer that is embedded in the mastoid cavity along with the implanted electronics. The other end of the tube is closed with a soft-walled balloon inserted into the round window niche. The balloon subsequently will pulsate with fluctuations in the fluid produced by the piezoceramic transducer.

Hüttenbrink (2001) reported that preliminary temporal bone studies using a "primitive" prototype of the device demonstrated efficient energy transmission, even at higher frequencies. He further noted that this device might be applicable to cases of ossicular damage in addition to sensorineural hearing loss, and that it precludes problems with efficient positioning on and stimulation of the ossicular chain that have been seen with some other MEIs.

Esteem (Formerly Envoy) (Envoy Medical Corp., St. Paul, MN) The Esteem (formerly Envoy) is another fully implantable MEI, which is intended for patients with moderate to severe sensorineural hearing loss. It was developed by St. Croix Medical (now Envoy Medical). The device incorporates two piezoelectric transducers. One transducer is used to obtain the acoustic signal from the malleus (the sensor), and, after processing in a replaceable subcutaneous

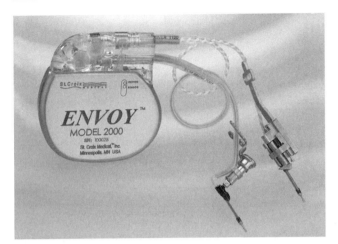

Figure 13–6 Shown is an early version of the Envoy (later renamed Esteem). This device places one piezoelectric transducer in contact with the malleus to detect sound impacting on the tympanic membrane. This provides the signal to the processor (shown on the left), which is placed beneath the skin behind the ear. A second piezoelectric transducer is placed in contact with the stapes and is driven by the processor. (Courtesy of www.stcroixmedical.com.)

component that contains the circuitry and battery, a second transducer is used to stimulate the stapes (the driver). Because the signal is obtained from and then resupplied to the ossicles, the ossicular chain must be made discontinuous to avoid feedback, which is accomplished by removal of a portion of the incus. Patients are supplied with a unit that allows transcutaneous selection of programs volume adjustment, and placement of the device on standby. The implanted sound processor component contains a lithium battery that is nonrechargeable and will require replacement every 3 to 5 years (Chen et al, 2004). An illustration of an early version of the Envoy is shown in **Fig. 13–6**.

After an animal trial phase, two human patients in Europe were reportedly implanted with an early version of this device. Subsequently, a multisite FDA phase I clinical trial was completed during 2002 on seven U.S. subjects. Candidacy criteria included bilateral sensorineural hearing loss with a speech recognition score of ≥ 60% and hearing thresholds in the implanted ear within the following ranges: 35 to 70 dB HL at 500 and 1000 Hz, 40 to 75 dB HL at 2000 Hz, and 40 to 85 dB HL at 4000 Hz. Reliability problems were reported, in that only three of the seven subjects showed benefit at initial activation. Three of the four subjects who did not initially benefit were reimplanted, but only two of these showed benefit at the second activation. Thus, only five of the original seven patients had working systems at the 2-month postactivation interval when key postoperative measurements were taken (Chen et al, 2004).

Using Abbreviated Profile of Hearing Aid Benefit (APHAB) questionnaires, all five recipients with working systems reported perceived benefit increases with the Envoy relative to a preoperative best-fit conventional hearing aid (Chen et al, 2004). The subjects commented that sound quality with the Envoy was more "natural." Functional gain was reportedly comparable at low and middle audiometric frequencies.

However, the. Envoy produced insufficient functional gain at and above 3000 Hz for the National Acoustic Laboratories–Revised (NAL-R) prescription formula (Byrne and Dillon, 1986).

Data labeled "pure-tone air-conduction thresholds" in Fig. 10 in Chen et al, 2004, appear to show unaided and aided sound-field thresholds. These data indicate that mean aided thresholds actually were poorer with the Envoy than a conventional amplifier despite the reported comparable functional gain. This is presumably due to individual decreases in unaided air-conduction thresholds postoperatively, so that more functional gain was needed to overcome the iatrogenic (implantation-related) sensitivity loss. Also, although Chen et al (2004) state that the Envoy showed word recognition performance that "improved significantly over hearing aid conditions," this appears to contradict the graphed data in their article, which show a mean percent correct score for the Envoy that is ~15 to 20% poorer than the mean preoperative hearing aid score. Because no standard deviations or individual data were reported, the degree of intersubject variability is unknown. Finally, it was reported that, due to breaches in the hermetic transducer enclosure, there were decreases in performance and further device failures by 6 months postactivation (Chen et al, 2004). Further work subsequently done by the manufacturer, including replacing the original conformal coating of the transducers with a laser-welded biocompatible metal enclosure, reportedly has made the devices more reliable and produced better high-frequency output. According to the Web site of the manufacturer (www.envoymedical. com), a phase II clinical trial is currently underway in the United States, and the device has received the CE mark and is being implanted in Europe.

Electromagnetic-Based Devices

Maniglia (SIMEHD, Wilson Greatbatch, Ltd.; Case Western Reserve, Ohio) In Cleveland, at Case Western Reserve University, Maniglia and his colleagues developed an MEI, which they called the Semi-Implantable Middle Ear Electromagnetic Hearing Device (SIMEHD; Gaverick et al, 1997; Maniglia et al, 1995, 1997). The device consists of a titanium encapsulated magnet glued to the ossicular chain, stimulated by an electromagnetic coil placed in close proximity in the attic of the middle ear, as shown in **Fig. 13–7**. A subcutaneous RF receiver is placed behind the ear. The target population for this device is patients with symmetrical moderate to severe sensorineural hearing loss and word recognition scores of ≥ 60%.

This device was implanted in seven cats and evaluated over approximately 9 months of in vivo operation (Maniglia et al, 1995). Results showed comparable ABR thresholds to those obtained with acoustic stimuli, and histological evaluation demonstrated no adverse effects. The results of this work led to FDA approval for limited clinical trials, in conjunction with Wilson Greatbatch Ltd. To the knowledge of the authors, however, there has only been preliminary evaluation of this device in one human subject, due to a finding of inadequate power output (personal communication, A. J. Maniglia, 1998).

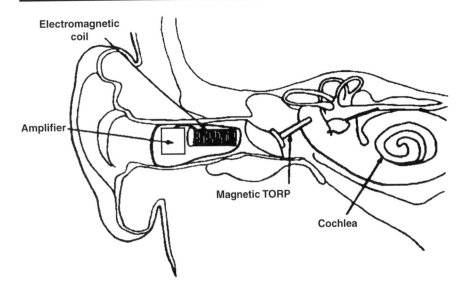

Figure 13–7 Schematic of the Tos and Kartush device. With this device, a partial ossicular replacement prosthesis (PORP) or a total ossicular replacement prosthesis (TORP) with an imbedded magnet replaces part or all of the ossicular chain. The magnet is then caused to vibrate by an electromagnetic coil housed inside an in-the-canal hearing aid shell. (From Tos, M., Salomon, G., & Bonding, P. (1994). Implantation of electromagnetic ossicular replacement device. Ear, Nose, and Throat Journal, 73(2), 92–103, with permission.)

Tos and Kartush (TORP/PORP, Michigan; Smith Nephew Richards Company Another variation of an electromagnetic device was that evaluated by Tos, Kartush, and colleagues at the Michigan Ear Institute (e.g., see Kartush and Tos, 1995; McGee et al, 1991; Tos et al, 1994). This semi-implantable device, evaluated in conjunction with Smith Nephew Richards Company, is intended for patients with mixed hearing loss. In this device, the magnet is encapsulated in a total ossicular replacement prosthesis (TORP) or a partial ossicular replacement prosthesis (PORP). The electromagnetic coil for stimulation of the magnet is placed in a custom earmold in the ear canal. The device is shown in **Fig. 13–8**.

In an FDA-approved pilot study in 1991, the device was placed in nine patients in whom surgical replacement of all or part of the ossicular chain was accomplished (Tos et al, 1994). According to Caye-Thomasen and colleagues (2002), three patients implanted could not be evaluated because one subsequently had a cerebral hemorrhage, one extruded the TORP, and the third had no contact of the TORP with the stapes footplate. Results from the other six patients demonstrated adequate functional gain and reduced feedback relative to a conventional hearing aid, and the patients all preferred the MEI. However, there were problems with obtaining a comfortable and stable fit of the electromagnetic driver in the ear canal, and Smith Nephew Richards company eventually discontinued their support of the project.

Spindel (RWEM; Virginia) Spindel and colleagues from UVA Health Sciences Center, Charlottesville, Virginia, investigated stimulation of the cochlear fluids via an electromagnetic device in which a magnet is placed on the round window membrane (Spindel et al, 1995). This placement is intended to minimize the impact of the device on the ossicular chain, so that residual hearing will be unaffected, and a reverse pathway creating feedback will be avoided.

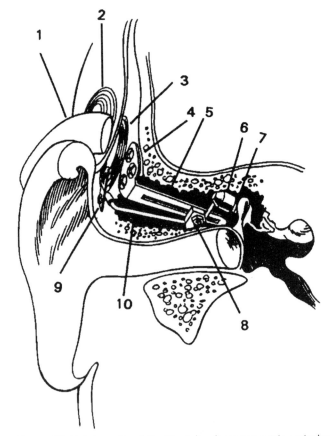

Figure 13–8 Schematic of the Maniglia electromagnetic ossicular stimulator: (1) external unit, (2) transmitting antenna, (3) receiving antenna, (4) horizontal support, (5) vertical support, (6) titanium encased electronics and electromagnetic coil, (7) titanium encased magnet attached to the incus, (8) locking system, (9) electrical feedthrough, (10) malleable titanium tubing. (From Maniglia, A., Ko, W., Garverick, S., et al. (1997). Semi-implantable middle ear electromagnetic hearing device for sensorineural hearing loss. Ear, Nose, and Throat Journal, 76(5), 333–338, 340, 341, with permission.)

Thirteen guinea pigs were implanted and stimulated via an external electromagnetic coil (Spindel et al, 1995). Results from ABR measurements were reported to be comparable for both magnetic and acoustic stimulation with a headphone. More recently, it was reported that the device, called the round window electromagnetic (RWEM) system, is still in preclinical research, now at James Madison University in Harrisonburg, Virginia (Spindel, 2002).

Soundtec Direct System (Hough; DDHS; Oklahoma City)
Hough and colleagues in Oklahoma City also developed an electromagnetic device (e.g., Baker et al, 1995; Hough et al, 1988, 2001a,b). This was the precursor to the Soundtec MEI that was originally called the DDHS (Direct Drive Hearing System) and later simply the Direct System. An early model was evaluated in guinea pigs via measurement of auditory nerve action potentials, and on some human patients undergoing surgery for otosclerosis and chronic tympanic membrane perforation. During the surgery, magnets were temporarily placed on the ossicular chain and stimulated with an electromagnetic coil situated in the external auditory canal. Positive results from these experiments led to FDA approval for a limited clinical trial. In that trial, patients implanted with neodymium iron boron magnets initially showed good results, but the magnets degraded over approximately 3 months' wearing time, and the units stopped functioning. To recover electromagnet function, the magnets were replaced with samarium cobalt magnets. A problem was that, because the samarium cobalt magnets had to be larger to provide the same magnetic strength as the neodymium iron boron magnets, mass damping of the ossicular chain resulted in decreased auditory pathway function.

After some redesign of the original device, Hough and colleagues, in conjunction with Soundtec, again moved forward with FDA human clinical trials. As shown in **Fig. 13–9,** like the Tos and Kartush device, this MEI places the energizing coil in a deep insertion earmold assembly in the ear canal, with a sound processor placed over the external ear. After temporary separation of the incudostapedial joint, a 27 mg neodymium iron boron magnet encased in a laser-welded titanium canister with a ring is slipped onto the stapes. An advantage is that this MEI can be implanted in an otology office using local anesthesia and an approach through the tympanic membrane (as the only implanted component is the magnet). The disadvantage, however, is the potential for problems caused by having an object in the ear canal.

The Direct System underwent phase I clinical trial on 5 subjects (Hough et al, 2001a) and phase II evaluation on an additional 103 patients with moderate to moderately severe bilateral sensorineural hearing loss (and word recognition scores of > 60%) across 10 U.S. sites (Hough et al, 2001b, 2002). In the phase II clinical trial, the subjects' hearing thresholds on average did not worsen significantly from preoperative to postoperative measurements, but it was noted that a few individual subjects did show significant decreases (10–15 dB or more) in air-conduction sensitivity and, more infrequently, in bone-conduction sensitivity. The Direct System showed a mean 7.9 dB increase in functional gain averaged across 500 to 4000 Hz at the 20-week assessment, and

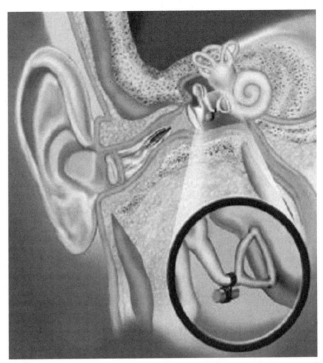

Figure 13–9 In the Soundtec Direct System, an electromagnetic coil replaces the acoustic output transducer (receiver) in an in-the-canal hearing aid. The electromagnetic field generated by this coil causes the magnet attached to the ossicular chain to vibrate, thus transmitting the acoustic energy to the middle ear. (Courtesy of www.depts. washington.edu/hearing.)

a 9.6 dB increase in functional gain at 2000 to 4000 Hz, compared with the preoperative conventional hearing aids. (Again, it is not possible to determine without aided threshold data whether the increase in functional gain was needed to compensate for decreases in air-conduction thresholds postoperatively, or if the increase in fact indicates that the MEI was better able to approximate prescribed gain than was the preoperative hearing aid.) There was a small but significant mean increase of 5.3% in word recognition in quiet with the Direct System versus the conventional amplifier, but the differences for sentences or listening in noise were not significant. Subjective tests using the APHAB (Cox and Alexander, 1995) and a custom-designed questionnaire showed significantly improved scores for the MEI relative to the preoperative hearing aid, including reduced feedback and occlusion effect, and improved sound quality.

In a retrospective case review, Silverstein et al (2005) assessed 64 patients who had been implanted with the Direct System, 4 of whom had bilateral systems implanted. These investigators reported an average functional gain with the MEI of 26 dB and high patient acceptance. The major problems encountered were magnet movement and noise complaints, but these were found to be improved by anchoring the magnet with fat and more careful processor placement.

After the phase II clinical trial, the Soundtec Direct System was approved in 2001 for introduction in a behind-the-ear (BTE) design, and later in an ITE design. After a period of time on the market, however, the Direct System was withdrawn, apparently for further redesign.

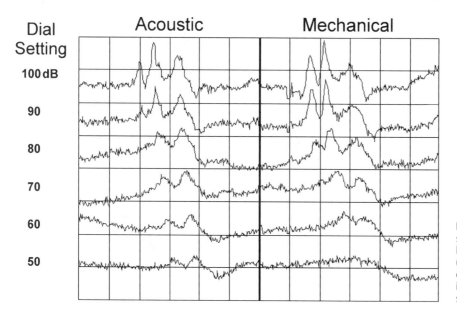

Figure 13–10 An example of auditory brainstem responses obtained from a rhesus monkey through acoustical versus mechanical (Fredrickson device/MET) stimulation of the ossicular chain with click stimuli. Note the similarities in amplitude, morphology, and response threshold.

Controversial Point

- There have been several reports of bilateral implantation with MEIs. At this point, this practice would generally be considered controversial, given that there are still no long-term safety and efficacy data on these devices, and in some MEIs the middle ear cannot be returned to its preimplant status should the device later be explanted. There is still a need to determine, however, whether a unilaterally implanted MEI worn with a contralateral acoustic hearing aid will result in the same binaural processing benefits that occur with bilateral conventional hearing aids.

Electromechanical-Based Devices

Otologics MET and Carina (Frederickson; Washington University School of Medicine, St. Louis; Otologics, LLC,[1] Boulder, Colorado)   Fredrickson and colleagues (including the first author of this chapter) Washington University School of Medicine in St. Louis developed an electromechanical MEI (Fredrickson et al, 1973, 1995), which was the precursor of the Otologics MET (Middle Ear Transducer) Ossicular Stimulator. An early version of the device was implanted in 12 rhesus monkeys for up to 2 years of in vivo evaluation. Results showed comparable morphology and thresholds for stimulation via the electromechanical device versus acoustically with headphones both for ABRs, as illustrated in **Fig. 13–10,** and for distortion product otoacoustic emissions (DPOAE), as illustrated in **Fig. 13–11** (unpublished data collected during the first author's tenure at Washington University School of Medicine). In addition, histological evaluation of chronically implanted ears indicated no deleterious effects from the implant being in place.

Under the auspices of Otologics, the Fredrickson concept was developed into the semi-implantable Otologics MET (Kasic and Fredrickson, 2001), which is intended for patients with bilateral moderate to moderate/severe sensorineural hearing loss. This device is shown in **Fig. 13–12**. The circular external piece, called the ButtonAudio Processor, connects transcutaneously to the implanted electronics and transducer. Internal electronics of the device are placed in a recess in the mastoid bone, and the pistonlike titanium transducer is placed in a hole bored into the long process of the incus, with expected osseointegration during the healing process.

Phase I clinical trials were completed on nine patients using the Otologics MET in the United States, followed by phase II clinical trials on ~77 patients across 11 U.S. sites (Jenkins et al, 2004; Kasic and Fredrickson, 2001). Clinical trial work was also done in Europe and Japan. Jenkins et al (2004) reported results on the U.S. phase II patients, and on an additional 205 patients implanted with the device in Europe. Patients in this study had hearing thresholds in the implanted ear within the following ranges: 15 to 75 dB HL at 500 Hz, 30.0 to 77.5 dB HL at 1000 Hz, 50 to 85 dB HL at 2000 Hz, and 55 to 90 dB HL at 4000 and 8000 Hz. The U.S. patients were evaluated preoperatively with a set of newly fitted digital hearing aids, as well as with their "walk-in" hearing aids, to serve as baseline comparison conditions. Results indicated that mean postoperative bone- and air-conduction thresholds did not decrease significantly relative to preoperative thresholds, although some individual subjects did develop larger postoperative air–bone gaps. Aided thresholds with the preoperative hearing aid were reported to be slightly better than with the MET at 3000 and 4000 Hz, but slightly better with the MET at 6000 Hz. Word recognition scores and APHAB questionnaire results indicated that the MET performed about the same as the preoperative digital hearing aids, and either the same or better than the patient's walk-in hearing aids.

[1]Both authors of this chapter previously worked for Otologics, LLC.

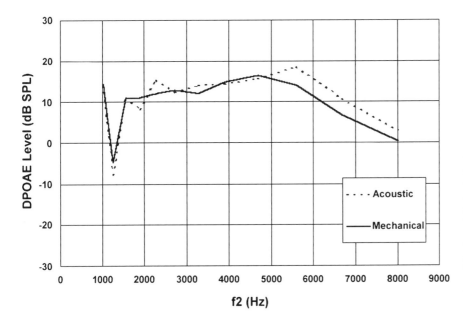

Figure 13–11 An example of distortion product otoacoustic emissions (DPOAE) obtained from a rhesus monkey. A DPOAE "audiogram" was generated using acoustic signals for the first and second primary tones. This was then compared with the DPOAE audiogram generated using the same signals but with the first tone presented acoustically and the second presented via mechanical (Fredrickson device/MET) stimulation of the ossicular chain. As can be seen, the DPOAE level produced by the two primary tones is similar for both modes of stimulation, plotted by frequency of the secondary tone, f2. SPL, sound pressure level.

Figure 13–12 The Otologics MET Ossicular Stimulator. Shown are the external processing unit (the Button Audio Processor), the internal receiving coil and electronics, the anchoring and positioning mechanism, and the transducer tip coupled to the incus. (Courtesy of Otologics LLC.)

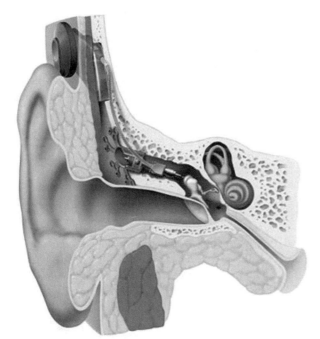

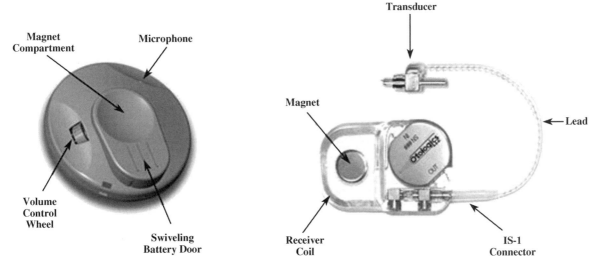

The MET received the CE mark in 2001 and was marketed in Europe, but the company withdrew the product from the FDA approval process in 2003. A fully implantable version of the device, called Carina also has been developed. This device was approved in February 2006 for phase I clinical trial in the United States, and patient recruitment for the study continues. The Carina also received the CE mark in October 2006 and is on the market in Europe. In this device, a capsule containing the microphone and the electronics is implanted in the skin behind the ear, and the implant battery is charged by placing a device over the skin at the location of the implant. No published data on the performance of this fully implantable MEI were available at the time this book chapter went to press, but reports are expected to appear soon.

Med-El Vibrant Soundbridge (Ball; California; Med-El, Austria)   Another semi-implantable device that is electro-mechanical in nature is theVibrant Soundbridge, developed by Ball and colleagues (e.g., Ball and Maxfield, 1996; Gan et al, 1997). This MEI was originally marketed by Symphonix, but is currently being marketed by Med-El (www.vibrant-medel.com). The Vibrant Soundbridge, shown in **Fig. 13–13**, uses a floating mass transducer (FMT) to transmit stimuli to the ossicular chain. The FMT is a small encapsulated magnet that is free to move longitudinally in its enclosure. A coil wound around the outside of the enclosure energizes the magnet, causing it to vibrate back and forth along its axis. This assembly is clipped to the long process of the incus, thereby transferring the motion of the magnet to the ossicle. Power and signal are transmitted via inductive coupling from the external disk-shaped unit to the implanted electronic receiver and transducer.

The Vibrant Soundbridge was given the CE mark in 1998 for marketing in Europe. In 2000, it became the first MEI to

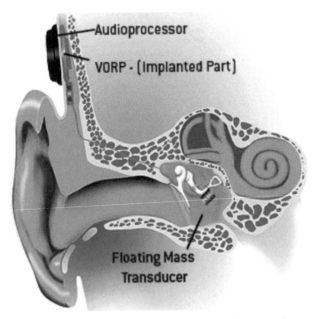

Figure 13–13 The Vibrant Soundbridge consists of an external component containing the processor, microphone and battery, and an implanted component consisting of a subcutaneously placed electronic unit and the floating mass transducer (FMT). The FMT is crimped onto the long process of the incus.

receive FDA approval for use in the United States. Nearly 80 patients were implanted in a phase II clinical trial, and an additional 53 in a phase III clinical trial (Luetje et al, 2002). In the phase III trial, subjects had sensorineural hearing loss in the implanted ear with thresholds within the following ranges: 30 to 65 dB HL at 500 Hz, 40 to 75 dB HL at 1000 Hz, 45 to 80 dB HL at 2000 Hz, and 50 to 85 dB HL at 4000 Hz, and > 50% word recognition scores. The poorer ear was implanted. Subjects were initially fitted with an analog processor (Vibrant P), then 50 of the 53 subjects were refitted with a digital processor (Vibrant D). The subjects, from 11 clinical sites, were followed over a 5-month period. Although a few subjects showed greater decreases, 96% of the subjects had ≤10 dB shift in PTA air-conduction thresholds with the device in place. There was also a significant increase in functional gain for the MEI relative to the preoperative hearing aid, although this did not translate into a significant improvement in phonemically balanced word scores or in Speech Perception in Noise (SPIN) test (Kalikow et al, 1977) low-predictability item scores. Aided thresholds were not reported in this study. Because the preoperative hearing aids were said to reach target prescription gain under the NAL-R formula, it is assumed that the additional functional gain seen for the MEI was needed to achieve target due to small postoperative air–bone gaps. Using a Profile of Hearing Aid Performance (PHAP; Cox and Gilmore, 1990) and a custom-designed questionnaire, a majority of the subjects reported improved sound quality, better speech perception in noise, and better own voice perception with the Vibrant Soundbridge compared with the preoperative hearing aid. There was also a reduction in reported feedback occurrences with the MEI. A negative finding was that patients felt it was harder to use the telephone with the MEI than with the preoperative hearing aid (Luetje et al, 2002).

A consistent finding in published studies that have compared the Vibrant Soundbridge to performance preoperatively with a hearing aid has been reports of improved sound quality and greater patient satisfaction with the MEI (e.g., Fraysse et al, 2001; Luetje et al, 2002; Sterkers et al, 2003; Uziel et al, 2003). Uziel et al (2003) reported that aided thresholds were comparable but that individual performance on speech test measures in quiet and in noise were either equivalent or superior to the MEI compared with a preoperative hearing aid.

One of the concerns expressed regarding many MEIs has been variability seen across individual patients in available gain. Sterkers et al (2003) noted finding the greatest variability in gain across 125 Vibrant Soundbridge recipients at 4000 Hz, a finding they suggested might be related to differences in attachment either due to surgical fixation issues or to patient anatomy. Snik et al (2001) reported acceptable agreement to NAL-R prescribed target values with the MEI for most recipients but relatively low gain for a subgroup of the subjects. For the latter group, the researchers believed this was related to suboptimal positioning and fixation of the transducer to the incus. Needham et al (2005) examined the issue of possible mass loading effects with the Vibrant Soundbridge using LDV measurements of stapes displacement before and after placement of the FMT on the ossicular chain in cadaver temporal bones. Results indicated that placement of the transducer usually did reduce stapes displacement during stimulation, but there were large variations in the degree of loss across temporal bones. Changes in stapes displacement ranged from 0 to 28 dB. The effect was largest at frequencies > 1000 Hz.

As of 2003, there were reportedly more than 800 patients implanted worldwide with the Vibrant Soundbridge (Sterkers et al, 2003). The manufacturer's Web site (www.vibrant-medel.com) reports that thousands of people have now been implanted with the device. Less than 2 years after its U.S. commercial introduction, however, this MEI was removed from the market when Symphonix announced its dissolution, reportedly at least partly due to slow sales. Subsequently, the technology was purchased by Med-El, and the device was again made available in the United States and Europe; however, at the time of this writing, it has been withdrawn from the U.S. market.

◆ Outstanding Issues

Research Design Considerations

At this time, relatively limited data overall have been published from human trials on most MEIs, and because different devices differ considerably, published research on one device may not apply to another MEI design. Thus, the real effectiveness of MEIs in human subjects is still not very clear. In the opinion of the authors, there have been substantial limitations in some of the published MEI studies to date. The following issues should be considered both in evaluating the published research and in planning stronger clinical efficacy evaluations of MEIs in the future.

Special Consideration

- Much of the published research to date on those MEIs that have reached clinical trials has been done either by the company marketing the device or in studies that are financially supported by that company, a situation that can sometimes lead to unconscious bias in research design and analysis. There has also been a paucity of involvement in this field by research audiologists, with much of the work to date accomplished by engineers and otolaryngologists. It is hoped that as MEIs see wider commercial availability, there will be more independent studies on their functioning and efficacy that are conducted by audiologists.

One important factor in studies of these types is the appropriateness of the comparison condition. Some studies have only compared an MEI to the preoperative unaided condition. It is important that the comparison be the nonsurgical alternative of conventional hearing aids. In those studies comparing performance with an MEI to preoperative performance with a hearing aid (similar to the preimplant trial with amplification done for cochlear implant candidates), it has not always been clear whether the preoperative amplification trial represented the "best" (most optimal) aided performance possible. Patients who

volunteer to participate in a study requiring invasive surgery are typically doing so because they are very dissatisfied with their current hearing aids. Obviously, it is important to ensure that their dissatisfaction is not due to a poorly functioning, poorly fitted, or poorly selected hearing aid rather than to poor performance with acoustic amplifiers per se.

Another serious research design problem has been the unfortunate practice of reporting only functional gain across the comparison conditions, without reporting aided (sound-field) thresholds. Because by definition functional gain is the difference between unaided and aided sound-field hearing thresholds at the time of testing, any changes in either measure resulting from the implant surgery will affect the comparison. Of most concern (and a relatively common finding) is when an air–bone gap develops postimplantation because of loss of air-conduction sensitivity via loading of the ossicular chain with the MEI transducer. When this occurs, more gain must be applied by the device to overcome the conductive component, leading to an artificial inflation of functional gain measured with the MEI compared with that measured with the conventional hearing aid. It is "artificial" because it does not represent aided thresholds, which may in fact be the same or better for the preoperative hearing aid condition compared with the MEI. In addition, the goals for both the conventional hearing aid and the MEI fitting should be consistent. If the preoperative hearing aid is expected to match gain prescribed with a formula, resulting in aided thresholds that allow sensitivity to low-level sounds of interest, then the postoperative MEI fitting should meet the same criteria, whether or not additional functional gain is needed to arrive there. The only difference of interest would be the case where an MEI was able to reach good aided threshold levels, and a best-fit hearing aid could not. Given relative parity in aided thresholds, any improvement in perceived performance or speech recognition with the MEI is then a true measure of its suprathreshold efficacy.

Pitfall

- Functional gain is not an appropriate comparison measure if a conductive gap has occurred due to placement of the MEI transducer. For example, a patient shows presurgery functional gain of 15 dB (at a particular frequency) with a conventional hearing aid but postsurgery functional gain of 25 dB with the MEI. Is the MEI "performing better"? Not necessarily. If the patient has developed a 10 dB postoperative air–bone gap due to the impact of the transducer on ossicular mechanics, aided thresholds for both devices are actually the same. If aided thresholds for both hearing devices are good (e.g., 25 dB HL), the fitting goal of good audibility for low-level sounds has been achieved, and additional functional gain is neither needed nor beneficial.

Another important consideration in MEI research is the use of objective measures versus subjective responses, the latter typically obtained from questionnaires. Some studies have placed great emphasis on the patients' subjective impressions of how well they understand speech or think they perform in a noisy listening environment. Although it is important to evaluate improvements in perception of MEI-transduced sound quality and to determine overall patient satisfaction with a device, questionnaire data should not replace objective evaluations of speech understanding in quiet and in background noise.

Special Consideration

- Patients in MEI studies may show a large "Hawthorne effect" because they cannot be blinded to the comparison conditions. That is, patients who have undergone a surgical implantation will want to believe the implanted device performs better than their previous hearing aid, to justify their decision to undergo an invasive implantation procedure. This effect, when present, will bias questionnaire results in favor of the MEI. However, it will only last for a period of time, so longer term studies should help in determining if patients are truly satisfied with their MEIs.

The last research design consideration is the need to report data in a manner that illustrates the range of individual performances that a given MEI can produce. There has been a notable failure to report individual data and indeed even variability statistics for group mean data (standard deviations or standard errors) in many published MEI studies to date. Given the known fairly high variability in intersubject performances found for some devices, this is not good research reporting. Although mean performance improvements with an MEI compared with a preoperative hearing aid are promising, it is also crucial to know whether all individual patients reflect the average trends. Appropriate parametric or nonparametric group statistical analysis methods should also be applied and reported to establish significance of findings.

Special Consideration

- It is unfortunate that many clinical studies in the field of MEIs have not reported individual data, standard deviations of means, or results of statistical analysis. This makes it difficult for the practicing audiologist to counsel individual patients who are interested in MEIs, because the potential risk of poor results for an individual patient is unknown. Consider, for example, that a slight mean performance improvement shown across a group of subjects for an MEI compared with a preoperative hearing aid can reflect two very different underlying scenarios: (1) half of the subjects have much better performance with the MEI, and the other half have poorer performance with the MEI; or (2) all the subjects show small but consistent benefit with the MEI compared with the preoperative hearing aid. Before recommending MEIs to their patients, audiologists should insist that clinical research results from manufacturers include data on individual performance variability in addition to group mean results.

Future Research Needs and Directions

For the potential advantages of MEIs to be fully realized, perhaps the most important need at this time is for a better understanding of the impact of middle ear transducers on the mechanics of the middle ear. Hüttenbrink (1999, 2001) provides a cogent, in-depth discussion of ossicular mechanics and potential problems with many of the available MEI transducer designs. He notes that nearly all available designs fail to maintain normal vibratory modes during stimulation and can produce excessive loading of the ossicular chain. In addition, he notes that a stable attachment of the transducer is necessary for good energy transmission, but that this can be difficult to achieve. Over time a once-solid attachment may degrade, due to normal displacement of the tympanic membrane with changes in ambient and middle ear pressure, the impact of ossicular vibration due to long hours of device stimulation, and the growth of connective tissue at the attachment point. More studies using LDV measurements in cadaver models and intraoperatively during MEI surgeries may assist in better transducer design and attachment techniques that will maximize efficient and stable energy transmission to the cochlea, and minimize damage to middle ear structures.

Even with a good transducer design and stable placement, there are likely to be differences in the manner in which sound is transmitted from an MEI to the cochlea versus how sound is transmitted in the unloaded ossicular chain via an acoustic amplifier. As knowledge is increased about differences between MEI-amplified sound and preoperative acoustic-amplified sound in frequency response and bandwidth, loudness dynamic range, and other parameters, modifications appropriate for MEIs can be made to prescriptive formulas developed for conventional hearing aids. Furthermore, unless it is determined that there is minimal intersubject performance variability with MEIs, which is not currently the case, then methods need to be developed for more accurate individualized fitting and evaluation of MEIs. In other words, ideally there needs to be a way to evaluate individual suprathreshold performance with an MEI that is akin to the use of probe microphone measurements in conventional hearing aid fittings. Some work has been done in this area by Otologics with development of a method to individually measure electromechanical thresholds, loudness, and dynamic range for use in more accurate fitting of the MET and Carina. Their measurement methods are device-specific, however, and not applicable to other MEIs.

Future developments in conventional air-conduction hearing aids may benefit MEI development as well. For example, higher processing speeds and lower power consumption of new digital signal-processing circuits provide greater flexibility in frequency shaping and permit a wider frequency response that may prove to be particularly beneficial with some MEIs. Additionally, multimicrophone and beamforming technologies now appearing in commercial conventional instruments and being evaluated in research laboratories for improvement of signal-to-noise ratio (SNR) may be applied to fully implantable MEIs, because more than one microphone could be implanted under the skin with less cosmetic concern than when external placement is needed.

Development of better battery and microphone technologies for fully implantable hearing devices is still needed and will likely build on work in other medical areas. For example, cardiac pacemaker companies have already produced prototype implantable rechargeable batteries that produce no by-products during charging and that remain functional for > 1000 charging cycles, making them suitable for use in the body. This is the approach used with the Envoy device. The disadvantage is that the battery eventually must be replaced. Batteries for other fully implantable MEIs developed to date require recharging every few days through a transcutaneous link. Higher capacity batteries and lower power circuits can be expected to evolve, increasing time of use between recharging.

Microphones that are constructed of biocompatible materials (or encased in them) are also being investigated for use in fully implantable MEIs. Techniques for placing these microphones to avoid a loss of sensitivity due to fibrosis or migration (movement) of the microphone are important considerations. The major challenge in developing an implantable microphone lies in enclosing a conventional, most likely electret, microphone in a biocompatible case in such a way as to not reduce its sensitivity or significantly affect its frequency response due to the enclosure. Alternatively, a microphone constructed completely of biocompatible materials might eventually be developed. For example, modern microchip technology could be used to construct a microphone from silicon, a ceramic material used successfully in the body for many years. Another important consideration will be to develop an implanted microphone that will not convey biological noise (e.g., blood flow) to the signal processor.

♦ Summary

At this time, it seems reasonable to conclude that semi-implantable MEIs would not generally be considered appropriate for patients with mild to moderate sensorineural hearing loss who perform satisfactorily with conventional hearing aids. Even though fully implantable models theoretically offer additional benefits that might arguably be applicable even to persons with milder hearing loss, it is the opinion of the authors that it is not reasonable at this point in development for this technology to be applied to patients who have viable nonsurgical alternatives. At the other end of the audiogram, as cochlear implants have evolved and are routinely providing good open-set speech recognition for many patients, they are becoming the intervention of choice for those in the severe hearing loss range (as well as for more profound hearing losses). Furthermore, MEIs to date have not been able to produce gain and output results initially hoped for, particularly without producing feedback. Finally, there are research efforts under way to develop fully implantable cochlear implants, and also hybrid devices that would combine cochlear implant and hearing aid technology into a single device for those patients who have residual low-frequency hearing but severe to profound high-frequency hearing loss. These latter efforts, combined with continuing improvements in conventional hearing aid technology, have resulted in candidacy ranges that significantly overlap the target population for those MEIs intended for sensorineural hearing loss. Much more research will need to be done before it becomes clear which type of hearing device will ultimately result in best patient performance for given degrees of hearing loss.

At this time, then, most MEIs are most applicable to a niche group—specifically, those with moderate to moderately severe sensorineural hearing loss who are not performing well or are dissatisfied with even the best conventional hearing aids, but whose hearing loss does not reach the degree needed for cochlear implant candidacy. In addition, MEIs that do not place anything in the outer ear canal may be a viable alternative for persons who should not have their ear canals occluded, for instance, because of chronic otitis externa or earmold irritation. Some of the special-purpose MEIs (e.g., Rion RDE) may also be a good alternative for patients who have mixed or conductive hearing loss that is not amenable to full surgical or medical correction, particularly if they can be placed during routine middle ear reconstruction surgery.

So, how well are MEIs performing to date? In the years since the authors wrote a chapter on MEIs for the first edition of this textbook, some investigational reports on MEIs have shown promising results, particularly in terms of the perceived quality and "naturalness" of MEI-transduced sound compared with that from a preoperative conventional hearing aid. However, there have been few findings of significant improvement in speech recognition with an MEI, and only some reports of inadequate gain and/or instability of device performance over time. The overall commercial viability of these devices is still a question given the market withdrawal of several devices due to poor sales and/or performance. In some ways, though, the technology is still in its infancy, and it is too early to know whether MEIs will eventually realize their full potential. There are many university research groups and private companies investing large amounts of money, time, and talent into the development of MEIs, so future research with redesigned devices may show better results. There is every reason to expect more MEI models to appear in the future, so the practicing audiologist will want to watch for and carefully evaluate the MEI literature as it emerges.

References

Baker, R. S., Wood, M., & Hough, J. (1995). The implantable hearing device for sensorineural hearing impairment: The Hough Ear Institute experience. Otolaryngologic Clinics of North America, 28(1), 147–153.

Ball, G., & Maxfield, B. (1996). Floating mass transducer for middle ear applications. Paper presented at the Second International Symposium on Electronic Implants, Gothenburg, Sweden.

Byrne, D., & Dillon, H. (1986). The National Acoustic Laboratories' (NAL) new procedure for selecting the gain and frequency response of a hearing aid. Ear and Hearing, 7(4), 257–265.

Caye-Thomasen, P., Hedegaard Jensen, J., Bonding, P., & Tos, M. (2002). Long-term results and experience with the first-generation semi-implantable electromagnetic hearing aid with ossicular replacement device for mixed hearing loss. Otology and Neurotology, 23, 904–911.

Chen, D. A., Backous, D., Arriaga, M., et al. (2004). Phase I clinical trial results of the Envoy system: A totally implantable middle ear device for sensorineural hearing loss. Otolaryngology–Head and Neck Surgery, 131(6), 904–916

Cox, R. M., & Alexander, G. (1995). The abbreviated profile of hearing aid benefit. Ear and Hearing, 16(2), 176–186.

Cox, R. M., & Gilmore, C. (1990). Development of the Profile of Hearing Aid Performance (PHAP). Journal of Speech and Hearing Research, 33(2), 343–357.

Dumon, T., Zennaro, O., Aran, J., & Bebear, J. (1995). Piezoelectric middle ear implant preserving the ossicular chain. Otolaryngologic Clinics of North America, 28(1), 173–187.

Fraysse, B., Lavieille, J., Schmerber, S., et al. (2001). A multicenter study of the Vibrant Soundbridge middle ear implant: Early clinical results and experience. Otology and Neurotology, 22(6), 952–961.

Fredrickson, J. M., Coticchia, J., & Khosla, S. (1995). Ongoing investigations into an implantable electromagnetic hearing aid for moderate to severe sensorineural hearing loss. Otolaryngologic Clinics of North America, 28(1), 107–120.

Fredrickson, J. M., Tomlinson, D., Davis, E., & Odkuist, L. (1973). Evaluation of an electromagnetic implantable hearing aid. Canadian Journal of Otolaryngology, 2, 53–62.

Gan, R. Z., Wood, M., Ball, G., et al. (1997). Implantable hearing device performance measured by laser Doppler interferometry. Ear, Nose, and Throat Journal, 76(5), 297–309.

Gaverick, S. L., Kane, M., Ko, W., & Maniglia, A. (1997). External unit for a semi-implantable hearing device. Ear, Nose, and Throat Journal, 76(6), 397–401.

Goode, R. L. (1970). An implantable hearing aid: State of the art. Transactions of the American Academy of Ophthalmology and Otolaryngology, 74(1), 128–139.

Goode, R. L. (1989). Current status of electromagnetic implantable hearing aids. Otolaryngologic Clinics of North America, 22(1), 201–209.

Hough, J., Dormer, K., Baker, R., et al. (1988). Middle ear implantable hearing device: Ongoing animal and human evaluation. Annals of Otology, Rhinology and Laryngology, 97, 650–658.

Hough, J. V., Dyer, R., Jr., Matthews, P., & Wood, M. (2001a). Semi-implantable electromagnetic middle ear device for moderate to severe sensorineural hearing loss. Otolaryngologic Clinics of North America, 34(2), 401–416.

Hough, J. V., Dyer, R., Jr., Matthews, P., & Wood, M. (2001b). Early clinical results: SOUNDTEC Implantable Hearing Device Phase II Study. Laryngoscope, 111(1), 1–8.

Hough, J. V., Matthews, P., Wood, M., & Dyer, R., Jr. (2002). Middle ear electromagnetic semi-implantable hearing device: Results of the Phase II SOUNDTEC Direct System clinical trial. Otology and Neurotology, 23(6), 895–903.

Hüttenbrink, K. B. (1999). Current status and critical reflections on implantable hearing aids. American Journal of Otology, 20(4), 409–415.

Hüttenbrink, K. B. (2001). Middle ear mechanics and their interface with respect to implantable electronic otologic devices. Otolaryngologic Clinics of North America, 34(2), 315–335.

Hüttenbrink, K. B., Zahnert, T., Bornitz, M., & Hofmann, G. (2001). Biomechanical aspects in implantable microphones and hearing aids and the development of a concept with a hydroacoustical transmission. Acta Otolaryngologica, 121(2), 185–189.

Javel, E., Grant, I., & Kroll, K. (2003). In vivo characterization of piezoelectric transducers for implantable hearing aids. Otology and Neurotology, 24(5), 784–795.

Jenkins, H. A., Niparko, J., Slattery, W., et al. (2004). Otologics Middle Ear Transducer Ossicular Stimulator: Performance results with varying degrees of sensorineural hearing loss. Acta Otolaryngologica, 124, 391–394.

Kalikow, D. N., Stevens, K. N., & Elliott, L. L. (1977). Development of a test of speech intelligibility in noise using sentence materials with controlled word predictability. Journal of the Acoustical Society of America, 61, 1337–1351.

Kartush, J. M., & Tos, M. (1995). Electromagnetic ossicular augmentation device. Otolaryngologic Clinics of North America, 28(1), 155–172.

Kasic, J. F., & Fredrickson, J. (2001). The Otologics MET ossicular stimulator. Otolaryngologic Clinics of North America, 34(2), 501–513.

Luetje, C. M., Brackman, D., Balkany, T., et al. (2002). Phase III clinical trial results with the Vibrant Soundbridge implantable middle ear hearing device: A prospective controlled multicenter study. Otolaryngology–Head and Neck Surgery, 126(2), 97–107.

Maassen, M. M., Lehner, R., Leysieffer, H., et al. (2001). Total implantation of the active hearing implant TICA for middle ear disease: A temporal bone study. Annals of Otology, Rhinology, and Laryngology, 110(10), 912–916.

Maniglia, A. J., Ko, W., Rosenbaum, M., et al. (1995). Contactless semi-implantable electromagnetic middle ear device for the treatment of sensorineural hearing loss: Short-term and long-term animal experiments. Otolaryngologic Clinics of North America, 28(1), 121–140.

Maniglia, A. J., Ko, W., Garverick, S., et al. (1997). Semi-implantable middle ear electromagnetic hearing device for sensorineural hearing loss. Ear, Nose, and Throat Journal, 76(5), 333–341.

McGee, T. M., Kartush, J., Heide, J., et al. (1991). Electromagnetic semi-implantable hearing device: Phase I clinical trials. Laryngoscope, 101(4, Pt. 1), 355–360.

Miller, D., & Fredrickson, J. (2000). Implantable hearing aids. In M. Valente (Ed.), Audiology: Treatment (pp. 489–510). New York: Thieme Medical Publishers.

Needham, A. J., Jiang, D., Bibas, A., et al. (2005). The effects of mass loading the ossicles with a floating mass transducer on middle ear transfer function. Otology and Neurotology, 26(2), 218–224.

Nunley, J. A., Agnew, J., & Smith, G. (1976). A new design for an implantable hearing aid. Biomedical Sciences Instrumentation, 12, 69–72.

Park, J. Y., Coticchia, J., & Clark, W. (1995). Use of distortion product otoacoustic emissions to assess middle ear transducers in rhesus monkeys. American Journal of Otology, 16(5), 576–590.

Rutschmann, J. (1959). Magnetic audition: Auditory stimulation by means of alternating magnetic fields acting on a permanent magnet fixed to the eardrum. IRE Transactions on Medical Electronics, 6, 22–23.

Silverstein, H., Atkins, J., Thompson, J., Jr., & Gilman, N. (2005). Experience with the Soundtec implantable hearing aid. Otology and Neurotology, 26(2), 211–217.

Snik, A. F., Mylanus, E., Cremers, C., et al. (2001). Multicenter audiometric results with the Vibrant Soundbridge, a semi-implantable hearing device for sensorineural hearing impairment. Otolaryngologic Clinics of North America, 34(2), 373–388.

Spindel, J. H. (2002). Middle ear implantable hearing devices. American Journal of Audiology, 11, 104–113.

Spindel, J. H., Lambert, P., & Ruth, R. (1995). The round window electromagnetic implantable hearing aid approach. Otolaryngologic Clinics of North America, 28(1), 189–205.

Sterkers, O., Boucarra, D., Labassi, S., et al. (2003). A middle ear implant, the Symphonix Vibrant Soundbridge: Retrospective study of the first 125 patients implanted in France. Otology and Neurotology, 24, 427–436.

Suzuki, J., Kodera, K., Nagai, K., & Yabe, T. (1994). Long-term clinical results of the partially implantable piezoelectric middle ear implant. Ear, Nose, and Throat Journal, 73(2), 104–107.

Suzuki, J., Kodera, K., & Yanagihara, N. (1985). Middle ear implant for humans. Acta Otolaryngologica, 99(3–4), 313–317.

Tos, M., Salomon, G., & Bonding, P. (1994). Implantation of electromagnetic ossicular replacement device. Ear, Nose, and Throat Journal, 73(2), 92–103.

Uziel, A., Mondain, M., Hagen, P., et al. (2003). Rehabilitation for high-frequency sensorineural hearing impairment in adults with the Symphonix Vibrant Soundbridge: A comparative study. Otology and Neurotology, 24(5), 775–783.

Welling, D. B., & Barnes, D. (1995). Acoustic stimulation of the semicircular canals. Otolaryngologic Clinics of North America, 28(1), 207–219.

Wilska, A. (1935). Ein methode zur bestimmung der horsch wellanamplituden des trommelfells bei verscheiden frequenzen. Skandinavisches Archiv für Physiologie, 72, 161–165.

Yanagihara, N., Aritomo, H., Yamanaka, E., & Gyo, K. (1987). Implantable hearing aid: Report of the first human applications. Archives of Otolaryngology–Head and Neck Surgery, 113(8), 869–872.

Yanagihara, N., Gyo, K., & Hinohira, Y. (1995). Partially implantable hearing aid using piezoelectric ceramic ossicular vibrator: Results of the implant operation and assessment of the hearing afforded by the device. Otolaryngologic Clinics of North America, 28(1), 85–97.

Yanagihara, N., Gyo, K., Suzuki, K., & Araki, H. (1983). Perception of sound through direct oscillation of the stapes using a piezoelectric ceramic bimorph. Annals of Otology, Rhinology, and Laryngology, 92(3, Pt. 1), 223–227.

Yanagihara, N., Sato, H., Hinohira, Y., et al. (2001). Long-term results using a piezoelectric semi-implantable middle ear hearing device: The Rion Device E-Type. Otolaryngologic Clinics of North America, 34(2), 389–400.

Zenner, H. P., & Leysieffer, H. (1998). Totally implantable hearing device for sensorineural hearing loss. Lancet, 352, 1751.

Zenner, H. P., & Leysieffer, H. (2001). Total implantation of the Implex TICA hearing amplifier implant for high-frequency sensorineural hearing loss: The Tübingen University experience. Otolaryngologic Clinics of North America, 34(2), 417–446.

Zenner, H. P., Limberger, A., Baumann, J., et al. (2004). Phase III results with a totally implantable piezoelectric middle ear implant: Speech audiometry, spatial hearing and psychosocial adjustment. Acta Otolaryngologica, 124, 155–164.

Chapter 14

Cochlear Implants in Children

Patricia M. Chute and Mary Ellen Nevins

The medical, audiologic, and educational management of children with severe to profound hearing loss has been dramatically altered by the introduction of cochlear implants. Children born with severe to profound deafness are now provided with technological options that can afford them better access to speech and language through audition. The process of receiving a cochlear implant involves the combined efforts of audiologists, speech-language pathologists, educators, and otologists for the implantation of the device.

This medical/surgical/educational treatment, however, requires monitoring throughout the lifetime of the child. Health care institutions that were once responsible solely for the diagnosis of hearing impairment are currently involved in the comprehensive (re)habilitation of children with hearing loss in an unprecedented manner. As implant technology has matured, the demands of time and money on health care systems has become greater. Although the impact of cochlear implant technology on the education of children with severe to profound hearing loss is still evolving, studies point to successful integration of implant recipients into the mainstream at younger ages (Chute and Nevins, 2006; Geers and Brenner, 2003; Niparko et al, 2001). As this generation of children with implants passes through the educational system, the outcomes of implantation appear promising. In general, overall performance of children and adults with cochlear implants has been impressive enough to support three manufacturers in the United States.

At present, cochlear implantation is an option available to profoundly deaf children between 12 and 24 months of age whose hearing levels are 90 dB hearing level (HL) or greater. For children older than 24 months, a severe sensorineural hearing loss (pure-tone average [PTA] 70 dB or greater) places them within the candidacy criteria. As more states in the United States embrace the concept of universal newborn hearing screening, the number of younger children who are identified as having a hearing loss will increase. Thus, an additional responsibility exists for providing a range of services for deaf and hard-of-hearing children, including not only cochlear implants but also hearing aids and other sensory devices.

In the final analysis, the number of children receiving cochlear implants will be most affected by (1) changes in hearing aid technology, (2) the comparison of hearing aid benefit to performance with cochlear implants, (3) financial and technical support of medical and government agencies, and (4) manpower issues as the need for qualified professionals increases. Any of these issues can have a direct effect on the number of children seeking and receiving cochlear implants. Each of these issues will be addressed as factors to be considered when choosing cochlear implantation for a child.

◆ Recent Advances in Hearing Aid Technology

Hearing aid technology has changed substantially over the last decade (see Chapters 1, 6, and 12) as devices have become smaller and have provided better performance in difficult listening situations. Advanced signal processing and programmability have provided hearing aid wearers with instruments that offer choices depending on the listening environment; multiple memory hearing aids that offer better hearing in a diversity of auditory conditions are currently available. Cosmetically, hearing aids have become smaller and more efficient. For a small segment of the hearing aid population, hearing aids can be implanted when warranted (see also Chapters 13 and 15).

Hearing aids and frequency modulation (FM) systems still support most individuals who have hearing loss. They are the preferred treatment alternative for children whose hearing loss is mild to moderate/severe. It should be noted that some children with severe to profound hearing loss are also capable of performance that enables them to develop good speech, language, and listening skills. Generally speaking,

however, the effectiveness of these sensory aids becomes compromised as the degree of impairment increases.

Although FM systems can provide children with more direct signal input (see Chapters 17 and 18), older children often feel stigmatized by their use. Recently, FM systems have become miniaturized and located in more traditional behind-the-ear (BTE) hearing instruments. This enables children to have access to improved signal-to-noise ratios (SNRs) without the need for cumbersome equipment. Despite good performance in some children with these devices, there remains a group of children who are still unable to obtain substantial benefit from these traditional types of amplification.

◆ Comparing Hearing Aid Benefit to Implant Performance

Predicted benefit from conventional amplification systems often was the criterion by which decisions regarding school placement and mode of communication were made (Moores, 1987; Quigley and Kretschmer, 1982). Children unable to develop acceptable spoken language skills were placed in educational systems that offered manual communication and therefore did not require the use of hearing aids. Those children demonstrating the ability to process some speech through their hearing aids were placed in oral schools recognized for their ability to use residual hearing for speech production. Researchers working with profoundly deaf children explored the wide spectrum of ability found in children in oral schools.

Children who were profoundly deaf with some measurable hearing were often capable of developing adequate speech and listening skills. Children with greater hearing losses (>110 dB HL) did the poorest of the group. Geers and Moog (1987) developed categories of speech perception in an effort to predict whether a deaf child would be capable of developing spoken language. They determined that children who were capable of better speech perception were more likely to develop understandable speech. In an attempt to provide a direct comparison between hearing aid benefit and cochlear implant performance, Osberger et al (1993) identified three distinct groups of hearing aid users within the profound hearing loss group. Subjects were categorized on the basis of PTA and were systematically compared with a group of children who received cochlear implants. These three groups consisted of children whose PTAs were (1) between 90 and 100 dB hearing threshold level (HTL), (2) between 101 and 110 dB HTL, and (3) >110 dB HTL. Overall, children with cochlear implants performed better than children within the two poorer hearing groups. Children with cochlear implants performed as well as and, in some cases, better than the children whose hearing losses were between 90 and 100 dB HTL. Results such as these coupled with steady improvement in processing strategies have driven the movement of audiologic requirements upward on the audiogram, from the corner audiogram to flat losses of 90 dB HL to eventually those with hearing loss in the 70 dB range. This, in effect, creates a larger pool of audiologic candidates and has resulted in an overall increase in children receiving cochlear implants. A list of audiologic candidacy guidelines follows:

1. The child must be between the ages of 12 months and 17 years, 11 months.

2. The child between 12 and 24 months of age must present with a profound bilateral sensorineural hearing loss. The child older than 24 months can present with a severe to profound bilateral sensorineural hearing loss.

3. The child must demonstrate little or no benefit from appropriate binaural hearing aids. A child may demonstrate some open-set speech recognition with traditional amplification and still be considered a cochlear implant candidate. The child must participate in a 3- to 6-month hearing aid trial if there has been no previous aided experience.

♦ Financial and Technical Support for Implants

With growing numbers of parents seeking implantation for their children, the financial support from third-party private and public insurers has become a critical consideration. Because implants are approved for use in children, most health care insurers support this technology. Although the amount of state and federal support in this country for this technology varies, patient access to implants is more widespread than a decade ago. Because a discrepancy often exists in gross charge billed by the implant facility and the actual payment issued from the insurance provider, in some circumstances, costs are borne by the consumer. However, support for cochlear implantation varies from state to state and country to country. For example, in Great Britain and Canada (Summerfield et al, 1997), the government supports the total cost of implantation through the national health ministries. As the trend toward bilateral implantation becomes more widespread, reimbursement both in this country and abroad may become more of an issue. With regard to access, the number of cochlear implant centers in the United States has grown to ~350 (personal communication, C. Menapace, Cochlear Americas, June 2005) from the initial 8 centers involved in the grassroots technology movement of the late 1970s and early 1980s. To become a cochlear implant center, it is recommended (but not required) that personnel attend a training workshop sponsored by the manufacturer. Implant companies support local centers by providing technological assistance and reimbursement services. Because technical and financial support is now available on a more extensive basis, the number of children receiving implants each year is increasing dramatically. However, estimates from the manufacturers suggest that there is still only 20% penetration of the pediatric market potential for this technology (personal communication, C. Menapace, Cochlear Americas, June 2005).

Manpower Issues as the Need for Qualified Professionals Increases

The rapid rise in the number of children with cochlear implants has placed a large burden on implant centers and educational programs as they grapple with identifying professionals with expertise in this area. Chute (2003) surveyed cochlear implant centers and graduate schools in the United States to determine the scope of the problem. The author found that seasoned cochlear implant centers were serving large numbers of recipients with a relatively small number of staff persons. Additionally, most graduate programs were providing limited to no exposure to cochlear implants in their curriculum. Financial issues in clinics following children with implants were also seen as reimbursement rates dropped. More efficient methods of providing services has been explored (Backous, 2005). As the health needs of the baby boomer population grow, the pressure on all aspects of health care will need to be reassessed.

♦ Response from the Deaf Community

It would be a grievous oversight to exclude mention of the response of the deaf community to implantation and how it has evolved over time. Deaf community leaders initially opposed implantation in children; a position paper issued by the National Association of the Deaf (NAD) deplored the cochlear implant process in young children. Some deaf advocates likened implantation to questionable practices in the past, such as reproductive regulation on deaf adults and medical experimentation on deaf children. Federal legislation preceding this technological advance influenced enrollment figures of children in schools for the deaf in the United States. In the 20-year period between 1975 and 1995, more than 50% of children left state residential schools for education in their home regions or districts (Gallaudet University, Center for Assessment and Demographic Studies, 1994). Concerned by this enrollment trend at state centers of deaf culture (i.e., state schools for the deaf), the deaf community viewed the implant as a further threat to its existence and actively urged parents to reject it for their children.

Acceptance of the cochlear implant by the deaf community can be viewed within the context of any new and emerging technology. Initial negative response has matured into tacit acknowledgment of the potential of the device to provide auditory access to those who value it as a communication tool. In fact, a growing number of deaf families are now seeking implants for their children in an effort to provide them with greater opportunities and choices for the future. Issues related to identity of the cochlear implant recipient within the larger deaf community continue to provide challenges in supporting a peaceful coexistence between the two groups. The passage of additional time, and the emergence of a new population of young deaf adults who are successful implant users, will likely shape the perspective of the deaf community in years to come.

When looking back at the developments in implantation over the past decade, there is much that has transpired. It is the purpose of this chapter to bring the reader through the various aspects of implantation: implant design, candidacy, surgical issues, device activation, care and maintenance, habilitation, parental and school roles, performance, educational achievements, implants in special populations, and future considerations. It is intended to provide a knowledge base for many of the issues that face parents, teachers, and allied health professionals who work in the field of deafness and (re)habilitation of children.

◆ Cochlear Implant Design

Basic Implant Function

A cochlear implant incorporates several internal and external components. The internal portion is composed of electrodes, a receiver stimulator, an antenna, and a magnet. Externally, there is a microphone, an external transmitter, cords, and a body-worn or BTE speech processor. Implants function in a manner similar to a hearing aid; however, the final transmission of the signal in the cochlea is markedly different. Incoming sounds are detected by a microphone that is worn by the recipient. Signals received from the microphone are transmitted to the speech processor, where they are analyzed using an algorithm specific to that device. The processed signal is then forwarded through a cord to the external transmitter that is placed in apposition over the internal receiver. The transmitter and receiver are held in place through external and internal magnets. The signal is sent by means of FM transmission through the skin to the internal receiver. The information is frequency analyzed and delivered to the electrodes in a manner that is specific to the speech-processing strategy of the particular device. Because the normal auditory system consists of a great number of functioning hair cells distributed throughout the cochlea, multiple sites of stimulation are more representative of the incoming signals than a single site. Therefore, any attempt at artificially stimulating the neural elements remaining in deafened cochleas is best accomplished at numerous locations.

History and Development

The cochlear implant first received approval from the U.S. Food and Drug Administration (FDA) for use in children in 1990. Its development began back in the mid-1960s with Dr. William House and evolved over the next five decades as the device transitioned from experimental technology to one supported by the manufacturing process. Interested readers are directed to Clark (2002) for a detailed account of the evolution of these devices.

Cochlear implants available today for the pediatric population represent the advances that were made in technology throughout the 2 decades since its approval. Each system differs from the other on several features, and decisions regarding the choice of a device should be made by well-informed parents. Features that need to be considered when choosing a cochlear implant include the following: reliability and performance, speech-processing platforms, flexibility, cosmetics, maintenance cost, and warranty. Additional factors that parents may consider pertain to the level of company support of the product and its projection of future product development.

Currently Available Devices

The three manufacturers in the United States of cochlear implant technology are Advanced Bionics Corp. (Sylmar, CA), Cochlear Americas (Englewood, CO), and Med-El Corp. (Research Triangle Park, NC). Each of these companies supports several generations of devices that have evolved as the industry has grown. There is no doubt that there will be additional generations or devices before this chapter is published. For that reason, the reader is directed to the companies' Web sites listed below to explore the latest technologies available. The main devices are the Nucleus Freedom (from Cochlear Americas), the HiRes 90K (from Advanced Bionics), and the Med-El Sonata (from Med-El). The various generations of these devices have secondary names that change with each new product introduction. For more specific information on each of the devices supported by the manufacturers, consult the following Web sites:

Advanced Bionics Corp.: www.bionics.com

Cochlear Americas: www.cochlearamericas.com

Med-El Corp.: www.medel.us.com

◆ Process of Implantation

Candidacy Selection

The process of implantation can be viewed as a series of stages through which the child and parents must pass: candidacy, surgery, device activation, and habilitation. The first of these stages, candidacy, is critical to the success of implantation in children. The proper selection of children for implantation should be performed by a multidisciplinary team of professionals with knowledge of deafness and childhood development for speech, language, and audition. Team members should include an audiologist, a speech-language pathologist, a surgeon, and, when possible, an educator of deaf children. Many teams also include a psychologist and a social worker. Although the fundamental criteria for implantation are based on audiologic performance, centers experienced with cochlear implants in children have identified other factors that can contribute to successful use of the implant (Chute and Nevins, 2002). These factors may include medical/radiological integrity, speech and language capabilities, educational environment, and parental/child expectations.

Audiologic criteria for implantation are driven by performance with traditional forms of amplification, such as hearing aids, FM systems, vibrotactile aids, and frequency transposition aids. Children must have had access to an adequate trial (at least 3–6 months) with these conventional forms of amplification, as well as adequate training with the aids, before an implant can be considered. Good preimplant listening experiences suggesting a history of consistent hearing aid use coupled with extensive opportunities for developing auditory skills contribute to the positive decision regarding implant candidacy. In other words, children being considered for implantation must be using amplification on a daily basis and be enrolled in programs that value audition.

Pearl

- Audiologic criteria are the first to be evaluated when considering a particular child for an implant. Once hearing testing confirms the child is audiologically a candidate, evaluation in other areas begins.

The role of vibrotactile aids during this candidacy period is sometimes considered for children with very profound losses. In a survey of 14 major implant centers in the United States, it was reported that more than 75% used this type of device during the preimplant training period; however, the percentage of children using vibrotactile aids within each center ranged from 1 to 6%. Approximately 40% of the centers used transpositional technology (high-frequency information is transposed into the low-frequency region, where there is some residual hearing). However, only 3.5% of the children at any given center had access to these devices. The most popular device used during the preimplant period was an FM system for children and hearing aids for adults (Chute, 1997).

Regardless of the device used in the preimplantation period, the measurement of hearing aid benefit from traditional amplification is the key factor considered when identifying an implant candidate. Linguistically appropriate test materials that assess auditory speech perception have been standardized on a population of deaf and hard-of-hearing children and assist in measuring hearing aid benefit and skill growth over time. Designed for children at a variety of language levels, tests were developed for youngsters using conventional hearing aids, tactile aids, and cochlear implants center. Test procedures fall into two basic categories known as closed-set and open-set measures of speech perception. Although the selection criteria for each implant center vary somewhat with respect to the particular tests used to assess benefit, the FDA now allows children with minimal open-set speech recognition to obtain a cochlear implant. Present guidelines permit a score of ≤ 30% on either the Multisyllabic Lexical Neighborhood Test (MLNT) or the Lexical Neighborhood Test (LNT).

Children with some residual hearing have also successfully received implants in the past, and although a range of performance has been seen in this group, the overall results have been impressive. Sehgal et al (2000) reviewed a group of children who had some residual hearing and found that despite variations in performance, most of the children were able to obtain a level of performance that surpassed their previous performance with hearing aids. As more children with residual hearing are implanted, there are growing numbers of them that now use a cochlear implant in one ear and a hearing aid in the other. Studies of Ching et al (2001) demonstrate improved benefit when using both devices together. In no case was a decrement in performance noted. In fact, many children who have been wearing cochlear implants alone are now being refit with a hearing aid in the contralateral ear.

However, for children who receive no benefit from a hearing aid in the opposite ear, there has been a growing trend toward bilateral implantation. Originally, bilateral implantation was not a consideration, as there was little or no indication of the efficacy of these devices. With outcomes that equal or surpass hearing aids, clinicians who fit bilateral hearing aids have begun to question the judiciousness of fitting only one implant. The number of children receiving bilateral implants both simultaneously or sequentially has risen substantially over the past few years (personal communication, C. Menapace, Cochlear Americas, June 2005). Studies have demonstrated improved listening in noise and in quiet as well as localization benefit. Further studies of speech production also indicate trends toward improved speech output by bilateral recipients. In the near future, it would not be unreasonable to think that bilateral implantation will be considered best practice for the field.

Pearl

- Bilateral cochlear implants demonstrate improved benefit and may be considered the new recommendation for families seeking implants for their children.

Special Considerations for Very Young Children

The dilemma presently facing implant teams is in trying to assess children who are younger than 2 years old for implantation. Although the FDA has approved implantation for children 12 months of age, once any device is approved, surgeons may go "off-label" and use the device in other populations. When a device is used off-label, it means that it is being used in a population for which approval has not been granted. For example, in cases of children who were deafened from meningitis and present with ossifying cochleas before the age of 12 months, the device can be implanted once medical necessity is demonstrated.

Audiologic assessment of very young children is performed in two ways: measurement of functional gain (unaided vs aided) afforded by the hearing aids and the use of questionnaires designed to assess daily listening and speaking experiences. Robbins and Osberger (1991) developed two qualitative instruments: the Meaningful Auditory Integration Scale (MAIS) and the Meaningful Use of Speech

Scale (MUSS) are questionnaires that use parental report across a wide range of subjects with respect to an individual child's hearing aid use and attempts at communication. Responses to these questionnaires help the implant team to make decisions about implantation for a particular child. The MAIS was later redesigned to focus on the younger child (the Infant-Toddler MAIS [IT-MAIS]) and is used widely for assessment for this group of implant candidates.

In addition to the measures previously discussed, the use of electrophysiological techniques to support the decision to implant, choose an ear for implantation, and measure the response of the auditory system has grown. Abbas and Brown (2000) have studied a variety of electrophysiological measures for monitoring device function, assessing neural responsivity, and estimating programming.

In many experienced centers, audiologic criteria for implantation serve as the gatekeeper for the child to gain entry to the implant process. Professionals at these centers have identified several additional elements that are evaluated in candidacy selection, including chronological age, duration of deafness, medical/radiological findings, multiple handicapping conditions, speech and language abilities, family structure and support, expectations of the family (parents and child), educational environment, and availability of support services. With the intent of providing an organized listing of all factors considered for candidacy, a tool known as the Children's Implant Profile (ChIP) was developed to aid in the decision-making process (Nevins and Chute, 1996). The ChIP is based on a retrospective review of a large number of implant recipients and is used as a counseling aid for both parents and professionals.

Decisions regarding candidacy should be made on the basis of input from each team member in his or her respective area of expertise so that an individual profile on the ChIP is generated. This profile identifies the areas that must be remediated before a child can be considered for cochlear implant surgery. Once a center recommends a child for candidacy, the final decision to implant any given child remains with the parents. Teams providing information and support to parents at the candidacy stage establish a solid foundation for the ongoing relationship required between families of implant recipients and implant centers during the postimplantation period.

Controversial Point

- If a child has good speech perception abilities in the unimplanted ear and a profound loss in the opposite ear, should he or she be considered a candidate in the profound ear?

Surgical Preparation for Implantation

The surgical stage of the implant process represents one of the most stressful periods for parents. Therefore, hospital procedures and the logistics of the hospital stay should be carefully reviewed with the family by the implant personnel.

In addition, children themselves should be counseled regarding the procedure using conceptually and linguistically appropriate materials. The Clarke School for the Deaf/Center for Oral Education (Northampton, MA) has developed a storybook that outlines the process using pictures. Each of the manufacturers listed earlier in this chapter provides coloring or sticker books for this purpose as well. Several teams use stuffed animals and/or dolls to role-play the events with the child. Every attempt should be made to include the child during this stage. Clearly, older children must be informed about the surgical aspects of the implant and the postoperative appearance of the wound.

Practical consideration concerning postoperative management should be reviewed immediately before and after surgery. Postoperatively, information about bathing, physical activities, and return appointments also needs to be addressed. It is recommended that this information be provided to the parents in both spoken and written form. Finally, parents are assigned an activation appointment approximately 2 to 4 weeks after surgery. More recently, some centers have begun activating the implant the day after surgery.

Cochlear Implant Activation

New methodologies are now available to the clinician to make the initial activation of the device one that is based on physiological responses rather than behavioral ones. All implants now incorporate a system that uses neural responses to identify some of the levels that are required to set the device. This provides a more precise set of values by which the implant will function. In addition to these physiological methods, "mapping" the cochlear implant system uses standard pediatric testing techniques incorporating traditional reinforcement paradigms. The procedure requires the child to respond to an electrical signal that is delivered to each electrode. The mapping or programming procedure requires the child's speech processor to be connected to an interface box that communicates with a computer. The headset (which includes the microphone and the transmitter coil) is placed on the child's head over the area of the internal receiver. Because profoundly deaf children often have a better perception of low-frequency sound, it is customary to begin with a low-frequency electrode. The initial task is to determine the threshold level for a particular electrode. Electrical pulses are delivered to a designated electrode at a particular current level determined by the audiologist, who adjusts the levels through the computer keyboard. The units used to measure these levels vary from one device to the next and do not equate with decibel levels.

Once the child acknowledges hearing a sound or is behaviorally observed to have heard one, an assessment of threshold is made. For very young children, standard observational procedures are used; play audiometry is used with older children. The lowest level at which a child consistently identifies sound sensation is designated at the threshold, or T level. These levels are obtained for each of the active electrodes. In some devices, however, T levels are not required and are estimated based on comfort levels.

An assessment of comfort level (known as a C or M level) provides information about the level at which sound is comfortably loud for the listener. Because many children do not have a well-developed concept of sound, assessing comfort may be too abstract a task, making C levels difficult to obtain. In an attempt to obtain an objective measure of the C level in children, research has been conducted using the electrically elicited stapedial reflex (also known as the electroacoustic reflex threshold, [EART]). Spivak and Chute (1994) used standard tympanometric recordings to measure middle ear muscle reflexes when stimulating the implanted ear. These measurements were successfully used to provide clinicians with a more objective assessment of C levels. It is possible to create a map with these levels and to ensure that the signal delivered to the electrode is not uncomfortable. More recently, the use of the neural responses permits the clinician to use an approved algorithm to set both the T and C levels so that children can obtain a functional map at the time of activation (Hughes et al, 2000).

A map is somewhat similar to the frequency specifications of a conventional hearing aid. However, it is much more specific to an individual recipient because it contains the T and C levels and the frequency boundaries for each of the programmed electrodes. Under no circumstances should one child be given another child's map, because it might cause an uncomfortable sensation. In some of the newer devices, this is virtually impossible, as the device will not function if it is placed on the ear of anyone other than the one for which it was programmed.

Implant systems support speech processors that can store more than one program. Multiple storage capacity enables the user to try different maps in different listening situations. These programs are accessed by means of control knobs or buttons, depending on the device. For example, one map may enhance higher frequencies, whereas another may delete some low-frequency information that may be perceived as noise. Multiple map storage capacity has allowed children to optimize some of the map features in a shorter period of time. This may contribute to better performance at earlier intervals. Multiple map storage capacity enables the mapping procedure to become a more interactive one, calling for the involvement of parents and teachers. Informed decisions regarding ideal map choices can be

made with input from the local educational professional or therapist who is following the child on a daily basis. Minor changes in current levels can be built into the stored programs so that children do not have to return to the implant center as frequently.

Responses at Activation

The range of performance that can occur after children have experienced their first stimulation with a cochlear implant can vary substantially. Some children are able to detect a wide range of speech signals in structured situations upon activation of the device. Others are able to discriminate patterns of speech immediately in structured situations. Yet others will wear the speech processor but will show no awareness to sound. The last group resists wearing the device even when it is turned off.

Setting early therapeutic goals directly after the tuning will be child driven and depend on the child's age, responsiveness, and cognitive/linguistic ability. Children who are capable of immediately detecting signals in structured situations can be taught using a variety of speech input techniques and begin training for pattern recognition. On the opposite end of the spectrum are those children who refuse to wear the device. These youngsters require the implementation of a wearing program in an attempt to get the device activated and begin sound introduction. Parental commitment to the management program suggested by the implant center is crucial; networking parents with others who have had similar experiences may be helpful.

Map Changes

Despite the availability of multiple map storage capacity, return to the implant center for readjustment of the implant is a required part of the postimplant process. Periodically, as a child's auditory perceptual performance changes, his or her map may also need adjustment. New T and C levels can be obtained, and new programs can be written to the microchip of the speech processor. Generally, most implant centers request that children return for frequent follow-up visits for the first 6 months of implant use. As the child's responses with the implant stabilize, the need for additional mapping sessions decreases. Additionally, as neural responses are now available with all devices, children may not have to return as often to the centers, because neural responses levels estimate final mapping levels quite well.

The linguistic constraints of very young children and their lack of auditory experience often prevent them from indicating when a remapping is necessary. In these instances, observations by the parents and teachers are invaluable in signaling when a mapping change is warranted. Certain signs indicate a need for remapping that teachers and parents should recognize. In an effort to hear better, children may suddenly begin to increase the sensitivity or volume from its designated setting. Changes in speech production, a decrease in vocalizations, and loss of speech features that the child was previously able to produce may all be indicators that remapping is necessary. Finally, if the child suddenly develops physical symptoms (e.g., an eye or facial twitch or sensation in the neck or tongue), an appointment with the implant center should be made immediately. Physical manifestations or unusual sensations may require the deletion of electrodes that are causing problems.

Parents, school personnel, and implant center facilities must work together to determine the need for remapping of any individual child. Without good communication, children may go for long periods with maps that are not appropriate and, in some cases, useless.

Care and Maintenance

In addition to monitoring the effectiveness of a child's individual map, it is important that parents and teachers become aware of methods to properly maintain the external components of the cochlear implant system. If the device is carefully maintained on a daily and weekly basis, many simple problems that can arise will be avoided. Many of the procedures used to maintain and care for cochlear implant equipment are similar to those used with conventional hearing aids. Although the burden of maintaining the unit generally rests on the child's parents and/or the child, teachers should also be aware of some of the issues of daily maintenance, especially for the very young child with an implant.

As with any electronic equipment, the foremost avoidable problems are related to physical abuse and moisture. Most school-age children wear their implants behind their ear like traditional hearing aids; therefore, the issue of loss during physical activity or damage from moisture (sweat) must be monitored. To prevent this, newer processors are now water resistant and can be kept on the ear through a traditional earmold or a built-in "lock" provided by the manufacturer. Some devices couple a pediatric battery pack that can be clipped to the back of the child's clothing, thereby affording the wearer the freedom of a BTE, the security of the device being tethered to their clothing, and longer battery life due to the larger battery. To decrease moisture from daily use, most manufacturers supply Dry & Store, from Ear Technology Corp. (Johnson City, TN), to assist in this process. It should be noted, however, that earlier generations of implant devices will not have many of these features, and it is best for the professional working with a child with an implant to seek additional information from the implant center or the manufacturer.

Although excessive moisture in the headset or speech processor will create certain problems with the units, extreme dryness with a subsequent buildup of electrostatic discharge (ESD) can also create problems. In classrooms or homes that are hot and dry, some simple precautions can be taken to help guard against problems caused by ESD. Carpeting can be sprayed with a solution of 50% fabric softener and 50% water. Humidifiers also can be used to increase moisture.

On the playground, buildup of ESD when using plastic equipment, specifically slides, has generated some concern. Although it is recommended that either the cochlear implant should be removed or the child should be counseled against playing on this equipment, the incidence of problems from static has been minimal. There have been some instances of map corruption or map loss after playing on some plastic apparatus. Because it is not a consistent finding, it is difficult to determine the exact combination of factors that may contribute to the problem. If a child has been in the playground and suddenly exhibits changes in his or functional ability with the implant, the teacher should notify the parents. The parents should be instructed to contact the implant facility to have the processor checked. Often all that is required is rewriting of the map to the speech processor.

Children using computers can use antistatic mats under the chair and the keyboard and an antistatic shield over the screen to reduce ESD. Van de Graaff generators that are often on display at science museums must be avoided because these generate a large amount of static electricity (Static Electricity and Cochlear Implants, 1996). An amusement park ride known as the Drop Zone must also be avoided because it uses a magnetic break system to stop the ride.

Troubleshooting the Device

Parents and teachers (and the child, if age appropriate) should have some familiarity with methods that are used to troubleshoot the implant. The amount and type of exposure may depend on the implant facility servicing the child. At the very least, literature on how to perform these procedures should be made accessible; booklets provided by the manufacturers are available on request. In addition, it is preferable that "hands-on" practice of troubleshooting techniques be provided.

Inevitably, the cochlear implant, like many other mechanical devices, will not function properly at some point or cease to function completely. Teachers and therapists must realize that they should not panic if this happens. Knowledge of how the system works should allow for troubleshooting the unit quickly and efficiently. It is important to remember that there can be more than one piece of equipment malfunctioning at any given time. Therefore, once a problem is found with one component, the troubleshooting process should continue to ensure the entire mechanism is functioning. Some devices provide a test wand that enables the teacher or parent to perform a quick check of the system without having to remove the device from the child's head. Minor problems can be easily solved using extra batteries and cords, which should be made available to assist the child during the school day.

Pearl

- When children stop responding to auditory input with their cochlear implants, the problem is most likely caused by low battery power. Replacing batteries is the most common form of troubleshooting to be performed on the implant system.

If the processor stops functioning entirely, it should be left on the child in the "off" position. This will prevent the unit from being lost or exposed to other damaging situations. For example, removing the unit and placing it in the child's backpack might subject it to abuse from other materials in the backpack. As long as the speech processor is in the "off" position, the child can continue to wear the nonfunctioning unit with no possibility of danger to the child or the unit.

In some instances, the external equipment is operating appropriately, but the child's auditory responsiveness deteriorates or is suddenly inconsistent. Although several circumstances may account for this behavior (e.g., a map change), a slight possibility also exists that there may be a problem with the function of the internal receiver. Therefore, it is important for the teacher to be aware of some of the "red flags" that may indicate a problem with the internal portion of the device. These include behaviors such as sudden, inconsistent auditory responses to sounds previously a part of the child's repertoire, deterioration in speech production, frequent equipment changes, and general lack of progress for no apparent reason. The presence of telemetry systems now makes it much easier to troubleshoot internal receiver malfunctions, and all of the newer devices have incorporated software that assesses device functionality each time the child is remapped. However, children with some of the original implant systems do not have access to this type of technology and cannot be routinely tested. Devices that are intermittent are extremely difficult to assess even with telemetry. Ongoing communication between the school and the implant center will help in identifying any potential external or internal equipment problems.

Several situations, both medical and environmental, should be avoided after implantation. Medically, implant recipients must take precautions during magnetic resonance imaging (MRI) because the internal receiver contains a magnet, and physical damage may result. Newer devices are considered MRI compatible; however, this often requires the removal of the magnet prior to having the procedure performed. It is best to check with the individual implant manufacturer and implant facility before undergoing an MRI. Any other type of x-ray procedure will not be problematic. Implant recipients should always inform physicians that they have a cochlear implant. Should the individual require any other type of surgery, it is important that the implanting surgeon be advised.

Implant users should be aware of possible interference from two-way radios and cellular telephones that may operate on the same frequency. Although this is rare, there are some isolated circumstances in which interference occurs. Airport security systems may be activated because of the presence of the implant magnet. If the speech processor must be placed through the x-ray system, it will not be damaged. As a general rule, the implant center should be contacted when questions about implant integrity arise.

Auditory Learning with a Cochlear Implant

Traditional approaches to teaching deaf children focused on training children to listen. This type of activity required listening practice in small group activities using nonspeech stimuli, such as musical instruments and environmental sounds. Exposure to speech occurred only after success was achieved with these gross stimuli. These training paradigms were seldom successful because children were not exposed to everyday spoken language. More recently, emphasis has been placed on the child's ability to learn through listening

and incorporates a more natural intervention that exposes the child to speech on an appropriate cognitive level using common, daily experiences (Chute and Nevins, 2006).

Pearl

- Because implant systems' processors are uniquely designed to process speech, meaningful spoken language is preferred over musical instruments or environmental sounds as input in developing listening skills.

(Re)habilitation for the Young Child

The precise method used to develop listening skills will vary depending on the age at the time of implantation and the level of linguistic sophistication the child exhibits. Because teams are now implanting children as young as 12 months of age, habilitation for the infant/toddler may often fall to the early interventionist. Using traditional paradigms that encourage the parents to become the first teachers, the early interventionist will focus on identifying routines of the child's day during which rich auditory narration will be provided. Listening, in these recurring events, has meaning and is required for completing tasks of interest. Language that is referenced to a household routine, such as having a snack or getting ready for bed, provides the child with a consistent activity using vocabulary that is meaningful and predictable. The overall habilitation goal for children in this group is the development of language. These activities can be adapted using new vocabulary and expanded language as the age of the child increases. Listening skills should be developed in a naturalistic manner by surrounding the child with speech appropriate to his or her level and sounds naturally occurring in the environment. As the child ages, there is also merit in providing an opportunity to participate in activities in which listening is the focus of the language-driven task. Nursery rhymes, songs, and finger plays that incorporate body movements can also accomplish a great deal with respect to auditory and linguistic input for the young child. Some children implanted at age 1 will show near-age-appropriate listening and language skills and may be ready for direct entry into local preschool programs with hearing peers. Others may continue to require small instruction classrooms that will allow them to accrue additional language and listening skills to support mainstream education in later years. In these small instruction classrooms, more formal listening activities may be provided. Auditory lessons can be constructed to practice a broad range of listening from discrete skills such as discrimination between words differing in length or the identification of words found within a concept category.

The ultimate goal of auditory learning activities is auditory comprehension or understanding through listening. The development of auditory skills is always framed in a language context. Chute and Nevins (2002) built upon Erber's (1982) identification of stages of auditory processing and conceptualize four broad stages of skill development:

detection, pattern perception, segmental identification, and comprehension.

Detection requires that the listener indicate that a sound has been heard. It is unnecessary for the sound to be identified, but to demonstrate this skill, the child's response must occur within a certain time limit. Children may indicate detection ability by turning to a sound in the environment or in a more structured task, such as placing beads on a string.

Pattern perception requires the child to recognize differences in words, phrases, sentences, or connected discourse based on suprasegmental features such as duration (e.g., syllable number within words or number of words within a sentence). Stimuli for these tasks are planned by the teacher and require the use of closed-set responses. Initially, opportunities should be provided to the child to recognize pattern differences using both auditory and visual cues. Once the child has demonstrated ability in the task on this level, the visual signal can be removed, and the child can be presented with the auditory signal alone.

In tasks of segmental identification, a child is asked to listen to one item presented from a group of similar items and choose the one presented. This task presents words, phrases, sentences, and connected discourse that have the same patterns so that more keen listening skill is required. Once again, the child should be provided with visual input before progressing to auditory-alone presentation of the stimuli. Linguistic levels of input should always be varied commensurate with the age and ability of the child and should not be restricted to single-word items. Not only is the activity itself driven by the language level of the child, but the directions for participating in the activity must be within the child's language capability as well.

The level of auditory skill referred to as "thinking while listening" (Robbins et al, 1995) demonstrates the auditory comprehension of language. This skill requires the child to process the auditory stimuli and produce a verbal response that is more than a repetition of the signal. Auditory comprehension tasks can also be created at a variety of linguistic levels, and professionals are encouraged to consider the linguistic environment of any auditory task (Nevins and Chute, 1996). As the age of the implant recipient increases, opportunities for listening at various levels can be incorporated into classroom routines and curriculum. Auditory lessons can be designed using content lessons from the standard curriculum, thereby offering the child information that is educational and meaningful. Although published auditory skills curricula are available to assist the speech and hearing professional in designing listening tasks across these four areas of skill development, others have suggested a method for adapting classroom curricula for this purpose (Nevins and Chute, 1996).

Controversial Point

- Should children and families who sign or speak a second language that is not English be told to stop using that language?

Rehabilitation for the Teenage Recipient

The adolescent implant recipient presents certain challenges that must be addressed to ensure continued implant use. For successful interaction with adolescents, some evaluation of identity, self-concept, and self-esteem must be obtained (Knoff, 1987). These issues become extremely important when addressing both the decision to implant and the rehabilitative needs of the teenage implant recipient. Traditional auditory training and speech production therapy should include a strong counseling component that addresses the teenager's ability to cope with change on a daily basis. Teenagers must be able to view their hearing loss as something that may be limiting but not devaluing. Training should include the acquisition of new social and coping skills that may help to minimize the effect of the hearing loss.

Pitfall

- Boredom with traditional adult therapy materials, adapted for use with the teenage population, may result in disinterest and disillusionment with the cochlear implant.

Postimplant habilitation should begin with the subject or aspect of sound that holds the most interest for the teenager. It may be advisable to begin with half-hour sessions to avoid the possibility of boredom. Oftentimes, despite their deafness, teenagers enjoy watching programs on music video television stations. Sessions that compare different musical styles in a listening-only task can be fun and teach pattern recognition with material of interest to the student. Subject information from class assignments can be introduced as well. The key to working with the adolescent is to maintain interest and a willingness to return to and participate in habilitation activities.

Because speechreading enhancement is one of the major benefits from use of a cochlear implant in the adolescent population, speech tracking (De Fillipo and Scott, 1978) may be useful. Speech tracking, a speechreading technique that requires the individual to repeat verbatim a paragraph that is being read, is probably the best technique to use with this population because it will maintain interest (as long as the materials are chosen carefully) and provides a speech model that uses continuous discourse.

The number of adolescents seeking implants has grown as these devices have become more cosmetically appealing and the signal from the devices more robust. However, depending on the degree of hearing loss, the use of amplification prior to implantation, and the amount of spoken language skill, performance in this group can vary widely.

Role of Parents

Regardless of the implanted child's age group, the parents' role in the (re)habilitation process is critical to success. Parents must be active participants in the entire implantation process and act as the interface between the school and the implant facility. They are responsible for monitoring the child's performance with individual maps and coordinating input to the programming audiologist. In addition, parents must adhere to the follow-up schedule recommended by the implant center and make adjustments in that schedule, depending on the child's response. Archbold (1994) reported that the child spends only 1% of his or her time at the implant center; most of the child's remaining time is split between home and school. If parents do not take responsibility for monitoring a child's implant use, the device will not be capable of allowing the child to reach his or her full potential.

Pearl

- Encouraging a strong parent, implant center, and school network increases the likelihood that a child will experience success with his or her implant and habilitation program.

The consistent use of speech and voice by parents of deaf children who receive implants is a critical aspect of communicating in the home. Parents are urged to speak to their children in full voice even if they are using simultaneous communication or cued speech. Cochlear implantation in children need not result in an alteration of whatever linguistic approach has been chosen by the family. Instead, the implant appears to supplement existing communication strategies. Robbins et al (1995) studied the language abilities of children who used total versus oral communication and found that children who used speech and sign language performed as well as and in some areas better than the oral children. Speech production abilities of the children who used total communication appeared to lag somewhat; it was suggested that this was due to the tendency by parents and educators not to challenge these children productively. Regardless of which mode of communication is adopted, good auditory input by the parents and heightened expectation for spoken language are crucial for success.

Parents also need to cooperate with the school or private therapist who is providing the child's auditory and speech training. Families who offer their children an enriched listening and language environment encouraging the use of speaking and listening skills generally support some of the most successful implant users. When parents are detached from the process and view a child's performance as the responsibility of the school and the therapist, the likelihood of the child maximizing his or her potential decreases. Conversely, when parents support the teachers and therapists by reinforcing skills that have been introduced, children appear to respond in a more positive fashion.

Role of the School

The school program can contribute substantially to a child's ability to develop good listening and speaking behaviors.

Educational environments that value the role of audition and use it as an integral part of teaching and learning can provide the proper support for developing auditory and speech skills of implant recipients. Conversely, classrooms cannot support children with cochlear implants when no voice is used and American Sign Language (ASL) is the designated language of instruction. To maximize school involvement, some facilities use an educational consultant model to maintain communication within the individual educational setting. These educational consultants offer guidance to the teacher/therapist regarding the importance of providing an environment that facilitates auditory learning while simultaneously acknowledging the demands and realities of a school day.

Pitfall

- Implant centers that do not include local school professionals as extended members of the implant team may lose a valuable resource for ensuring implant success.

As noted earlier, school personnel should be well versed in the care and maintenance of the cochlear implant equipment so that any malfunction can be assessed and remediated as soon as possible. Liaison with the implant facility through a team educator can easily provide this information to the school staff. In addition, multiple storage capacity speech processors permit school staff to become active participants in the remapping process by providing input about the child's performance with a particular program.

Finally, school professionals should also work in a cooperative effort with parents to ensure good follow-up of a child's speech, language, and auditory program. A proactive communication philosophy will drive teacher reports of progress, plateaus, or equipment problems that can help parents in making decisions regarding a return to the implant center or the direction that home training should take. Issues of educational management of the child with an implant do not end at any specified time after the child receives the device. Rather, new management concerns surface as the child moves through the educational system.

Controversial Point

- Should the school have to bear the financial burden of paying for mappings?

◆ Performance of Children with Cochlear Implants

Measurement of performance with cochlear implants has changed as the devices have changed. Although aided thresholds can be obtained, they do not provide enough information about overall function of the implant. Thresholds with an implant usually occur at ~30 dB HL throughout frequencies 250 to 4000 Hz. In some cases, these may be slightly better, and in others, slightly poorer. Regardless of threshold level, some assessment of speech perception should be obtained. Early reports of outcomes focused on basic skills of pattern recognition and closed-set word recognition. As speech processing improved, open-set speech recognition became the gold standard on which success was measured. As more children were able to demonstrate this ability, children with residual hearing were brought into the process. Data from these children suggested that their performance was also impressive. As the speech-processing strategies continue to evolve, outcomes with implants will also improve in the areas of speech perception, speech production, language development, and educational achievement.

Speech Perception

Assessing the degree of benefit from any sensory aid requires outcome measures that reflect changes in performance over time. The special considerations for testing speech perception in deaf children include the type of stimuli, the vocabulary and linguistic level of the child, the motoric and attention abilities of the child, the test–retest reliability of the materials, and the need for stimuli that provide analytic information. As the average age of children being implanted decreases, it becomes more challenging to measure early changes in perception because these children most often lack the linguistic sophistication necessary to assess benefit. As a result of implantation, there has been a new emphasis on developing methods to assess changes in auditory perception in young children. These tests fall into two basic categories: standardized measures and questionnaires.

Tests of Speech Perception

In developing tests that can be used for the pediatric population, researchers must address certain issues that can affect performance and inadvertently provide misinformation. Although some studies use nonspeech or synthetic speechlike stimuli for adults (Dorman, 1993), speech is more meaningful and can be attended to for longer periods of time in young children.

Speech perception measures for children can be classified in a manner similar to that used for adults (i.e., open- and closed-set tasks). Closed-set tests of speech perception assess environmental sound awareness, timing, and intensity cues or segmental discrimination. Tests administered must be within the language and vocabulary level of the child to obtain a proper assessment of auditory ability. In addition, to maintain the attention of the child, tests for very young children often use brightly colored pictures or actual toys (Geers and Moog, 1989; Ross and Lerman, 1971); video games are now also available.

A complete speech perception battery that evaluates the perception of phonemes, words, and phrases, known as Evaluation of Auditory Responses to Speech (EARS; Allum,

1997), was developed in Europe to be used with children of different countries and is available in 14 languages. Closed-set tests, such as the Word Intelligibility by Picture Identification (WIPI; Ross and Lerman, 1971) and the Northwestern University Children's Perception of Speech (NU-Chips; Elliot and Katz, 1980), provide clinicians with information regarding an individual child's ability to identify words that have similar phonetic content. For the youngest implant users, the Early Speech Perception (ESP) test (Geers and Moog, 1989), which also has a low verbal version, can begin to assess some of the earlier detection and pattern recognition abilities in younger children. In most cases, young children require a live-voice presentation for testing because recorded speech does not hold their attention. Generally, tests using recorded speech are preferred; monitored live-voice (MLV) presentation using an unfamiliar speaker is acceptable. In all cases, several speech perception measures are required for each child to obtain a more complete picture of his or her abilities. When possible, these tests should reflect a variety of stimuli and performance levels.

Tests of open-set speech recognition should be used for children who have some functional vocabulary. Initially, traditional single-word open-set tests, such as the Phonetically Balanced Kindergarten (PBK) test (Haskins, 1949), may be too difficult for this population because of the lack of vocabulary. For this reason, the MLNT and LNT were developed (Kirk et al, 1995) using vocabulary more likely to be in the repertoire of the deaf or language-impaired child. As the results of implantation have become more impressive, children are now being assessed using more traditional audiologic tests, such as the PBK.

For older children, assessment of conversational speech is recommended. Sentence material for this population includes the Hearing in Noise Test–Children (HINT-C) and the Bamford-Kowal-Bench (BKB) sentences (Bench and Bamford, 1979). Tests using single sentences have high validity because humans communicate in sentences; however, the effects of vocabulary, syntax, grammar, and coarticulation must be considered.

For the very young implant recipient, formal assessment is limited. In an attempt to obtain information regarding this group's use of audition and speech, a series of questionnaires was developed. Robbins and Osberger (1991) devised the MAIS, which was later revised to account for younger children (the IT-MAIS), and the MUSS, both of which obtain information through parental report regarding a child's ability to use auditory and speech stimuli. An interviewer administers the questionnaires by providing a sequence of prompts and examples with respect to specific auditory or speech activities. Parents are asked to scale ability on a continuum from "never" to "always." These tests are administered at various intervals before and after implantation.

Results of Speech Perception Testing

As newer speech-processing strategies have been incorporated into cochlear implant systems, the performance of individuals with these devices has shown marked improvement. Depending on which generation of software and hardware is being investigated, outcomes show performance in superior ranges for a large majority of the recipients. However, it should be remembered that no implant can override central processing problems or other disabilities that will impact learning. Clearly, the age at implantation and the duration of deafness still have the greatest effect on the results.

Speech and Language Performance

The speech and language gains made by children who have been implanted early underscore what has been known for decades of research about the critical age for language learning. With the age of implantation dropping to early infancy, more children are receiving cochlear implants within the first year of life. This phenomenon coupled with better speech processing has been able to provide an improved signal to the developing child so that he or she can advance alongside typically developing peers. Studies of phonological processing in these children have demonstrated near-normal abilities or those with only a slight delay (Chin and Pisoni, 2000).

Special Consideration

- Performance with a cochlear implant is most sensitive to age at implantation and duration of deafness. Children who are implanted at early ages are likely to show greater and more rapid auditory, speech, and language benefit than children implanted later with longer duration of deafness. However, progress of the latter group, although occurring at a slower rate, may still be impressive over time.

The performance of children who use cochlear implants can vary widely across subjects and devices. The magnitude of the change in both speech perception and speech production may vary according to physiologic and environmental factors. Long-term follow-up is required to determine the impact these devices will have on implanted children's educational achievements and lifestyle.

Educational Achievements of Children with Cochlear Implants

A continuum of school placements is available for deaf children driven by historical and political ideals. Children can be placed in residential schools for the deaf, self-contained classrooms, resource rooms, inclusive classrooms, or in the mainstream. Residential schools for the deaf that embrace auditory/oral goals have proven to be effective placements for children with cochlear implants. Conversely, schools using ASL and deemphasizing speaking and listening will be poor environments for children with implants. However, as implants have now become more acceptable across the deaf community, many schools for the deaf are incorporating cochlear implant tracks to assist in educating this group of children. Gallaudet University, in Washington, DC, for example, now has a preschool program within the Kendall Demonstration Elementary School that has been designed for children with cochlear implants. Many other schools have followed suit.

Self-contained or small instruction classrooms may be found in local school districts, allowing children to be educated in separate classes within the confines of a hearing school environment. This situation allows social mainstreaming of deaf/hard-of-hearing children by providing them with contact with hearing children during nonacademic periods. Academic mainstreaming is also available for children whose skills and abilities warrant access to curricula and instruction in regular classrooms. Resource rooms may be the first step in accessing the mainstream by providing small group, replacement instruction for particular academic areas, such as language arts and reading, subjects traditionally challenging for children with hearing loss. The recent trend toward inclusion has resulted in small groups of children with hearing loss placed in regular classrooms. There, they receive instruction from a teacher of the deaf who collaborates with the classroom teacher. Full mainstreaming represents the ability of deaf children to achieve academically alongside their hearing peers. Most often a secondary goal of implantation for many parents is the desire for the integration of their child into a regular classroom.

Paul and Quigley (1984) and Ross et al (1991) note that mainstream placement may be the most appropriate setting for the hard-of-hearing child. Because children with implants appear to be achieving at levels that are similar to moderately or severely impaired children, it is a logical conclusion that these children be considered for mainstream placement. Pflaster (1980) and Allen and Osborn (1984) suggest that students in the mainstream attain higher levels of performance on standardized tests of achievement than do their nonmainstreamed peers. Therefore, in an effort to provide children with cochlear implants the opportunity to perform at levels near their hearing age mates, mainstream placement is considered an important decision for these children's academic careers.

Pitfall

- The use of a cochlear implant does not necessarily guarantee readiness for mainstream education. The decision to mainstream a child with an implant must be made using several criteria, only one of which is auditory perceptual ability.

Nevins and Chute (1996) suggest a "whole child" approach in recommending children for the mainstream. Both formal and informal measures can be used to assist in this decision. Formal measures should include assessment in the areas of language and reading, in addition to audition and speech production. Academically, children being considered for mainstream placement should be at the top of their small instruction class in their present school setting and, of course, have the desire to be mainstreamed.

The school receiving the child must also share some responsibilities by providing the appropriate educational and support services that will be needed for success. Modification of teaching style and physical setting may be necessary to ensure the best acoustic environment for the child. A commitment by the classroom teacher to communicate with the implant center and the parents regarding the child's progress is also necessary.

Francis et al (2000) tracked school-age children with implants and observed progress toward educational independence starting at 20 months postimplantation. Hasenstab et al (2000) surveyed parents of children who received the Nucleus 22 channel implant. Although only 30% of the questionnaires were returned, parents reported that most of these children were at least partially mainstreamed. Tyler et al (1997) followed 30 prelinguistically deafened children who were using total communication and were implanted with the Nucleus device for 3 to 5 years. They reported only a "few" children who experienced changes in educational placement and noted that these children demonstrated the largest gains in language and the highest speech perception scores.

Monitoring children's performance once they are in the mainstream has received very little attention. It is important to recognize that once placed in the mainstream, children require constant monitoring to ensure success. A new tool known as the Assessment of Mainstream Progress (AMP) was developed to determine success in the mainstream as well as placement there (Chute and Nevins, 2002). This questionnaire uses teacher input across several areas to determine performance in typical classroom behaviors. Summerfield et al (1997) adapted an earlier version of this scale for use with children in Great Britain to assist in demonstrating how cochlear implants can alleviate some of the financial burden on the educational system.

The final analysis of the success of children with cochlear implants in educational settings will require years of monitoring and necessitate that large groups of children progress through the entire educational sequence. Certainly, there will always be a group of children who are challenged academically. However, it is believed that children who receive implants at early ages can begin their academic careers in regular school settings and achieve at levels similar to their hearing peers. Further study in the area of the educational impact of the implant will serve to document its efficacy.

Performance of Special Populations

The number of implants performed in children has grown steadily through the years as devices have changed and performance has improved. For this reason, implants are now being used in children who previously may not have been considered ideal candidates for implantation. These are children with abnormal cochleas, secondary noncognitive handicaps, cognitive handicaps, auditory neuropathy, and "soft" neurologic signs.

Abnormal Cochleas

Although children with abnormal cochleas have received implants throughout the period of device investigation, performance has not been predictable or consistent. Children with either Mondini's deformities or ossified cochleas are part of this group receiving implants. Performance studies of these children vary depending on several factors. These may include variables such as the depth of insertion, the overall current levels required for stimulation, the age at implantation, and the duration of deafness. For children with Mondini's malformations, the degree of the malformation has an impact on the number of electrodes that can be inserted. Waltzman (2000) notes that even as the degree of malformation increases, children are still capable of using the signal from the implant to obtain an enhancement in speechreading ability. If a full insertion is possible, these children should perform similarly to other children with the same age at time of implant and duration of deafness.

Children with ossified cochleas demonstrate much more variability, and no consensus with regard to performance has emerged. Some researchers report poorer performance, whereas others report equivalent performance. All studies note, however, that children with ossified cochleas often require longer periods of device use before substantial changes in performance are observed (Waltzman, 2000).

Noncognitive and Cognitive Handicaps

The effect of noncognitive secondary handicaps, such as blindness, mild cerebral palsy, and spina bifida, in children who receive cochlear implants has been studied in very small numbers of children. Results would indicate the primacy of factors that are related to the age of implantation and duration of deafness in predicting performance and not the nature of the additional handicap (Chute and Nevins, 1995). In contrast, children with secondary handicaps that are cognitive in nature tend to achieve at the lower end of the performance continuum, with most obtaining only sound detection and a smaller number obtaining pattern perception (Bertram et al, 2000). The poorest group of performers was autistic children, and the authors suggest that these children do not perform well enough to warrant implantation.

Auditory Neuropathy

Children who have some form of auditory neuropathy (dyssynchrony) have been investigated as diagnosis of this group became more clinically available. The larger group of these children tends to perform well (Peterson et al, 2003); however, a subgroup of them demonstrate poor overall levels of performance. The hypothesis is that the first group of children likely includes those with auditory dys-synchrony, whereas the latter group includes those with a true neuropathy. Unfortunately, there is no method of distinguishing between these two groups at the candidacy stage.

"Soft" Neurologic Signs

The final group represents a population that is difficult to diagnose because they are being implanted at early ages. These children demonstrate "soft" neurologic signs in that they have an inability to maintain eye contact, have poor or immature play skills, and also exhibit underdeveloped motor control. Because these children are receiving implants at early ages and represent some of the more recent implant recipients, it is unclear as to how this device will affect their overall growth and development.

◆ Cochlear Implants and Other Assistive Devices

With interference from background noise identified as the main problem for any individual with hearing loss, the use of an FM system to improve the SNR is especially important in the classroom. These devices, along with implants, have evolved technologically and now offer more compatible, cosmetically appealing options that perform extremely well. BTE speech processors can now boot directly into personal FM systems that fit snugly into the device. The benefits of using these systems have long been recognized, and as more school-age children enter the mainstream, the number of them being fit with FMs has markedly increased. However, as good as these devices are, they are subject to some minor difficulties, and it is suggested that they be fit only on children who have experience with their cochlear implant and are able to explain verbally if the sound is distorted. For this reason, children without listening experience or linguistic ability often use the desktop or classroom systems to enhance the primary signal. In this case, proper management of the equipment should also be stressed. The role of educational audiologists cannot be overstated in these cases, as they are the primary professionals in the schools with the knowledge and skill to ensure proper function of devices.

Pearl

- Personal FM use should be provided only in children who have the requisite experience with their implant as well as language skills to express any problems with the clarity of the signal.

As implant recipients have enjoyed improved speech perception ability, many have turned their attention to the enjoyment of music. As newer speech-processing strategies are developed to improve this perception, many current recipients still find pleasure in listening to compact discs and MP3 players. Recipients can directly connect to these external devices through patch cords that are provided by the individual manufacturers. In some cases, individuals have also used these patch cords to obtain direct input from the television. Precautions are necessary when interfacing cochlear implant equipment into a source that is plugged directly into an electrical outlet. In these circumstances, users are required to have a surge protector in-line with the outlet and the equipment.

Some implant manufacturers may provide telephone adapters that offer direct input into the telephone and deliver a slightly enhanced signal for many users. Experienced implant recipients who are capable of telephone use often find this accommodation helpful because it provides better speech recognition for some. Implant recipients are cautioned about using adapters during electrical storms because they are connected directly into the telephone line. Many of the newer systems have telecoils incorporated into the device that are easily accessible. Generally speaking, children should not be interfaced with any additional external equipment unless they are sophisticated users of the implant, can provide appropriate feedback, and take responsibility for their actions.

◆ Future Directions

The cochlear implant of the future will be smaller and/or all implantable and provide better speech understanding in noise. It will also provide musical perception that far surpasses what is available today. More children with residual hearing will be implanted as the performance with these devices exceeds that which was obtainable with hearing aids. Hybrid devices that use both acoustic and electrical stimulation are being investigated now and hold great promise for the future of individuals with different levels of hearing loss.

The paradigms that are used to map the processors will change. Implants can now be mapped using levels that are obtained while the child is undergoing surgery, thereby making the process one that has greater fluidity and provides better sound earlier. Remote mapping will expand to more facilities that are distant from the implant center. Mapping in this manner is now being performed in some centers in the United States (Franck, 2006). As more implants are performed, it will become a customary part of audiologic services with which all professionals are familiar. Mapping will move into the school systems as the software becomes more user-friendly. Speech pathologists and educators will have more training in this area as the curriculum of implantation makes its way into the graduate programs. Cochlear implant centers will grow, and the larger established centers will become centers of excellence for problem cases. Bilateral implantation will become best practice, thereby affording implanted children more access to softer sounds and sounds that occur in a background of noise.

In addition to all the technological and candidacy changes that will occur, one of the greatest impacts on the industry may come from the health care system itself. Cochlear implants are currently financed through private third-party insurers and managed care systems. Oftentimes restrictions by some carriers exist with regard to the type of device and investigational status with the FDA. Although it is hoped that financing of implants by insurers will continue, it is worrisome if the industry decides to view these devices as hearing aids and designate them as exclusionary. Even now, there are often problems obtaining funding for follow-up visits to the implant center. Managed care providers may not pay for services at a center outside their network even though it may have more experience and is the recipient's choice. In addition to making decisions regarding which implant facility a patient must use, there may come a time when the decision regarding which device is implanted will be made by the managed care company and not the recipient or his or her parents. Despite these concerns surrounding managed care, the future for implantation remains exciting and promises to surpass the impact that hearing aid technology had in the field of deafness and hearing loss in the 1950s.

References

Abbas, P. J., & Brown, C. J. (2000). Electrophysiology and device telemetry. In S. Waltzman & N. Cohen (Eds.), Cochlear implants (pp. 219–221). New York: Thieme Medical Publishers.

Allen, T. E., & Osborn, T. I. (1984). Academic integration of hearing-impaired students: Demographic, handicapping and achievement factors. American Annals of the Deaf, 129, 100–113.

Allum, D. J. (1997). Experience in evaluating children with cochlear implants using a multi-language test battery (EARS). Paper presented at the meeting of the Fifth International Cochlear Implant Conference, New York.

Archbold, S. (1994). Implementing a paediatric cochlear implant programme: Theory and practice. In: B. McCormick, S. Archbold, & S. Sheppard (Eds.), Cochlear implants for young children (pp. 25–59). London: Whurr.

Backous, D. (2005). Lean solutions. In J. P. Womack & D. T. Jones (Eds.). New York: Free Press.

Backous, D. (2006). Methodology for improved cochlear implant patient access, safety and program viability, 9th International Conference on Cochlear Implants, June 14–17, Vienna.

Bench, J., & Bamford, J. (1979). Speech-hearing tests and the spoken language of hearing-impaired children. London: Academic Press.

Bertram, B., Lenarz, T., & Lesinski, A. (2000). Cochlear implants for multi-handicapped children: Pedagogic demands and expectations. In S. Waltzman & N. Cohen (Eds.), Cochlear implants (pp. 247–249). New York: Thieme Medical Publishers.

Chin, S. B., & Pisoni, D. B. (2000). A phonological system at 2 years after cochlear implantation. Clinical Linguistics and Phonetics, 14, 53–73.

Ching, T. Y., Psarros, C., Hill, M., et al. (2001). Should children who use cochlear implants wear hearing aids in the opposite ear? Ear and Hearing, 22(5), 365–380.

Chute, P. M. (1997). Timing and trials of hearing aids and assistive devices. Otolaryngology–Head and Neck Surgery, 117, 208–213.

Chute, P. M. (2003, April). Manpower issues effecting cochlear implantation. Paper presented at the Eighth Conference on Cochlear Implants in Children, Washington, DC.

Chute, P. M., & Nevins, M. E. (1995). Cochlear implants in people who are deaf/blind. Journal of Visual Impairment and Blindness, 89, 297–300.

Chute, P. M., & Nevins, M. E. (2002). A parent's guide to cochlear implants. Washington, DC: Gallaudet University Press.

Chute, P. M., & Nevins, M. E. (2006). School professionals working with children with cochlear implants. San Diego, CA: Plural Publications.

Clark, G. (2002). Cochlear implants: Fundamentals and applications. New York: Springer-Verlag.

De Fillipo, C. L., & Scott, B. (1978). A method for training and evaluating the reception of ongoing speech. Journal of the Acoustical Society of America, 63, 1186–1192.

Dorman, M. (1993). Speech perception in adults. In R. S. Tyler (Ed.), Cochlear implants: Audiological foundations (pp. 145–190). San Diego, CA: Singular Publishing Group.

Elliot, L., & Katz, D. (1980). Development of a new children's test of speech discrimination. St. Louis: Auditec.

Erber, N. (1982). Auditory training. Washington, DC: AG Bell.

Francis, H. W., Koch, M. E., Wyatt, R., & Niparko, J. K. (2000) Trends in educational placement and cost benefit consideration in children with cochlear implants. In S. Waltzman & N. Cohen (Eds.), Cochlear implants (pp. 266–268). New York: Thieme Medical Publishers.

Franck, K. (2006). Cochlear implant programming using telemedicine at the Children's Hospital of Philadelphia. Volta Voices, 13, 16–19.

Gallaudet University, Center for Assessment and Demographic Studies. (1994). Annual survey of deaf and hard of hearing children and youth. Washington, DC: Author.

Geers, A., & Brenner, C. (2003). Background and educational characteristics of prelingually deaf children implanted before five years of age. Ear and Hearing, 24, 2S–14S.

Geers, A. E., & Moog, J. S. (1987). Predicting spoken language acquisition in profoundly deaf children. Journal of Speech and Hearing Disorders, 52(1), 84–94.

Geers, A. E., & Moog, J. S. (1989). Evaluating speech perception skills: Tools for measuring benefits of cochlear implants, tactile aids, and hearing aids. In E. Owen & D. K. Kessler (Eds.), Cochlear implants in young deaf children (pp. 227–256). Boston: College-Hill Press.

Hasenstab, S., Vanderark, W. D., & Kastetter, S. K. (2000). Parent report of support services for their children using cochlear implants. In S. Waltzman & N. Cohen (Eds.), Cochlear implants (pp. 250–251). New York: Thieme Medical Publishers.

Haskins, H. A. (1949). A phonetically balanced test of speech discrimination for children. Unpublished master's thesis, Northwestern University, Evanston, IL.

Hughes, M. L., Brown, C., Abbas, P. L., et al. (2000). Comparison of EAP thresholds with MAP levels in the Nucleus 24 cochlear implant: Data from children. Ear and Hearing, 21, 164–174.

Kirk, K. I., Pisoni, D. B., & Osberger, M. J. (1995). Lexical effects on spoken word recognition by pediatric cochlear implant users. Ear and Hearing, 16, 470–481.

Knoff, H. M. (1987). Assessing adolescent identity, self-concept and self-identity. In R. G. Harrington (Ed.), Testing adolescents: A reference guide for comprehensive psychological assessments (pp. 51–81). St. Louis: Westport Publishers.

Moores, D. F. (1987). Educating the deaf: Psychology, principles and practices (3rd ed.). Boston: Houghton Mifflin.

Nevins, M. E., & Chute, P. M. (1996). Children with cochlear implants in educational settings. San Diego, CA: Singular Publishing Group.

Niparko, J., Kirk, K., Mellon, N., et al. (2001). Cochlear implants: Principles and practices. Philadelphia: Lippincott Williams & Wilkins.

Osberger, M. J., Maso, M., & Sam, L. K. (1993). Speech intelligibility of children with cochlear implants, tactile aids or hearing aids. Journal of Speech and Hearing Research, 36, 186–203.

Paul, P., & Quigley, S. (1984). Language and deafness. San Diego, CA: College-Hill Press.

Peterson, A., Shallop, J., Driscoll, C., et al. (2003). Outcomes of cochlear implantation in children with auditory neuropathy. Journal of the American Academy of Audiology, 14, 188–201.

Pflaster, G. (1980). A factor analysis of variables related to the academic performance of hearing-impaired children in regular classes. Volta Review, 82, 71–84.

Quigley, S. P., & Kretschmer, R. E. (1982). The education of deaf children. Baltimore: University Park Press.

Robbins, A. M., & Osberger, M. J. (1991). Meaningful use of speech scales. Indianapolis: University of Indiana School of Medicine.

Robbins, A. M., Osberger, M. J., Miyamoto, R., & Kessler, K. (1995). Language development in young children with cochlear implants. Advances in Otorhinolaryngology, 50, 160–166.

Ross, M., Brackett, D., & Maxon, A. (1991). Assessment and management of mainstreamed hearing-impaired children. Austin, TX: Pro-Ed.

Ross, R., & Lerman, J. (1971). Word intelligibility by picture identification. Pittsburgh, PA: Stanwix House.

Sehgal, S. T., Kirk, K. I., Pisoni, D. B., & Miyamoto, R. T. (2000). Effect of residual hearing on children's speech perception abilities with a cochlear implant. In S. Waltzman & N. Cohen (Eds.), Cochlear implants (pp. 219–221). New York: Thieme Medical Publishers.

Spivak, L. G., & Chute, R. M. (1994). The relationship between electrical acoustic reflex thresholds and behavioral comfort levels in children and adult cochlear implant patients. Ear and Hearing, 15, 184–192.

Static electricity and cochlear implants. (1996). Englewood, CO: Cochlear Corp.

Summerfield, A. Q., Marshall, D. H., & Archbold, S. (1997). Cost-effectiveness consideration in pediatric cochlear implantation. American Journal of Otology, 18, S166–S168.

Tyler, R. S., Fryauf-Bertschy, H., Kelsay, D. M., et al. (1997). Speech perception by prelingually deaf children using cochlear implants. Otolaryngology–Head and Neck Surgery, 117, 180–187.

Waltzman, S. (2000). Variables affecting speech perception in children. In S. Waltzman & N. Cohen (Eds.), Cochlear implants (pp. 199–206). New York: Thieme Medical Publishers.

Chapter 15

Cochlear Implants in Adults

Susan B. Waltzman and William H. Shapiro

Cochlear implants have developed into an accepted treatment for severe to profound deafness in patients who derive minimal benefit from conventional amplification. The implants consist of an internally implanted electrode array and a receiver/stimulator. The external portion of the device consists of a microphone, a speech processor, and a transmitter coil. Although a hearing aid amplifies incoming sound, a cochlear implant replaces the function of the damaged hair cells by converting acoustic energy into electrical pulses that enervate the remaining fibers of the eighth cranial nerve (CN VIII). The microphone converts incoming sound into electrical signals that are shaped and amplified by the processor. The signal is then transmitted to the coil and transferred to the internal receiver/stimulator through a transcutaneous system. The electrodes are stimulated in a manner that is determined by the processing strategy available in a particular prosthesis. Despite the fact that the basic structure of cochlear implants has remained relatively stable over a 35-year development period, significant changes and modifications have been made to both the design and the information transfer schemes. The devices had either single or multiple electrodes and channels, and the electrode array could be either intracochlear or extracochlear.

The processing schemes vary according to several factors, including analog versus pulsatile stimulation, simultaneous or sequential stimulation, and the pattern of speech representation and conversion. In addition to the evolution of the prostheses themselves, criteria for candidacy of hearing-impaired adults have also changed over the years. Past history, design, speech-encoding strategies, and results of cochlear implants in adults have been well documented in other publications. The intent of this chapter is to focus on current issues and devices.

♦ Devices and Processing Strategies

Currently, there are three devices that are approved by the Food and Drug Administration (FDA) for use in the United States: HiRes90K from Advanced Bionics Corp. (Valencia CA; www.advancedbionics.com), Nucleus Freedom from Cochlear Ltd. (Lane Cove, Australia; www.cochlear.com), and Pulsar from Med-El Hearing Technologies GmbH (Innsbruck, Austria; www.medel.com). At a minimum, each of the devices implements one or more variations of the following coding strategies: continuous interleaved sampling (CIS), number of maxima (n of m), and simultaneous analog strategy (SAS).

CIS uses a nonsimultaneous pulsatile pattern in which the stimuli, although interleaved, are not overlapping and can be delivered at very rapid rates and sequentially to minimize electrode interaction while maximizing data transmission (Wilson et al, 1990). The acoustic signal is filtered into frequency bands analogous to the number of electrodes in a given device. Successful transmission of spectral information can be done by extracting frequency specific amplitude modulations or by using the Hilbert transform (Med-El). All three manufacturers implement some version of CIS.

SAS is a derivative of a previously used strategy: compressed analog (CA). Briefly, CA, as implemented in the defunct Ineraid device, compressed the incoming wide acoustic stimulus into a narrower electrical signal using automatic gain control (AGC). SAS enhanced CA by using AGC following the filtering and by using current steps that change in small intervals. Although this approach preserved aspects of the fine structure of the signal, the simultaneous transmission affected channel interaction, thereby limiting the efficiency of the strategy. Research is currently under way to explore several aspects of simultaneous stimulation that would reduce and/or eliminate electrical channel interaction. SAS is currently employed in the Advanced Bionics device.

When the Nucleus 22 (Cochlear Ltd.) device was initially introduced, it used a speech-encoding strategy in which fundamental and formant frequency information was conveyed. Initially, F0F2 (fundamental frequency + first formant) and then F0F1F2 (F0F1 + second formant) information was extracted from the incoming speech signal and transmitted to the electrodes with pulsatile, nonsimultaneous bipolar stimulation. In 1990, the Multi Peak (MPEAK) strategy was introduced in which a filter bank circuit was added to the existing speech coding, allowing three electrodes to be dedicated to high-frequency bands ranging from 2000 to 6000 Hz. In 1994, the spectral peak coding strategy (SPEAK) superseded MPEAK. The SPEAK strategy is an implementation of n of m, which shares some similarities with CIS. Twenty bandpass filters with center frequencies between 250 and 10,000 Hz were the basis for coding; electrodes were selected and stimulated on the basis of the highest spectral peaks (not exceeding using 10 channels) of the incoming stimulus. Although more rapid than previous strategies in the Nucleus device, the rate at which the electrodes could be stimulated is 250 pulses per second/channel, a relatively slow rate.

In 1996, the Nucleus 24 device manufactured by Cochlear Ltd. was introduced. For the first time, the Cl24 incorporated modifications to the internal electronics package to accommodate newer processing strategies. The device implements three encoding modes: SPEAK, CIS, and ACE (advanced combined encoder). The ACE strategy functions much like SPEAK but simulates at a faster rate. ACE incorporates elements of SPEAK and CIS by assigning electrodes on the basis of the stimulus and allowing for more variable and rapid stimulation to increase efficient transmission of timing cues. The Cochlear Nucleus Freedom device currently implements ACE, CIS, and SPEAK, and the Med-El Pulsar offers the choice of two strategies: CIS and an implementation of the n of m coding system.

It is important to note that current devices are being designed to incorporate numerous trial schemes in an attempt to improve the devices' ability to replicate the ear. One such attempt relates to stimulating one group of electrodes with one strategy (SAS) and the remainder of the array with a second strategy (CIS) to make use of fine temporal information while reducing channel interaction. Furthermore, software upgrades have been designed to improve performance in quiet and noise without the need for additional surgery to replace the implanted portion. Research is ongoing to develop more effective coding strategies and modify existing schemes to improve communication possibilities for a wider population. In addition, until several years ago, electrodes were uniformly straight and flexible, but upon insertion were found to sit against the outer wall of the cochlea, causing trauma, including osseous spiral lamina fracture, stria vascularis damage, and basilar membrane penetration. Perimodiolar electrode arrays were subsequently developed to reduce the trauma and increase the possibility of (1) preserving residual hearing, (2) lowering power consumption and stimulation levels by placing the electrode closer to the simulated elements, and (3) achieving more selective cell population stimulation (Roland, 2005). Although many of these goals have not been realized on the basis of electrode design alone, the interactions of coding schemes and electrode array design have substantially increased the possibilities of improved performance. Please visit the manufacturers' Web sites for current information.

♦ Criteria for Implantation

The criteria for implantation have changed substantially since adults began receiving cochlear implants as a treatment for deafness. Initially, in the late 1970s and early to mid-1980s, the clinical trials required that only adults who were postlingually bilaterally profoundly deafened and received no benefit from appropriate hearing aids would be candidates for implantation. "No benefit from amplification" was most often defined as a score of 0% on monosyllabic words in the best aided condition. Several factors contributed to the relatively conservative criteria for implantation. First, too few published data were available that could confirm substantial benefit with an implant. Basically, it was not known what was realistic in terms of expectations or what the upper limits of the expectations could be. It was wise, then, to begin by implanting those individuals who would be most likely to gain, that is, adults who heard before and whose onset of deafness occurred after the development of speech and language. Second, to ensure that no loss of functional hearing was occurring, only those adults who had no measurable benefit from hearing aid(s) were deemed to be candidates. As the numbers of patients increased, along with more advanced speech-processing strategies, the level of auditory-only speech perception being reported in adults was quite good and exceeded expectations. Over the years, the increasingly better results have led to an expansion of the criteria for implantation in adults to include those with considerable amounts of residual hearing and/or preoperative speech perception skills and those with prelingual or congenital deafness.

Currently, the newest Advanced Bionics device, the HiResolution Bionic Ear System: HiRes90K, is approved by the FDA for adults with the following indications: severe or profound hearing loss and limited benefit from appropriate amplification, described as 50% or less on Hearing in Noise Test (HINT) sentences (Nilsson et al, 1994). Adult inclusion criteria for the Cochlear Ltd. Nucleus Freedom are as follows: (1) bilateral severe to profound sensorineural hearing loss, (2) no useful benefit from hearing aids, and (3) aided scores of 50% or less on sentence recognition tests in the ear to be implanted and 60% or less in the nonimplanted ear or bilaterally. Similar inclusion criteria exist for the Med-El Pulsar device: bilateral severe to profound sensorineural hearing loss and a best aided score of < 40% on HINT sentences presented in the noise condition.

It is important to point out that once a device receives postmarket approval (PMA) from the FDA, the indications for use often serve only as guidelines, and individual practitioners frequently implant patients outside the recommended criteria.

In addition to changes in the inclusion criteria for adult implantation, new configurations and designs have led to further expansion of potential implant candidates. Standard cochlear implantation often causes any residual hearing in the implanted ear to become irrelevant, and only electrical hearing is available. Individuals with substantial levels of low-frequency hearing often choose or are counseled not to proceed with implantation because of the potential consequences, including the loss of the pleasing quality of sound and the ability to appreciate music, perhaps associated with a decrement in pitch perception. Investigations have begun to explore the possible benefits of combining low-frequency acoustic hearing with high-frequency electrical stimulation via a cochlear implant. Shortened electrode arrays have been developed in an attempt to eliminate damage to the apical portion of the scala tympani when the electrode is positioned in the basal portion. Results to date have been promising, with some patients showing (1) preservation of residual hearing, (2) increased speech understanding in noise, and (3) improved music recognition and appreciation (Gantz et al, 2005). The technology, however, has not been without difficulties. Some patients have lost their residual low-frequency hearing immediately following surgery or after several months, which substantially reduced the benefits from the short electrode device. In addition, some recipients have complained about the nature of the sound despite ostensibly "good" results. Further exploration into the design of this technology is continuing in

an attempt to rectify the shortcomings and maximize the potential to patients with low-frequency hearing.

♦ Assessment

The preoperative assessment determines whether the patient is medically and audiologically appropriate for implantation and, if so, assists in the choice of ear to be implanted. Furthermore, the preoperative results serve as a baseline to which postoperative performance is compared; therefore, the postoperative audiologic assessment is virtually identical to the preoperative test battery.

The medical evaluation includes a physical examination and clearance for surgery and radiological studies. The cause of the hearing loss is determined, and treatment options are discussed based on the results. Computed tomography (CT) scans and magnetic resonance imaging (MRI) are a routine part of the preoperative assessment. The results are used to view anatomical abnormalities that might affect ear choice and determine whether modifications to the surgical technique are necessary to ensure proper placement of the electrode array. Intraoperatively, device monitoring and plain films are advisable to confirm device functioning and proper placement. Postoperatively, if a change is noted in the performance of the implant recipient, radiological studies are sometimes needed to determine whether electrode migration or damage has occurred. Under these conditions, preoperative and intraoperative radiological studies are particularly helpful for comparison purposes.

Pearl

- Device monitoring confirms proper functioning and patient stimulation and can provide baseline data for programming.

The audiologic test battery is designed to determine the type and degree of hearing loss and the speech perception capabilities of the person unaided, aided (preoperatively), and with the implant postoperatively. Audiologic testing includes unaided and aided pure-tone air and bone thresholds, speech reception thresholds, and speech recognition scores where possible. These measurements should be obtained both under earphones and in the sound field, preoperatively and postoperatively. Immittance measurements, otoacoustic emissions, and electrophysiological testing are often used to further confirm the extent of the hearing loss and provide additional diagnostic information. On occasion, a patient may present with inappropriate amplification because of an increase in hearing loss and/or the use of inappropriate amplification, thereby requiring a trial period with appropriate hearing aids (usually on loan) before administration of the test battery to determine implant candidacy.

The measurement of speech recognition and the acoustic cues that determine the level of recognition is central to the preoperative and postoperative assessments. Preoperatively, the information is used to determine whether the individual fulfills the predetermined guidelines for implantation; that is, would this patient be likely to perform better with an implant than with a hearing aid? The results also serve as a baseline to which postoperative results are compared to determine device efficacy. Postoperatively, speech recognition measures not only provide data on absolute performance but also assist in determining the signal-processing scheme most beneficial to the patient, the setting of the best "program" within a given strategy, and the perceptual areas most in need of auditory rehabilitation. It is important to note that over time and with listening experience, significant changes occur in the auditory percepts defined by the implant. Although one expects to see improvement in auditory recognition with increased length of implant use, a decrease in perceptual skills could indicate the need for adjustments, device failure, or other issues.

Speech recognition depends on the ability to integrate a variety of acoustic cues, which are dynamic in nature, including frequency, temporal, and intensity information. As an example, vowel identification is predicated on the presence of the first three formant frequencies (F0F1F2), yet the same formant frequencies can allow for the recognition of several various speech sounds because the range of frequencies necessary for the identification of one vowel overlaps the range necessary for the determination of several other vowels (Denes and Pinson, 1963). The same applies to the identification of consonants: recognition depends on a variety of cues. For example, fricative sounds are distinguished from other consonants by virtue of the turbulent sound that is produced, but sounds within that category are distinguished from one another by virtue of intensity and spectral cues. The /s/ and /sh/ sounds can be differentiated from other fricative sounds such as /f/ and /v/ by the fact that they are more intense, but they can be differentiated from one another because of the difference in spectral composition: most of the energy of /s/ is in the area of 4000 Hz, whereas the concentration of energy for /sh/ is in the vicinity of 2000 to 3000 Hz (Denes and Pinson, 1963; Dorman, 1993). Although the importance of these varying acoustic cues is undeniable, the identification of speech is accomplished by incorporating the acoustic cues with the linguistic cues attached to a given language. It is our knowledge of the language, semantics, and other nonlinguistic cues that assist us in recognizing speech and deciphering the message. This is true whether the hearing is through the normal auditory channels or a cochlear implant. The assessment of speech perception pre- and postimplantation is based on the concept of characterizing the ability of the individual to recognize speech at the phoneme, word, and sentence levels.

Before the onset of cochlear implants as a treatment for profound deafness, few standardized tests were available to assess all levels of speech recognition pre- and postimplantation. In 1981, Owens et al developed the minimum auditory capabilities (MAC) battery. The battery included tests that evaluate suprasegmental and segmental aspects of the speech signal in both closed- and open-set configurations. Tests of prosodic characteristics included accent, noise/voice, and question/statement, in which the patient was not required to identify the stimulus but merely to address whether it was a noise or a human voice or a question or statement, and so on. Closed-set tests assessed vowel recognition and spondee identification. Open-set tests included Northwestern University 6 (NU-6) monosyllabic words (Tillman and Carhart, 1966) and CID sentences presented in an auditory-only condition (Silverman and Hirsh, 1955). The battery also included measures to assess speechreading and speechreading plus audition skills. In 1983, Tyler et al developed a battery that added an assessment of speech in noise to the MAC. In 1986, the battery became available on laser disc to eliminate speaker bias on the visual and audiovisual segments of the battery (Tyler et al, 1986).

In 1984, Boothroyd proposed a different concept for the assessment of acoustic cues delivered by means of a cochlear implant. He was concerned that any stimulus that had linguistic content could potentially enhance the perception of acoustic cues being transmitted by the implant. He developed the Speech Pattern Contrast (SPAC) test, which concentrated on assessing the ability of the implant to transmit the prosodic and phonemic features of the speech signal. The SPAC subtests included the following: rise/fall, roving stress, initial consonant manner, final consonant manner, vowel place, vowel height, initial consonant place, final consonant place, and phoneme recognition. Although the battery appeared to provide useful speech feature information that was potentially beneficial for both adjusting an implant and providing useful data regarding the development of processing strategies (Filson et al, 1992; Waltzman and Hochberg, 1990), the test was lengthy and cumbersome to administer and, therefore, not widely used clinically. The SPAC was part of a larger battery of 26 audiologic tests that were used in a study to differentiate between cochlear implants (Cohen et al, 1993; Waltzman et al, 1992a). Analyzing the results from this study, Filson and colleagues (1992) showed that a shorter battery of tests could describe individual patient performance, document improvement over time, and distinguish between devices and subjects. This further discouraged widespread clinical use of the SPAC.

As devices became more technologically advanced and patient performance improved dramatically after implantation, the speech recognition test battery was condensed to include only measures of open-set phoneme, word, and sentence recognition presented in the auditory-only condition. There are, however, some patients whose postoperative performance requires a lower level of data accumulation. Long-term deafened adults may still obtain only minimal benefit

Table 15–1 Assessment of Speech Recognition

Phoneme level
  Vowel confusion test
  Consonant confusion test
Word recognition level
  NU-6 monosyllabic word test
  CNC test
Sentence recognition level
  CID sentence test
  BKB sentence test
  HINT sentence test

BKB, Bamford-Kowal-Bench; CID, Central Institute for the Deaf; CNC, consonant-nucleus-consonant; HINT, Hearing in Noise Test; NU-6, Northwestern University 6.

from an implant or require an extended period of use to demonstrate open-set speech recognition. In this situation, it is important to use closed-set or speechreading plus audition ability to show communication benefit.

At present, the more typically clinically used measures include a monosyllabic word test scored as both words and phonemes correct and a sentence recognition test **(Table 15–1)**. The more frequently used monosyllabic test is the consonant-nucleus-consonant (CNC) test (Peterson and Lehiste, 1962), and the most frequently used sentence recognition tests are the CUNY (Boothroyd et al, 1988) and HINT sentences (Nilsson et al, 1994). Both sentence tests have versions that allow for presentation in quiet and noise, a very important aspect of the evaluation because testing in quiet does not reflect true functioning in noncontrolled listening situations, and patients often experience ceiling effects on speech recognition due to high levels of functioning.

As cochlear implant use became increasingly widespread and additional processing strategies became available, further standardization of a clinical test battery became necessary to allow for data comparison across centers, patients, devices, and strategies. In 1997, a group of professionals representing implant centers and manufacturers drafted a minimum speech test battery for adult cochlear implant patients (Luxford and Ad Hoc Subcommittee of the Committee on Hearing and Equilibrium of the American Academy of Otolaryngology–Head and Neck Surgery, 2001). The battery included CNC word lists and HINT sentences. It was designed not to exclude other tests but to ensure that all implant centers are, at the very least, administering a given monosyllabic word test and sentence test. The manufacturers split the cost of creating compact disc versions of the test, and the discs were made available to implant centers nationwide.

Vowel and consonant confusion tests provide yet another avenue for assessing perception at the phonemic level (Tyler et al, 1986). These tests were designed to isolate the ability of the patient to obtain manner, place of articulation, and voicing information through the implant itself. Theoretically, one could adjust processor programs that might facilitate

the auditory percept of these cues. Although often lengthy to administer, consonant confusion measures provide valuable information and are the tools of choice for those involved with signal-processing development.

Standardization of stimuli presentation level has also been attempted. Although test stimuli were routinely presented at a level of 70 dB sound pressure level (SPL), Skinner et al (1997) and Firszt et al (2004) recommended that the presentation level be reduced to 60 dB SPL to better simulate conversational speech. They believed that the higher level artificially inflated the speech perception capabilities, preoperatively and postoperatively, of implant recipients, and 60 dB SPL has now become the accepted standard. In addition, lowering the SPL further can provide additional information and tax the system to determine skill level. No matter what presentation level is used, it remains imperative to specify the level at which a test is administered and the signal-to-noise ratio (SNR).

In addition to the medical and audiologic preoperative assessments, the prospective candidate should be fully informed as to the devices available so that he or she can make an informed decision regarding surgery and recovery, postoperative programming and evaluations, and potential postoperative benefits. Patient expectations often play a large role in perceived success following implantation. Therefore, based on the candidate's profile and baseline characteristics, the cochlear implant team should summarize the expected and possible outcomes. It is wise not to be too specific either negatively or positively because, despite available data, performance is often not predictable.

◆ Speech Recognition with Cochlear Implants

Several factors, including advanced speech-coding strategies and the broadening of eligibility criteria, have contributed to substantially improved performance in adult implantees. This evolution and development of more sophisticated coding strategies over the past 20 years has enabled patients to obtain increasingly better outcomes. In 1981, with the Nucleus Wearable Speech Processor (WSP) using a fundamental frequency + second formant (F0F2) strategy, the average open-set speech understanding was ~12% following 6 months of usage; by 1999, with the ACE strategy in the Sprint processor (Cochlear Ltd), the average score was 85%. Although numerous other changes, including less restrictive inclusion criteria, occurred during this period, the effects of strategy development have been instrumental in improving outcomes. On average, the postlingually deafened adult patient, with currently available cochlear implant devices, can obtain high levels of speech recognition in quiet with scores of 90% on sentences and ~50% on monosyllabic word recognition. Despite this, scores on both word and sentence recognition tests still range from 0 to 100%, and the ability to function in less ideal listening situations, such as noisy backgrounds, reduces the competence of the listeners substantially, although bilateral implantation may offer advantages to some patients (Das and Buchman, 2005).

Special Consideration

- Bilateral simultaneous and sequential implantation is becoming more frequent because of the possibility of increased speech understanding in the presence of background noise and improved localization. Recent investigations have confirmed that many adults do show substantial improvement in both areas following bilateral implantation.

A wide range of performance can also be found in congenitally, prelinguistically, and other long-term deafened adults. Current devices have enabled these groups to obtain significantly better speech recognition results than those reported with prior speech processors; however, the maximum performance achieved does not necessarily reach the highest levels of functioning of the postlinguistically and short-term deafened adult patient. Other adult hearing-impaired populations have also benefited from implantation. Several investigators have studied the impact of cochlear implantation in the geriatric population. Uniformly, these studies have shown no problems related to the surgical procedure, significant improvements in speech understanding in quiet and noise, and highly positive effect on quality of life (Haensel et al, 2005; Kelsall et al, 1995; Leung et al, 2005; Waltzman et al, 1993).

Pitfall

- Postimplantation sound-field audiometric results are not necessarily indicative of speech recognition: they represent loudness only.

Pitfall

- Absolute scores on speech recognition tests administered in quiet are not indicative of functioning in noncontrolled listening situations.

Comparisons between devices on the basis of data collected across institutions, however, often remain problematic. Different patient selection criteria, test measures, methodology, and data analysis make comparisons extremely difficult. However, one recurrent theme occurs: most adult cochlear implant patients do extremely well with cochlear implants. In fact, as Dorman (2006) correctly points out, the majority of adults score between 80 and 100% on open-set sentence recognition tests, enabling these patients to communicate well in a variety of situations, including telephone use (Cohen et al, 1989; Cray et al, 2004; Dorman et al, 1991). Although these results are very impressive, there still remains a large segment of people who do not derive substantial benefit from implantation either in quiet or under difficult listening situations; the factors that might account for the variable performance need to be explored.

◆ Factors Affecting Performance

Despite the numerous advances in cochlear implant technology, which is the key factor affecting implant performance, the variability of performance still exists within and between devices. Open-set recognition scores continue to range between 0 and 100%, although, as technology has improved, the number of patients achieving higher end scores has increased dramatically over time. In addition to technology and the other confounding issues already covered in this chapter, including selection criteria and candidacy modifications, other variables need to be included to possibly account for this heterogeneity.

Surviving Neural Population

Undoubtedly, the number and place of surviving ganglion cells and how they are clustered play a significant role in outcome. Despite the pervasive logic of this assertion, a preliminary histopathological account of temporal bones from four Nucleus multichannel cochlear implant users provided conflicting reports. In 1997, Linthicum and Otto (1997) reported that a subject with the second-lowest cell count had the highest performance score, whereas a subject with the highest cell count had the poorest score. However, complicating issues were present: the patient with the most remaining fibers had the shortest electrode array insertion. Morphological studies are continuing that will hopefully provide meaningful correlations between neural element survival and performance. Clinically, the capability of guesstimating cell survival remains elusive despite attempts to quantify the data. The use of auditory evoked potentials and other methods are being explored in an effort to assess neural integrity. In fact, clinical investigations into the utility of stimulation between actual electrodes through either the creation of virtual channels or current steering are currently being conducted. The formation of these stimulation areas may allow for surviving neural elements to be stimulated, which in turn could translate into increased pitch perception, speech understanding, and so on.

Length of Deafness (Plasticity of the Auditory System) and Age at Implantation

Numerous reports have shown that adults with congenital and/or prelingual deafness obtained no measurable open-set speech recognition after implantation (Brimacome et al, 1989; Waltzman et al, 1992b; Zwolan et al, 1996). These studies, however, reflected performance with older speech-processing strategies rather than currently available, more technologically advanced coding schemes. More recently, investigators have shown that prelingually and/or congenitally long-term deafened adults can obtain substantial speech recognition (Moody-Antonio et al, 2005; Schramm et al, 2002; Waltzman and Cohen, 1999; Waltzman et al, 2002). Despite these encouraging results, length of deafness continues to affect outcome, although perhaps not to the same degree as reported a decade ago.

Device Programming

Crucial to patient performance is programming, which requires manipulation of device-specific coding strategy parameters to obtain maximum speech recognition for each recipient. Traditionally, two essential basic values, common to all devices, that must be measured are electrical thresholds and comfort levels. In fact, newer model implants are capable of objective programming methods, which can help to shorten programming sessions and assist with the difficult-to-program patient: The Advanced Bionics and Med-El devices permit the programmer to measure comfort levels only; the software can then automatically set threshold levels. In addition, Neural Response Telemetry (NRT) in the Nucleus, Neural Response Imaging (NRI) in the Advanced Bionics HiRes90K, and Auditory Nerve Response Telemetry (ART) in the Med-El Pulsar are helpful tools in assessing the functioning of the device and assisting in the establishment of electrical thresholds. Other device-specific parameters that can be controlled are input dynamic range, frequency boundary and gain adjustments, maximum, pulse rate, and pulse width.

Accurate electrical thresholds and comfort levels in a given strategy remain the main factors that contribute to an accurate program. Fluctuations in these and other measures can cause a variety of patient complaints. A programming schedule that incorporates regularly planned visits is prudent, particularly until the patient can accurately detect changes in hearing that signify the need for remapping. For the first year following initial stimulation, approximately five visits should be planned, with intermediate visits occurring if problems arise. After the first year, patients typically reduce the number of regularly scheduled follow-up sessions to two per year (Shapiro, 2006; Skinner, 2003).

Controversial Point

- Should adults routinely receive auditory habilitation following implantation?

Device Failures

Patient complaints, including intermittency, reduced speech recognition, buzzing, pain, and noise in the device, are often signs of a need for remapping. There is, however, another possibility: device failure. Although the percentage of failures remains small, the absolute numbers are increasing.

Failures can be total and sudden in nature or can be gradual in nature, with some of the above-mentioned symptoms being precursors to a total failure. Yearly evaluations are critical to the process of diagnosing a failure. If a patient's performance on routinely administered speech recognition tests decreases, and no improvement is noted following equipment changes, remapping, and so on, a device failure should be considered. Following a definitive diagnosis, reimplantation should occur as quickly as possible so that performance is not compromised (Alexiades et al, 2001; Balkany et al, 2005; Waltzman et al, 2004).

Other Factors

Additional contributors to outcome include etiology of deafness, preoperative speech recognition scores, anatomical and surgical issues, psychological factors, family support, and expectations. As time goes on, professionals will no doubt learn more about the level of contribution of all possible variables. It is most important to remember, however, that as technology evolves, the influence of the many variables on results will no doubt change, and what may have considerable effect under the current scheme of things may have less significance in the future.

Pearl

- It is important to remember that selection criteria are guidelines and that all factors must be considered on a case-by-case basis when determining candidacy and discussing possible outcomes.

Pitfall

- Unrealistic expectations on the part of the patient can lead to disappointment and nonuse of the implant. It is vital that the candidate and family understand the range of postoperative performance.

♦ Summary

Cochlear implants in adults have come a long way since they were first introduced. Implants have evolved from single-channel devices providing little or no speech recognition to multichannel implants using advanced signal-processing strategies. The hearing-impaired adult has truly benefited from the cooperative efforts of researchers and clinicians who have collaborated on numerous investigative endeavors in all areas of cochlear implantation. The results have been remarkable. Adults who have lost their hearing or never heard have been provided with different degrees of hearing that have enabled them to communicate with family and friends, resume or begin education and professional careers, enjoy music and other forms of entertainment, and maintain more independent lifestyles. Gratifying as these results may be, the task is not complete. There still remain hearing-impaired adults population who do not benefit from the current technology, nor have professionals reached the maximum capability for existing and future implant users. The field is extremely dynamic and the future very promising.

References

Alexiades, G., Roland, J. T., Fishman, A., & Waltzman, S. (2001). Cochlear reimplantation: Surgical techniques and functional results. Laryngoscope, 111, 1608–1613.

Balkany, T. J., Hodges, A., Buchman, C., et al. (2005). Cochlear implant soft failures consensus development conference statement. Otology and Neurotology, 26, 815–818.

Boothroyd, A. (1984). Auditory perception of speech contrasts by subjects with sensorineural hearing loss. Journal of Speech and Hearing Research, 27, 134–144.

Boothroyd, A., Hnath-Chisolm, T., & Hanin, L. (1988). Voice fundamental frequency as an auditory supplement to the speech reading of sentences. Ear and Hearing, 9, 306–312.

Brimacome, J., Beiter, A., & Barker, M. (1989). Cochlear implant results in pre/perilinguistically deafened adults. Paper presented at the annual meeting of the American Academy of Otolaryngology–Head and Neck Surgery, Washington, DC.

Cohen, N. L., Waltzman, S., & Fisher, S. (1993). A prospective, randomized study of cochlear implants. New England Journal of Medicine, 328, 233–237.

Cohen, N. L., Waltzman, S., & Shapiro, W. (1989). Telephone speech comprehension with use of the Nucleus cochlear implant. Annals of Otology, Rhinology, and Laryngology, 98, 8–11.

Cray, J. W., Allen, R., Stuart, A., et al. (2004). An investigation of telephone use among cochlear implant recipients. American Journal of Audiology, 13, 200–212.

Das, S., & Buchman, C. (2005). Bilateral cochlear implantation: Current concepts. Current Opinion in Otolaryngology and Head and Neck Surgery, 13, 290–293.

Denes, P., & Pinson, E. (1963). Speech recognition. In P. Denes & E. Pinson (Eds.), The speech chain (pp. 124–146). Murray Hill, NJ: Bell Telephone Laboratories.

Dorman, M. F. (1993). Speech perception in adults. In R. Tyler (Ed.), Cochlear implants (pp. 145–190). San Diego, CA: Singular Publishing Group.

Dorman, M. F., & Spahr, A. J. (2006). Cochlear implants in adults. In S. Waltzman & J. T. Roland (Eds.), Cochlear implants (pp. 199–204). New York: Thieme Medical Publishers.

Dorman, M. F., Dove, H., Parkin, J., et al. (1991). Telephone use by patients fitted with the Ineraid cochlear implant. Ear and Hearing, 12, 368–369.

Filson, K., Fisher, S., Weston, S., & Shapiro, W. (1992). Evaluation and adaptation of a cochlear implant test battery. Seminars in Hearing, 13, 208–217.

Firszt, J. B., Holden, L., Skinner, M., et al. (2004). Recognition of speech presented at soft to loud levels by adult cochlear implant recipients of three cochlear implant systems. Ear and Hearing, 25, 375–387.

Gantz, B. J., Turner, C., Gfeller, K., & Lowder, M. (2005). Preservation of hearing in cochlear implant surgery: Advantages of combined electrical and acoustical speech processing. Laryngoscope, 115, 796–802.

Haensel, J., Ilgner, J., Chen, Y., et al. (2005). Speech perception in elderly patients following cochlear implantation. Acta Otolaryngologica, 125, 1272–1276.

Kelsall, D. C., Shallop, J. K., & Burnelli, T. (1995). Cochlear implantation in the elderly. American Journal of Otology, 16, 609–615.

Leung, J., Wang, N., Yeagle, J., et al. (2005). Predictive models for cochlear implantation in elderly candidates. Archives of Otolaryngology–Head and Neck Surgery, 131, 1049–1054.

Linthicum, F., & Otto, S. (1997). Functional histopathology of four 22-electrode cochlear implant temporal bones. Paper presented at the Association for Research in Otolaryngology, St. Petersburg Beach, FL.

Luxford, W. M. & Ad Hoc Subcommittee of the Committee on Hearing and Equilibrium of the American Academy of Otolaryngology–Head and Neck Surgery. (2001). Minimum speech test battery for postlingually deafened adult cochlear implant patients. Otolaryngology–Head and Neck Surgery, 124, 125–126.

Moody-Antonio, S., Takayanagi, S., Masuda, A., et al. (2005). Improved speech perception in adult congenitally deafened cochlear implant recipients. Otology and Neurotology, 26, 649–654.

Nilsson, M., Soli, S., & Sullivan, J. (1994). Development of the Hearing in Noise Test for the measurement of speech reception thresholds in quiet and in noise. Journal of the Acoustical Society of America, 95, 1085–1099.

Owens, E., Kessler, D., & Schubert, E. (1981). The minimum auditory capabilities (MAC) battery. Hearing Aid Journal, 34, 9–34.

Peterson, G. E., & Lehiste, I. (1962). Revised CNC lists for auditory tests. Journal of Speech and Hearing Disorders, 27, 62–70.

Roland, J. T. (2005). A model for cochlear implant electrode insertion and force evaluation: Results with a new electrode design and insertion technique. Laryngoscope, 115, 1325–1339.

Schramm, D., Fitzpatrick, E., & Seguin, C. (2002). Cochlear implantation for adolescents and adults with prelinguistic deafness. Otology and Neurotology, 23, 698–703.

Shapiro, W. (2006). Device programming. In S. Waltzman & J. J. Roland (Eds.), Cochlear Implants (pp. 133–145). New York: Thieme Medical Publishing.

Silverman, S. R., & Hirsh, I. (1955). Problems related to the use of speech in clinical audiometry. Annals of Otology, Rhinology, and Laryngology, 64, 1234–1244.

Skinner, M. W. (2003). Optimizing cochlear implant speech performance. Annals of Otology, Rhinology, and Laryngology, 191, 4–13.

Skinner, M. W., Holden, L., Holden, T., et al. (1997). Speech recognition at simulated soft, conversational and raised-to-loud vocal efforts by adults with cochlear implants. Journal of the Acoustical Society of America, 101, 3766–3782.

Tillman, T., & Carhart, R. (1966). An expanded test for speech discrimination utilizing CNC monosyllabic words (Northwestern University Auditory Test No. 6 [USAF School of Aerospace Medicine Tech. Report]). Brooks Air Force Base, TX: USAF School of Aerospace Medicine.

Tyler, R., Preece, J., & Lowder, M. (1983). Iowa cochlear implant tests. Iowa City: University of Iowa.

Tyler, R., Preece, J., & Tye-Murray, N. (1986). The Iowa phoneme and sentence tests. Iowa City: University of Iowa, Department of Otolaryngology–Head and Neck Surgery.

Waltzman, S.B., & Hochberg, I. (1990). Perception of speech pattern contrasts using a multichannel cochlear implant. Ear and Hearing, 11, 50–55.

Waltzman, S. B., & Cohen, N. (1999). Implantation of patients with prelingual long term deafness. Annals of Otology, Rhinology, and Laryngology, 177, 84–87.

Waltzman, S. B., Cohen, N., & Fisher, S. (1992a). An experimental comparison of cochlear implant systems. Seminars in Hearing, 13, 195–207.

Waltzman, S. B., Cohen, N., & Shapiro, W. (1992b). Use of a multichannel cochlear implant in the congenitally and prelingually deaf population. Laryngoscope, 102, 395–399.

Waltzman, S. B., Cohen, N., & Shapiro, W. (1993). The benefits of cochlear implantation in the geriatric population. Otolaryngology–Head and Neck Surgery, 108, 329–333.

Waltzman, S. B., Roland, J. T., & Cohen, N. (2002). Delayed implantation in congenitally deaf children and adults. Otology and Neurotology, 23, 333–340.

Waltzman, S. B., Roland, J. T., Waltzman, M., et al. (2004). Cochlear reimplantation in children: Soft signs, symptoms and results. Cochlear Implants International, 5, 138–145.

Wilson, B., Lawson, D., & Finley, C. (1990). Speech processors for auditory prostheses (Fourth Quarterly Progress Report on NIH Project N01-DC-9-2401: 4–24).

Zwolan, T. A., Kileny, P., & Telian, S. (1996). Self-report of cochlear implant use and satisfaction by prelingually deafened adults. Ear and Hearing, 17, 198–210.

Chapter 16

Audiologic Rehabilitation Intervention Services for Adults with Acquired Hearing Impairment

Jean-Pierre Gagné and Mary Beth Jennings

Audiologic rehabilitation has been recognized as a domain of audiology ever since the emergence of audiology as an allied health discipline. Since its beginnings, the importance of audiologic rehabilitation services within the discipline of audiology, the types of services that can be provided by rehabilitative audiologists, and the service delivery models used to organize and define the scope of practice in rehabilitative audiology have been in constant evolution. At present, the scope of practice and the panoply of services provided by rehabilitative audiologists are more diversified than they have been at any time in the past. In recent years, conceptual models of rehabilitation have been developed and proposed. Those models have served to (re)define the goals of audiologic rehabilitation and to organize the manner in which rehabilitative services are provided to patients.

This chapter focuses on audiologic rehabilitative services for adults and elderly persons with acquired hearing loss. The intervention activities available and most frequently provided to this population are presented. Then a conceptual framework of audiologic rehabilitation is proposed. The framework serves to (re)define the goals and the organization of rehabilitation services and to place the various intervention strategies within a context of a comprehensive intervention program. The application of the framework to one specific model of intervention, defined as a solution-centered problem-solving intervention process, is presented. A case presentation that illustrates the application of this model of intervention is provided.

◆ Overview of Audiologic Rehabilitation

The Origins and Development of Audiologic Rehabilitation Services

It is widely recognized that in North America the field of audiologic rehabilitation for persons with acquired hearing impairment emerged as a formal professional discipline after World War II. Veterans Administration (VA, now Veterans Affairs) services developed extensive rehabilitative programs for military personnel who had acquired hearing loss during the war. Intensive audiologic rehabilitation services, provided over a period of several weeks, included hearing aid fitting, hearing aid orientation, information counseling, auditory and speechreading training (provided individually or in groups), speech correction, and, when required, occupational and vocational training (Ross, 1997). Despite the reported success of those programs, audiologic rehabilitation services failed to expand in a significant way beyond the VA settings. This is primarily because during the same period, major breakthroughs occurred in hearing measurement techniques and diagnostic audiology. The market economy and career opportunities encouraged many professionals (and professional training programs) to specialize in the area of medical (diagnostic) audiology rather than in rehabilitative services. Also, provisions in the professional

code of ethics prevented audiologists from dispensing hearing aids (with the exception of audiologists employed by the VA services). This constituted a major obstacle to professionals interested in audiologic rehabilitation because it excluded audiologists from being directly involved in the provision of an important component of rehabilitation services designed for persons with hearing impairment. Over the years, the high cost of providing comprehensive audiologic rehabilitative services (particularly compared with diagnostic services), as well as the poor reimbursement schedule for audiologic rehabilitation services (at least in the United States) and the confusion concerning whether or not audiologists are able to bill for rehabilitation services (in the United States), contributed to a general decline in interest in audiologic rehabilitation. Finally, there is a lacunae of experimental data to demonstrate the effectiveness of audiologic rehabilitation services.

Services Related to Amplification and Other Technological Devices

At present, few public institutions in the United States offer comprehensive audiologic rehabilitation services. Where they are available, audiologic rehabilitation services are often limited to activities related to the recommendation of hearing aids and post–hearing aid fitting evaluation. In some settings, hearing aid orientation services are provided to individuals who acquire those devices (see Chapter 12). Results of surveys conducted among audiologists practicing in the United States have shown that only a minority of professionals provide group audiologic rehabilitation services. The majority of respondents stated they provide hearing aid orientation; they advise patients concerning hearing assistive technology (HAT), and information related to communication strategies, on an individual basis (Prendergast and Kelley, 2002).

Technological advances in the field of electronics in the mid-1960s (i.e., the miniaturization of electronic components used in hearing aids and the development of aids with flexible electroacoustic characteristics) and the development of programmable and digital hearing aids in the 1980s and 1990s made it possible to design hearing aids that allowed customized adjustments of the devices provided to patients with hearing loss. The expertise of audiologists was sought to select appropriate models and types of hearing aids and to adjust the amplification devices according to the characteristics of the patients' hearing loss. Thus, at present, a major focus of the activities provided by rehabilitative audiologists centers on various technical aspects of the hearing aid fitting process (see Chapters 4 and 5). Also, particularly in the United States, a major milestone in the organization of audiologic rehabilitation services occurred in 1979, when the American Speech-Language-Hearing Association (ASHA) removed its restriction on allowing audiologists to dispense hearing aids (ASHA, 1979). At present, audiologists are recognized as the professionals who have the competency to provide all aspects of the rehabilitation services required by persons with hearing loss.

Pitfall

- For many audiologists, the focus of audiologic rehabilitation begins and ends with the prescription and fitting of hearing aids. The hearing aid fitting process is an important intervention strategy. However, the scope of audiologic rehabilitation extends beyond hearing aid fitting.

Since the last decade, the development and availability of auxiliary aids (frequently referred to as HAT) have provided rehabilitative audiologists with additional armamentaria to respond to some of the needs expressed by persons with hearing loss (see Chapter 17). Audiologists are often consulted for the selection, evaluation, and instruction on how to install, operate, and use auxiliary devices. The introduction of Public Law No. 101–336 (Americans with Disabilities Act [ADA], 1991; Dewine, 1992) constitutes another major milestone in the development of rehabilitative audiology. This law was enacted to provide a national mandate to eliminate discrimination against all persons with disabilities (including those with hearing disabilities) in the areas of employment, access to public accommodations, transportation, state and local government services, and telecommunications. In each of those areas, the availability and use of auxiliary aids can provide important solutions to many of the difficulties encountered by individuals with hearing loss (Dewine, 1992). However, with the exception of frequency modulation (FM) amplification systems, audiologists are still not fully recognized as the professionals most competent to provide expert advice and consultation concerning the selection, installation, and use of services related to auxiliary aids that are required by the law. This aspect of rehabilitative audiology has yet to be fully exploited by audiologists, yet it represents an opportunity for the growth of the profession.

♦ Speech Perception Training

Since the establishment of audiologic rehabilitation as a discipline, it has been recognized that amplification systems alone do not provide solutions to all the speech perception difficulties encountered by persons with hearing loss. Speech perception training programs have always been considered a cornerstone of audiologic rehabilitation programs for adults with acquired hearing loss. Generally, these services are grouped under three categories: auditory training, speechreading (lipreading) training, and auditory-visual speech perception training. Several types of programs have been developed and proposed. Regardless of the perceptual modality in which they are dispensed, the goal of speech perception training programs is to overcome the speech perception deficits that result from permanent hearing loss.

Initially, the programs developed by the VA served as a model for many of the speech perception training programs incorporated into rehabilitation services for individuals with acquired hearing loss. The introduction of commercially available tactile devices and cochlear implants for persons with profound hearing loss in the 1980s spawned a renewed interest in many of the initial activities traditionally associated with audiologic rehabilitation. Specifically, clinical procedures were developed to assess the auditory, visual, and auditory-visual speech perception performances of persons who were potential candidates for those devices (see Chapters 14 and 15). Postfitting training programs have been modified and redesigned to optimize the receptive speech perception performances of persons with profound hearing loss. Some of the rehabilitative procedures developed primarily for tactile aid and cochlear implant users were redesigned for patients with a less severe degree of hearing loss. Also, several studies were designed to evaluate the effectiveness of speech perception training programs provided to persons who sought these rehabilitative services (Alcantara et al, 1990; Lesner et al, 1987; Walden et al, 1977, 1981). Generally, there is little evidence to support the claim that speech perception training programs are effective. However, there is some evidence that such programs can be efficacious and effective (Sweetow and Palmer, 2005). Furthermore, there is evidence to suggest that the speech perception performances of cochlear implant and hearing aid users can be improved by taking part in an auditory training program.

Pearl

- Excellent auditory, visual, and auditory-visual speech perception testing protocols have been developed for patients who are candidates for, or users of, cochlear implants and tactile aids. Also, several speech perception training programs were developed for the same patients. Those materials can easily be adapted to testing and training speech perception among patients with less severe acquired hearing impairment.

Computer applications to speech perception training have been developed. Examples of these programs include the Dynamic Audio Video Interactive Device (DAVID; Sims et al, 1979), Computer Assisted Speech Perception Evaluation and Training (CASPER; Boothroyd, 1987), Auditory-Visual Laser Videodisc Interactive System (ALVIS; Kopra et al, 1987), Computerized Laser Videodisc Programs for Training Speechreading and Assertive Communication Behaviors (Tye-Murray et al, 1988), Computer-Aided Speechreading Training system (CAST; Pichora-Fuller and Benguerel, 1991), and the Computer-Assisted Tracking Simulation (CATS; Dempsey et al, 1992). Programs that use CD-ROM technology include Conversation Made Easy (Tye-Murray, 2002), Learning to Lipread (Allen, 2000), Seeing and Hearing Speech (2001), Sound and Beyond (2003), and Listening and Auditory Communication Enhancement (LACE: NeuroTone Inc., 2007). **Appendix 16–1** provides a listing of some of the interactive speech perception training programs that have been developed and the names and addresses of the persons who can be contacted for additional information. These programs make it possible to provide intensive speech perception training to patients while minimizing the amount of preparation and direct intervention time (and their related costs) normally required by the clinician.

Several issues must be considered when designing or selecting a speech perception training program. Among these issues are decisions concerning the implementation of analytic-based or synthetic (global)-based training programs, the selection of the sensory modality in which to provide training, and decisions on whether the intervention program should be provided on an individual (one-to-one) basis or in a group setting.

Controversial Point

- Several computerized programs have been developed to provide intensive speech perception training opportunities for patients with hearing impairment. In general, those programs have not provided the panacea that was expected in terms of significantly improving the speech perception competencies of their intended patients. In the opinion of the authors, computerized training programs have not replaced the role of an experienced clinician in speech perception training. However, an appropriate use of those programs may be the provision of additional training for individuals who are both familiar with computer technology and highly motivated to improve their speech perception performance.

Analytic versus Synthetic Speech Perception Training

Erber (1996) described a general framework that can be applied to speech perception training (**Fig. 16–1**). The matrix considers two aspects of speech perception training: the type of stimuli used and the type of responses required to perform the task. Each cell of the matrix corresponds to a different speech perception task. All possible speech perception training tasks are incorporated into the matrix. However, some cells are more commonly applied than others.

	Speech unit	Syllable	Word	Phrase	Sentence	Narrative
Detection	A	A				
Discrimination	A	A	A			
Identification	A	A	A	A/S	S	
Comprehension				S	S	S

Figure 16–1 Stimulus-response matrix summarizing various speech perception competencies. Each cell represents a specific type of speech perception training task. The cells with a symbol indicate tasks most often incorporated into speech perception training programs for persons with an acquired hearing impairment. The cells containing the symbol *A* describe primarily analytic speech perception tasks, whereas those containing the symbol *S* describe primarily synthetic speech perception tasks. (Adapted from Erber, N. P. (1996). Communication therapy for hearing-impaired adults (2nd ed.). Melbourne, Australia: Clavis Publishing, with permission.)

Traditionally, speech perception training has been considered under two broad categories: analytic and synthetic (or global). Analytic training programs involve dividing the speech signal into small components and training these components independently (Blamey and Alcantara, 1994). Typically, the types of activities grouped under analytic speech perception training tasks include the detection of vowels; the discrimination of consonants; and the identification of various speech stimuli, including suprasegmental features of speech sounds (e.g., prosody and accent) and speech elements (e.g., vowels, consonants, and words) (**Fig. 16–1**). Examples of analytic speech perception training activities are described in **Table 16–1**. Slight changes in test procedures or changes in the test stimuli

---

Table 16–1 Analytic Speech Perception Training Activities

Syllables in words
    Words are contrasted by several syllables. A stimulus word is presented by the clinician. The patient is asked to identify the stimulus word within a closed-set response format (e.g., *beach* vs *baseball* vs *telephone*).

Sentence that differ in number of syllables
    Sentences that differ n the number of syllables they contain are presented in a closed-set format (e.g., "The boy is crying," vs "The kangaroo is jumping"). The clinician produces one of the sentences, and the patient is asked to identify the stimulus-sentence.

Discrimination of vowels
    Words or nonsense syllables (CVC) that differ only in their vowel content are contrasted (e.g., *beet, bit, bat, but, boot*). The clinician presents sequences of two test stimuli. The patient is asked whether the two stimuli are the same or different.

Identification of vowels, consonants, words, or syllabic pattern
    Selected stimuli are presented in a closed-set format with a minimum number of two foils presented (e.g., *bite* vs *kite* vs *fight*). One of the stimuli is presented by the clinician. The patient must indicate which stimulus was presented from the set of possible responses.

CVC, consonant-vowel-consonant.
Note: All of these activities can be auditorily-alone, visually-alone, or audiovisually.

Table 16–2 Examples of Ways to Modify the Level of Difficulty in Analytic Training Activities

- Training can begin with a detection task, followed by a discrimination task, and finally an identification task.
- In any identification task, the level of difficulty can be decreased by reducing the number of alternatives available in the response foils. The level of difficulty can be increased by increasing the number of alternatives available in the response foils.
- Initially, within a given task, the stimuli used should include the speech elements that are the most distinctive. Gradually, the task can be modified to include speech elements that are more similar in the sensory modality in which the activity is conducted. (e.g., in an auditory training activity, begin with *beet* vs *bat* contrasts, later include *beet* vs *bit* contrasts).
- Text support can be provided to decrease the difficulty of the task. Text support can be removed to increase the difficulty of the task.
- Initially, a slightly exaggerated production of the test stimulus can be presented to emphasize the speech element targeted. Later, a more natural production of the test stimulus can be presented.
- Initially, the test stimuli can be presented in isolation. Later, the test stimuli can be presented in a carrier phrase or in a sentence context. For example, the stimulus word *pepper* could be presented in isolation or in the context of a facilitating phrase, such as "Please pass the salt and ____."

used can modify the level of difficulty of a speech perception task. Suggestions of ways to modify an analytic speech perception task to vary the level of difficulty associated with the activity are provided in **Table 16–2**. Over the years, several authors have described speech perception training activities on the basis of an analytic approach. Examples of some of those programs are Jeffers and Barley (1971), Erber (1982), Plant (2004), Spitzer et al (1993), Jennings (1994), and Tye-Murray (1997).

Synthetic speech perception training focuses on helping the patient apply his or her implicit knowledge of linguistics, to make use of inferences, to use contextual and situational cues, and to apply his or her "knowledge of the world" to the interpretation and understanding of the speech message. Generally, synthetic programs are designed to teach patients to make optimal use of the linguistic redundancies available in ongoing speech. Boothroyd (1988) described several levels of linguistic redundancies that are available in speech. These include phonological, lexical, syntactic, semantic, topical, and pragmatic constraints **(Table 16–3)**. Knowledge and use of the linguistic rules that govern a spoken language can improve a patient's

ability to understand a spoken message (Erber, 1996). Training activities may be designed to foster the use of any of those sources of linguistic redundancies. However, synthetic speech perception activities typically include the identification or comprehension of phrases, sentences, and continuous discourse (i.e., narrative; **Fig. 16–1**). Examples of activities that have been designed to train synthetic speech perception skills are described in **Table 16–4**. Examples of ways to modify the level of difficulty of synthetic training activities are provided in **Table 16–5**.

Training activities based on continuous discourse material have been developed by DeFilippo and Scott (1978) and Erber (1996). Speech tracking is a procedure developed by DeFilippo and Scott (1978) as a method for training and evaluating the reception of ongoing speech. Speech tracking requires that the patient (i.e., the receiver) listen to a segment of ongoing speech, usually taken from a written passage and spoken by a communication partner (i.e., the sender), and then repeat the utterance verbatim **(Table 16–6)**. DeFilippo (1988) provides a detailed account of how speech tracking can be applied to speech perception training in any perceptual modality.

Table 16–3 Levels at which Linguistic Rules Can Be Applied to Enhance Speech Perception

Phonological constraints
  Refers to the fact that rules govern how speech acts (e.g., phonemes) can be grouped together to produce words. For example, within any English word, the phoneme /z/ is not likely to be preceded by the phoneme /t/.

Lexical constraints
  Refers to the fact that in any given language, the number of words that exist is finite. Moreover, some words are more familiar than others, and some words are used more frequently than others. For example, during a conversation, the word *telephone* is more likely to be uttered than the word *xylophone*.

Semantic constraints
  Refers to the fact that the words used in a sentence are usually related to each other in a meaningful way. For example, although the sentence "Put the salt on the cloud" is syntactically correct, semantically it is highly improbable.

Topical constraints
  Refers to the fact that language usually takes place within a physical and social context. Generally, the use of language bears some relationship with the context in which it is used. For example, in a stadium, during a football game, it is more likely that the topic of discussion will center on sports-related activities than on religious beliefs and values.

Pragmatic constraints
  Refers to the fact that language is governed by social norms that determine how it is used within a given community or situation. These rules are employed to make the use of language more efficient for the purpose of exchanging ideas and to avoid confusion. For example, during a conversation, generally only one person at a time speaks, and there are rules that govern turn taking.

Definitions and examples inspired by the work of Boothroyd, A. (1988). Linguistic factors in speechreading [monograph]. Volta Review, 90(5), 77–88; and Erber, N. P. (1996). Communication therapy for hearing-impaired adults (2nd ed.). Melbourne, Australia: Clavis Publishing.

Table 16–4 Examples of Synthetic Speech Perception Training Activities

Category activities
   A semantic category is selected (e.g., animals). The clinician presents words from the category, and the patient is asked to recognize the items.

Fill-in-the-blank activities
   Sentences are presented to the patient with text support. In each written sentence, one or two words are replaced by a blank. The clinician presents the entire sentence (including the missing word[s]), and the patient is asked to identify the missing word(s).

Question–answer activities
   The patient is provided with a series of questions related to a topic of conversation. The patient presents a question to the clinician, who then provides the answer. The patient must repeat the answer to the question before moving to the next question (see Erber, 1996).

Topic–sentence activities
   The patient is presented with a topic. The clinician then presents sentences related to that topic, and the patient is asked to repeat the sentences.

Direction-following activities
   The patient is presented with directions and is required to carry out the actions requested by the clinician.

Speech-tracking activities
   The clinician presents a phrase from a written passage. The patient is asked to repeat the utterance of speech verbatim (see DeFilippo, 1988).

Conversation activities
   The patient and the clinician carry out a conversation. The clinician assesses the fluency of the conversation, and the patient and clinician discuss the general success of the conversation, identifying difficulties and possible solutions (see Erber, 1996).

Note: These activities can be auditorily-alone, visually-alone, or audiovisually.

Erber (1996) described a procedure entitled QUEST?AR. This activity is a conversational-based training procedure that provides interactive practice with common question–answer sequences. The patient asks a communication partner (e.g., the clinician) a series of 30 prepared questions **(Table 16–7)**. The patient must either repeat the answer or indicate in some fashion that the response was understood. When a communication breakdown occurs, the patient and/or the communication partner must find ways to resolve the communication breakdown before proceeding to the next question. One advantage of this activity is that it is the patient who initiates each new question. Thus, that person has some insights into the possible responses that can be provided. This procedure is an effective approach to developing synthetic speech perception abilities. Erber (1996) provides a detailed account of the different ways that the QUEST?AR procedure can be adapted to practice various aspects of synthetic speech perception skills.

In addition to the two clinical procedures presented previously, several other authors have described speech perception training activities that can be used to practice synthetic abilities. Examples of those programs are Jeffers and Barley (1971), Spitzer et al (1993), Jennings (1994), Erber (1996), Plant (1996ab, 2002), Strachan et al (1997), and Tye-Murray (1997).

It is important to note that a speech perception training program designed for an individual is seldom limited to one training approach. Typically, during a given session, a patient may complete both analytic and synthetic training activities and activities designed to develop conversational fluency and communication management skills (see the following section). Also, analytic and synthetic speech perception training activities can be conducted in any perceptual modality (auditory only, visual only, or audiovisual). In some instances, the stimuli used to conduct the activity may be degraded in some fashion to make the task more

Table 16–5 Examples of Ways to Modify the Level of Difficulty in Synthetic Training Activities

- Selecting topics that are familiar to the patient will make the task easier; selecting topics that are less familiar to the patient will make the task more difficult.

- The use of test material that is written in simple language (in terms of vocabulary words, syntactic structures, and semantic contents) will reduce the level of difficulty of the task; the use of linguistically more complex test material will increase the level of difficulty of the task.

- Informing the patient of the topic to be discussed before completing an activity will make the task easier; discussing the topic with the patient before completing the task (e.g., identifying key words and concepts) will further facilitate the task.

- The use of partly scripted (i.e., written) test materials during an activity will make the task easier; removing the text support will increase the level of difficulty of the task.

- Increasing the number of test items or the length of the utterances to which the patient must attend will increase the level of difficulty of a task; decreasing the number of test items or length of the utterances to which the patient must attend will decrease the level of difficulty of a task.

- Practicing the task under ideal environmental conditions (e.g., in quiet and under good lighting conditions) and presenting the stimuli in an audiovisual mode will facilitate the task; degrading the quality of the environmental conditions (e.g., adding background noise, increasing the distance between the clinician and the patient and degrading the lighting conditions in the room) will make the task more difficult.

- The use of clear speech and emphasis on key words or phrases will facilitate the task; the use of conversational (natural) speech without any special emphasis will make the task more difficult.

Table 16–6 Example of the Speech-tracking Procedure*

Clinician [reading from a written text]: He lit the lamp on the secretary . . . and began to write to his wife.†
Patient: He bit the lamp . . .

Clinician: He . . . *LIT* . . . the lamp [emphasizing the word in italics].
Patient: He lit?

Clinician: He lit the lamp . . .
Patient: He lit the lamp.

Clinician [nodding in agreement]: On the secretary.
Patient: And he was lazy?

Clinician: ON THE SECRETARY [repeated slowly using clear speech].
Patient: He lit the lamp on the. . .

Clinician: SE-CRE-TARY [repeated with emphasis].
Patient: Secretion.

Clinician: SE-CRE-TARY . . . a table to write on . . . a desk . . . a *SE-CRE-TARY* [using paraphrase and synonym].
Patient: A table to write on?

Clinician: Yes, *SE-CRE-TARY* [a confirmation and repetition of the misperceived word, with emphasis].
Patient: A secretary?

Clinician [nodding to approve the response]: He lit the lamp on the secretary . . .
Patient He lit the lamp on the secretary.

Clinician: And began to write to his wife.
Patient: And began to write his life.

Clinician [facial expression indicating that the response was a close approximation]: and began to write *TO his WIFE* . . .
Patient: And began to write to his wife.

Clinician [nods to indicate a correct response and then proceeds with the next sentence]

* Based on speech-tracking procedure developed in DeFilippo, C. L. & Scott, B. L. (1978). A method for training and evaluating the reception of ongoing speech. Journal of the Acoustical Society of America, 634, 1186–1192.
† Passage from Bellow, S. (1947). The victim. New York: Vanguard Press.

Table 16–7 Topics and Questions from QUESTions for Aural Rehabilitation (QUEST?AR)

Where did you go?	Museum, restaurant, post office, shopping, camping, doctor, zoo, beach, airport, swimming, mountains, picnic, music lesson, Mars, supermarket, and so forth
Questions	1. Why did you go there?
	2. When did you go there?
	3. How many people went with you?
	4. Who were they [names]?
	5. What did you take with you?
	6. Where is [the place where you went]?
	7. How did you get there?
	8. What did you see on the way?
	9. What time did you get there?
	10. What did you do first?
	11. What did you see?
	12. How many? What color? And so on.
	13. What happened at [the place you went]?
	14. What else did you do?
	15. What were other people doing at [the place where you went]?
	16. What was the most interesting thing that you saw?
	17. What was the most interesting thing that you did?
	18. What did you buy?
	19. What kind? What flavor? What color? And so on.
	20. How much did it cost?
	21. Did anything unusual happen? What?
	22. How long did you stay?
	23. What did you do just before you came home?
	24. When did you leave?
	25. How did you get home?
	26. What happened on the way home?
	27. What time did you get home?
	28. How did you feel then?
	29. When are you going back?
	30. Do you think that I should go sometime?

Source: From Erber, N. P. (1996). Communication therapy for hearing-impaired adults (2nd ed.). Melbourne, Australia: Clavis Publishing, with permission.

difficult for the patient. Several strategies can be used to degrade the auditory signal in a clinical setting. These include low-pass filtering of the signal, reduction of the overall level of the signal, and introduction of background noise so the task is conducted at a poor signal-to-noise ratio (SNR). Depending on the objectives of the program, the task can be conducted with or without the patient's personal speech perception aid (i.e., hearing aid). Similarly, some strategies can be used to degrade the quality of the visual-speech signal during a visual or an audiovisual speech perception training activity. For example, the distance and the viewing angle between the clinician and the patient can be increased, the overall illumination of the room can be reduced, and the lighting contrast between the background visual field and the clinician's face can be increased.

Perceptual Modalities

When designing a speech perception training program for a patient, it is important to determine under which perceptual modalities to conduct the training activities. Traditionally, speech perception training was conducted in a unisensory modality: either auditory training or visual speech perception training (lipreading or speechreading). In recent years, it has been recognized that in most instances speech perception is a multisensory activity. That is, except for some rare instances where the visual signal is not available (e.g., communicating by telephone or conversing with someone who is in another room), the persons involved in a conversation have access to both the auditory and the visual signals provided by the interlocutor. Thus, in most instances, the ultimate goal of speech perception training for patients with acquired hearing loss should be to improve their auditory-visual speech perception competencies. However, the question remains: In which perceptual modality should training be conducted to optimize audiovisual speech perception performances? This question is particularly relevant because recent investigations have shown that auditory-visual speech perception does not necessarily involve the simple addition of the cues extracted from the visual signal with the cues extracted from the auditory signal. At present, for adults with acquired hearing loss, no clear evidence in the literature indicates whether training should be conducted in a unisensory modality (auditory or visual) or in a multisensory modality (audiovisual).

One way to determine in which perceptual modality to focus training is to assess the patient's speech perception competency in each of the unisensory modalities (auditory and visual). An analysis of the results of auditory-speech perception tests and the results of visual-speech perception tests will indicate whether the patient is functioning optimally in each of those two sensory modalities. Training should focus on practicing speech perception in the perceptual modality in which the patient is least proficient. For example, the results of an assessment test battery may indicate that in quiet, with his or her speech perception aid, the patient performs as would be expected (considering the person's hearing loss) in the auditory-only modality. However, the results of visual-speech perception evaluation procedures may reveal that the patient fails to use visual cues optimally. For this person, speech perception training should focus on speechreading activities.

At present, the tendency is to emphasize training in the patient's nondominant sensory modality (Erber, 1979). For most patients with acquired moderately severe hearing loss, audition remains the primary sensory modality for speech perception (especially after they have been fitted with an appropriate amplification system and once they have fully acclimatized to using the device). For those individuals, speech perception training programs should be designed to help fully exploit the visual information available in the speech signal. Training programs may be conducted in a visual-only mode. Alternatively, speech perception activities may be conducted audiovisually but under conditions in which the auditory signal is degraded to foster the integration of the available visual cues and the degraded audio signal. The following example will serve to illustrate this latter training condition. First, a speech perception activity is initiated in an auditory-only mode. Second, a masking noise, such as speech babble, is introduced, and the level of the noise is adjusted until the patient's performance declines substantially (i.e., but remains slightly above chance level). Then, under that acoustic condition (audition in noise), visual speech cues are provided, and the same training activity is completed. Under this latter condition, the patient will have access to some auditory cues, but that information will be insufficient to perform the task optimally. Providing visual information will train the patient to combine the degraded audio signal with the available visual-speech cues. This training paradigm can be incorporated into analytic and synthetic training activities.

Group versus Individual Speech Perception Training

Many of the training activities described previously can be conducted with patients on an individual basis or in a small group. Individual speech perception training provides the clinician with the opportunity to tailor the programs to the specific skills, goals, and interests of the individual. Group speech perception training may be performed in small groups of individuals who are closely matched in their speech perception competencies and for whom similar rehabilitative goals have been established. According to Blamey and Alcantara (1994), costs can be reduced through the use of group training, but it may be at the expense of the effectiveness of the training program. Moreover, in a group setting, the clinician must be aware of (and able to cater to) the program objectives of each of the individuals in the group. Effective group training programs usually require that the clinician be very alert and experienced at coordinating speech perception training activities.

A patient may be involved in both group and individual sessions. Individualized intervention programs constitute an efficient approach for the practice and development of specific speech perception competencies. Group intervention programs provide the participants with an opportunity to practice their communication skills in a more realistic (yet somewhat controlled or safe) environment. Groups also provide camaraderie and an opportunity for the participants to share their experience and expertise. In general, individual intervention programs are best suited for training analytic skills. On the other hand, group intervention programs are most appropriate for practicing communication management skills and for addressing the psychosocial effects of hearing loss.

Ideally, when group intervention programs are conducted, the minimum number of group members should be 5, and the maximum number of participants should not exceed 10. Groups should consist of participants with similar functional skills and for whom the objectives retained as part of their rehabilitation program are compatible with each other rather than constituted strictly on the basis of their audiometric characteristics. Also, when possible, efforts should be made to regroup participants who share a similar socioeconomic status and educational level and who have similar work-related responsibilities. This will ensure that the discussions held within the group will be more homogeneous and of interest to all the group members. It is recommended that patients who have difficulty communicating in the language in which the group will be conducted, who are not cognitively intact, or who display behaviors that might be disruptive within a group setting should not be invited to take part in a group intervention program. Those individuals will be better served within an individually based intervention program.

Group and individual training programs vary in their duration and in the length of each session. Typically, programs extend over a period of 8 to 12 sessions. Sessions, 60 to 90 minutes in duration, are usually held once or twice a week over this period of time, with assignments for home practice to be performed between sessions. In a program that combines analytic, synthetic, and communication management training, the analytic portion of the training program should rarely exceed 25% of the total time within a given session. Intensive group intervention programs may also be provided. For example, participants may attend daily sessions over a period of 1 or 2 weeks. In this case, daily sessions may include several 45- to 60-minute training activities, separated by coffee breaks and meals. Patient progress can be more easily monitored when the clinician uses work sheets for each exercise.

Telephone Training

The telephone is an important means of communication for most patients. However, communicating over the telephone can prove to be a challenge for persons with hearing loss. The acoustic signal received over the telephone will not be the same as a live-voice signal. The telephone may degrade the signal by narrowing the audio-frequency range available to the listener and by introducing background noise and distortion. An increasing number of persons with hearing loss use a cellular phone in conjunction with hearing aids. For those patients, the problem of interfering noise and acoustic distortion associated with telephone communication is exacerbated (Levitt et al, 2005). Also, visual information is not available to supplement the auditory information in the speech signal. Thus, communication by telephone may constitute an important rehabilitative need for many individuals with acquired hearing loss.

Telephone training may be provided to individuals with hearing loss who use hearing aids or cochlear implants. The goal of the training program may be different, depending on the device used and the benefit the patient receives from the device in auditory-only communication. The goal of telephone training will vary according to the individual. For some patients with acquired hearing loss, the goal of an intervention program may be to allow them to carry out a conversation for business or personal purposes. For others, the goal of an intervention program may be limited to the transmission of essential information.

An important component of all telephone training programs consists of identifying the most appropriate coupling system to use for telephone communication. This will be determined by the types of phones most often used by the patient, by the person's hearing loss, and by the type of personal hearing amplification system worn. There are exciting new developments related to the use of cellular phones that are beneficial for persons with hearing loss (Tchorz and Schulte, 2005). For example, in some instruments, the telecoil is automatically activated whenever the telephone is within the range of the stationary magnetic field of the device. For more information on telephone compatibility, refer to Chapter 17 in this volume. The recent introduction of telecoils that automatically turn on when in range of the stationary magnetic field of the telephone and of FM amplification systems that use wireless Bluetooth technology to connect to cellular phones are exciting developments in improving accessibility of cellular telephones for persons with hearing loss (Tchorz and Schulte, 2005). Also, some patients will require information on how to use a teletypewriter (TTY) and operator-assisted services. Often, when this is the case, the provision of information concerning these forms of telephone communication will not be sufficient. Instructions and systematic practice on how to use a TTY and operator-assisted services will be required (**Table 16–8**). Currently, these patients may choose to use newer technologies, such as text messaging, rather than a TTY.

Erber (1985) developed an intervention program for telephone use that consists of three phases. Initially, information concerning the individual's auditory abilities and communication goals is collected. This information is obtained from case history questionnaires and audiologic test results. Also, interviews are used to assess the individual's auditory abilities/difficulties, need for telephone communication, and goal in seeking this type of rehabilitative service. The second stage involves practicing simulated conversations. The results of this activity serve to define the specific goals for the intervention program. On the basis of this information, training exercises are designed to develop specific skills. Finally, the individual participates in conversations in practical, real-life situations over the telephone. Examples of training activities that may be incorporated into a telephone training program are outlined in **Table 16–8**. Few published comprehensive telephone training programs exist for persons with hearing loss. Two noteworthy exceptions are Erber (1985) and Castle (1988).

Table 16–8 Activities that Can Be Included in Rehabilitation Programs Designed to Improve Communication by Telephone

Orientation to telephone devices
The clinician provides information concerning auxiliary devices that are commercially available for use with the telephone (e.g., built-in amplifiers, in-line amplifiers, portable amplifiers, use of hardwired and wireless auxiliary devices that can be used with a telephone, and telephones specifically designed for individuals with hearing loss). The patient may be oriented to other systems used for telephone communication, such as devices that provide visual information (e.g., teletypewriter and voice carryover, fax, and e-mail). Also, information may be provided on the existence and use of telephone relay services.

Hearing aids and telephones
The clinician provides information on the different ways to couple telephones and hearing aids (i.e., hearing aid microphone, hearing aid tele-coil, and hearing aid hooked up to other types of assistive devices). For more information on this topic, the reader is referred to Chapter 17 in this volume. Practice sessions would be conducted to teach the patient how to use the telephone with the coupling system that is most suitable for the patient.

Development of strategies
The clinician provides an orientation to, and practice in, the use of anticipatory and repair strategies that can be used during telephone conversations. Some repair strategies that may be particularly applicable to telephone conversations are the use of spelling, code words, alphabet, numbers, counting, and key words (Castle, 1988). For those individuals who have great receptive difficulties over the telephone, training activities may focus on the use of code systems, such as speech codes, number codes, International Morse code, and touch-tone telephone code (Castle, 1988).

Conversational practice
Role-playing activities may be performed to simulate various conversations that might be held over the telephone (e.g., calling to make an appointment and calling to obtain information about schedules for plays and movies). At first, fully scripted scenarios can be used. Later, the scenarios may be modified so that the conversations are only partially scripted. Finally, the scenarios may include open-ended conversations (Erber, 1985). At each stage, the level of difficulty of the activities can be gradually increased. For example, initially the participants may conduct a face-to-face conversation. Then, the visual cues provided by the communication partner (often the clinician) can be gradually obscured (e.g., increasing the distance between the partners or decreasing the amount of lighting in the room). Eventually, one of the communication partners can move to a different room. Finally, conversations can be held from remote locations by means of commercially available telephones (Erber, 1985).

Carrying out real conversations
Patients can also carry out real conversations within the clinical setting. At first, they would call persons with whom they are familiar, such as friends and family members. Later, patients can carry out conversations with unknown individuals. For example, they can call the local transit company to ask for schedule or fare information.

Special Consideration

- Most patients with hearing impairment will require assistance from their audiologist to identify the type of coupling system that would best suit their needs for telephone use. In addition, many individuals, particularly elderly persons, may require assistance in learning how to adjust and how to use the coupling system that they acquire to communicate by telephone. Furthermore, some individuals may benefit from some specific training in the use of communication management strategies that can be applied during telephone conversations. Comprehensive rehabilitation programs should include the provision of all the services related to the use of the telephone by persons with hearing impairment.

◆ Communication Management Training

Over the years, expert clinicians observed that some persons with limited speech perception competencies were proficient communicators, whereas others with better speech perception competencies experienced communication difficulties in many situations. Beginning in the early 1980s, interest was renewed in designing audiologic rehabilitation programs that extended beyond speech perception training.

Those programs centered on the development of strategies aimed at facilitating communication, rather than focusing strictly on speech perception competencies. These programs incorporated many aspects of linguistic and sociolinguistic models of communication, such as the pragmatics of verbal exchanges. Also, these programs were based on a broader conception of communication that considered the effects of the type of information exchanged during conversations and the effects of the physical and social environment in which communication takes place (**Fig. 16–2**). An important dimension of those programs was a recognition that communication is an interactive process between individuals and that communication partners are an integral part of this process. The attitudes and behaviors of individuals who communicate with persons who have hearing loss can have an impact on the success (or failure) of a conversational exchange. On the basis of this knowledge, many rehabilitation programs were designed to help patients with hearing loss and their communication partners manage communication more effectively. Components of communication management training programs include communication strategies, conversational fluency, assertiveness training, stress management, and personal adjustment.

Communication Strategies

Broadly defined, communication strategies include any verbal or nonverbal behaviors that can be used to improve the effectiveness of communication. Tye-Murray (1994) grouped

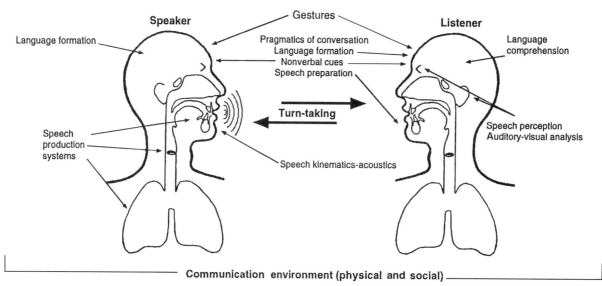

Figure 16–2 Simplified model of the communication process. (Adapted from an unpublished figure by McFarland and Gagné, personal communication, September 1998.)

communication strategies under two general categories: facilitation strategies and repair strategies. According to the author, facilitation strategies include behaviors used to prepare for and manage an ongoing conversation. Repair strategies are behaviors that are applied when a breakdown in communication occurs.

Facilitation strategies such as anticipatory strategies and attending strategies are used to optimize the recognition and comprehension of the verbal message. For example, preparing a list of potential vocabulary words, phrases, or sentences that may be used during an upcoming conversation (e.g., with a bank teller) would constitute a form of anticipatory strategy. Attending to the facial characteristics of a talker to obtain information concerning the emotional state of the person (e.g., anxious, happy, or sad) constitutes a form of attending strategy because facial expressions are almost always consistent with the content of the message.

Managing the physical environment in which a conversation takes place is another form of facilitation strategy. Patients can be taught to recognize physical properties of a given environment (e.g., living room, kitchen, restaurant, or meeting room) that are not ideal for communication (e.g., noise, reverberation, and poor lighting). Moreover, patients can be informed of, and taught, strategies that can be used to manage or modify environmental conditions to maximize their speech recognition performance. Instructional strategies are used to inform the communication partner of speaking behaviors that will facilitate speech understanding. For example, it has been shown that the use of clear speech can significantly improve a person's auditory-speech and visual-speech intelligibility (Gagné et al, 2002). Communication partners can improve their ability to be understood by persons with hearing loss if they use clear speech (Schum, 1997). In some cases, communication partners might benefit from training in the production of clear speech. According to Schum (1997), the production of clear

speech simply requires that the person talk naturally slower and louder, articulate accurately, use voice inflection to stress key words, and use pauses between phrases and sentences. Clinical experience has shown that even without extensive instructions or training, almost everybody can modify their speech articulation patterns to produce clear speech that will improve their speech intelligibility. However, most persons without training in the use of clear speech will tend to revert to their usual speaking patterns after a short period of time. During a conversation, patients may need to periodically remind their communication partners to use clear speech.

Message-tailoring strategies are also effective facilitation strategies. For example, Erber (1988) has shown that patients with hearing loss have less difficulty answering questions requiring a closed-set response than general open-ended questions (e.g., "Should we walk or take a bus to the concert?" rather than "How do we get there?"). Teaching patients with hearing loss to use and solicit these types of facilitation strategies constitutes an effective way of preventing or minimizing the number of communication breakdowns that may occur during a conversation.

Repair strategies are behaviors used to overcome a communication breakdown between communication partners. A communication breakdown occurs when one of the communication partners fails to understand a message that was intended for that person. Repair strategies can be used by the person who is providing the information (expressive strategies) or by the person for whom the message is intended (receptive strategies). The most frequently used repair strategy consists of simply asking the talker to repeat the message (Tye-Murray et al, 1992). Yet it has been demonstrated that other types of strategies may be more effective in repairing a communication breakdown (Gagné and Wyllie, 1989). Other types of repair strategies are asking the talker to rephrase the statement, simplifying the message, elaborating the message, providing the topic of the message, using natural gestures, and spelling or writing the misperceived message (Kaplan et al, 1987; Tye-Murray, 1994). Studies have shown that with some training, patients with hearing loss can be taught to request a wider range of repair strategies (Erber, 1996).

Examples of programs that include activities designed to optimize the use of appropriate communication strategies are Erber (1988, 1996), Jennings (1993), Jennings et al (1991), Kaplan et al (1987), Spitzer et al (1993), Tye-Murray (1994, 1997, 2002), Tye-Murray and Schum (1994), and Wayner and Abrahamson (1996).

Conversational Fluency

Conversation constitutes an important social behavior that involves more than the simple exchange of information between two or more individuals. During a conversation, several factors influence the degree of satisfaction experienced by the participants. Erber (1988, 1996) identified several factors that contribute to the degree of satisfaction experienced by the participants during a conversation. These include temporal aspects/rhythm of interchange, metacommunication/clarification, topic, intimacy/sensitivity, information, time/direction/fantasy, attitude, honesty, and power/control. These factors may differ in their importance to various communication partners. Other issues identified include the relationships among the communication partners, the expectations of the communication partners, the purpose of the conversation, and the outcomes of the conversation. For a detailed discussion of the factors that influence conversational fluency and satisfaction and a description of clinical procedures that can be used to assess and train conversational fluency, the reader is referred to Erber (1996, especially Chapter 9, pp. 203–223). When one of the communication partners has hearing loss, the general fluency of a conversation is often affected. This can cause dissatisfaction for all the persons participating in the conversation.

Pitfall

- Many communication management intervention programs focus exclusively on the elimination (or minimization) of communication breakdowns that occur during conversations. Other factors related to the goal and the processes involved in verbal communication are neglected. At best, those programs will increase the amount of information exchanged during a conversation. However, the motivation of the communication partners to communicate and their degree of satisfaction related to the conversation may be severely compromised. As Erber (1996) pointed out, several relevant variables must be considered when training conversational fluency.

Erber (1988, 1996) identified three basic correlates of conversational fluency. They are clarification ratio (the proportion of time devoted to successful exchanges of information), turn rate (the speaking turn-per-minute rate), and time sharing (the proportion of time each communication

partner talks during a conversation). On the basis of this information Erber (1988, 1996) and a colleague (Erber and Yalland, 1998) proposed two procedures that can be used to analyze aspects of conversational fluency. CONAN (Erber and Yelland, 1998) consists of a procedure that can be used to collect, store, and analyze temporal aspects of a communication exchange while a conversation is in progress. DYALOG (Erber, 1996, 1998) is a computer-based program devised to measure the occurrences of communication breakdowns and the amount of time devoted to repairing those breakdowns during a conversation.

Erber and his collaborator (Erber, 1988, 1996; Erber and Yelland, 1998) have proposed several activities that can be used to train conversational fluency. Among them is an activity named TOPICON (Erber, 1988, 1996). In this activity, the patient or clinician chooses a topic of interest from a prepared list. Next, the patient and clinician carry out a conversation. The clinician assesses the fluency of the conversation on the basis of several preselected variables known to influence conversational fluency and satisfaction. For example, the clinician may count the number of conversational turns between the dyad, the amount of speaking time taken by each person involved in the conversation, and the number of communication breakdowns that occur within a predetermined period. After the conversation is completed, the patient and clinician discuss the success of the conversation, determine the sources of difficulties encountered, and identify possible solutions that might be implemented to overcome those difficulties. Other activities include viewing and analyzing specific segments of videotaped conversations, identifying the global characteristics of the conversation, and judging the level of satisfaction experienced by the participants. In addition, Erber (1988, 1996) described conversational activities, such as speech-tracking procedures, question–answer activities, and topic-centered conversations, that can be used to improve conversational fluency. During those activities, initially the participants take part in controlled (scripted) conversations. Later, the participants take part in conversations that involve an increasing number of topic changes. Other training programs that may be used to assess and train conversational fluency include Spitzer et al (1993), Jennings (1994), and Plant (1996a,b, 2002).

Assertiveness Training

Many persons with hearing loss learn to use appropriate communication strategies in a clinical environment where they feel secure. However, they may feel uncomfortable using those same strategies when they interact with persons with whom they communicate on an everyday basis outside the clinical setting. In such cases, assertiveness training may be provided to overcome these obstacles. According to Tye-Murray (1994) and Trychin (1986), the goal of assertiveness training is to increase the cooperation of communication partners while maintaining an equality among all the participants in a conversation. Patients can learn to use effective (neutral, nonaggressive) strategies that will enable them to solicit assistance from their communication partners without diminishing their own self-esteem (or the esteem others have of them) and maintain an appropriate role within a conversational framework. Important aspects of assertiveness training include requesting modifications in the physical environment and informing the communication partner of some difficulties experienced and the reason for those difficulties (e.g., "I have a hearing loss that makes it very difficult for me to follow a conversation when there is a lot of noise in the background. Would you mind if we continue our conversation in the living room, where it is quieter?"). Providing communication partners with appropriate (positive and constructive) feedback is also an important component of assertiveness training. Such behaviors will lead the patient and his or her communication partners to use and, over time, maintain good communication practices. Examples of programs that include assertiveness training are Jennings (1993) and Wayner and Abrahamson (1996).

Stress Management

Most people at some point experience stress in their work or personal lives. Some individuals may have difficulty adapting to prolonged stressful situations. Training in stress management has become popular among the general population. Most persons with an acquired hearing loss will experience the added stress of having to function in a hearing society. For example, they worry that they will not be able to detect, recognize, and react appropriately to sounds and warning signals (e.g., alarm clock, microwave oven, doorbell, and fax machine), that they will not know when someone speaks to them, or that they will not correctly understand the information provided by their communication partners.

The effects of stress may manifest themselves in several different ways. Stress may be the cause of headaches, upset stomach, disturbed sleep pattern (including nightmares), decreased productivity at work, disorganization, anxiety, depression, excessive worrying, and withdrawal (Trychin, 1986). Typical physiological responses to stress include an increase in muscle tension, pulse rate, blood pressure, perspiration, and shallow breathing (Trychin, 1986). Stress management training programs have been developed for persons with hearing loss. In these programs, participants are shown how to recognize stressful situations related to their hearing loss and identify their physical and psychological reactions to these situations. They are taught strategies to manage stressful situations. Additionally, they are taught relaxation procedures to cope with the physical and psychological responses they exhibit. Examples of programs that include training in stress management are Trychin (1986), Jennings (1993), and Wayner and Abrahamson (1996).

Special Consideration

- Patients who report many symptoms of stress attributable to their hearing impairment may benefit from a stress management course. Ideally, courses should be adapted to the specific needs of persons with hearing impairment. However, if such courses are not available, patients may be referred to any reputable stress management course offered in the community where the facilitator is made aware of the hearing needs of the participant with hearing loss.

Personal Adjustment

Persons with hearing loss must learn to adapt and cope with all aspects of their lives, including their physical safety, basic communication needs, affective and social relationships, work or vocational performances, and sporting and other leisure activities. The process of adaptation to hearing loss is still not well understood (Hyde and Riko, 1994). However, it is recognized that it may take several years before those with acquired hearing loss are able to adapt completely to the effects of their hearing loss and (re)develop functional life habits (Hétu, 1996; Hyde and Riko, 1994).

Hearing loss is not simply a physical impairment. A comprehensive rehabilitative program must cater to all the consequences of hearing loss on a patient's life. Persons with hearing loss may request help from their rehabilitative audiologist regarding various aspects of the adjustment process. Intervention in this area of rehabilitation may address many different domains of personal adjustment, including the person's behavioral, emotional, cognitive, physical, and interpersonal reactions to the hearing loss (Schum, 1994). Interventions centered on issues related to aspects of personal adjustment should not be considered different (or distinct) from any other form of rehabilitation services provided to persons with hearing loss.

A panoply of intervention approaches exists to address personal adjustment difficulties. Counseling, a term used to describe strategies designed to help patients adjust to specific or situational problems, is often employed when referring to intervention approaches designed to address personal adjustment difficulties. Erdman (1993) provides an excellent review of counseling approaches that can be applied to rehabilitative audiology. Programs that specifically explore aspects of intervention related to personal adjustment among persons with hearing loss are Trychin (1986), Jennings (1993), and Wayner and Abrahamson (1996).

Individual versus Group Intervention Programs

An important issue that has yet to be resolved empirically is whether audiologic rehabilitation services are more effective when provided on an individual basis or when they are incorporated into a group intervention program. The results obtained from self-rated questionnaires indicate that patients taking part in group communication training programs experience a reduction in the deleterious impact of hearing loss. Furthermore, the participants with hearing loss report an increase in their use of hearing aids as well as a better use of appropriate communication strategies (Hawkins, 2005). Current clinical practice favors the use of group intervention programs for services related to communication strategies, conversational fluency, assertiveness training, stress management, and personal adjustment. Several reasons may account for this tendency. First, group intervention programs are more time efficient because several participants receive services at once. Second, some intervention activities are more easily conducted within a group setting. For example, role-playing activities involving several participants can be easily completed in a group setting. Third, group sessions provide a relatively secure environment in which participants can practice newly acquired skills. An individual can practice a specific intervention strategy with other group members and with the audiologist. Fourth, groups provide excellent opportunities for discussions. Groups allow participants to describe difficulties they and other group members may encounter or that other members of the group may not have recognized as such. For example, a participant with hearing loss may express a feeling of insecurity when he or she is alone because of not always being able to hear the doorbell. Other participants with hearing loss may express a similar feeling, whereas still others, including participants without hearing loss (e.g., accompanying persons), may become aware that this situation is truly problematic for someone with hearing loss. Participants without hearing loss may learn this difficulty is not unique to their communication partner. Another example would be a participant with normal hearing who reports he or she feels lonely because his or her social life has been severely curtailed on account of the partner's unwillingness to attend social gatherings because of his or her hearing loss. Again, participants with hearing loss and those without hearing loss may be able to relate this experience to their own situation.

In many societies, a negative stigma is attached to persons who have a hearing impairment (e.g., cognitive limitations, old age, and senility). The complex process of stigmatization associated with hearing loss is beyond the scope of the present chapter. Interested readers should refer to Hétu (1996) and Jennings (2005a) for their excellent treatments of this topic. For the purpose of this discussion, suffice it to say that on learning (or acknowledging) they have hearing loss, individuals must reconstruct the image that they have of themselves. Hearing loss brings about changes in a person's physiological system. More importantly, it changes that person's perception of self and social identity. This process invariably leads to a diminishment of self-image and self-esteem. This is not only due to the stereotype that society holds of hearing loss but also because often the person's own view of hearing impairment, before learning of his or her hearing loss, may in many respects be consistent with the negative image that society in general holds of hearing impairment. This often leads to feelings of guilt and shame. In some cases, this process leads to the development of maladaptive behaviors (e.g., denial, withdrawal, isolation, and aggressiveness), and it almost always, at least for some period of time, constitutes an obstacle to the person's ability to manage his or her rehabilitative needs.

At the community level, whether or not hearing impairment is a stigmatizing characteristic may depend on the social environment as well as on the persons present in that environment. For example, coworkers may make fun of and tease a colleague with hearing impairment. If so, that person may experience stigma (or feel stigmatized) in his or her work environment. However, the same person may not feel stigmatized at home in the presence of family members or when he or she participates in a group communication training program that is attended by other persons who have hearing loss. In order for an individual to be stigmatized, there must be an agreement that the individual is different from others and that the difference is undesirable (Coleman, 1997). The psychological literature has shown that group intervention programs constitute an effective approach to reconstructing self-image. Groups help the participants realize

they are not the only ones to experience specific hearing disabilities and that their situation is not unique. Groups provide a forum to discuss feelings, behaviors, and problematic situations attributable to hearing impairment. Group discussions and activities can serve to explain and describe the causes and consequences of hearing impairment for the persons with hearing loss and for their communication partners. Also, groups offer opportunities to overcome feelings of ineptness in dealing with the problems they experience. For those reasons alone, group programs constitute an important intervention approach to certain aspects of rehabilitative audiology. That is not to say that in certain cases a person's rehabilitative needs may not be better served by an individual or combined individual and group intervention program.

Group intervention programs should include a small number of persons (usually fewer than 10 participants) who share similar predicaments and rehabilitative needs. The participants with hearing loss do not necessarily need to be matched by degree or type of hearing loss. Groups should also involve the participation of persons who interact with the participants that have hearing impairment (i.e., accompanying persons, including spouse and other family members, friends, relatives, and coworkers). Activities should involve both the persons with hearing loss and their communication partners. In some cases, activities can involve separating the participants into two groups, one consisting of persons with hearing loss and the other consisting of the persons who accompany them. However, such activities should be kept to a minimum, given that an important objective of group intervention programs is to allow both groups of participants to mutually inform each other of their experiences.

Typically, group intervention programs run for 8 to 12 sessions. Sessions are held once or twice a week, with assignments for home practice to be performed between sessions. Each session is usually ~60 to 90 minutes. Group programs may also be provided on a more intensive basis, such as in full- or half-day sessions over a period of 1 or 2 weeks.

Group intervention programs may be organized in a comprehensive manner to provide a wide range of information and training to the participants. These programs may include information regarding hearing loss and devices, speechreading training, and communication management training. Examples of this type of program are Getty and Hétu (1991), Giolas (1982), Jennings et al (1991), Spitzer et al (1993), and Wayner and Abrahamson (1996).

Communication Partners

In the audiologic rehabilitation literature, the term *communication partners* usually refers to all individuals who communicate on a regular basis with persons who have hearing loss (e.g., spouses, other family members, close friends, relatives, and colleagues). In recent years, interest in involving communication partners in audiologic rehabilitation programs has increased. This is equally so for individual and group intervention programs.

Many intervention programs designed for adults and elderly persons with acquired hearing loss address issues related to communication difficulties experienced in certain situations. Communication necessarily involves the participation of more than one person. Communication breakdowns attributable to hearing loss result in an experience that is less than satisfactory for all the persons involved in the exchange, that is, the person with hearing loss and his or her communication partners (Erber, 1996). As discussed in previous sections, strategies to avoid or overcome communication breakdowns can be used by both persons with hearing loss and their communication partners (e.g., expressive communication repair strategies).

Communication partners play an important role throughout the personal and emotional adjustment processes that persons with acquired hearing loss undergo as they adapt to their new life situation. In addition to being empathetic and supportive of their companion, communication partners may be invited to play an active role in the intervention program. For example, they may be asked to complete exercises or activities designed to improve communication between persons with hearing loss and the persons with whom they interact (see Erber, 1996; Tye-Murray and Schum, 1994). The participation of communication partners in an intervention program may facilitate the rehabilitation of their partners with hearing loss. Following participation in a group audiologic rehabilitation program, some elderly participants report a significant reduction in handicap. The results of the investigation revealed that the participants who were accompanied by a support person, such as a spouse or a peer, reported the greatest amount of reduction in handicap. Moreover, their involvement in an intervention program will make communication partners more aware of some of the difficulties experienced by persons with hearing loss.

It has been documented that spouses and other communication partners may experience their own difficulties because of their interactions with persons who have hearing loss (Hétu et al, 1993). A person with hearing loss may choose to listen to the television at a very high volume. This may be very annoying to the other members of the household who do not have hearing loss. Or, always having to act as the "unofficial interpreter" at social gatherings may be burdensome for the spouse of a person with hearing loss. A couple's intimate and sexual relationship can suffer when one of the partners has hearing loss (Hétu et al, 1993). In sum, communication partners also experience difficulties associated with the fact that they interact with a person who has hearing loss. Those problems are legitimate and should not be neglected. Intervention programs in rehabilitative audiology should cater to the needs of those persons.

Controversial Point

- The contribution of communication partners in group intervention programs for persons with hearing impairment is multifaceted. On the one hand, they may be a resource available to assist individuals with hearing impairment overcome some of the difficulties they experience. On the other hand, it has been demonstrated that communication partners may be candidates for rehabilitation services in their own right. Comprehensive rehabilitation programs should cater to the specific needs of communication partners.

◆ Foundations of Audiologic Rehabilitation

Definitions

Many definitions of rehabilitative audiology exist (**Table 16–9**). Some of those definitions describe the activities that comprise intervention services or treatment programs associated with rehabilitative audiology (see ASHA, 1984). Others define audiologic rehabilitation as a process that aims primarily to resolve the communication disabilities experienced by persons with hearing loss (ASHA, 1984; Hull, 1982; McCarthy and Culpepper, 1987). Still others define the goal of rehabilitative audiology as the alleviation (or minimization) of handicaps created by hearing impairment (ASHA, 2001; Erdman, 1993; Gagné, 1998; McKenna, 1987; Ross, 1997). Generally, those definitions are based on the theoretical orientation that the respective authors have concerning audiologic rehabilitation. Since the 1980s, dramatic changes have taken place in the way rehabilitation in general (and rehabilitative audiology in particular) has been conceptualized. This section will outline a contemporary conceptual model of audiologic rehabilitation.

Models of Rehabilitative Audiology

In all disciplines that involve the use and application of knowledge, the way in which a concept is conceived has an influence on how the available information is applied to the discipline. A conceptual model provides a framework that is used to organize, describe, and investigate various elements of knowledge and factors related to a concept of interest. Hyde and Riko (1994) argue that one important function of conceptual models is to provide precise and comprehensive definitions of concepts and domains. They state that "terminology is more than labels; it reflects and affects its underlying constructs and it provides the vehicle for debate and research" (Hyde and Riko, 1994, p. 347). Moreover, models guide the way clinical services are dispensed to patients who seek these services. Conceptual models are rarely static; these evolve over time. As elements of the concept are investigated, a better understanding of the general model is developed, and refinements are made to the original model or the model is rejected and replaced by other, more comprehensive models.

Not unlike other disciplines, research and clinical services in audiologic rehabilitation are model driven. Over the years, our conception of rehabilitation has evolved, and the practice of audiologic rehabilitation has been greatly influenced by this evolution. It has been recognized (the pioneers of our discipline might say "rediscovered") that audiologic rehabilitation must involve more than fitting patients with appropriate amplification devices, in some cases supplemented by hearing aid orientation information and sometimes complemented by speechreading and auditory training sessions.

Professionals and academics recognize the need to provide more comprehensive services to their patients. There is a greater awareness of the effects of hearing impairment on communication and on other aspects of life (including the

Table 16–9 Examples of Definitions of Rehabilitative Audiology

---

Hull (1982, p. 6)
"Aural rehabilitation is an attempt at reducing the barriers to communication resulting from hearing impairment, and facilitating adjustment relative to the possible psychosocial, occupational and educational impact of that auditory deficit."

ASHA (1984, p. 37)
"Aural rehabilitation refers to services and procedures for facilitating adequate receptive and expressive communication in individuals with hearing impairment."

Erdman (1993, p. 374)
"The ultimate goal of [r]ehabilitative [a]udiology is to facilitate adjustment to the auditory and nonauditory consequences of hearing impairment."

McKenna (1987, p. 5)
"Ultimately the aim of rehabilitation must be the restoration of the individual to as high a level of functioning as possible."

McCarthy and Culpepper (1987, p. 305)
"The purpose of an aural rehabilitation program is to focus on assisting hearing-impaired individuals in the realization of their optimal potential in communication, which is needed in educational, vocational, or social settings."

Ross (1997, p. 19)
"[Aural rehabilitation] . . . Includes . . . any device, procedure, information, interaction, or therapy which lessens the communicative and psychosocial consequences of a hearing loss."

Gagné (1998, p. 70)
"The goal of audiological rehabilitation is to eliminate or reduce the situations of handicap experienced by individuals who have a hearing impairment and by persons with normal hearing who interact with those individuals."

ASHA (2001)
"Audiologic/aural rehabilitation is an ecological, interaction process that facilitates one's ability to minimize or prevent the limitations and restrictions that auditory dysfunctions can impose on well-being and communication, including interpersonal, psychosocial, educational, and vocational functioning."

Gagné (2000, p. 65)
"The goal of audiological rehabilitation is to restore or optimize participation in activities considered limitative by persons who have a hearing impairment or by other individuals who partake in activities that include persons with a hearing impairment."

---

impact hearing impairment may have on persons with normal hearing who interact with individuals who have hearing loss). Since the early 1970s, several models of service delivery in rehabilitative audiology have been proposed. Most noteworthy for their contribution to the development of rehabilitation services provided to persons with acquired hearing loss are the models proposed by Goldstein and Stephens (1981), Giolas (1982), Alpiner (1987), McKenna (1987), Hyde and Riko (1994), and Erber (1996). Each of these presents a model of service delivery that is consistent with the authors' views of rehabilitative audiology. All these models are similar in that they insist on the need for a systematic approach to the delivery of services in audiologic rehabilitation. In general, the approaches consist of a process that includes procedures to evaluate patients' competencies and needs, the selection of intervention strategies designed to respond to those needs, an implementation of the intervention program retained, and a postintervention evaluation. On the basis of the results of the postintervention evaluation, patients are either discharged or encouraged to pursue the same or different rehabilitation objectives. One important contribution of those service delivery models is that they differentiate the acts of rehabilitation (treatment programs, e.g., as the use of amplification, speech perception training, or communication management training) from the process of rehabilitation programs (assessment, intervention, and evaluation). Conceptually, this was an important advancement in the evolution of the profession.

International Classification of Impairments, Disabilities and Handicaps

In the 1980s, a concerted effort was initiated to develop a generic conceptual model of rehabilitation that would be accepted internationally and that would apply to all forms of rehabilitation services, regardless of the discipline (**Fig. 16–3**). A main objective of the *International Classification of Impairment, Disabilities and Handicap* (*ICIDH*) developed by the World Health Organization (WHO, 1980) was to propose definitions for concepts that could be used by all professionals involved in rehabilitation. Specifically, the WHO classification scheme of rehabilitation is based on the concepts of impairment, disability, and handicap. These concepts are well defined and have guided our interpretation of what rehabilitation is; what the goal of rehabilitation services ought to be; and how rehabilitation services should be conceived, organized, and dispensed. **Table 16–10** gives definitions of *impairment, disability,* and *handicap* provided by the *ICIDH* (WHO, 1980). The following examples illustrate how these three concepts apply to audiologic rehabilitation. A loss of external hair cells in the cochlea is an example of an auditory impairment. A person's inability to hear speech normally because of an auditory impairment would constitute a hearing disability. The person's inability to perform activities considered normal for the society, such as communicating by telephone, would be considered a handicap. It is important to recognize that the progression from impair-

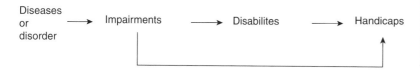

Figure 16–3 The relationship between the different components of the World Health Organization's *International Classification of Impairments, Disabilities and Handicaps* (*ICIDH*). (From World Health Organization. (1980). International classification of impairments, disabilities and handicaps. Geneva: WHO Press, with permission.)

ment to disability and handicap is not always simple. An impairment may not always cause a disability, and a disability does not necessarily cause a handicap (Hyde and Riko, 1994). The types and extent of the handicaps experienced by two persons with the same type and degree of hearing loss and similar hearing disabilities may differ. For example, reduced sound localization abilities in noise (a disability) may be very handicapping for a person who works outdoors on noisy construction sites and who must attend appropriately to the warning signals placed on mobile equipment. The same disability may not constitute a handicap for another person who works in a quiet business office and whose responsibilities do not require the localization of sounds. Also, two persons with different magnitudes of impairment may experience a similar handicap. For example, the construction worker cited above may have a moderately severe hearing loss, and his colleague may have a severe hearing loss. Yet both workers may experience a similar handicap on the construction site. Stephens and Hétu (1991) described how the concepts of impairment, disability, and handicap apply to rehabilitative audiology.

The *ICIDH* (WHO, 1980) and its adaptation to audiologic rehabilitation is helpful in defining the goal of audiologic rehabilitation. Audiologic rehabilitation rarely addresses the domain of hearing impairment. Audiologic rehabilitation services for a person with a sensorineural hearing loss do not focus on eliminating or reducing that person's hearing impairment (i.e., the person's hearing loss will not change as a result of rehabilitation services). Some aspects of rehabilitation programs are designed to reduce or eliminate hearing disabilities. For example, wearing hearing aids may help the person understand speech under several communicative conditions (i.e., in quiet and noisy environments). Speechreading training programs are designed to enhance audiovisual speech perception

performance in a variety of communicative settings. In some instances, intervention programs in audiologic rehabilitation address specific problems. For example, some patients consult an audiologist because they experience difficulties in performing certain activities that have a direct impact on their everyday activities (e.g., responding appropriately when the doorbell rings and conversing with clients on the telephone). In those cases, the intervention program may focus on addressing the patient's specific handicaps that are attributable to hearing loss. Also, professionals may choose to focus an intervention program on certain specific activities that are deemed important by their patient. For example, a person may report having difficulty adapting to a new work environment. Hence, the intervention program may be designed to solve specific problems that manifest themselves in that particular environment.

An important contribution of the *ICIDH* (WHO, 1980) was to provide a framework of rehabilitation that differed from medical models of health. The conceptual framework incorporated into the *ICIDH* was better suited to deal with chronic disorders such as a sensorineural hearing impairment, and it provided a novel approach concerning how rehabilitation services can be conceived, organized, and dispensed. Over the years, a few of this model's shortcomings were identified. Primary criticism related to the fact that the *ICIDH* did not provide a clear distinction among the constructs of impairment, disability, and handicap. Moreover, in many circles, the model was used to describe a unidirectional (causal) relationship among the three constructs (i.e., impairments lead to disabilities, which lead to handicaps, without allowing for the movement from handicaps back to disabilities and impairments). As well, the *ICIDH* was criticized because it did not adequately account for the role of social and physical environments in the creation of handicaps (WHO, 2001).

Table 16–10 WHO Definitions of Impairment, Disability, and Handicap

Impairment
Any loss or abnormality of psychological function or anatomical structure or function.

Disability
Any restriction or inability (resulting from an impairment) to perform an activity in the manner or within the range considered normal for a human being.

Handicap
Any disadvantage for a given individual, resulting from an impairment or a disability, that limits or prevents the fulfillment of a role that is normal (depending on age, sex, and social and cultural factors) for that individual.

Source: Definitions from World Health Organization. (1980). International classification of impairments, disabilities and handicaps. Geneva: WHO Press.

International Classification of Functioning, Disability and Health

After 2 decades of use, major changes in health care provision systems, and a new social understanding of impairment, there was a need to revise the original *ICIDH* (WHO, 1980). In 2001, the WHO proposed a revised classification system: the *International Classification of Functioning, Disability and Health,* commonly referred to as the *International Classification of Functioning (ICF; WHO, 2001).* This classification system is recognized internationally, and the treatment approaches underlying this conception of health are being applied in many disciplines of rehabilitation. Adherence to the *ICF* changes how intervention services are conceived, organized, and dispensed. Given the importance of the system, this section provides a brief description of the model and attempts to point out how it may be applied to clinical intervention services in audiologic rehabilitation.

The overall aim of the *ICF* (WHO, 2001) is to provide a common framework for describing consequences of health conditions, specifically for understanding the dimensions of health and functioning. The main elements of the *ICF* appear in **Fig. 16–4,** and they are defined in **Table 16–11.** The ICF has two parts, each with two components. One part incorporates aspects of functioning and disability (body functions and structures; activities and participations). The other part incorporates aspects of contextual factors (environmental and personal). According to the *ICF* (WHO, 2001), an individual's state of health is determined by the dimensions of functioning and disability; these dimensions interact with each other. The schematic representation of the model indicates that the dimensions of health (body functions and body structures, activities, and participations) may be influenced by environmental and personal factors. The model also indicates that these contextual factors may be influenced by the dimensions of health. Thus, in this model, one's health condition is seen as a result of a complex relationship between functioning and disability in interaction with two categories of contextual factors.

Pearl

- In providing rehabilitation services, the audiologist should always consider that the patient's difficulties are the result of a complex interaction between functioning and disability, on the one hand, and environmental and personal factors, on the other. Conceiving audiologic rehabilitation from this perspective will make it easier to identify solutions to the specific problems experienced and expressed by the patient.

The conceptual framework underlying the *ICF* (WHO, 2001) differs from the original classification system in some fundamental ways. An important characteristic of the *ICF* model is the recognition that a health condition may be caused by complex interactions of functioning at many levels: the body (impairments), the person (activity/activity limitation), and society (participation/participation restrictions). In this model, an impairment may or may not lead to activity limitations or participation restrictions. For example, a person with hearing loss (impaired body function) due to damaged outer hair cells (impaired body structures) may refrain from attending the bridge club meetings (a participation restriction) because of the hearing difficulties experienced while playing cards (an activity limitation). However, the same person may not experience an activity limitation when watching/listening to the television at home because in that situation he or she uses an auxiliary aid (e.g., an infrared amplification system) to pick up the audio signal. The same individual may stop attending a social dance class because of the difficulties experienced in

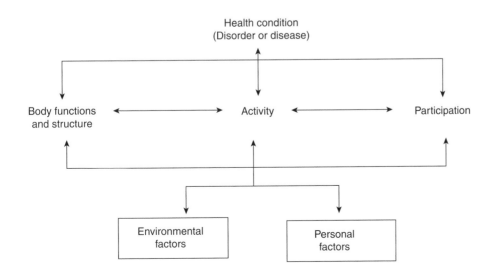

Figure 16–4 Illustration of the interactions of the concepts incorporated into the *ICIDH.* (From World Health Organization. (2001). International classification of functioning, disability and health. Geneva: WHO Press, with permission.)

Table 16–11 Definitions of Terms Related to the *International Classification of Functioning, Disability and Health*

Health condition: An alteration or attribute of the health status; it may be a disease (acute or chronic), disorder, injury, or trauma.

Functioning: An umbrella term encompassing all body functions, activities, and participation.

Disability: An umbrella term for impairment, activity limitations, or participation restrictions.

Body functions: The physiological functions of body systems (including psychological functions).

Body structures: Anatomical parts of the body such as organs, limbs, and their components.

Impairments: Problems in body function or structure as a significant deviation or loss; may be temporary or permanent; progressive, regressive, or static; intermittent or continuous. The deviation from the population norm may be slight or severe and may fluctuate over time.

Activity: The execution of a task or an action by an individual; used in the broadest sense to capture everything that an individual does, at any level of complexity, from simple activities to complex skills and behaviors.

Activity limitation: Difficulties an individual may have in executing activities; refers to a difficulty in the performance, accomplishment, or completion of an activity at the level of the person.

Participation: Involvement in a life situation.

Participation restriction: Problems an individual may experience in involvement in life situations.

Contextual factors: The complete context of an individual's life and living. They include two components: environmental factors and personal factors. Both of these types of factors may have an impact on the individual with a health condition and that individual's health and health-related states.

Environmental factors: Make up the physical, social, and attitudinal environment in which people live and conduct their lives. These factors are external to individuals and can have positive or negative influence on the individual's performance as a member of society, or on an individual's capacity to execute actions or tasks, or on the individual's health and health-related states. Environmental factors are classified according to individual or societal level:

    Individual level: The immediate environment of the individual, including settings such as home, workplace, and school. Included at this level are the physical and material features of the environment that an individual comes face to face with, as well as direct contact with others, such as family, acquaintances, peers, and strangers.

    Societal level: Formal and informal social structure, services, and overarching approaches or systems in the community or society that have an impact on individuals. This level includes organizations and services related to the work environment, community activities, government agencies, communication and transportation services, and informal social networks, as well as laws, regulations, formal and informal rules, attitudes, and ideologies.

Personal factors: The particular background of an individual's life and living. Personal factors are composed of features of the individual that are not part of a health condition or health states. These factors may include gender, race, other health conditions, fitness, lifestyle, habits, upbringing, coping styles, social background, education, profession, past and current experience, overall behavior pattern and character style, individual psychological assets, and other characteristics, all or any of which may play a role in disability at any level.

Source: http://www3.who.int/icf/icftemplate.cfm?myurl=introduction.html%20&mytitle=Introduction. Reprinted with permission from the World Health Organization.

that context. In that situation, the person's participation in the latter activity is restricted. However, other persons with similar hearing impairment may not experience the same level of difficulty in the same setting. For those persons, participating in that activity (social dance class) would not be restrictive.

Examples of how personal factors may or may not contribute to a person's participation in an activity are as follows. Imagine two older persons with a similar hearing loss who participate in the same social gathering of friends. One person is very shy/introverted, and the other is very assertive/extroverted. The latter person may request that communication partners face him or her when they are engaged in a conversation. This strategy may significantly reduce (or eliminate) the problems associated with communicating in that difficult listening environment. The shy/introverted person may not use any effective communication strategies when he or she does not understand the interlocutor. As a result, the involvement of the shy/introverted person may be restricted in that activity (i.e., the social gathering), whereas the assertive/extroverted person with a hearing loss may be able to participate fully in the discussions that occur during the gathering. It is fairly easy to imagine how factors related to the physical environment

may restrict one's participation in a given activity. For example, two friends, one of whom has a hearing impairment, may have difficulty conversing on a noisy street corner. However, the same two persons may be able to partake in a satisfying conversation when they are sitting in a quiet and well-lit living room.

The *ICF* model indicates that the social environment may also cause an activity limitation or a participation restriction. For example, it may be very acceptable for a person who has a hearing loss to request that his or her communication partner, who has a soft voice, speak more loudly in many social environments, such as in the person's living room, a park, and a shopping mall. The same request would be inappropriate in other social environments, such as in a romantic restaurant or a funeral home. Finally, it is worth noting that, according to the *ICF* model (WHO, 2001), a person without hearing loss may experience activity limitations and participation restrictions because someone in his or her environment has an impairment. For example, a spouse without hearing impairment may stop attending the bridge club because her husband, who has a hearing impairment, is no longer able to participate with her in that activity because he has difficulty hearing in that environment. As a result, the spouse is also restricted.

Many contemporary models of audiologic rehabilitation are consistent with the *ICF* conceptual framework (WHO, 2001). First, the fact that personal and environmental factors must be considered in assessing one's health condition has been recognized by several authors (Gagné, 1998; Gagné et al, 1999; Hyde and Riko, 1994; Stephens and Hétu, 1991). For example, the concept of personal factors as it is intended in the ICF model is closely related to the concept of predicament described by Hyde and Riko (1994). The importance of considering the physical and social environment in evaluating the difficulties experienced by someone who has a hearing impairment (or by someone with normal hearing who interacts with a person who has a hearing impairment) has been addressed by Gagné and colleagues (1999). As well, the notion that a "situation of handicap" (similar to the concept of health condition in the *ICF* model) is the result of an interaction among impairment and personal and environmental factors was incorporated into the conceptual models of audiologic rehabilitation proposed by several authors (see Gagné, 1998; Gagné et al, 1999).

Some approaches to audiologic rehabilitation (e.g., Stephens and Hétu, 1991) are compatible with the conceptual framework provided by the *ICF* (WHO, 2001). Based on those models, Gagné (2000) proposed that the goal of audiologic rehabilitation be redefined as intervention procedures designed "to restore or optimize participation in activities considered limitative by persons who have a hearing impairment or by other individuals who partake in activities that include persons with a hearing impairment"

(p. 65s). Accepting the conceptual framework underlying the *ICF* and this definition of audiologic rehabilitation has many implications for the way that rehabilitation services should be conceived, designed, organized, and dispensed. Some of those implications are presented in **Table 16–12**.

Rehabilitation as a Process

It is recognized that rehabilitation is a process that takes place over a long time (Erdman, 1993; Hyde and Riko, 1994; Schum, 1994). Rehabilitation does not occur only during the limited period of time during which the patient takes part in a structured audiologic rehabilitation program. Investigators have shown that a person's awareness of having hearing difficulties and the impact of the impairment on the person's life is part of a process that evolves from the time the hearing impairment is acknowledged to the time the individual has reached an optimal restoration of his or her normal life habits (Hétu, 1996; Hyde and Riko, 1994). This process may extend over a period of several years. During that time, a person's perception and description of the problems encountered because of the hearing loss, and his or her reactions to those problems, evolve (Hétu, 1996). A person's predicament (including auditory demands, beliefs, resources, attitudes, aptitudes, behaviors, perceptions, and lifestyle) and his or her communication needs also change as a function of time. Intervention programs must recognize this evolutionary process of rehabilitation. Moreover, those programs must cater to the

Table 16–12 Implications for Intervention Programs Based on Optimizing Participation in Activities

- An important component of all intervention programs should be to identify and describe, in a precise manner, the activities in which specific difficulties arise because one of the individuals participating in this activity has a hearing loss.

- All the factors that may contribute to the production of an activity limitation or a participation restriction must be identified, including the personal factors of all the persons involved and the environmental factors present in the setting in which the activity limitation or participation restriction occurs.

- A very personal and subjective dimension is present in what constitutes an activity limitation or participation restriction. An activity limitation and/or a participation restriction can only be described and defined by the persons who participate in that activity. That is, capturing the individuals' perspective and perception of the problem is essential to the intervention process.

- The major focus of intervention services must be placed on real-life situations. Accordingly, objectives of the intervention programs must be individualized and contextualized.

- Each activity is unique. Hence, the solution to each problem must also be unique and adapted to all the persons involved in the activity, as well as to the context in which the difficulties are experienced.

- Solutions to an activity limitation generally include more than the individual with hearing impairment. Hence, the participants in an intervention program should include all the persons who are involved in, and committed to, resolving the targeted activity limitation or participation restriction. The description of the activity limitation or participation restriction and the possible solutions to the difficulties experienced must take into account the perspectives of all those involved in the intervention program.

- Possible solutions to the problems must take into account the uniqueness of activity limitation and identify solutions that are possible, and acceptable, for all the persons involved in the intervention program.

- The clinician and all the other participants must be involved in identifying and selecting the intervention strategy that is most likely to succeed in resolving the targeted activity limitation. The intervention strategy retained must take into account the personal factors of all the participants and the environmental factors (individual and societal) associated with the activity limitation. Furthermore, only those solutions that are acceptable to all the participants should be considered as possible intervention strategies. This implies that for each intervention program, the solution retained as an intervention strategy must be negotiated with the participants.

- Generic intervention programs (e.g., wearing hearing aids and participating in a communication management training program) constitute potential intervention strategies that may be applied to resolve activity limitations or participation restrictions. However, the goal of the intervention program must center on optimizing the participation of all the persons involved in the activity and not on the application of (or compliance with) the intervention strategy per se.

- Only the persons who are involved in an activity in which there is a limitation or a participation restriction are able to describe what would constitute a satisfactory outcome as a result of taking part in an intervention program.

specific problems expressed by the individual at a given point during this process of rehabilitation.

A recognition that rehabilitation is a process implies that solutions to problems associated with hearing loss are not likely to be solved by a one-shot intervention program, such as wearing hearing aids or participating in a communication management program. The rehabilitation needs of patients change as a function of time. Their ability to manage problematic situations also changes as a function of time. At any given time during the process of rehabilitation, a proposed intervention strategy may or may not be acceptable to a patient. The acceptability of an intervention strategy is closely linked to the patient's predisposition in terms of the process of rehabilitation. Typically, early in the process of rehabilitation, patients will more readily comply with intervention strategies that are not intrusive to their communication partners (e.g., they will agree to wear a hearing aid, use auxiliary aids at home, use visual cues to optimize their speech perception competencies, and use receptive communication strategies). Later on, sometimes years later, patients may be able and willing to apply intervention strategies that require the cooperation of others (e.g., informing communication partners that they have a hearing loss and asking others to use clear speech or other specific expressive communication repair strategies).

Pitfall

- Both for the clinician and the patient, it is unrealistic to imagine that all the rehabilitative needs of a person with acquired hearing loss can be met within one intervention program. Rehabilitation is a process that extends over a long period of time (it may be as long as 5, 10, or even 15 years), and the rehabilitative needs of patients evolve as a function of time. Every intervention program should be confined to resolving specific hearing-related problems that are reported by the patient at the time he or she consults for rehabilitation services.

In selecting an intervention strategy to resolve a specific hearing-related problem, consideration must be given to solutions that are possible and acceptable to the patient. That is, professionals must take into account the patient's predisposition in terms of the process of rehabilitation. To comply with this principle of rehabilitation, all the components of an intervention program must be openly discussed and negotiated with the patient. Intervention programs that fail to respect this condition of intervention are not likely to succeed. Experimental data or clinical experience may suggest that a given intervention strategy is well suited to overcome specific problems due to hearing loss. However, if the patient is not able or willing to implement this strategy to address the problem under consideration, that strategy should not be incorporated into the intervention program. Patients are not likely to participate in an intervention program that does not cater to their specific needs. Also, they are unlikely to implement solutions that are retained as intervention strategies if they are not comfortable with those strategies. A failure to respect these conditions of intervention may lead the patient to withdraw from the rehabilitation program altogether.

Rehabilitation as a Solution-centered Intervention Process

In an earlier section, it was stated that the goal of rehabilitative audiology is to restore or optimize participation in an activity considered limitative because of the hearing difficulties experienced by one of the persons involved in that activity. The implication of this perspective on intervention programs was discussed. Given this perspective and consistent with the acknowledgment that rehabilitation is a process, intervention programs in rehabilitative audiology can be viewed as a solution-centered problem-solving process (Erdman, 1993; Gagné, 1998; Hyde and Riko, 1994; McKenna, 1987). As it relates to intervention programs in rehabilitative audiology, the general sequence of events involved in problem solving are outlined in **Table 16–13**.

Table 16–13 General Sequence of Events that Apply to Problem Solving in Audiologic Rehabilitation

1. Recognize that a problem exists.
2. Identify the problem.
3. Describe the problem (analyze the problematic activity).
4. Set the objectives and define the desired outcome while taking into account:
   - The problem (i.e., the activity limitation or the participation restriction)
   - The personal factors of all the persons involved in the activity limitation or participation restriction
   - The environmental factors (individual and societal level) in which the activity limitation or participation restriction occurs
5. Identify the possible solutions.
6. For each solution identified, analyze and evaluate the implications of choosing that solution (in terms of potential benefits, feasibility, and acceptability).
7. Select one or more acceptable solutions.
8. Implement the solution(s).
9. Evaluate the effects of applying the solution(s) (regarding outcome, impact, and consequences).
10. Identify the factors that facilitated or constituted an impediment to the implementation of the solution(s).

Source: From Gagné, J. P. (1998). Reflections on evaluative research in audiological rehabilitation. Scandinavian Audiology Supplementum, 49, 69–79. Adapted with permission.

For this problem-solving process to be successful and relevant, it is essential that the patient participate in all aspects of the intervention program. Specifically, the patient must be involved in the recognition, identification, and description of the limitations and/or restrictions experienced when attempting to participate in certain activities; the negotiation and definition of the objectives of the intervention program; the identification, selection, and implementation of the intervention strategy; the definition of the desired outcome (including the criteria used to evaluate the success of the intervention program); the identification of the factors (positive and negative) that contributed to the outcome; and the evaluation of the effects, impact, and consequences of the intervention program.

A solution-centered, problem-solving approach to intervention incorporates a phenomenological dimension (Erdman, 1993). Consideration of the patient's perspective is essential to capture the personal meaning of what it is like to experience an activity limitation or a participation restriction because at least one person participating in the activity has hearing difficulties, to identify potential ways to solve the problems, and to evaluate the process and success of the negotiated intervention program. The procedures used to obtain this information must make it possible for the patient to provide his or her perception of all the facets of the intervention program. The most effective method to achieve these goals is to use open-ended interviews.

Pearl

- The more a patient is involved in the definition of the objective, the implementation, and the evaluation of his or her intervention program, the more likely it is that the program will correspond to the patient's rehabilitative needs. Also, increasing a patient's involvement in all aspects of the management of his or her intervention program will increase the likelihood the intervention program will be successful.

Perhaps the most critical components of a solution-centered problem-solving approach to intervention consist of identifying as precisely as possible the activity limitation and/or participation restriction to be addressed by the intervention program and defining the specific objectives of the program. A thorough understanding of the problem encountered by the patient in a given environment (i.e., both at the individual level and at the societal level) will enable the clinician and all the other participants to clearly identify the objective of the intervention program. As mentioned previously, the description of the activity limitation and/or participation restriction can only be provided by the persons involved in that activity. The clinician's role is to ensure that all the dimensions of the activity have been identified. On the basis of this information, the specific objective of the intervention program can be formulated.

Goal Attainment Scaling (Kiresuk et al, 1994) has been used widely with a variety of populations. The technique discussed

Table 16–14 Defining the Objective of an Intervention Program

The process of defining a specific objective should

1. Include all the individuals involved in the pursuit of the objective
2. Define the role and responsibilities of each person involved in the intervention program
3. Describe the conditions under which the stated objective will be accomplished (personalized and customized according to the expressed needs, willingness, and capabilities of each participant)
4. Specify the criteria that will be used to evaluate whether the objective has been reached (i.e., the outcome measure)
5. Provide a time frame within which the objective should be reached

Source: From McKenna, L. (1987). Goal planning in audiological rehabilitation. British Journal of Audiology, 21, 5–11, with permission.

in this text provides a framework for organizing the process of rehabilitation by involving the patient, clinician, and significant others in setting goals for rehabilitation that are unique to the individual involved. *Goal Attainment Scaling* also provides a means for quantitative and qualitative documentation of change in performance following rehabilitation programs. It is believed that when individuals are involved in selecting personal goals, they have a greater responsibility for working toward meeting the goals. Based on *Goal Attainment Scaling*, McKenna (1987) provided a useful framework for defining the objectives of an intervention program in audiologic rehabilitation. According to the author, each specific objective should state clearly (in an unambiguous fashion and in quantifiable terms) how the participants will behave if the intervention program is successful. Some essential components of defining the objective of an intervention program are provided in **Table 16–14**.

Once defined, the objective of the intervention program constitutes a form of agreement (i.e., a contract) among the clinician and the participants. The objective states who will do what and under what circumstance. Also, it specifies the time frame for the implementation of the intervention strategy. Objectives that are well defined will help the participants (including the clinician) identify possible solutions that could be implemented to attain the objectives. An example of an objective formulated according to the criteria specified by McKenna (1987) is provided in **Table 16–15**.

Evaluating the outcome of the intervention program is a critical component of a solution-centered problem-solving

Table 16–15 Example of an Intervention Objective

Mr. King and his poker partners will use appropriate repair strategies whenever a communication breakdown occurs during their weekly card-playing evening. As a result of an 8-week communication management program, in which Mr. King and all of his partners will participate, Mr. King will be able to understand the messages intended for him after no more than two repair strategies have been provided to him.

Source: Criteria based on McKenna, L. (1987). Goal planning in audiological rehabilitation. British Journal of Audiology, 21, 5–11.

approach to rehabilitation. That is, once the intervention component of the program has been completed, it is important to evaluate whether the objective of the program has been met. Clearly defined objectives will greatly facilitate outcome evaluation. A component of problem solving that is often overlooked is the evaluation of the process, impacts, and consequences of the intervention program. Throughout an intervention program, and especially at the conclusion of the program, time should be taken to evaluate the process of the intervention program. For example, the clinician and the participants should discuss the frequency and the duration of individual sessions, the length of the intervention program, and the nature of the activities included in the program. Information regarding these and other aspects of the intervention process may provide the clinician and the participants with useful insights concerning the application of specific intervention strategies. Also, it may suggest modifications that could be implemented to existing intervention strategies to make them more effective and appropriate for solving certain activity limitations and/or participation restrictions.

Almost always, participation in an intervention program has some impact and consequences that are not directly related to the specific objective or the desired outcome of the program. The consequences of taking part in an intervention program may be positive or negative. For example, Mrs. Smith may participate in an intervention program to learn communication strategies that could be used to solve problems she encounters during family gatherings. Later, she may report having used those same strategies (successfully) in other activities (e.g., during business meetings). Mr. Jones reports that he has difficulty understanding coworkers in the lunch room. The negotiated intervention strategy (i.e., asking his colleagues to face him when they speak to him) has proven to be very successful in terms of the stated objective of the program (i.e., when he applies the strategy, he does not have any difficulty understanding his coworkers). However, the implementation of this strategy has had a negative impact (e.g., revealing to his colleagues that he has difficulty understanding speech because of hearing loss). Specifically, he has to bear the brunt of all the jokes about persons with hearing loss, and he finds this very demeaning. The important point to be retained from these examples is that the evaluation of an intervention program should extend beyond the measurement of outcome (i.e., beyond measuring if the specific objective was attained). An evaluation of the impact and consequences of an intervention program is essential to evaluate the patient's satisfaction with the treatment. This information also provides a more comprehensive evaluation of the effectiveness of an intervention program. Data concerning the possible impact and consequences of an intervention program can be used by the clinician and the patient to evaluate the advantages and disadvantages of implementing a given intervention strategy. This information may serve to modify or adapt intervention programs for other patients who experience similar situations of handicap.

The implementation of a solution-centered, problem-solving approach to rehabilitation represents a major change from traditional approaches to rehabilitation. First,

the relationship between the clinician and the participants is altered. In traditional rehabilitation programs, the clinician assumes the role of the "expert." The expert diagnoses the problems, informs the patient of the causes and the consequences of the problems, selects an intervention strategy judged to be appropriate to "fix the patient's problem," and informs and trains the patient in the application of the intervention strategy retained. Often, the clinician decides when to terminate the intervention program. In a solution-centered problem-solving approach to rehabilitation, during the course of an intervention program, the role of the expert is often assumed by the patient (who else can truly describe the activity limitations and/or participation restrictions that are experienced, express the desired outcome, determine which of the possible intervention strategies is acceptable, and evaluate the success of the intervention program?). Throughout most of the intervention program, the clinician and the participants are equal partners with a common goal: identifying solutions to the activity limitations and/or participation restrictions that are experienced. As mentioned earlier, the involvement of the participants is essential in all phases of the intervention program. Second, the selection of an intervention strategy is negotiated between the clinician and the participants, and it is always guided by the objective of the program. That is, the intervention strategy retained, whether novel or generic, must always be tailored to the specific objective of the program.

Third, and perhaps most important, the focus of the intervention program is shifted. Often, the implicit goal of many rehabilitation programs is to solve the problems experienced by the person with hearing loss. The source of the problem is deemed to be the hearing loss. The focus of the rehabilitation program is on the disabilities of the patient, and the responsibility of overcoming the problems rests with the person with hearing loss. In a solution-centered problem-solving approach to rehabilitation, the focus is placed on resolving the activity limitations and/or participation restrictions that are experienced (i.e., not necessarily to overcome the hearing impairment). This change in perspective has implications for intervention. Solutions to problems must consider changes that can be made to the environment in which an activity limitation or a participation restriction occurs. Also, possible solutions should consider all the persons, including those individuals with no hearing disabilities, who participate in the problematic activity. Changing the perception of the rehabilitation process will serve to reestablish the role and responsibility of all the persons involved in the activity. It recognizes that the burden of solving a problem does not rest solely on the person with hearing loss (the consequences of this change in perception will most likely have a positive impact on the person's self-esteem). Also, it clearly indicates that other persons involved in that activity have a role in creating some restrictions to participation. Moreover, it offers those individuals an opportunity to participate in the resolution of problems that they may themselves experience in that situation.

Finally, two additional issues concerning the implementation of a solution-centered problem-solving approach will be addressed briefly. First, an intervention program will rarely include only one objective. Generally, patients will be able to identify several activity limitations and/or participation restrictions that they encounter in their daily lives. A given intervention program may include more than one objective. However, to attend appropriately to each of the objectives selected, the number of objectives retained should be limited. Typically, an intervention program will cover two or three objectives. However, this may vary considerably depending on the patient's predicament, the nature of the activity limitations, the clinician's competency and motivation, and the amount of time available to provide rehabilitation services. The negotiated objectives must be realistic, and there should be indications that those objectives can be reached within the time period established for the intervention program. In this regard, the clinician's role in negotiating objectives for an intervention program is critical.

It is best to select objectives that can be attained within a period of 2 or 3 months. Objectives that require a longer period of intervention should be broken down into smaller components that can be evaluated within this time frame. Once the period of time negotiated to attain an objective has been reached, an evaluation of the process, outcome, impact, and consequences of the intervention program should be conducted. On the basis of the results of the evaluation, the initial objective may be redefined (if the goal was not reached), other objectives may be pursued, or the patient may decide to suspend his or her participation in a structured intervention program.

Second, patients should learn to implement the problem-solving process independently. This could be included as one of the negotiated objectives of an intervention program (with the approval of the patient, of course). The process of problem solving is systematic and fairly simple to learn, and it can be applied to all problematic situations. Patients can be taught the different steps and the sequence involved in problem solving (outlined in **Table 16–13**). They can be trained on how to address each component of this process. Initially, the clinician may play a more active role in the implementation of the process. Gradually, patients should be encouraged to implement the sequence of problem solving themselves, first with the support of the clinician and eventually independently. With some guidance and training, most patients will be able to apply the problem-solving process by themselves. In doing so, they will become much more independent in managing their own rehabilitation needs.

Jennings (2005b) provided evidence that adults who attended group audiologic rehabilitation programs, participated in *Goal Attainment Scaling* (Kiresuk et al, 1994), and were trained in using a problem-solving process successfully attained goals that were set prior to attending the program. In addition, the participants increased their daily use of hearing aids as well as the number of assistive devices they owned. Participants continued to make gains in all of these areas when followed up to 6 months after having completed the program. These results suggest that once adults with hearing loss have set personal goals and gained skills required to tackle these goals, they adopt the behaviors needed to manage their communication difficulties, and they maintain these behaviors beyond the duration of their participation in the intervention program.

Pearl

- The principles and application of a problem-solving process are simple and can be applied to all problematic situations. Most patients can learn to apply the process of problem solving to resolve difficulties they encounter in their everyday lives. In doing so, they will become more proficient at managing their rehabilitative needs. They are also more likely to increase their self-confidence and improve their self-esteem.

♦ Case Presentation

The final section of this chapter will illustrate how a solution-centered, problem-solving approach can be applied to rehabilitative audiology. This will be accomplished in the form of a fictitious case presentation.

Background Information

Five years ago, C.D., a 50-year-old man, had bilateral hearing loss develop over a period of approximately 6 weeks. His hearing loss was attributed to a virus. Initially, the hearing loss was profound. Gradually, over a period of 6 months, his hearing sensitivity improved slightly. Since then, C.D.'s hearing tests have been stable and indicate he has severe hearing loss bilaterally. Audiologic test results indicate he has poor auditory–word recognition abilities in quiet bilaterally. Within 2 months of acquiring his hearing loss, C.D. was fitted binaurally with behind-the-ear (BTE) hearing aids. Both aids are equipped with a telecoil and a direct audio input. Also, he owns an FM system that he uses primarily for meetings at work. C.D. has not been able to use a telephone successfully, even with auxiliary devices. He relies on the use of a TTY, e-mail, and fax for distance communication, both at home and at work.

C.D. actively participated in audiologic rehabilitation programs for a period of 2 years after the onset of his hearing loss. Those programs consisted of hearing aid orientation, individualized speech perception training, and communication management training. C.D.'s wife has been very supportive throughout the process of rehabilitation. She was actively involved in the rehabilitation programs. Also, since the onset of his hearing loss, C.D. participates in a support group for individuals with sudden hearing loss.

C.D. is employed by a large consulting firm in computer applications. His employer and coworkers are aware of C.D.'s hearing loss. In fact, he was given a 1-year disability leave at the time he acquired his hearing loss. When he returned to work, his ability to perform his regular duties was reassessed, and he was informed that he could resume his previous position within the company. Primarily, his responsibilities involved debugging commercial software application programs.

C.D. contacted his rehabilitation audiologist 3 years after he had completed his previous intervention program. He reported that he had recently been promoted to a new position within the company. The position involved working in a team of six professionals, serving clients both on- and off-site.

Description of the Activity Limitations and Participation Restrictions

Discussions with the clinician revealed that C.D.'s new position involved regular team meetings both with and without clients. Those meetings often centered on very technical aspects of computer applications, and the information discussed was essential for C.D. to do his work. C.D. was concerned because frequently he was not able to follow the discussion in those meetings. Recently, he failed to complete work that he was responsible for because he was unaware that he had been assigned those tasks. When asked to describe specific activities in which he experienced problems because of his hearing difficulties, C.D. identified two different activities in which he had problems participating: during the team's weekly meeting and when he met with clients in their workplace. It was decided that initially the intervention program would focus on resolving the participation restrictions experienced during the team's weekly meetings.

C.D. was asked to identify the possible causes for the difficulties experienced during the weekly meetings. Specifically, he was asked to consider (1) factors related to himself, (2) factors related to the other members of the team who took part in the meetings, and (3) factors related to the environment in which the meetings were held. During discussions with the clinician, several possible causes for the difficulties experienced were identified for each of the factors. With regard to himself, C.D. reported that his speechreading abilities had "slipped" somewhat over the years. He found it difficult to speechread in a group that involved six or more participants. Also, he observed that the meetings were held late in the afternoon when he was tired. He believed that this made it more difficult for him to concentrate and follow the discussions.

Concerning the other members of the team, C.D. noted that his coworkers empathized with his situation. He remarked that they tried to be helpful because they realized that "a team's accomplishments are only as good as the sum of its members." However, he reported that they often forgot that he has hearing loss. Frequently, several persons would talk at the same time, most of the individuals forgot to let him know when they were the one talking, and some of the team members had weak voices yet didn't make an effort to speak up. C.D. stated that he used his FM system during the meetings, but he observed that his lapel microphone failed to pick up the voices of all the participants.

Concerning factors related to the environment, C.D. reported that the conference room was equipped with a long rectangular table. He sat on one side of the table, which made it difficult for him to see everyone around the table. He was aware that sitting at the end of the table would offer better speechreading opportunities, but that place was taken by the team leader. C.D. also reported that there was a coffee machine in the conference room. Periodically, the machine generated noise, but the frequency of occurrence and the duration of the noise were unpredictable.

Negotiated Objective and Structure of the Intervention Program

When asked what his objective was in seeking rehabilitative services, C.D. reported he would like to be able to follow the discussions perfectly during the meetings, but stated that this was not a realistic goal. He added, "I guess my goal would be to communicate to my optimum level during the meetings." Discussions with the clinician focused on identifying a tangible indicator that could be used to measure whether he was communicating optimally during the meetings. The indicator retained was that C.D. would no longer miss completing tasks that were assigned to him during the meetings.

It was agreed that the first part of the intervention program would concentrate on identifying possible solutions for the difficulties C.D. encountered during the meetings. The second part of the program would be devoted to exploring and implementing the solutions retained. Furthermore, it was agreed that for those two components of the intervention program, C.D. and the clinician would meet twice weekly over a period of 1 month. Also, it was agreed that once the intervention strategies had been implemented, the overall success of the intervention program would be evaluated over a period of 3 months.

Intervention Program

C.D. was asked to identify possible strategies that could be used to improve his ability to understand conversations during the team meetings. The strategies identified by the clinician and C.D. are listed in **Table 16–16.** Discussions ensued on the potential benefit, feasibility, and acceptability of each of the strategies identified. Two strategies were discarded. First, the possibility of requesting that the meetings be held in another (more quiet) conference room was discussed. However, according to C.D., this request was not realistic because no other room was available for meetings in the building. Likewise, C.D. stated that no oval or round conference table was available. He rejected the idea of requesting that the company purchase a new conference table. He thought that request would be exaggerated.

C.D. stated that he would continue to use his FM system during the meetings. Also, C.D. agreed that he would meet with his team leader to discuss the implementation of some of the other strategies identified. Specifically, he would (1) request that strategies involving the participation of the other team members be discussed during a team meeting, (2) request that he sit at the end of the conference table so that he could more easily speechread all the team members, (3) suggest that the coffee machine be moved to a different room, (4) investigate the possibility that the company would purchase a conference microphone for his FM system, and (5) investigate the possibility that the company would purchase a computerized note-taking system.

Several sessions were devoted to preparing C.D. for his upcoming meetings with his team leader and his coworkers.

Table 16–16 List of Possible Strategies Identified to Resolve the Situation of Handicap

Strategies related to the patient
 Sharpen speechreading skills
 Increase level of self-confidence and not hesitate to request a clarification when he has not understood
 Inform and remind other team members of patient's communication needs*
 Reestablish a set of communication rules that should be followed during meetings*
 Always use FM system during meetings
 Select/request a better place to sit in the conference room*

Strategies that involve the cooperation/participation of other team members
 Follow the established communication rules:
  Only one person speaks at a time*
  Talker signals that he or she is talking
 Use appropriate communication strategies:
  Members look at patient when they talk*
  Provide cueing for patient when necessary
  Use clear speech*
 Hold meetings at an earlier time of day when the patient is less tired and it is easier for him to concentrate on the discussion at hand*

Strategies related to the physical environment
 Hold meetings in a different (more quiet) conference room
 Alternatively, remove the coffee machine from the conference room*
 Change present rectangular table for an oval or round table

Other possible solutions
 Replace the existing FM system microphone with a conference microphone*
 Make use of a computerized note-taking system

* Indicates strategies that were incorporated into the intervention program (see discussion in text).

For example, activities were designed to enable C.D. to describe to his coworkers the types of hearing difficulties he experienced during team meetings. Ways of presenting this information in a factual, nonaccusatory fashion and without appearing to rely on self-pity or somehow diminishing his contribution to the group were discussed and practiced during sessions. Other activities were designed to identify approaches that could be used to solicit the active participation of his coworkers in implementing strategies that could be used by all team members during the weekly meetings (without appearing to be aggressive or accusatory and taking into account the personality of the team members and the dynamics of the group). Different communication management strategies were identified. Ways that they could be integrated into the weekly team meetings were discussed. Also, approaches to providing feedback to his coworkers to reinforce their use of facilitating strategies were discussed and practiced. Many of the activities incorporated into this part of the intervention program were accomplished through role-playing activities, first with the clinician, and then with his spouse assuming the role of the team members. Also, the clinician guided C.D. on where to obtain information on a conference microphone for his FM system and a computerized note-taking system, including addresses, costs, and advantages/disadvantages of each system. Practice sessions were devoted to finding ways to present this information to his superiors at work.

After approximately 1 month of attending his rehabilitation sessions on a regular basis, C.D. met with his team leader. As a result of this meeting, the following actions were agreed on and initiated:

1. The team leader agreed to change seating positions with C.D. during the weekly meetings (he did not see this as a big issue, and he was unaware that sitting at the end of the conference table would be advantageous for C.D.).

2. Ways to improve the exchange of information that would enable C.D. to understand better and participate more actively in the meetings would be discussed during an upcoming team meeting. The team leader would include an item on the meeting agenda that would be entitled "Optimizing Communication Flow within the Group." Furthermore, the team leader would introduce the topic to the team members and ask C.D. to preside over the discussion on this topic.

3. The team leader and C.D. agreed that the option of scheduling the meetings at an earlier time of the day would be discussed with the other group members.

4. The team leader would inquire about the possibility of relocating the coffee machine. This was done, and within a week the coffee machine was moved to another room.

5. The team leader set up a meeting with the company's budget director, C.D., and himself. The purpose of the meeting was to discuss the possibility of acquiring a computerized note-taking system and a conference microphone for the FM system. The budget for the computerized note-taking system was not granted, but funds were made available to purchase a conference microphone. C.D. was responsible for ordering the microphone.

The group discussion on how to optimize communication during team meetings was held approximately 3 weeks after C.D. met with the team leader. During the meeting, C.D. described to his coworkers some of the difficulties he encountered during team meetings because of his hearing loss. Many of the team members reported that they were aware that C.D. had hearing loss but that they did not realize that he had difficulty following group discussions, especially because he did so well during one-to-one conversations. According to them, overall, C.D.'s participation and performance during the team meetings did not seem to present any problems. ("You seem to be doing so well!" was a common response.) C.D. described the conference microphone and showed how it could be used during team meetings. It was agreed that team members would face C.D. when they spoke during meetings, they would speak clearly without overexaggerating their pronunciation, and only one person would speak at a time. Whenever those rules were not followed, it would be every team member's responsibility (including C.D.) to remind the group of the communication rules that were agreed on.

The team members agreed to hold the meetings in the morning rather than late in the afternoon. Also, everybody agreed that it would be helpful to have a written record of the topics discussed during the meetings. Those notes would specifically include a list of actions to be completed by each team member. It was decided that, on a rotating basis (excluding C.D.), one team member would take notes on a laptop computer. Immediately after the meeting, the notes would be sent to all team members via e-mail. Finally, it was agreed that this agenda item (optimizing communication during team meetings) would be rediscussed by the group in approximately 2 months.

After the initial series of regular sessions that took place during the first month of the intervention program, C.D. and the rehabilitation audiologist met on four different occasions. For each of those meetings, the primary topics of discussion were as follows: session 1, postmortem of C.D.'s meeting with his team leader; session 2, postmortem of C.D.'s meeting with the team members; session 3, preparation for review meeting with team members that was held 2 months after the implementation of strategies to improve communication during team meetings; and session 4, postintervention evaluation of the intervention program with the rehabilitation audiologist.

Outcome, Impact, and Consequences of the Intervention Program

Three months after the intervention program was initiated, C.D. met with the rehabilitation audiologist to evaluate the outcome, impact, and consequences of the program. C.D. reported that, overall, the action plan established with his team members was beneficial. Related to the objective of the program, C.D. reported that he had not missed any assignments since the intervention program had been implemented. On the basis of those results, both C.D. and the rehabilitation audiologist agreed that the intervention program was successful. According to C.D., removing the coffee machine from the conference room, changing his seating position during meetings, and changing the meetings to an earlier time during the day all contributed to the success of the program. The implementation of communication rules negotiated with his team members was somewhat successful. However, C.D. reported that not everybody always followed the rules. Also, the other team members did not

always remind the "culprits" that they were contravening the established procedures. C.D. did not feel that he should be the only person to remind others of the agreement, so he was not consistent in asking his teammates to follow the established procedures. C.D. always used his FM system and the conference microphone during the meetings. This proved to be of some help.

C.D. reported that the single most beneficial component of the intervention program was the implementation of a note-taking system. This strategy was extremely useful for C.D. because it provided him, in writing, some of the important information he had missed (in fact, it made C.D. realize how much information he missed during meetings). During the team meeting devoted to evaluate the success of the communication rules established within the team, all the participants reported that they benefited personally from the note-taking system. The notes served as an archive for the discussions and decisions made during the meetings. Notes from previous meetings were often retrieved and used to remind the team members of past decisions and the rationale underlying those decisions. The team leader reported that the note-taking strategy had significantly improved the efficacy of the group meetings. As a result, he had incorporated this strategy in other group meetings that he coordinated.

Based on C.D.'s own admission, one negative impact of implementing the note-taking system was that he played a less active role during the meetings. Specifically, he was less attentive to the group discussions because he knew he could rely on the notes to obtain the important information. However, by doing so, he felt that he missed out on some of the details that were discussed during the meetings. Also, because he could rely on the notes, C.D. was not consistent in requesting that his coworkers use the communication rules whenever he did not follow what was being discussed during the meetings.

On the basis of the postintervention evaluation, C.D. and the rehabilitation audiologist agreed that the intervention program would be pursued further. One aspect of the program would focus on improving the use of communication strategies during team meetings. Another aspect of the program would consider solutions to difficulties that C.D. encountered when he met with clients in their own offices.

◆ Summary

The process of adapting to hearing loss is long, complex, and yet to be fully understood. Most adults and elderly persons with acquired hearing impairment could benefit from the expertise of rehabilitation audiologists to help facilitate this process of adaptation. In this chapter, we have described some of the tools of rehabilitation (intervention strategies) that can be integrated into a comprehensive rehabilitation program (e.g., speech perception and communication management training). Special consideration was given to the process of intervention (e.g., identifying problems in terms of activity limitations and participation restrictions, defining objectives, implementing intervention strategies, and evaluating the success of the program). A solution-centered, problem-solving approach to intervention was described. The approach is based on the belief that the goal of rehabilitative audiology is to restore or optimize participation in activities considered limitative because of hearing difficulties experienced by one of the persons involved in those activities. This approach differs from traditional rehabilitative audiology. It

clearly defines the goal and the process of intervention. Moreover, it redefines the role of the clinician and patients in the intervention process. More importantly, it provides concrete solutions to real problems experienced by patients in their everyday lives. It has been shown that the successful application of a solution-centered, problem-solving approach to rehabilitative audiology is not only beneficial to patients but also gratifying to clinicians (Dillon et al, 1997).

Appendix 16–1

Information on Computer Applications to Speech Perception Training

Dynamic Audio Video Interactive Device (DAVID)
Donald G. Sims
Department of Communication Research
National Technical Institute for the Deaf
Rochester Institute of Technology
Rochester, NY 14623–0887

Computer-assisted Speech Perception Evaluation and Training (CASPER)
Nancy Plant
c/o Arthur Boothroyd
City University Graduate Center
Department of Speech and Hearing Sciences
33 West 42nd Street
New York, NY 10036

Auditory-visual Laser Videodisc Interactive System (ALVIS)
Lennart L. Kopra
c/o Department of Communication Sciences and Disorders
The University of Texas at Austin
CMA 7.202
Austin, TX 78712

Computerized Laser Videodisc Programs for Training Speechreading and Assertive Communication Behaviors
Richard S. Tyler
Department of Otolaryngology,
Head and Neck Surgery
The University of Iowa Hospitals
Iowa City, IA 52242

Computer-aided Speechreading (CAST)
M.-K. Pichora-Fuller, Director
Human Communication Lab
University of Toronto, Mississanga
3359 Mississanga Road North
5B - 2037B
Mississanga, Ontario L5C 1C6
Canada

Computer-assisted Tracking Simulation (CATS)
James J. Dempsey
Department of Communication Disorders
Southern Connecticut State University
501 Crescent Street
New Haven, CT 06515–1355

Sound and Beyond
Cochlear Americas
400 Inverness Parkway, Suite 400
Englewood, CO 80112
www.cochlearamericas.com

Learning to Lipread: An Introductory Course
M J. Allen
P.O Box 412
Marden, S.A. 5070, Australia
Sales@lipread.com.au

Seeing and Hearing Speech
Sensimetrics Corporation
48 Grove Street
Somerville, MA 02144–2500
www.sens.com

Conversation Made Easy
CID Publications
4560 Clayton Avenue
St. Louis, MO 63110
www.cid.edu/home/publications/books.htm

Listening and Auditory Communication Enhancement (LACE)
NeuroTone Inc.
2317 Broadway, Suite 205
Redwood City, CA 94063
www.lacecentral.com

References

Alcantara, J. I., Cowan, R. S. C., Blamey, P. J., & Clark, G. M. (1990). A comparison of two training strategies for speech recognition with an electrotactile speech processor. Journal of Speech and Hearing Research, 33, 195–204.

Allen, M. J. (2000). Learning to lipread: An introductory course. Marden, Australia: M. J. Allen.

Alpiner, J. (1987). Rehabilitative audiology: An overview. In J. G. Alpiner & P. A. McCarthy (Eds.), Rehabilitative audiology: Children and adults (pp. 3–17). Baltimore: Williams & Wilkins.

American Speech-Language-Hearing Association. (1979). Legislative council changes ASHA's name, ratifies ERA motion, adopts code changes. ASHA, 21, 33–35.

American Speech-Language-Hearing Association. (1984). Committee on Rehabilitative Audiology: Definition of and competencies for aural rehabilitation. ASHA, 26, 37–41.

American Speech-Language-Hearing Association. (2001). Knowledge and skills required for the practice of audiologic/aural rehabilitation [Knowledge and Skills]. Available from www.asha.org/policy

Bellow, S. (1947). The victim. In Rehabilitative audiology. New York: Vanguard Press.

Blamey, P., & Alcantara, J. I. (1994). Research in auditory training. Journal of the Academy of Rehabilitative Audiology, 27, 161–191.

Boothroyd. A. (1987). CASPER, computer-assisted speech-perception evaluation and training. In Proceedings of the 10th Annual Conference of the Rehabilitation Society of North America (pp. 734–736). Washington, DC: Association for Advancement of Rehabilitation Technology.

Boothroyd, A. (1988). Linguistic factors in speechreading [monograph]. Volta Review, 90(5), 77–88.

Castle, D. L. (1988). Telephone strategies. Bethesda, MD: Self Help for Hard of Hearing People.

Coleman, L. M. (1997). Stigma: An enigma demystified. In L. J. Davis (Ed.), The disability studies reader (pp. 216–231). New York: Routledge.

DeFilippo, C. L. (1988). Tracking for speechreading training [monograph]. Volta Review, 90 (5), 215–239.

DeFilippo, C. L., & Scott, B. L. (1978). A method for training and evaluating the reception of ongoing speech. Journal of the Acoustical Society of America, 63, 1186–1192.

Dempsey, J. J., Levitt, H., Josephson, J., & Porrazzo, J. (1992). Computer-assisted tracking simulation (CATS). Journal of the Acoustical Society of America, 92, 701–710.

Dewine, L. (1992). Americans with Disabilities Act: A declaration of opportunities. Audecibel, 41, 7–10.

Dillon, H., James, A., & Ginis, J. (1997). Client Oriented Scale of Improvement (COSI) and its relationship to several other measurements of benefit and satisfaction provided by hearing aids. Journal of the American Academy of Audiology, 8, 27–43.

Erber, N. P. (1979). Auditory-visual perception of speech with reduced optical clarity. Journal of Speech and Hearing Research, 22, 212–223.

Erber, N. P. (1982). Auditory training. Washington, DC: Alexander Graham Bell Association for the Deaf.

Erber, N. P. (1985). Telephone communication and hearing impairment. San Diego, CA: College-Hill Press.

Erber, N. P. (1988). Communication therapy for hearing-impaired adults. Melbourne, Australia: Clavis Publishing.

Erber, N. P. (1996). Communication therapy for hearing-impaired adults (2nd ed.). Melbourne, Australia: Clavis Publishing.

Erber, N. P. (1998). DYALOG: A computer-based measure of conversational performance. Journal of the Academy of Rehabilitative Audiology, 31, 69–76.

Erber, N. P., & Yelland, J. (1998). CONAN: A system for analysis of temporal factors in conversation. Journal of the Academy of Rehabilitative Audiology, 31, 77–86.

Erdman, S. A. (1993). Counseling hearing-impaired adults. In J. G. Alpiner & P. A. McCarthy (Eds.), Rehabilitative audiology: Children and adults (2nd ed., pp. 374–413). Baltimore: Williams & Wilkins.

Gagné, J. P. (1998). Reflections on evaluative research in audiological rehabilitation. Scandinavian Audiology Supplementum, 49, 69–79.

Gagné, J. P. (2000). What is treatment evaluation research? What is its relationship to the goals of audiological rehabilitation? Who are the stakeholders of this type of research? Ear and Hearing, 21(4), 60s–73s.

Gagné, J. P., McDuff, S., & Getty, L. (1999). Some limitations of evaluative investigations based solely on normed outcome measures. Journal of the American Academy of Audiology, 10, 46–62.

Gagné, J. P., Rochette, A. J., & Charest, M. (2002). Auditory, visual and audiovisual clear speech. Speech Communication, 37, 213–230.

Gagné, J. P., & Wyllie, K. A. (1989). The relative effectiveness of three communication strategies on the visual-identification of misperceived words. Ear and Hearing, 10, 368–374.

Getty, L., & Hétu, R. (1991). Development of a rehabilitation program for people affected with occupational hearing loss: 2. Results from group intervention with 48 workers and their spouses. Audiology, 30, 317–329.

Giolas, T. G. (1982). Aural rehabilitation: An orientation. In T. G. Giolas (Ed.), Hearing handicapped adults (pp. 78–105). Englewood Cliffs, NJ: Prentice Hall.

Goldstein, D. P., & Stephens, S. D. G. (1981). Audiological rehabilitation: Management model I. Audiology, 20, 432–452.

Hawkins, D. B. (2005). Effectiveness of counseling-based adult group aural rehabilitation programs: A systematic review of the evidence. Journal of the American Academy of Audiology, 16(7), 485–493.

Hétu, R. (1996). The stigma attached to hearing impairment. Scandinavian Audiology Supplementum, 43, 12–24.

Hétu, R., Jones, L., & Getty, L. (1993). The impact of acquired hearing impairment on intimate relationships: Implications for rehabilitation. Audiology, 32, 363–381.

Hull, R. H. (1982). What is aural rehabilitation? In R. H. Hull (Ed.), Rehabilitative audiology (pp. 3–11). New York: Grune & Stratton.

Hyde, M. L., & Riko, K. (1994). A decision-analytic approach to audiological rehabilitation [monograph]. Journal of the Academy of Rehabilitative Audiology, 27, 337–374.

Jeffers, J., & Barley, M. (1971). Speechreading (lipreading). Springfield, IL: Charles C. Thomas.

Jennings, M. B. (1993). Aural rehabilitation curriculum series: Hearing help class 2. Coping with hearing loss. Toronto: Canadian Hearing Society.

Jennings, M. B. (1994). Service delivery models for older adults with hearing impairments: Individual sessions. In P. B. Kricos & S. A. Lesner (Eds.), Hearing care for the older adult: Audiologic rehabilitation (pp. 227–265). Boston: Butterworth-Heinemann.

Jennings, M. B. (2005a). Audiologic rehabilitation needs of older adults with hearing loss: Views on assistive technology uptake and appropriate support services. Journal of Speech-Language Pathology and Audiology, 29(3), 112–124.

Jennings, M. B. (2005b). Factors that influence outcomes from aural rehabilitation of older adults: The role of perceived self-efficacy. Unpublished doctoral dissertation, University of Western Ontario, London.

Jennings, M. B., Sheppard, A., & Sutherland, G. (1991). Aural rehabilitation curriculum series: Hearing help class. 1. Help for hearing aid users. Toronto: Canadian Hearing Society.

Kaplan, H., Bally, S., & Garretson, C. (1987). Speechreading: A way to improve understanding (2nd ed.). Washington, DC: Gallaudet University Press.

Kiresuk, T. J., Smith, A., & Cardillo, J. E. (1994). Goal attainment scaling: Applications, theory, and measurement. Hillsdale, NJ: Lawrence Erlbaum.

Kopra, L., Kopra, M., Abrahamson, J., & Dunlop, R. (1987). Lipreading drill and practice software for an auditory-visual interactive system. Journal of Comprehensive Users Speech Hearing, 3, 58–68.

Lesner, S. A., Sandridge, S., & Kricos, R. (1987). Training influences on visual consonant and sentence recognition. Ear and Hearing, 8, 283–287.

Levitt, H., Kozma-Spytek, L., & Harkings, J. (2005). In-the-ear measurements of interference in hearing aids from digital wireless telephones. Seminars in Hearing, 26(2), 87–98.

McCarthy, P., & Culpepper, B. (1987). The adult remediation process. In J. G. Alpiner & R. A. McCarthy (Eds.), Rehabilitative audiology: Children and adults (pp. 305–342). Baltimore: Williams & Wilkins.

McKenna, L. (1987). Goal planning in audiological rehabilitation. British Journal of Audiology, 21, 5–11.

Pichora-Fuller, M. K., & Benguerel, A. (1991). The design of CAST (Computer-Aided Speechreading Training). Journal of Speech and Hearing Research, 34, 202–212.

Plant, G. (1996a). SYNTREX: Synthetic training exercises for hearing-impaired adults. Somerville, MA: Hearing Rehabilitation Foundation.

Plant, G. (1996b). TACTRAIN: Tactaid VII training program for hearing impaired adults. Somerville, MA: Hearing Rehabilitation Foundation.

Plant, G. (2002). SpeechTrax. Innsbruck, Austria: Med-El Medical Electronics.

Plant, G. (2004). Analytika (2nd ed.). Innsbruck, Austria: Med-El Medical Electronics.

Prendergast, S. G., & Kelley, L. A. (2002). Aural rehab services: Survey reports who offers which ones and how often. Hearing Journal, 55(9), 30–35.

Ross, M. (1997). A retrospective look at the future of aural rehabilitation. Journal of the Academy of Rehabilitative Audiology, 30, 11–28.

Schum, D. (1997). Beyond hearing aids: Clear speech training as an intervention strategy. Hearing Journal, 50(10), 36–40.

Schum, R. L. (1994). Personal adjustment counseling [monograph]. Journal of the Academy of Rehabilitative Audiology, 27, 223–236.

Seeing and hearing speech. (2001). Somerville, MA: Sensimetrics Corp.

Sims, D., Von Feldt, J., Dowaliby, F., et al. (1979). A pilot experiment in computer assisted speechreading instruction utilizing the Data Analysis Video Interactive Device (DAVID). American Annals of Deafness, 124, 618–623.

Sound and beyond. (2003). Englewood, CO: Cochlear Corp.

Spitzer, J. B., Leder, S. B., & Giolas, T. G. (1993). Rehabilitation of late-deafened adults: Modular program manual. St. Louis: Mosby.

Stephens, D., & Hétu, R. (1991). Impairment, disability and handicap in audiology: Towards a consensus. Audiology, 30, 185–200.

Strachan, S., Scullino, M. L., & Jennings, M. B. (1997). Aural rehabilitation curriculum series: Hearing help class 3 and 4: Speechreading. Toronto: Canadian Hearing Society.

Sweetow, R., & Palmer, C. V. (2005). Efficacy of individual auditory training in adults: A systematic review of the evidence. Journal of the American Academy of Audiology, 16(7), 494–504.

Tchorz, J., & Schulte, M. (2005). Utilizing Bluetooth for better speech understanding over the cell phone. Hearing Review, 12(2), 50–51.

Trychin, S. (1986, January/February). Stress management 3: Self-help for hard of hearing people. SHHH Journal, 7(1), 12–13.

Tye-Murray, N. (1994). Communication strategies training [monograph]. Journal of the Academy of Rehabilitative Audiology, 27, 193–207.

Tye-Murray, N. (1997). Communication training for older teenagers and adults: Listening, speechreading and using conversational strategies. Austin, TX: Pro-Ed.

Tye-Murray, N. (2002). Conversation made easy: Speechreading and conversation training for individuals who have hearing loss (adults and teenagers). St. Louis: Central Institute for the Deaf.

Tye-Murray, N., Purdy, S. C., & Woodworth, G. (1992). The reported use of communication strategies by members of SHHH and its relationship to client, talker, and situational variables. Journal of Speech and Hearing Research, 35, 708–717.

Tye-Murray, N., & Schum, L. (1994). Conversation training for frequent communication partners [monograph]. Journal of the Academy of Rehabilitative Audiology, 27, 209–222.

Tye-Murray, N., Tyler, R., Bong, B., & Nares, T. (1988). Using laser videodisc technology to train speechreading and assertive listening skills. Journal of the Academy of Rehabilitative Audiology, 21, 143–152.

Walden, B. E., Erdman, S. A., Montgomery, A. A., et al. (1981). Some effects of training on speech recognition by hearing-impaired adults. Journal of Speech and Hearing Research, 24, 207–216.

Walden, B. E., Montgomery, A. A., Scherr, C. K., & Jones, C. J. (1977). Effects of training on the visual recognition of consonants. Journal of Speech and Hearing Research, 20, 130–145.

Wayner, D. S., & Abrahamson, M. A. (1996). Learning to hear again: An audiologic rehabilitation curriculum guide. Austin, TX: Hear Again.

World Health Organization. (1980). International classification of impairments, disabilities and handicaps. Geneva: WHO Press.

World Health Organization. (2001). International classification of functioning, disability and health. Geneva: WHO Press.

Chapter 17

Hearing Assistance Technology (HAT)

A. U. Bankaitis

Hearing assistance technology (HAT) refers to a broad array of devices designed to facilitate reception of auditory information via amplification, vibrotactile stimulation, and/or visual display (Thibodeau, 2004). HAT may function alone as independent communication devices or in conjunction with hearing instruments. The term *hearing assistance technology* is often used interchangeably with the more common term *assistive listening device* (ALD). However, as clarified by Thibodeau (2004), both HAT and ALD represent terms with inherently different connotations; whereas ALD implies assisting or improving listening, HAT represents a more inclusive term and is associated with the goal of optimizing communication.

The point created by Thibodeau (2004) is not a trivial one, nor is the use of the acronym HAT an issue of preference or semantics. A primary role of audiologists is to manage nonmedical aspects of hearing loss. Because most forms of hearing loss are not medically manageable, the role and

influence of audiologists on communication quality are exceptionally significant. Although hearing instruments represent a vital component in the aural rehabilitation process, these devices should not necessarily serve as end points in the process.

♦ Benefits of HAT

The decreased ability to understand speech represents a major consequence of sensorineural hearing loss, particularly in noisy and/or reverberant environments (Killion, 1997; Moore, 1997). The characteristic attenuation of sound associated with conductive impairment poses similar communication difficulties. In simplistic terms, HAT bridges the distance between speaker and listener, providing individuals with hearing loss an optimal environment to listen to speech and/or to be alerted to environmental sounds. Products categorized under this technology umbrella are designed to transmit sound as directly as possible to the individual with hearing loss. As a result, HAT offers several distinct advantages over traditional amplification achieved with hearing instruments. First, HAT significantly improves signal-to-noise ratios (SNRs). Whereas hearing instruments with directional microphones improve SNR by as much as +8 dB under ideal listening conditions (Ricketts and Dahr, 1999), some HAT services can improve SNR by +15 dB (Hawkins and Van Tassel, 1982). Second, HAT inherently minimizes the influence of poor room acoustics, eliminating or at least minimizing the negative effects of reverberation. Third, many forms of HAT can virtually eliminate background noise. Although exposure to environmental and background noise is critical from an auditory training perspective, in some situations, the application of HAT will provide the most favorable strategy for optimizing communication.

Controversial Point

- Some products advertised as HAT devices or ALDs have built-in hearing instrument capabilities. For example, some new wireless headsets designed to improve cell phone communication by amplifying incoming calls for non–hearing instrument users come equipped with additional program settings that enable "customization" of sound quality when the phone is not in use. Marketed as ALDs, some wireless headsets are packaged with fitting software that necessitates access to a computer and a Hi-PRO box (GN-Otometrics). Although incorporating wireless headset technology into hearing instruments would be beneficial, the converse may create opportunities for unlicensed and unqualified individuals to fit patients with products designed to function as hearing instruments.

◆ Clinical Need for HAT

It has been estimated that nearly 30 million people in the United States exhibit some degree of hearing loss (National Institutes of Deafness and Communication Disorders [NIDCD], 2005), a figure representing 10% of the current population (Kochkin, 1999). Fortunately, hearing instruments have greatly improved the quality of life (QoL) of individuals with hearing loss. Hearing instrument wearers have been found more likely to report perceived improvements in their physical, emotional, mental, and social well-being, exhibiting more socially active lifestyles with minimal reports of depression, worry, paranoia, and insecurity, as compared with non–hearing instrument wearers (Kochkin and Rogin, 2000). Perceived improvements were further magnified when users were fit with dual-microphone technology. For instance, Schuchman et al (1999) documented 400 to 500% improvement in hearing instrument satisfaction in noisy situations using dual-microphone technology compared with omnidirectional

technology. Kuk (1996) also showed that dual-microphone technology doubled customer satisfaction with hearing instrumentation in noisy situations. In a 10-year patient satisfaction study assessing trends in the U.S. hearing instrument market, Kochkin (2002) substantiated these earlier findings, observing a definite patient perceptual advantage with dual-microphone technology. Patients perceived greater satisfaction in large group interactions, workplace communication, outdoor activities, and entertainment situations when using dual-microphone technology in difficult listening situations.

Despite the benefits of hearing instruments and perceived increase in user satisfaction with dual-microphone technology, a significant percentage of patients remain unsatisfied with hearing instruments. The degree of dissatisfaction increases in more challenging listening situations where background noise is present. In general, slightly less than 50% of hearing instrument wearers are not satisfied with hearing instruments (Kochkin, 1999). Poor perceived benefit in noise represents the most common reason why consumers do not wear hearing instruments (Kochkin, 2000). Prominent industry researchers have identified hearing instrument performance in noise as a key barrier to industry growth (Kochkin and Strom, 1999). This has shifted some of the hearing industry's focus toward more sophisticated multiple microphone technology (Kochkin, 2000); however, HAT is currently available and readily accessible to those seeking a supplemental communication solution beyond hearing instrumentation alone. Finally, with the historically low 20% market penetration of hearing instruments (Kochkin, 1999), HAT can serve as the point of entry for individuals with hearing loss initially reluctant to pursue amplification in the form of hearing instrumentation.

◆ Barriers to HAT Integration

The extent to which audiologists educate patients on HAT remains unknown, but most likely it is fairly low due to known barriers impeding successful integration of HAT into current audiology practices. From an educational perspective, the extent to which HAT is routinely incorporated into graduate and doctoral curricula is unknown. Although many audiology training programs may include an overview of HAT as part of an amplification or professional management course, rarely has the topic been taught extensively. As a result, audiologists are not adequately prepared in presenting HAT options to prospective patients.

Assuming a working knowledge of HAT, the majority of audiologists report not having the time to educate patients about HAT (Servedio, 2000). Traditionally, amplification orientation focuses mainly on hearing instruments, leaving little or no time for HAT. One solution would involve allocating additional resources to assist with HAT orientation. Unfortunately, most clinicians report lack of resources availability as yet another barrier to integrating HAT into clinical practice (Prendergast and Kelley, 2002). Not surprisingly, given the number of HAT products available in the market, most audiologists report not having the time or energy to acquire product knowledge (Ross, 2004). Finally, from a financial perspective, many audiologists view HAT as not profitable (Servedio, 2000). These combined factors generate professional apathy and disinterest that further perpetuate barriers hindering an increased presence of HAT in the audiology clinic.

Special Consideration

- Many audiologists view HAT as unprofitable and therefore may not incorporate this technology into current clinical practice (Servedio, 2000). Although the margins are significantly lower than hearing instrumentation, generating awareness and advocating the use of HAT in conjunction with hearing instruments not only can increase the potential for optimizing communication for hearing-impaired patients but also can facilitate the likelihood of success with amplification. Furthermore, HATs will help leverage audiologists as *the* communication experts for hearing-impaired patient populations.

In the event HAT options are presented to patients by audiologists, the literature suggests that most patients do not recall discussions about such products. There is a discrepancy between what clinicians reportedly communicate to patients and what information patients recall. An overwhelming majority (78%) of clinicians report that HAT options are discussed with patients the majority of the time (Prendergast and Kelley, 2002). However, when patients are asked to recall the various amplification options that were presented, only 30% indicate that technology beyond traditional hearing instruments was reviewed (Stika et al, 2002). Many factors can influence this discrepancy. For example, clinicians may not respond honestly, patients may simply be overwhelmed and unable to retain information, or they simply do not remember. Regardless of the reason, the research suggests that consumer awareness about HAT remains poor.

From these perspectives, the primary goal of this chapter is to provide foundational information on HAT, including an overview of the technology and practical suggestions on how to generate consumer awareness of such products. Specifically, this chapter will provide current and future audiologists with (1) an introduction of telecommunications technology; (2) a review of cell phone technology; (3) a presentation of HAT systems, including frequency modulation (FM), infrared (IR), alerting, and personal listening systems; and (4) recommendations on how to effectively integrate HAT into existing clinical practices.

◆ Technology Overview

In the absence of standardized categories, HAT information will be presented as four technology types: telecommunications, cell phone, HAT systems, and miscellaneous.

Telecommunications Technology

Amplified Telephones

Amplified telephones work in the same manner as standard telephones and are designed to increase the volume of the incoming caller's voice when needed. Most amplified telephones may be set to either return to the nonamplified default setting or stay in the amplified mode once the user hangs up the handset. In general, the majority of amplified telephones are essentially the same, with the number of features integrated into a specific telephone representing the only differentiating factor between models. For example, some amplified telephones feature volume and tone control buttons only. Other amplified telephones include additional features such as caller ID, call waiting, memory dial buttons, and adjustable telephone ring signalers, still others offer additional features, such as a built-in answering machine, bedshaker, and strobe light or remote lamp flasher. As a result, each manufacturer has introduced numerous models of amplified telephones, creating a seemingly unlimited number of available products. Because most patients are familiar with telephone functions, and most amplified telephones do not differ significantly from one another, audiologists should be familiar with factors influencing the amplified telephone purchase process.

Four amplified telephone issues influence the consumer purchase process. First, amplified telephones are either corded or cordless. Patients typically have a preference for one type. Because feature density, or the number of features available on a particular amplified telephone, is the same for corded and cordless models, the audiologist should simply determine the patient's preference.

Second, feature density must be matched to the patient's need and capabilities. For example, some amplified telephones have minimal features, basically providing only the ability to increase the volume of the caller's voice and manipulate a tone control. Low feature density telephones work well for those patients intimidated by additional buttons, indicator lights, and switches beyond basic telephones and/or with limited experience or capabilities. In contrast, high feature density telephones equipped with caller ID, call waiting, built-in alarm clocks, and optional bedshakers or remote lamp flashers offer patients a more sophisticated product.

Third, cost must be taken into consideration because amplified telephone prices vary. Based on the manufacturer's suggested retail price, basic amplified telephone models generally cost about $79, whereas more advanced models approach $300. Although price influences the purchase process, it is critical to ensure that the ultimate needs of the patient are met and that product recommendations are not solely price driven. For example, a patient concerned about hearing the telephone while sleeping should minimally consider investing in a moderately priced amplified telephone equipped with a bedshaker accessory instead of a less expensive amplified telephone equipped only with an adjustable audible ringer.

Fourth, although most patients know how to use a telephone, the ability for patients to experience the benefits and/or features offered by an amplified telephone remains

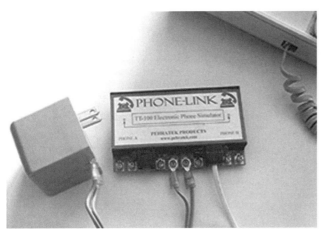

Figure 17–1 The Phone-Link telephone simulator from Pehratek Products. (Courtesy of Pehratek Products.)

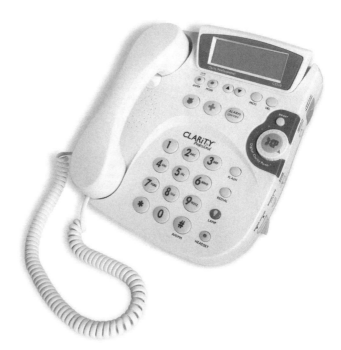

Figure 17–2 The Clarity Professional C2210 corded amplified telephone with intelligent amplification. (Courtesy of Clarity, a Division of Plantronics, Inc.)

critical. Most clinical offices do not provide access to multiple phone lines enabling direct telephone hook-up for demonstration purposes; however, relatively inexpensive phone-linking devices are available that allow two phones to be linked to one another in such a way that consumers can hear the phone ring, manipulate telephone features, and converse over the telephone without requiring access to a phone jack or tying up an existing telephone line. When the handset of one linked telephone is picked up, the phone-linking device will cause the other linked amplified telephone to ring. The telephone will continue to ring until the handset is picked up, at which time the consumer can experience the benefits of the demonstration phone and make a more informed decision as to whether the phone will meet his or her needs. **Figure 17–1** shows a popular telephone simulator from Pehratek Products (Chaska, MN) that costs slightly less than $200.

Advanced Telephone Technology   Although most amplified telephones feature similar technology, innovative applications of existing technology have recently emerged. For example, Clarity, a division of Plantronics, Inc. (Chattanooga, TN), offers models that feature what the company refers to as "intelligent amplification" **(Figs. 17–2** and **17–3).** The concept of intelligent amplification is based on the application of a proprietary digital signal processing (DSP) chip that amplifies incoming signals via wide dynamic range compression (WDRC) while providing both noise and acoustic echo reduction strategies. Although this technology is not new, it is the first time hearing aid technology has been incorporated into amplified telephones. Furthermore, Clarity models offer unique tone control settings using a proprietary algorithm identified as most beneficial to those with moderate sensorineural hearing loss, as determined by unpublished research conducted at Washington University School of Medicine's Department of Adult Audiology (Clarity Valued Partner Conference, May 2005).

The Clarity Professional C2210 Corded Amplified Telephone
The C2210 is a corded telephone that provides up to 50 dB of amplification with a choice of two tone settings **(Fig. 17–2).** The first tone setting provides standard linear frequency

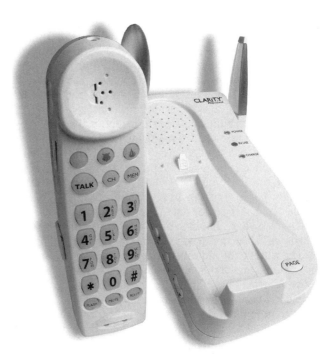

Figure 17–3 The Clarity Professional 4210 cordless amplified telephone with intelligent amplification. (Courtesy of Clarity, a Division of Plantronics, Inc.)

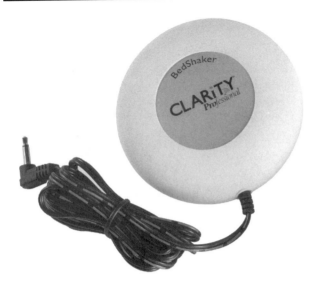

Figure 17–4 Standard bedshaker accessory designed to work with amplified telephones and other hearing assistive technology. (Courtesy of Clarity, a Division of Plantronics, Inc.)

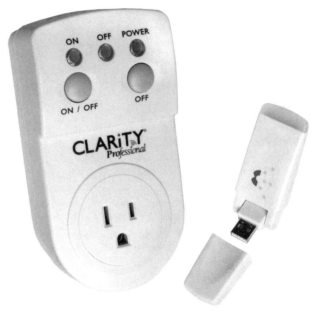

Figure 17–5 Remote lamp flasher accessory designed specifically for the Clarity Professional C2210 amplified telephone. A transmitter sends a signal to a remote receiver, which flashes a lamp sequentially on and off, providing a visual indication that the telephone is ringing. (Courtesy of Clarity, a Division of Plantronics, Inc.)

shaping. The tone setting engages a multiband compressor on the DSP chip. The user has access to a 15 dB amplification range via the volume dial located on the right-hand portion of the telephone base. As needed, the telephone user may increase the volume by turning the dial clockwise. When the dial is positioned in the maximum clockwise position, the telephone provides up to 15 dB of amplification. Additional amplification is accessed by pressing and releasing the boost button located above the volume dial. The boost button will illuminate, indicating that it has been activated. While the boost button is activated, the volume dial will increase to a 15 to 50 dB range. When the volume dial is positioned in the full-on clockwise position with the boost button engaged, the telephone provides 50 dB of amplification. The boost button feature may be deactivated by pressing and releasing the button again. In addition to call waiting and caller ID with 50 name and number history, this telephone is equipped with a built-in alarm clock. Optional accessories include a bedshaker and a remote lamp flasher.

A bedshaker is a standard accessory available for use with many amplified telephones, not just the C2210. As shown in **Fig. 17–4,** the Clarity model resembles a small, corded disk. It is slightly less than 4 inches in diameter and weighs 6.5 oz. The bedshaker is plugged into the appropriate socket of the telephone base and then placed under a pillow. When a call comes in, the bedshaker vibrates fairly vigorously, providing a vibrotactile indication that the telephone is ringing. The stimulus generated by the bedshaker is sufficient to arouse a sleeping individual. The bedshaker is also activated by the alert from the built-in alarm clock.

The remote lamp flasher is a second accessory specifically designed for the C2210 corded telephone described above. As illustrated in **Fig. 17–5,** this accessory consists of two separate components: a transmitter and a receiver. The smaller of the two components is the transmitter. It plugs into the base of the C2210 amplified telephone via a special jack. The receiver is plugged into a wall socket, allowing for a standard lamp to be plugged into the receiver base. When a call arrives, the transmitter sends a signal to the receiver, which responds by flashing a lamp sequentially on and off, providing a visual indication that the telephone is ringing. The lamp flasher is also activated by the alert within the built-in alarm clock. The telephone and lamp do not need to be in the same room; however, they must be within 30 feet of one another for the remote lamp flasher to activate.

The Clarity Professional C4210 Cordless Amplified Telephone
As shown in **Fig. 17–3,** the C4210 cordless telephone provides 50 dB of amplification. As with the C2210, the phone has a volume dial and boost button. The amplification range is identical to that of the C2210. Instead of two tone control settings, the C4210 provides the user with three tone settings. The first two tone settings are identical to those of the C2210, whereas the third setting engages a more aggressive version of the multiband compressor. The three tone settings allow users to customize the listening experience. This phone operates on 2.4 GHz, reducing interference experienced with many cordless telephones operating in lower frequency ranges. In addition, this specific frequency allows the user to maintain a farther distance from the base with less signal interference. Instead of the lamp flasher and bedshaker options, the C4210 offers visual ringers in the handset and base, as well as a vibrating finder in the handset. In those instances when the handset is out of the base, these vibrating features provide the user with a supplemental sensory notification to the auditory ring. Finally, The Clarity Professional C4210 is equipped for call waiting and caller ID.

Other Telephone Options   Individuals with more severe degrees of hearing loss or those with severe speech impairments will be unable to effectively use amplified or traditional telephones (Crandell and Smaldino, 2002). In these cases, Voice Carry Over (VCO) and teletypewriter (or text telephone, TTY), or telecommunications device for the deaf (TDD), systems may be appropriate.

Voice Carry Over Telephone   A VCO telephone transmits incoming calls as text, providing the ability to read what the caller is communicating. This device resembles and is used in the same manner as a traditional telephone. Unlike traditional phones, the verbal conversation relayed by the other party is transcribed into written text by a relay service operator. The transcribed text is then sent by the relay service operator over the phone line, where it slowly scrolls across the VCO's screen. No typing is required by the VCO user. The only requirement is to make arrangements with the local relay service to facilitate telephone calls.

Pearl

- Local relay service may be contacted by dialing 711 anywhere in the United States. The 711 call is free; long-distance charges are applied where appropriate.

Teletypewriter   A TTY device receives and transmits text or typed speech via standard telephone lines. The acronym TTY is often used interchangeably with TDD; however, TTY is probably a more appropriate term because it describes the actual device rather than referring to the specific population who may need to use the device (E-Michigan Deaf and Hard of Hearing People, 2005). A TTY consists of a keyboard, a display screen, a modem, and a handset cradle. It connects to a phone line directly, by plugging the TTY's phone cord into the phone jack, or indirectly, by placing the handset of a traditional telephone onto the TTY's handset cradle. Using a sound-based coding system, the TTY converts text into audible beeps, which are then transmitted over the telephone line. When both parties are using a TTY, users take turns sending text messages using a special text-code system. The user code signifies whose turn it is to communicate and whose turn it is to listen. The sent messages appear as written text across the TTY display screen. Messages may be read or printed out.

When only one party is a TTY user, as with VCO telephones, the telephone conversation must be facilitated by a relay service. This service involves a third-party operator who serves as the intermediary between the TTY user and the non-TTY user. The relay operator is responsible for transmitting a text message of what the non-TTY user is verbally communicating to the TTY user via the operator's own TTY. In the event the TTY user responds nonverbally to the operator, the operator verbalizes the communication to the non-TTY user.

Telephone Amplifiers

Telephone amplifiers are devices used with existing telephones for purposes of amplifying the incoming volume of the caller's voice. These devices offer some advantages over amplified telephones. Because telephone amplifiers connect directly to existing phones, amplified conversation will take place using a telephone that the patient is already accustomed to using. Also, because telephone amplifiers are less sophisticated devices than amplified telephones, they represent a more economical option. Finally, telephone amplifiers are portable and easy to connect, although some involve less installation preparation prior to initial use. Several different types of telephone amplifiers are currently available and may be grouped into distinct categories accordingly: in-line amplifiers and strap-on amplifiers.

In-line Amplifiers   In-line amplifiers refer to telephone amplification devices that attach to existing corded telephones, amplifying the incoming volume of the caller's voice. An example of an in-line amplifier from ClearSounds Communications (Burr Ridge, IL) is shown in **Fig. 17–6**. These devices are not compatible with cordless phones or with corded telephones with the dial pad in the handset. From an engineering perspective, in order for in-line amplifiers to work, the telephone's signal processing must occur prior to the amplification produced by the telephone amplifier. With most corded telephones, the telephone processing occurs at the phone's base; because the in-line amplifier attaches between the base and the receiver, the in-line amplifier receives the signal after it has been processed, enabling the device to amplify the signal. In the case of corded telephones with the dial pad in the handset, the processors are located in the handset, with the base of the telephone serving only as a handset cradle. Unprocessed signals routed to the in-line amplifier from the base will not be recognized by the in-line amplifier; therefore, the signal routed from

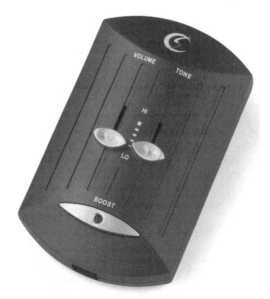

Figure 17–6 The ClearSounds IL-40 in-line telephone amplifier (Courtesy of ClearSounds Communications.)

the in-line amplifier to the handset will not be amplified. For this reason and in the absence of a cord connecting the base and the handset, in-line amplifiers will not work with cordless telephones.

In-line amplifiers are typically powered by a 9 V battery. During use, when the handset of the phone is off the cradle, an indicator light will illuminate, indicating acceptable battery levels for operation. When the handset is replaced on the cradle, the battery indicator light will turn off. In the event the battery is drained, the battery indicator light will not illuminate, indicating the need for a new battery. Depending on how much the in-line amplifier is used and how loudly it is adjusted, batteries will last, on average, ~6 to 12 months. Depending on the specific model and user settings, in-line amplifiers may amplify telephone signals by 18 to 40 dB.

Strap-On Amplifiers Strap-on amplifiers are designed to strap onto a telephone handset **(Fig. 17–7)**. Proper use requires positioning the amplifier directly over the earpiece of an existing telephone handset. Unlike in-line amplifiers, strap-on amplifiers do not connect to existing phones via cords, making these amplifiers more portable. In addition, this type of amplifier works with most telephones, including cordless phones, telephones with the dial pad in the handset, and pay phones. Depending on the model, strap-on amplifiers amplify signals from 20 to ~30 dB.

Telephone Ring Signalers

Telephone ring signalers function as supplemental ringers for existing telephones. These devices do not amplify the volume of the caller's voice; rather, they enhance only the incoming ring of the telephone, making it easier to hear the phone ring. They represent an appropriate solution for those individuals who have difficulty hearing the telephone ring but have little or no difficulty conversing over the phone.

Telephone ring signalers are available as direct phone line devices and direct telephone connect devices. Direct phone line devices connect directly into the wall phone jack and do not require disconnection and rerouting of telephone cords from the existing telephone. These devices are designed to function independently and do not allow interfacing with an existing phone. In contrast, direct telephone connect devices may connect to a phone line as described above or directly into an existing telephone. This type provides installation flexibility. For some patients, installing a ring signaler that does not require disconnecting and rerouting existing telephone cords may be more appropriate.

In terms of installation, some devices run on AA or AAA batteries, and others come equipped with alternating current (AC) power adapters. Once the power source is appropriately installed, direct phone line telephone ring signalers are connected to the wall socket via a separate telephone cord. Because the existing telephone must be plugged into the telephone wall socket, this type of telephone ring signaler requires access to either a dual telephone jack or the use of a T-adapter. The T-adapter is comparable to a power strip; it plugs into a single telephone jack to provide access to two telephones. The T-adapter is included with most models and is also available at most hardware stores and home centers.

Direct telephone connect devices can be installed in a similar fashion as described above, or they can be connected directly to existing telephones. The line from the existing phone must be disconnected from the wall jack and rerouted to the line-out jack of the telephone ring signaler. A separate phone cord included with the product is plugged into the line-in jack of the telephone ring signaler, with the other end plugged into the wall outlet.

Most telephone ring signalers include audible ringers with adjustable volume controls that can generate approximately a 95 dB sound pressure level (SPL) signal measured at 1 m. Depending on the model, some telephone ring signalers, such as the Ringmax from Williams Sound Corp. (Eden Prairie, MN; **Fig. 17–8**), are equipped with adjustable frequency settings ranging from a lower tone of 500 Hz to a higher frequency tone of ~1300 Hz, allowing the user to choose between up to four different telephone ring pitches. Other telephone ring signalers provide visual and/or vibrotactile signaling options. For example, the ClearSounds CL1 telephone ring signaler in **Fig. 17–9** comes equipped with a strobe flasher and a special jack that will accommodate a bedshaker.

Cell Phone Technology

Over the past several years, cell phones have dominated the U.S. phone market, with reported penetration rates of nearly 50% as of December 2002 (Federal Communications Commission [FCC], 2005a) and with more than 55% of

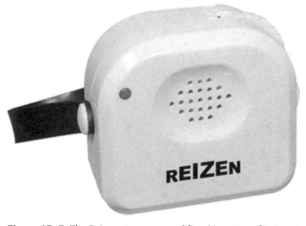

Figure 17–7 The Reizen strap-on amplifier. (Courtesy of Reizen Inc.)

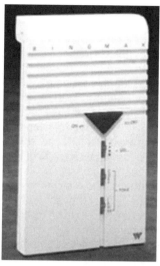

Figure 17–8 The Williams Sound Corp. Ringmax telephone ring signaler. (Courtesy of Williams Sound Corp.)

Americans between the ages of 15 and 59 using cell phones (FCC, 2003). Taking into consideration the demographics of hearing loss and the demographics of cell phone users, the proportion of the hearing-impaired population who will need to wear hearing instruments and use cell phones will continue to increase, creating a greater need for audiologists to effectively counsel and address cell phone interference issues with hearing instrument wearers.

The Hearing Aid Compatibility Act of 1988 required most telephones manufactured in or imported into the United States to be hearing aid compatible. When the law was first passed, cell phones were exempt because Congress considered this technology as a complement to, not a substitute for, essential telephones (47 USC § 610(b)(2)(A)) . In 1988,

cell phones were mainly business tools (FCC, 2005a), although the law was written to allow the FCC to "periodically assess the appropriateness of continuing exemptions" (47 USC § 610(b)(2)(C)).

Technological advancements quickly led to an increased demand for digital wireless technology, resulting in a decrease in costs and the subsequent emergence of a cellular phone mass market. Analog cell phones were slowly becoming obsolete as more consumers purchased digital cell phones. Unfortunately, these market trends adversely affected individuals with hearing loss, who started experiencing significant cell phone interference issues when attempting to use the cell phone with hearing instruments. Whereas analog cell phones do not cause cell phone interference for hearing instrument users (American National Standards Institute [ANSI] ASC C63 SC8, 1996), digital cell phones do. The potential for experiencing interference while using a cell phone is magnified in the presence of conventional analog-type hearing instruments, although not all digital devices are immune to such interference (Kozma-Spytek, 2005). The interference manifests in the form of an audible buzzing noise, which may become distracting enough to negatively interfere with cell phone communication (Berger and TEM Consulting, 2005).

Sources of Cell Phone Interference for Hearing Instrument Wearers

Three primary sources contribute to potential cell phone interference: cell phone radio-frequency (RF) transmission, cell phone transmission technology, and baseband, magnetic interference (Kozma-Spytek, 2005).

Cell Phone Radio-Frequency Transmission   Basically, the cell phone is actually a radio. When using a digital cell phone, conversations are transmitted from the digital cell phone by a wireless network in the form of radio waves. The radio waves emitted from and by the cell phone are called RF emissions (Kozma-Spytek, 2005). RF emissions create a pulsating electromagnetic field within the vicinity of the cell phone's antenna that may be detected by the hearing instrument when set in the telecoil (T) or microphone/telecoil (MT) positions (FCC, 2005a). The hearing instrument's microphone and other components will also pick up the electromagnetic energy when the hearing instrument is switched from the T mode to M mode only (FCC, 2005a; Kozma-Spytek, 2005).

Cell Phone Transmission Technology   Cell phone transmission technology is generally represented by one of three types: Time Division Multiple Access (TDMA), Code Division Multiple Access (CDMA), or Global System for Mobile Communications (GSM). Each technology transmits information via the cellular network differently. For example, CDMA transmission technology codes digital cell signals emitted from the cell phone as distinct strings by applying a unique coded multiplier to the digital string. As the coded string circulates throughout the entire frequency range of the network with other coded strings emitted from other cell phones, the receiver of the other cell phone identifies the

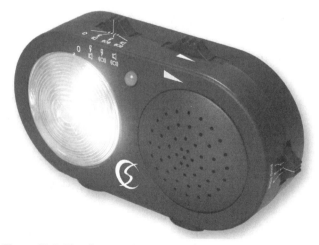

Figure 17–9 The ClearSounds CL1 telephone ring signaler. (Courtesy of ClearSounds Communications.)

unique coded multiplier applied to the digital string and extracts the signal from the network (Noll, 1998). This technology is used primarily in the United States (e.g., Verizon Wireless and Sprint PCS), Canada, and South Korea (Kozma-Spytek, 2005).

TDMA transmission technology, also used primarily in North America, works differently. It actually divides the network frequency band into specific carrier frequencies. Multiple phones share the same carrier frequency but only for a designated portion of time. TDMA transmits cell phone conversations by sequentially relaying portions of each conversation one short burst at a time (Mann, 2005). Instead of a mathematically coded approach, TDMA transmits cell phone activity across a time domain. The largest TDMA carrier in the United States currently is AT&T Wireless.

GSM is a variant of TDMA technology. The biggest difference between the two transmission technologies is that GSM can handle both voice calls and data, whereas TDMA can handle only voice calls (Noll, 1998). GSM is considered the world's most common digital technology for cell phones, introduced in 1992 as the European Union (EU) standard (Mann, 2005). This transmission technology is also used extensively throughout Asia and Africa. GSM carriers in the United States include T-mobile, and Cingular & AT&T (Cellular Abroad, 2007).

Currently, most digital cellular phones are designed to work with only one of these technologies. For example, Verizon digital cellular phones will transmit cell phone conversations using CDMA transmission technology, whereas an AT&T digital cellular phone will transmit cell phone conversations using TDMA transmission technology. The specific interference generated by each of these technologies maintains different spectral characteristics, resulting in the experience of more or less interference by the hearing instrument user depending on the specific transmission technology used.

Baseband, Magnetic Interference   For hearing instruments containing telecoils, users may experience interference originating from the cell phone's electronics, including the key pad, display window, backlighting, battery, and circuit board, referred to as baseband, magnetic interference (Kozma-Spytek, 2005).

Legislative Developments Addressing Cell Phone Interference

Recent legislative developments should eventually resolve cell phone interference for hearing instrument wearers. The government has responded to the communication needs of hearing-impaired individuals by partially lifting the exemption of cell phones from the Hearing Aid Compatibility Act of 1988, mandating compliance with ANSI C63.91.

ANSI C63.91   Adopted by the FCC, ANSI C63.91 is a technical standard that provides guidelines related to measuring the RF emission levels produced by cell phones and measuring immunity levels of hearing instruments to RF emissions (ANSI, 1996; FCC, 2005a). The standard provides rating categories for cell phones and hearing instruments. The intent of the rating categories is to assist consumers in choosing a cell

phone that will successfully operate with a particular hearing instrument. Digital wireless telephones will be assigned a rating of U1 through U4, where U1 represents a cell phone emitting the highest RF emissions and U4 a phone emitting the least amount of RF emissions. Similarly, the degree to which a hearing instrument is susceptible to cell phone interference will be assigned an immunity rating of U1 through U4. A hearing instrument rated as U1 is the most susceptible (or least immune) to RF emission interference, whereas a hearing instrument rated as U4 is the least susceptible (or most immune to RF emission interference; FCC, 2005a).

Compatibility between cell phones and hearing instruments is determined by combining U-rating scores. The higher the summed total, the better the performance. For example, a U2 rated cell phone paired with a hearing instrument with an immunity rating of U2 yields a combined score of 4 (i.e., U2 + U2 = U4). A sum of 4 indicates that the wireless cell phone is usable; a sum of 5 or 6 indicates the cell phone will provide normal or excellent performance, respectively (ANSI, 1996; FCC, 2005a). As of September 2005, the FCC has required each digital cell phone manufacturer to make available at least two cell phones, or 25% of the total phone models it offers, whichever is greater, for each transmission technology with reduced RF emissions. By definition, reduced RM emissions refer to cell phones rated as U3 or higher (FCC, 2005a).

Furthermore, ANSI C63.91 stipulates satisfactory operation of digital cell phones with telecoils in the absence of the application of accessory devices such as neckloops. In other words, cell phones must be compatible with hearing instruments when switched to the T mode. Cell phone compatibility with a hearing instrument's telecoil will be determined using the same rating scale previously described. For example, the cell phone's magnetic field quality, reported as U1T through U4T, is combined with the hearing instrument's magnetic field immunity, also reported as U1T through U4T. Again, a sum of 4 indicates that the wireless cell phone is usable; a sum of 5 or 6 indicates the cell phone will provide normal or excellent performance, respectively (ANSI, 1996; FCC, 2005a). By September 2006, the FCC required each digital cell phone manufacturer to make available at least two cell phones for each transmission technology it offers with telecoil ratings of U3T or higher (FCC, 2005a).

By February 18, 2008, 50% of digital cell phones offered by manufacturers must be compliant with a U3 and U3T reduced RF emission requirement. After February 18, 2008, the Analog Sunset Order will take effect, whereby cell phone manufacturers will no longer be required to provide analog cell phone service (FCC, 2005a,b).

Practical Solutions to Current Cell Phone Interference Issues

Although the legislative progress described above will assist in reducing cell phone interference for hearing instrument users, individuals with hearing loss using hearing instruments are currently experiencing cell phone interference, and more immediate solutions are necessary. It is important for individuals with hearing loss to be made aware of potential cell phone and hearing instrument incompatibilities. Patients must be prompted to try out cell phones with current instrumentation prior to investing in a long-term cell phone plan. This will allow them to try phone models using different cell phone transmission technologies to determine which phone seems most compatible with current hearing instruments. Because increased distance between the hearing instrument and digital cell phone antenna reduces the potential for a cell phone user to hear the interference, patients may consider two options: purchasing a flip-phone handset or investing in an induction ear hook cell phone accessory.

Cell phones come in a variety of styles, including flip phone and standard handset. As the name suggests, flip-phone handsets flip open and closed. In the closed position, the screen, dial pad, and other buttons cannot be seen. When the cell phone is flipped open, the components of the telephone are revealed. In contrast, standard handsets do not flip open, exposing the cell phone's screen, dialing pad,

and function buttons at all times. This particular handset style maintains the cell phone's antenna and earpiece in relatively close proximity to one another. In contrast, a flip-phone handset positions the cell phone antenna farther away from the ear as compared with the standard cell phone style (Kozma-Spytek, 2005). As such, flip phones are less prone to generating interference with hearing instrumentation.

The use of a relatively inexpensive induction earhook cell phone accessory can alleviate most of the interference experienced by hearing instrument users. The NoiZfree Telephone Induction earhook (Earcare NoiZfree, Athens, Greece; **Fig. 17–10A**) is a 30 inch cord with a lightweight induction earhook on one end and a 2.5 mm jack on the other. The 2.5 mm jack plugs directly into the cell phone via the headset port, and the earhook is placed behind the ear. To use the cell phone, the hearing instrument must be switched to either T or MT. Sound from the cell phone is routed along the wire to the induction earhook, which

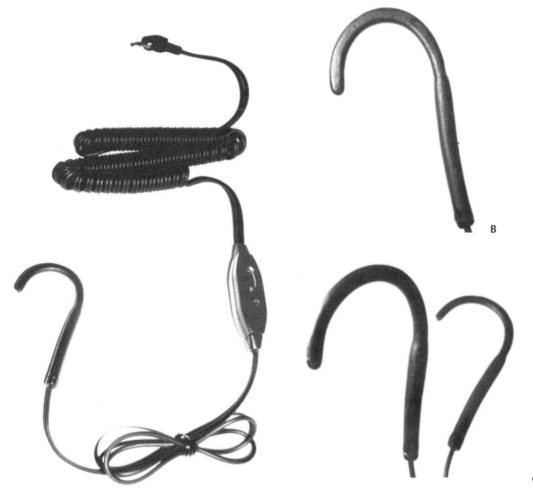

Figure 17–10 (A) The NoiZfree Telephone Induction Ear Hook interfaces with cell phones. The inherent design of this product increases the distance between the cell phone antenna and the hearing instrument, significantly reducing the potential for the hearing instrument wearer to perceive cell phone interference. **(B)** The NoiZfree Telephone Induction Ear Hook, monaural style, for routing cell phone signals electromagnetically to one hearing instrument. **(C)** The NoiZfree Telephone Induction Ear Hook, binaural style, for routing cell phone signals electromagnetically to both hearing instruments. (Courtesy of Earcare NoiZfree.)

sends the information electromagnetically directly to the hearing instruments. Because a microphone is located on the cord, not far from the induction earhook, it is not necessary for the user to hold the cell phone in the traditional location. The distance between the cell phone antenna and the hearing instrument should be sufficient to eliminate the potential for cell phone interference. The earhook is available in monaural (**Fig. 17–10B**) and binaural (**Fig. 17–10C**) configurations. In addition, an earhook/earbud configuration is available to allow individuals with unilateral hearing loss to hear the cell phone conversation in stereo.

HAT Systems

A variety of HAT systems are commercially available, including FM, IR, and alerting systems. These systems have been grouped together because each requires similar components to function: audio source, transmitter, receiver, and coupling method.

Audio Source

The audio source of an HAT system is the sound of interest ultimately routed to the listener(s). Depending on the product, the audio source may involve a TV, iPod, MP3 player, radio, computer, or telephone. The audio source may also involve an individual or individuals, such as a teacher, lecturer, colleague at a business meeting, or person at a party, restaurant, or other venue. When the audio source involves another person, the HAT system will require some type of microphone, whether handheld, lapel, or head-worn (Bengtsson and Brunved, 2000).

Transmitter and Receiver

The transmitter routes the signal from the audio source to the receiver. The mode of signal transmission will differ across the various HAT systems. FM systems transmit signals via radio waves, whereas IR systems transmit similar signals via light waves. The receiver accepts signals routed by the transmitter and directs the signal to the listener. Both the transmitter and the receiver rely on compatible technologies to work together. An FM transmitter will not work with a receiver from an IR system; an FM transmitter must be paired with a compatible FM receiver in order for the system to work.

Coupling Method

Coupling method refers to the manner in which auditory signals are routed from the receiver to the ear. There are different coupling methods available. For example, auditory signals may be routed to the ear via any type of headphone (traditional over-the-head style, earbuds, and under-the-chin style), neckloop, or silhouette inductor. In addition, signals may be sent directly to a hearing instrument using direct audio input (DAI). Given the variety of coupling methods, some of the more common methods will be reviewed in a little more detail.

Silhouette Inductor   A silhouette inductor is essentially the same thing as an induction earhook, described above. It is a thin, flat, hook-shaped device designed to fit behind the ear. The silhouette inductor plugs directly into a compatible HAT. Signals are ultimately routed electromagnetically from the silhouette induction hook directly to the telecoil of the hearing instrument.

Neckloop   A neckloop is a transducer resembling a thick necklace that is worn around the neck. Neckloops may connect directly with many HATs. Similar to the silhouette inductor, the neckloop transmits signals from the HAT in the form of electromagnetic energy directly to the telecoil of the individual's hearing instrument.

Direct Audio Input   DAI refers to circuitry within behind-the-ear (BTE) hearing instruments that enable HAT to directly connect to the instrument. A manufacturer-specific adapter, referred to as an audio boot, is needed to allow for an electrical connection between the BTE hearing instrument and the HAT (Thibodeau, 2003). The audio boot attaches to the bottom of the BTE, where it connects with the hearing instrument's DAI contacts (Bengtsson and Brunved, 2000), thereby routing the signal into the individual's ear via the hearing instrument.

FM Systems

FM portable systems broadcast signals from the speaker to the listener via radio waves. The audio source for most FM systems is a microphone, worn by the speaker. A transmitter connected to the microphone wirelessly sends radio waves to a receiver typically worn by the listener. The receiver may deliver the auditory signal to the listener's ears via a sound-field speaker, an interface with a hearing instrument, or a headphone (Thibodeau, 2003). In addition, a neckloop may be used by the listener, delivering the signal directly to the telecoil of the hearing instrument. **Figure 17–11** illustrates a popular FM personal system available from Williams Sound Corp.

Because the transmission mode of FM signals involves radio waves, the FCC has designated specific frequency bands for HAT use. FM systems operate at frequency bands ranging from 72 to 76 MHz and 216 to 217 MHz (Bengtsson and Brunved, 2000). Recently, the higher frequency band of 216 to 217 MHz was designated primary status in the United States, restricting the use of this higher frequency band to FM systems directly connected to hearing instruments (Launer, 2003). The frequency bands are divided into several channels. An FM transmitter and receiver pair must be tuned to the same channel within the same frequency band in order for the auditory signal to be routed appropriately. Wider band FM systems, which maintain a smaller overall number of channels, are more prone to interference from other FM or broadcasting systems than the newer narrowband systems, which have 3 times as many usable channels (Bengtsson and Brunved, 2000). In contrast to the lower frequency band, the 216 to 217 MHz band has been found to significantly reduce the potential for transmitter interference, noise interference, and distortions (Launer, 2003).

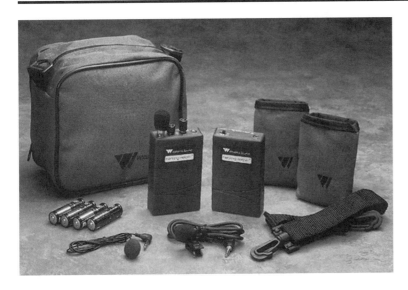

Figure 17–11 The Williams Sound Corp. Hearing Helper Wireless FM System (PFM 300) from Williams Sound Corp. (Courtesy of Williams Sound Corp.)

FM systems offer several advantages to those with hearing loss. First, these systems are suitable for any degree of hearing loss. Second, as previously mentioned, FM systems can significantly improve SNR by as much as +15 dB, providing individuals with optimal listening situations (Crandell and Smaldino, 2002; Hawkins and Van Tassel, 1982). Depending on the environment and specific system, the range of signal transmission is not a limiting factor, ranging from 15 to 100 feet (Launer, 2003). In certain situations, this advantage can serve as a potential disadvantage, as the signal is not limited within the confines of a room.

Infrared Systems

IR systems wirelessly transmit signals via infrared light. The transmitter plugs directly into the sound source and is responsible for sending signals to a receiver headset worn by the patient via invisible light waves. For many models, the transmitter also serves as the recharging base for the receiver headset. In general, batteries fully recharge within 3 hours, allowing for up to 8 hours of continuous TV viewing, for example.

The receiver is housed within the headset worn by the user. The headset is designed to be worn either under the chin or over the head. Once the receiver converts IR light waves to the original auditory signal, the signal is routed to the headphone. **Figure 17–12A** shows a traditional IR system from Senneiser Electronic GmbH & Co. KG (Wennebostel, Germany) with an under-the-chin receiver headset. Other available models interface with a neckloop **(Fig. 17–12B),** enabling the user to route signals electromagnetically from the receiver directly to hearing instruments without necessitating the use of an under-the-chin headset.

As with FM systems, IR systems operate on several different subcarrier frequencies. Earlier versions of IR systems primarily used the 95 kHz subcarrier frequency. During the mid-1990s, however, the electronic ballasts used with fluorescent lights created a source of interference for 95 kHz

systems (Bengtsson and Brunved, 2000). The interference was perceived by the listener as a fairly loud hum, buzzing, or static-like artifact. To resolve the interference issue, manufacturers have switched to 2.3 MHz and/or 2.8 MHz subcarrier frequencies, although 95 kHz systems are still commercially available. Because different IR systems are tuned to different frequency bands, both the transmitter and the receiver must operate on the same frequency in order for the device to work. For example, a 95 kHz receiver will not pick up signals emitted by a 2.3 MHz transmitter; only a 2.3 kHz receiver will be capable of picking up signals from the 2.3 MHz transmitter.

For maximum reception, users should position themselves directly in front of the transmitter, particularly when using a more interference-prone 95 kHz system. Although IR light is invisible, it behaves like visible light, reflecting off light-colored walls and ceilings and being absorbed by darker colored surfaces (Bengtsson and Brunved, 2000). IR transmissions will not pass through walls; therefore, the system will function only when the transmitter and the receiver are in the same room.

Pitfall

- IR systems are designed to broadcast on either the 95 kHz or the 2.3 MHz frequency. Patients can potentially use the receiver (headset) of their personal IR system in public facilities; however, the receiver will only work in facilities that operate IR transmitters of the same frequency. For example, a receiver tuned to the 95 kHz frequency will not pick up sound in facilities equipped with IR transmitters broadcasting on the 2.3 MHz frequency.

Alerting Systems

Alerting systems use any combination of transmitters and receivers to alert individuals of incoming auditory signals.

Devices feature amplified signals and/or vibrotactile and visual indicators. The components of an alerting system are connected electronically and are relatively inexpensive, providing individuals with an economical solution to specific communication needs. These systems are flexible and customizable, allowing users to build up the system as needed. Alerting systems may be very basic or very complex, depending on the needs and capabilities of the user.

Basic Alerting System For illustrative purposes, an alerting system incorporating one transmitter (**Fig. 17–13A**) and one receiver (**Fig. 17–13B**) may be considered basic. The transmitter shown in **Fig. 17–13** from Sonic Alert Inc. (Troy, MI) is a typical baby monitor, designed to detect the sounds of a baby's crying. It plugs directly into a standard electrical socket and is placed in the child's bedroom. The remote receiver shown in **Fig. 17–13B** detects incoming signals from the transmitter and generates an alerting signal. The receiver also plugs into a standard electrical socket and should be placed in the room occupied by the hearing-impaired individual. As shown in **Fig. 17–13B,** the bottom portion of this particular remote receiver has an outlet socket. A lamp plugged into the socket of the remote receiver will turn on and off in response to signals sent by the transmitter, visually signaling to the hearing-impaired individual that the baby is crying. Because both the transmitter and the remote receiver are plugged into the wall socket, the communication between the two components occurs via the home's electrical system. As long as these two components are plugged in, they will communicate with one another anywhere throughout the house.

Advanced Alerting System

As described above, basic alerting systems use only one transmitter and one receiver. Basic systems can be built up with additional transmitters and/or receivers, resulting in more advanced alerting systems. Advanced alerting systems incorporate at least two transmitters and/or receivers. The combination of transmitters and receivers is nearly limitless.

To illustrate the flexibility of alerting systems, the basic alerting system designed to allow the parent to hear the baby cry can be expanded to also alert the parent that the phone is ringing. A second transmitter (i.e., telephone ring signaler) must be added to the basic system. The second transmitter is designed to detect incoming phone calls. It plugs directly into the phone as well as a standard electrical socket. As described in the previous example, in the event the baby cries, the transmitter in the baby's room will send a signal to the remote receiver in the room occupied by the parent. The remote receiver will cause the lamp to flash on and off, visually indicating to the parent that the baby is crying. In addition, in the event the telephone rings, the second transmitter, located in the room with the phone, will send a signal to the same remote receiver that resides in the room occupied by the hearing-impaired person, causing the same lamp to flash on and off; however, the flash

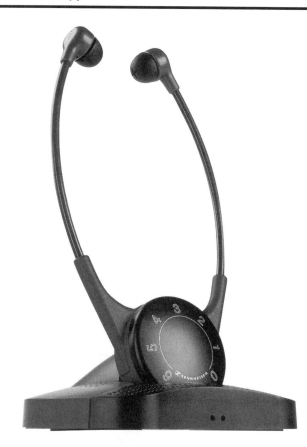

A

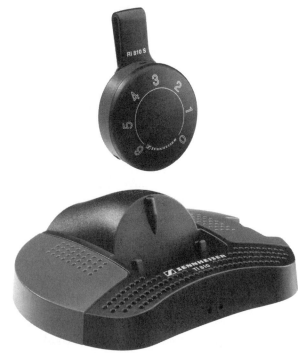

B

Figure 17–12 (A) Sennheiser Set 810 infrared system with standard under-the-chin receiver headphone. **(B)** Sennheiser Set 810 infrared system with special receiver designed to connect to a neckloop. This arrangement allows signals to be routed electromagnetically from the neckloop to the telecoil of the user's hearing instrument(s). (Courtesy of Sennheiser Electronic GmbH & Co. KG.)

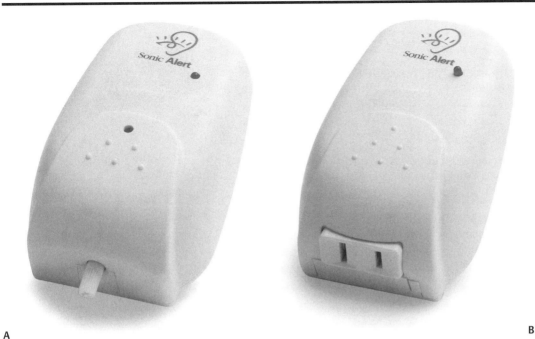

A   B

Figure 17–13 (A) The Sonic Alert BC400 Sonic Sitter. **(B)** The Sonic Alert SA101 Basic Remote Receiver. (Courtesy of Sonic Alert Inc.)

pattern of the lamp will differ depending on which transmitter sent the signal. This arrangement helps the hearing-impaired individual know when the phone is ringing versus when the baby is crying.

Personal Listening Systems

Personal listening systems refer to hard-wired, single-component devices. In contrast to FM, IR, and alerting systems, personal listening systems do not rely on separate transmitter and receiver components. These systems connect the sound source to the listener via a wire or cable. Obviously, one of the immediate disadvantages of personal listening systems is the listener must maintain close proximity to the sound source at all times. Nevertheless, these devices are relatively inexpensive and versatile, providing individuals with hearing loss the ability to improve communication on a one-to-one basis, in small group situations, while listening to the TV or radio, or while riding in the car.

As shown in **Fig. 17–14,** personal listening systems, such as the Pocketalker from Williams Sound Corp., consist of a standard base and earphone. The base incorporates the microphone, earphone connection, and tone and volume controls. The microphone will pick up the audio source and must be placed as close to the source as possible. During one-to-one conversations, the speaker should hold the personal listening device and speak into the microphone. In larger groups, the listener can hold the personal listening device and direct the microphone toward the sound source or place it on a table or other surface close to the speakers of interest. An extended cord is usually available with most personal listening systems to provide additional flexibility.

Signals from the microphone are amplified and routed to the listener via headphones or earbuds. Most devices increase the volume for a maximum gain of ~40 dB or allow neckloop interface so that signals may be electromagnetically routed to the listener's hearing instrument(s).

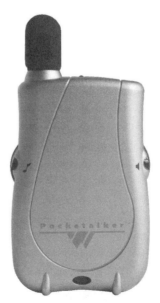

Figure 17–14 The Williams Sound Corp. Pocketalker. (Courtesy of Williams Sound Corp.)

Miscellaneous HAT Products

Microphone Arrays

Patients with hearing loss have access to products designed to interface with hearing instruments for purposes of improving speech intelligibility in noise. For example, the LINK-IT from Etymotic Research Inc. (Elk Grove Village, IL) is a wireless directional microphone array worn behind the ear that transmits sound to either a BTE or in-the-ear (ITE) device via the hearing instrument's telecoil. As shown in **Fig. 17–15,** the LINK-IT resembles a silhouette inductor with a 2 inch microphone bar extending forward from the top of the device. It is designed to reside behind the ear, between the user's BTE and/or eyeglass temples. The microphone bar contains three directional microphones that work in conjunction with one another to provide +7 dB improvement in SNR monaurally with an additional +2 to +3 dB improvement in SNR when used binaurally (Etymotic Research Inc., 2006).

Signals detected by the LINK-IT are transmitted electromagnetically from the LINK-IT's induction hook and routed to the telecoil of the hearing instrument. This product was designed to be used in those difficult listening situations when hearing instruments do not provide sufficient directivity for speech understanding (Etymotic Research Inc., 2006).

Alarm Clocks

Alarm clocks designed specifically for individuals with hearing loss allow users to wake to amplified auditory signals and vibrotactile and/or visual stimulation. Most alarm clocks are designed to generate a 113 dB SPL alarm, may be

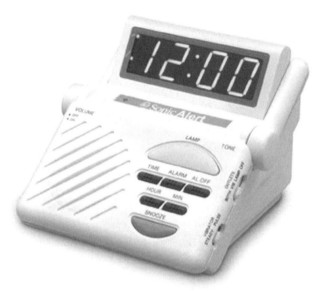

Figure 17–16 The Sonic Alert SB1000 Sonic Boom Classic 1000 Alarm Clock. (Courtesy of Sonic Alert Inc.)

used with optional bedshakers, and accommodate lamps that may be plugged into the clock to generate a visual lamp flash during the alarm cycle. Alarm clocks are available in standard (**Fig. 17–16**) and travel models (**Fig. 17–17**). **Figure 17–16** shows a popular alarm clock from Sonic Alert designed for the hearing-impaired market. One of the unique features of this particular model is that the alarm clock acts as a remote receiver. Alarm watches are also available to provide audible and/or vibrating alarms without disturbing others.

Pearl

• The alarm clock shown in **Fig. 17–16** may be used as a remote receiver in a basic or advanced alerting system. For example, hearing-impaired patients can use the Sonic Alert model in conjunction with a baby monitor.

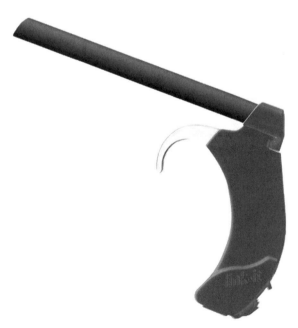

Figure 17–15 The LINK-IT microphone array. (Courtesy of Etymotic Research Inc.)

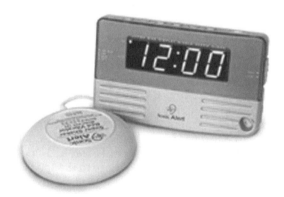

Figure 17–17 The Sonic Alert SBT200ss Sonic Boom travel alarm clock. (Courtesy of Sonic Alert Inc.)

Smoke Detectors

Amplified smoke detectors operate like standard detectors but provide a much louder auditory signal (usually 90–95 dB SPL). The auditory signal is supplemented with a strobe signal.

◆ Integrating HAT Into Clinical Practice

To gain a better understanding of how audiologists can more efficiently integrate HAT into current practices, the Division of Adult Audiology at Washington School of Medicine in St. Louis conducted a pilot HAT program designed to identify potential techniques that would generate consumer awareness about HAT. Specifically, the goal was simply to observe which strategies were most effective in making patients aware of the availability of HAT with minimal investment of time and money on the part of the clinic. A second goal of the project was to identify those strategies considered least obtrusive to the established, daily routine of the clinic.

HAT products were displayed in two different patient counseling rooms in the Division of Adult Audiology at Washington University School of Medicine. Each of these rooms showcased nearly 20 different HAT products, with some of them set up as working models, whereby patients could actually experience using the product. The working models were accompanied by step-by-step instructions on how to use the product. The remaining HAT products were on dislplay but not actively functioning. Educational HAT brochures were made available to patients in the reception area and clinical rooms. Finally, a postcard advertising the availability of HAT was developed and mailed to an established patient base at the Division of Adult Audiology and also to patients from the Division of Geriatrics at Washington University Medical Center.

Much more research in the form of carefully controlled studies is needed to assess the efficacy of HAT awareness-generating strategies; however, valuable insight was gained as a result of observations made by the audiology staff at Washington University School of Medicine. The following anecdotal observations and initial trends serve as preliminary guidelines for the audiologist to take into consideration in terms of attempting to effectively generate patient awareness about HAT.

The Right Kind of Training Is Critical

Product benefits, uses, and limitations are important for audiologists to know; however, they also must be aware of product characteristics that may potentially create barriers to successful use. For example, how to set up the HAT correctly represents the most common source of frustration to patients; if audiologists cannot guide patients on how to properly set up a specific HAT at home, the likelihood of product return significantly increases.

Working Product Demonstrations Must Be Set Up and Readily Accessible to Consumers

Patients must be able not only to touch, feel, and manipulate a product, but also to actually use that product. This experience will independently educate patients regarding the benefits of HAT and also lead them to initiate further discussion about the product with audiologists. More importantly, patients with access to working demonstrations will make a purchase decision more quickly. For example, in the Washington University study, IR systems that were initially displayed but not connected to TVs generated some interest from curious patients. Once the IR systems were connected to TVs and patients were able to experience the product, sales of IR systems increased by over 1000%. To put this in perspective, prior to installation of an interactive demonstration station, three IR systems were dispensed in the entire preceding year. Currently, on average, three systems are dispensed each month.

"How to" Instructions Should Be Available

Working demonstrations and display models must be accompanied by product images and simple instructions, along with contact information. This enables patients to try products on their own, without prompting or oversight by an audiologist or other staff member. In addition, it helps to alleviate patients' fears that the products are complicated or difficult to use.

More HAT Products Are Not Necessarily Better

Initially, the goal of the HAT product displays in the Washington University study was to exhibit approximately 20 different products. Based on subjective feedback from the audiology staff, it was evident that many patients were overwhelmed rather than intrigued by the number of choices. Throughout the course of phase 1, product choices were pared to 10 products. When there were fewer HAT choices, audiologists reported that patients were more willing to approach the demonstration models.

Special Consideration

- Exposure to too many products may be overwhelming to patients. Paring down options may be more effective in converting patients to HAT users.

Eliminating Poorly Selling HAT Products May Not Be the Answer

Surprisingly, despite the availability of a working amplified telephone that patients could use to make outgoing calls, sales in amplified telephones in the Division of Adult Audiology at Washington University School of Medicine clinic have not changed significantly from sales prior to the initiation of the HAT project. At first, it was thought that amplified telephones should be eliminated from the HAT display line. However, it was observed that most patients seemed to approach amplified telephone technology first, before exploring any other HAT product. Amplified telephones represent the most familiar HAT devices to novice patients and are most likely the least threatening. Despite poor sales in amplified telephones, these products are considered critical in generating patient interest in HAT and ultimately result in interest in other products.

HAT Mailings Do Not Necessarily Bring in a Return on Investment

Although many factors influence the effectiveness of a mass mailing, initial results of the Washington University project indicate that a mass mailing announcing the availability of HAT was not effective in generating awareness in the clinic's established patient base. This topic will be further explored throughout the research project, but the current impression is that the most effective "point of purchase" for HAT devices is during the initial discussion of hearing loss and hearing instrument options.

Integrate Flexibility into the Product Line

New HAT products are constantly being introduced to the market. Although it is not productive or necessary for audiologists to expend significant time and energy on identifying and learning about all new products, it is important that they periodically reassess HAT offerings within the clinical environment.

Application of Lessons Learned in Clinical Practice

Based on the information learned from phase 1 of the HAT research project at Washington University, audiologists should consider developing a small-scale, interactive HAT display either in the reception area or in a counseling room in the audiology clinic. Although the display does not have to involve a significant number of products, ideally, two working amplified telephones, at least one cell phone product, and at least one working demonstration model of an IR system should be considered for display. These four products will probably be the most effective in piquing patient curiosity and generating interest in HAT technology. In choosing amplified telephones, it is a good idea to include one corded and one cordless model. This will effectively communicate to patients that choices in amplified telephone models are available. In addition, it is critical to set up the telephones to allow patients to hear the different tones and to experience using them. This may be accomplished by investing in a relatively inexpensive phone-linking device, described above (**Fig. 17–2**). Because phone-linking devices place two linked telephones in close proximity to one another, the most effective demonstration strategy is to link a cordless phone to a corded model. In doing so, patients using the cordless telephone can walk away from the corded telephone being used by another party. This flexibility not only allows patients to test the cordless telephone's reception range but also eliminates the potential of overhearing the conversation from the other party.

Given the increased demand for eliminating interference associated with cell phone use, audiologists should be prepared to offer patients a solution. Audiology clinics should have available at least one cell phone product for patients to try. Because most cell phone users have a cell phone on hand, a cell phone induction hook, for example, can be plugged into the patient's cell phone. A phone call can then be placed by the clinic to the cell phone user to enable the patient to assess whether or not a particular product works well.

Finally, at least one IR system should be installed in the clinic to allow patients to experience the benefits of this form of technology. Because these types of devices are most commonly used at home with a TV, investing in a dedicated TV for product demonstration would be beneficial. IR systems also can be effectively showcased by hooking the transmitter to other audio sources, including a CD or DVD player.

◆ Summary

HAT represents an underutilized technology in audiologic practice. The technology itself is not complicated; however, effectively integrating HAT into the audiology practice requires familiarity with general product lines and an effective strategy for showcasing the technology in the clinical setting. The information covered in this chapter should provide audiologists with a basic understanding of HAT and initial guidelines on effectively generating product awareness to patients.

References

American National Standards Institute. (1996). Methods of measurement of compatibility between wireless communication devices and hearing aids (ANSI ASC C63 SC8). Retrieved November 4, 2005 from http://grouper.ieee.org/groups/emc/private/asc-c63/sc_8/hac/c6319b23.doc

Bengtsson, P. O., & Brunved, P. B. (2000). When hearing aids are not enough: The need for assistive devices. In M. Valente, H. Hosford-Dunn, & R. Roeser (Eds.), Audiology treatment (pp. 581–599). New York: Thieme Medical Publishers.

Berger, H. S., & TEM Consulting. ANSI C63.19 hearing aid/cellular telephone compatibility. Retrieved November 8, 2005, from http://www.ou.edu/engineering/emc/projects/CDG.html

Cellular Abroad. (2007). Retrieved August 8, 2007, from http://www.cellularabond.com/q_as.html*gsm

Crandell, C. C., & Smaldino, J. (2002). Room acoustics and auditory rehabilitation technology. In J. Katz J (Ed.), Handbook of clinical audiology (5th ed., pp. 607–630). Philadelphia: Lippincott Williams & Wilkins.

E-Michigan Deaf and Hard of Hearing People.(2005). TTY or TDD: The text telephone. Retrieved November 6, 2005, from http://www.michdhh.org/assistive_devices/text_telephone.html

Etymotic Research Inc. (2006). Frequently asked questions. Retrieved February 27, 2006, from http://www.etymotic.com/pdf/linkit-brochure.pdf

Federal Communications Commission. (2003). Eighth annual CMRS competition report, sections II.C.1.b.(i) and II.C.1.d. Retrieved November 2, 2005, from http://hraunfoss.fcc.gov/edocs_public/attachmatch/FCC-03-150A1. pdf

Federal Communications Commission.(2005a). Technology access program. Retrieved November 6, 2005, from http://tap.gallaudet.edu/fcc/analogelim.htm

Federal Communications Commission. (2005b). Section 68.4(a) of the commission's rules governing hearing aid-compatible telephones. Retrieved November 8, 2005, from http://hraunfoss.fcc.gov/edocs_public/attachmatch/FCC-03-168A1.pdf

47 U.S.C. § 610(b)(2)(A). Retrieved November 4, 2005, from http://wireless.fcc.gov/releases/011114-hearing.txt

47 U.S.C. § 610(b)(2)(C). Retrieved November 4, 2005, from http://www.fcc.gov/Bureaus/Wireless/Notices/2001/fcc01320.doc

Hawkins, D., & Van Tassel, D. (1982). Electroacoustic characteristics of personal FM systems. Journal of Speech and Hearing Disorders, 47, 355–362.

Killion, M. (1997). SNR loss: I can hear what people say but I can't understand them. Hearing Review, 4(12), 8–14.

Kochkin, S. (1999). Baby boomers spur growth in potential market, but penetration rate declines. Hearing Journal, 52(1), 33–48.

Kochkin, S. (2000). MarkeTrak V: Why my hearing aids are in the drawer—the consumers' perspective. Hearing Journal, 53(2), 34–42.

Kochkin, S. (2002). MarkeTrak VI: 10-year customer satisfaction trends in the US hearing instrument market. Hearing Review, 9(10), 14–25.

Kochkin, S., & Rogin, C. (2000). Quantifying the obvious: The impact of hearing instruments on quality of life. Hearing Review, 7(1), 6–35.

Kochkin, S., & Strom, K. (1999). Battling noise. Hearing Review, 3 (Suppl.), 1.

Kozma-Spytek, L. (2005). Digital wireless telephones and hearing aids: Frequently asked questions (and answers). Retrieved July 7, 2005, from http://www.tap.fallaudet.edu/DigitalCellFAQ.htm

Kuk, F. (1996). Hearing aid survey tests user satisfaction. Hearing Instruments, 49(1), 24–29.

Launer, S. (2003). Wireless solutions: The state of the art and future FM technology for the hearing impaired consumer. In D. Fabry & C. DeConde Johnson (Eds.), Access: Achieving clear communications employing sound solutions (pp. 31–38).

Mann, M. Mobile phone basics. Retrieved November 8, 2005, from http://www.socketcom.com/pdf/TechBriefMobilePhone.pdf#search='mobile%20phone%20basics%20and%20Socket'

Moore, B. (1997). An introduction to the psychology of hearing (4th ed.). San Diego, CA: Academic Press.

National Institutes of Deafness and Communication Disorders. Statistics about hearing disorders, ear infections, and deafness. Retrieved November 1, 2005, from http://www.nidcd.nih.gov/health/statistics/hearing.asp

Noll, A. M. (1998). Introduction to telephones and telephone systems (3rd ed.). Boston: Artech House.

Prendergast, S., & Kelley, L. (2002). Aural rehab services: Survey reports who offers which ones and how often. Hearing Journal, 55(9), 30–35.

Ricketts, R. A., & Dahr, S. (1999). Aided benefit across directional and omni-directional hearing aid microphones for behind-the-ear hearing aids. Journal of the American Academy of Audiology, 10(4), 180–189.

Ross, M. (2004). Hearing assistance technology: Making a world of difference. Hearing Journal, 57(11), 12–17.

Schuchman, G., Valente, M., Beck, L. B., & Potts, L. (1999). User satisfaction with an ITE directional hearing aid. Hearing Review, 6(7), 12–22.

Servedio, D. (2000). ALDs: It's time to take full advantage of this valuable, but underused, technology. Hearing Journal, 53(8), 38–39.

Stika, C., Ross, M., & Cuevas, C. (2002, May/June). Hearing aid services and satisfaction: The consumer viewpoint. Hearing Loss, 25–31.

Thibodeau, L. (2003). Terminology and standardization. In D. Fabry & C. DeConde Johnson (Eds.), Access: Achieving clear communications employing sound solutions (pp. 75–86).

Thibodeau, L. M. (2004). Hearing assistance technology (HAT) can optimize communication. Hearing Journal, 57(11), 11.

Chapter 18

Room Acoustics for Listeners with Normal Hearing and Hearing Impairment

Joseph J. Smaldino, Carl C. Crandell, Brian M. Kreisman, Andrew B. John, and Nicole V. Kreisman

To ensure that children with disabilities have equal access to free and appropriate public education in the United States, four major federal laws have been enacted: the Education for All Handicapped Children Act of 1975 (the original Public Law [P.L.] 94–142); a revised version of P. L. 94–142 entitled the Education of the Handicapped Act Amendments of 1986 (P.L. 99–457); the most recent revision of the Individuals with Disabilities Education Act (IDEA) Amendments of 1997 (P.L. 105–117); and the Rehabilitation Act of 1973 (Section 504), which focuses on accessibility. Since publication of the first edition of this book, it has become clear that adequate classroom acoustics is such a powerful prerequisite for learning that it must be considered as fundamental for all children, instead of simply a solution for children with disabilities. The Technology-Related Assistance for Individuals with Disabilities Act Amendments of 1994 (P. L. 103–218) and the No Child Left Behind Act of 2001 (P. L. 107–110) provide impetus for creating desirable listening and learning classroom environments.

Understanding the problems associated with inadequate classroom acoustics, the impact of undesirable acoustics on all students, and modern solutions to the problem of inadequate acoustics remains the central focus of this chapter (Bess et al, 1996; Crandell, 1991, 1992; Crandell and Smaldino, 1995; Crandell et al, 2005; Flexer, 1992; Smaldino, 1997).

Because classroom instruction primarily involves a teacher communicating to students, accurate recognition of the teacher's speech signal by the students is important. To the extent that the acoustic characteristics of the classroom listening environment interfere with accurate speech recognition, the acoustics of the room may be a barrier to learning. Acoustic barriers to listening and learning have been extensively studied over the past 25 years (see Crandell et al, 2005, for a review). From this research, it is clear that the acoustic factors that most often affect accurate speech recognition in a room include (1) the relative intensity of the information-carrying components of the speech signal to all competing signals or noise (i.e., signal-to-noise ratio, SNR), (2) the degree to which the temporal aspects of the information-carrying components of the speech signal are preserved, and (3) the interaction among these variables. In addition, speech recognition in a room can be influenced by linguistic and articulatory factors. Linguistic factors include the word familiarity and vocabulary of the listener, the context, the number of syllables in words, and the linguistic competency of the listener. Articulatory factors include the gender, articulatory abilities, and dialect of the speaker. This chapter will focus on the acoustic factors that influence speech recognition in rooms, with a primary emphasis on classrooms. For discussions of the linguistic or articulatory variables that influence speech recognition, the reader is directed to Ferrand (2001).

◆ Intensity of the Speaker's Voice

For optimal speech recognition to occur in a room, the speaker's voice must be heard clearly above the individual listener's threshold of audibility and the background noise level of the room. The intensity of a speaker's voice varies with the amount of pressure developed by the lungs, the length of time the vocal folds are closed, and the resonances of the vocal tract (which change with the position of the tongue). The degree of mouth opening is also an important factor for appropriate projection of the voice. The human voice has relatively limited acoustic power. The vowels are the strongest components of speech, and consonants are the weakest. The average sound pressure level (SPL) produced by a speaker (at 1 m) during quiet, normal, and loud speech is 45, 65, and 85 dB SPL, respectively (Ferrand, 2001; Hawkins and Yacullo, 1984). The range of speech is ~30 dB (+12 dB to −18 dB above and below the average speech spectrum).

Because of the limited power of the human voice and the acoustic environment in an enclosure (noise, reverberation, and distance), many rooms will require the use of an amplification device to ensure a high level of speech recognition. Speaking loudly in many rooms will not improve speech recognition because loud speech generally increases the

intensity of the vowel phonemes but not the consonant phonemes. As will be discussed in a later section, most cues important for accurate speech recognition are carried by consonant phonemes, not vowels (French and Steinberg, 1947). Moreover, speaking with a high vocal output for extended periods can often lead to various forms of vocal pathosis, such as chronic hoarseness and vocal nodules. Gotaas and Starr (1993) reported that 80% of public school teachers, who often have to speak loudly during an entire school day, reported vocal fatigue compared with 5% of the general population. In addition, it appears that many speakers cannot sustain loud levels of speech for extended periods. Ottring et al (1992) investigated the potential of training teachers to increase their speaking levels behaviorally in the classroom. Results indicated that it was possible to train teachers to increase their speaking level from 3 to 5 dB, but continual training was necessary to sustain the level enhancement. It was concluded that classroom amplification is the most consistent means to increase teachers' voice levels above their normal speaking level.

◆ Background Room Noise

In addition to the power of the speaker's voice, background (or ambient) noise in a room may compromise speech recognition. The term *background noise* refers to any auditory disturbance that interferes with what a listener wants or needs to hear (Crandell et al, 2005). Background noise in a room can emanate from several possible sources. These sources include external noise (noise that is generated from outside the building, e.g., airplane traffic, local construction, automobile traffic, and playgrounds), internal noise (noise that originates from within the building but outside the room, e.g., in rooms adjacent to cafeterias, lecture rooms, gymnasiums, and busy hallways), and room noise (noise that is generated within the room; Crandell and Smaldino, 1995, 1996b). Sources of room noise include individuals talking, sliding chairs or tables, and shuffling hard-soled shoes on noncarpeted floors, as well as instructional equipment motors and fans, such as those from computers and data projectors. Heating, ventilation, and air-conditioning systems may also significantly contribute to room noise levels.

Measurement of Room Noise

The acoustic characteristics of background noise in a room often vary considerably as a function of time because of the changing activities taking place in that room. This variability often makes it difficult to measure room noise and its effects in a simple manner. Despite this difficulty, most measures of room noise continue to be single-number descriptors. One of the most common single-number descriptors of room noise is the measurement of the relative SPL of the noise at a specific point or points in time on an A-weighting scale. A device called a sound level meter is used to measure the amplitude of sound. Sound level meters range from compact, inexpensive, battery-operated units to computer-based devices that can measure and record numerous properties of a signal. They are classified according to standards set forth in American National Standards Institute (ANSI) S1.14 (1983). Type I sound level meters meet the most rigorous standards, whereas type II are for general purpose and type III are for hobby use. Most serious measurement of room noise would require at least a type II model, preferably a type I. Many sound level meters incorporate weighting filter networks. The A-weighting network, referred to as dB(A), is designed to simulate the sensitivity of the average human ear under conditions of low sound loudness (40 phons). The B-weighting network, referred to as dB(B), simulates loud sound (70 phons), and the C-weighting, referred to as dB(C), approximates how the ear would respond to very loud sound. The convention for room and factory noise measurements is the A-weighting network. One alternative to the traditional sound level meter is an audio analysis system. One such affordable system is the IE-45 from Ivie Technologies Inc. (Lehi, UT), a handheld system that is coupled to a Samsung Q1 tablet personal computer. A type II microphone comes standard with the system; type I microphones with preamplifiers are available. Extension cables are also available, so the individual performing the measurements can be as far away as 25 feet from the microphone. Besides functioning as a sound level meter, the IE-35 is a real-time analyzer that can store measurements and compare these measures to established

recommended sound spectral levels for communication called noise criteria (NC) curves, record seat-to-seat SPL variations, and provide recordings of SPL over time. An optional reverberation time (RT) program can be used to measure how long it takes a loud sound level to decrease 60 dB in intensity (RT-60).

The single number obtained from a sound pressure measurement performed with the A-weighting scale can be obtained with a variety of very different spectra. A more thorough way to measure noise in an enclosure is to conduct a spectral analysis of the noise. Spectral analysis of the noise (usually 63–8000 Hz) requires an octave band, or one-third octave band filter network associated with the sound level meter. Another way of evaluating the effects of noise on speech communication is through the use of noise criteria (NC) curves (Beranek, 1954). The NC curves are a family of frequency/intensity curves based on octave band sound pressure across a 20 to 10,000 Hz band and have been related to successful use of an acoustic space for a variety of activities. When using NC curves (see **Fig. 18–1**), sound levels are plotted across eight octave frequencies from 63 to 8000 Hz. The NC value that characterizes a room is determined by the highest octave band SPL that intersects the NC family of curves. Thus, in **Fig. 18–1,** the NC curve would be 50 dB. The NC rating is generally 8 to 10 dB below the dB(A)

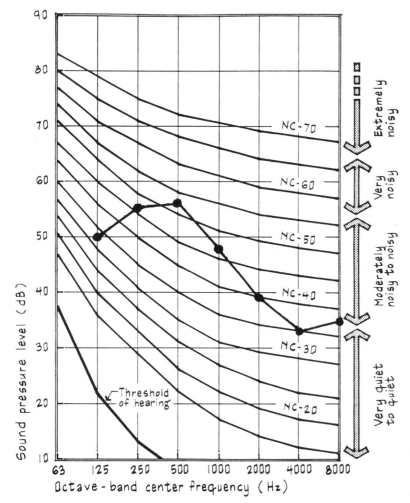

Figure 18–1 Example of noise criteria (NC) curves. (Adapted from Egan, M. (1987). Architectural acoustics. New York: McGraw-Hill, with permission. Reprinted by J. Ross Publishing.)

Table 18–1 Appropriate NC Units and Computed Equivalent dB(A) Readings for Various Environments

Type of Space	NC Units	Computer Equivalent dB(A) Readings
Broadcast studios	15–20	25–30
Concert halls	15–20	25–30
Theaters (500 seats, no amplification)	20–25	30–35
Music rooms	25	35
Schoolrooms (no amplification)	25	35
Television studios	25	35
Apartments and hotels	25–30	35–40
Assembly halls (amplification)	25–30	35–40
Homes (sleeping areas)	25–30	35–40
Movie theaters	30	40
Hospitals	30	40
Churches (no amplification)	25	35
Courtrooms (no amplification)	25	30–35
Libraries	30	40–45
Restaurants	45	55
Coliseums for sports only (amplification)	50	60

NC, noise criteria.
Source: From Egan, M. (1987). Architectural acoustics. New York: McGraw-Hill. Reprint by J. Ross Publishing. Reprinted with permission.

level of that room. To illustrate the advantages of this method over a single-number descriptor, assume that a significant amount of low-frequency noise was present in a room. This noise would have a great impact on the NC value assigned to the room; however, a single-number measure such as dB(A) would not provide sufficient detail to identify and reduce offending frequency bands. It is recommended that background noise levels in rooms be measured by means of NC curves whenever possible, because this method provides the examiner additional information regarding the spectral characteristics of the noise. Specifically, with this information, the audiologist or acoustic consultant can isolate and modify sources of excessive noise in the room. Appropriate NC units for various rooms are found in **Table 18–1**. **Table 18–2** presents the effects of different NC units on communicative efficiency. A similar concept to NC curves is room criteria (RC) curves. In the development of RC curves, NC curves were modified at very low and very high frequencies to include frequencies commonly associated with mechanical noises, such as heating and air-conditioning units. The reader is

directed to Beranek (1954) and Egan (1987) for further details concerning the measurement of noise.

Background Noise Levels in Rooms

Background noise levels have been reported in many enclosures, such as classrooms, malls, transportation settings, and homes (Bess et al, 1984; Crandell, 1992; Crandell and Smaldino,1995; Pearsons et al, 1977; Sanders, 1965). Sanders (1965) measured the noise levels in 47 occupied and unoccupied classrooms in 15 different school buildings. Mean occupied noise levels ranged from an average of 69 dB(B) in kindergarten classrooms to 52 dB(B) in classrooms for children with hearing loss. Unoccupied classroom noise levels were ~10 dB lower than the occupied classroom settings, ranging from 58 dB(B) for kindergarten classrooms to 42 dB(B) in classrooms used for children with hearing impairment. Pearsons et al (1977) reported that noise levels averaged 45 dB(A) for suburban residential settings and 55 dB(A) for urban dwellings. Mean

Table 18–2 Effects of Different NC Units on Communicative Efficiency

NC Units	Communication Environment	Typical Applications
20–30	Very quiet office; telephone use satisfactory; suitable for large conferences	Executive offices and conference rooms for 50 people
30–35	"Quiet" office; satisfactory for conferences at a 15 foot table; normal voice 10 to 20 feet; telephone use satisfactory	Private or semiprivate offices, reception rooms, and conference rooms for 20 people
35–40	Satisfactory for conferences at a 6 to 8 foot table; telephone use occasionally slightly difficult; normal voice 3 to 6 feet	Medium-sized offices and industrial business offices
40–50	Satisfactory for conferences at 4 to 5 foot table; telephone use slightly difficult; normal voice 1 to 2 feet, raised voice 3 to 6 feet	Large engineering and drafting rooms
50–55	Unsatisfactory for conferences of more than two or three people; telephone use slightly difficult; normal voice 1 to 2 feet, raised voice 3 to 6 feet	Secretarial areas (typing), accounting areas (business machines), blueprint rooms, etc.
Above 55	Very noisy; office environment unsatisfactory	Not recommended for any type of room

NC, noise criteria.
Source: From Egan, M. (1987). Architectural acoustics. New York: McGraw-Hill. Reprint by J. Ross Publishing. Reprinted with permission.

outdoor noise levels were 2 to 10 dB more intense than indoor settings. Noise levels were measured at 54 dB(A) for department store environments and 77 dB(A) in transportation locales (train and aircraft noise). Bess et al (1984) measured background noise levels in 19 classrooms for children with hearing loss. Median unoccupied noise levels were 41 dB(A), 50 dB(B), and 58 dB(C). When the classroom was occupied with students, background noise levels increased ~15 dB to 56 dB(A), 60 dB(B), and 63 dB(C). Crandell and Smaldino (1995) reported that background noise levels in 32 unoccupied classroom settings were 51 dB(A) and 67 dB(C). As will be shown later, noise levels of the magnitude measured in many rooms make accurate speech recognition difficult, if not impossible, particularly for listeners with hearing impairment.

General Effects of Noise on Speech Recognition

Background noise in a room deleteriously affects a listener's speech recognition by reducing, or masking, the highly redundant acoustic and linguistic cues available in the signal. *Masking* refers to the phenomenon in which the threshold of a signal, such as speech, is raised by the presence of another sound, such as room noise. For example, a listener may be able to understand a speaker who is speaking at normal conversational levels comfortably in a quiet room. However, if other persons begin to talk, the data projector is turned on, and/or the ventilation system begins to generate noise, the speaker will now have to raise the level of his or her voice for the listener to hear what is being discussed. If the speaker does not raise his or her voice, the noise in the room will mask much of the important acoustic information presented by the speaker.

In general, because the spectral energy of consonant phonemes is considerably less intense than vowel phonemes, background noise in a room often masks the consonants more than the vowels. Loss of consonant information has a great effect on speech recognition because most of the cues important for accurate speech recognition are carried by the consonants (French and Steinberg, 1947). Several variables affect the ability of a noise to mask speech. These variables include the long-term acoustic spectrum of the noise, the average intensity of the noise relative to the intensity of speech, and fluctuations in the intensity of the noise over time (e.g., Beranek, 1954; Crandell et al, 2005; Nabelek and Nabelek, 1994). Low-frequency noise in a listening environment tends to be a more effective masker of speech than high-frequency noise because of upward spread of masking. Upward spread of masking is the phenomenon in which a masking noise produces greater masking at frequencies above the frequency of the masker than at frequencies below the masker. For example, a 500 Hz noise would more effectively mask a 1000 Hz signal than would a 4000 Hz masker. The fact that low-frequency noise has a greater effect on speech recognition than high-frequency noise is important because the predominant spectra of noise found in typical listening environments are low frequency (Crandell and Smaldino, 1995; Crandell et al, 2005). The most effective masking noises are commonly those with spectra similar to the speech spectrum because all speech frequencies are

masked to some degree. In general, noises that are continuous in nature are more effective maskers than interrupted or impulse noises, because continuous noises reduce a greater amount of the spectral-temporal information available in the speech signal. Continuous noises in the room include the hum of air-conditioning and heating systems, faulty fluorescent lighting, and the long-term spectra of individuals talking.

In most listening environments, the fundamental determinant for speech recognition is not the overall level of the room noise, but rather the relationship between the intensity of the signal and the intensity of the background noise at the listener's ear. This relationship is referred to as the signal-to-noise ratio (SNR) or message-to-competition ratio (MCR). To illustrate, if a speech signal is presented at 75 dB SPL, and a noise is 70 dB SPL, the SNR (or MCR) is 75 minus 70 dB, or +5 dB. For listeners with normal hearing and listeners with hearing loss, speech recognition ability tends to be the highest at favorable SNRs and decreases as the SNR within the listening environment is reduced (Crandell et al, 2005; Crum, 1974; Finitzo-Hieber and Tillman, 1978; Nabelek and Nabelek, 1994). For example, Crum (1974) examined the word recognition of adults with normal hearing at various SNRs (SNR = +12 dB, +6 dB, and 0 dB). Word recognition scores reached a plateau at high SNRs (95% at +12 dB SNR) but diminished as the SNR became less favorable (80% and 46% at +6 dB SNR and 0 dB SNR, respectively). Generally speaking, speech recognition in adults with normal hearing is not severely degraded until the SNR approximates 0 dB (speech and noise are at equal intensities). As discussed in the next section, this SNR depends on many factors, such as the type of noise, type of speech stimuli, and articulatory abilities/dialect of the speaker.

Signal-to-Noise Ratios in Various Enclosures

Because of high background noise levels, relatively poor SNRs have been reported in many settings. Pearsons et al (1977) reported that average SNRs were +14 to +9 dB in suburban and urban residential settings, respectively. In outdoor settings, SNRs decreased to approximately +8 to +5 dB. Additional measurements indicated that in department store settings, the average SNR was +7 dB, whereas transportation settings yielded an average SNR of −2 dB. Plomp (1986) reported that the average SNR found at parties ranged from +1 dB to −2 dB. In classroom environments (Table 18–3), the range of SNRs has been reported to be from +5 dB to −7 dB (e.g., Crandell et al, 2005; Sanders, 1965).

Table 18–3 A Summary of Studies Examining Classroom Signal-to-Noise Ratios

Investigation/Year	Signal-to-Noise Ratio (dB)
Sanders (1965)	+1 to +5
Blair (1977)	−7 to 0
Markides (1986)	+3
Finitzo-Heiber (1988)	+1 to +4

Effects of Noise on Speech Recognition in Listeners with Hearing Impairment and Normal Hearing

It has been amply demonstrated that the speech recognition performance of listeners with sensorineural hearing loss (SNHL) is reduced in noise when compared with listeners with normal hearing (Finitzo-Hieber and Tillman, 1978; Killion, 1997; Nabelek and Nabelek, 1994). In general, it appears that listeners with SNHL require the SNR to be improved by 4 to 12 dB (Crandell et al, 2005; Killion, 1997) and by an additional 3 to 6 dB in rooms with moderate levels of reverberation (Hawkins and Yacullo, 1984) to obtain speech recognition scores equal to listeners with normal hearing. The degree of SNHL apparently influences the SNR required by the individual with hearing loss. Killion (1997) reported that a listener with a 30 dB SNHL requires a +4 dB greater SNR than an adult with normal hearing to maintain equivalent speech recognition. With a 90 dB SNHL, the required SNR is +18 dB. Despite the speech recognition deficits seen in the hearing impaired, the specific auditory, cochlear, central, and/or cognitive mechanisms to explain these difficulties remain unclear. The reader is directed to Crandell and Smaldino (1992) and Killion (1997) for reviews of possible hypotheses to explain speech recognition difficulties in the hearing impaired.

Although it is recognized that listeners with SNHL experience greater speech recognition deficits in noise than normal hearers, several populations of children with normal hearing sensitivity also experience significant difficulties recognizing speech in noise (Boney and Bess, 1984; Crandell, 1991, 1992, 1993, Crandell & Smaldino, 1992, 1995, 1996a,b; Crandell et al, 2005; Nabelek and Nabelek, 1994). These listeners, as shown in **Table 18–4,** adapted from Crandell et al (2005), include children with fluctuating conductive hearing loss (or a history of recurrent otitis media with effusion), learning disabilities, articulation, language, and/or reading (dyslexia) disabilities, (central) auditory processing deficits, minimal degrees of SNHL (pure-tone sensitivity 15–25 dB hearing level [HL]), unilateral SNHL, developmental delays, and attention deficit disorders, as well as English as a second or other language (ESOL) children. For example, Crandell (1993) examined the speech recognition abilities of children with minimal degrees of SNHL at commonly reported classroom SNRs ranging from +6 to –6 dB. The children with minimal hearing loss exhibited pure-tone averages (500–2000 Hz) from 15 to 25 dB HL. Speech recognition was assessed via sentence stimuli with multitalker babble serving as the noise competition. Results from this investigation are presented in **Fig. 18–2** and indicate that children with minimal degrees of SNHL performed more poorly than normal hearers across most listening conditions.

Table 18–4 Populations of Children with Normal Hearing Who May Experience Difficulty Recognizing Speech in Noise

- Young (< 15 years old)
- Conductive hearing loss
- History of recurrent otitis media
- Language disorder
- Articulation disorder
- Dyslexia
- Learning disabilities
- Non-native English speaking
- Central auditory processing deficit
- Minimal degree of bilateral SNHL
- Unilateral SNHL
- Development delays
- Attentional deficits

SNHL, sensorineural hearing loss.

Moreover, the differences in recognition scores between the two groups increased as the listening environment became more unfavorable. For example, at an SNR of +6 dB, both groups obtained recognition scores in excess of 80%. At an SNR of –6 dB, however, the group with minimal hearing impairment was able to obtain < 50% correct recognition compared with ~75% recognition ability for the group of normal hearers.

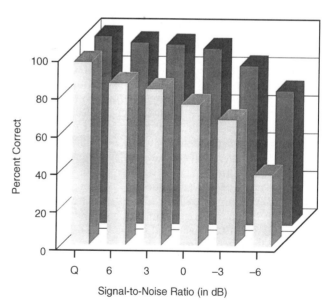

Figure 18–2 Mean speech recognition scores (percentage correct) of children with normal hearing (*dark shaded bars*) and children with minimal degrees of sensorineural hearing loss (*light shaded bars*) in quiet (Q) and at various signal-to-noise ratios.
(Adapted from Crandell, C., Smaldino, J., & Flexer, C. (2005). Sound field amplification: Applications to speech perception and classroom acoustics (2nd ed.). Clifton Park, NY: Thomson Delmar Learning, with permission.)

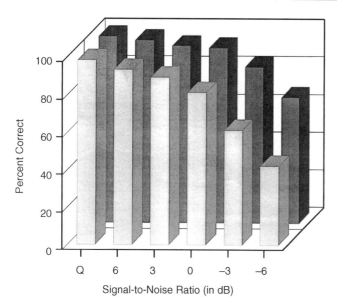

Figure 18–3 Mean speech recognition scores (percentage correct) of native-English-speaking children (*dark shaded bars*) and normative-English-speaking children (*light shaded bars*) in quiet (Q) and at various signal-to-noise ratios.
(Adapted from Crandell, C., Smaldino, J., & Flexer, C. (2005). Sound field amplification: Applications to speech perception and classroom acoustics (2nd ed.). Clifton Park, NY: Thomson Delmar Learning, with permission.)

Crandell and Smaldino (1996a) examined the speech recognition of 20 non-native-English-speaking children and 20 normative-English-speaking children under classroom SNRs of +6, +3, 0, –3, and –6 dB. Speech recognition was assessed via sentence stimuli, with multitalker babble serving as the noise competition. The same trends in speech recognition as demonstrated for the minimally hearing-impaired children were shown for these populations (see **Fig. 18–3**). That is, although both groups obtained essentially equivalent speech recognition scores in quiet, the non-native-English-speaking group performed significantly worse as the listening environment became less favorable. Similar findings have been reported for adult ESOL listeners (Bergman, 1980). Bergman (1980), for example, examined the speech recognition of adult native-Hebraic listeners under various conditions of acoustic degradations, including noise (SNR = +3 dB), reverberation (RT = 2.5 seconds), and split-band dichotic listening. Results indicated that the ESOL subjects obtained significantly poorer speech recognition scores than the native-English speakers across all listening conditions. Interestingly, these results were obtained even though the native-Hebraic listeners had been speaking English for more than 50 years.

Another group of normal-hearing children is young listeners. Prior research has indicated children require higher SNRs than adult listeners to achieve equivalent speech recognition scores (Crandell and Bess, 1986; Elliot, 1982; Nabelek and Nabelek, 1994). Elliot (1982) reported that young listeners require an additional 10 dB of signal strength to produce equivalent recognition scores to those of adults. Moreover, adultlike ability to recognize speech in

noise is not reached until ~13 to 15 years of age (Crandell and Bess, 1986; Elliot, 1982; Nabelek and Nabelek, 1994). Presumably, the additional signal strength is necessary to provide adequate acoustic cues to the immature auditory and linguistic system. On the basis of the aforementioned data, it is reasonable to assume that commonly reported levels of classroom noise have the potential of adversely affecting speech recognition in all pediatric listeners. To examine this assumption, speech recognition data from the germinal article by Finitzo-Hieber and Tillman (1978) can be examined. In their study, they compared the word recognition ability of 12 normal-hearing children and 12 children with mild to moderate binaurally symmetrical SNHL under varying conditions of SNR and RT. The results of the speech recognition in noise aspect of this study are summarized in **Table 18–5**. The word recognition scores for the children with normal hearing decreased to 60% at an SNR of 0 dB (a commonly reported SNR in the classroom). At the same SNR, word recognition scores for the children with SNHL were only 42%. Certainly, it is reasonable to assume that learning, attention, and behavior could be adversely affected if such reduced amounts of the acoustic signal were available to either child (particularly the child with hearing loss).

Criteria for Appropriate Signal-to-Noise Levels

Several acoustic, linguistic, and articulatory factors influence the determination of appropriate SNRs in a room. Acoustic factors include the spectrum of the noise, fluctuations in the noise over time, the type of signal that is being presented (sentences, words, nonsense syllables, vowels, and consonants), and the power of the speaker's voice. Linguistic factors include word familiarity and vocabulary size of the listener, the context, the number of syllables in a word, and linguistic competency. Articulatory factors incorporate the gender of the speaker and the articulatory abilities and dialect of the speaker or listener. Unoccupied classroom noise levels to achieve optimal SNR and maximal speech recognition scores in normal-hearing and hearing-impaired children are well known. **Table 18–6** shows noise levels recommended by various studies, over

Table 18–5 Mean Speech Recognition Scores (Percentage Correct) by Children with Normal Hearing and with SNHL for Monosyllabic Words in Quiet and at Various SNRs

| SNR | Groups | |
	Normal Hearing (*n* = 12)	Hearing Impaired (*n* = 12)
Quiet	94.5	87.5
+ 12 dB	89.2	77.8
+ 6 dB	79.7	65.7
0 dB	60.2	42.2

SNHL, sensorineural hearing loss; SNR, signal-to-noise ratio.
Source: Adapted from Finitzo-Hieber, T., & Tillman, T. (1978). Room acoustics effects on monosyllabic word discrimination ability for normal and hearing-impaired children. Journal of Speech and Hearing Research, 21, 440–458. Reprinted with permission.

Table 18–6 Recommended Unoccupied Classroom Noise Levels to Achieve Optimum Speech Recognition for Children with Normal Hearing and with Hearing Impairment

Investigator/Year	Unoccupied Noise Level (dB(A))	Population
Niemoeller (1968)	30	Hearing impaired
Gengel (1971)	30	Hearing impaired
Ross (1978)	35	Hearing impaired
Knudsen & Harris (1978)	35	Normal hearing
Borrild (1978)	35	Normal hearing/
	25	hearing impaired
Fourcin et al (1980)	35	Hearing impaired
Bradley (1968)	30	Normal hearing
Finitzo-Hieber (1988)	35	Hearingimpaired
Portuguese School Standard	35	Normal hearing/ hearing impaired
German Performance/ Design Standard (1989)	30	Normal hearing/ hearing impaired
Swedish Board of Housing, Building, and Planning (1994)	30	Normal hearing/ hearing impaired
Berg (1993)	35–40	Normal hearing
ASHA	30	Normal hearing/ hearing impaired
Crandell et al (1995)	30–35	Normal hearing/ hearing impaired
Crandell & Smaldino	30–35	Normal hearing/ hearing impaired

Source: Adapted from Access Board. (1998). Retrieved from http://www.access-board.gov. Reprinted with permission.

nearly 30 years, and is remarkable for the consistency of the recommended levels.

In 2002, the American National Standards Institute (ANSI, 2002) issued standard S12.6, which stipulated a background noise level of no more than 35 dB. As noted previously, speech recognition in adults with normal hearing is not severely compromised until the SNR of the listening environment is ~0 dB. However, normal-hearing children who are learning speech and language and those with listening deficits due to hearing loss or other listening and learning risk factors require a much better SNR. For listeners with SNHL, investigators have suggested that SNRs in learning environments should exceed a minimum of +15 dB (ANSI, 1995, 2002; Crandell, 1991, 1992; Crandell and Smaldino, 1992, 1995, 1996a,b; Crandell et al, 2005; Finitzo-Hieber and Tillman, 1978; Niemoeller, 1968). This recommendation is based on the finding that the speech recognition of listeners with hearing impairment tends to remain relatively constant at SNRs in excess of +15 dB but deteriorates at poorer SNRs. In addition, when the SNR decreases below +15 dB, persons with hearing loss have to spend so much effort on listening to the message that they often prefer to communicate through other modalities (e.g., sign language and written materials).

To accomplish a +15 SNR, in most settings, it appears that unoccupied room noise levels cannot exceed 30 to 35 dB(A) or approximately an NC 25 curve (ANSI, 1995, 2002; Crandell, 1991, 1992; Crandell and Smaldino, 1992, 1995, 1996a,b; Crandell et al, 2005; Finitzo-Hieber and Tillman,

1978; Niemoeller, 1968). Studies have reported that these acoustic criteria are infrequently achieved in the academic setting (Crandell, 1992; Crandell and Smaldino, 1995; Knecht et al, 2002; McCroskey and Devens, 1975). McCroskey and Devens (1975) demonstrated that only one of nine elementary classrooms actually met these acoustical recommendations. Crandell and Smaldino (1995) reported that none of 32 classrooms met recommended criteria for background noise. Similarly, applying the ANSI (2002) classroom acoustics standard, Knecht et al (2002) found that most of the 32 elementary school classrooms they studied did not meet the recommended background noise level of 35 dB(A).

Noise Effects on Academic and Teacher Performance

In addition to affecting speech recognition deleteriously, background noise can also compromise academic performance, reading and spelling skills, concentration, attention, and behavior in children (Green et al, 1982; Ko, 1979; Koszarny, 1978; Lehman and Gratiot, 1983). Koszarny (1978) reported that noise levels tend to more seriously affect concentration and attention in children with lower intelligence quotients (IQs) and high anxiety levels. Green et al (1982) found that classroom noise alone accounted for ~50 to 75% of the variance in reading delays of 1 year or more in elementary school children. Lehman and Gratiot (1983) reported that reductions in classroom noise (by means of acoustical modification) had a significant effect, increasing concentration, attention, and participatory behavior in children. Interestingly, the noise levels were reduced from typically reported noise levels of 35 to 45 dB(A) to the suggested guideline of 30 dB(A). Classroom noise has also been shown to affect teacher performance (Ko, 1979). For example, Ko (1979) obtained information from more than 1200 teachers concerning the effects of noise in the classroom. Results indicated that noise related to classroom activities and traffic, as well as airplane noise, was correlated with teacher fatigue, increased tension and discomfort, and an interference with teaching and speech recognition. In a 1998 survey of school administrators, the General Accounting Office (GAO) found that inappropriate classroom acoustics was the most commonly cited problem that affected the learning environment (Access Board, 1998). Additional studies (Crandell et al, 2005; Sapienza et al, 1999) have reported that teachers exhibit a significantly higher incidence of vocal problems than the general population. It is reasonable to assume that these vocal difficulties are caused, at least in part, by teachers having to increase vocal output to overcome the effects of classroom noise during the school day.

♦ Reverberation

Reverberation refers to the prolongation or persistence of sound within an enclosure as sound waves reflect off hard surfaces (bare walls, ceilings, windows, and floors) in the room. Operationally, RT refers to the amount of time it takes for a sound, at a specific frequency, to decay 60 dB (or one millionth of its original intensity) after termination of the signal. For example, if a 110 dB SPL signal at 1000 Hz took 1 second to decrease to 50 dB SPL, the RT of that enclosure at 1000 Hz would be 1 second. A common formula used to estimate RT was suggested by Sabine (1964):

$$RT_{60} = \frac{0.049V}{\Sigma S\alpha}$$

where RT_{60} = reverberation time in seconds; 0.049 is a constant (use 0.161 if room volume is stated in meters); V = room volume in cubic feet; and $\Sigma S\alpha$ = the sum of the surface areas of the various materials in the room multiplied by their respective absorption coefficients at a given frequency. If one reviews the variables in the RT formula just described, it is apparent that two basic factors influence the RT in a room. The first is the room volume. The larger the room volume, the longer the RT will be. The second variable is the amount of sound absorption in the room. The greater the area and sound absorptive characteristics of such materials, the shorter the RT. Reverberation is decreased when surfaces in the room have a large sound absorption coefficient, or α (alpha), calculated as the amount of sound energy absorbed by surfaces in the room divided by the total sound energy from the signal source. The α of a room varies with the thickness, porosity, and mounting configuration of materials in a room and the frequency of the signal (Siebein et al, 1997). Materials with α less than 0.2 are considered to be sound-reflective; materials with α greater than 0.2 are considered to be sound-absorbent. For instance, a brick wall has α ranging from 0.03 at 125 Hz to 0.07 at 4000 Hz, whereas a carpeted concrete floor ranges from 0.02 at 125 Hz to 0.65 at 4000 Hz. Use of absorbent materials can decrease noise by 3 to 8 dB (Siebein et al, 1997). Although not apparent in the formula, room shape may also influence the level of reverberation. Rooms with irregular shapes, such as oblong, often exhibit higher RTs than rooms with more traditional quadrilateral dimensions.

The Sabine formula assumes that the room is of relatively normal proportions and that absorbent surfaces and objects are evenly distributed throughout, creating a diffuse reverberant sound field. The latter assumption is often unmet in small rooms. A room may have only one or two absorbent surfaces (e.g., a carpeted floor or acoustically tiled ceiling), causing RT to vary substantially throughout the room. To account for this, Fitzroy (1959) created a modified RT formula that may be more appropriate for such small rooms as classrooms:

$$RT_{60} = \left(\frac{0.049V}{S^2}\right)\left[\left(\frac{2XY}{\alpha_{xy}}\right)+\left(\frac{2XZ}{\alpha_{xz}}\right)+\left(\frac{2YZ}{\alpha_{yz}}\right)\right]$$

where S = surface area of the room in square feet; α = absorption coefficient; X = room length; Y = room width; and Z = room height. Fitzroy predicated this formula on the idea that the three axes of a room could each generate multiple reflections with different characteristics. This method produces RT values very close to measured values in classrooms with carpeted floors, sound-absorbent ceilings, and highly reflective walls.

The RT of small rooms can also be estimated using the Norris-Eyring (Eyring, 1930) method, which takes into account the directivity (directional characteristics) of the sound source:

$$L_p = L_w + 10\log\left[\left(\frac{Q}{4\pi D^2}\right)+\left(\frac{4}{R}\right)\right]+10$$

where L_p = SPL in dB; L_w = sound power level in watts; Q = directivity of the signal source (1 = omnidirectional, 2 = hemispherical); D = distance from the signal source to the receiver; and R = room constant in Sabines of absorption.

Measurement of Reverberation

Reverberation time is usually measured in the classroom by presenting a high-intensity, broadband stimulus, such as white or pink noise, into an unoccupied room and measuring the amount of time required for that signal to decay 60 dB at various frequencies (Nabelek and Nabelek, 1994; Sabine, 1964; Siebein et al, 1997). Commercially available instruments for the recording RT vary from inexpensive, compact, battery units that allow the audiologist to do rudimentary measures of RT to highly technological, computer-based devices that can measure and record numerous aspects of the acoustic decay properties of an environment.

RT can also be estimated from formulas similar to those presented earlier by means of commercially available software programs that calculate the dimensions, volume, and absorption characteristics of an enclosure. Because the primary energy of speech is between 500 and 2000 Hz, RT is often reported as the mean decay time at 500, 1000, and 2000 Hz. Unfortunately, such a measurement paradigm may not adequately describe the reverberant characteristics of a room because high RTs may exist at additional frequencies. Room reverberation varies as a function of frequency and should therefore be measured at discrete frequencies. Generally, because most materials do not absorb low frequencies well, room reverberation is shorter at higher frequencies and longer in lower frequency regions. It is recommended that RT be measured at discrete frequencies from 125 to 8000 Hz whenever possible. Such information could significantly aid the audiologist in determining the appropriate degree and type of absorptive materials needed for reduction of RT in that environment. The reader is directed to ANSI (2002), Beranek (1954), Crandell et al (2005), Egan (1987), and Siebein et al (1997) for further details concerning the measurement of reverberation.

Reverberation Times in Rooms

Essentially all rooms exhibit some degree of reverberation. Audiometric test booths usually exhibit RTs of ~0.2 second. Living rooms and offices often have RTs between 0.4 and 0.8 second (Nabelek and Nabelek, 1994). As can be seen in

Table 18–7 A Summary of Studies Examining Classroom RTs

Investigation/Year	RT (seconds)
Kodaras (1960)	0.40–1.10
Nabelek & Pickett (1974a)	0.50–1.00
McCroskey & Devens (1975)	0.60–1.00
Bradley (1986)	0.39–1.20
Crandell & Smaldino (1994)	0.35–1.20

RT, reverberation time.

Table 18–7, RTs for classrooms are usually reported to range from 0.4 to 1.2 second (Crandell, 1992; Crandell and Smaldino, 1995; Crandell et al, 2005; McCroskey and Devens, 1975; Nabelek and Nabelek, 1994). Auditoriums, churches, and assembly halls often have RTs in excess of 3.0 seconds (Crandell, 1992; Nabelek and Nabelek, 1994; Siebein et al, 1997). The presence of people in a room further affects RT. A room full of people will have an RT that is 0.05 to 0.1 second lower than when it is empty (Crandell et al, 2005).

General Effects of Reverberation on Speech Recognition

It is well documented that excessive reverberation can adversely influence speech recognition (see Nabelek and Nabelek, 1994). Reverberation degrades speech recognition through the masking of direct and early reflected energy by reverberant energy (Bolt and MacDonald, 1949; Nabelek and Nabelek, 1994). The reverberant speech energy reaches the listener after the direct sound and overlaps with that direct signal, resulting in a "smearing" or masking of speech. **Figure 18–4** presents a spectrograph of the phrase "the beet again" in reverberant (RT = 1.2 seconds) and nonreverberant (RT = 0.0

second) listening environments. In this figure, time (in milliseconds) is presented on the abscissa, whereas frequency (in kilohertz) is shown on the ordinate. Amplitude, or intensity, of the speech sample is indicated by the relative density or darkness of the pattern. As can be seen, reverberation causes a prolongation or "spread" of the spectral energy of the vowel sounds, which tends to mask succeeding consonant phonemes, particularly those consonants in word final positions. It is reasonable to expect that the masking effect for reverberation would be greater for vowels than for consonants because vowels exhibit greater overall power and are of longer duration than consonants.

Note too that in **Fig. 18–4,** the reverberant sound energy of the /i/ phoneme in the word *beet* has extended over the energy of the final /t/ consonant, making recognition of that consonant (and consequently the entire word) more difficult. In highly reverberant environments, words may actually overlap with one another, thus causing reverberant sound energy to fill in temporal pauses between words. Moreover, in highly reverberant environments, such as auditoriums and gymnasiums, temporal pauses between sentences may be obliterated, causing difficulty in distinguishing where one sentence ends and another sentence begins.

Effects of Reverberation on Speech Recognition in Listeners with Hearing Impairment and Normal Hearing

Speech recognition tends to decrease as the RT of the environment increases (Crandell et al, 2005; Finitzo-Hieber and Tillman, 1978; Gelfand and Silman, 1979; Kreisman, 2003; Moncur and Dirks, 1967; Nabelek and Nabelek, 1994). Moncur and Dirks (1967) examined the monosyllabic word recognition of adult listeners with normal hearing at four different RTs (RT = 0.0, 0.9, 1.6, and 2.3 seconds) in monaural (near ear) and binaural listening

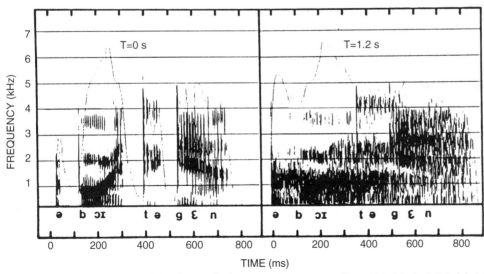

Figure 18–4 A spectrograph of the phrase "the beet again" in nonreverberant (RT = 0.0 second) and reverberant (RT = 1.2 seconds) conditions. RT, reverberation time.

(From Nabelek, A.. & Nabelek, I. (1994). Room acoustics and speech perception. In: J. Katz (Ed.), Handbook of clinical audiology (4th ed., pp. 624-637). Baltimore: Williams & Wilkins, with permission.)

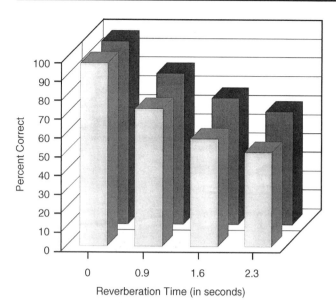

Figure 18–5 Monaural (*light shaded bars*) and binaural (*dark shaded bars*) speech recognition at various reverberation times.
(Adapted from Moncur, J., & Dirks, D. (1967). Binaural and monaural speech intelligibility in reverberation. Journal of Speech and Hearing Research, 10, 86–195, with permission.)

conditions. Results indicted that speech recognition ability was markedly reduced as RT increased **(Fig. 18–5).** In addition, results indicated that binaural recognition scores were significantly higher than monaural perceptual abilities. Improved binaural speech recognition in reverberation with and without hearing aids has been documented in other studies as well (see Nabelek and Nabelek, 1994, for a review of these studies).

Speech recognition in adults with normal hearing is often not compromised until the RT exceeds ~1.0 second (Crum, 1974; Gelfand and Silman, 1979; Moncur and Dirks, 1967; Nabelek and Nabelek, 1994). As with background noise, however, several acoustic, linguistic, and articulatory factors determine the degree to which reverberation affects speech recognition. Listeners with SNHL, however, need considerably shorter RTs (i.e., 0.4 to 0.5 second) for maximum speech recognition (Crandell, 1991, 1992; Crandell and Bess, 1986; Crandell et al, 2005; Finitzo-Hieber and Tillman, 1978; Niemoeller, 1968). Additional studies have also indicated that the populations of normal-hearing children discussed previously also have greater speech recognition difficulties in reverberation than do young adults with normal hearing. Boney and Bess (1984), for example, demonstrated that children with minimal degrees of SNHL (pure-tone thresholds 15–30 dB HL at 500–2000 Hz) experience greater difficulty understanding speech degraded by reverberation than children with normal hearing sensitivity. Specifically, speech recognition scores were obtained in nonreverberant (RT = 0.0 second) and reverberant (RT = 0.8 second) environments. Results from this investigation indicated that the children with minimal hearing loss performed significantly worse than the control group, particularly within the reverberant listening condition **(Fig. 18–6).**

Reverberation and Subjective Sound Quality

Excessive reverberation can also affect subjective sound quality. For example, the subjective quality of music has been shown to improve with the addition of reverberation. Formulas to derive optimum RTs, as a function of room characteristics and various forms of music, have been developed for theaters and auditoriums (Siebein et al, 1997). Often, these formulas suggest RTs of 2 or 3 seconds to add "liveliness" or "coloration" to music. The effect of reverberation on speech quality, however, tends to not be as well recognized. Haas (1972) indicated that early reflections and some reverberation enhance the quality of speech, causing an increase in loudness, "liveliness," and "growth in body." Overall, it appears that short to moderate RTs increase the subjective quality of speech, whereas excessive reverberation causes speech to sound muffled and less understandable.

In addition to measurable effects of reverberation on speech perception, this distortion of the signal has an impact on the perceived quality of speech, including clarity and listening effort. Early reflections increase the perceived loudness of a signal at the ear and assist with localization, increasing perceptual quality of the signal (Roberts, 2003). This explains a contradictory finding in research into reverberation. Several studies have demonstrated that speech perception decreases as RT is increased above zero, indicating that the absence of reverberation (RT = 0 second) provides the optimal listening environment (Finitzo-Hieber and Tillman, 1978; Nabelek and Nabelek, 1994).

In most real-world environments, a small degree of reverberation is likely to be more beneficial for speech perception than a nonreverberant environment. There are two principal reasons for this. First, early reflections increase the level of the signal at the ear, making low-intensity

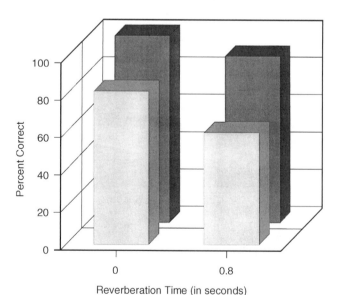

Figure 18–6 Mean speech recognition scores (percentage correct) of children with normal hearing (*dark shaded bars*) and children with minimal degrees of sensorineural hearing loss (*light shaded bars*) in a non-reverberant (RT = 0.0 second) and reverberant (RT = 0.8 second) listening condition. RT, reverberation time.

sounds and certain parts of speech, such as low-intensity but high-information consonants, more audible. This is the primary benefit of a small amount of reverberation in diffuse field theory. In the presence of any noise, increases in early reflections increase the intensity level of the signal and thus improve the SNR (Hodgson and Nosal, 2002). Second, as stated previously, the presence of early reflections improves localization ability. This improvement may assist the listener in segregating a signal emanating from a single source (e.g., the voice of one speaker) from a diffuse noise field. In addition to the objective benefits of small amounts of reverberation for speech perception, studies of individual preferences for listening environments find that most listeners report a more natural sound when listening in rooms where early reflections are present as compared with an anechoic environment (Crandell et al, 2005; Hodgson and Nosal, 2002).

Recommended Criteria for Reverberation Time

As previously discussed, speech recognition in adults with normal hearing is not significantly affected until the RT exceeds ~1.0 second. For listeners with SNHL, most investigators have recommended that listening environments should not exceed ~0.4 second (through the speech frequency range: 500, 1000, and 2000 Hz) to provide optimum communicative efficiency. A summary of suggested guidelines for RTs in the classroom can be found in **Table 18–8**. In 2002, ANSI issued S12.6, which recommended an RT of 0.6 second for moderately sized learning environments. A review of the literature suggests that appropriate RTs for the hearing impaired are rarely achieved (Crandell, 1992; Crandell and Smaldino, 1995; McCroskey and Devens, 1975). Crandell and Smaldino (1995) reported that only 9 of 32 classrooms (27%) displayed RTs of 0.4 second or less.

Table 18–8 Recommended Classroom RT to Achieve Optimum Speech Recognition for Children with Normal Hearing and with Hearing Impairment

Investigator/Year	RT (second)	Population
Niemoeller (1968)	0.4–0.6	Hearing impaired
Gengel (1971)	0.7	Hearing impaired
Knudsen & Harris (1978)	0.75	Normal hearing
Ross (1978)	0.4	Hearing impaired
Borrild (1978)	0.9	Normal hearing/
	0.4	hearing impaired
Fourcin et al (1980)	0.5	Hearing impaired
Bess & McConnell (1981)	0.4	Hearing impaired
Bradley (1986)	0.4	Normal hearing
Egan (1987)	0.5	Hearing impaired
Finizo-Hieber (1988)	0.4	Hearing impaired
Portuguese School	0.6–0.8	Normal hearing/
Standard (1988)	0.4–0.6	Hearing impaired
ASHA (1995)	0.4	Normal hearing/
		hearing impaired
Crandell et al (1995)	0.4	Normal hearing/
		hearing impaired
Crandell & Smaldino	0.4	Normal hearing/
		hearing impaired

Source: Adapted from Access Board. (1998). Retrieved from http://www.access-board.gov. Reprinted with permission.

Knecht et al (2002), applying the ANSI (2002) criteria for reverberation, found that most of the 32 elementary school classrooms they studied did not meet the 0.6 second maximum reverberation time recommended in the standard.

Effects of Noise and Reverberation on Speech Recognition

Thus far, the isolated effects of background noise and reverberation have been discussed. However, these acoustic events do not occur separately in a room. In most enclosures, noise and reverberation combine in a synergistic manner to adversely effect speech recognition (Crandell and Bess, 1986; Crandell and Smaldino, 1995; Crandell et al, 2005; Crum, 1974; Finitzo-Hieber and Tillman, 1978; Kreisman, 2003; Nabelek and Nabelek, 1994). Synergistic theory suggests that the sum of the two variables is greater than one would expect by simply adding the two variables together. For example, imagine two specially designed test rooms that have only noise or reverberation. When testing an individual in the noisy room, the audiologist may see recognition scores diminish 10% (from scores obtained in quiet). In the reverberant room, assume the audiologist sees a similar 10% decrease in recognition. If, however, the audiologist places this individual in a room that contains both noise and reverberation, the audiologist may not see a 20% decrease in recognition (i.e., 10% for noise, 10% for reverberation), but perhaps a 30 or 40% reduction. It appears that this synergistic effect occurs because reverberation fills in the temporal gaps in the noise, making the noise more steady state in nature and a more effective masker. As with noise and reverberation in isolation, research indicates that listeners with hearing impairment and normal-hearing children experience greater speech recognition difficulties in noise and reverberation than adult normal listeners (Crandell and Bess, 1986; Crandell and Smaldino, 1995, 1996a,b; Crandell et al, 2005; Finitzo-Hieber and Tillman, 1978; Nabelek and Nabelek, 1994).

This finding of an interactive effect among distortions has also been demonstrated for other types of signal modification. For example, Stuart and Phillips (1998) found that, even for listeners with normal hearing with a simulated high-frequency hearing loss, the presence of multiple temporal distortions is greater than the sum of those distortions alone. In this study, individuals with normal hearing were given word recognition tasks with stimuli time-compressed or reverberated. For some test conditions, the test subjects were given a simulated high-frequency hearing loss by low-pass filtering the stimuli at 2000 Hz. Each of these distortions (time compression, reverberation, and simulated hearing loss) caused a significant decrease in word recognition ability. When distortions were combined, an interactive effect was seen, causing greater decreases in word recognition than the sum of these distortions alone.

An example of the synergetic effect of noise and reverberation on the monosyllabic word recognition of children with normal hearing and SNHL is shown in **Table 18–9**. Note that even at the best SNR and RT (SNR = +12 dB, RT = 0.4 second), children with normal hearing do not recognize speech perfectly (83%), and children with hearing impairment

Table 18–9 Mean Speech Recognition Scores (Percentage Correct) by Children with Normal Hearing and with SNHL for Monosyllabic Words across Various SNRs and RT

Testing Condition	Groups	
	Normal Hearing (*n* = 12)	Hearing Impaired (*n* = 12)
RT = 0.0 second		
Quiet	94.5	83.0
+12 dB	89.2	70.0
+6 dB	79.7	59.5
0 dB	60.2	39.0
RT = 0.4 second		
Quiet	92.5	74.0
+12 dB	82.8	60.2
+6 dB	71.3	52.2
0 dB	47.7	27.8
RT = 1.2 second		
Quiet	76.5	45.0
+12 dB	68.8	41.2
+6 dB	54.2	27.0
0 dB	29.7	11.2

RT, reverberation time; SNHL, sensorineural hearing loss; SNR, signal-to-noise ratio.
Source: Adapted from Finitzo-Hieber, T., & Tillman, T. (1978). Room acoustics effects on monosyllabic word discrimination ability for normal and hearing-impaired children. Journal of Speech and Hearing Research, 21, 440–458.

perform even more poorly (60%). As the SNR becomes poorer or as RT gets longer, speech recognition decreases to the worst case studied (SNR = +0 dB, RT = 1.2 second), where children with normal hearing achieve a 30% score, and children with hearing loss recognize virtually none of the speech (11%). It should be noted that each of these listening conditions has been commonly reported in classroom environments. Imagine trying to succeed in school, perceiving only 11% of what is presented by the teacher.

The synergistic effect of noise and reverberation is likely to be related to the fact that noise and reverberation mask signals in different ways. For example, stop consonants in word-final position are particularly susceptible to reverberation, which can be explained by the tendency of reverberation to smear the acoustic signal into the temporal pause that is a feature of stops as the articulators are closed. Final fricatives, particularly high-frequency sounds such as /f/, /v/, and /Θ/, are especially susceptible to noise due to their low-intensity and high-frequency spectral content, but are fairly resistant to reverberation. In addition, although noise masks both initial and final phonemes of words about equally, final phonemes are particularly affected by reverberation (Helfer, 1994; Nabelek and Nabelek, 1994). This effect is diminished for rapid connected speech, in which energy from the final phoneme of one word can mask the initial phoneme of the next word. Nasal and semivowel consonants also show very different effects of noise and reverberation (Helfer, 1994). The pattern of errors in the combination of noise and reverberation is different from either alone. Although reverberation alone has its greatest effect on the low-frequency features of consonants such as voicing, the interaction of noise and reverberation increases the distortion of all features of consonant

sounds—voicing, manner, and place—as a result of reverberant noise energy obscuring phonemic cues (Gelfand and Silman, 1979; Helfer, 1994). Helfer (1994) also found that final stop consonants are most susceptible to reverberation due to loss of temporal information, whereas final fricatives are most susceptible to noise due to masking of high-frequency energy, characteristic of many fricatives, by noise.

◆ Speaker–Listener Distance

In most rooms the acoustics of a speaker's speech signal changes as it travels to the listener. **Figure 18–7** shows some of the paths of direct and reflected sounds from a speaker to a listener in a room. The direct sound is that sound that travels from the speaker to a listener without striking other surfaces within the room. The direct sound is usually the first sound to arrive at the listener's ears because it travels the shortest path between the speaker and the listener. The power of the direct sound decreases with distance because the acoustic energy is spreading over a larger area as it travels from the source. Specifically, the direct sound decreases 6 dB SPL with every doubling of distance from the sound source. This phenomenon, called the inverse square law, occurs because of the geometric divergence of sound from the source. According to the inverse square law, if a speaker's voice is 65 dB SPL at 1 m (average conversational level), then his or her voice will be 59 dB SPL at 2 m, 53 dB SPL at 4 m, and so on. Because the direct sound energy decreases so quickly, only those listeners who are seated close to the speaker will be hearing direct sound energy. It should be noted that the inverse square law does not pertain to sound beyond the critical distance in a room (see below).

At slightly farther distances from the speaker, early sound reflections will reach the listener. Early sound reflections are those sound waves that arrive at a listener within very short time periods (~50 msec) after the arrival of the direct sound. They are often combined with the direct sound and may actually increase the perceived loudness of the sound (Nabelek and Nabelek, 1994). This increase in loudness may actually improve speech recognition in listeners with normal hearing. In a typical room, most of the early reflections strike minimal room surfaces on their path from speaker to listener.

As a listener moves farther away from a speaker, reverberation dominates the listening environment. As discussed in an earlier section, reverberation consists of the sound waves that strike multiple room surfaces as they move from speaker to listener. As sound waves strike multiple room surfaces, they are generally decreased in loudness as a result of the increased path length they travel and the partial absorption that occurs at each reflection with the room surfaces. Some reverberation is necessary to reinforce the direct sound and to enrich the quality of the sound. However, reverberation can lead to acoustic distortions of the speech signal, including temporal smearing and masking of important perceptual cues.

Another way of viewing sound distribution in an enclosure is shown in **Fig. 18–8**. In this figure, line DS_{SPL} represents

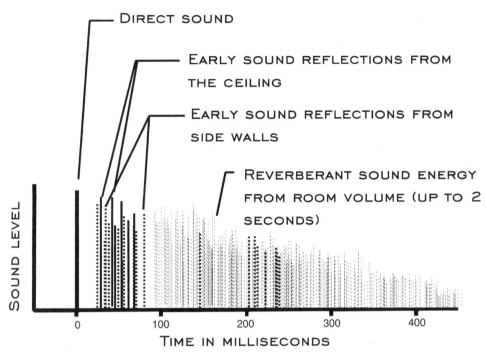

Figure 18–7 Components of sound (direct sound, early reflections, and late reflections) in a room. (From Siebein, G., Crandell, C., & Gold, M. (1997). Principles of classroom acoustics: Reverberation. Educational Audiology Monographs, 5, 32–43, with permission.)

the relative SPL of the direct sound in the room. Curve TOT_{SPL} depicts the total sound pressure in the room. The total sound pressure is the summation of reflected and direct sound energy in the enclosure. Stated otherwise, the total sound pressure is that sound energy that a listener will hear in a room at various distances. Curve TOT_{SPL} shows that

sound decay in accordance with the inverse square law only occurs in free-field environments because no surfaces reflect sound and reinforce that sound wave. Point D_c shows the critical distance (D_c) of the room, which refers to that point in a room in which the intensity of the direct sound is equal to the intensity of the reverberant sound (Puetz,

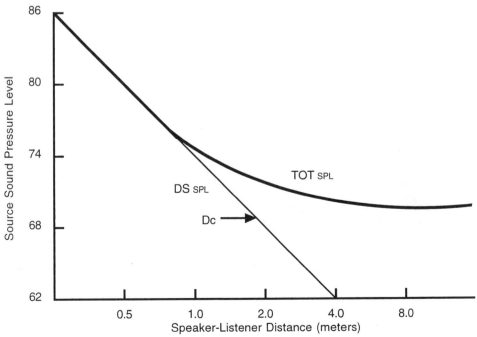

Figure 18–8 The distribution of sound within a room as a function of speaker-to-listener distance. Dc, critical distance; DS_{SPL}, relative SPL of the direct sound in the room; TOT_{SPL}, total sound pressure in the room.

(From Nabelek, A., & Nabelek, I. (1994). Room acoustics and speech perception. In J. Katz (Ed.), Handbook of clinical audiology (4th ed., pp. 624–637). Baltimore: Williams & Wilkins, with permission.)

1971). Within the D_c, the effects of reverberation on the speech signal would be minimized. Operationally, critical distance (D_c) is defined by the following formula:

$$D_c^x = 0.02\sqrt{VQ/nRT}$$

where V = volume of the room in m³, Q = directivity factor of the source (the human voice is approximately 2.5), n = number of sources, and RT = reverberation time of the enclosure at 1400 Hz. In an average-sized classroom with a commonly reported level of reverberation, the critical distance of the room would be approximately 3 m.

As noted previously, the inverse square law does not apply to enclosures such as classrooms or theaters. Thus, one cannot determine the SPL of the speaker's voice by simply deducting 6 dB for every doubling of distance from the source. To estimate the SPL (and thus the SNR) at any given location in a room (in meters), the following formula can be used:

$$SPL = Ps + 10\log[(1/4p\rho2) + (4/A)]$$

where Ps = the sound power of the source and A = the total sound absorption of the room.

Effects of Distance on Speech Recognition

Speech recognition in many rooms depends on the distance of the listener from the speaker (Crandell, 1991; Crandell and Bess, 1986; Crandell and Smaldino, 1995; Crandell et al, 2005; Leavitt and Flexer, 1991; Puetz, 1971). If the listener is within the critical distance of the room (relatively close to the speaker), reflected sound waves have minimal effects on speech recognition. Beyond the critical distance, however, the reflections can compromise speech recognition if enough of a spectrum and/or intensity change in the reflected sound is present to interfere with the recognition of the direct sound.

Overall, speech recognition scores tend to decrease until the critical distance of the room is reached. Beyond the critical distance, recognition ability tends to remain essentially constant unless the room is very large (e.g., an auditorium). In such environments, speech recognition may continue to decrease as a function of increased distance. These findings suggest that speech recognition ability can be maximized by decreasing the distance between a speaker and a listener within the critical distance of the room.

Pearl

- To improve auditory speech recognition, the listener must be within the critical distance of the room at all times. Positioning of teacher and listener within this distance also allows the listener to augment the auditory speech signal with visual cues from speechreading. In classrooms, the critical distance is often no more than 6 to 8 feet from the teacher. In large rooms or where the teacher moves around the room during instruction, hearing assistive technologies (HATs) such as personal frequency modulation (FM) or infrared sound-field systems may be necessary to keep listeners within the critical distance.

In a series of studies, Crandell and Bess (1986) examined the effects of distance on the speech recognition of children with normal hearing in "typical" classroom environments (SNR = +6 dB; RT = 0.45 second). They recorded monosyllabic words at speaker–listener distances often encountered in the classroom (6, 12, and 24 feet). The multitalker babble was used as the noise competition. Subjects consisted of children 5 to 7 years of age. Results from this investigation, shown in **Fig. 18–9,** indicate a decrease in speech recognition ability as the speaker–listener distance was increased.

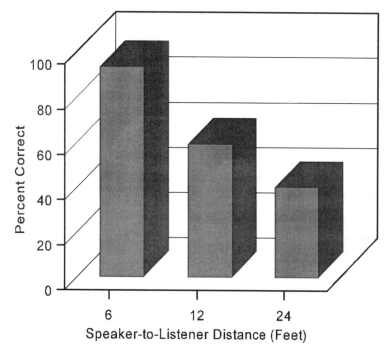

Figure 18–9 Mean speech recognition scores (percentage correct) of children with normal hearing in a "typical" classroom environment (SNR = +6 dB; RT = 0.6 second) as a function of speaker-to-listener distance. RT, reverberation time; SNR, signal-to-noise ratio. (Adapted from Crandell, C., Smaldino, J., & Flexer, C. (2005). Sound field amplification: Applications to speech perception and classroom acoustics (2nd ed.). Clifton Park, NY: Thomson Delmar Learning, with permission.)

Specifically, mean word recognition scores of 89, 55, and 36% were obtained at 6, 12, and 24 feet, respectively. These results suggest that children with normal hearing who are seated in the middle to rear of a typical classroom setting have greater difficulty understanding speech than is commonly suspected.

Before concluding this section, it is important to note that several theoretical considerations and resulting acoustic formulas have been developed to estimate speech recognition in rooms of varying acoustical qualities at different locations with the room. These formulas include the (1) Speech Intelligibility Index (SII), (2) Speech Transmission Index (STI), (3) early-to-late ratios (ELRs), (4) early decay time (EDT_{10}), (5) early-to-late energy ratios (EL_t), (6) useful-to-detrimental energy ratio (U_{80}), (7) early energy fraction (D_{50}), (8) relative loudness or relative strength, and (9) articulation loss of consonants. Unfortunately, most of these indices were developed for adult listeners with normal hearing and may not be applicable for children or listeners with SNHL. For a discussion of these formulas, the reader is directed to Siebein et al (1997).

◆ Methods to Improve Room Acoustics

The remaining sections of this chapter will address procedures for reducing the effects of noise, reverberation, and distance in rooms, particularly classrooms. These procedures include (1) acoustic modifications of the room, (2) using "clear" speech procedures, (3) reduction of speaker–listener distance, (4) optimizing visual communication, and (5) personal and group amplification systems.

Acoustic Modifications of the Room

The speech recognition difficulties experienced by listeners with hearing impairment and children with normal hearing highlight the need to provide an appropriate listening environment for these populations. Recall that the ANSI (2002) criteria for such populations indicate that SNRs should exceed +15 dB; unoccupied noise levels should not exceed 35 dB(A), and RT_{60} should not surpass 0.6 second for moderately sized rooms (through the speech frequency range). These acoustic recommendations, however, are rarely achieved in most listening environments. As recently as 2002, Knecht et al surveyed 32 different unoccupied classrooms and found that most did not meet the ANSI (2002) criteria for either SNR or reverberation. Recall also that background room noise can originate from external and internal sources. To conduct the most appropriate modification of the room, it must first be determined which specific noise source or sources need to be reduced. Following are common procedures for reducing various types of noise in rooms, such as classrooms. For more complete discussions on acoustic modifications and noise reduction the reader is directed to Egan (1987) and Crandell et al (2005).

Special Consideration

• Background noise levels and RTs are constantly interacting in a room. Although improving one often improves the other, this is not always true. Both noise and reverberation must be thoroughly evaluated when establishing the adequacy of a room for communication. This evaluation includes a spectral analysis of both the background noise (e.g., NC and RC curves) and the reverberant characteristics of the room.

Reduction of External Noise Levels

1. Rooms used for both hearing-impaired and normal-hearing listeners must be located away from high-noise sources, such as busy automobile traffic, railroads, construction sites, airports, and furnace/air-conditioning units. The most effective way to achieve this goal in a school is through appropriate planning with contractors, school officials, architects, architectural engineers, audiologists, and teachers for the hearing impaired before the design and construction of the building. Such consultation should include strategies for locating rooms away from high external noise sources. Moreover, acoustic modifications, such as the placement of vibration reduction pads underneath the supporting beams of the building to reduce structure-borne sounds, can be implemented. Unfortunately, acoustic planning before building construction is rare (Crandell and Smaldino, 1995; Crandell et al, 2005).

2. A sound transmission loss (STL) of at least 45 to 50 dB is often required for external walls. STL refers to the amount of noise that is attenuated as it passes through a material. If an external noise of 100 dB SPL is reduced to 60 dB SPL in the room, the exterior wall of that room has an STL of 40 dB SPL. A 7 inch concrete wall provides ~53 dB attenuation of outside noise, whereas windows and doors provide only 24 and 20 dB attenuation, respectively. Therefore, doors and windows on the external wall should be avoided in situations of high external noise levels. Average STL values for different structures can be found in most books published on acoustics. Methods to increase the STL of an external wall include (1) the placement of absorptive materials (e.g., fiberglass material) between the wall studs, (2) the use of thick or double-concrete construction on the exterior wall, and (3) the addition of several layers of gypsum board (at least $5/8$ inch) or plywood material. See the ANSI (2002) standard for performance criteria and design suggestions.

3. All exterior walls must be free of cracks or openings that would allow extraneous noises into the room. Even small openings in external walls can significantly reduce the STL.

4. If windows are located on the external wall, they must be properly installed, heavy weighted, or double-paned (e.g., storm windows) and remain closed (whenever possible) if

high external noise sources exist. In addition, existing windows can be sealed with nonhardening caulk to increase the STL. Of course, safety regulations must be checked before sealing outside windows.

5. Landscaping strategies can also attenuate external noise sources. These strategies include the placement of trees or shrubs (that bloom all year long) and earthen banks around the school building.

6. Solid concrete barriers with an STL of 30 to 35 dB can be placed between the school building and the noise source to reduce external noise entering into the room.

Reduction of Internal Noise Levels

1. Often, the most cost-effective procedure for reducing internal noise levels in the classroom is to relocate the children in that room to a quieter area of the building. Rooms used for communication must not be located next to a high-noise source, such as the gymnasium, metal shop, cafeteria, or band room. At least one quiet environment, such as a storage area or closet, should separate rooms from each other or from high-noise sources in the school building.

2. If suspended ceilings separate the room from another room, sound-absorbing materials should be placed in the plenum space above the wall.

3. Double-wall or thick-wall construction should be used for the interior walls, particularly those walls that face noisy hallways or rooms. Additional layers of gypsum board or plywood and/or the placement of absorptive materials between wall studding can also increase the attenuation characteristics of interior wall surfaces. Moreover, all cracks between rooms should be sealed.

4. Acoustic ceiling tile and/or carpeting can be used in hallways outside the room.

5. All rooms should contain acoustically treated or well-fitting (preferably with rubber or gasket seals) high-mass-per-unit-area doors. Hollow-core doors between rooms, and facing the hallway, should not be used. Doors (or interior walls) should not contain ventilation ducts that lead into the hallways.

6. Heating or cooling ducts that serve more than one room can be lined with acoustic materials or furnished with baffles to decrease noise emitting from one room to another.

7. Permanently mounted blackboards can be backed with absorptive materials to reduce sound transmission from adjacent rooms.

Reduction of Room Noise Levels

1. The simplest procedure to reduce the effects of room noise is to position children away from high-noise sources, such as fans, air conditioners, heating ducts, faulty lighting fixtures, and doors or windows adjacent

to sources of noise. Often, however, room noise sources are so intense that no location in the room is appropriate for communication. In these cases, acoustic modification of the room must be conducted.

2. Malfunctioning air-conditioning/heating units and ducts should be replaced or acoustically treated. Heating ducts, for example, can be lined with acoustic materials or fit with silencers to reduce both vibratory and airborne noise. In addition, rubber supports and flexible sleeves or joints should be used to reduce the transmission of structural-borne noise through the ductwork system. Moreover, all fans and electrical motors in air-conditioning/heating units must be lubricated and maintained on a regular basis.

3. Installation of thick, wall-to-wall carpeting (with adequate padding) to dampen the noise of shuffling of hard-soled shoes, the movement of desks/chairs, and so forth can reduce room noise levels.

4. Acoustic paneling can be placed on the walls and ceiling. Wall paneling typically should be placed partly down the wall and not on walls parallel to one another.

5. The placement of some form of rubber tips on the legs of desks and chairs can decrease room noise. This recommendation is particularly important if the room is not carpeted.

6. Acoustically treated furniture can be purchased for rooms. It must be noted that such furniture can be expensive and may present hygiene problems.

7. Hanging of thick curtains or acoustically treated Venetian blinds over window areas to dampen room noise levels can be effective.

8. Avoid open-plan rooms for children because it is well recognized that such rooms are considerably noisier than regular rooms.

9. Instruction should not take place in areas separated from other teaching areas by sliding doors, thin partitions, or temporary walls. Walls between instruction areas must be of sufficient thickness and continuous between the solid ceiling and floor. Walls that are not continuous allow for significant sound transmission between rooms.

10. Fluorescent lighting systems, including the ballast, need to be regularly maintained and replaced if faulty.

11. Typewriter or computer keyboard noise can be lowered by the placement of rubber pads or carpet remnants under such instruments. Whenever possible, such instruments (and any other office equipment) should be located in separate rooms. Rubber pads to reduce vibratory noise should be placed under all office equipment in the school.

12. Children can be encouraged to wear soft-soled shoes.

13. Of course, classroom management is also important to limit noise. Students should be encouraged to limit talking when it is not contributing to the lesson being taught.

Reduction of Room Reverberation

The presence or absence of absorptive surfaces within a room will affect the reverberant characteristics of that environment. Materials with hard, smooth surfaces, such as concrete, cinder block, and hard plaster, are poor absorbers, whereas materials with soft, rough-surfaced, and/or porous surfaces (e.g., cloth, fiberglass, and corkboard) tend to be good absorbers of sound. Hence, rooms with bare cement walls, floors, and ceilings tend to exhibit higher RTs than rooms that contain absorptive surfaces such as carpeting, draperies, and acoustic ceiling tile. A useful index in determining the reverberant characteristics of a room is the absorption coefficient. Absorption coefficient (α) refers to the ratio of unreflected energy to incident energy present in a room. A surface with an absorption coefficient of 1.00 would technically absorb 100% of all reflections, whereas a surface structure with an absorption coefficient of 0.00 would reflect all of the incident sound. A summary of absorption coefficients for different materials is found in **Table 18–10**. Note that the absorption coefficients, which are typically indicated from 125 to 4000 Hz, are frequency dependent.

Specifically, most surface materials in a room do not absorb low-frequency sounds as effectively as higher frequencies. Because of these absorption characteristics, room reverberation is often shorter at higher frequencies than in lower frequency regions. Generally, surfaces are not considered absorptive until they reach an absorption coefficient of 0.20. When excessive reverberation occurs, the tendency is to treat most or all of the surfaces in a room with sound-absorbing materials. If all of the surfaces become sound absorbent, then the speaker is effectively speaking in an anechoic or nonreverberant environment. The speaker will have to raise his or her voice or use an amplification system to overcome the lack of reflected sounds that would normally be present in a room. Several procedures to reduce reverberation in a room include the following:

1. Reverberation can be reduced by covering the hard reflective surfaces in a room with absorptive materials, such as acoustic paneling. To reduce reverberation, ceilings should be covered with acoustic tiles. The tiles should be suspended from the structural deck and have an absorption coefficient of at least 0.65. This will absorb multiple order sound reflections from the corners of the room and reduce the RT to acceptable levels. Acoustic panels may also be placed on walls but typically not on walls parallel to one another. Cork bulletin boards, carpeting, and bookcases can also be strategically placed on the walls; however, such materials are not as absorptive as acoustic paneling. Interestingly, the installation of absorptive materials not only will reduce reverberation in the environment but also will decrease the noise level in the room by 5 to 8 dB.

2. Thick carpeting on the floors can significantly reduce reverberation and noise in a room. Rooms with both acoustic ceiling tile and carpets have ~60% of room surfaces covered with absorptive material. However, rooms

Table 18–10 Absorption Coefficients for Various Materials

Material	Frequency (Hz)					
	125	250	500	1000	2000	4000
Ceilings						
Plaster or gypsum	0.14	0.10	0.06	0.05	0.04	0.03
Acoustic tiles, $^2/_3$ inch (suspended 16 inches from ceiling)	0.25	0.28	0.46	0.71	0.86	0.93
Acoustic tiles, $^1/_2$ inch (suspended 16 inches from ceiling)	0.52	0.37	0.50	0.69	0.79	0.78
Acoustic tiles, $^1/_2$ inch (cemented directly to ceiling)	0.10	0.22	0.61	0.56	0.74	0.72
High-absorbent panels, 1 inch (suspended 16 inches from ceiling)	0.58	0.88	0.75	0.99	1.00	0.96
Walls						
Brick	0.03	0.03	0.03	0.04	0.05	0.07
Concrete painted	0.10	0.05	0.06	0.07	0.09	0.08
Window glass	0.35	0.25	0.18	0.12	0.07	0.04
Marble	0.01	0.01	0.01	0.02	0.02	0.00
Plaster or concrete	0.12	0.09	0.07	0.05	0.05	0.04
Plywood	0.28	0.22	0.17	0.09	0.10	0.11
Concrete block (coarse)	0.36	0.44	0.31	0.29	0.39	0.25
Heavyweight drapery	0.14	0.35	0.55	0.72	0.70	0.65
Fiberglass wall treatment, 1 inch	0.08	0.32	0.99	0.76	0.34	0.12
Fiberglass wall treatment, 7 inches	0.86	0.99	0.99	0.99	0.99	0.99
Wood paneling on fiberglass blanket	0.40	0.99	0.80	0.50	0.40	0.30
Floors						
Wood parquet on concrete	0.04	0.04	0.07	0.60	0.06	0.07
Linoleum	0.02	0.03	0.03	0.03	0.03	0.02
Carpet on concrete	0.02	0.06	0.14	0.37	0.60	0.65
Carpet on foam rubber padding	0.08	0.24	0.57	0.69	0.71	0.73

with just the ceiling and floor covered are prone to acoustic defects, such as flutter echoes. Flutter echoes are the continued reflection of sound waves between two opposite parallel surfaces. This is a particular problem in small rooms, such as classrooms. It can be heard as a distinctive "slapping" or "ringing" sound. Absorbing materials can be placed on the walls, or the walls can be splayed slightly to reduce this problem. Sound-absorbent acoustic panels (1 inch thick minimum) can be placed on the sidewalls at the front of the room to reduce flutter in the area where the teacher speaks.

3. Curtains or thick draperies can be placed to cover the hard reflective surfaces of windows. Even when the curtains are open, they will serve to minimally reduce the RT of the enclosure.

4. Positioning of mobile bulletin boards and blackboards at angles other than parallel to opposite walls will also reduce the reflected sound in an enclosure.

5. Some teachers have used creative artwork from egg cartons or carpet scraps attached to walls or suspended from ceilings to help absorb noise and reduce reverberation. Safety regulations must be checked before placing potentially non-fire-retardant materials in the room.

6. Recall that as room size increases, so does RT. Therefore, keeping classrooms small and designing rooms with moderate ceiling heights are important considerations. A ceiling height of ~10 to 13 feet is usually acceptable.

7. In rooms where greater teacher-to-student distances are encountered, such as middle schools and high schools, it is useful to provide a surface to reflect sound waves to the students. This becomes relatively easy in rooms that are used for conventional lecture-style teaching. An area of the room can be designated as the "teaching" area. This is the location from which the teacher will speak. The acoustic design issue is to provide early sound reflections from the ceiling to seats in the room. The front part of the ceiling should be gypsum board, plaster, or other sound-reflecting material. This will allow early sound reflections from the teacher's voice as she or he speaks to reinforce the direct sound and increase the loudness of sound reaching students in the room.

Pitfall

- When making modifications to reduce the reverberation in a room, care must be taken to avoid overapplication of acoustic materials that absorb the low-intensity, high-frequency components of speech. Overapplication may reduce speech recognition and affect sound quality.

Present Status of Acoustic Modification in Classrooms

Despite the numerous strategies for treating the acoustic environment, classrooms often exhibit minimum degrees of acoustic modifications. Bess et al (1984) reported that although 100% of the rooms in their study had acoustic

ceiling tiles, only 68% had carpeting, and only 13% had draperies. None of the classrooms contained any form of acoustic furniture treatment. Crandell and Smaldino (1995) reported that although all the 32 classrooms examined had acoustic ceiling tiles, only 14 (54%) contained carpeting. Moreover, only one of the classrooms (3%) had drapes, whereas none of the rooms had acoustic furniture treatments.

"Clear" Speech

"Clear" speech procedures may also facilitate speech recognition in many enclosures. The term *clear speech* refers to a process in which the speaker focuses attention on a clearer pronunciation of speech while using a slightly reduced rate of speaking and a slightly higher intensity (Picheny et al, 1985). Several investigations have demonstrated that clear speech can significantly augment speech recognition in noisy and reverberant environments (Crandell et al, 1998; Payton et al, 1994; Schum, 1996). Payton et al (1994), for example, demonstrated that the average improvement in speech recognition when using clear speech was 20% for listeners with normal hearing and 26% for listeners with SNHL. Crandell et al (1998) found that recognition scores in a typical classroom environment (SNR = 0 dB; RT = 0.6 second) improved 18% when using clear speech procedures. It is not unreasonable to expect speakers, such as teachers, to learn clear speech procedures because talkers can be trained to continuously produce clear speech after a minimal amount of instruction and practice (Schum, 1996).

Pearl

- Meeting acoustic guidelines in a room does not necessarily ensure high speech recognition for all listeners in that room. To ensure optimal speech recognition, the speaker may still need to decrease speaker–listener distance (physically or through room amplification systems), provide ample visual information, and use speaking techniques such as clear speech.

Reducing Speaker–Listener Distance

Another consideration in reducing the adverse effects of noise and reverberation is to ensure that the listener receives the speaker's voice at the most favorable speaker–listener distance possible. That is, for optimum speech recognition to occur, the listener needs to be in a face-to-face situation and in the direct sound field of the speaker. Recall that speech recognition can only be improved within the critical distance of the room. Beyond the critical distance, recognition ability tends to remain essentially constant. Therefore, in any listening environment, the speaker–listener distance should not exceed the critical distance of the room. Unfortunately, the critical distance in many rooms is present only at speaker–listener distances relatively close to the speaker. Thus, the simple recommendation of preferential seating is often not adequate to ensure an appropriate listening environment. Rather, to remain within the critical distance of a room, restructuring of the room may need to be considered. For example, whenever possible, small group instruction (where the speaker addresses one small group at a time) should be recommended over more traditional room settings (where the speaker instructs in front of numerous rows of listeners). Crandell et al (1998) showed that recognition scores for children in normal classroom settings were 92% when they were instructed in small group settings.

Optimizing Visual Communication

Proximity to the speaker and face-to-face contact will also aid the listener with hearing impairment in maximizing speechreading skills. Optimal speaker–listener distance for maximum speechreading has been shown to be approximately 5 feet (Schow and Nerbonne, 1996). Speechreading ability tends to decrease significantly at 20 feet. Investigators have reported that speechreading benefit increases as a function of decreasing SNR (Rosenblum et al, 1996). That is, listeners often obtain significantly more information visually as the acoustic environment becomes more adverse. Rosenblum et al (1996) noted that speechreading can improve the SNR in typical classroom noise levels by more than 17 dB. However, the task of speechreading becomes much more difficult if the students must take notes as well.

Personal and Group Amplification Systems

Another potential procedure for reducing speaker–listener distance is through the use of a personal or group amplification systems. Before any amplification system is recommended in a room, physical modifications of the room must first be conducted. Unfortunately, it is often the case that significant acoustic modifications of a room cannot be accomplished because of excessive cost. A variety of personal and group amplification systems have been used to improve speech recognition in rooms. These systems include personal hearing aids and room amplification systems.

Hearing Aids

Hearing aids often offer little to no benefit in noisy or reverberant environments (Crandell, 1991; Crandell et al, 2005; Duquesnoy and Plomp, 1983; Plomp, 1986). Simple amplification in and of itself often does little to improve the SNR of the listening environment. Plomp (1986) reported that hearing aids offered limited speech recognition benefit when background noise level exceeded 50 dB(A). Duquesnoy and Plomp (1983) indicated that minimum benefit occurred from personal amplification when background noise levels reached 60 dB(A). Certainly, a review of everyday background noise levels (see discussion above) would suggest that most environments exhibit background noise levels in excess of 50 to 60 dB(A). Clearly, these data suggest that children should not use *just* hearing aids in the classroom setting. Several potential SNR-enhancing options for hearing aids may help listeners separate the signal from noise. The following section reviews several of these strategies. For more complete discussions of these technologies, the reader is directed to Chapters 1 and 17 in this volume.

Use of Directional Microphones

Because of the design of directional microphones, specific frequency spectra coming from various azimuths around the head (usually the front) are amplified more than other spectra coming from different azimuths (usually the sides and back). Thus, if a speaker is in front of the listener, the hearing aid microphone will pick up much of the speech from the speaker while not amplifying the background noise. This differential sensitivity to sound, if used wisely by the hearing aid wearer, can improve the SNR in a particular situation as much as 3 to 4 dB (Hawkins and Yacullo, 1984).

Directional microphones appear to be the single most effective option available in hearing aids today to improve the SNR if the signal is coming from the front of the listener and the noise from the rear of the listener. It must be noted, however, that in a classroom, the technology must be used cautiously, because if the wearer is not well schooled in how to position the directional microphones, the wanted signal may be attenuated in favor of background noise. In an environment such as a classroom, reception of signals all around the listener's head may be desirable, such as during classroom discussion. In a highly reverberant room, the advantages offered by the microphone may be reduced or negated (Hawkins and Yacullo, 1984). Improvements in directional microphone technology continue. Recently, dual-microphone designs coupled with digital signal-processing technology appear to be able to offer even greater improvements in SNR than conventional dual-microphone designs. In the future, multiple-microphone arrays of up to five microphones, working in concert with digital algorithms, may be able to improve the SNR by 11 to 13 dB.

Binaural Amplification

The advantages of listening to speech in noise through two ears (as opposed to one) or binaural amplification (compared with one hearing aid) are well recognized (Nabelek and Nabelek, 1994). The advantages stem primarily from head shadow effect and binaural interaction factors. The term *head shadow effect* refers to the acoustic effects of the head on speech and noise when these sources are at different locations in a room. Specifically, the listener with two ears, or two hearing aids, has the capability of favorably placing one ear toward the desirable sound (speech) and positioning the head to partially block the acoustics of an undesirable signal (noise). The term *binaural interaction* refers to the various central auditory processing phenomena known to exist when listening with two ears. These phenomena include analysis of time and intensity curves arriving at the ears (localization), binaural summation, and binaural release from masking (masking level differences). Head shadow effect and binaural interaction are believed to be the basis, at least partially, for a listener with binaural hearing (or binaural hearing aids) to demonstrate greater abilities to localize, focus attention, and perceive speech in a background of noise.

Modification of Frequency Response

One of the earliest strategies for reducing the upward spread of masking effects of low-frequency noise is shaping the frequency response of the hearing aid so that the high frequencies (encompassing the consonants) are emphasized and the low frequencies are deemphasized. In a room with abundant steady-state low-frequency noise, such as air-conditioning/ventilator noise, the ability to shift the frequency response of the amplification system in this way can effectively improve the SNR. As the interfering noise spectrum becomes more speechlike, the effectiveness of this strategy is diminished because important speech frequencies are removed. Modification of the frequency response has been available for many years in hearing aids through the nonadaptive high-pass filter setting. In recent years, digitally programmable instruments have been made available that offer up to eight programs or memories, which are user selectable either through a remote control unit or a button or switch on the instrument itself. For a discussion of these issues, see Chapter 17 in this volume.

Adaptive Signal-Processing Strategies

Many of the hearing aids available today use some form of adaptive signal processing in an attempt to enhance the SNR of the listening environment. Adaptive signal-processing strategies are those strategies that alter the electroacoustic characteristic(s) of the hearing aid in response to the listener's specific environment. These include (1) conventional single-channel automatic gain control; (2) adaptive compression; (3) multichannel compression; (4) bass increases at low levels (BILL) strategies, such as the DigiFocus circuitry from Oticon A/S (Smørum, Denmark); and (5) treble increases at low levels (TILL) strategies, such as the K-Amp from Etymotic Research Inc. (Elk Grove Village, IL). Research has demonstrated that these strategies benefit some listeners in noise, but not others. The reader is directed to Valente (1996a,b) for a review of these investigations and to Chapters 1, 4, and 5.

Digital Noise Reduction

Considerable research has been conducted to develop digital signal-processing methods that can enhance a desired speech signal while reducing the background noise. Many of the methods require a great deal of computing power to implement, which has not been feasible in a wearable device. The recent development and implementation of digital signal processing in a form that can be placed in a wearable device has rekindled research interest in digital noise reduction methods. For example, strategies that use both one and multiple microphones are currently being researched. Single-microphone designs attempt to identify the speech spectrum versus the noise spectrum and to selectively filter the noise spectrum, thus improving the SNR. Typical multiple-microphone designs are of two general types. One type involves a scheme to adaptively subtract a noise (received from one microphone) from a noise plus signal (received by another microphone) to derive a signal minus most of the noise component. The second type (referred to as adaptive beam forming) involves adaptively changing the sensitivity of an array of multiple microphones, so that the sensitivity pattern of the microphones is maximum for a forward-occurring speech signal and minimal for surrounding noise (Levitt, 1993).

Use of FM, Direct Audio Input, and Inductance Coupling

Certainly, the most effective procedure for improving the SNR for a hearing aid user is through hearing assistive technologies, such as direct audio input (DAI), inductance coupling, or FM technology. These technologies will be briefly discussed in the next section. For a more complete discussion, see Chapter 17 in this volume.

Room Amplification Systems

If placed correctly, room amplification systems can significantly enhance the SNR of the listening environment. Studies concerning room amplification systems in classrooms have shown that such systems can improve speech recognition, listening, attention, academic performance, and on-task behaviors (see Lewis, 1991, and Crandell et al, 2005, for reviews). Several forms of room amplification systems are commonly used. These include (1) personal FM amplification, (2) sound-field FM amplification, (3) induction loop, and (4) infrared.

Personal FM Amplification With a personal FM system (often called an auditory trainer), the teacher's voice is picked up through an FM wireless microphone located near his or her mouth (thus decreasing the speaker–listener distance), where the detrimental effects of reverberation and noise are minimal. The acoustic signal is converted to an electrical waveform and transmitted by an FM signal to a receiver. The electrical signal is then amplified, converted back to an acoustic waveform, and conveyed to one or more listeners in the room. The listeners can receive the signal through headphones, earbuds, or directly through their hearing aids through induction loop or DAI technology. Because of the high SNR provided by this arrangement (often 15–25 dB), personal FM systems are an essential recommendation for students with hearing loss or with normal hearing who exhibit significant speech recognition difficulties in classroom settings. Personal FM systems have recently become available for both children with SNHL and children with normal hearing in behind-the-ear models. Such models have been shown to be particularly useful for students in junior or senior high school who may not want to use personal FM systems because of the potential stigma associated with such devices. Currently, FM systems on the market permit a personal FM receiver to be added to, and become part of, a regular hearing aid. It is likely that FM systems of this type will be widely available as options on more hearing aids in the future.

Sound-Field Amplification A sound-field amplification system is similar to a personal FM system; however, the speaker's voice is conveyed to listeners in the room through one or more strategically placed loudspeakers. Sound-field systems are generally used to assist normal-hearing children in the classroom. The objectives when placing a sound-field system in a classroom are twofold: to amplify the speaker's voice by ~8 to 10 dB, thus improving the SNR of the listening environment, and to provide amplification uniformly throughout the classroom regardless of teacher or student position. Sound-field systems vary from compact, portable, battery-powered single-speaker units to more permanently placed, alternating current (AC)-powered speaker systems that use multiple (usually four) loudspeakers.

Numerous investigations have shown that when sound-field amplification systems are positioned within the classroom, psychoeducational and psychosocial improvements occur for children with normal hearing sensitivity (see Crandell and Smaldino, 1996b, and Crandell et al, 2005, for a review of these studies). In what is considered the original investigation on sound-field amplification, the Mainstream Amplification Resource Room Study (MARRS) examined the following educational strategies on academic achievement: (1) children receiving regular classroom instruction supplemented by resource room instruction and (2) children educated in the regular classroom with sound-field amplification (Sarff, 1981). Study participants were children with normal hearing and children with minimal degrees of SNHL. Results indicated that both groups of children, particularly the minimally hearing-impaired children, demonstrated significant improvements in academic achievement, especially in reading, when receiving amplified instruction. Younger children tended to demonstrate greater academic improvements than older children. Furthermore, academic gains in the amplified group were obtained at a faster rate, to a higher level, and with reduced cost, when compared with the unamplified group. Several studies have reported similar findings (see Crandell et al, 2005, for a review).

It is reasonable to assume that these academic improvements were the result of the improved listening environment offered by the sound-field amplification system. Crandell and Bess (1986) examined the effects of sound-field FM amplification on the speech recognition of children with normal hearing in a classroom environment (SNR = +6 dB; RT = 0.45 second). Sentence stimuli were recorded in amplified and unamplified listening conditions at speaker–listener distances of 6, 12, and 24 feet. Multitalker babble was used as the noise competition, and subjects consisted of 20 children, ages 5 to 7 years. Results from this investigation **(Fig. 18–10)** showed that sound-field FM amplification improved speech recognition at every speaker–listener distance, particularly at 12 and 24 feet. Numerous studies have reported similar improvements in speech recognition with the use of sound-field technology (see Crandell et al, 2005, for a review).

Sound-field amplification systems in the classroom have been shown to be extremely cost-effective for several reasons. First, such systems are typically the most inexpensive of all the available classroom amplification systems. Second, sound-field systems provide benefit for every child in the

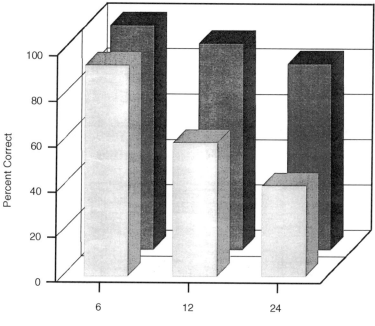

Figure 18–10 Mean speech recognition scores (percentage correct) of children with normal hearing in a "typical" classroom environment (SNR = +6 dB; RT = 0.6 second) with (*dark shaded bars*) and without (*light shaded bars*) sound-field frequency modulation (FM) amplification. RT, reverberation time; SNR, signal-to-noise ratio. (Adapted from Crandell, C., Smaldino, J., & Flexer, C. (2005). Sound field amplification: Applications to speech perception and classroom acoustics (2nd ed.). Clifton Park, NY: Thomson Delmar Learning, with permission.)

classroom, whereas personal FM systems or personal hearing aids only offer benefit to the individual user. In addition, because sound-field systems provide amplification for all children in the classroom, these systems do not stigmatize certain children, which can be the situation with auditory trainers or hearing aids. Third, sound-field systems are often the most inexpensive procedure of improving classroom acoustics. Acoustic modifications, such as acoustic ceiling tile, wall panels, or acoustically modified furniture, can be cost-prohibitive for some schools. As noted, however, essentially all classrooms will require at least a minimal degree of acoustic modification before the installation of sound-field amplification. Finally, the use of sound-field amplification systems has been shown to reduce the number of children requiring resource room assistance (Crandell et al, 2005; Flexer, 1992).

The average cost of a sound-field system is $700. Based on a class size of 25 students, the cost per pupil is $28. Dividing this figure over 10 years (the estimated life span of a sound-field system), the unit cost per child is only $2.80. Because sound-field systems significantly improve the classroom listening environment, additional cost-effectiveness may be obtained by reducing the number of children requiring resource room assistance. For selection procedures to determine whether a child is a candidate for personal or sound-field technology, the reader is directed to Crandell et al (2005) and Bess et al (1996) for a thorough discussion of amplification options in the pediatric population.

Controversial Point

- Numerous investigations have demonstrated that sound-field amplification improves academic, psychoeducational, and psychosocial achievement in normal-hearing children. To date, there remains limited information to support the use of this technology for children with mild to profound degrees of SNHL. Because of this paucity of data and because personal FM systems offer a substantially better SNR (15–25 dB) than sound-field FM systems (8–10 dB), it is recommended that personal FM systems be used by children with SNHL whenever possible. It is also important to remember that hearing aids alone will often offer limited benefit to children in classrooms.

Electromagnetic Induction Loop System   An induction loop system consists of a microphone connected by means of a cord or an FM radio signal to an amplifier. A length of wire, which is wound around a magnetic core under its installation, extends from the amplifier. This wire is placed either around the head of an individual (neckloop) or around a designated area, such as a classroom or theater. When an electrical current flows through the wire loop, it creates a magnetic field, which can be picked up through the telecoil of a hearing aid. Generally speaking, induction loop systems require a hearing aid to have a telecoil that is sensitive enough to pick up the magnetic field throughout the room

for good speech recognition to occur. Moreover, speech recognition tends to decrease as the listener moves away from the induction loop.

Infrared Light Wave Systems   Infrared systems consist of a wireless microphone, infrared converter, and infrared receiver. The microphone converts the acoustic signal to an electrical signal, which is then transmitted to the converter. The converter transduces the electrical signal to an invisible infrared signal and transmits it to a receiver that is worn by the listener. The receiver then transduces the infrared signal back into electrical energy. The electrical signal is changed into acoustic energy and routed to the listener through an induction loop/hearing aid telecoil setup or through headphones. For optimum sound quality with such systems, the listener must be in a direct line with the transmitter. For large rooms, such as theaters and auditoriums, arrays of transmitters must be used to ensure that all listeners are appropriately placed with the infrared light beam. Infrared systems cannot be used outside, because they are susceptible to interference from sunlight.

One distinct advantage that infrared systems have over traditional FM sound-field systems is the lack of "bleed-through" to adjacent classrooms. This is especially beneficial when schools have multiple classroom amplification systems operating at the same time. Because the infrared system cannot send a signal except in a direct line of sight of the transmitter, there is little risk of the signal being carried and heard outside of a given classroom.

Sound-field amplification has been shown to benefit many populations of children who are at risk of listening and learning in adverse acoustic environments, including normal-hearing children who are still acquiring language and normal-hearing children for whom English is a second language (Crandell et al, 2005). Because of the very positive cost/benefit ratio, it has been suggested that our goal should be to make classrooms acoustically accessible for all children (a universal design element; see Flexer's chapter in Crandell et al, 2005). This goal can be accomplished by using infrared wireless microphones and receiver/amplifiers, because there is no restriction as to the number of systems that can operate in adjacent classrooms without interference.

◆ Efficacy Measures for Interventions to Improve Room Acoustics

On the basis of an evaluation of the acoustic status of a room (see Crandell et al, 2005, for a step-by-step protocol), a decision may be made to improve the acoustic situation. No matter how the improvement is attempted, whether it is through physical modifications or the use of assistive technology, a measurable outcome of the intervention will be required to prove that the intervention was effective. Conversely, outcome measures can show that the intervention was not effective and that a different intervention may be more appropriate.

Many rooms, such as classrooms, are difficult places in which to conduct efficiency studies. Not only are teachers often reluctant to conduct intrusive and lengthy test procedures, but measures must often be conducted during the school day with all of the students in the classroom. The logistics can be intimidating. Despite this, several different approaches have been used to document the effects of intervention to improve acoustics on speech recognition, listening, and learning in the classroom.

Some of the earliest efforts involved observing global changes in academic achievement or "on-task" behavior. Because these measures were so global and possibly influenced by factors unrelated to the acoustic interventions, it is difficult to use these measures to establish unambiguous cause-and-effect relationships. In an attempt to resolve the ambiguities, researchers have used a variety of speech recognition measures with stimuli ranging from nonsense syllables, words, and sentences to establish efficacy of acoustic interventions. Some of the more analytical speech test materials even allowed researchers to pinpoint specific problems not only with the acoustics of the room but also with perceptual differences between students in the classroom. Although speech recognition materials are intuitively pleasing, the linkage between speech recognition, listening, and learning is not well established. In addition, speech recognition testing is awkward to do in the confines of the school day, and many of the test protocols are simply too complex or too lengthy to be practical in the classroom setting. Because of these difficulties, researchers have turned to subjective report questionnaires to obtain specific information concerning variables known to directly influence learning in the classroom.

The trend toward the use of report inventories parallels the increased use of hearing handicap inventories by audiologists as a primary vehicle to document successful hearing aid fittings in adults. Several of these subjective questionnaires can be completed by the teacher. The most prominent of these questionnaires is the Screening Instrument for Targeting Educational Risk (SIFTER; Anderson, 1989) (**Appendix 18-1**), in which the teacher observes and rates each student (or classroom of students) in five content areas: academics, attention, communication, class participation, and school behavior. The total score in each content area is then categorized as pass, marginal, or fail. A preschool version of the SIFTER (**Appendix 18-2**) can be used to evaluate younger children (3 years through kindergarten)

(Anderson and Matkin, 1996). Although originally intended as a tool to help identify students at risk for listening problems, it has proven to be useful in establishing efficacy of intervention in the classroom. When used in a pretest/posttest experimental design, any change in student performance as a result of classroom acoustic intervention can be documented. An extension of the SIFTER called the Listening Inventories for Education (LIFE; Anderson and Smaldino, 1998) (**Appendixes 18-3 and 18-4**) retains a teacher self-report questionnaire but also adds a self-report questionnaire that is completed by the student. By obtaining direct input from the student regarding listening difficulties in the classroom, the overall validity of the subjective approach to efficacy should be improved. The Children's Home Inventory of Listening Difficulties (CHILD, Anderson and Smaldino, 2001) is a further extension of LIFE; using CHILD, teachers in the classroom environment, as well as parents and children at home, can assess the adequacy of the environment for listening and observe changes as a result of intervention. Samples of LIFE, SIFTER, and Preschool SIFTER are provided in the appendixes. CHILD is available as a free download (www.phonak.com).

◆ Summary

Audiologists have a significant role to play in ensuring that acoustic barriers to communication are minimized. With that consideration in mind, the purpose of this chapter is to review known acoustic barriers to listening and learning in rooms, particularly classrooms. SNR, RT, speaker–listener distance, and combination effects have been discussed in light of their effects on accurate speech recognition for children with normal hearing and with hearing impairment. On the basis of considerable research, the ANSI (2002) standard recommends a background noise level not to exceed 35 dB(A) and an RT_{60} of 0.6 second for average-sized classrooms, (curve = ~25, SNR = +15 dB or better). Methods have been suggested to improve room acoustics, including acoustic modifications of the room, reduction of speaker–listener distance, enhancement of visual communication, and use of "clear" speech procedures. Technological suggestions include personal FM, induction loop systems, and infrared sound-field amplification devices. Finally, approaches have been outlined that have been used for documenting the efficacy of acoustic modifications and use of amplification in the classroom environment.

Appendix 18–1

Screening Instrument for Targeting Educational Risk (SIFTER)

By Karen L. Anderson, Ed.S., CCC-A

STUDENT _____ TEACHER _____ GRADE _____

DATE COMPLETED _____ SCHOOL _____ DISTRICT _____

The above child is suspect for hearing problems which may or may not be affecting his/her school performance. This rating scale has been designed to sift out students who are educationally at risk possibly as a result of hearing problems.

Based on your knowledge from observations of this student, circle the number best representing his/her behavior. After answering the questions, please record any comments about the student in the space provided on the reverse side.

1. What is your estimate of the student's class standing in comparison of that of his/her classmates?	UPPER 5　4	MIDDLE 3　2	LOWER 1
2. How does the student's achievement compare to your estimation of her/her potential?	EQUAL 5　4	LOWER 3　2	MUCH LOWER 1
3. What is the student's reading level, reading ability group or reading readiness group in the classroom (e.g., a student with average reading ability performs in the middle group)?	UPPER 5　4	MIDDLE 3　2	LOWER 1

ACADEMICS

4. How distractible is the student in comparison to his/her classmates?	NOT VERY 5　4	AVERAGE 3　2	VERY 1
5. What is the student's attention span in comparison to that of his/her classmates?	LONGER 5　4	AVERAGE 3　2	SHORTER 1
6. How often does the student hesitate or become confused when responding to oral directions (e.g., "Turn to page . . .")?	NEVER 5　4	OCCASIONALLY 3　2	FREQUENTLY 1

ATTENTION

7. How does the student's comprehension compare to the average understanding ability of her/her classmates?	ABOVE 5　4	AVERAGE 3　2	BELOW 1
8. How does the student's vocabulary and word usage skills compare with those of other students in his/her age group?	ABOVE 5　4	AVERAGE 3　2	BELOW 1
9. How proficient is the student at telling a story or relating happenings from home when compared to classmates?	ABOVE 5　4	AVERAGE 3　2	BELOW 1

COMMUNICATION

10. How often does the student volunteer information to class discussions or in answer to teacher questions?	FREQUENTLY 5　4	OCCASIONALLY 3　2	NEVER 1
11. With what frequency does the student complete his/her class and homework assignments within the time allocated?	ALWAYS 5　4	USUALLY 3　2	SELDOM 1
12. After instruction, does the student have difficulty starting to work (looks at other students working or asks for help)?	NEVER 5　4	OCCASIONALLY 3　2	FREQUENTLY 1

CLASS PARTICIPATION

13. Does the student demonstrate any behaviors that seem unusual or inappropriate when compared to other students?	NEVER 5　4	OCCASIONALLY 3　2	FREQUENTLY 1
14. Does the student become frustrated easily, sometimes to the point of losing emotional control?	NEVER 5　4	OCCASIONALLY 3　2	FREQUENTLY 1
15. In general, how would you rank the student's relationship with peers (ability to get along with others)?	GOOD 5　4	AVERAGE 3　2	POOR 1

SCHOOL BEHAVIOR

Additional copies of this form are available in pads of 100 each from
The Educational Audiology Association
4319 Ehrlich Road, Tampa, FL 33624
ISBN 0-8134-2845-9

TEACHER COMMENTS

Has this child repeated a grade, had frequent absences or experienced health problems (including ear infections and colds)? Has the student received, or is he/she now receiving, special support services? Does the child have any other health problems that may be pertinent to his/her educational functioning?

The S.I.F.T.E.R. is a SCREENING TOOL ONLY

Any student failing this screening in a content area as determined on the scoring grid below should be considered for further assessment, depending on his/her individual needs as per school district criteria. For example, failing in the Academics area suggests an educational assessment, in the Communication area a speech-language assessment, and in the School Behavior area an assessment by a psychologist or a social worker. Failing in the Attention and/or Class Participation area in combination with other areas may suggest an evaluation by an educational audiologist. Children placed in the marginal area are at risk for failing and should be monitored or considered for assessment depending upon additional information.

SCORING

Sum the responses to the three questions in each content area and record in the appropriate box on the reverse side and under Total Score below. Place an **X** on the number that corresponds most closely with the content area score (e.g., if a teacher circled 3, 4 and 2 for the questions in the Academics area, an **X** would be placed on the number 9 across from the Academics content area). Connect the **X**'s to make a profile.

CONTENT AREA	TOTAL SCORE	PASS						MARGINAL		FAIL				
ACADEMICS		15	14	13	12	11	10	9	8	7	6	5	4	3
ATTENTION		15	14	13	12	11	10	9	8	7	6	5	4	3
COMMUNICATION		15	14	13	12	11		10	9	8	7	6	5	4	3
CLASS PARTICIPATION		15	14	13	12	11	10	9	8	7	6	5	4	3
SOCIAL BEHAVIOR		15	14	13	12	11	10	9	8	7	6	5	4	3

Appendix 18–2

Screening Instrument for Targeting Educational Risk in Preschool Children (age 3–kindergarten) (Preschool SIFTER)

By Karen L. Anderson, Ed.S., CCC-A, and Noel Matkin, Ph.D.

Child _____ Teacher _____ Age _____

Date Completed ____/____/____ School _____ District _____

The above child is suspect for hearing problems which may affect his/her ability to listen, pay attention, develop language, follow teacher instruction and learn normally. This rating scale has been designed to sift out children who are at risk for educational delay and who may need further evaluation. Based on your knowledge of this child, circle the number that best represents his/her behavior. If the child is a member of a class that has students with special needs, comparisons should be made to normal learning classmates or normal developmental milestones. Please share additional comments about the child on the reverse side of this form.

1. How well does the child understand basic concepts when compared to classmates (e.g., colors, shapes, etc.)?	ABOVE AVERAGE BELOW 5 4 3 2 1	**PRE-ACADEMICS**	☐
2. How often is the child able to follow two-part directions?	ALWAYS FREQUENTLY SELDOM 5 4 3 2 1		
3. How well does the child participate in group activities when compared to classmates (e.g., calendar, sharing)?	ABOVE AVERAGE BELOW 5 4 3 2 1		
4. How distractible is the child in comparison to his/her classmates during large group activities?	SELDOM OCCASION FREQUENT 5 4 3 2 1	**ATTENTION**	☐
5. What is the child's attention span in comparison to classmates?	LONG AVERAGE SHORTER 5 4 3 2 1		
6. How well does the child pay attention during a small group activity or story time?	ABOVE AVERAGE BELOW 5 4 3 2 1		
7. How does the child's vocabulary and word usage skills compare to classmates?	ABOVE AVERAGE BELOW 5 4 3 2 1	**COMMUNICATION**	☐
8. How proficient is the child at relating an event when compared to classmates?	ABOVE AVERAGE BELOW 5 4 3 2 1		
9. How does the child's overall speech intelligibility compare to classmates (i.e., production of speech sounds)?	ABOVE AVERAGE BELOW 5 4 3 2 1		
10. How often does the child answer questions appropriately (verbal or signed)?	ALMOST ALWAYS FREQUENTLY SELDOM 5 4 3 2 1	**CLASS PARTICIPATION**	☐
11. How often does the child retain information during group discussions?	ALMOST ALWAYS FREQUENTLY SELDOM 5 4 3 2 1		
12. How often does the child participate with classmates in group activities or group play?	ALMOST ALWAYS FREQUENTLY SELDOM 5 4 3 2 1		
13. Does the child play in socially acceptable ways (i.e., turn taking, sharing)?	ALMOST ALWAYS FREQUENTLY SELDOM 5 4 3 2 1	**SOCIAL BEHAVIOR**	☐
14. How proficient is the child at using verbal language or sign language to communicate effectively with classmates (e.g., asking to play with another child's toy)?	ABOVE AVERAGE BELOW 5 4 3 2 1		
15. How often does the child become frustrated, sometimes to the point of losing emotional control?	NEVER SELDOM FREQUENTLY 5 4 3 2 1		

TEACHER COMMENTS: (frequent absences, health problems, other problems or handicaps in addition to hearing?)

The Preschool S.I.F.T.E.R. is a SCREENING TOOL ONLY. The primary goal of the Preschool S.I.F.T.E.R. is to identify those children who are at-risk for developmental or educational problems due to hearing problems and who merit further observation and investigation. Analysis has revealed that two factors, expressive communication and socially appropriate behavior, discriminate children who are normal from those who are at-risk. The greater the degree of hearing problem, the greater the impact on these two factors and the higher the validity of this screening measure. If a child is found to be at-risk then the examiner is encouraged to calculate the total score in each of the five content areas. Analysis of the content area score may assist in developing a profile of the child's strengths and special needs. The profile may prove beneficial in determining appropriate areas for evaluation and developing an individual program for the child.

SCORING

There are two steps to the scoring process. First, enter scores for each of the indicated questions in the spaces provided and sum the total of the 6 questions for the expressive communication factor and then the 4 questions for the socially appropriate behavior factor. If the child's scores fall into the At-Risk category for either or both of these factors, then sum the 3 questions in each content area to develop a profile of the child's strengths and potential areas of need.

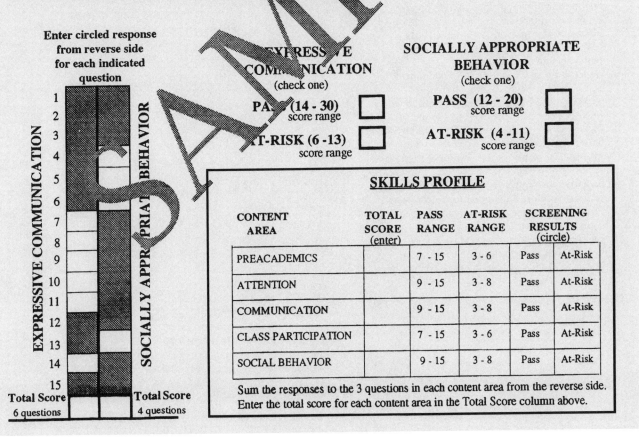

Enter circled response from reverse side for each indicated question

EXPRESSIVE COMMUNICATION (check one)

PASS (14 - 30) score range ☐

AT-RISK (6 -13) score range ☐

SOCIALLY APPROPRIATE BEHAVIOR (check one)

PASS (12 - 20) score range ☐

AT-RISK (4 -11) score range ☐

SKILLS PROFILE

CONTENT AREA	TOTAL SCORE (enter)	PASS RANGE	AT-RISK RANGE	SCREENING RESULTS (circle)	
PREACADEMICS		7 - 15	3 - 6	Pass	At-Risk
ATTENTION		9 - 15	3 - 8	Pass	At-Risk
COMMUNICATION		9 - 15	3 - 8	Pass	At-Risk
CLASS PARTICIPATION		7 - 15	3 - 6	Pass	At-Risk
SOCIAL BEHAVIOR		9 - 15	3 - 8	Pass	At-Risk

Sum the responses to the 3 questions in each content area from the reverse side. Enter the total score for each content area in the Total Score column above.

Appendix 18–3

Listening Inventory for Education (LIFE): An Efficacy Tool

Teacher Appraisal of Listening Difficulty

By Karen L. Anderson, Ed.S., CCC-A, and Joseph J. Smaldino, Ph.D.

Name _____ Grade_____Date_____
(Complete only for trial periods with individuals)

School _____ Teacher _____

Whole Classroom Sound Field Amplification Trial Period Y / N   Class Trial Period Length____Weeks
Individual Amplification Trial Period **Y** / **N**   Hearing Aid User **Y** / **N**   Trial Period Length____Weeks
Type of Hearing Technology Used With Individual: _____

Instructions: Circle the number which best describes student listening and learning behaviors. See reverse for suggestions to aid students in listening and understanding classroom instruction.

The student's:

	AGREE	NO CHANGE	Not Observed		DISAGREE
1. Focus on instruction has improved (more tuned in to instruction).	(2)	(1)	(0)	(-1)	(-2)
2. Appears to understand class instruction better.	(2)	(1)	(0)	(-1)	(-2)
3. Overall attention span has improved (less fidgety and/or less distracted).	(2)	(1)	(0)	(-1)	(-2)
4. Attention has improved when listening to directions presented to whole class.	(2)	(1)	(0)	(-1)	(-2)
5. Stays on task longer with less need for redirection.	(2)	(1)	(0)	(-1)	(-2)
6. Follows directions more quickly or easily (less hesitation before beginning work).	(2)	(1)	(0)	(-1)	(-2)
7. Answers questions in a more appropriate way or answers appropriately more often.	(2)	(1)	(0)	(-1)	(-2)
8. Improved understanding of instructional videos and/or morning announcements.	(2)	(1)	(0)	(-1)	(-2)
9. More involved in class discussions (volunteer more, follow better).	(2)	(1)	(0)	(-1)	(-2)
10. Improved understanding of answers or comments by peers during discussions.	(2)	(1)	(0)	(-1)	(-2)
11. Improved attention and understanding when noise is present (ventilator fan, transitions).	(2)	(1)	(0)	(-1)	(-2)
12. Improved ability to discriminate similar words or sounds (hat vs back, page 11 vs page 7).	(2)	(1)	(0)	(-1)	(-2)
13. Attention improved when listening in groups (small group/cooperative learning activities).	(2)	(1)	(0)	(-1)	(-2)
14. Socially more confident with other children or more comfortable in peer conversations.	(2)	(1)	(0)	(-1)	(-2)
15. Rate of learning seems to have improved (quicker to comprehend instruction).	(2)	(1)	(0)	(-1)	(-2)
16. Based on my knowledge and observations I believe that the amplification system is beneficial to the student's overall attention, listening and learning in the classroom.	(5)	(2)	(0)	(-2)	(-5)

Comments: (e.g., absences, equipment use problems)

Total Appraisal Score _____

APPRAISAL SUMMARY (circle one)

Highly Successful   26 - 35

Successful   16 - 25

Minimally Successful   5 - 15

Distributed by the Educational Audiology Association
4319 Ehrlich Rd, Tampa FL 33624 1-800-460-7322

LISTENING INVENTORY FOR EDUCATION
SUGGESTIONS FOR ACCOMMODATING STUDENTS WITH AUDITORY DIFFICULTIES

Students with auditory problems face extra challenges learning in a typical classroom setting. Typically, they can hear the teacher talk, but miss parts of speech or do not hear clearly, especially if noise is present. Students usually do not know what they didn't hear because they didn't hear it. They often may not know that they "misheard" a message unless they have already had experience with the language and topic under discussion. Use of amplification, having fluctuating hearing ability, hearing loss in just one ear, permanent hearing loss of any degree or central auditory processing disorders all compromise a student's ability to focus on verbal instruction and comprehend the fragments of speech information that are heard. The following items are suggestions for accomodating these student's special auditory needs and helping them learn their best in your classroom.

1. Seat the student close to where you customarily teach.
Sound weakens as it crosses distance. If a student has any auditory difficulties, how close you are to him/her will make a big difference on how well the student can hear and understand you.
- Can the student be moved to the front of the room?
- Can the student be allowed flexible seating so they can move to a better vantage point as classroom activities change? (e.g. move close to TV during movies)
- If your teaching style causes you to move around the room when you talk, is it possible to stay in close proximity to the student with auditory problems?
- When giving test directions, can you see the student's face clearly? Are you standing near the student's desk? Is the lighting on your face and not from a window behind you? Be sure the student is watching you.
- Develop a signal the student can use if he or she does not understand or has missed critical information.

2. Be aware of the benefits and limitations of lipreading.
- Only about 30-40% of speech sounds are visible on the lips. Lipreading supplements a student's hearing but is most helpful when the topic of conversation and vocabulary are known. New concepts and new vocabulary words have little meaning using lipreading.
- Is the student seated so they can see your face clearly? Too close and they view your face from a skewed angle, too far and the quick, tiny mouth movements are imperceptible.
- Lipreading is only possible if you are facing the student. If you use the chalkboard, do not provide verbal instruction while writing or be prepared to summarize or repeat that information for the student.
- Reading aloud to the class with your face downward makes lipreading very difficult. Hold the book below your chin so your face is easily visualized.
- Students cannot lipread and take notes at the same time. Classroom notetakers can use carbonized (NCR) paper and share notes easily. The student can use these notes from other students to fill in gaps in understanding.
- The extra demands of trying to understand using only speech fragments and of constantly trying to lipread can be very fatiguing. Listening breaks are natural, especially after rapid class discussions, lectures or new information.

3. Noise is a barrier to learning.
- Adults and children with normal hearing usually can tolerate a small amount of background noise without having their speech understanding compromised. Students with auditory problems are already missing fragments of what is said, especially if a message is spoken farther than from 3-6 feet away. Noise covers up word endings and brief words, reverberation smears the word fragments that are perceived.
- Can the student be allowed flexible seating so they can move away from noise sources? (e.g. lawn mower)
- Overhead projectors allow the student to clearly view the teacher's face, however, their fan noise interferes with understanding. If the student has a poorer hearing ear, face that one toward the overhead projector (or noisy ventilator, etc.) and seat close, but not next to the projector.
- If possible, eliminate or dampen unnecessary noise sources. Sometimes apsorbtive material, such as styrofoam or a thick bathtowel placed under an aquarium heater or animal cage will absorb some noise. Seat the student away from animal distractions.
- Keep your classroom door closed, especially when classes pass in the hall, gym or lunchroom activities are audible.
- One of the main causes of noise in the classroom is due to the activity of students. Seat away from peers who are very active or habitually noisy. Allow student's time to search their desks so that the noise generated will not occur during verbal instruction. Inform the custodian of especially squeaky desks.

4. Control or allow for distance.
- During group discussion, students with auditory problems typically can understand the students seated next to them but cannot understand students who are answering from more distant seats.
- Use a student's name when calling on them to answer a question. This will allow the student with hearing needs a chance to turn to face the answering student and to lipread if at all possible.
- Summarize key points given by classmates, especially brief messages like numeric answers, yes/no, etc.
- Allow or assign a student buddy that the student with auditory problems can ask for clarification or cueing.

Appendix 18–4

Listening Inventory for Education (LIFE): An Efficacy Tool

Student Appraisal of Listening Difficulty

By Karen L. Anderson, Ed.S., CCC-A, and Joseph J. Smaldino, Ph.D.

Name _____ Grade _____ Date _____

School _____ Teacher _____
Hearing Aid User Y / N   **Trial Period**   **Type of Classroom**
Trial Period Y / N   Length ____Weeks   **Hearing Technology** _____

Instructions: Circle the item which best describes the student's difficulty listening in the situations shown on picture card items 1-10. Optional items 11-16 can be scored if these situations are encountered in the listening environment. See reverse for intervention suggestions to improve listening and understanding.

Classroom Listening Situations	ALWAYS		SOMETIMES		NEVER
1. Teacher talking in front of room Comments:	(10)	(7)	(5)	(2)	(0)
2. Teacher talking during transition time Comments:	(10)	(7)	(5)	(2)	(0)
3. Teacher talking with back turned Comments:	(10)	(7)	(5)	(2)	(0)
4. Listening with hallway noise present Comments:	(10)	(7)	(5)	(2)	(0)
5. Other students making noise Comments:	(10)	(7)	(5)	(2)	(0)
6. Student answering during discussion Comments:	(10)	(7)	(5)	(2)	(0)
7. Listening with overhead projector fan on Comments:	(10)	(7)	(5)	(2)	(0)
8. Teacher talking while moving Comments:	(10)	(7)	(5)	(2)	(0)
9. Word recognition during a test or directions Comments:	(10)	(77)	(5)	(2)	(0)
10. Watching a video movie in classroom Comments:	(10)	(7)	(5)	(2)	(0)

Additional Listening Situations

11. Cooperative small group learning	(20)	(15)	(10)	(5)	(0)
12. Listening in gym (inside & outside)	(20)	(15)	(10)	(5)	(0)
13. Listening in school assembly	(20)	(15)	(10)	(5)	(0)
14. Listening to students during lunch	(20)	(15)	(10)	(5)	(0)
15. Students talking while coats are hung up	(20)	(15)	(10)	(5)	(0)

Scoring

		PRE-TEST		POST-TEST
Sum of Items 1 - 10	(100 possible)			
Sum of Items 11-16	(100 possible)	_____	CLASSROOM LISTENING SCORE	_____
Total Score of Items	(200 possible)	_____	ADDITIONAL SITUATIONS SCORE	_____

LISTENING INVENTORY FOR EDUCATION
SUGGESTIONS FOR IMPROVING CLASSROOM LISTENING

Mark an X next to each statement that corresponds with the situations indicated on the reverse side in which the student is experiencing any difficulty.

Classroom Difficult Listening Situations

_X_ 1. Let the teacher know that you cannot understand. Develop a signal system with your teacher.

_X_ 1. Be sure that you are seated near the teacher. Ask to move if needed.

_____ 2. Ask a student buddy to explain the directions ("Did she say page 191?).

_____ 2. Before the teacher hands out a test to the class, ask what kind of test it is and how you take it (fill in all blanks, true/false, multiple choice).

_____ 3. Have another student or two in your class that will share their class notes with you; the teacher can help to arrange this and provide carbonized paper. It is still your job to listen very carefully as your teacher talks. Notes can help you fill in gaps you may have missed as you study later.

_____ 3. Be sure that the teacher is aware of how important it is for you to see his/her face. Ask your parent to send a note to the teacher. Ask for the teacher to repeat information, ask a neighbor, use your signal.

_____ 4. If there is noise in the hall, ask for door to be closed. Arrange with your teacher ahead of time to have permission to get up and close the door whenever it's noisy.

_____ 5. Let your teacher know that noise from classmates is interfering with your understanding; use your signal system to alert your teacher that it's too noisy.

_____ 6. Ask your teacher to say student's names when calling on them to answer questions. Watch her face and listen carefully for names so you can quickly turn to face the talking student.

_____ 6. If you miss information from student answers or discussion: 1) ask answering student to repeat the information, 2) ask the teacher to repeat, 3) ask a neighbor

_____ 7. If you did not hear all of the announcements, ask the teacher or a neighbor what they were about.

_____ 8. If you cannot understand what the teacher is saying as he or she talks when the class is getting out books or papers it is important to be sure you are ready and watching the teacher during these times. If you miss a page number or other information be sure to raise your hand and ask - you are probably not the only one who didn't hear the teacher clearly in all the noise of changing activities.

_____ 9. Spelling tests are easiest if you really know the word list and can tell the difference between similar words (e.g., champion and trampoline have similar sounds but have different endings). Sit close and watch the teacher's face carefully. If you are not sure you clearly heard a word, let the teacher know immediately (you could use your signal).

_____ 10. Hearing speech clearly in a movie can be hard because of the background music on some videos. Sit close to the TV even if it means sitting in a different seat. If used, ask the teacher to put the FM microphone next to the TV. Have a note taker. Request closed captioned videos be used.

Additional Difficult Listening Situations

_____ 11. In small group work, be sure to sit close to other students and try to be able to see all of their faces. If used, pass the FM microphone from student to student. Ask students to repeat what you missed. It helps if your group could meet in a quieter spot of the class or in the hall while you work.

_____ 12. While in the gym, stand close to the teacher for directions and ask other children for directions you may have missed. Ask the teacher to repeat what you missed. Use a signal system to let your teacher know you didn't understand.

_____ 13. To hear in an assembly it is important to be near the front. If you have a personal FM the person speaking should wear the transmitter.

_____ 14. Ask your friends to repeat or clarify when something is missed (Did you say tomorrow night?"). Sit where you can easily see their faces and try to sit away from noisier children or noisy areas of your classroom. Remind your friends they may need to tap you to get your attention when it's really noisy and if you are not watching their faces.

_____ 15. You need to depend on your friends to catch your eye, tap you or for them to wait until they see you looking at them before they talk to you. Ask them to repeat what you have missed (Practice is at what time? You called Suzy when?).

References

Access Board. (1998). Retrieved from http://www.access-board.org

American National Standards Institute. (1983). Specifications for sound-level meters (ANSI S1.14–1983). New York: Author.

American National Standards Institute. (2002). Acoustic performance criteria, design requirements and guidelines for classrooms (ANSI S12.6–2002). New York: Author.

American Speech-Language-Hearing Association. (1995). Guidelines for acoustics in educational environments. ASHA, 37(Suppl.14), 15–19.

Anderson, K. (1989). Screening instrument for targeting education risk (SIFTER). Tampa, FL: Educational Audiology Association.

Anderson, K., & Matkin, N. (1996). The preschool screening instrument for targeting education risk. Tampa, FL: Educational Audiology Association.

Anderson, K., & Smaldino, J. (1998). The listening inventories for education (LIFE). Tampa, FL: Education Audiology Association.

Anderson, K., & Smaldino, J. (2001). Children's Home Inventory of Listening Difficulties (CHILD). Retrieved from www.Phonak.com

Beranek, L. (1954). Acoustics. New York: McGraw-Hill.

Bergman, M. (1980). Aging and the perception of speech. Baltimore: University Park Press.

Bess, F., Gravel, J., & Tharpe, A. (1996). Amplification for children with auditory deficits. Nashville, TN: Bill Wilkerson Center Press.

Bess, F. H., Sinclair, J., & Riggs, D. (1984). Group amplification in schools for the hearing-impaired. Ear and Hearing, 5, 138–144.

Bolt, R. H., & MacDonald, A. (1949). Theory of speech masking by reverberation. Journal of the Acoustical Society of America, 21, 577–580.

Boney, S., & Bess, F. (1984). Noise and reverberation effects in minimal bilateral sensorineural hearing loss. Paper presented at the American Speech-Language-Hearing Association Convention, San Francisco.

Crandell, C. (1991). Classroom acoustics for normal-hearing children: Implications for rehabilitation. Educational Audiology Monographs, 2, 18–38.

Crandell, C. (1992). Classroom acoustics for hearing-impaired children. Journal of the Acoustical Society of America, 92(4), 2470.

Crandell, C. (1993). Speech recognition in noise by children with minimal degrees of sensorineural hearing loss. Ear and Hearing, 14, 210–216.

Crandell, C., & Bess, F. (1986). Sound field amplification in the classroom setting. Paper presented at the American Speech-Language-Hearing Association Convention, New Orleans.

Crandell, C., Siebein, G., Gold, M, et al. (1998). Classroom acoustics: 4. Speech perception of normal- and hearing-impaired children. Journal of the Acoustical Society of America, 103(5), 3063.

Crandell, C., & Smaldino, J. (1992). Sound field amplification in the classroom. American Journal of Audiology, 1(4), 16–18.

Crandell, C., & Smaldino, J. (1995). An update of classroom acoustics for children with hearing impairment. Volta Review, 1, 4–12.

Crandell, C., & Smaldino, J. (1996a). The effects of noise on the speech perception of non-native English children. American Journal of Audiology, 5, 47–51.

Crandell, C., & Smaldino, J. (1996b). Sound field amplification in the classroom: Applied and theoretical issues. In F. Bess, J. Gravel, & A. Tharpe (Eds.), Amplification for children with auditory deficits (pp. 229–250). Nashville, TN: Bill Wilkerson Center Press.

Crandell, C., Smaldino, J., & Flexer, C. (2005). Sound field amplification: Applications to speech perception and classroom acoustics (2nd ed.). Clifton Park, NY: Thomson Delmar Learning.

Crum, D. (1974). The effects of noise, reverberation, and speaker-to-listener distance on speech understanding. Unpublished doctoral dissertation, Northwestern University, Chicago.

Duquesnoy, A. J., & Plomp. R. (1983). The effect of a hearing aid on the speech-reception threshold of hearing-impaired listeners in quiet and in noise. Journal of the Acoustical Society of America, 73, 2166–2173.

Education for All Handicapped Children, P.L. 94–142. (1977). Federal Register, 42(163), 42474–42518.

Education of the Handicapped Act Amendments of 1986, P.L. 94–457. (1986). United States Statutes at Large, 100, 1145–1177.

Education of the Handicapped Act Amendments of 1990, P.L. 101–476. (1990). United States Statutes at Large, 104, 1103–1151.

Egan, M. (1987). Architectural acoustics. New York: McGraw-Hill.

Elliot, L. (1982, December). Effects of noise on perception of speech by children and certain handicapped individuals. Sound Vibrations, 9–14.

Eyring, C. F. (1930). Reverberation time in "dead" rooms. Journal of the Acoustical Society of America, 1, 217–241.

Ferrand, C. (2001). Speech science. Boston: Allyn & Bacon.

Finitzo-Hieber, T., & Tillman, T. (1978). Room acoustics effects on monosyllabic word discrimination ability for normal and hearing-impaired children. Journal of Speech and Hearing Research, 21, 440–458.

Fitzroy, D. (1959). Reverberation formula which seems to be more accurate with non-uniform distribution of absorption. Journal of the Acoustical Society of America, 31, 893–897.

Flexer, C. (1992). Classroom public address systems. In M. Ross (Ed.), FM auditory training systems: Characteristics, selection and use (pp. 189–209). Timonium, MD: York Press.

French, N., & Steinberg, J. (1947). Factors governing the intelligibility of speech sounds. Journal of the Acoustical Society of America, 19, 90–119.

Gelfand, S., & Silman, S. (1979). Effects of small room reverberation upon the recognition of some consonant features. Journal of the Acoustical Society of America, 66(1), 22–29.

Gotaas, C., & Starr, C. (1993). Vocal fatigue among teachers. Folia Phoniatrica (Basel), 45, 120–129.

Green, K. B., Pasternak, B., & Shore, B. (1982). Effects of aircraft noise on reading ability of school age children. Archives of Environmental Health, 37, 24–31.

Haas, H. (1972). The influence of a single echo on the audible speech. Journal of the Audiological Engineering Society, 20(2), 146–159.

Hawkins, D. B., & Yacullo, W. (1984). Signal-to-noise ratio advantage of binaural hearing aids and directional microphones under different levels of reverberation. Journal of Speech and Hearing Disorders, 49, 278–286.

Helfer, K. S. (1994). Binaural cues and consonant perception in reverberation and noise. Journal of Speech and Hearing Research, 37(2), 429–438.

Hodgson, M., & Nosal, E. (2002). Effect of noise and occupancy on optimal reverberation times for speech intelligibility in classrooms. Journal of the Acoustical Society of America, 111(2), 931–939.

Individuals with Disabilities Education Act (P. L. 105–117). (1998). Retrieved from http://www.edlaw.net/ptabcont.htm

Killion, M. (1997). SNR loss: I can hear what people say, but I can't understand them. Hearing Review, 4(12), 8–14.

Knecht, H. A., Nelson, P., Whitelaw, G., & Feth, L. (2002). Background noise levels and reverberation times in unoccupied classrooms: Predictions and measurements. American Journal of Audiology, 11, 65–71.

Ko, N. (1979). Response of teachers to aircraft noise. Journal of Sound Vibrations, 62, 277–292.

Koszarny, Z. (1978). Effects of aircraft noise on the mental functions of school children. Archives of Acoustics, 3, 85, 86.

Kreisman, B. (2003). The effects of simulated reverberation on the speech-perception abilities of listeners with normal hearing. Unpublished doctoral dissertation, University of Florida, Gainesville.

Leavitt, R., & Flexer, C. (1991). Speech degradation as measured by the Rapid Speech Transmission Index (RASTI). Ear and Hearing, 12, 115–118.

Lehman, A., & Gratiot, A. (1983). Effets du bruit sur les enfants à l'école [Effects of noise on schoolchildren]. Proceedings of the Fourth Congress on Noise as a Public Health Problem (pp. 859–862). Milan: Centro Ricerche e Studi Amplifon.

Levitt, H. (1993). Digital hearing aids. In G. Studebaker & I. Hochberg (Eds.), Acoustical factors affecting hearing aid performance (pp. 317–335). Boston: Allyn & Bacon.

Lewis, D. (1991). FM systems and assistive devices: Selection and evaluation. In J. Feigin & N. Stelmachowicz (Eds.), Pediatric amplification (pp. 115–138). Omaha, NE: Boys Town National Research Hospital.

McCroskey F, Devens J. (1975). Acoustic characteristics of public school classrooms constructed between 1890 and 1960. Proceedings of Noise Expo, National Noise and Vibration Control Conference (pp. 101–103). Bay Village, OH: Acoustical Publications.

Moncur, J. P., & Dirks, D. (1967). Binaural and monaural speech intelligibility in reverberation. Journal of Speech and Hearing Research, 10, 186–195.

Nabelek, A., & Nabelek, I. (1994). Room acoustics and speech perception. In J. Katz (Ed.), Handbook of clinical audiology (4th ed., pp. 624–637). Baltimore: Williams & Wilkins.

Niemoeller, A. (1968). Acoustical design of classrooms for the deaf. American Annals of Deafness, 113, 1040–1045.

No Child Left Behind Act of 2001 (P. L. 107–110), 20 USC 6301 et seq. (2001).

Ottring, S., Smaldino, J., Plakke, B., & Bozik, M. (1992). Comparison of two methods of improving classroom S/N ratio. Paper presented at the American Speech-Language and Hearing Association Convention, San Antonio, TX.

Payton, K. L., Uchanski, R., & Braida, L. (1994). Intelligibility of conversational and clear speech in noise and reverberation for listeners with normal and impaired hearing. Journal of the Acoustical Society of America, 95(3), 1581–1592.

Pearsons, K., Bennett, R., & Fidell, S. (1977). Speech levels in various noise environments (EPA 600/1–77–025). Washington, DC: Office of Health and Ecological Effects.

Picheny, M. A., Durlach, N., & Braida, L. (1985). Speaking clearly for the hard of hearing: 1. Intelligibility differences between clear and conversational speech. Journal of Speech and Hearing Research, 28, 96–103.

Plomp, R. (1986). A signal-to-noise ratio model for the speech reception threshold for the hearing impaired. Journal of Speech and Hearing Research, 29, 146–154.

Puetz, V. (1971). Articulation loss of consonants as a criterion for speech transmission in a room. Journal of the Audiological Engineering Society, 19, 915–929.

Roberts, R. A. (2003). Effects of noise and reverberation on the precedence effect in listeners with normal hearing and impaired hearing. American Journal of Audiology, 12(2), 96–105.

Rosenblum, L. D., Johnson, J., & Saldana, H. (1996). Point-light facial displays enhance comprehension of speech. Journal of Speech and Hearing Research, 39, 1159–1170.

Sabine, W. (1964). Collected papers on acoustics. Mineola, NY: Dover Publications. (Original work published 1927)

Sanders, D. A. (1965). Noise conditions in normal school classrooms. Exceptional Children, 31, 344–353.

Sapienza, C., Crandell, C., & Curtis, B. (1999). Effect of sound field FM amplification on vocal intensity in teachers. Journal of Voice, 13(3), 375–381.

Sarff, L. (1981). An innovative use of free field amplification in regular classrooms. In R. Roeser & M. Downs (Eds.), Auditory disorders in school children (pp. 263–272). New York: Thieme-Stratton.

Schow, R., & Nerbonne, M. (1996). Introduction to audiologic rehabilitation (3rd ed.). Boston: Allyn & Bacon.

Schum, D. J. (1996). Intelligibility of clear and conversational speech of young and elderly listeners. Journal of the American Academy of Audiology, 7(3), 212–218.

Siebein, G., Crandell, C., & Gold, M. (1997). Principles of classroom acoustics: Reverberation. Educational Audiology Monographs, 5, 32–43.

Smaldino, J. (1997). Room acoustics. Paper presented at the Acoustical Society of America Conference on Acoustical Barriers to Listening and Learning, Los Angeles.

Stuart, A., & Phillips, D. P. (1998). Recognition of temporally distorted words by listeners with and without a simulated hearing loss. Journal of the American Academy of Audiology, 9(3), 199–208.

Valente, M. (1996a). Hearing aid standards, options, and limitations. New York: Thieme Medical Publishers.

Valente, M. (1996b). Strategies for selecting and verifying hearing aid fittings. New York: Thieme Medical Publishers.

Chapter 19

Vestibular Rehabilitation

Alan L. Desmond

Vestibular disorders, responsible for complaints of vertigo and disequilibrium, are a common complaint in the adult and geriatric population. Dizziness is among the three most common complaints encountered in the primary care setting, sharing equal time with headaches and low back pain, and may affect half the population in the United States during their lifetime. After the age of 65, dizziness is one of the most frequent reasons for a doctor visit and hospital admission. As the elderly population increases, so will the number of complaints regarding balance disorders. The world population of citizens older than 60 years is expected to double between 1990 and 2030. The need and opportunity for audiologists trained in the assessment and treatment of vestibular disorders are obvious.

The audiology scope of practice includes "the conduct and interpretation of behavioral, electroacoustic, or electrophysiologic methods used to assess hearing, balance, and neural system function," and "consultation and provision of rehabilitation to persons with balance disorders using habituation, exercise therapy and balance retraining" (American Speech-Language-Hearing Association [ASHA], 1996). A position statement by the American Academy of Audiology (AAA, 2000) recommends that audiologists "participate as full members of the vestibular and treatment teams to . . . carry out goals of vestibular rehabilitation therapy."

♦ Definitions

Although terms such as *vestibular rehabilitation, adaptation, compensation,* and *habituation* seem to be used interchangeably in the literature, important distinctions need to be made. For the purposes of this chapter, the author will use the following definitions.

Vestibular rehabilitation refers to the process of training the patient in the techniques for recovery from vestibular weakness. *Rehabilitation,* in general, is defined as the process of "putting back in good condition, bringing or restoring to a normal or optimal state of health by medical treatment and . . . therapy."

Vestibular adaptation refers to the response of the central nervous system (CNS) to asymmetrical peripheral vestibular afferent activity and resulting sensory conflicts. This implies a gradual decrease in neuronal response to constant abnormal stimuli (Curthoys and Halmagyi, 1996).

Vestibular compensation encompasses the entire repertoire of strategies used by the patient to reduce symptoms and improve overall balance function and stabilize gaze. This includes neuronal adaptation of the vestibulo-ocular reflex (VOR), sensory substitution, and alternative predictive and cognitive strategies used to overcome the symptoms of vestibular deficit.

Vestibular habituation is "the long-term reduction in a neurologic response to a particular stimulus that is facilitated by repeated exposure to the stimulus. In the vestibular system, the unpleasant response is usually a vertiginous sensation, often associated with nausea, in response to certain head movements" (Shepard and Telian, 1996, p. 29). In this context, vestibular rehabilitation involves maximizing vestibular compensation and promoting the learning and formation of habits (habituation) to promote reduction of symptoms and enhance postural and gaze stability.

◆ Past Approaches to the Patient with Dizziness

Treatment for vestibular disorders has historically fallen into three categories: (1) medical treatment of symptoms and underlying pathological conditions; (2) surgical stabilization of the end organ or vestibular nerve through reparative or ablative techniques; and (3) observation, reassurance, and counseling to "learn to live with it."

Medical treatment most often involves prescribing vestibular or CNS sedating medications. The most common medication prescribed is meclizine (Antivert). The use of vestibular suppressant and CNS sedative medications in the treatment of vestibular disorders has been questioned because vestibular compensation and rehabilitation may be delayed by these medications. Kroenke et al (1990) reported that only 31% of patients treated for dizziness with prescription medication believed this therapy to be helpful. Side effects of CNS sedative and vestibular suppressant medications include drowsiness and slowing of reaction

time, potentially leading to an increased risk of falling (Manning et al, 1992).

Surgical approaches to vestibular pathological conditions are applicable only to unstable or progressive peripheral lesions. Conditions such as endolymphatic hydrops, Meniere's disease, perilymphatic fistula, and superior canal dehiscence are sometimes treatable through reparative surgeries. Ablative procedures may be recommended for intractable benign paroxysmal positional vertigo (BPPV) or Meniere's disease. Conditions such as acoustic neuroma and vestibular schwannoma frequently require surgical intervention and often result in permanent loss of vestibular input from the affected side. These conditions represent a minority of patients with vestibular complaints.

Observation, reassurance, and counseling that the condition is not life threatening may be appropriate and helpful in many cases but do not address the needs of symptomatic patients seeking some relief. Physicians tend to focus more on potential mortality as opposed to the patient's quality of life (Sloane et al, 1994). Many patients cannot or do not wish to "learn to live with it." Vestibular loss often leads to restriction, disability, and reduced quality of life, and patients with chronic balance disorders often persist in seeking diagnosis and treatment. It is not uncommon for a patient with a chronic balance problem to see several different specialists with little or no coordination between specialists, often resulting in duplication of tests.

Vestibular rehabilitation offers an alternative form of treatment to many patients previously falling into one of the three aforementioned categories. Treatment of vestibular disorders through exercise and repositioning techniques has gained popularity over the last 2 decades, and recent literature supports the efficacy of these approaches. The concept of an exercise or rehabilitation approach to dizziness and balance disorders is not new. British otolaryngologist Terrance Cawthorne is the earliest documented proponent of an exercise approach in treating patients with vestibular symptoms. Cawthorne (1945) described the complexity of the balance system and the relationship between the vestibular system and visual and somatosensory inputs. He noted that after unilateral labyrinthectomy, active patients seemed to recover faster and more completely than more sedate patients.

Cawthorne, along with physiologist Dr. F. S. Cooksey, developed a series of exercises, known as Cawthorne-Cooksey exercises, thought to promote central compensation and habituation through repetition of symptom-provoking maneuvers. These exercises laid the basic framework of current vestibular rehabilitation programs. Concepts such as critical periods of compensation after injury, the need to provide the patient with progressively more difficult exercises, and the need to reduce functional disability are all addressed (Cooksey, 1945).

McCabe (1970, pp. 1430–1431) expanded on Cawthorne's and Cooksey's ideas and described "labyrinthine exercises" as "our most useful single tool in the alleviation of protracted recurrent vertigo." He advocated the importance of patient education and the need for proper stimulus to allow the brain to "get over" vestibular losses. McCabe described the two peripheral vestibular apparatuses as "partners," and his explanation regarding vestibular exercises is worth repeating:

"1. Explain to the patient the nature of his or her disorder using the analogy of partners:

   a. The disorder is a disease of the balance center, which is made up of two TK parts that act as partners, working together to maintain balance.

   b. In the disorder, one partner cannot carry his or her share of the balancing load.

   c. At certain times, a comparison of partners occurs, and one is found wanting; then trouble (vertigo) ensues.

   d. The longer the two partners ignore each other, the worse the trouble is going to be when they meet.

   e. The closer and more often the two partners confront each other with the problem they mutually want to solve (disequilibrium), the more quickly it will be solved.

   f. When the partners reach an agreement that is mutual, balance results.

2. Give to the patient, on the basis of the above description, a series of instructions pertinent to the nature and severity of his or her symptoms and disease.

3. Reassure the patient, saying something along the following lines: "You do not have a life-threatening illness. Your symptoms are only as important as the degree to which they annoy you. You will in time master them; when you do, they will disappear."

McCabe (1970) went on to note that medications strong enough to suppress symptoms may also prevent or delay the reparative process.

Margaret Dix (1984, p. 477) promoted the concept of vestibular rehabilitation. She emphasized encouragement, motivation, and patient education as critical factors for success. She based her therapy program on the original Cawthorne-Cooksey exercises, but added, "The rationale, then, of head exercises in vestibular disorders is to provoke deliberately and systematically as many spells of vertigo as can be tolerated."

A common bond between most of the published reports from this period is the emphasis on intentionally provoking symptoms by creating an error signal or sensory conflict. In theory, cerebellar, or "adaptive," plasticity works to integrate what is initially perceived as abnormal and through repetition and motor learning (habituation) interprets the vestibular signals as normal. Adaptive plasticity refers to the brain's ability to modify the amount (or gain) of the vestibular ocular reflex to minimize visual-vestibular conflict. Sensory conflicts occur when disagreement exists between incoming (afferent) information regarding movement, balance, and orientation. This can occur when an asymmetrical response occurs between the two labyrinths in response to head movement or when a disagreement (or conflict) exists between vestibular, visual, or proprioceptive input. An example of sensory conflict would be the frequently described sensation of movement or disorientation that occurs while sitting in a car next to a large truck or bus. The size of the truck or bus allows for full-field stimulation. When the truck or bus moves forward, a brief illusory sensation that one is moving backward occurs. Those with a healthy vestibular system quickly prioritize the incoming information and rely on the vestibular response, indicating lack of movement. Patients with vestibular weakness may not react quickly or appropriately and lose balance or orientation.

♦ Physiological Basis for Recovery

Static Symptoms

The tonic, or resting, state of the paired vestibular labyrinths is a delicate balance that can be disrupted by a sudden injury to one or both labyrinths. Conditions responsible for unilateral vestibular injury include vestibular neuronitis and labyrinthitis, as well as surgical procedures, such as eighth nerve section or labyrinthectomy. After a sudden loss or reduction in the function of one labyrinth, a predictable set of clinical signs and symptoms occurs. These "static" symptoms include spontaneous nystagmus following Alexander's law, a subjective sensation of vertigo, postural instability, ataxia, and ocular tilt reaction (Curthoys and Halmagyi, 1996; Leigh and Zee, 1999). These symptoms result from a sudden profound asymmetry in resting activity between the two vestibular nuclei. Whenever an imbalance exists in the output of the vestibular nuclei, a sense of rotation toward the vestibular nuclei with the higher resting potential is perceived. Alexander's law refers to the pattern of nystagmus typically seen during the acute phase of peripheral vestibular asymmetry. The intensity of nystagmus increases when gaze is directed toward the fast phase of nystagmus (away from the lesioned side) and decreases when gaze is directed toward the slow phase (toward the lesioned side). Ocular tilt reaction indicates tonic imbalance of the activity of the VOR (the VOR may be defined as reflexive eye movement in response to head movement) and consists of skew deviation (vertical misalignment) and ocular counter-rolling (fixed torsion) of the eyes and head tilt toward the lower eye. The reader is referred to Leigh and Zee (1999) for a complete review.

Over a period of hours to days, these symptoms diminish considerably through the process of vestibular adaptation. Because evidence suggests that labyrinthine receptors and peripheral neurons do not regenerate, the process of adaptation is thought to be a result of plasticity within the CNS. The exact mechanism is not understood, but most researchers believe that the process of vestibular adaptation is a function of alterations in activity of the vestibular nuclei. Smith and Curthoys (1989) and Curthoys and Halmagyi (1996) offer thorough reviews of studies pertaining to "tonic rebalancing" after unilateral labyrinthine loss.

It is estimated that human peripheral vestibular afferent fibers have resting potentials of up to 100 spikes per second. Considering that ~18,000 vestibular afferents are in each labyrinth, the resting activity being received by each vestibular nucleus may be more than 1 million spikes per second (Curthoys and Halmagyi, 1996). Any head movement results in a change in this resting potential, and the vestibular nuclei receive asymmetrical inputs from the two vestibular labyrinths. Earlier reports of vestibular physiology described a simple "push-pull" arrangement, in which a head movement would cause an excitatory response in one vestibular nucleus and a corresponding, but not necessarily equal, inhibitory response in the contralateral vestibular nucleus. It is now believed that for each head movement, both inhibitory and excitatory responses occur in both vestibular nuclei, and that the inhibitory responses are the result of inhibitory commissural connections from the contralateral vestibular nucleus (Curthoys and Halmagyi, 1996). It is these commissural connections that help explain the process of tonic rebalancing.

After the sudden loss of or reduction in function of one labyrinth, an immediate dramatic decrease occurs in the resting activity of the ipsilateral vestibular nucleus. An immediate increase in resting activity also occurs in the contralateral vestibular nucleus, which is likely the result of the loss of inhibitory commissural connections normally received from the lesioned side (Smith and Curthoys, 1989). Simply stated, the two vestibular nuclei are interactive and depend on each other to maintain equal resting outputs. Each exerts some inhibitory influence on the other. When the function of one is lost, the other temporarily responds with an increase in activity over and above its normal resting level of activity. This creates a sudden profound asymmetry in the two vestibular nuclei and leads to the above-mentioned signs and symptoms of sudden unilateral vestibular deafferentation (UVD).

The CNS responds by reducing the resting level of the intact side (a process known as "cerebellar clamp") and gradually restores activity in the vestibular nucleus on the lesioned side. This process leads to tonic rebalancing and a reduction in static symptoms. Restoration of activity in the vestibular nucleus on the lesioned side should not be confused with restoration of response from the lesioned peripheral labyrinth. This process of tonic rebalancing and the time course for reduction of static symptoms such as spontaneous nystagmus and ocular tilt do not appear to depend on visual or physical exercise stimulation.

The rebalancing of neural activity between the two vestibular nuclei becomes evident when a subject with previous unilateral vestibular loss, after a period of adaptation, has a loss in the contralateral labyrinth. Because the symptoms of sudden unilateral vestibular loss as described previously are believed to be a result of sudden asymmetry in the resting potentials of the vestibular nuclei, common sense would dictate that a loss of function in the remaining labyrinth would result in the absence of, but symmetrical output from, the two vestibular labyrinths. However, in such a case, the subject responds behaviorally as if the loss of the remaining labyrinth results in a sudden asymmetry, with the well-known pattern of static symptoms of acute unilateral loss. This reaction, known as *Bechterew's phenomenon,* provides evidence of restoration of activity in the vestibular nucleus on the lesioned side. The role of the commissural connections has been described by Bienhold and Flor (1978). To determine the role of these connections in vestibular compensation, the researchers surgically destroyed commissural connections in the frog at various stages of compensation after unilateral labyrinthectomy. They noted (1) an immediate return of symptoms of unilateral labyrinthectomy, (2) that the level of symptoms was independent of the time allowed and level of compensation, and (3) that no recompensation could be observed. This indicates that without these commissural connections allowing for information from the contralateral labyrinth to be received by the lesioned side vestibular nucleus, vestibular adaptation could not take place. The restoration of activity in the vestibular nucleus of the lesioned side may play an important role in the recovery from static symptoms but does not appear to contribute significantly to the reduction of dynamic symptoms (Smith and Curthoys, 1989).

Dynamic Symptoms

Dynamic symptoms include those symptoms that occur as a result of head movement resulting from dysfunction of the VOR. The role of the VOR is to allow for stable gaze or focus while the head is moving. The VOR performs this function by causing eye movements that are equal and opposite of head movements, in effect visually canceling out head movement (**Fig. 19–1**). Although the static symptoms of acute unilateral vestibular loss are quite predictable and easily identified, dynamic symptoms of VOR dysfunction are more subtle, and recovery of VOR function is more dependent on external influences.

Symptoms of VOR dysfunction typically do not include complaints of vertigo but, rather, visual blurring with head movement (oscillopsia) and visual-provoked and motion-provoked disequilibrium and disorientation. Brandt (1991, glossary, p. xviii) defines oscillopsia as "apparent movement of the visual scene due to involuntary retinal slip in acquired ocular oscillations or deficient VOR." In this context, "acquired ocular oscillations" would be nystagmus, which should be evident to the examiner. Nystagmus is involuntary eye movement associated with tonic imbalance within the peripheral or central vestibular system. When nystagmus is present, this eye movement may prohibit accurate visual fixation or visual following, leading to oscillopsia without head movement. Patients without nystagmus but with a deficient VOR will typically experience oscillopsia only when they are moving. Some patients with confirmed (by calorics) bilateral vestibular loss experience no more than mild disequilibrium, whereas others complain of blurred vision and "bouncing" with any head movement. Patients with oscillopsia tend to be asymptomatic when they are not moving. To varying degrees, head movement causes a decrease in visual acuity, which can be easily documented with a standard Snellen eye chart.

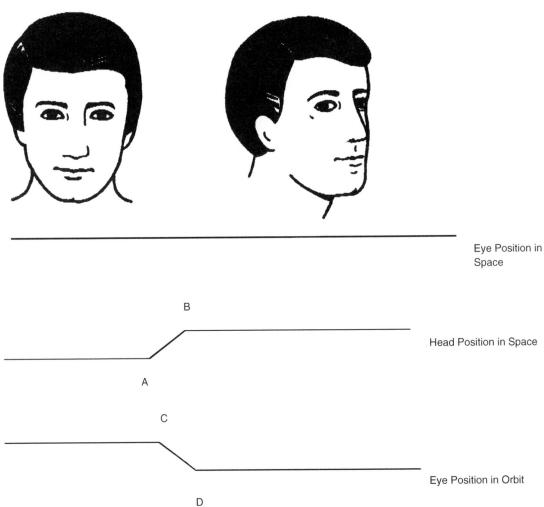

Eye Position in Space

Head Position in Space

Eye Position in Orbit

Figure 19–1 The role of the vestibulo-ocular reflex is to maintain eye position in space as the head moves. Point A represents the onset of head movement, and point C represents the onset of reflexive eye movement in the orbit (typically < 16 msec after onset of head movement). This minimal duration of retinal slip accounts for maintenance of gaze stability with head movement. Points B and D represent a 30-degree excursion of head movement and eye movement in opposite directions, demonstrating a gain of 1, and in effect visually canceling out the effect of head movement.(Adapted from Leigh, R. J. & Zee, D. S. (1999). The neurology of eye movements (3rd ed.). New York: Oxford University Press, with permission.)

Pearl

- Many equipment manufacturers are offering computerized dynamic visual acuity (DVA) measurement devices. These often involve a target that is visible only when the head is moving above a predetermined velocity or head speed. Head speed is measured through a head-worn accelerometer. Herdman et al (1998) report DVA is highly sensitive and specific for differentiating normal patients from patients with vestibular dysfunction. Successful vestibular rehabilitation is often accompanied by noted improvements in DVA.

The basis for these complaints is termed *retinal slip,* or the inability to maintain focused, centered vision (foveal vision) with head movements. Retinal slip occurs when the VOR cannot adequately compensate for head movement, and images do not remain stable on the retina. Visual acuity is best when an image is centered and stable on the retina. A gradual decline in visual acuity is noted as visual images move across the retina at increasing speeds. No significant decrease is noted when images move across the retina at speeds of 2 to 3 degrees per second, but at 4 to 5 degrees per second and above, gaze stability and visual acuity are compromised (Leigh and Zee, 1999). *Gaze stability* may be defined as the ability to maintain foveal vision during head movements.

It is estimated that the range of head speeds encountered in real life is from 0.5 to 5.0 Hz, and the VOR normally responds efficiently to head speeds up to 8 Hz (Gresty et al, 1977). A variety of voluntary cerebellar-generated eye movements may allow for gaze stability at speeds < 1 Hz, but only the VOR can allow for gaze stability and clear vision to head movements > 2 Hz. It is impossible to voluntarily move the eyes at speeds needed to maintain visual acuity during typical head movements. The latency of response for the VOR is < 16 msec, whereas the latency for a voluntary eye movement is ~76 msec for a predictable target and 150 to 250 msec for an unpredictable target (Leigh and Zee, 1999).

When retinal slip occurs, and visual acuity is compromised, a sensory conflict between perceived visual, vestibular, and somatosensory information can occur. Patients with vestibular deficits tend to become more reliant on accurate visual and somatosensory feedback for maintenance of equilibrium, orientation, and balance. In the early stages after vestibular injury, a notably greater reliance on visual information is seen (Keshner, 1994). Gaze instability leads to inaccurate visual feedback, affecting appropriate sensory integration of the incoming information.

Recovery of the VOR is believed to occur primarily as a result of CNS and cerebellar plasticity and is possibly part of the process of cerebellar clamp. The retinal slip caused by VOR dysfunction leads to an "error signal" in that images would be blurred during locomotion. CNS plasticity uses this error signal and gradually recalibrates the output or gain of the VOR in an effort to enhance stable and clear vision. (*Gain* may be defined as the ratio of eye movement amplitude to head amplitude. A 10 degree head movement should result in a 10 degree eye movement in the opposite direction, for a perfect gain of 1.) It has been demonstrated that VOR gain and direction can be modified by subjecting patients with normal vestibular function to error signals (Demer et al, 1989). It is believed that the error signal induced by VOR dysfunction triggers an adaptive response from the CNS. Several investigators report that visual and somatosensory deprivation delays may ultimately limit vestibular compensation in animals, and delays in initiation of vestibular therapy in humans may negatively affect long-term disability (Bamiou et al, 2000; Smith et al, 1986).

Some authors have described the short latency neuronal connections between the peripheral vestibular sensory receptors and the extraocular muscles that control eye movements as a simple three-neuron arc (Shepard and Telian, 1996). Discussions of this short latency network responsible for the VOR do not explain its adaptive capabilities when faced with an error signal.

The primitive nature of this three-neuron arc appears to allow for such short latencies in eye movement response to head movement. Any adaptation or recalibration in response to reduced visual acuity appears to take place higher in the brainstem. In other words, one part of the neural network is responsible for short latencies, whereas another part is responsible for accurate eye movements. (See Chapter 4 in *Audiology: Diagnosis* for a comprehensive overview of the vestibular system.)

As noted earlier, a gradual reduction in resting activity in the vestibular nuclei occurs on both sides after UVD. Regarding dynamic symptoms, a noted reduction in gain of the VOR also occurs in both directions immediately after unilateral labyrinthectomy. Over a period of days to weeks, a gradual increase in the gain of the VOR in response to head movements toward the lesioned side occurs. The gain of the VOR for head movements toward the intact labyrinth remains reduced compared with its preoperative level. This increase of gain on the lesioned side and reduction in gain on the intact side results in a reduction in asymmetrical

response to horizontal head movements (Smith and Curthoys, 1989).

Restoration of VOR function plays a large role in the recovery of dynamic visual acuity after unilateral vestibular injury. For slow to moderate head movements, the intact labyrinth can provide sufficient stimulation to both vestibular nuclei to allow for adequate VOR response (therefore clear vision). The inhibitory response from the intact labyrinth provides the necessary stimulus for these slow to moderate head movements. Because of the nonlinearity of the excitatory versus inhibitory responses of the sensory receptors (cristae) on the intact side, the faster the head movement, the less useful the inhibitory information from the intact side becomes when the head moves away from the intact side. There does not appear to be a measurable limit to the range of excitatory response, and the VOR responds normally to head movements toward the intact side up to 8 Hz. The inhibitory response saturates at zero spikes per second at moderate speed head movements, which prohibits the intact labyrinth from accurately responding to faster head movements away from the intact side. This deficit appears to be permanent and results in retinal slip with faster head movements toward the lesioned side (Curthoys and Halmagyi, 1996).

♦ Adaptive Strategies

Patients with loss of vestibular function, either unilateral or bilateral, adopt several strategies to increase gaze stability with head movement. In addition to the described recovery of the VOR through plasticity of the CNS, some behavioral changes and substitutions of vestibular responses take place.

Cervical-Ocular Reflex Input

The input of the cervical-ocular reflex (COR) has been recognized since Robert Barany's work in the early 1900s. The COR is thought to be a compensatory reflexive eye movement in response to stimulation from the ligaments, muscles, and joints in the neck. The COR's input for gaze stabilization in patients with normal vestibular function is insignificant (Bronstein and Hood, 1986). This is probably also true of patients with unilateral vestibular loss. In patients with bilateral loss of labyrinthine function, the COR has been shown to provide a small contribution to eye–head coordination at very low speeds of head movement.

Bronstein and Hood (1986, p. 407) reported that, "in the absence of vestibular function, the COR appears to take on the role of the vestibulo-ocular reflex in head-eye coordination in a) the initiation of the anti-compensatory saccade which takes the eyes in the direction of the target, and b) the generation of the subsequent slow compensatory eye movements." Kasai and Zee (1978) concluded that central preprogramming played a large role in COR functioning. The COR operates only at very low frequencies in normal subjects (maximum gain at 0.025 Hz, negligible at 0.4 Hz); however, significant contribution from the COR is noted in patients with vestibular loss up to 0.5 Hz (Kasai and Zee, 1978).

Modification of Saccades

Saccades are the fastest eye movements and may be voluntary or involuntary (as in the fast phase of nystagmus). Saccades allow us to refixate our gaze with minimal duration of retinal slip. The speed of initiation of a saccade is 150 to 250 msec when the target is unpredictable and ~76 msec with a predictable target (Leigh and Zee, 1999). Research indicates that saccades are amenable to increased efficiency through practice. Fischer and Ramsperger (1986) reported that daily practice results in a small but significant reduction in response latency and an increase in accuracy. Because response latency is significantly decreased when the target is predictable, it is likely that some central preprogramming of eye movements occurs when a patient with vestibular loss moves his or her head. These patients may make a voluntary saccade contralateral to the direction of head movement to compensate for the inefficient VOR response (Kasai and Zee, 1978). Through repetitive conditioning and feedback, patients tend to predict the necessary saccade in response to head movement. Modification of saccades is noted in both unilateral and bilateral patients.

Modification of Smooth Pursuit

Smooth pursuit tracking, or visual following, allows for gaze stability on objects moving through the field of vision. This type of eye movement is generated in the cerebellum and can either function alone while the head is still or can interact with the VOR to assist in gaze stability while moving. Smooth pursuit tracking ability does not appear to improve in well-compensated individuals with adult-onset vestibular loss. Smooth pursuit abilities tend to break down around 1 Hz in both normal individuals and labyrinthine-deficient patients.

Substitution of Sensory Inputs and Decreased Head Movements

After the loss of vestibular function bilaterally, a "reweighting" of priority and dependency on visual and somatosensory inputs occurs for the maintenance of balance and postural control. Initially, a shift toward visual dependency occurs. While walking, patients may visually lock on to targets and use this to provide information regarding relative motion. Gradually, these patients learn to more equally distribute their dependency on proprioceptive and visual information as well as remaining vestibular function.

A deficient VOR is not an issue when the head is not moving; therefore, some patients develop a strategy of avoiding any rapid head movements to prevent the symptoms of retinal slip. This strategy does not allow for the natural compensation process to take place and does not alter the fact that when the head is inevitably moved quickly, symptoms will ensue.

♦ Vestibular Rehabilitation Therapy Planning

In establishing reasonable goals and planning a therapy program suitable for a patient, the therapist must take into consideration several variables that include the following:

1. The patient's specific complaints and concerns regarding lifestyle limitations

2. Any permanent impairments not amenable to therapy

3. A realistic expected level of improvement

4. The therapist's concern regarding patient safety and the risk of falling

The therapist must base his or her recommendation of home-based exercises on the patient's risk of falling. In many cases, a family member can be trained to assist the patient while he or she exercises at home. Younger, healthier patients may not be at risk of falling and can complete most of the therapy program at home. It is not uncommon for patients to modify their exercises (usually by slowing down required movements) to avoid symptoms. To ensure that the patient has improved satisfactorily and to obtain outcome data, the patient is asked to attend one follow-up session several weeks later.

Controversial Point

• There has been much discussion over the past several years regarding the audiologist's role in vestibular rehabilitation. The Academy of Audiology (2000) position statement on diagnosis and treatment of vestibular disorders states that audiologists "participate as full members of the balance treatment team." It is recognized that there are patients who require the expertise and training of other allied health professionals. But where do you draw the line? Which patients can be managed by audiology alone? Which need to be referred, and to whom?

There is general agreement that canalith repositioning is within the scope of practice for audiologists. Other professionals, including physical therapists, primary care physicians, and chiropractors, also do canalith repositioning. There are two main groups of patients who are candidates for vestibular rehabilitation: those with stable vestibular dysfunction but no other contributory problems affecting their balance and mobility, and those with stable vestibular dysfunction, in addition to other contributory factors. Those in the first group can be managed by audiology alone. These patients tend to be younger, better able to understand and follow instructions, and less likely to fall and injure themselves during therapy exercises. It is the author's practice to send these patients home with an exercise program and follow up with them at 4 and 8 weeks.

The second group of patients tend to be older and in need of more hands-on guidance. Often there are other issues, such as weakness, joint instability, and visual deficits. The author refers these patients to physical therapy. It has been the author's experience that physical therapists add components to the therapy that audiologists would not have been able to address. A good physical therapist is invaluable in managing elderly patients with multifactorial balance problems.

Pitfall

- Many patients beginning therapy, as in any exercise program, feel worse before they begin to feel better. It is the practice of the author to ask patients to commit to 4 weeks of therapy before judging its effectiveness.

◆ Treatment Strategies

The goals of vestibular rehabilitation are as follows:

1. To minimize symptoms and functional disability

2. To increase mobility and independence

3. To reduce the risk of falls and injury

Treatment strategies are determined by the results of the vestibular evaluation, patient symptoms and complaints, pretherapy assessment, and general health and physical abilities of the patient. Patients may have specific functional limitations on which they wish to focus. The patient's general health and residual vestibular function may dictate reasonable therapy goals. In designing a program for vestibular rehabilitation, it is important to keep in mind that each patient will compensate in a different way. Vestibular rehabilitation exercises will assist the patient in developing compensatory strategies, but the specific compensatory technique each patient develops is unpredictable.

General guidelines to optimize the benefits of vestibular rehabilitation are as follows:

1. Make every effort to have the patient decrease the use of centrally sedating or vestibular-suppressant medications, such as diazepam and meclizine.

2. Exercises must provoke symptoms and create an "error signal." Adopt a "no pain, no gain" approach, educating the patient that the VOR will only modify its gain and symmetry when the brain recognizes a conflict or error signal situation.

3. Extensive counseling before initiating therapy may enhance patient compliance. Patients who understand their condition and its limitations and understand how their symptoms are provoked may be less fearful and more willing to continue therapy.

4. Therapy should be initiated as soon as possible.

5. Therapy sessions should be performed frequently to foster carryover and motor learning.

6. Exercises should be varied in speed and direction and should simulate real-life conditions when possible.

7. Once therapy goals have been reached, a general conditioning program and maintenance exercises are necessary to prevent a return of symptoms.

8. Patients should be counseled that they may experience periods of decompensation and may require further intensive therapy.

Treatment of Unilateral Vestibular Loss

Therapy designed to treat the patient with one normal functioning labyrinth and a loss or reduction in function in the other labyrinth is termed *adaptation therapy.* The goals of adaptation therapy are the following:

1. To promote tonic rebalancing of the vestibular nuclei

2. To decrease symptoms associated with head movements through habituation therapy

3. To increase gaze stability through modification and enhancement of oculomotor abilities

4. To increase postural stability through sensory integration training

Treatment of Bilateral Vestibular Loss

Therapy designed for the patient with bilateral vestibular loss is based on the premise that no remaining peripheral vestibular response to head movement exists, and therefore no VOR function exists. Appropriate therapy for the patient with absence of VOR function is termed *substitution therapy.* The goals of substitution therapy are as follows:

1 To promote the use of alternative sensory inputs, such as visual and somatosensory information, when vestibular function is lost

2. To promote alternative gaze stabilization strategies by enhancing oculomotor abilities and potentiating the COR

3. To teach the patient to recognize situations where alternative sensory information is unavailable or unreliable

4. To provide information regarding fall hazards and techniques to minimize the risk of falling

Some therapists may wish to design a therapy plan directed more toward the patient's specific complaints, which may not always correspond to vestibular tests results. Using this strategy, patients may be divided into three categories: gaze stabilization (for complaints of visual disorientation and blurring associated with head movement), motion sensitivity (for complaints of motion-induced nausea), and postural and gait stability (for complaints of unsteadiness).

Limits of Vestibular Rehabilitation

In designing a vestibular therapy program, the therapist must keep in mind that balance is a multisensory function, and impairments in any of the sensory systems involved in balance can limit the potential benefits of vestibular rehabilitation. As noted in the section on dynamic symptoms, a permanent impairment in the VOR response to rapid head movements in the direction of the damaged labyrinth can exist. Years after vestibular injury, horizontal VOR gain to rapid impulsive head movement toward the lesioned side may remain significantly less than normal. At head speeds > 2 Hz, no efficient strategies for correcting retinal slip exist, and in many well-compensated patients, this accounts for their only lasting complaint.

Unstable Lesions

Unstable lesions do not respond well to vestibular rehabilitation. Unstable lesions include conditions such as Meniere's disease and perilymph fistula. CNS adaptation depends on a stable asymmetry in the vestibular nuclei. Vestibular rehabilitation has been shown to be helpful in patients with Meniere's disease if their episodes are infrequent (i.e., several weeks minimum between episodes), but intensive therapy would need to be reinstituted after each episode. Ablative procedures are sometimes recommended to create a stable asymmetry. In these cases, vestibular rehabilitation should be started as soon as possible after the procedure.

Cerebellar Dysfunction

Cerebellar dysfunction as the result of stroke or degeneration inhibits vestibular rehabilitation. Tonic rebalancing and modifications to the gain of the VOR are believed to depend on plasticity within the cerebellum. If the cerebellum is dysfunctional, the adaptation process may be slower and limited. CNS abnormalities (e.g., cerebrovascular accident [CVA]) do not necessarily inhibit vestibular compensation if the lesion is not located within the vestibular pathways, although historically these patients require longer therapy programs. It is important to keep in mind that cerebellar dysfunction can be caused by vestibular or centrally sedating medications, because the goal of these medications is to reduce the asymmetry in activity by inhibiting the cerebellar response and activity within the vestibular nuclei. It is this same asymmetry that serves as a stimulus for adaptation and compensation.

Compromised Visual or Somatosensory Inputs

Compromised visual or somatosensory inputs are not uncommon in the elderly population. The potential, then, for sensory substitution is limited if a patient has decreased vision or proprioception. Normal visual changes with aging include reduced night vision resulting from yellowing of the cornea and a slowing of pupillary reaction to lighting changes. Binocular vision plays a role in depth perception and visual feedback of relative motion. Patients with monocular or asymmetrical vision are not uncommon,

particularly those in the process of having cataract surgery. Patients relying on visual feedback can be hampered by bifocal lenses. It is well known that magnifying lenses induce changes in VOR gain. Each time patients change their gaze through different lenses, they experience a change in magnification, which can lead to oscillopsia and visual disturbance. The constant alterations in spectacle magnification experienced with use of bifocals may inhibit appropriate changes in VOR gain.

To maximize recovery of the VOR, a visual stimulus for retinal slip is needed. If the patient is visually impaired, he or she may not be able to adequately see targets during therapy. Visual deprivation has been demonstrated to impede recovery of horizontal VOR function (Smith et al, 1986). Admittedly, these patients most likely do not relate visual blurring only in response to head movements.

Patients with peripheral sensory neuropathy or decreased leg strength as a result of injury may have limited use of proprioceptive feedback. Muscle mass is reduced by as much as 50% in the elderly, and leg strength is necessary for efficient use of ankle strategy.

Patient Compliance

Patient compliance is the key to a successful vestibular rehabilitation program. Desmond and Touchette (1998) reported that 35% of patients for whom vestibular rehabilitation was recommended elected not to participate in a therapy program. They found that most of these patients stated that they were "not interested" even though they apparently felt a need to undergo vestibular evaluation. The authors interpreted this as a lack of motivation or confidence on the part of patients that they could benefit from therapy. Physicians who do not understand, or accept, the concept of vestibular rehabilitation may reinforce this attitude.

Vestibular Therapy and "Central" Lesions

Patients with persistent complaints regarding postural stability of "central" origin have long been considered to have limited potential benefit from vestibular therapy and have been eliminated from most studies of vestibular rehabilitation. Because the actual process of adaptation is believed to take place in the cerebellum and brainstem, injuries to the central region may reasonably limit vestibular adaptation and ultimately impair overall compensation from vestibular injury. Patients with migraine-related vertigo have been shown to benefit from vestibular rehabilitation (Whitney et al, 2000). However, patients with migraine in addition to peripheral vestibulopathy do not benefit from therapy as much as those with pure vestibular dysfunction (Wrisley et al, 2002).

✦ Fall Prevention

Falls occur frequently and are the leading cause of injuries and injury deaths in the elderly population. Almost 40% of the geriatric population of the United States experiences a fall each year (Hausdorff et al, 2001). Falls leading to hip fracture often result in premature institutionalization and death, as well as enormous health care costs. Approximately 40% of elderly American patients with hip fractures die within 1 year or are placed in long-term care. Clearly, this is a staggering health care problem, which will increase dramatically as the elderly population increases. No one argues that we, as health care and medical professionals, should intervene. The questions, rather, are What should we do? and Will it actually make a difference?

Much attention has been paid to this subject in recent years, and systematic evaluation and intervention are on the rise in the United States. In fact, the Elder Fall Prevention Act of 2003 (H.R. 3513) which was passed in August of 2007, sought "to expand and intensify programs with respect to research and related activities concerning elder falls."

Poor balance and instability in the elderly have been described as part of a "geriatric syndrome," because the specific causes of these complaints are often not obvious to the examiner. This is primarily because poor balance in the elderly is most often multifactorial, with no single clinical abnormality responsible. The risk factors for increased likelihood of falling have been identified, and intervention for these risk factors has been shown to significantly reduce the risk of falling. Obviously, intervention cannot eliminate the possibility of an injurious fall, but research indicates that systematic evaluation and intervention can dramatically reduce the likelihood of a fall.

Tinetti et al (1994) studied a group of elderly (at least 70 years old) subjects with known risk factors for falling. By applying interventions aimed at specific risk factors, the intervention group had significantly fewer falls than the untreated control group. Specifically, subjects identified with "balance impairment" had the greatest reduction in falls (over 50% fewer). Close et al (1999) followed a group of elderly (65 years+) patients who had presented to an emergency room after a fall injury. After medical and occupational therapy assessment, the intervention group received care for identified risk factors for falling. At 1 year follow-up, the control group had more than twice as many falls as the intervention group.

Jacobson (2002) expanded on these findings by developing an assessment protocol to identify risk factors in patients who had fallen or had fear of falling. At the author's facility (Blue Ridge Hearing and Balance Clinic, Bluefield, WV), the author has modeled the Fall Prevention Clinic (FPC) after the protocol outlined by Jacobson. With the cooperative effort of otolaryngology and physical therapy departments, the author began a program to identify at the primary care level those at risk of falling, provide assessment for known risk factors for falling, and provide education, intervention, and environmental modification when indicated.

Screening in Primary Care

Elderly patients may not be aware they are at increased risk of falling. Unfortunately, examinations to determine the cause of fall injuries, if done at all, typically take place after the fact. The known risk factors often develop independently and insidiously. A simple screening procedure at the primary

care level may identify some of the known risk factors, and intervention can begin. The questionnaire in Appendix 19–1 was developed for use by primary care physicians. Because some physicians may be unfamiliar with the implications of a positive response to some of the questions, the author developed a physician's guide (see Appendix 19–1) to help physicians interpret the answers to the screener questions.

Assessment

When a patient is referred for a fall risk assessment at FPC, the author follows an evaluation protocol to assess many of the known risk factors. Following a thorough history interview, the patient undergoes a series of tests of hearing and vestibular function: audiogram, electronystagmography (ENG), rotary chair test, and posturography. Evaluation for orthostatic hypotension and a review of medications and interactions are performed. The author works with physical therapists in the region to provide a comprehensive assessment of known risk factors that are out of the scope of audiology practice. Examination for strength, sensation, and range of motion of the lower extremities is performed. Screening tests for depression and cognition are completed. The patient's lifestyle, concerns, and goals are reviewed. A report is then forwarded to the referring physician with recommendations for intervention. The primary care physician is provided with a checklist (Appendix 19–2) of applicable risk factors, along with suggestions for intervention. This checklist quickly allows the physician to view risk factors that have been identified in that particular patient, a brief description of how and why that factor affects balance, and a suggestion on intervention strategy. With the multifactorial nature of disequilibrium of aging, the primary care physician must be the center point of coordinated intervention.

Physical Therapy Assessment of Multifactorial Balance Disorders

See **Table 19–1** for tests to assess balance disorders.

◆ Benign Paroxysmal Positional Vertigo

BPPV represents the single most likely diagnosis in a patient complaining of vertigo and accounts for up to 30% of patients with peripheral vestibular dysfunction (Epley, 1992a). Diagnosis and treatment of BPPV do not require sophisticated or expensive equipment. The theory behind treating BPPV is unlike that of other vestibular pathological conditions. Whereas most vestibular rehabilitation strategies use repetition, motor learning, and CNS plasticity in hopes of relieving symptoms, treatment for BPPV typically includes none of these.

Pathophysiology of BPPV

General agreement exists that the site of lesion in BPPV is the ampulla of the offending semicircular canal, with the posterior canal of one labyrinth involved in 90% of cases.

Table 19–1 Physical Therapy Assessment of Multifactorial Balance Disorders

Manual muscle test
  Muscle groups are tested for strength and symmetry (i.e., right leg vs left leg). Resistance against the therapist's hand is subjectively judged on a 0 (minimum) to 5 (maximum) performance scale.
Range of motion
  Evaluation is performed for reduced mobility of ankle, knee, and hip joints. This is objectively measured using an instrument known as a goniometer that measures changes in joint position referenced to baseline.
Sensation
  Lower extremity sensation can be assessed using subjective responses to pin prick, vibration, and sharp/dull discrimination.
Coordination
  Subjective assessment of the patient's ability to perform smooth, rhythmic movements of the upper and lower extremities provides assessment of gross motor control.
Posture
  Subjective observation of head position on spine, spinal alignment, and position of trunk is performed.

Typical diagnostic signs include the following:

1. A provoking position (lying supine with affected ear down)

2. A short latency before vertigo and nystagmus occur (usually 3–15 seconds)

3. Severe subjective vertigo accompanied by nystagmus (typically geotropic rotary nystagmus when the posterior canal is involved)

4. A short duration of symptoms (usually < 1 minute)

5. Fatigability (repeated provocation results in a reduced response)

6. A reversal in the direction of nystagmus on rising (sometimes)

BPPV is by far the most common cause of episodic vertigo and has historically been found to be frequently misdiagnosed and ineffectively treated at the primary care level (Li et al, 2000). Von Brevern et al (2002) estimate that only 4% of BPPV patients are offered canalith repositioning treatment. Patients typically report brief episodes (< 1 minute) of intense vertigo, usually brought on by lying down, rolling over in bed, or tilting the head back. BPPV is a mechanical dysfunction of the inner ear and does not usually represent an ongoing disease process. It is relatively easily diagnosed and treated. BPPV does not respond to medication, but rather is most effectively treated by canalith repositioning procedures. The typical pattern of BPPV is one of intermittent episodes. The vertigo (spinning sensation) may occur frequently for weeks at a time, disappear for months, then reappear with no warning.

BPPV is believed to be a result of a plug of calcium carbonate and protein crystals (otoconia) that have become dislodged from the utricle, settling most frequently in the posterior semicircular canal. Otoconia cause no problem until the patient moves in a manner stimulating the offending semicircular canal. The otoconia then begin moving, causing abnormal stimulation of the motion sensor in the affected ear. While the otoconia are in motion (typically 15–45 seconds), the patient is experiencing conflicting signals from the two labyrinths of the inner ear.

BPPV can be diagnosed by performing the Dix-Hallpike maneuver (see Chapter 25 in *Audiology: Diagnosis*). If this maneuver makes the patient vertiginous, the eyes are simultaneously inspected for nystagmus. The direction of the nystagmus allows for identification of the specific offending canal. Once this has been accomplished, the patient can be treated.

Many patients with BPPV will also complain of associated disequilibrium and postural instability. Some speculation exists that there may be abnormal responses from the affected semicircular canal or that the otolith structures (particularly the utricles) are no longer functioning symmetrically as a result of displaced otoconia. Blatt et al (2000) determined that simple canalith repositioning treatments improved complaints of postural instability and improved posturography scores in patients complaining of postural instability associated with BPPV.

Schuknecht (1969) first proposed the theory of cupulolithiasis, in which he suggested that BPPV was the result of otoconial debris attached to the cupula of the offending posterior semicircular canal. Epley (1992a) offered an alternative theory of canalithiasis that more thoroughly explains the source of the above-mentioned typical signs and symptoms of BPPV. The theory of canalithiasis proposes that there are free-floating particles (otoconia) that have gravitated from the utricle and collect near the cupula of the posterior canal. When the head is moved into a position that causes the particles to move away from the cupula, the resulting hydrodynamic drag causes cupular deflection (and asymmetrical stimulation), resulting in vertigo and nystagmus until the particles come to rest in the now gravitationally dependent section of the canal. It is likely that both of these conditions exist, and treatments have been proposed for both.

Treatment for Cupulolithiasis

Brandt and Daroff (1980) found that the symptoms of BPPV were quickly relieved by repeatedly provoking symptoms through head-positioning exercises. They speculated that the noted rapid improvement was not a result of habituation, but rather a means of dispersion of otolithic debris from the cupula. The liberatory or Semont maneuver **(Fig. 19–2)** was described in detail by Semont et al (1988). Semont and his colleagues, over an 8-year period involving 711 cases, reported an 84% success rate after one maneuver and a 93% success rate after two maneuvers. Theoretically, the movement required to displace otoconia from the cupula must be relatively rapid and may be contraindicated in elderly patients or patients with a history of back or neck problems.

Treatment for Canalithiasis

The canalith repositioning procedure for canalithiasis was introduced by John Epley of the Portland Otologic Clinic in Portland, Oregon. This procedure has undergone several modifications and is known by a variety of names:

1. Canalith repositioning procedure (CRP)

2. Canalith repositioning maneuver (CRM)

3. Particle repositioning maneuver

4. Epley maneuver

All these procedures are based on the belief that free-floating otoconia in the posterior canal are responsible for BPPV. The goal of each maneuver is to cause the otoconia debris to migrate out of the posterior canal, through the common crus, and into the vestibule. Yamane et al (1984) proposed that "dark cells" of the utricle absorb and dissolve the otoconia, whereas others (Mira et al, 1996) suggest that the otoconia harmlessly dissolve in the endolymph. The natural course of BPPV, with spontaneous remission within a few weeks, may be a confounding factor in determining precisely the success rate of CRP, but there is general agreement that CRP is a safe and effective treatment for BPPV.

Epley's original description of CRP is as follows:

Preliminary   Identification of offending canal and noted latency and duration of nystagmus response

Preparation   Premedication with transdermal scopolamine or diazepam

Maneuvers   Commencement of maneuvers as described in **Fig. 19–3,** changing head positions when the nystagmus response has ceased. If no nystagmus is appreciated, an estimate of latency plus duration of previous response (typically 6–13 seconds) dictates when the head is moved to the next position. Complete cycles are performed until no nystagmus response is present.

Oscillation   A handheld oscillator with a frequency of ~80 Hz is applied to the mastoid process of the affected side.

Follow-up   Patients are advised to keep their head upright for 48 hours after the procedure. CRP may be repeated weekly until the patient is asymptomatic and no nystagmus is noted in the Hallpike position (Epley, 1992b).

The procedure for CRP has undergone some modifications since it was introduced by Epley. Many practicing clinicians do not use any type of oscillation, with results similar to those of Epley (1992b). The length of time the patient needs to remain upright after treatment has also been modified. Some period of time has been recommended to keep the free-floating otoconia from gravitating back into the posterior canal. Although most published reports recommend 48 hours, it is the author's practice to simply ask the patient to refrain from any bending or tilting of the head for 24 hours and to sleep with two or three pillows for one night. The success rate for this procedure is similar to previous reports of efficacy. Several recent reports (Cohen and Kimball, 2004; Marciano and Marcelli, 2002; Roberts et al, 2005) indicate that no post-treatment restrictions may be necessary.

Variant Forms of BPPV

BPPV can also occur in the anterior and horizontal semicircular canals. Anterior canal BPPV is extremely rare, but horizontal canal BPPV is common. Both canalithiasis and

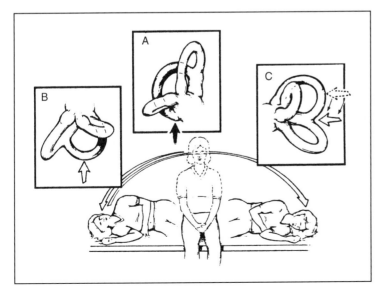

Figure 19–2 The Semont maneuver. The patient is moved quickly from sitting **(A)** into the position that provokes vertigo **(B)** and is kept in that position for 2 to 3 minutes. She is then turned rapidly to the opposite ear-down position **(C),** with the therapist maintaining the alignment of the neck and head on the body. The patient must stay in this position for 5 minutes. The patient is then slowly taken into a seated position. She must remain in the vertical position for 48 hours and avoid the provoking position for 1 week. The position of the right labyrinth is shown in each head position, and the posterior canal is shaded. The solid arrow indicates the location of the cupula of the posterior canal; the open arrow indicates the location of debris free-floating in the long arm of the posterior canal during the different stages of the treatment. (From Herdman, S. J., Tusa, R. J., Zee, D. S., et al. (1993). Single treatment approaches to benign paroxysmal positional vertigo. Archives of Otolaryngology–Head and Neck Surgery, 119, 450–454, with permission.)

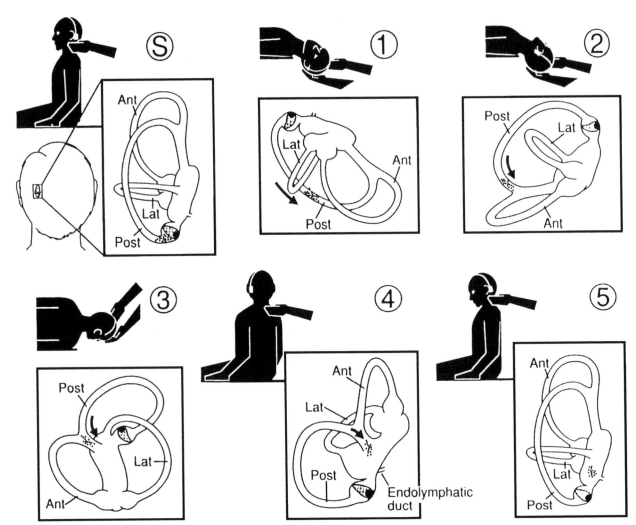

Figure 19–3 Positions of the left posterior semicircular canal (PSC). **(S)** Starting position. **(1)** Patient is brought into the offending left Hallpike position, causing flow of debris away from the cupula of the left PSC. **(2)** While the patient remains in the supine position, the head is rotated to the right side. **(3)** With the orientation of the head to the right shoulder unchanged, the patient is rolled over onto his right shoulder and hip, looking down toward the floor. **(4)** The head remains to the right, tilted down, as the patient rises to the sitting position. **(5)** The head is rotated forward, chin tilted down. The patient should be kept in each of these positions until nystagmus has ceased or for a period of time at least equal to the duration of time from initiation of provoking (Hallpike) maneuver to the cessation of nystagmus. Nystagmus should be viewed in all positions because a change in the direction of nystagmus indicates possible failure to deposit all the debris in the vestibule. Ant, anterior; Lat, lateral; post, posterior. (From Epley, J. (1992). The camalith repositioning procedure: for treatment of benign paroxysmal positional vertigo. Otolaryngology–Head and Neck Surgery, 107(3), 399–404, with permission.)

cupulolithiasis have been implicated as causative factors and may be the determining factors in the direction of nystagmus noted. Anterior canal BPPV is most typically provoked by a Hallpike maneuver with the affected ear on the up side. Because the same position can trigger posterior canal BPPV of the down-side ear, differentiating canal involvement is done by observing the direction of nystagmus while the patient experiences vertigo. As noted earlier, posterior canal BPPV is marked by geotropic (beating toward the earth) rotary nystagmus; in anterior canal BPPV, the nystagmus is primarily ageotropic (beating away from the earth). Treatment of anterior canal BPPV may be accomplished by performing CRP as if treating posterior canal BPPV in the opposite ear.

Horizontal canal BPPV may be elicited during the Hallpike maneuver, but it is best provoked by having the patient lie in the supine position or in the 30 degree elevated position, then move the head quickly to the ear-down position, both to the right and to the left. Horizontal canal BPPV may be diagnosed by observing horizontal geotropic nystagmus while the patient is vertiginous. The patient is typically more vertiginous, and the intensity of the nystagmus is greater, when the affected ear is down. As in other forms of BPPV, there is a short latency and a transient response, with a duration typically longer than that observed in BPPV of the other two canals. Repositioning technique for horizontal canal BPPV involves having the patient, starting in the supine position, rotate 360 degrees in the direction away from the affected canal. The author has found that simply performing a modification of the Epley maneuver with the patient's head elevated to 30 degrees will often clear the horizontal canal of free-floating debris.

Home Treatment of BPPV

Some patients present with a history consistent with BPPV; however, Hallpike tests on the day of examination fail to provoke an episode of vertigo. One option in this instance is to have the patient reschedule, with instructions to avoid any head tilt for a few hours prior to the reexamination. If an episode of BPPV can be provoked at a later date, appropriate repositioning can be completed. The author (Desmond, 2002) has found that in a series of 101 consecutive patients presenting with histories consistent with BPPV, ~50% had a negative Dix-Hallpike at the time of exam. Of those willing to return for repeat testing, 40% had a positive Dix-Hallpike and received treatment. Occasionally, a patient will not be willing or able to return, or may have a negative Dix-Hallpike test a second or third time. In these instances, home-based exercises may be recommended.

Brandt-Daroff Exercises

Home provocation exercises intended to relieve BPPV have been used since they were introduced by Brandt and Daroff in 1980. Prior to this, many patients with symptoms of BPPV were advised to avoid the offending position. Brandt and Daroff (1980) speculated that repeated provocation of the positional vertigo would promote loosening and ultimate dispersion of the otolithic debris from the cupula. They reported that 66 of 67 patients experienced complete relief of the positional vertigo within 14 days, with most requiring 7 to 10 days. Positional nystagmus also was absent. The Brandt-Daroff exercises, as described in **Fig. 19–4,** are designed to intentionally provoke episodes of BPPV repeatedly in a controlled safe manner. The positions are strikingly similar to

those used in the Semont maneuver (discussed earlier in this chapter). The movements differ in that in the Brandt-Daroff exercises, the patient comes back to the sitting position and rests before continuing with additional movements.

Modified Epley Procedure

Radtke et al (1999) compared the efficacy of Brandt-Daroff exercises with a modified canalith repositioning procedure intended for self-treatment of BPPV **(Figs. 19–5** and **19–6).** Their modified Epley procedure (MEP) is very similar to the previously described repositioning procedure of Epley, with the exceptions of no oscillation, no antiemetic medication, and no follow-up period of keeping the head erect after repositioning. The patient is instructed to perform the modified procedure 3 times a day, daily, until he or she is free of positional vertigo for 24 hours. Radtke et al (1999) reported that after 1 week, 18 of 28 patients (64%) using the MEP were asymptomatic compared with 6 of 26 patients (23%) using the Brandt-Daroff exercises. Although these data indicate that the MEP may be more effective than the Brandt-Daroff exercises, neither is nearly as effective as single-treatment CRP, as described earlier. In the author's clinic, the author has used the exercises described by Radtke et al (1999). Over 90% of patients at the clinic complaining of positional vertigo but having negative vestibular function tests, including Dix-Hallpike, have resolution of positional vertigo symptoms at 2-week follow-up using these exercises.

Although success rates of CRP are impressive, several patients with intractable positional vertigo do not respond to repositioning procedures. These patients may be candidates for surgical intervention. Surgical procedures to relieve the symptoms of BPPV include sectioning of the posterior nerve (singular neurectomy) to eliminate response from the ampulla of the posterior canal and occlusion of the posterior canal (canal plugging) to preclude loose otoconia from entering the posterior canal.

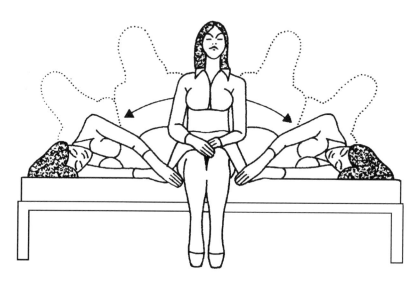

Figure 19–4 Brandt-Daroff exercises for benign paroxysmal positional vertigo are performed by having the patient repeatedly move from a sitting position to the affected side, waiting until the vertigo stops, then resuming the sitting position. The movement can then be repeated in the opposite direction if the affected side is unknown. (From Brandt, T., & Daroff, R. (1980). Physical therapy for benign paroxysmal positional vertigo. Archives of Otolaryngology, 106, 484–485, with permission.)

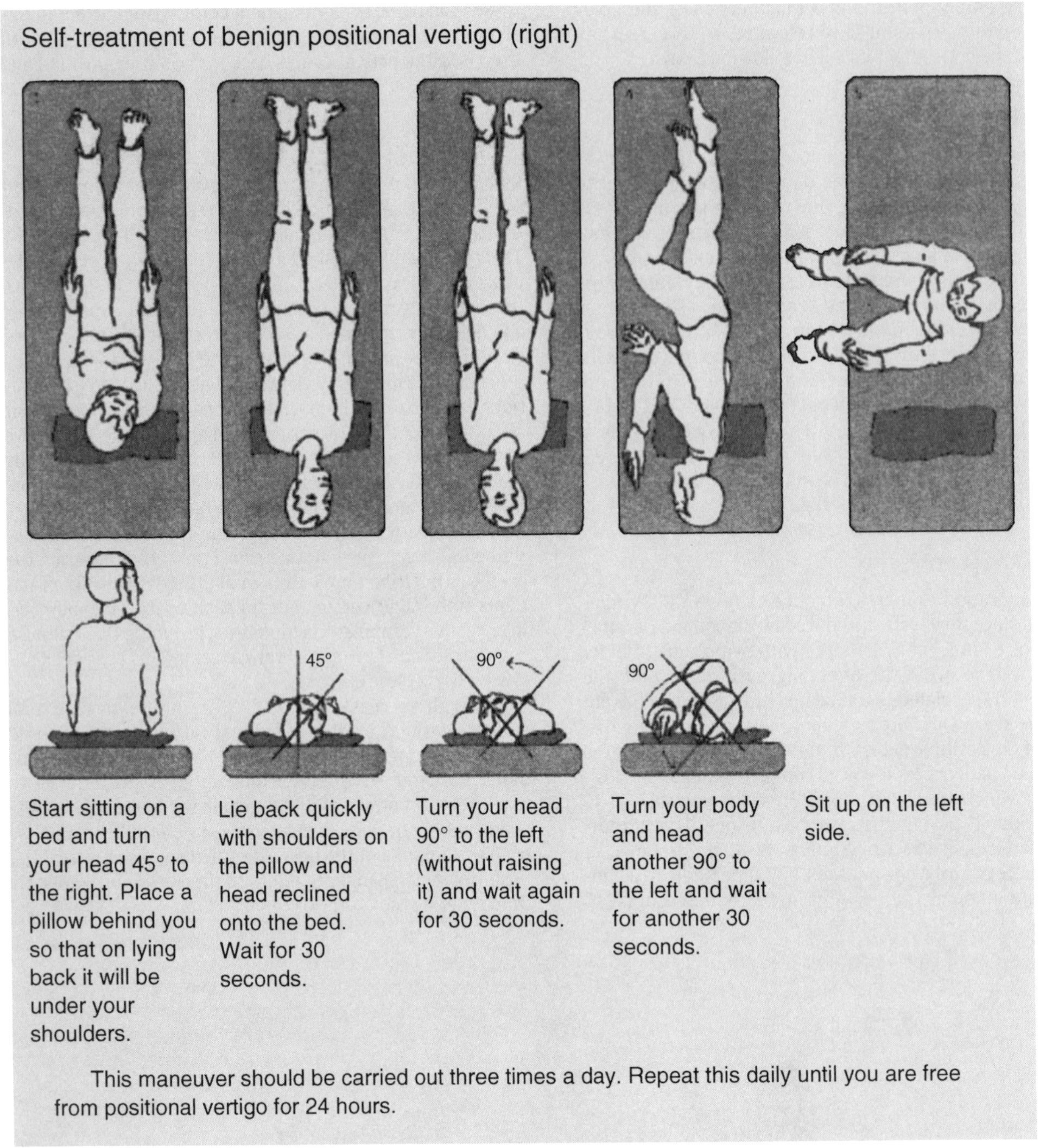

Self-treatment of benign positional vertigo (right)

Start sitting on a bed and turn your head 45° to the right. Place a pillow behind you so that on lying back it will be under your shoulders.

Lie back quickly with shoulders on the pillow and head reclined onto the bed. Wait for 30 seconds.

Turn your head 90° to the left (without raising it) and wait again for 30 seconds.

Turn your body and head another 90° to the left and wait for another 30 seconds.

Sit up on the left side.

This maneuver should be carried out three times a day. Repeat this daily until you are free from positional vertigo for 24 hours.

Figure 19–5 Right benign paroxysmal positional vertigo self-treatment technique. (From Radtke, A., Neuhauser, H., Von Brevern, M., et al. (1999). A modified Epley's procedure for self-treatment of benign paroxysmal positional vertigo. Neurology, 53, 1358–1360, with permission.)

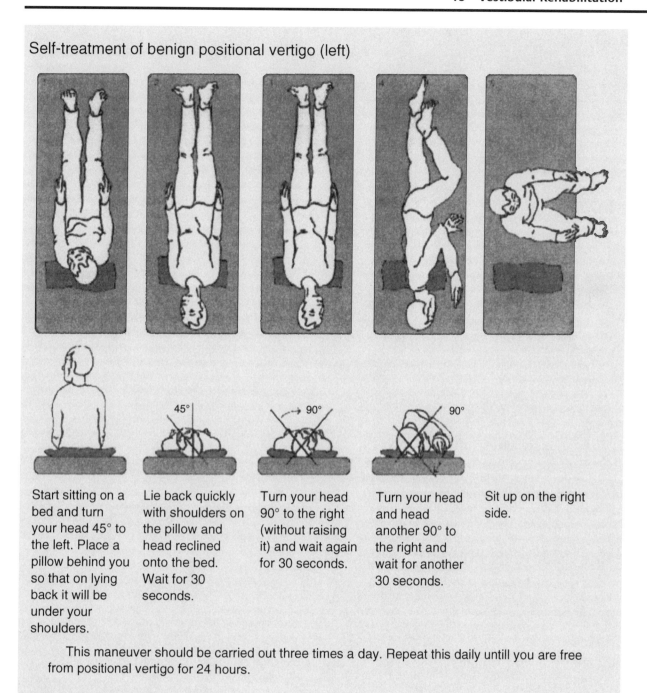

Self-treatment of benign positional vertigo (left)

Start sitting on a bed and turn your head 45° to the left. Place a pillow behind you so that on lying back it will be under your shoulders.

Lie back quickly with shoulders on the pillow and head reclined onto the bed. Wait for 30 seconds.

Turn your head 90° to the right (without raising it) and wait again for 30 seconds.

Turn your head and head another 90° to the right and wait for another 30 seconds.

Sit up on the right side.

This maneuver should be carried out three times a day. Repeat this daily untill you are free from positional vertigo for 24 hours.

Figure 19–6 Left BPPV self-treatment technique. (From Radtke, A., Neuhauser, H., Van Brevern, M., et al, (1999). A modified Epley's procedure for self-treatment of benign paroxysmal positional vertigo. Neurology, 53; 1358–1360, with permission.)

♦ Summary

Research and clinical experience indicate that a large number of patients with vestibular dysfunction can benefit from vestibular therapy. Past approaches to treating patients with dizziness have been shown to be less effective than a customized intensive therapy program. However, vestibular rehabilitation is still in its early stages. The goal of this chapter is to review the clinical evidence, explain the basis for vestibular adaptation and compensation, and give the reader some practical tools to begin a vestibular rehabilitation program.

Acknowledgments   There are aspects of the assessment for risk of falls that are clearly out of the scope of practice and expertise of audiology. Kim Slemp, PT, Smyth County Community Hospital, Marion, VA, contributed the information regarding physical therapy assessment of the multifactorial balance disordered patient.

Appendix 19–1

Fall Risk Questionnaire

Name _____ Date _____

Please answer all questions.

Yes No

1. ☐ ☐ Have you had a fall or near-fall in the past year?
2. ☐ ☐ Do you have a fear of falling that restricts your activity?
3. ☐ ☐ Do you experience dizziness or a sensation of spinning when you lie down, tilt your head back, or roll over in bed?
4. ☐ ☐ Do you feel uneasy or unsteady when walking down the aisle of a supermarket, for instance, or in an area congested with other people?
5. ☐ ☐ Do you have difficulty walking in the dark or on uneven surfaces, such as gravel or a sloped sidewalk?
6. ☐ ☐ Do your feet or toes frequently feel unusually hot or cold, numb or tingly?
7. ☐ ☐ Do you wear bifocal or trifocal glasses, or is your vision notably better in one eye?
8. ☐ ☐ Do you experience loss of balance or a lightheaded/faint feeling when you stand up?
9. ☐ ☐ Do you take medication for depression, anxiety, nerves, insomnia (lack of sleep), or pain?
10. ☐ ☐ Do you take four or more prescription medications daily?
11. ☐ ☐ Do you feel as if your feet just won't go where you want them to go?
12. ☐ ☐ Do you feel as if you can't walk a straight line or are pulled to the side while walking?
13. ☐ ☐ Has it been longer than 6 months since you participated in a regular exercise program?
14. ☐ ☐ Do you feel that no one really understands how much dizziness and balance problems affect your quality of life?
15. ☐ ☐ Are you interested in improving your balance and mobility?

Physician's Guide to the Fall Risk Questionnaire

Questions 1 and 2: A previous fall may indicate increased risk for future falls. Inquire as to the circumstances of the fall. Fear of falling can lead to restricted activity.

Questions 3, 4, and 5: A positive response to any of these questions indicates the possibility of a vestibular disorder. Patients with BPPV are at risk of falling if they tilt their head back. Patients with vestibular disorders tend to be more reliant on vision for postural control. When the visual feedback is unreliable (moving visual scene) or unavailable (dark), patients are at risk of loss of balance and falling. Vestibular evaluation may be indicated (e.g., ENG, posturography, and rotary chair test).

Questions 5 and 6: The sense of touch is an important contributor to balance and orientation. The stretch receptors in the legs, the fingertips, and the soles of the feet provide sensory feedback for balance. An assessment for peripheral neuropathy may be indicated.

Question 7: Vision plays an important role in balance, and patients with visual deficits have greater risk of falls. Visual problems associated with decreased postural stability include visual acuity less than 20/50, asymmetric vision-impairing binocular vision and depth perception, slow pupillary reaction causing increased adaptation time when going from a lighted to a dark room, and vice versa, and impaired peripheral vision.

Multifocal glasses have been shown to increase the risk of falling. Ophthalmology evaluation may be indicated.

Question 8: Orthostatic hypotension may result in an increased risk of falling when assuming the upright position. Diabetes and many medications used to regulate heart rate and blood pressure can lead to orthostatic hypotension.

Questions 9 and 10: The use of four or more daily prescription medications and the use of tricyclic antidepressants and/or benzodiazepines are associated with increased risk of falls.

Questions 11 and 12: Poor motor control is a sign of possible cerebellar dysfunction. The integration of vestibular, visual, and somatosensory information takes place in the cerebellum. Cerebellar dysfunction can result in slow or inappropriate reaction to self-movement or external visual stimuli.

Question 13: Inactive patients may have accelerated decrease in muscle mass and decreased reaction time when faced with a possible fall.

Question 14: Physicians often underestimate (compared with the patient) the impact that a balance problem has on the patient's quality of life.

Question 15: Therapy for improved balance requires motivation and commitment. Patient compliance is important to a successful fall prevention program.

Appendix 19–2

Risk Factors and Intervention Suggestions

Intervention

Name _____ Date _____

Referring Physician _____

The following have been identified as possible factors in increasing this patient's risk of future falls.

___**Vestibular pathology:** An impairment of the vestibular system can cause the patient to become dizzy or off-balance; associated with certain movements and certain visual environments. Vestibular rehabilitation can minimize the effects of this impairment.

___**Polypharmacy:** The use of four or more prescription medications or the initiation of a new medication or dosage has been associated with an increased risk of falling. A review of all medications by the primary care physician is indicated.

___**Use of tricyclic antidepressants or benzodiazepines:** Associated with increased risk of falls. Selective serotonin reuptake inhibitor (SSRI) antidepressants may have fewer side effects, but it is not clear that they result in a reduced risk of falling compared with tricyclics and benzodiazepines. A review of the patient's medications is indicated.

___**Orthostatic (postural) hypotension:** Postural presyncope associated with orthostatic hypotension may result in an increased risk of falling when assuming the upright position. Diabetes and many medications used to regulate the heart rate and blood pressure can suppress the carotid sinus reflex and result in temporary cerebral hypoperfusion. Increased fluids, support hose, and/or brief exercise (fist clenching, etc.) before standing can reduce the effect of orthostatic hypotension. A review of medications is indicated.

___**Impaired proprioception (somatosensation):** The sense of touch is an important contributor to balance and orientation. The stretch receptors in the legs, the fingertips, and the soles of the feet provide feedback. Balance retraining therapy can help the patient use vestibular and visual feedback to compensate for loss of proprioceptive information. Vestibular rehabilitation is recommended.

___**Cerebellar dysfunction:** The integration of vestibular, visual, and proprioceptive information takes place in the cerebellum. Cerebellar dysfunction can result in slow or inappropriate reaction to self-movement and external visual stimuli. Vestibular rehabilitation can maximize the patient's potential, but benefit is often limited. Environmental assessment and reduction of fall hazards are recommended.

___**Hearing loss:** Hearing loss reduces one's orientation and awareness of one's surroundings. A person with hearing loss is more likely to be startled by movement in the visual field, as he or she has fewer auditory warning signals. Amplification may be helpful.

___**Impaired vision:** Vision plays an important role in balance, and patients with visual deficits have greater risk of falls. Visual problems associated with decreased postural stability include visual acuity less than 20/50, asymmetric vision-impairing binocular vision and depth perception, slow pupillary reaction causing increased adaptation time when going from a lighted to a dark room, and vice versa, and impaired peripheral vision. Ophthalmologic or optometric evaluation is recommended.

___**Depression:** Depressed patients may be more internally (therefore less externally) aware. The use of antidepressant and anxiolytics increases the risk of falling. Psychiatric or psychological evaluation is recommended.

___**Impaired cognition:** Patients with impaired cognition may be less aware of their surroundings or more likely to engage in risky activities. Neurologic evaluation is recommended.

___**Impaired reaction time:** Many fall avoidance strategies are dependent on reaction time when postural stability is challenged. Slower reaction time may increase the risk of falls when the patient's limits of stability are exceeded. Neurologic evaluation is recommended.

References

American Academy of Audiology. (2000). Position statement on the audiologist's role in the diagnosis and treatment of vestibular disorders. Retrieved from http://www.audiology.org/professional/positions/vestibular.php

American Speech-Language-Hearing Association. (1996). Scope of practice in audiology. ASHA Supplement, 16(38), 2, 12–15.

Bamiou, D. E., Davies, R., McKee, M., & Luxon, L. (2000). Symptoms, disability and handicap in unilateral peripheral vestibular disorders: Effects of early presentation and initiation of balance exercises. Scandinavian Audiology, 29(4), 238–244.

Bienhold, H., & Flor, H. (1978). Role of commissural connections between vestibular nuclei in compensation after unilateral labyrinthectomy. Journal of Physiology, 284, 178P.

Blatt, P. J., Georgakakis, G., Herdman, S., et al. (2000). The effect of the canalith repositioning maneuver on resolving postural instability in patients with benign paroxysmal positional vertigo. American Journal of Otology, 21(3), 356–363.

Brandt, T. (1991). Medical and physical therapy. In T. Brandt (Ed.), Vertigo: Its multisensory syndromes (pp. 15–17). New York: Springer-Verlag.

Brandt, T., & Daroff, R. (1980). Physical therapy for benign paroxysmal positional vertigo. Archives of Otolaryngology, 106, 484–485.

Bronstein, A. M., & Hood, D. (1986). The cervico-ocular reflex in normal subjects and patients with absent vestibular function. Brain Research, 373, 399–408.

Cawthorne, T. (1945). The physiological basis for head exercises. Chart Social Physiotherapy, 30, 106–107.

Close, J., Ellis, M., Hooper, R., et al. (1999). Prevention of falls in the elderly trial (PROFET): A randomized controlled trial. Lancet, 353(9147), 93–97.

Cohen, H. S., & Kimball, K. (2004). Treatment variations on the Epley maneuver for benign paroxysmal positional vertigo. American Journal of Otolaryngology, 25(1), 33–37.

Cooksey, F. S. (1945). Rehabilitation in vestibular injuries. Proceedings of the Royal Society of Medicine: Section of Otology, 273–278.

Curthoys, I. S., & Halmagyi, G. M. (1996). How does the brain compensate for vestibular lesions? In R. W. Baloh & G. M. Halmagyi (Eds.), Disorders of the vestibular system (pp. 145–154). New York: Oxford University Press.

Demer, J. L. Porter, F. I., Goldberg, J., et al. (1989). Adaptation to telescopic spectacles: Vestibulo-ocular reflex plasticity. Investigative Opthalmology and Visual Science, 30(1), 159–170.

Desmond, A. (2002). Reduce false negatives in BPPV diagnosis. Advance for Audiologists, 4(4), 27.

Desmond, A. L., & Touchette, D. A. (1998). Balance disorders: Evaluation and treatment; a short course for primary care physicians. Micromedical Technologies. Available at http://www.micromedical.com/book.htm

Dix, M. (1984). Rehabilitation of vertigo. In M. R. Dix & J. D. Hood (Eds.), Vertigo (pp. 467–479). New York: John Wiley & Sons.

Epley, J. (1992a). BPPV diagnosis and management: Vestibular update. Micromedical Technologies, 8, 1–4.

Epley, J. (1992b). The canalith repositioning procedure: For treatment of benign paroxysmal positional vertigo. Archives of Otolaryngology–Head and Neck Surgery, 107(3), 399–404.

Fischer, B., & Ramsperger, E. (1986). Human express saccades: Effects of randomization and daily practice. Experiments in Brain Research, 64, 569–578.

Gresty, M. A., Hess, K., & Leech, J. (1977). Disorders of the vestibulo-ocular reflex producing oscillopsia and mechanisms compensating for loss of labyrinthine function. Brain, 100, 693–716.

Hausdorff, J. M., Rios, D., & Edelberg, H. (2001). Gait variability and fall risk in community-living older adults: A 1 year prospective study. Archives of Physical and Medical Rehabilitation, 82(8), 1050–1056.

Herdman, S. J., Tusa, R., Blatt, P., et al. (1998). Computerized dynamic visual acuity test in the assessment of vestibular deficits. American Journal of Otology, 19, 790–796.

Jacobson, G. (2002). Development of a clinic for the assessment of risk of falls in elderly patients. Seminars in Hearing, 23(2), 161–178.

Kasai, T., & Zee, D. (1978). Eye-head coordination in labyrinthine-defective human beings. Brain Research, 144, 123–141.

Keshner, E. A. (1994). Postural abnormalities in vestibular disorders. In S. J. Herdman (Ed.), Vestibular rehabilitation (pp. 47–67). Philadelphia: F. A. Davis Co.

Kroenke, K., Arrington, M. E., & Mangelsdorff, A. D. (1990). The prevalence of symptoms in medical outpatients and the adequacy of therapy. Archives of Internal Medicine, 150, 1685–1689.

Leigh, R. J., & Zee, D. S. (1999). The neurology of eye movements (3rd ed.). New York: Oxford University Press.

Li, J. C., Li, C., Epley, J., & Wienberg, L. (2000). Cost-effective management of benign positional vertigo using canalith repositioning. Otolaryngology–Head and Neck Surgery, 122(3), 334–339.

Manning, C., Scandale, L., Manning, E. J., & Gengo, F. M. (1992). Central nervous system effects of meclizine and dimenhydrate: Evidence of acute tolerance to antihistimines. Journal of Clinical Pharmacology, 32, 996–1002.

Marciano, E., & Marcelli, V. (2002). Postural restrictions in labyrintholithiasis. European Archives of Otorhinolaryngology, 259(5), 262–265.

McCabe, B. F. (1970). Labyrinthine exercises in the treatment of diseases characterized by vertigo: Their physiologic basis and methodology. Laryngoscope, 80, 1429–1433.

Mira, E., Valli, S., Zucca, G., & Valli, P. (1996). Why do episodes of benign paroxysmal positioning vertigo recover spontaneously? Journal of Vestibular Research: Equilibrium and Orientation, 6(4s), S49.

Radtke, A., Neuhauser, H., von Brevern, M., & Lempert, T. (1999). A modified Epley's procedure for self-treatment of benign paroxysmal positional vertigo. Neurology, 53, 1358–1360.

Roberts, R. A., Gans, R., Deboodt, J., & Lister, J. (2005). Treatment of benign paroxysmal positional vertigo: Necessity of postmaneuver patient restrictions. Journal of the American Academy of Audiology, 16, 357–366.

Schuknecht, H. F. (1969). Cupulolithiasis. Archives of Otolaryngology–Head and Neck Surgery, 90, 765–778.

Semont, A., Freyss, G., & Vitte, E. (1988). Curing the BPPV with a liberatory maneuver. Advances in Otorhinolaryngology, 42, 290–293.

Shepard, N. T., & Telian, S. A. (1996). Practical management of the balance disorder patient. San Diego, CA: Singular Publishing Group.

Sloane, P. D., Dallara, J., Roach, C., et al. (1994). Management of dizziness in primary care. Journal of the American Board of Family Practice, 7, 1–8.

Smith, P. F., & Curthoys, I. S. (1989). Mechanisms of recovery after unilateral labyrinthectomy: A review. Brain Research/Brain Research Reviews, 14, 155–180.

Smith, P. F., Darlington, C. L., & Curthoys, I. S. (1986). The effect of visual deprivation on vestibular compensation in the guinea pig. Brain Research, 364, 195–198.

Tinetti, M. E., Baker, D., McAvay, G., et al. (1994). A multifactorial intervention to reduce the risk of falling among elderly people living in the community. New England Journal of Medicine, 331(13), 821–827.

Von Brevern, M., Lezius, F., Tiel-Wilk, K., & Lempert, T. (2002). Medical management of patients with benign paroxysmal positional vertigo. Nervenarzt, 73(6), 538–542.

Whitney, S. L., Wrisley, D., Brown, K., & Furman, J. (2000). Physical therapy for migraine-related vestibulopathy and vestibular dysfunction with history of migraine. Laryngoscope, 110, 1528–1534.

Wrisley, D. M., Whitney, S., & Furman, J. (2002). Vestibular rehabilitation outcomes in patients with a history of migraine. Otology and Neurotology, 23, 483–487.

Yamane, H., Imoto, T., Nakai, Y., et al. (1984). Otoconia degradation. Acta Otolaryngologica Supplementum, 406, 263–270.

Chapter 20

Hearing Protection

Marshall L. Chasin

Hearing protection devices (HPDs) are available in a variety of shapes, sizes, and models with different attenuation characteristics and purposes. In part, these characteristics are inherent and related to the laws of physics; however, judicious use of modifications of acoustic networks and/or electronic circuitry can allow HPDs to take on almost any attenuation configuration. There are several drawbacks to traditional forms of HPDs. These relate to the occlusion effect, user comfort, ability to recognize speech in noise, and problems associated with localization and user safety. Solutions to these problems will be discussed. Methods to assess HPDs, along with single-number rating schemes, also will be discussed, along with their strengths and weaknesses.

Increased public awareness of the potential hazards of noise exposure has led to more prevalent use of HPDs. Unfortunately, many earlier models more effectively attenuated high-frequency input signals, which provide crucial cues for the recognition of speech (American National Standards Institute [ANSI] 2002). Moreover, given that most hazardous industrial noise is predominantly low frequency and typical HPD attenuation characteristics favor the higher frequencies, these HPDs were limited in their effectiveness in preserving hearing. It is not surprising, then, that early HPDs never attained widespread popularity or acceptance.

Major progress was made in the late 1980s with the introduction of "tuned" HPDs (Killion, DeVilbiss, and Stewart, 1988). Electroacoustic modifications, using compression or phase cancellation techniques combined with wireless communication technology, have resolved many problems inherent to early HPDs, namely, inadequate attenuation of hazardous low frequencies and overattenuation of high-frequency speech. For example, hunters can now wear HPDs that function as hearing aids to amplify low-level input signals and as attenuators for higher input level signals.

♦ Types of Hearing Protection Devices

There are essentially two major types of HPDs: earplugs and earmuffs. Earplugs are usually one size fits all and can be made of foam or premolded plastic. These are typically rolled up and expand once inserted in the user's ear. Depending on how deeply these earplugs are seated in the ear canal, varying degrees of attenuation and occlusion will be obtained. Premolded plugs can be seated deeply or in a more shallow position in the ear canal; this relates more to the size of the ear canal than to insertion depth per se. For these reasons, earplug HPDs tend to have more variabilities than earmuff models. In contrast, earmuff HPDs are circumaural and are connected either to a spring-loaded headband or to a safety helmet. Because insertion depth and individual variability in ear canal size are not factors with this type of HPD, the attenuation variability associated with this style is not as great as that with earplug HPDs (**Table 20–1**).

Table 20–1 Noise Reduction Ratings of Three Typical HPDs along with Their Octave-band Attenuations and Associated Standard Deviations

	NRR (dB)	Frequency (Hz)	125	250	500	1000	2000	4000	8000
AearoE.A.R. earplug	31	Mean attenuation	35.7	41.5	46.2	42.4	37.7	44.7	46.4
		SD	7.4	8.5	6.2	5.3	2.4	3.5	4.5
4000 earmuff	27	Mean attenuation	15.5	25.1	35.0	41.0	36.5	36.9	39.8
		SD	2.7	2.9	2.5	3.2	2.8	2.4	2.4
"Combat" earplug	8	Mean attenuation	4.4	4.0	10	17.6	24.6	24.0	22.2
		SD	3.4	2.7	2.6	3.1	3.2	4.5	4.7

Note: The E.A.R. earplug (Aearo Corp., Indianapolis, IN) is a typical industrial foam earplug HPD. The 4000 earmuff (Aearo Corp., Indianapolis, IN) is commonly used in industry. The "combat" earplug (Aearo Corp., Indianapolis, IN) is a premolded HPD for military use that provides hearing protection while allowing users to hear many environmental noises.
HPD, hearing protection device; NRR, noise reduction rating; SD, standard deviation.
Source: Data courtesy of Aearo Corp.

◆ Attenuation Characteristics

Considerable research has been focused on refining the attenuation properties of HPDs (e.g., Berger et al, 2003; Shaw and Theissen, 1958; Zwislocki, 1957). The degree to which HPDs attenuate environmental sound energy across frequencies can be affected by many factors. Such factors pertain not only to the thickness and density of the material used in hearing protectors but also to the level of bone-conducted sound transmission.

Typical HPDs, without acoustic design modifications, attenuate high-frequency sounds more effectively than low-frequency sounds. **Figure 20–1** reports the frequency-dependent characteristics of a typical industrial foam plug inserted deeply into the ear canal. As can be seen in **Fig. 20–1A,** as frequency increases, attenuation increases and is essentially asymptotic above 2000 Hz. Without deep insertion, low-frequency attenuation (up to 750 Hz) would be compromised to only 15 to 20 dB. This is because low-frequency sound energy would more freely enter the space between the ear canal wall and the earplug. This would not be an issue with circumaural earmuff HPDs. **Figure 20–1B** shows typical foam earplugs.

Three acoustic phenomena account for this frequency dependence. The first phenomenon is that all frequencies with a half wavelength less than the diameter of an obstruction (e.g., an HPD) are attenuated. As a result, low-frequency sounds, which have longer wavelengths, more easily pass through obstructions, whereas high-frequency sounds, with shorter wavelengths, are greatly attenuated. This is why walls in lecture halls attenuate higher frequency consonants more than lower frequency vowels. For example, a high-frequency consonant such as /s/ as in *sign* has energy at 4000 Hz and above. The wavelength for 4000 Hz is 8.5 cm, so that any obstruction with a diameter in excess of 4.25 cm will attenuate this sound. Lower frequencies have much longer wavelengths, and larger diameter obstructions are required for significant attenuation of these sounds. The second phenomenon involves the impact of stiffness and mass. Details are beyond the scope of this chapter; however, it is sufficient to say that the greater the mass of the HPD, the greater the overall attenuation it provides. The greater its mass, though, the less likely an HPD will be worn. The third phenomenon pertains to the resonator characteristics of the ear canal. The human ear canal, which is ~25 to 28 mm (1 inch) long, is closed medially at the tympanic membrane and open at the lateral side. Thus, the ear canal

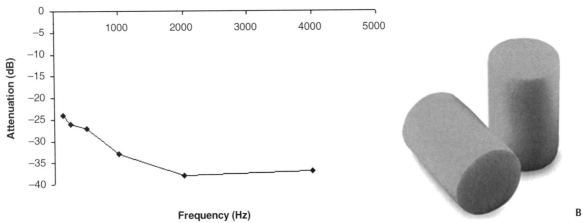

Figure 20–1 (A) Attenuation of a deeply inserted hearing protection device typically used in industry. Note that the attenuation is the greatest in the higher frequency region. **(B)** Photograph of typical industrial foam earplugs. (Courtesy of Elliott Berger, Aearo Corp., Indianapolis, IN.)

acts as a quarter-wavelength resonator that has a maximum resonance of ~17 dB at around 2700 Hz. This resonance is well known when measuring hearing aids using real-ear measures and is referred to as the real ear unaided gain (REUG). Whenever the ear canal is occluded (with a hearing aid or an HPD), this naturally occurring resonance is lost (or, more specifically, moved beyond 10 kHz, where it has minimal value). Loss of this natural ear resonance would reduce sound pressure levels (SPLs) by 10 to 15 dB in the 4000 Hz region. Subsequently, with earplug HPDs, an additional high-frequency insertion loss is caused by this destruction of the 2700 Hz resonance. In contrast, earmuff HPDs do not destroy the natural ear resonance in the 2700 Hz region, and as such, there is less relative high-frequency attenuation than if earplugs were used. Earmuffs do, however, yield greater attenuation in the 500 to 1000 Hz region. Nevertheless, it cannot be stated definitively that earmuffs yield improved intelligibility in noise compared with earplugs, because hearing loss configuration and wide subject variability (see, e.g., the standard deviations (SDs) in **Table 20–1**) are confounding factors (Abel et al, 1982).

Pearl

- Earmuff HPDs provide a flatter attenuation than conventional earplug HPDs because the real ear unaided response (REUR) is not destroyed. In addition, subject variability is less with earmuff HPDs than with earplug HPDs.

Generally, ear canals are conical and are wider at the lateral opening and narrower toward the tympanic membrane. Conical tubes (e.g., oboes and saxophones) acoustically behave as half-wavelength resonators with higher frequency

resonances at integer multiples of the first resonance. There is some evidence that for some patients, the second resonance of the REUG at ~5500 Hz is merely another manifestation of the ear canal resonance and not simply the resonance of the concha bowl of the pinna (Chasin, 2005).

Berger et al (2003) reviewed the methods to assess the attenuation of HPDs and noted that at 2000 Hz, the bone-conduction limit for hearing protection was the lowest (40 dB). That is, attenuation of > 40 dB in the 2000 Hz region is an artifact of the objective measuring system. At this input level, sound is conducted through the temporal bone directly to the cochlea, bypassing the air-conduction route. One can measure an attenuation in excess of 40 dB at 2000 Hz by using artificial test fixtures (ATFs) or a real-ear probe microphone measurement technique (e.g., microphone in real ear [MIRE]), but these values would not correspond with real-ear performance. The only exception is found in Schroeter (1986), who constructed an ATF with as much inherent self-insertion loss as possible, then accounted for the bone-conduction route by postmeasurement computational corrections. **Figure 20–2** (Berger et al, 2003) shows the bone-conduction limits across frequency for hearing protector attenuation.

Pearl

- The maximum possible attenuation in the 2000 Hz region is ~40 dB because sound enters directly by bone conduction above this level.

There are two equally valid real-ear measurement approaches for the assessment of HPDs. In both approaches, the real-ear measurement device should be calibrated in the normal fashion to equalize the probe and the room characteristics:

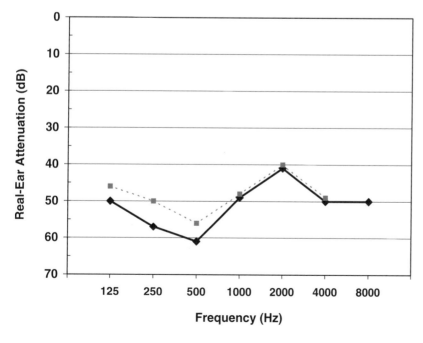

Figure 20–2 The bone-conduction limits for sound transmission for hearing protection devices indicating that the maximum attenuation is 40 dB at 2000 Hz. The dotted line represents previous data. (Adapted from Berger, E. H., Kieper, R. W., & Gauger, D. (2003). Hearing protection: Surpassing the limits to attenuation imposed by the bone-conduction pathways. Journal of the Acoustical Society of America, 114(4, Part 1), 1955–1967, with permission.)

Internal stimulus technique This approach uses the built-in stimuli (either warble tone or broadband complex noise) of the real-ear measurement device. With the probe tube situated in the ear canal (as close to the tympanic membrane as possible), using a higher level stimulus (e.g., 70–80 dB SPL), an REUG is measured. The HPD (earplug or earmuff) can then be fitted, and a real ear insertion gain (REIG) can be measured. The negative deviation from 0 dB (as opposed to a positive deviation from 0 dB for hearing aid gain) on the real-ear measurement device is a frequency-by-frequency measure of real-ear attenuation of the HPD. The reason for the higher stimulus level is to ensure that one is above the noise floor of the real-ear measurement system, which, depending on the manufacturer and frequency, can be approximately 30 dB.

External stimulus technique This approach uses an external complex stimulus, such as music or an industrial noise spectrum. After calibrating the real-ear measurement system in the normal fashion, the probe tube is situated as close to the eardrum as possible. However, prior to assessing the REUG and the subsequent REIG, both the reference microphone and the loudspeaker of the real-ear measurement system need to be disabled. Depending on the manufacturer, this may involve setting the stimulus level to "off" or to 0 dB. Using a well-controlled complex stimulus (e.g., broadband music or industrial noise) as input, the REUG is measured. The HPD can then be fitted in the normal fashion and the REIG measured. As with the first approach, the stimulus level needs to be sufficiently intense to ensure that the attenuated measured values are sufficiently above the noise floor of the real-ear measurement device. A caveat with this technique is that monitoring of the external stimulus must be performed (e.g., by using a sound level meter) to ensure that the stimulus level is the same for both the REUG and the REIG responses.

> **Pitfall**
>
> - When performing an REIG test on an HPD, ensure that the REUG level is sufficiently intense so that the internal noise of the real-ear measurement device does not alter the (high-frequency) attenuation results.

◆ Limitations

Workers in industrial and construction settings do not always wear recommended HPDs. For example, in a survey by Neitzel and Seixas (2005), construction workers used hearing protection less than one quarter of the time that they were exposed to noise > 85 dB(A). There are many reasons why workers choose not to wear HPDs, among them the occlusion effect, poor sound localization, variable audibility of warning sounds with potentially dangerous consequences, poor speech communication in noise, comfort concerns,

and an overall perceived lack of usefulness. In the study by Neitzel and Seixas (2005), construction workers obtained < 3 dB of protection from their HPDs. The following section deals with some of the reasons for this.

The Occlusion Effect

The occlusion effect is the improvement in low-frequency bone-conduction thresholds on closing the ear canal. This results in the amplification of internal physiological noise that masks the low-frequency unoccluded thresholds. The essential characteristics of this phenomenon were first delineated by Zwislocki in the 1950s (Zwislocki, 1957). The occlusion effect is well known in audiology and typically results in an echo, as reported by hearing aid users. One way to minimize the occlusion effect is by extending the bore of the hearing aid canal into the bony portion of the external ear canal. The extent of the occlusion effect can be measured clinically with real-ear measurement equipment (using the external stimulus technique outlined above). Because the occlusion effect is the enhancement of low-frequency sounds, such as those from the voice of the HPD wearer, high vowels (or close vowels, in which the tongue is positioned as close as possible to the roof of the mouth without creating a constriction that would be classified as a consonant), such as /i/ as in *beet* and /u/ as in *boot*, will have energy transferred from the mouth, through the condyle of the jaw, to the bony medial portion of the outer ear canal. Plugging one's ears or using an earplug while voicing these vowels will clearly demonstrate the deleterious enhancement of the first formant (low-frequency resonance).

The method to obtain the estimate of the occlusion effect is similar to the external stimulus technique described above to obtain real-ear attenuation. Once the real-ear measurement device is calibrated in the normal fashion to account for room and probe tube characteristics, the speaker and reference microphone are disabled. With the probe tube deeply inserted in the ear canal (as close to the eardrum as possible), the subject is asked to utter the vowel [i] as in *beet*. Attention should be paid to the low-frequency sound energy of the spectrum of this vowel. The identical procedure should be repeated with the HPD in place. The difference between the two measures is an estimate of the occlusion effect.

Figure 20–3 demonstrates a real-ear measurement of the SPL of the first formant region of [i] with and without occlusion of the ear canal with an earplug. Note the significant increase in SPL below 1000 Hz, which is a manifestation of the occlusion effect. The effect would be minimal for some lower vowels, such as [a] as in *father*, that have minimal low-frequency energy to magnify. **Figure 20–3** also demonstrates the improvement (lessening of the occlusion effect) with a deeply seated earplug that terminates 2 mm past the second bend in the ear canal. This long-bore earplug (usually custom made) sits against the bony portion of the ear canal, preventing it from vibrating, thereby preventing the build-up of low-frequency sound. A long-bore earplug (or a hearing aid with a long-bore canal) will typically minimize the occlusion effect. For

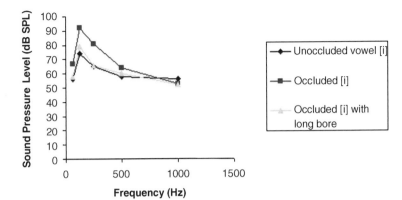

Figure 20–3 The occlusion effect (increase in low-frequency sound pressure level) for the first formant region of the high vowel [i], as in *beet*, when a shallow earplug is used. Note the lack of occlusion effect for this same earplug when it is deeply inserted (past the second bend) into the ear canal.

many wearers, a potential disadvantage of a long-bore earplug (or hearing aid) is discomfort.

Another way to minimize the occlusion effect is to use an acoustic vent (an air hole) that allows predominantly low-frequency sound energy to escape. However, vents in earplugs or earmuffs reduce the attenuation characteristics for lower frequency environmental sounds, thereby compromising the effectiveness of any HPD. To minimize the occlusion effect for a long-bore earplug, a 1.4 mm internal diameter vent is required; for a shorter bore earplug, the internal diameter vent needs to be larger, at 4 mm (Killion, Wilber, & Gudmundsen, 1988). This larger vent would certainly compromise the safety benefit of HPDs in most situations. However, it is quite possible that the smaller 1.4 mm vent would be useful in some other situations, especially if there is minimal low-frequency environmental noise present. Therefore, use of a small vent and/or a long-bore (custom-mold) earplug could be an effective way to minimize the occlusion effect, depending on the environmental noise.

Horizontal Localization of Sound

Although the primary purpose of HPDs is to preserve hearing, attention is being focused on the potential hazards associated with front–back and left–right localization confusions that can occur with HPDs worn in industrial environments. There have been many studies about auditory localization confusions in the horizontal plane (Brungart et al, 2004; Simpson et al, 2005) with the use of HPDs. These reports indicate that left–right sound localization deteriorates as the HPD system provides greater overall attenuation. Such a system may be when two HPDs are worn concurrently, such as an earplug and earmuff. The increased attenuation provided by the earplug and earmuff may provide improved attenuation, but localization is compromised by such a degree that the utility of such an HPD system is questionable. Brangart et al. (2004) found that this was the case if the signal to be located was > 500 Hz, but that the localization ability was not too poor with signals < 250 Hz. These results are consistent with findings that, at < 250 Hz, attenuation is minimal (Berger et al, 2003) and as such poses no great difficulty with localization. At higher frequencies, such as 2000 to 4000 Hz warning sounds commonly found in industry, horizontal localization ability would be quite deleteriously affected. In some cases, a high-frequency warning sound may be inaudible with an HPD system that provides excessive (high-frequency) attenuation.

Chasin and Chong (1999), studied horizontal warning sound confusions on 10 normal-hearing subjects with a 4000 Hz signal, using three different HPD conditions, as well as the open ear. The three HPD conditions were (1) E.A.R. foam earplugs from Aearo Co. (Indianapolis, IN), (2) ER-15 earplugs (Etymotic Research Inc., Elk Grove Village, IL), and (3) modified ER-15 earplugs (ER-15 SP) that yielded less high-frequency attenuation than the standard ER-15 earplugs. Attenuation of these three earplugs is reported in **Fig. 20–4**. The E.A.R. earplug, which is considered standard in the hearing conservation industry, consists of a foam cylinder that is compressed and inserted into the ear. The foam expands to take the shape of the ear canal. Depending on the degree of insertion, as with any noncustom product, there can be a wide range of variability. The ER series of earplugs, discussed later in this chapter, provide uniform attenuation, and therefore less attenuation, at 4000 Hz than does the foam E.A.R. earplug. For the purposes of this study by Chasin and Chong (1999), the modified ER-15 earplug was altered to provide even less attenuation than the ER-15 earplug. (The ER-15 SP provides a similar attenuation as the modified ER-15 earplug).

Although the acoustic and perceptive etiologies of such localization confusions are rather complex, a major factor is the audibility of high-frequency spectral cues. Chasin and Chong (1999) therefore hypothesized that the modified ER-15 earplug would have the fewest localization confusions, and the E.A.R. foam earplug would have the most. Their hypothesis was confirmed, and it was recommended that earplugs with minimal high-frequency attenuation (either by design or by modification) can be used in moderate industrial environments (up to 100 dB(A)) to reduce

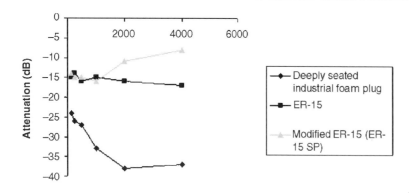

Figure 20–4 Attenuation of an industrial earplug (ER-15) and a modified ER-15 earplug (ER-15 SP).

the number of front–back localization confusions of high-frequency warning signals. Results for the localization scores are shown in **Table 20–2** as a function of attenuation at 4000 Hz.

Pearl

• The greater the HPD attenuation at 4000 Hz, the greater the horizontal sound localization problem.

Speech Communication

There is general agreement that as the noise level is increased (with a subsequent degradation in signal-to-noise ratio [SNR]), speech communication ability (as measured by word recognition tasks) decreases. In most cases, it is the SNR that is the primary factor in determining speech recognition, although other factors, such as reverberation and auditory processing skills, can be equally important. Speech errors caused by a low input level for speech input are similar to those caused by a higher input level for noise. In industry, the SNR is inherently poor, and the presence of reverberation further decreases speech recognition. A study by Abel et al (1982) demonstrated that, while speech recognition decreased as the SNR decreased, HPDs had minimal effect on normal-hearing subjects. The concern, especially among younger workers, that HPDs will alter their ability to

communicate in noise may be baseless. Casali et al (2004) also reported that there was no evidence that, for normal-hearing workers in relatively quiet occupational settings, HPDs compromise their ability to understand. Nevertheless, most workers in occupational settings do have some sensorineural hearing loss, whether from noise exposure, presbycusis, or other causes, such as recreational noise/music exposure. Abel et al (2000) reported poorer consonant discrimination ability was correlated with poorer high-frequency hearing thresholds ($r = 0.72$). Using HPDs that attenuate higher frequency sounds greater than low-frequency sounds is equivalent (at least in terms of consonant confusions and a decrease in intelligibility) to having an artificially created high-frequency hearing loss. Because the attenuation patterns of most forms of "untuned" HPDs function as low-pass filters (creating a high-frequency loss of sensitivity), it is understandable that many workers feel that they cannot communicate effectively while wearing HPDs.

Tufts and Franks (2003) demonstrated that communication in noisy environments is further exacerbated when earplugs are worn, as a speaker's voice is typically less intense, with an overall poorer SNR, and has correspondingly less high-frequency speech energy. They concluded that "talkers wearing earplugs (and consequently their listeners) are at a disadvantage when communicating in noise" (p. 1069).

There are three strategies to improve speech communication (and localization of warning signals) in noise: active noise reduction, use of HPDs with built-in communication systems, and use of HPDs with less high-frequency attenuation. The first approach, active noise reduction, was proposed over 70 years ago. Depending on its various forms, it uses phase cancellation to attenuate lower frequency signals in the environment. These devices have found wide acceptance in a range of nonoccupational listening environments, including on airplanes. Because active noise reduction techniques use phase cancellation (generating a sound that is 180 degrees out of phase so that cancellation occurs), it is more useful for frequencies below 1000 Hz, although there is no reason why its range cannot be wideband. Typical low-frequency attenuation using these devices is 10 to 15 dB. Using such devices would significantly improve the SNR by reducing the low-frequency environmental noise while maintaining the mid- to high-frequency consonant

Table 20–2 Percentage of Both Front–Back and Back–Front Localization Confusions as a Function of the Attenuation at 4000 Hz for Three Different Earplugs

Earplug	Front–Back (%)	Back–Front (%)	4000 Hz Attenuation (dB)
E.A.R.	42	24	31
ER-15	31	22	15
Modified ER-15	28	16	7
Open ear condition*	16	12	0

* Shown for comparison purposes.

sounds that are so crucial to speech recognition. Active noise reduction HPDs have not yet gained widespread acceptance in industry primarily because of cost, yet studies such as Casali et al (2004) attest to the potential benefits in terms of improved speech recognition and vehicle backup alarm detection in noise.

The second approach involves the use of HPDs with built-in communication systems. It should be pointed out that even with communication systems, HPDs should still provide adequate hearing protection. A study by Powell et al (2003) reported that, although such devices can be useful, precautions must be taken to ensure that the output of the communication device is limited to prevent temporary threshold shift (TTS) and other acoustic trauma from the transduced signal. Plyler and Klumpp (2003) reported that when a flat or uniform earplug (e.g., the ER-15) was compared with a commercially available electronic communication system, the acoustic ER-15 performed much better on the Hearing in Noise Test. This is not to suggest, however, that an electronic communication system, if coupled with an HPD of adequate attenuation, would not be superior. Clearly, more work needs to be performed in this area before definitive and optimal electroacoustic characteristics of such devices are delineated. Also, depending on the occupational environment, use of HPDs that provide less overall attenuation, especially at higher frequencies, may be beneficial for speech communication, minimizing horizontal localization confusions and increasing worker acceptance (Chasin and Chong, 1999).

Special Consideration

- Precautions must be taken to ensure that the output of any electronic communication device is limited to prevent TTS.

Wear and Tear

Earmuff HPDs appear to be more susceptible than earplug HPDs to the effects of aging and ambient environmental conditions. Noncustom earplugs are disposable, so there is understandably no long-term concern. Custom-made earplugs can degrade over time; this is primarily a function of earmold

material as well as any physiological change in the ear, such as a significant loss of body weight. Kotarbinska (2005) studied the long-term effect of earmuff HPDs over a 3-year period and found that the attenuation could be seriously degraded due to usage, storage, and the various exposures to ambient work conditions. He found that the deterioration in attenuation was directly related to the contact area of the HPD cushion with the user's head. Stiffening or cracking of the cushion was the main factor. Starck et al (2005) studied the effects of cold on the cushions of HPDs and found that in conditions below 7°C, the HPD cushion ring was too stiff to provide adequate low-frequency attenuation (especially below 125 Hz). However, when a worker wore the HPD, the temperature of the cushion ring quickly rose above 7°C, and the original attenuation characteristics were obtained. It was suggested that if a worker takes breaks from the noise when working in a cold climate, he or she should continue to wear the HPD or otherwise keep the cushion rings warm.

◆ Acoustically Tuned Alternatives

As mentioned earlier, the presence of a significant occlusion effect and the high-frequency attenuation characteristics of hearing protection can create a major concern for the wearer. Issues relating to sound localization of warning signals and degraded speech communication in noise frequently cause workers to either remove HPDs or wear them in a nonoptimal fashion. The occlusion effect can be used in some cases to benefit performing artists and to artificially reduce vocal strain, but, as a general rule, the effect should be minimized. Rarely is the high-frequency attenuation characteristic of HPDs beneficial.

Before 1988, all HPDs were "untuned," in the sense they attenuated higher frequency sound energy more effectively than low-frequency sound energy. Killion, DeVilbiss, and Stewart (1988) devised a custom earplug with ~15 dB of attenuation over a wide range of frequencies. This model was based on earlier work by Elmer Carlson. The earplug, named the ER-15, has become widely accepted by musicians as well as industrial workers who operate in relatively quiet environments (< 100 dB(A)). **Figure 20–5** shows the attenuation characteristics of the ER-15 earplug, an ER-25 (i.e.,

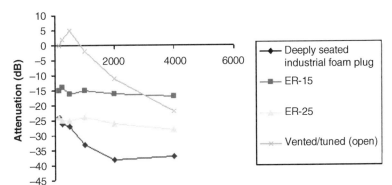

Figure 20–5 Attenuation characteristics of the ER-15, ER-25, and vented/tuned earplug. An industrial-type foam plug from **Fig. 20–1** is illustrated for comparison purposes.

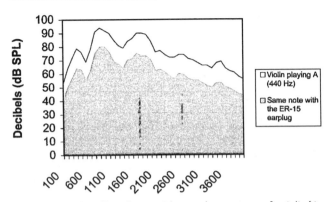

Figure 20–6 The effect the ER-15 has on the spectrum of a violin [A₄ (440 Hz)] played at a mezzo forte level. Note that the attenuated spectrum is essentially parallel to the unattenuated one.

25 dB wideband attenuation) earplug, a vented/tuned earplug, and an industrial-type foam plug. **Figure 20–6** shows the effect the ER-15 has on the spectrum of a violin [A₄ (440 Hz)] played at a mezzo forte level. Note that the attenuated spectrum is essentially parallel to the unattenuated one, suggesting that the music is attenuated from a potentially damaging level to a nondamaging level.

Pearl

• Musicians require flat attenuation HPDs, such as the ER series of earplugs, to hear the proper relationship between low-frequency fundamental energy and high-frequency harmonic energy.

The design of the ER-15 and ER-25 earplugs is remarkably simple. Essentially, a button-sized element that functions as an acoustic compliance is connected to a custom earmold, with the volume of air in the sound bore acting as an acoustic mass. The resulting resonance between the compliance and the mass is in the 2700 Hz region and is designed to offset the insertion loss caused by the earplug. The high-frequency resonance is sufficiently broad to compensate for

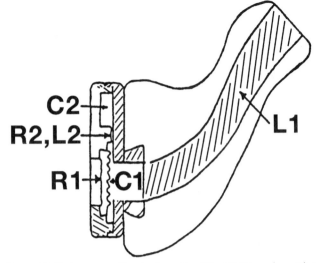

Figure 20–7 A cross-sectional schematic of the ER-15 earplug with a custom earmold showing capacitances (C), resistances (R), and inductances (L). (Courtesy of Etymotic Research Inc., Elk Grove Village, IL)

the relatively high-frequency attenuation. The compliance value of the ER element is constant. Earmold laboratories use a mass meter to verify that the custom earmold has the correct volume of air in the sound bore to establish an essentially flat attenuation pattern. A schematic of the ER-15 is shown in **Fig. 20–7**. In addition, an ER-9, with only 9 dB of flat attenuation, is available, but this model should be used only in quieter environments (< 95 dB(A)). As with any HPD, real-ear measurements can be made to verify the function of the ER series of earplugs.

Because earmolds are custom made, the length of the sound bore should be adjusted to fit. As pointed out by Zwislocki (1957) and shown in **Fig. 20–3,** the deeper the end of the earmold is situated in the ear canal, the smaller the occlusion effect. Research with completely-in-the-canal hearing aids indicates that this can be achieved if the earmold terminates 2 to 3 mm inside the bony portion of the ear canal (Chasin, 1997).

A noncustom-made (and less expensive) earplug called the ER-20/HI-FI **(Fig. 20–8)** essentially uses the folded horn

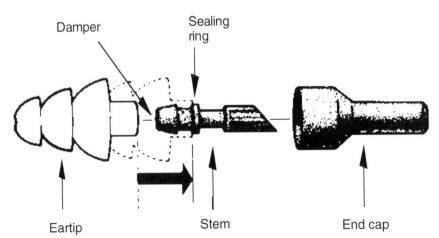

Figure 20–8 The ER-20/HI-FI earplug. (Courtesy of Elliott Berger, Aearo Corp.)

concept to enhance higher frequencies, thereby reducing the high-frequency attenuation seen in most HPDs. The folded horn concept is a modification of the acoustic transformer effect, where the flaring tube is folded on itself because of space limitations, but high-frequency enhancement is maintained (Killion et al, 1992). This concept was used in the mid-1980s, albeit unsuccessfully, to obtain some of the horn benefits for in-the-ear hearing aids. The other purpose of the folded horn is to relocate the sound entry point for the earplug from a position ~15 mm outside the entrance of the ear canal to the floor of the concha, where there is significant high-frequency amplification. There have been other attempts in the HPD industry to create noncustom devices that can provide a more uniform attenuation across the frequency range. An example is Bilsom's Natural Sound Technology (NST) earplug (Howard Leight/Bilson, owned by Bacon-Daldoz, Smithfield, RI). Another is the E.A.R. 9000 earmuff (Aearo Corp., Indianapolis, IN), which was the first design to offer a flat attenuation of ~25 dB (Allen and Berger, 1988).

The ER-20/HI-FI earplug **(Fig. 20–8)** has a noise reduction rating (NRR) of 12 dB. A newer version has an NRR of 16 dB. Unlike the ER-15 and ER-25 earplugs, the ER-20/HI-FI has a slight high-frequency roll-off, with attenuation ranging from 15 dB for the lower frequency signals to 22 dB for the higher frequency signals.

An alternative to uniformly attenuating HPDs is an earplug that has minimal effect at lower frequencies with a significant high-frequency attenuation. This type, called the vented/tuned earplug (Chasin, 1996), is custom made with a Select-A-Vent (SAV) drilled within the main sound bore. In its most open position, it is acoustically transparent below 2000 Hz, with a significant high-frequency attenuation (up to 28 dB, with a typical maximum attenuation of 20 dB). It can easily be simulated by removing the attenuator element on the ER-series earplugs.

A vented/tuned earplug allows the wearer to hear low- and mid-frequency sound energy but provides significant attenuation for the high-frequency stimuli in the immediate vicinity. Such an earplug can be used by dentists, for example, to minimize the sound of dental drills, while allowing communication with patients.

Placing the SAV cover over the sound bore increases the overall attenuation, ultimately creating the equivalent of an industrial earplug. Many musicians use this type of earplug in the completely open position. The attenuation pattern of the vented/tuned earplug in its most open SAV state is shown in **Fig. 20–5,** along with the attenuation pattern of other earplug. There is a small (4–5 dB) resonance in the 500 Hz region, an acoustic inertance caused by vibration of the mass of air in the vent. Such a vent-associated resonance is frequently observed by audiologists who prescribe hearing aids. This small resonance can be used to improve the monitoring ability of musicians and vocalists. It also can be used as part of a program to reduce vocal strain (Chasin, 1996). Cox (1979) delineated the physics behind vent-associated resonance. It is important to note that the frequency of this resonance is proportional to the length of the bore/cross-sectional area (Chasin, 1996). To keep this resonance as low as possible (e.g., for improved vocal monitoring in noise), one needs to ensure that the earmold has a long bore and a narrow cross-sectional area. Typically, both of these modifications need to be made, because the vent-associated resonance is proportional to the square root of the above dimensions.

Modifications of the vented/tuned earplugs are also available that use acoustic resistors in or in front of the vent. Earmold laboratories have different names for these "filtered" vented/tuned earplugs, and the attenuation characteristics will vary depending on the filter used as well as on the sound bore dimensions. **Figure 20–9** illustrates the increased attenuation as the filter value (in ohms [Ω]) increases. Similar results can be obtained with successively narrower SAVs; the narrower the SAV, the greater the attenuation, especially in the mid- to high-frequency range.

Sonomax Hearing Healthcare Inc. (Montreal, Canada) has developed a new technology to address some of the issues that undermine effective use of hearing protectors (see **Fig. 20–10**). A medical-grade silicone generic earmold "envelope" of appropriate size is selected, inserted in the ear canal, and filled with a self-curing liquid silicone compound to achieve an acoustic seal. The two-part liquid cures to a firm but flexible solid state in about 4 minutes, enabling

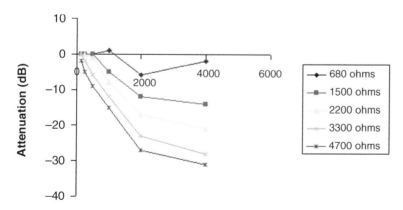

Figure 20–9 Attenuation characteristics of a vented earplug with various filters in the vent showing the increase in attenuation as the filter value increases from 680 to 5500 Ω.

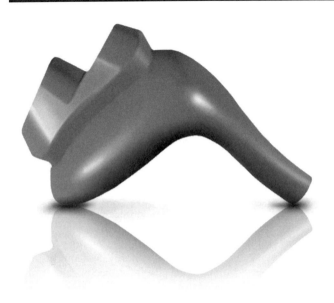

Figure 20–10 The custom E.A.R. earplug from Sonomax Hearing Healthcare Inc. features various filters in a vent. The high-frequency attenuation increases as the filter value (in ohms) increases. (Courtesy of Sonomax Hearing Healthcare Inc., Montreal, Canada.)

delivery of a comfortable custom-fit earplug in a single session (Voix et al, 2002).

The Sonomax earmold (now called the custom E.A.R.) features a transverse sound bore that provides a well-engineered and controlled open channel through the length of the earplug. Each earplug is tested for performance using a modified MIRE or real-ear measurement technique. A dual-element microphone is inserted in the sound bore of the finished earplug; while in the subject's ear, a noise field is generated, and the SPL is measured inside and outside the earplug simultaneously. The noise reduction measured across the two microphone diaphragms is converted to an equivalent attenuation value by the use of computer software. On removal of the microphone probe, the sound bore may be fully blocked, or acoustical dampers of various resistances may be inserted to permit adjustment to the attenuation to match earplug performance to the needs of the individual. The sound bore may also be used to interface the completed earmold with electronic communication devices, such as in-plant radios, personal entertainment devices, and in-ear sound monitors.

It should be noted that this form of HPD is essentially a filtered earplug. Depending on the degree of the resistor that is inserted in the sound bore, there will be various amounts of high-frequency attenuation. Such earplugs potentially provide a similar attenuation to conventional HPDs (i.e., greater high-frequency attenuation), but they have the added benefit of not providing excessive attenuation, which degrades speech recognition and localization cues. Unlike the ER series of HPDs, the custom E.A.R. does not provide a flat or uniform attenuation pattern and is therefore not intended for musicians and those in the performing arts.

◆ Electronic Alternatives

Advancements in technology have made it possible to develop HPDs that depend on electronic rather than acoustic characteristics. One important innovation is active noise reduction (ANR), which is based on the principle that two identical signals, which when added together out of phase, will cancel each other. Although it is difficult to assess a quickly varying signal and to generate another with the identical spectrum but 180 degrees out of phase, it is a relatively easy task for steady-state signals, especially if the signals are low frequency (i.e., long wavelength). ANR hearing protection has not gained wide acceptance because of its high cost, its limitation to low-frequency attenuation, and, until recently, its limitation to relatively steady-state signals.

In contrast, active sound transmission hearing protection, using a form of electronic sound transmission, has gained acceptance. In this type of HPD, a modified hearing aid circuit is used that allows for amplification at low input levels but attenuation or peak clipping at higher input levels. An external monitoring microphone is used to assess the environmental noise level, and the amplification stages are reduced or disabled completely above a certain preselected level.

There are some reports regarding the use of level-dependent circuits, such as the K-Amp from Etymotic Research (Killion, 1993), as well as the use of hearing aids that have been turned off (Berger, 1988; Hetu et al, 1992). These approaches have been shown to be useful for workers with mild hearing losses, as long as there is no vent in the custom product or earmold attached to a behind-the-ear aid. Because most hearing aid fittings use an acoustic vent, hearing aids that are to be used in this fashion should be constructed with SAVs. During noise exposure, the worker can plug the vent or open the vent to the desired degree for everyday speech communication.

Specialized devices can serve as both hearing aids and active hearing protectors. In the hearing aid mode, such a device can provide as much as 40 dB of gain, with peak gains as little as 15 dB. When the device is turned off, the shell provides attenuation of 35 dB in the lower frequencies and 40 dB in the higher frequencies. The NRR associated with the shell of a turned-off hearing aid is ~27 dB. Given the significant advantages of this versatility, it is only a matter of time before more hearing aid manufacturers offer such devices. HPD manufacturers have also realized the potential for devices that are level dependent or multifunctional. HPDs now exist that allow wearers to push a button to hear speech; when the button is released, the full attenuation characteristics are reestablished.

An inherent aspect of these devices, especially those using input compression, is that there is a short attack time before the circuit is activated and a corresponding attenuation of the noise source. When one examines the specification sheets on these devices, attack times of 1 to 5 msec are typical, but it should be pointed out that these values are artifacts of the method used to assess nonlinear hearing aids. The ANSI measure for attack time involves increasing the input level from 55 to 90 dB SPL, with an equivalent decrease for the release time (ANSI, 2003). The 1 to 5 msec values are those obtained from this paradigm. Much shorter attack times would be measured (on the order of microseconds) if the increase was from 55 to 110 dB SPL, for example, which is more typical of the impulse sound levels that would be experienced by hunters who wear HPDs to protect against the sound of gunfire. In addition, for these more realistic values, the release times would be significantly longer than those found on a typical ANSI specification sheet (W. A. Cole, personal communication, 2005).

Pearl

- Electronic HPDs have compression systems using very rapid attack times.

The music and entertainment industry has adopted active sound transmission. Many performers, for example, now wear ear monitors that look like hearing aids connected to a cable. The earpiece houses one or more receivers and, depending on the model, a preamplifier. These ear monitors are connected directly to the sound engineer's rack or by way of a wireless frequency modulation (FM) route. In both cases, such a device allows the wearer to receive only the sound that is desired. At the same time, the wearer is not be subjected to other potentially harmful environmental sounds. Some versions use in situ microphones that can continually measure the noise level in the wearer's immediate environment. **Figure 20–11** shows such a custom device. Ear monitors are made in both custom (requiring an earmold impression) and noncustom (one-size-fits-all) formats. Such monitors are gradually finding use outside of the entertainment industry. For example, such devices can be found embedded in earmuff-style HPDs, and many use Bluetooth wireless technology to assist communication over short distances.

♦ Assessment Techniques

To determine whether HPDs are meeting their intended goals, objective assessment techniques are required. Although one may expect such measures to focus on attenuation, this term, as pointed out by Berger et al (2003), is rather

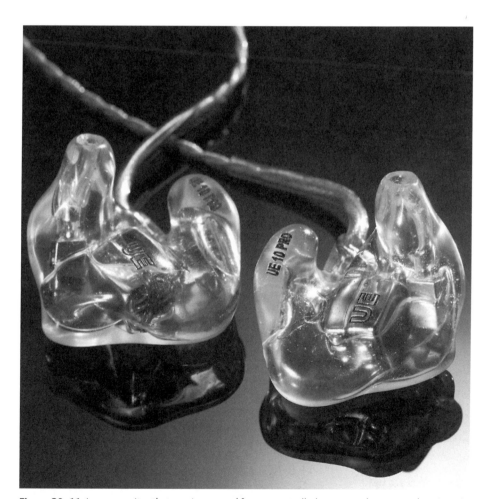

Figure 20–11 In-ear monitor that receives sound from a controlled source such as a sound engineer's console or via a wireless form of transmission. The monitor also serves to attenuate noise in the immediate vicinity. (Courtesy of Ultimate Ears.)

poorly defined; instead, there should be a discussion of insertion loss and noise reduction. Insertion loss is similar to insertion gain in that two consecutive measures are made with miniature microphones. Insertion loss can be assessed using the MIRE technique. One measure is made in the ear canal without the HPD, and the other is made in the identical location with the HPD in place. The difference is the insertion loss. Because the location of the microphone is identical in both conditions, all factors that affect the SPL, other than the decrease in SPL caused by the HPD, are subtracted. A potential problem with the insertion loss measure is the inadvertent contribution of the bone-conduction route. This can become a problem for those hearing protectors with significant measured attenuations (i.e., > 40 dB at 2000 Hz).

Noise reduction is a simultaneous measure made by two separate microphones: one on the outside of the HPD and the other on the medial side in the ear canal. A noise reduction measure can be affected by the precise location of the microphone in the ear canal as well as by diffraction effects from the external portion of the ear canal. Yet this measure can be useful in high noise environments and can use an actual industrial spectrum as the stimulus.

Subjective techniques can be categorized as threshold or suprathreshold based. Threshold-based techniques are the oldest and in most cases provide a high degree of reliability. In any subjective technique, the individual's ability to respond is a factor; this contributes an inevitable source of error. For this reason, SD scores tend to be higher for subjective techniques than for objective techniques.

Real ear attenuation at threshold (REAT) is a subjective technique that assesses the change in the hearing threshold of a patient with and without hearing protection. This measure is analogous to functional gain as used with hearing aid amplification. REAT can be assessed under earphones or binaurally in the sound field. Two potential problems with REAT, especially if measured in the sound field, are an inability to attain a sufficiently quiet environment to achieve a "true" unprotected condition, and low-frequency masking, which may occur as a result of physiological noise that overestimates the degree of low-frequency attenuation. These potential problems are the same for functional gain testing of hearing aids. When REAT is assessed under earphones, the first factor is rarely an issue, but corrections need to be made for a slightly smaller volume, as part or all of the concha is occupied by an earplug.

Suprathreshold-based techniques tend to have poorer test–retest reliability than REAT and are not commonly used. They include measures of midline lateralization, speech reception thresholds, and other psychophysical tests. For an excellent review of these techniques, the interested reader is referred to Alberti (1982) and Berger at al (2003).

◆ Single-value Attenuation Rating Schemes

Several single-number attenuation rating schemes are used today. The most commonly used scheme in the United States is the NRR. Other common schemes are the octave-band method and the single number rating (E. H. Berger, personal communication, 2004). Most provinces in Canada use the ABC scheme, which categorizes hearing protectors as class A, B, or C, depending on their octave-band attenuation values and the measured L_{eq}—a time-weighted average (Behar and Desormeaux, 1994).

The NRR is a relatively simple method that can be used to characterize the attenuation of HPDs. The innovation came from the work of Botsford (1973), who found that the environmental noise measured in dB(C) (dB C-weighted) and the noise level measured in dB(A) (dB A-weighted), when assessed in the ear canal with the hearing protector in place, were constants and could be used to characterize the HPD.

NRR calculations, as identified by Preves and Pehringer (1983), rest on some assumptions and require the use of various correction factors. The validity of these assumptions has led to some criticism of the NRR technique. One such assumption is that the environmental noise spectrum is a constant pink noise—equal octave-band levels across the spectrum. An example of a correction factor is taking into consideration that some users do not wear their HPDs as specified, so a "correction" must be made. In addition, the spectral uncertainty may lead to an inaccurate estimate. For these reasons, a 3 dB correction factor is included along with a statistical estimate incorporating 95% of the population (2 SDs).

To understand the potential problem with the assumption that the spectrum is a constant pink noise, it may be useful to review and compare the C- and A-weighting networks. The C-weighting network is essentially no weighting at all—less than a 1 dB effect to 6000 Hz. However, the A-weighting network attempts to simulate human hearing sensitivity—a significant low-frequency roll-off of 16 dB at 125 Hz, with no effect at and above 1000 Hz. Thus, if an environmental noise spectrum has significant low-frequency energy, the dB(C) measure will be much greater than the dB(A) measure. In contrast, if there is minimal low-frequency noise, there will be minimal difference between a dB(A) and a dB(C) noise measurement.

When comparing C- and A-weighted measurements, a preliminary form of spectral analysis is performed. Clearly, accepting the NRR without reference to the spectral shape of the environmental noise can be a major source of error. The work of the National Institute for Occupational Safety and Health (NIOSH) yielded a correction factor of 3 dB in the calculation of the NRR for reasons pertaining to spectral uncertainties. Johnson and Nixon (1974) argued that this correction factor should be 5 or 6 dB. If this figure were to be subtracted from the calculation, the NRR would be a "worst case scenario." The NRR for each hearing protector is a measure based on the results of several subjects. Subsequently, a 2 SD pad is included as "a statistical adjustment so that the mean values are modified to reflect what some larger proportion of the population will actually achieve" (E. H. Berger, personal communication, 2004). This 2 SD range covers approximately 95% of the population. The NRR formula, where N = noise, is:

$$\text{NRR} = N\,(\text{C-weighted}) - N\,(\text{A-weighted}) + \text{attenuation}\,(\text{A-weighted}) - 3\,\text{dB} - 2\,\text{SDs}$$

As can be seen in this equation, if the true noise spectrum has no low-frequency energy, then the first two terms are identical, and the NRR is simply the attenuation and associated wearing and statistical factors. For a musician's ER-15 uniform attenuator earplug, the octave-band attenuation is ~15 dB, with the calculated NRR being only 7 dB. Johnson and Nixon (1974) noted that the NRR tends to be artificially high if there is minimal low-frequency attenuation and artificially low if there was a flat attenuation characteristic.

Pitfall

• The NRR is affected by many factors and tends to underestimate true attenuation for flat attenuation HPDs.

Table 20–1 shows the NRR along with octave-band attenuations and associated SDs for three HPDs. The first is for a typical industrial-type foam earplug HPD, and the second is for a typical earmuff HPD. Note the lower SDs inherent with earmuff-style HPDs. The third HPD in **Table 20–1** is a low attenuation preformed (i.e., a shaped plastic insert) earplug HPD used in combat. This type of HPD allows soldiers to hear most environmental sounds while providing significant hearing protection. It is a widely held view that the higher the NRR, the better the hearing protector. Depending on the noise or music level, the spectral shape, and the individual's communication or musical requirements, this may not be true.

Using only NRR scores as a guideline may lead to users being under- or overprotected. This is because conventional HPDs tend to maximally attenuate high-frequencies critical for speech audibility while minimally attenuating potentially harmful low-frequency environmental noise. As an alternative to the NRR, the audibility reduction rating (ARR) has been proposed. Whereas the NRR is essentially the average attenuation – 2 SDs – 3 dB, the ARR is the average attenuation + 2 SDs + 3 dB. Killion (1993) has suggested that HPDs should have two ratings: NRR and ARR. Because much of the mid- and high-frequency speech cues are lost when HPDs are worn, the audibility of speech is

seriously degraded. The ARR is an attempt to indicate how poor an HPD can be for speech communication. However, in today's environment, with active sound transmission and wireless technology, speech intelligibility can be significantly improved over that which would be expected from conventional HPDs.

Controversial Point

• Single-number rating schemes tend to oversimplify attenuation characteristics.

In practice, HPDs tend to be selected based on their NRR values: the higher, the better. However, in the vast majority of situations, the selected HPD provides excessive attenuation at the expense of wearing comfort, localization of warning sounds, and speech communication. Selection strategies for HPDs need to be based on the actual noise spectrum as well as the requirements of the individual worker and workplace. Solutions that involve in situ measurement of attenuation, a flat or uniform attenuation pattern, or electronic innovations that seek to improve speech intelligibility and localization, while maintaining sufficient noise attenuation, are all major steps forward. Significant progress is being made toward the goal of optimal attenuation with maintenance of optimal sound awareness, but much research still needs to be done.

◆ Summary

HPDs are an imperfect solution to imperfect work environments. They can cause the occlusion effect, degrade speech recognition, and alter the wearer's perception of warning signals. However, innovations such as electronic signal processing and uniform attenuation strategies can improve the usability of HPDs and reduce costs. Both subjective and objective assessment techniques are used to gauge the effectiveness of HPDs.

References

Abel, S. M., Alberti, P. A., Haythornthwaite, C., & Riko, K. (1982). Speech intelligibility in noise: Effects of fluency and hearing protector type. Journal of the Acoustical Society of America, 71(3), 708–715.

Abel, S. M., Sass-Kortsak, A., & Naugler, J. J. (2000). The role of high-frequency hearing in age-related speech understanding deficits. Scandinavian Audiology, 29(3), 131–138.

Alberti, P. W. (Ed.). (1982). Personal hearing protection in industry. New York: Raven Press.

Allen, C. H., & Berger, E. H. (1988). Development of a unique passive hearing protector with level-dependent and flat attenuation characteristics. NCEF, 34(3), 97–105.

American National Standards Institute. (2002). Methods for calculation of the speech intelligibility index (ANSI S3.5–1997). New York: Author.

American National Standards Institute. (2003). Specification of hearing aid characteristics (ANSI S3.22–2003). New York: Author.

Behar, A., & Desormeaux, J. (1994). NRR, ABC or . . . . Canadian Acoustics, 22(1), 27–30.

Berger, E. H. (1988). Tips for fitting hearing protectors: E.A.R. LOG 19. Indianapolis, IN: Cabot Safety Corp.

Berger, E. H., Kieper, R. W., & Gauger, D. (2003). Hearing protection: Surpassing the limits to attenuation imposed by the bone-conduction pathways. Journal of the Acoustical Society of America, 114(4, Part 1), 1955–1967.

Botsford, J. H. (1973). How to estimate dBA reduction of ear protectors. Journal of Sound and Vibration, 6, 32–33.

Brungart, D. S., Kordik, A. J., & Simpson, B. D. (2004). The effects of single and double hearing protection on the localization and segregation of spatially-separated speech signals. Journal of the Acoustical Society of America, 116(4, Part 1), 1897–1900.

Casali, J. G., Robinson, G. S., Dabney, E. C., & Gauger, D. (2004). Effect of electronic ANR and conventional hearing protectors on vehicle backup alarm detection in noise. Human Factors, 46(1), 1–10.

Chasin, M. (1996). Musicians and the prevention of hearing loss. San Diego, CA: Singular Publishing Group.

Chasin, M. (1997). The acoustics of CIC hearing aids. In M. Chasin (Ed.), CIC handbook (pp. 69–81). San Diego, CA: Singular Publishing Group.

Chasin, M. (2005). The etiology of the REUG: Did we get it completely right? Hearing Journal, 58(12), 22–24.

Chasin, M., & Chong, J. (1999). Localization problems with modified and non-modified ER-15 musician's earplugs. Hearing Journal, 52(2), 32–34.

Cox, R. M. (1979). Acoustic aspects of hearing aid-ear canal coupling systems. Monographs in Contemporary Audiology, 1(3), 1–44.

Hetu, R., Tran Quoc, H., & Tougas, Y. (1992). Can an inactivated hearing aid act as a hearing protector? Canadian Acoustics, 20(3), 35–36.

Johnson, D. L., & Nixon, C. W. (1974). Simplified methods for estimating hearing protector performance. Journal of Sound and Vibration, 7, 20–27.

Killion, M. C. (1993). The parvum bonum, plus melius fallacy in earplug selection. In L. Beilin & G. R. Jensen (Eds.), Recent developments in hearing instrument technology (pp. 415–433). Kolding, Denmark: Scanticon.

Killion, M. C., DeVilbiss, E., & Stewart, J. (1988). An earplug with uniform 15-dB attenuation. Hearing Journal, 41(5), 14–16.

Killion, M. C., Stewart, J. K., Falco, R., & Berger, E. H. (1992). Improved audibility earplug (U.S. Patent 5,113,967).

Killion, M. C., Wilber, L. A., & Gudmundsen, G. I. (1988). Zwislocki was right.... Hearing Instruments, 39(1), 14–18.

Kotarbinska, E. (2005). The influence of aging on the noise attenuation of ear-muffs. Noise and Health, 7(26), 39–45.

Neitzel, R., & Seixas, N. (2005). The effectiveness of hearing protection among construction workers. Journal of Occupational and Environmental Hygiene, 2(4), 227–238.

Plyler, P. N., & Klumpp, M. L. (2003). Communication in noise with acoustic and electronic hearing protection devices. Journal of the American Academy of Audiology, 14(5), 260–268.

Powell, J. A., Kimball, K. A., Mozo, B. T., & Murphy, B. A. (2003). Improved communications and hearing protection in helmet systems: The communications earplug. Military Medicine, 168(6), 431–436.

Preves, D. A., & Pehringer, J. L. (1983). Calculating individuals' NRRs in situ using subminiature probe microphones. Hearing Instruments, 33(3), 10–14.

Schroeter, J. (1986). The use of acoustical test fixtures for the measurement of hearing protector attenuation: 1. Review of previous work and the design of an improved test fixture. Journal of the Acoustical Society of America, 79, 1065–1081.

Shaw, E. A. G., & Theissen, G. J. (1958). Improved cushion for ear defenders. Journal of the Acoustical Society of America, 30, 24–36.

Simpson, B. D., Bolia, R. S., McKinley, R. L., & Brungart, D. S. (2005). The impact of hearing protection on sound localization and orienting behavior. Human Factors, 47(1), 188–198.

Starck, J., Toppila, E., & Laitinen, H. (2005). Effects of coldness on the protective performance of earmuffs. Noise and Health, 7(26), 47–53.

Tufts, J. B., & Franks, T. (2003). Speech production in noise with and without hearing protection. Journal of the Acoustical Society of America, 114(2), 1069–1080.

Voix, J., Laville, F., & Zeidan, J. (2002). Filter selection to adapt earplug performances to sound exposure. Canadian Acoustics, 30(3), 122–123.

Zwislocki, J. (1957). In search of the bone-conduction threshold in a free sound field. Journal of the Acoustical Society of America, 29, 795–804.

Chapter 21

Mechanisms and Treatment of Tinnitus

Robert L. Folmer and William Hal Martin

♦ Definition and Epidemiology

Tinnitus is the perception of sound that does not have an external source and is distinguished from auditory hallucinations in schizophrenia or other forms of psychosis. Tinnitus can be constant or intermittent and perceived as ringing, buzzing, hissing, sizzling, roaring, chirping, or other sounds in the ears or head.

Seidman and Jacobson (1996) estimated that 40 million people in the United States experience chronic tinnitus. The prevalence of tinnitus increases with age: 27% of males and 15% of females 45 years or older experience the symptom (Adams et al, 1999). Tinnitus is rare in children who have

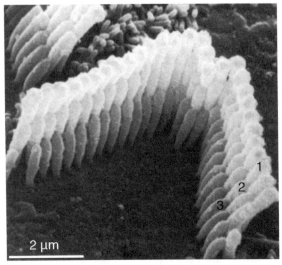
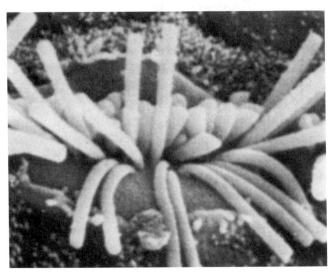
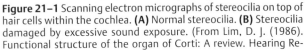

Figure 21–1 Scanning electron micrographs of stereocilia on top of hair cells within the cochlea. **(A)** Normal stereocilia. **(B)** Stereocilia damaged by excessive sound exposure. (From Lim, D. J. (1986). Functional structure of the organ of Corti: A review. Hearing Re-search, 22, 124, with permission; and from Slepecky, N. (1986). Overview of mechanical damage to the inner ear: Noise as a tool to probe cochlear function. Hearing Research, 22, 310, with permission.)

normal hearing (Stouffer et al, 1992). However, the prevalence of tinnitus in children with significant hearing loss has been reported as 33% (Drukier, 1989) or 64% (Graham, 1981). More males than females experience tinnitus because men traditionally had a greater amount of noise exposure in military service, in the workplace, and during recreational activities. Consequently, hearing loss and tinnitus are both more prevalent among men 45 years or older compared with women in the same age group (Adams et al, 1999).

◆ Mechanisms of Tinnitus

Acute tinnitus, which can last days or weeks, may be caused by ear infection, medications, head or neck injury, excessive exposure to loud sounds, impacted earwax, and changes in blood pressure or metabolism. With appropriate evaluation, such underlying conditions usually can be identified and treated, often with resultant resolution of tinnitus.

Chronic tinnitus (persistence for 6 months or more) can also result from these conditions and is more likely to occur in people who have hearing loss. Even though a true "cure" for most cases of chronic tinnitus is not available, patients can obtain relief from the symptom with assistance from clinicians who are familiar with tinnitus management strategies.

Objective tinnitus, which can be heard by people in proximity to the patient's ear, can be caused by vascular abnormalities (including congenital arteriovenous fistula, acquired arteriovenous shunt, glomus jugulare, high-riding carotid artery, carotid stenosis, persistent stapedial artery, dehiscent jugular bulb, and a vascular loop such as the anterior-inferior communicating artery [AICA] or posterior-

inferior communicating artery [PICA] compressing the auditory nerve) or mechanical disorders (including abnormally patent eustachian tube, palatal myoclonus, temporomandibular joint disorder, and stapedial muscle spasticity). However, objective tinnitus is rare, accounting for less than 1% of all cases. The vast majority of tinnitus cases are subjective: sounds are perceived only by the patient.

Subjective tinnitus is most commonly caused by exposure to excessively loud sounds such as gunfire, power tools, machinery, and music. Ringing in the ears occurs because of damage to stereocilia within the cochlea. Moderate sounds (80 dB sound pressure level [SPL] or lower) normally cause stereocilia to make tiny movements, triggering the release of neurotransmitter molecules from the basal end of hair cells that activate auditory neurons in the eighth cranial nerve (CN VIII). Excessive sound exposure (85 dB SPL or louder) causes stereocilia to bend more than they should **(Fig. 21–1)**. People then perceive high-pitched ringing tinnitus because hair cells that respond to higher frequency sounds are located at the base of the cochlea and are the first to be damaged by loud noise. Normal, undamaged stereocilia are shown in **Fig. 21–1A;** stereocilia damaged by excessive sound exposure are shown in **Fig. 21–1B.**

If the damage is modest and infrequent, stereocilia can recover, returning to their normal function in a few minutes or hours. The patient's hearing will be restored, and the tinnitus will stop. However, repeated exposure to hazardous sounds eventually causes irreparable damage to stereocilia and hair cells, resulting in permanent sensorineural hearing loss (SNHL) and possibly chronic tinnitus.

In addition to noise exposure, any condition that causes hearing loss or damages the auditory system can contribute to the generation of tinnitus **(Table 21–1)**. Imaging studies using functional magnetic resonance imaging (fMRI) (Folmer et al, 2002) or positron emission tomography (PET) (Arnold et al, 1996) demonstrated that the perception of

Table 21–1 Common Causes of Tinnitus

Presbycusis: hearing loss due to aging
Prolonged noise exposure: noise-induced hearing loss
Acoustic trauma: one-time exposure to high intensity sound
Otosclerosis: abnormal accumulation of calcium on middle ear ossicles or cochlea
Infections: bacterial, viral, fungal
Autoimmune hearing loss
Meniere's disease or endolymphatic hydrops: abnormally high inner ear pressure
Tumors/growths (e.g., acoustic neuroma and cholesteatoma)
Genetic predisposition
Ototoxicity
 • Medications: aminoglycoside antibiotics (e.g., gentamicin), valproate, quinine, cisplatin, loop diuretics (e.g., furosemide)
 • Heavy metals (e.g., lead)
Vascular problems:
 • Hypertension, arteriosclerosis, cerebral aneurysm, cerebrovascular accident
Metabolic problems:
 • Anemia, hypothyroidism, hyperthyroidism, diabetes mellitus
Head or neck injury

chronic tinnitus usually occurs as a result of hyperactivity within central auditory areas of the human brain, especially the auditory cortex (**Fig. 21–2**). As portions of the auditory system degenerate during the aging process or acquire damage from noise exposure, disease, and accidents, the natural balance of central auditory excitation versus inhibition is disrupted. In patients who hear tinnitus, excitatory pathways within the auditory system are active when they should not be: in quiet environments. This gives patients the perception of tinnitus sounds.

◆ Patient Evaluation

It is important to identify and treat any active disease processes that might contribute to the generation of tinnitus. Therefore, audiologists should work with experienced otolaryngologists as part of a tinnitus management team. The first step is to collect as much information as possible about the patient and his or her condition.

Tinnitus History

First, determine the duration of tinnitus and whether circumstances such as upper respiratory infection, otalgia, noise exposure, head trauma, sudden hearing loss, or vertigo occurred at the time of tinnitus onset. Ask the patient to describe the tinnitus: Is it intermittent or constant? High- or low-pitched? Unilateral or bilateral? Pulsatile or steady?

Unilateral tinnitus and unilateral hearing loss may provide preliminary evidence for acoustic neuroma or cerebrovascular accident. High-pitched tinnitus is usually associated with high-frequency hearing loss caused by presbycusis or excessive noise exposure. Low-pitched roaring tinnitus is sometimes associated with low-frequency hearing loss exhibited by patients

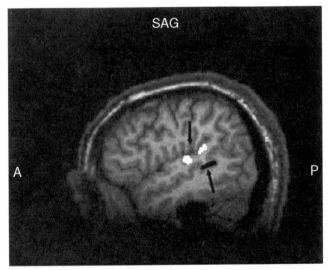

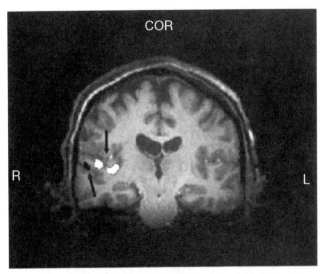

Figure 21–2 Functional magnetic resonance imaging (MRI) of brain activity responsible for tinnitus (this patient perceives tinnitus on the right side only). White areas: Masking sounds (white noise) played through a headphone to the left ear activate the auditory cortex primarily on the right side of the brain. Black area: This brain region (also the auditory cortex) is active when the patient hears tinnitus (and the masking sound is off). A, anterior; COR, coronal view; P, posterior; SAG, sagittal view.

with Meniere's disease. Pulsatile tinnitus, especially if it is synchronous with the patient's pulse, can indicate vascular abnormalities in the patient's head or neck.

Ask the patient if fatigue, stress, noise exposure, or any medications exacerbate the tinnitus. Also ask if masking sounds (e.g., water running in the shower), medications, or any other factors provide relief from tinnitus. This information can be used to formulate a tinnitus management program.

Assess the severity of the patient's tinnitus using an instrument such as the Tinnitus Severity Index (see **Appendix 21–1;** Meikle et al, 1995). A score of 36 or higher indicates bothersome tinnitus. Higher scores indicate that patients perceive their tinnitus to be a significant, even debilitating, problem.

Hearing History

Determine the presence and type of hearing loss (congenital, sudden, sensorineural, conductive, or mixed). Note the patient's history of ear infections, surgeries, noise exposure (occupational or recreational), otalgia, otorrhea, and vertigo or other balance problems. Ask whether immediate family members have experienced hearing loss or tinnitus.

Health History

Look particularly for conditions that can contribute to hearing loss and tinnitus, such as hypertension, hypothyroidism, diabetes mellitus, arteriosclerosis, and autoimmune disorders (e.g., lupus or rheumatoid arthritis). Also consider ototoxic medications, such as aminoglycoside antibiotics, cisplatin, furosemide, valproic acid, and high doses of quinine-containing compounds. When possible, patients with hearing loss or tinnitus should be given alternative medications free from ototoxicity. Excessive use of alcohol, caffeine, and aspirin or other nonsteroidal antiinflammatory drugs can exacerbate tinnitus for some patients. However, moderate use of these products is often possible.

Psychosocial History

Inquire about the patient's marital and occupational status. Unemployed patients living alone often perceive tinnitus to be more severe than do employed patients who have supportive social networks. Also ask about any history of insomnia, anxiety, depression, obsessive-compulsive disorder, or psychosis. A questionnaire such as the abbreviated Beck Depression Inventory (Beck and Beck, 1972) can be used to assess the presence and severity of depression.

Physical Exams and Testing

Patient evaluations should include the following physical examinations and tests.

Otolaryngologic–Head and Neck Exam

Otoscopic examination can detect infections such as otitis media, which will usually be accompanied by complaints of ear pain or fullness, and possibly hearing loss in combination with tinnitus. Otoscopy can also detect impacted earwax (cerumen), which can occlude the ear canal or cause immobilization of the tympanic membrane, resulting in conductive hearing loss, tinnitus, and a feeling of fullness in the ear. Symptoms usually resolve when the earwax is removed.

If the tinnitus is synchronous with the patient's pulse, it suggests a vascular contribution for the symptom. Auscultation of blood vessels in the neck can reveal venous hums or other types of bruits audible to the patient. Venous hum can be diagnosed by temporarily blocking blood flow through the jugular vein on the side where tinnitus is perceived.

Neurologic Exam

A complete neurologic exam should include Romberg's test, Dix-Hallpike maneuver (if the patient experiences vertigo), gait testing, and cranial nerve function tests.

Audiologic Testing

Audiologic tests should include pure-tone air- and bone-conduction thresholds, speech recognition testing, immittance, and most comfortable level (MCL) and loudness discomfort level (LDL) tests. Abnormal tympanograms and significant differences between air- and bone-conduction thresholds can indicate otitis media, otosclerosis, or cholesteatoma. See Chapter 9 in this volume for additional information on middle ear disorders.

MCL and LDL tests are used to assess the dynamic range of patients' hearing. Patients with LDLs that are only 5 to 20 dB above their MCLs have a reduced dynamic range of hearing that can be caused by recruitment or hyperacusis. The output from the audiometer can also be used to match the tinnitus for pitch and loudness and to test the effects of masking sounds on the patient's tinnitus.

Tinnitus Testing

Tinnitus evaluations can include the following:

- *Matching tinnitus to sounds played through headphones or earphones* Patients are asked to match the pitch and loudness of their tinnitus in the louder ear to sounds delivered to the contralateral ear. The pitch match is completed first. Next, the patient's threshold for that auditory stimulus (pure tone, mixed tones, noise band, or tone + noise) is established. Finally, the intensity of the stimulus is increased until the patient indicates that it is the same approximate loudness as tinnitus perceived in the contralateral ear. The matched loudness of tinnitus is then reported in dB above threshold (i.e., sensation level [SL]). Audiometers or specialized computer programs, such as Quiescence from SVD Inc. (Fredericton, New Brunswick, Canada), can be used for this purpose. SVD markets Quiescence as both a tinnitus evaluation tool and a treatment program. However, the authors of this chapter do not endorse Quiescence for tinnitus treatment. Several studies have shown that the matched loudness of tinnitus is not correlated with measures of tinnitus severity (Folmer, 2002; Meikle et al, 1984).

♦ *Determination of minimum masking level (MML)*   MML is the lowest intensity of broadband (200–12,000 Hz) or white noise that will completely mask the patient's tinnitus. Andersson (2003) reported that MML was positively correlated with tinnitus severity.

♦ *Measurements of residual inhibition (RI)*   RI is tinnitus suppression or temporary disappearance following patients' exposure to masking noise. To make RI assessments in our clinic, the authors present wideband (1800–12,000 Hz) noise 10 dB above the MML for 1 minute through headphones. For some patients who experience complete RI during clinical testing, it is the first time in months or years they have been able to enjoy silence. Unfortunately, the duration of RI is usually brief—often less than 1 minute.

See Johnson (1998) for more detailed descriptions of tinnitus testing procedures.

Additional Evaluations

Results of patient examinations and history collection might warrant additional evaluations. For example, asymmetrical hearing loss (15 dB or greater asymmetry at two or more consecutive test frequencies) and unilateral tinnitus can indicate a retrocochlear lesion such as acoustic neuroma (also known as vestibular schwannoma).

One test for retrocochlear pathology is the auditory brainstem response (ABR). See Chapter 20 in Volume 1 of this series for information on ABRs. Abnormal ABR waveforms can indicate retrocochlear lesion (e.g., acoustic neuroma) as a possible cause of ipsilateral hearing loss and tinnitus. If positive ABR results are obtained, MRI evaluation of the cerebellopontine angle with contrast material (e.g., gadolinium) should be performed.

Low-pitched roaring, ringing, or hissing tinnitus; hearing loss, which may be temporary or permanent; vertigo; and a feeling of pressure or fullness in the ear can indicate endolymphatic hydrops or Meniere's disease. Symptoms usually occur in the form of "attacks" that increase in frequency during the first few years of the disease, then decrease in frequency as hearing thresholds stabilize. See Chapter 10 in this volume for information on management of SNHL. Electrocochleography testing is one way to diagnose endolymphatic hydrops. See Chapter 19 in Volume 1 of this series for information on electrocochleography.

Patients who exhibit vestibular disorders should undergo electronystagmography testing to assess the severity and characteristics of their symptoms. Pulsatile tinnitus associated with abnormalities of blood vessels in the neck can be evaluated with sonography, conventional angiography, or magnetic resonance angiography. Conditions such as a dehiscent jugular bulb or stenosis of carotid arteries can sometimes be treated surgically. However, many forms of pulsatile tinnitus are not caused by these conditions. Pulsatile tinnitus is often a consequence of hearing loss, arteriosclero-

sis, weight loss or weight gain. These physiologic changes can cause patients to hear blood pulsing or "swishing" in vessels—sounds they did not perceive previously. Surgery is not recommended for most cases of pulsatile tinnitus.

Sudden hearing loss, especially if bilateral, may indicate autoimmune inner ear disease. Diagnostic tests include the Western blot immunoassay.

♦ Treatment of Active Disease Processes

Many contributors to tinnitus can be treated surgically or with medication.

Otitis Media

Successful treatment of the infection with oral antibiotics usually resolves all auditory symptoms. See Chapter 9 in this volume for additional information on middle ear disorders.

Allergies, Sinus Congestion, or Infection

When inflammation subsides, tinnitus associated with these conditions usually resolves.

Otosclerosis

Abnormal accumulations of calcium on middle ear ossicles (especially the stapes) or the cochlea can result in slowly progressing conductive or SNHL, tinnitus, and vestibular disturbances. Stapedectomy surgery—including implantation of ossicular prostheses—is often successful for advanced cases associated with significant hearing loss. A conventional hearing aid or bone-anchored hearing aid (Baha, formerly BAHA) can also benefit some patients. See Chapter 13 in this volume for information on implantable hearing aids.

Meniere's Disease or Other Forms of Endolymphatic Hydrops

Meniere's disease, characterized by abnormally high fluid pressure within the cochlea, has an estimated prevalence of 1% in the United States (da Costa et al, 2002). Management includes meclizine, antiemetics, and diuretics, as well as a low-sodium diet. If patients do not respond to meclizine, diazepam can be prescribed to reduce the severity of vertigo attacks. Surgical intervention, including installation of an endolymphatic shunt, labyrinthectomy, or vestibular neurectomy, or transtympanic injections of gentamicin are options in severe cases.

Autoimmune Inner Ear Disease

This disease has an estimated prevalence of 0.1% in the United States (Hain, 2004). Symptoms include sudden hearing loss in one ear that usually progresses to the opposite ear. Patients may also feel fullness in the ear and experience vertigo, as well as ringing, hissing, or roaring tinnitus. Most patients with autoimmune inner ear disease respond to initial treatment with oral prednisone.

Abnormal Auditory Growths

Growths such as acoustic neuroma and cholesteatoma can cause tinnitus. Acoustic neuroma (or vestibular schwannoma) is a benign neoplasm that arises from the vestibular division of CN VIII. Symptoms include unilateral hearing loss, tinnitus, and vestibular disturbances. Surgical resection or radiation treatment of the tumor can resolve these symptoms, especially if the neoplasm is detected while it is small.

Cholesteatoma is a benign epithelial cell mass that grows in the middle ear cavity. Over time, cholesteatomas can enlarge and destroy middle ear ossicles. Hearing loss, tinnitus, dizziness, and facial muscle paralysis can result from continued cholesteatoma growth. Early detection and surgical resection of auditory neoplasms can reduce the likelihood of residual symptoms.

Hyper- or Hypotension

Of these two disorders, hypertension is more likely to contribute to tinnitus. Maintenance of blood pressure within the optimum range can decrease or resolve tinnitus for some patients.

Metabolic Disorders

Disorders such as diabetes mellitus, hyperthyroidism, and hypothyroidism can contribute to tinnitus. Successful management of these conditions can reduce or resolve the patient's tinnitus.

◆ Managing Chronic Tinnitus

Successful treatment of the disorders discussed previously can resolve or reduce tinnitus. However, if tinnitus continues to bother the patient after other diseases have been treated, shift the clinical focus from treatment to management of the symptom. At this point, the clinician should do one of two things: spend the time necessary to help the patient manage tinnitus using strategies described in the following sections of this chapter, or refer the patient to a comprehensive tinnitus management program with experienced personnel who are willing and able to spend a substantial amount of time with each patient.

Like other neurologic symptoms, tinnitus can be considered chronic if it persists for 6 months or more. Approximately 90% of cases of chronic tinnitus are associated with some degree of SNHL (Meikle, 1997). Because SNHL is irreversible, most cases of chronic tinnitus cannot be "cured." Duckro et al (1984, p. 460) wrote: "As with chronic pain, the treatment of chronic tinnitus is more accurately described in terms of management rather than cure."

Special Consideration

- The goal of management is not necessarily to mask or remove the patient's perception of tinnitus. In many cases, this is not possible. Successful management enables patients to pay less attention to their tinnitus. An effective management program helps patients to understand and gain control over their tinnitus, rather than allowing it to control them. The ultimate goal is to reduce the severity of tinnitus. Clinicians should strive to help patients progress to where tinnitus is no longer a negative factor in their lives.

Establishing Tinnitus Severity

Only 25% of people who experience chronic tinnitus consider the symptom to be a significant problem (Seidman and Jacobson, 1996). These are the patients most likely to seek treatment. If a patient is not bothered by tinnitus, and no active disease processes are detected, no treatments are necessary. The clinician should reassure such patients that tinnitus is a harmless perception of sound and does not usually portend more serious medical conditions.

What differentiates the majority of patients not bothered by tinnitus from the minority who perceive it as a significant, even debilitating, problem? Is it the matched loudness, pitch, or other qualities of the sound(s) they hear? Several studies have concluded that tinnitus severity is not correlated with any of these psychoacoustic parameters (Folmer, 2002; Meikle et al, 1984).

Tinnitus severity can be defined and quantified several ways: by how much or how often a patient is bothered by tinnitus, by how much or how often tinnitus detracts from the patient's enjoyment of life, or by how disabling patients perceive their tinnitus to be. Instruments such as the Tinnitus Severity Index (see **Appendix 21–1**; Meikle et al, 1995) can be used to assess tinnitus severity.

◆ Tinnitus Management Strategies

Once underlying conditions have been treated or ruled out, reassure and counsel patients regarding factors that could exacerbate or improve their condition. If patients understand that tinnitus is nothing more than a perception of sound, they will be better able to pay less attention to it. This process of patient education and counseling helps to "demystify" the symptom of tinnitus and encourages patients to view their tinnitus with a more realistic perspective.

The severity of tinnitus is often associated with problems such as insomnia (Folmer and Griest, 2000), anxiety (Folmer et al, 2001), and depression (Folmer et al, 1999). Such issues can form a vicious circle, with each one exacerbating the

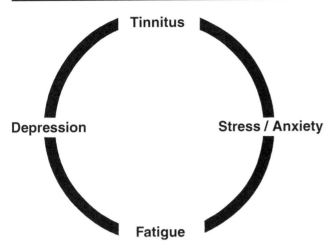

Figure 21–3 A vicious circle of symptoms. (From Tyler, R. S. (Ed.). (2006). Tinnitus treatment: Clinical protocols. New York: Thieme Medical Publishers, with permission.)

others (**Fig. 21–3**). Tinnitus is not always the starting point of this cycle—many patients experience depression, insomnia, or anxiety before tinnitus. Medication or psychotherapy will often reduce the severity of these symptoms and associated tinnitus (Folmer, 2002; Folmer and Shi, 2004). Because each patient has a unique medical, psychological, and social history, management programs should be individualized. In fact, the most successful tinnitus management programs employ multimodal strategies designed to address the specific needs of each patient (Roy and Chopra, 2002; Sullivan et al, 1994).

Acoustic Therapy

Acoustic therapy is a vital component of effective tinnitus management. One definition of acoustic therapy is *using external sounds to provide relief from tinnitus*. This is not a new concept.

- Alexander of Tralles (A.D. 525–605) suggested that tinnitus sufferers could obtain relief by walking in "sondry places."

- The Salerno school (12th–13th centuries) recorded the following line of reasoning: "Why is it that buzzing in the ears ceases if one makes a sound? Is it because a greater sound drives out the less?"

- Johan Jakob Wepfer (1620–1695) gave this account of one patient's technique: "He banged two pebbles together next to his ear so that the sound made by these stones would solve his problem."

- Jean Marie Gaspard Itard (1774–1838) wrote, "Producing a roaring fire in the grate considerably relieves the disturbance resulting from tinnitus which sounds like the distant murmuring of wind and a river in flood. The same approach can be adopted with whistling tinnitus by putting green or slightly damp wood on the fire. When the tinnitus is like the sound of bells, as long as it is not

too loud, it may be masked by the resonance of a large copper bowl into which falls a trickle of water from a vase. Finally, in the case of tinnitus resembling the sound of a set of wheels turning, one can place alongside the bed a noisy spring-driven motor adapted to a mechanical organ, or a large watch, of which the movements are speeded up by removal of the regulator" (Stephens, 1987, p. 11.).

Over the last two centuries, numerous techniques and devices have been developed to deliver acoustic therapy to tinnitus sufferers. Urbantschitsch (1883) used tuning forks. Wilson (1893) tried a telephone transducer. Spaulding (1903) played a violin. Porter and McBride (1916) suggested that tinnitus patients should place a loud ticking clock near their beds. Saltzman and Ersner (1947) recommended hearing aids for tinnitus relief.

The rationale for all of these strategies is the same: increase the level of external sounds in the patient's environment to decrease the patient's perception of tinnitus. In **Fig. 21–4A,** the tinnitus signal is prominent, and the level of background sound (or noise) is low. There is a large tinnitus signal-to-background-noise ratio.

This phenomenon was demonstrated by Heller and Bergman (1953). They asked 80 adults who had normal hearing and no tinnitus to enter a sound booth (one at a time) and make notes of the sounds they heard while in the booth. The interior of the booth had a maximum background sound level of 18 dB SPL. While they were in the booth, 75 (94%) of these subjects reported that they heard sounds such as buzzing, humming, ringing, insects, or pulsations. Heller and Bergman (1953, p. 82) concluded:

> It appears that tinnitus is present constantly, but is masked by the ambient noise which floods our environment. This ambient noise level for ordinary quiet living conditions usually exceeds 35 dB SPL and is of sufficient intensity to mask physiological tinnitus which remains subaudible. It would appear, then, that tinnitus will not be eliminated by any treatment but at best can only become subaudible.

One of the goals of acoustic therapy is to increase the level of background sound to decrease the tinnitus signal-to-noise ratio (SNR, as shown in **Fig. 21–4B**). Notice that the amplitude of the tinnitus signal has not changed. Background sound has been increased to make tinnitus less noticeable. An analogy: Bothersome tinnitus can be thought of as a candle burning in a dark room. Even a small candle flame seems bright in a dark room. However, when overhead light fixtures are turned on, the same candle flame becomes much less noticeable than it had been in the dark.

As illustrated in **Fig. 21–5,** many of our patients report that their tinnitus makes it uncomfortable to be in a quiet room. For this reason, the authors turn on a tabletop fountain in the lobby of our clinic while patients are waiting for their appointment. Many of the same patients say that their tinnitus is less bothersome when they are outdoors walking, working, or recreating. However, the reality is that patients have to come inside eventually.

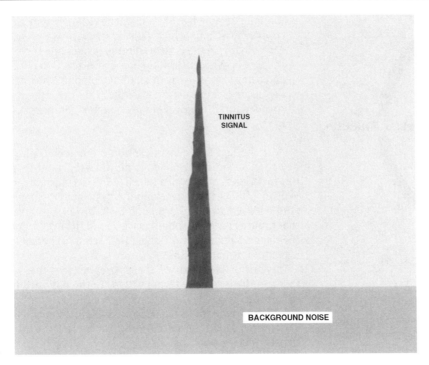

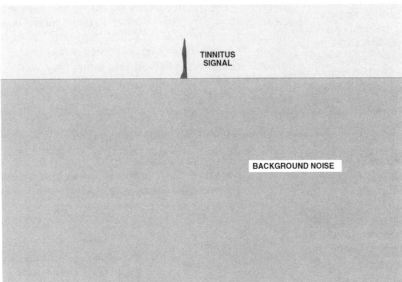

Figure 21–4 (A) Large tinnitus signal-to-background-noise ratio in a quiet environment. **(B)** Increased background sound decreases the perception of tinnitus. (From Tyler, R. S. (Ed.). (2006). Tinnitus treatment: Clinical protocols. New York: Thieme Medical Publishers, with permission.)

Pearl

- Provide this recommendation to every patient who experiences bothersome tinnitus: add pleasant sounds to any environment that is too quiet.

Sound Sources

Some tinnitus patients have already learned to employ acoustic therapy and routinely turn on a radio or television when they are at home. Of course, this is not always possible away from home, especially in the workplace. Another problem with radio or television is the variability of sounds emanating from these devices over time: music versus talk versus commercials. During the day, this variety of sounds might provide a welcome distraction from a patient's tinnitus. However, if patients want to add sounds to the bedroom to improve their sleeping patterns, the authors recommend a more consistent and less distracting sound source such as the following.

Tabletop Sound Machines   Various brands are available that play different types of sounds, such as rain, wind, waterfall, brook, ocean waves, and summer night. Some of these machines also have an input jack for headphones or auxiliary devices, such as the Sound Pillow (Phoenix Productions, San Antonio, TX).

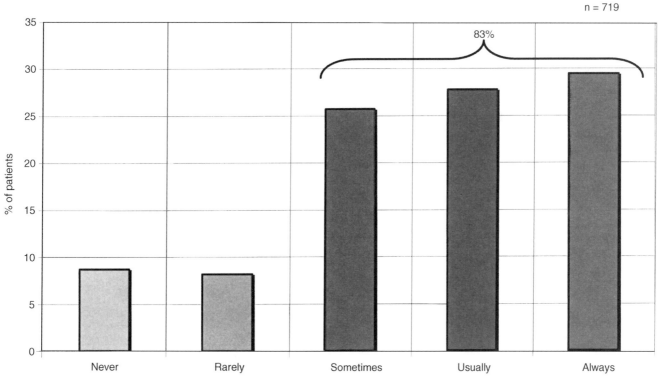

Figure 21–5 Patient responses to the question, "Does your tinnitus make it uncomfortable to be in a quiet room?"

Cassette Tapes and CDs Many different recordings of nature and environmental sounds (e.g., ocean waves, rain forest, and summer night) are available. However, some patients are distracted by the sounds of bird calls, crickets, and thunder included in the recordings. For these patients, the authors recommend compact discs (CDs) with continuous types of water or masking sounds with no other sound effects added (available at www.purewhitenoise.com).

Tabletop Water Fountains Many types are available in a variety of styles and price ranges, including those at www.Homedics.com.

Fans Some patients turn on a fan to help them sleep. However, some patients do not like to feel air blowing in the bedroom all night.

Air Purifiers Some patients find that the sound of the fan in their air cleaner provides them relief from tinnitus.

Insomnia is a common problem among tinnitus patients (Folmer and Griest, 2000). Improvements in sleep patterns are often associated with reductions in tinnitus severity (Folmer, 2002). Before resorting to medications, adding pleasant sounds to the bedroom is a good way to improve sleep patterns. In addition to the sound generators mentioned previously, the authors recommend the following sound delivery devices.

Pillows with Speakers Regular pillows with speakers embedded inside, such as the Sound Pillow (www.soundpil-low.com), help to make tinnitus less noticeable by adding background sounds to the bedroom. The pillow's cord can be connected to any sound machine or tape or CD player that has a stereo jack for headphones. Patients can then play any sort of pleasing or comforting sounds to help them sleep. For many patients, delivering these sounds close to their ears is more effective than playing sounds through a machine that sits on top of a nightstand or dresser.

Pillow Speakers For people who like to use a particular kind of pillow (or none at all), a pillow speaker can be used instead of a pillow with embedded speakers. These small, flat speakers plug into a sound machine or tape or CD player and deliver sounds near the patient's ears.

Headband Speakers A cloth headband with two small speakers sewn inside the band is available from MemoryTime (www.memorytime.com). Originally designed for runners and skiers, the Syke headband plugs into a sound machine or tape or CD player and can be worn to bed. For patients who also like to wear a mask while they sleep, the front of the headband can be pulled over their eyes.

Headphones and Earpieces Some patients wear these devices to bed and plug them into a sound machine (CD or tape player, radio, television, or tabletop sound generator). However, many patients find headphones and earpieces uncomfortable or impractical when they are trying to sleep.

Delivering sound directly into the ear canal is an efficient way to obtain relief from tinnitus. For this reason, the authors encourage our patients to listen to comforting sounds through headphones or earphones when possible. Limitations of these devices include the following:

♦ Patients' movements are restricted because they are attached to the sound machine by a cord. Mobility can be increased by using a portable radio, CD, iPod, or MP3 player.

♦ Headphones and earpieces are conspicuous and are not practical for many patients to wear, especially in their workplace. For patients who can afford them, ear-level devices are the best alternative.

Ear-level Devices

Sound Generators Ear-level sound generators (sometimes called "maskers") are available from General Hearing Instruments Inc. (Harahan, LA), Starkey Laboratories Inc. (Eden Prairie, MN), and Hansaton Akustik GmbH (Hamburg, Germany). These devices deliver a broadband of sound frequencies (typically 100–8000 Hz) and can provide several immediate benefits for tinnitus patients:

♦ Sound generators can make tinnitus less noticeable by decreasing the tinnitus SNR.

♦ Sound generators can muffle the piercing quality of high-pitched tinnitus, making the tinnitus more tolerable and easier to ignore.

♦ Sound generators give patients some control over their tinnitus. Part of the frustration for patients comes from the fact that they cannot escape from their tinnitus, and, if they have not yet employed acoustic therapy, they cannot reduce its loudness.

♦ Sound generators are the most portable and inconspicuous ways for patients to receive this type of acoustic therapy almost anytime, anywhere.

♦ Because sound generators deliver sound directly into the ear canal, the devices provide effective acoustic therapy using relatively low levels of sound.

♦ Some patients report improvement in their ability to concentrate (especially when reading) while wearing sound generators.

♦ Some patients experience RI after using sound generators. Even though RI is usually brief (30–60 seconds), for some patients it is the first time in years their tinnitus has been absent, and they are able to experience silence. For a small number of fortunate patients, RI can last hours, days, or weeks.

Ear-level sound generators can also contribute to long-term improvements in tinnitus severity:

♦ Sound generators can facilitate patients' habituation to tinnitus. That is, the devices are tools that can help patients learn to pay less attention to their tinnitus.

♦ The continuous sound exposure provided by these devices can increase blood flow to the inner ear (Quirk et al, 1992). This helps nourish and maintain auditory structures and may also contribute to healing processes when possible.

♦ Over time, it is possible that continuous sound exposure provided by ear-level devices can contribute to reductions in neural activity responsible for tinnitus generation and perception.

Complete masking of tinnitus is a phenomenon that sometimes occurs as a result of acoustic therapy. However, complete masking is not necessarily the goal unless the patient prefers this type of tinnitus relief. For patients who perceive their tinnitus at relatively low sensation levels (e.g., 0–2 dB SL), almost any sound delivered to their ears completely masks their tinnitus. The authors let their patients set the level of sound delivered by ear-level devices to obtain maximum relief from tinnitus. We instruct patients to set the level of sound generators to a comfortable, unobtrusive level. We also tell patients not to monitor their sound generators throughout the day. Otherwise, some patients substitute hypervigilance to their tinnitus with hypervigilance to their sound generators. Patients should set the level of sound generators once, then leave them alone and forget about them as much as possible. Sound generators are tools that give patients relief from tinnitus and can help them to pay less attention to tinnitus. We encourage our patients to wear the devices as much as possible during waking hours. Patients sometimes ask the following questions about ear-level sound generators:

Q: What if my tinnitus becomes louder? Is it okay to turn up the volume of the sound generator?

A: Yes. Even if most sound generators are turned all the way up, they cannot do physical harm to the auditory system. The maximum output for most ear-level sound generators is 80 dB SPL. Most patients do not want or need this level of sound for tinnitus relief. However, they may increase the volume if they so desire. Again, patients should keep the number of volume adjustments per day to a minimum.

Q: What if my tinnitus goes away for a while or becomes so faint that I don't feel the need to wear my sound generator? Should I still wear it? If I don't wear it every day, will the habituation process take longer?

A: If a patient does not want or need to wear a sound generator for one or more days, that is his or her prerogative. Patients will not necessarily have to use sound generators for the rest of their lives. One of the goals of tinnitus management is for patients to eventually be able to ignore their tinnitus most of the time without using any devices. To our knowledge, there is no evidence to indicate that curtailing sound generator use for 1 or more days interferes with the habituation process.

Q: How long will it take for me to habituate to my tinnitus?

A: As long as the patient continues to ask this question, he or she is not there yet; instead, the patient is still monitoring the tinnitus. Some people habituate to tinnitus very quickly. We usually do not see these people in our clinic, because their tinnitus is not bothersome, and they are not compelled to seek treatment for it. Some patients with bothersome tinnitus seem to believe that habituation is something that will be given to them by a clinician, a device, a medication, or a surgical procedure. In fact, habituation is a set of behaviors that patients must learn to cultivate within themselves. Clinicians provide information, tools, and strategies that can facilitate this process. However, patients must take responsibility for their own improvement.

> **Pitfall**
>
> • Ear-level sound generators do not have a good reputation among some clinicians because of the traditionally low success rate and high return rate reported for these devices.

Some clinicians choose not to promote or demonstrate ear-level sound generators for any of their tinnitus patients. Reasons for this include clinician unfamiliarity with sound generators, confusion about how to use them effectively, and the perception that the devices have a low success rate. A low success rate of ear-level sound generators can usually be attributed to one or more of the following pitfalls:

♦ Lack of an integrated, multimodal tinnitus management program. Some clinicians spend a minimal amount of time with patients, place sound generators into the patients' ears, then ask if there was any improvement. This approach has a low likelihood of success.

♦ Patients were not provided with the variety of reasons (as described in previous sections of this chapter) for wearing sound generators.

♦ Complete masking of tinnitus was mistakenly identified as the only goal; when this goal was not achieved, sound generators were deemed failures.

♦ The volume of sound generators was set so high that it was unpleasant for patients.

♦ Patients did not understand how substituting another sound for their tinnitus was supposed to be beneficial.

♦ The sounds generated by the devices were described to patients in negative terms, such as "masking noise" and "static."

To increase the acceptability and perceived benefits of ear-level sound generators, the authors recommend the following:

♦ Use the devices as one facet of a multimodal tinnitus management program. In-the-ear (ITE) devices represent only one type of acoustic therapy. Acoustic therapy is only one component of a comprehensive tinnitus management program.

♦ If possible, demonstrate ear-level devices before patients order them. Give patients time to walk around the clinic while wearing the devices.

♦ Describe the devices and the sounds they produce in positive terms. For example, if a patient reports that the

sound of water running in the shower provides relief from tinnitus, tell him or her that the sound generator makes a similar sound. Draw comparisons between the sound produced by the devices and positive experiences with external sounds reported by patients (e.g., with the sound of rain, a waterfall, the ocean, a brook, or the wind). Do not use words such as *noise* and *static*, because these words have negative connotations for many people.

♦ Instruct patients to adjust the volume of sound generators to a "comfortable" or "pleasant" level.

♦ Thoroughly explain the rationale for recommending a 30-day trial with ear-level devices. The 30-day trial period should allow patients to evaluate the physical comfort and acceptability of sound generators. Most patients should not expect to achieve habituation to tinnitus during this short amount of time.

♦ Explain each of the immediate and long-term reasons for wearing sound generators. Remind patients that complete masking of tinnitus is not always necessary and is not a measure of success.

Criteria for recommending a trial with ear-level sound generators include the following:

♦ Patients with normal or nearly normal hearing who are not candidates for hearing aids

♦ Otolaryngologic exam and clearance by an ear, nose, and throat (ENT) specialist physician

♦ During the demonstration of these devices, the patient reports that the sound from the device is at least tolerable and might provide some relief from (or reduced perception of) tinnitus.

♦ Patients are interested in using the devices as tools to facilitate improvements in their ability to habituate to tinnitus.

♦ Patients are interested in the possibility of changing patterns of neural activity responsible for tinnitus generation and perception.

♦ Patients with sound hypersensitivity who want to use the devices to desensitize their auditory system

Folmer and Carroll (2006) conducted a follow-up study of 50 tinnitus patients who purchased and used ear-level sound generators. Compared with responses on initial questionnaires, this group of patients exhibited significant improvements in tinnitus severity and self-rated loudness of tinnitus after using the devices for an average of 18 months.

Hearing Aids

Hearing aids are usually beneficial for tinnitus patients who also have significant hearing loss. Some patients blame their tinnitus for communication difficulties that are actually caused by their hearing loss. This is understandable, because hearing loss often progresses slowly over time, and patients do not always realize what they are missing. Tinnitus, in contrast, is the addition of an unpleasant perception that sometimes has a sudden onset. Many patients pay more attention to the addition of tinnitus than to their gradual loss of hearing.

Pearl

- It is important for patients to understand the relationship between hearing loss and tinnitus and to appreciate the differences between them.

The authors stress the following points with our patients:

- Tinnitus does not cause hearing loss, but hearing loss makes it more likely for a person to hear tinnitus.

- Even if their tinnitus stopped completely, patients with significant hearing loss would still have communication difficulties.

- Hearing aids do not amplify tinnitus. In fact, hearing aids usually reduce the loudness of tinnitus by amplifying external sounds.

- Hearing aids improve speech recognition for patients with significant hearing loss. This should relieve some of the frustration, isolation, and depression experienced by these patients.

- If hearing could be restored to pretinnitus thresholds, many cases of tinnitus would be cured. At the moment, the most practical way to restore hearing is by using hearing aids.

- Hearing aids are beneficial for the maintenance of central auditory pathways of patients with significant hearing loss. If these patients do not stimulate as many parts of their auditory systems as possible (at safe levels), the neural pathways are more likely to degenerate.

- Using hearing aids to stimulate the auditory system may contribute to permanent reductions in neural activity responsible for tinnitus generation and perception.

Some patients are in denial about the extent of their own hearing loss. That is one of the reasons the authors encourage spouses, significant others, relatives, or friends to accompany patients during their appointment in our clinic and to participate during the interview session. These companions supply important information that would otherwise be missed. The loved ones can also help clinicians to convince resistant patients about the extent of their communication difficulties and associated problems. Some patients require a great deal of encouragement before they are willing to try hearing aids.

Criteria for recommending a trial period with hearing aids include the following:

- Appropriate hearing loss determined by audiometric testing

- Otolaryngologic exam and clearance by an ENT specialist

- Patient admits communication difficulties.

- During a demonstration of programmable behind-the-ear (BTE) devices in the clinic, the patient reports that hearing aids improve his or her hearing sensitivity and/or reduce his or her perception of tinnitus.

- The patient is willing to pay for the devices and to use them regularly.

Fitting tinnitus patients with hearing aids is similar to fitting anyone with hearing aids. See Chapters 4 and 5 in this volume for additional information. The following factors should be addressed:

- Circuitry (conventional, programmable, digital)

- Style and size (BTE, ITE, completely-in-the-canal (CIC), etc.)

- Cost

- Care and maintenance

- Follow-up appointments

Programmable hearing aids provide audiologists the opportunity to adjust the pattern of amplification for optimal sound processing and tinnitus relief. For this reason, the authors recommend programmable hearing aids for patients who are able to afford them.

In order for tinnitus patients to receive maximum benefits from hearing aids, the following strategies should be employed:

- All patients should receive education about the relationship between hearing loss and tinnitus. Understanding this relationship and the mechanisms of tinnitus generation helps patients to place the symptom into perspective. Patients are then less likely to blame tinnitus for communication difficulties resulting from hearing loss.

- The nature of each patient's hearing loss and its effects on communication and socialization should be identified and discussed in detail.

- All patients should be informed about effective communication strategies that are useful for people with significant hearing loss. See Chapter 11 in this volume for information on these communication strategies.

Patients receive multiple benefits from hearing aids, including improved sound localization and identification, improved speech recognition, and reduced perception of tinnitus. Many patients who use hearing aids report reductions in feelings of frustration, social isolation, and depression. Improvements in these areas can also contribute to reductions in tinnitus severity.

Folmer and Carroll (2006) conducted a follow-up study of 50 tinnitus patients who purchased and used hearing aids for the first time. Compared with responses on initial questionnaires, this group of patients exhibited significant improvements in tinnitus severity and self-rated loudness of tinnitus after using hearing aids for an average of 18 months.

Combination Instruments

These devices combine two circuits, hearing aid and sound generator, into one wearable unit. Combination instruments are currently available from General Hearing Instruments, Starkey, and Hansaton. The authors' criteria for recommending a trial period with combination instruments are the same as our criteria for recommending hearing aids, with one additional variable: if patients already tried hearing aids and experienced some benefits from amplification but believe they might receive additional tinnitus relief from a sound generator, a trial period with combination instruments is considered.

Patients with One "Dead" Ear

Patients with severe to profound hearing loss and tinnitus in the same ear often present a challenge for clinicians attempting to use acoustic therapy. It is difficult to bring external sounds into the nonfunctioning ear to reduce the patient's perception of tinnitus. The authors' advice is to try everything. Try the most powerful hearing aid available. Even if these strategies do not improve the patient's speech recognition, it might provide some relief from tinnitus. Try an ITE or BTE sound generator or a single ear jack attached to a sound machine. If the sound generator does not work in the nonfunctioning ear, try the device in the opposite ear. Some patients receive tinnitus relief from the contralateral ear due to crossover pathways in the central auditory system. If the patient's better ear can benefit from amplification, try a hearing aid or a combination instrument in that ear. Finally, if patients are interested in improving their sound localization abilities, they could try a CROS (contralateral routing of signals), BICROS (bilateral contralateral routing of signals), or MultiCROS (multiple contralateral routing of signals) aid.

Other Devices to Improve Hearing

Any devices or procedures (including cochlear implants, brainstem implants, middle ear amplifiers, and prostheses) that improve patients' ability to hear external sounds have a good probability of making their tinnitus less noticeable. See Chapter 13 in this volume for information on implantable hearing aids. Future innovations in hearing aid technology, auditory prostheses, and surgical techniques will continue to improve the communication abilities of patients who have significant hearing loss. Many of these innovations will also reduce the loudness of tinnitus for patients who experience this symptom as a result of auditory dysfunction.

Cochlear Implants   Patients with severe to profound bilateral hearing loss usually cannot follow the authors' general recommendation for acoustic therapy: use external sounds to obtain relief from tinnitus. Fortunately, several studies have reported that cochlear implants reduce or suppress tinnitus for a majority of patients who experience tinnitus prior to implantation (Dauman, 2000; Ito, 1997). Cochlear implants are therefore a viable option for some patients who experience tinnitus and bilateral hearing loss of this severity. See Chapters 14 and 15 in this volume for additional information on cochlear implants.

Nearly all of the authors' tinnitus patients use acoustic therapy in one form or another. Because sound enrichment is just one component of a multimodal tinnitus management program, it is impossible to determine the effectiveness of acoustic therapy alone. However, counseling patients about how to use external sounds to reduce their perception of chronic tinnitus usually helps to reduce the severity of their condition.

♦ Lifestyle Management

The goal of tinnitus management is to reduce the severity of tinnitus until it is no longer a negative factor in the patient's life. Appropriate lifestyle changes can facilitate this process.

To recommend specific lifestyle changes that will help tinnitus patients to improve their overall condition, an effective tinnitus management program should include the following:

- The willingness to spend a substantial amount of time (up to several hours) with each patient

- Analysis of detailed health and psychosocial profiles of patients

- An interview/education session. In the authors' clinic, we review medical, hearing, tinnitus, and psychosocial histories, and conditions with our patients. During this process, patients supply additional information that might not be included in questionnaires or medical records. This interview/education session also gives clinicians time to ask questions and to discuss pertinent issues with patients. Patients receive education about how the auditory system works, how it is damaged by specific disease processes, and possible causes of their tinnitus, as well as reassurance and counseling regarding factors that could exacerbate or improve their condition.

- When possible, inclusion of spouses, significant others, relatives, or friends in the evaluation and treatment processes.

Before recommendations for lifestyle changes can be formulated, factors contributing to tinnitus severity must be identified for each patient. The authors' clinic staff mails detailed questionnaires to patients prior to their initial tinnitus clinic appointment. Three of the questionnaires request information about patients' health, hearing, and tinnitus histories (see Johnson, 1998, for questionnaire format and content). Twelve of the questions constitute a Tinnitus Severity Index (Meikle et al, 1995; see **Appendix 21–1**) that assesses the negative impacts of tinnitus upon patients. Patients also fill out the State-Trait Anxiety Inventory (STAI; Spielberger, 1998) and an abbreviated version of the Beck Depression Inventory (Beck and Beck, 1972).

After reviewing the patient's medical records and responses to questionnaires, the authors spend 1 to $1\frac{1}{2}$ hours interviewing each patient. This interview session serves several important purposes:

- It gives patients the opportunity to clarify and elaborate on their questionnaire responses.

- It gives clinicians the opportunity to ask additional questions.

- If patients are accompanied by spouses, friends, or relatives, these companions often provide important details about the patient's physical and emotional state, social and work history, communication difficulties, and so on.

- During the interview, clinicians identify specific problem areas and discuss them with the patient.

- When possible, clinicians suggest strategies, protocols, or devices that are likely to reduce the severity of the patient's tinnitus. Diagnostic testing is sometimes required before specific tinnitus management strategies are suggested.

- Part of the interview session is spent educating patients about possible causes of their tinnitus, as well as reassuring and counseling them regarding factors that could exacerbate or improve their condition. If patients understand that their tinnitus is nothing more dangerous than a perception of sound, they will be able to pay less attention to it.

◆ Recommended Lifestyle Changes

Adjust Patient Expectations and Perspective

Pearl

- Inform patients that clinicians usually cannot "cure" chronic tinnitus. Adjusting patient expectations is an important step in the process of reducing tinnitus severity.

Helping patients to gain perspective on their tinnitus and to adjust their expectations of a "cure" is an important step in reducing the severity of the condition. However, as Tyler et al (2001) suggested, it is also important to provide patients with hope. Even though a "cure" for most cases of chronic tinnitus is not currently available, there are many ways for patients to obtain relief from this symptom. The following observations have been made about patients who suffer from severe tinnitus:

- They tend to be very somatically aware and internally directed (Newman et al, 1997).

- They often resent the persistence of the noises, wish to escape them, and worry excessively about their health and sanity (Hallam et al, 1988).

- They have maladaptive coping strategies (this includes patients who attempt to avoid tinnitus, pray that their tinnitus will go away, and fantasize about not having

tinnitus). Maladaptive coping strategies also include dwelling on tinnitus, talking to others about how unpleasant the noises are, and catastrophizing about the consequences of tinnitus (Budd and Pugh, 1996). Catastrophic thinking is reflected in such statements by patients as "My entire life has been disrupted, and it is a daily struggle" and "There is never any peace or escape" (Neher, 1991).

- A study by Budd and Pugh (1995) demonstrated that patients who believe tinnitus is beyond their control are more likely to experience severe tinnitus, anxiety, and depression than patients who believe they can exert some control over their symptoms and other life events.

House (1981) made the following observations:

- Tinnitus as a symptom can become a scapegoat.

- Conflicts and needs are displaced on this symptom.

- Tinnitus can be a chief concern and often an obsession.

- This obsession leads to other neurotic behavior, such as social withdrawal, isolation, and difficulty with reality contact.

- In some cases, the tinnitus seems to take on the role of secondary gain. Tinnitus can relieve the guilt associated with job failure or social conflicts.

It is important for patients to recognize that not all of their problems are necessarily attributable to tinnitus. Patients should be encouraged to identify problems that can be treated apart from their tinnitus. For example, some patients blame tinnitus for difficulties that are actually caused by hearing loss, such as difficulty understanding speech in noisy environments. Amplification will improve speech recognition for many of these patients and can also reduce the loudness of their tinnitus.

Pearl

- Identification and treatment of problems mistakenly or disproportionately attributed to tinnitus can result in a reduction of importance patients assign to tinnitus. This will ultimately facilitate a reduction of tinnitus severity.

Rizzardo and colleagues (1998, p. 24) stated that there appears to be a "link between psychological distress and tinnitus in a potential somatopsychological and psychosomatic vicious circle (a psychological predisposition to react emotionally to events, tinnitus as a source of distress that reinforces the symptom, accentuating hypochondriac fears)."

Because patients with severe tinnitus sometimes develop cognitive distortions, including catastrophic thinking, cognitive behavioral therapy can be useful (Andersson et al, 2001). Some patients who exhibit maladaptive coping strategies improve when they are provided with cognitive coping strategies that are designed to help them interpret stressful situations and their disorder in more positive, adaptive ways (Kirsch et al, 1989).

Clinicians should strive to improve patients' understanding of tinnitus and their perspective about the symptom, and provide strategies for coping with tinnitus during the education and counseling portions of appointments. However, a series of ongoing psychotherapy sessions is sometimes necessary for patients to make significant improvements in these areas. When appropriate, encourage patients to pursue psychological counseling that is likely to help them. When possible, provide referrals to mental health professionals who practice near the patient's home.

Improve Sleep Patterns

Patients who experience insomnia tend to experience more severe tinnitus than patients who do not have trouble sleeping (Folmer and Griest, 2000). Improvements in sleep patterns are often associated with reductions in tinnitus severity (Folmer, 2002). If patients are not sleeping long enough or restfully enough, the authors recommend the following:

- Patients should bring pleasant sounds into the bedroom to reduce their perception of tinnitus. Demonstrate pillows embedded with flat speakers that can be connected to any sound source. The patient can then play any sort of pleasing or comforting music or sounds to help with sleep. Tabletop sound generation machines can also be demonstrated. These sound machines play various tranquil sounds and also have an input jack for the speaker pillows.

- If necessary, patients could try using an over-the-counter sleep medication, such as Alluna, Sominex, melatonin, Tylenol P. M., or Benadryl.

- If necessary, patients should talk to their physician about using prescription sleep medication, such as Ambien or trazodone. Sleep medications should be used as needed, not necessarily every night. After sleep patterns stabilize, patients should try to reduce their usage of sleep medications.

- Patients should follow the list of recommendations provided by the National Sleep Foundation (www. sleepfoundation.org).

- Patients should pursue activities and develop strategies that promote stress reduction and relaxation. If necessary, patients should pursue relaxation/stress management therapy.

- If insomnia persists, patients should make an appointment with a specialized sleep clinic for evaluation and treatment.

If patients report they usually get enough restful sleep, yet they still feel tired while they are awake, recommend they have a complete physical examination, including blood tests of thyroid function and hemoglobin concentration. Successful treatment of hypothyroidism or anemia often relieves fatigue experienced by patients who have these disorders.

Reduce Anxiety

Tinnitus severity is positively correlated with patients' level of anxiety (Folmer et al, 2001). Therefore, stress reduction is imperative for anxious patients. The authors use STAI (Spielberger, 1998) to assess anxiety levels in our tinnitus patients. The average STAI score (20 questions; minimum score 20, maximum score 80) for working adults is 35.5 ± 10.5 (Spielberger et al, 1983). If a patient scores 46 or higher on the STAI, anxiety management strategies should be recommended.

Like many psychological cosymptoms, anxiety is associated with other factors, such as insomnia, depression, communication difficulties, and employment, financial, or social problems. For patients who exhibit anxiety disorders, the authors recommend evaluation by a psychiatrist, preferably one who specializes in stress management. Other patients might benefit from stress reduction or relaxation techniques taught by licensed therapists or counselors. The Anxiety Disorders Association of America (www.adaa.org) can help patients locate a qualified therapist.

Some patients benefit from hypnosis; some benefit from biofeedback; others benefit from an exercise program, yoga, meditation, or regular massage. Almost anything that reduces the patient's level of stress or anxiety may decrease the severity of the tinnitus and will also help the patient to relax and sleep. Anxiolytic medication is necessary for some patients with severe anxiety.

Evaluate and Treat Depressed Patients

Depressed patients perceive their tinnitus to be more severe than do nondepressed patients (Folmer et al, 1999). In fact, the severity of tinnitus is positively correlated with the severity of patients' depression (Folmer et al, 2001). Identification and treatment of depression are essential elements of an effective tinnitus management program. The U.S. Preventive Services Task Force (2002) recommended screening adult patients for depression. In its simplest form, this screening can be accomplished by asking patients two questions: During the past 2 weeks, have you felt down, depressed, or hopeless? and During the past 2 weeks, have you felt little interest or pleasure in doing things? Affirmative responses to these questions should be followed by a more comprehensive analysis of depressive symptoms.

The authors use an abbreviated version of the Beck Depression Inventory (aBDI), consisting of 13 multiple-choice questions, to assess depression in tinnitus patients (Beck and Beck, 1972). A score between 5 and 7 indicates mild depression, a score between 8 and 15 indicates moderate depression, and a score of 16 or more indicates severe depression. The aBDI is a useful instrument because it is easy to administer and it can identify depression in patients who do not recognize or admit the severity of their own depression. If a patient scores 8 or more on the aBDI, the authors recommend that he or she receive effective treatment for depression. If the patient has not yet received any treatment for depression, we first recommend evaluation by a psychiatrist. This should be followed by an ongoing series of psychotherapy sessions and possibly antidepressant medication.

Folmer (2002) analyzed the association between aBDI scores and Tinnitus Severity Index scores for 190 patients 6 to 36 months after their initial appointment in a tinnitus clinic. Patients whose aBDI score decreased 3 or more points at follow-up exhibited significant reduction in Tinnitus Severity Index scores. Patients whose follow-up aBDI score stayed within 0 to 2 points of their initial score exhibited a smaller degree of improvement in tinnitus severity. However, patients whose initial aBDI score increased 3 or more points on the follow-up questionnaire did not exhibit significant changes in Tinnitus Severity Index scores. These results illustrate the importance of effective treatment for depression when it is present in tinnitus patients.

Reduce Anxiety/Break the Vicious Circle

As illustrated in **Fig. 21–3,** tinnitus, fatigue, anxiety, and depression can form a vicious circle and exacerbate each other (Folmer et al, 2001). A combination of medication and psychotherapy will typically reduce the severity of these symptoms and associated tinnitus. Patients should be encouraged to show **Fig. 21–3** to psychiatrists or psychologists during their initial session with these clinicians. The diagram will help clinicians to understand the relationships among these symptoms associated with severe tinnitus. Specific tinnitus expertise is not required of mental health professionals in order for them to help patients.

Pearl

- If clinicians can facilitate reductions in patients' levels of insomnia, anxiety, and depression, the severity of tinnitus should also decrease.

Address Communication Problems

Approximately 90% of all tinnitus patients have some degree of hearing loss (Meikle, 1997). Many of these patients report significant problems understanding conversations, television programs, movies, and so on. For patients who might benefit from amplification, recommend a trial period with appropriate hearing aids. See Chapters 4 and 5 in this volume for information on fitting of hearing aids. Also provide information to patients regarding hearing assistive technology (HAT) and effective communication strategies. See Chapter 17 in this volume for information on HAT.

Evaluate and Modify Medications

Few, if any, mediations are particularly effective for reducing the severity or perception of chronic tinnitus. When appropriate, recommend that patients consult with their physician about prescription medications to treat insomnia, anxiety, depression, phobias, obsessive-compulsive tendencies, or other psychological problems.

Controversial Point

- For complex problems such as anxiety disorders or major depression, medication alone seldom provides a complete solution.

In a systematic review of 16 randomized clinical trials, Pampallona and colleagues (2004) concluded that psychological treatment combined with antidepressant medication is more effective than medication alone. Some tinnitus patients certainly benefit from using antidepressant medications. Patients might also benefit from occasional, short-term use of anxiolytic or hypnotic medications. However, patients will not necessarily need to use any of these medications for the rest of their lives. Give all patients the goal of eventually improving to the point where they no longer need to take such medications. In some cases, effective psychotherapy can help patients progress so that prescription medications for sleep, anxiety, or depression are no longer required.

Anything that affects a patient's metabolism can affect his or her hearing or tinnitus. For this reason, medical conditions such as hyper- or hypothyroidism, hyper- or hypoglycemia, hyperlipidemia, and hypertension must be identified and treated with appropriate medications or other methods.

Some patients take potentially ototoxic medications without knowing it. For example, patients take quinine-based medications for a variety of conditions, including leg cramps and restless leg syndrome. Patients with a history of epileptic activity sometimes take the antiseizure medication valproic acid. Some patients have taken furosemide (Lasix) for years as a diuretic to control hypertension. These medications may or may not exacerbate hearing loss or tinnitus for a particular patient. However, because *Physicians' Desk Reference* (2007) lists hearing loss and tinnitus as common side effects of quinine, valproic acid, and furosemide, we recommend that patients talk to their physician about the possibility of switching to an alternative medication that does not have the same ototoxic potential.

Pitfall

- Do not discourage patients from using a non-ototoxic medication just because *Physicians' Desk Reference* lists tinnitus as one of its potential side effects.

Almost every antidepressant, anxiolytic, or hypnotic medication has the potential to trigger tinnitus for a small percentage of patients taking it. In the vast majority of cases, tinnitus resolves after the patient stops taking the medication. For patients who already experience chronic tinnitus, this should not be a reason for them to avoid medications that could benefit them. For example, patients with a history of cardiovascular or cerebrovascular disease should not avoid taking 81 mg of aspirin daily if

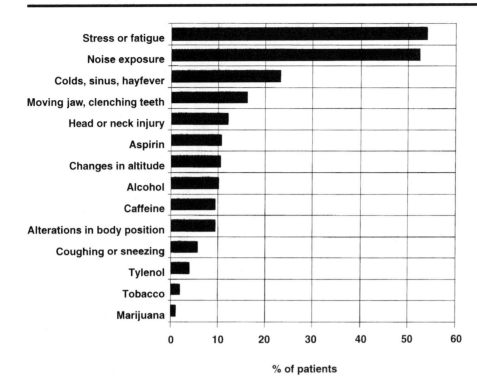

Figure 21–6 Factors that can increase the loudness of tinnitus. (From Tyler, R. S. (Ed.). (2006). Tinnitus treatment: Clinical protocols. New York: Thieme Medical Publishers, with permission.)

it is recommended by their physician. This small amount of aspirin is unlikely to increase the loudness of their tinnitus (see **Fig. 21–6**). However, the anticoagulant and anti-inflammatory properties of aspirin could save their lives. Even if a patient's tinnitus increases after taking a particular medication, the tinnitus should return to its premedication level after he or she stops taking the medication.

Some tinnitus patients have a long list of medications they are currently taking. If the medications being taken by a patient seem excessive, redundant, or potentially hazardous, recommend that each of the prescribing physicians review the entire regimen and decide if the present combination/dosage of medications is appropriate.

Dietary Considerations

Most patients report that low to moderate consumption of caffeine does not affect their tinnitus. Do not recommend a moratorium on caffeine for these patients. They may continue to enjoy coffee, tea, caffeinated soft drinks, or chocolate. As shown in **Fig. 21–6,** only ~9% of patients report that caffeine increases the loudness of their tinnitus. In most of these cases, relatively high levels of caffeine consumption are responsible for increases in tinnitus. The authors recommend that these patients reduce their intake of caffeine by switching to decaffeinated beverages as needed.

The authors make few other dietary recommendations for tinnitus patients. A small percentage of patients report that consumption of sugar, salt, dairy products, or other particular foods can increase the loudness of their tinnitus.

As a result, patients voluntarily restrict their intake of these foods. Because such food sensitivity is relatively rare in the tinnitus patient population, make dietary recommendations on an individual basis. Most patients are free to enjoy a varied, sensible diet.

Alcohol

Low to moderate consumption of alcohol is not a problem for most patients (see **Fig. 21–6**). In fact, many patients report that a drink or two helps them relax and to be less bothered by tinnitus. Usually a greater volume of alcohol is required to increase tinnitus. A rule of thumb: When a patient has consumed enough alcohol to initiate hangover symptoms (including headache), this seems to be the amount of alcohol that will also increase his or her tinnitus. If a patient consumes this much alcohol on a regular basis, it is probably excessive, and the patient should be evaluated for alcoholism. Using alcohol as a sleep aid is not recommended because metabolites of alcohol often interrupt sleep a few hours after drinking.

Dietary Supplements

Controversial Point

- There are no dietary supplements or herbal or homeopathic preparations that are particularly effective at reducing the severity of tinnitus.

In a double-blind, placebo-controlled study of 1121 tinnitus patients, Drew and Davies (2001) reported that ginkgo biloba was not more effective than placebo at reducing the severity of tinnitus. Therefore, do not recommend this supplement for tinnitus relief.

The authors recommend that most patients take a multivitamin/mineral supplement daily after eating. These supplements alone will probably not reduce the loudness or severity of a patient's tinnitus. However, supplements can help to maintain or improve the patient's general health, including the integrity and functioning of the auditory system. Taking appropriate dietary supplements can also improve the patient's sense of well-being. Patients who take an active role in their own health maintenance feel they have greater control over their condition. This positive perspective can contribute to increased optimism and ultimately to reductions in tinnitus severity.

Encourage Exercising

Some patients reduce their level of physical activity because exercising increases the loudness of their tinnitus. This increase in tinnitus is almost always temporary and is related to increased blood pressure during exertion. Because the benefits of regular exercise (including stress reduction, improved cardiovascular health, muscle tone, mood, and sleep patterns) far outweigh a temporary increase in tinnitus, the authors recommend that patients engage in a variety of physical activities when possible.

Reduce Unprotected Noise Exposure

As shown in **Fig. 21–6,** more than 50% of our patients report that excessive noise exposure can increase the loudness of their tinnitus. Encourage patients to wear earplugs or earmuffs as protection against harmful sounds (gunfire, gas lawn mowers, leaf blowers, chain saws, circular saws, heavy machinery, loud music, etc.) because noise-induced hearing loss (NIHL) will compromise patients' communication abilities and may also contribute to permanent increases in their tinnitus. (See Chapter 20 in this volume for additional information on hearing loss prevention.) Educate patients about the mechanisms and permanent nature of NIHL by using ear models and photomicrographs of hair cells damaged by excessive noise exposure (e.g., **Fig. 21–1B**). Clinicians should show patients evidence of NIHL when discussing results of audiometric tests.

Desensitize the Patient's Auditory System

Hypersensitivity to sound causes some patients to develop aversions to restaurants, movies, sporting events, concerts, parties, or church services and to abhor the sounds of a vacuum cleaner, sirens, bus brakes, or silverware striking plates or drinking glasses. Explain to patients that their increased sensitivity to sounds is a reflection of damage to outer hair cells that results in a form of recruitment. There is a real physiological reason, damage to the auditory system, that some sounds bother patients. However, some patients develop extreme phonophobia and wear earplugs most of

the time. These patients often withdraw from the workplace and all forms of socialization. Fear of sound exposure can cause them to become recluses. This exaggerated response is a reflection of the patient's mental state and coping skills. In these cases, make the following recommendations:

- Counsel patients to stop wearing hearing protection unless they are exposed to hazardous levels of sound. Overuse of earplugs or muffs can contribute to hypersensitization of the auditory system.

- To desensitize their auditory system, encourage patients to listen to pleasant sounds (e.g., music or masking sounds) at comfortable levels. Patients can listen to these sounds through headphones or from speakers, or by using ear-level sound generators. In addition to desensitizing the auditory system, this can help to reduce patients' fear of sounds.

- Encourage patients to increase socialization, resume employment if they are able, and rejoin society as soon as possible. It is true that the urban environment is often noisy, but becoming a recluse because of phonophobia is not a healthy lifestyle.

- When appropriate, recommend mental health evaluations and psychotherapy to help patients break their cycle of fearful thoughts and behaviors.

Modify Employment Status or Responsibilities

Most patients say their tinnitus is less bothersome when they are busy. Even if patients are retired or physically or mentally disabled, it is important for them to occupy their time with enjoyable and rewarding activities such as hobbies and volunteer work. Patients will then have less time to focus on their tinnitus. Encourage patients to seek employment or to continue working if they are able to do so. Employment can provide patients with a sense of purpose, increased self-esteem, optimism, and financial stability. In addition to experiencing depression and having low self-esteem and few financial resources, unemployed patients often exaggerate the magnitude of their auditory symptoms. If the patient is too young to retire and is physically and mentally able to work, he or she should be encouraged to do so. Even a relatively simple part-time job is preferable to staying home every day, often alone.

The authors provide a copy of the *Newsweek* article "Healing Myself with the Power of Work" (Norlen, 1999) to patients who need encouragement to seek employment. The author of the article was an attorney who stopped practicing law after 6 years because of severe depression. A job he took delivering morning newspapers helped him to regain his self-esteem and perspective. He concluded,

> One day soon I'll be ready to leave this job behind, but I'll never again view work as just a paycheck or a daily obligation. It will always be a part of my therapy, my healing. I don't know where my next job will be; in the courtroom, the classroom or the office. But wherever it is, my work will be a

weapon in my arsenal against the attacks I know will come again and again.

Many of the observations in the article apply to tinnitus patients who have stopped working and socializing because of depression and despair. As it did for the article's author, gainful employment can help tinnitus patients to feel more productive and hopeful. The article evokes another common theme: some patients dislike their present job and feel stressed about going to work every day. Remember that House (1981, p. 198) observed that "tinnitus as a symptom can become a scapegoat . . . it can relieve the guilt associated with job failure or social conflicts." Some patients use tinnitus as an excuse for quitting a job they do not like because their work or workplace elicits unacceptable levels of stress for them. It is beneficial for such patients to realize that tinnitus is not the major problem at their workplace. Clinicians should help patients to make this distinction whenever possible. The authors do not usually encourage patients to quit their current job, because such an action has financial and personal consequences that go beyond our clinical responsibilities. However, if it is clear that a patient does not want to continue in his or her current position, the authors help him or her to explore other possibilities. State vocational rehabilitation agencies can assist patients in this process.

Tinnitus and hearing loss can interfere with patients' abilities to perform some jobs. Information about different types of hearing aids, effective communication strategies, and HATs such as telephone amplifiers and frequency modulation (FM) systems should be given to patients who complain about communication problems at work.

Patients who are exposed to noise on their jobs must take precautions to protect their hearing. In some cases, tinnitus patients need to modify their work environment or duties to minimize occupational noise exposure. When necessary, patients should seek employment in a quieter environment within their current company or with a new employer.

Cultivate Personal Relationships/Increase Socialization

Personal relationships can suffer because of tinnitus or sound sensitivity. Some patients reduce socialization because of discomfort in noisy environments or because they are not sure how they might feel on a given occasion. Encourage patients to continue employment and participation in social activities as much as possible for the following reasons:

- When patients are busy, their tinnitus is less noticeable and less bothersome.

- Social contact can help patients to achieve or maintain a healthy perspective about their auditory symptoms.

- If patients stop working and socializing, they often give in to counterproductive feelings of hopelessness and despair. They then attribute a disproportionate amount of importance to their auditory symptoms.

- Friends, family members, and coworkers are more likely to be sympathetic and lend support to the patient if he or she gives realistic descriptions of his or her symptoms and makes efforts to persevere in spite of them.

- Patients feel better about themselves and more optimistic about the future if they remain active members of society.

Patients with supportive social and family relationships usually have more success coping with chronic medical conditions. Sullivan et al (1994) reported that patients who sought social support and those who had positive interactions with their spouses exhibited less tinnitus-related dysfunction than patients who did not experience supportive personal relationships.

Offer Referrals to Other Health Care Professionals

If any additional medical conditions that require evaluation or treatment are detected, patients should be referred to their primary care physicians or to clinical specialists. For example, depressed or anxious patients should be referred to psychiatrists or psychologists for evaluation and treatment. Patients who have trouble sleeping because they snore or experience sleep apnea should be referred to a specialized sleep clinic. Patients who experience severe headaches in addition to tinnitus should be referred to specialists such as neurologists who can help them manage their symptoms.

Pearl

- If coincident conditions improve, this will facilitate reductions in tinnitus severity, even if the patient's physical perception of tinnitus does not change.

♦ Formulation and Presentation of Recommendations

After patient evaluations, education, and device demonstrations are completed, a list of recommendations should be formulated, written, and explained to the patient. Recommendations can include appropriate acoustic therapy; use of hearing protection (all patients should wear earplugs or earmuffs when they are exposed to excessively loud sounds); and strategies for management of insomnia, anxiety, or depression. As appropriate, provide patients with referral and contact information for physical or psychiatric evaluations, psychological counseling, and other recommended services or products.

♦ Follow-up

In our practice, patients are encouraged to contact us during business hours if they have questions or concerns. Patients who order ear-level devices require follow-up appointments for fittings and adjustments. If we do not hear from them first, we call patients 1 month after their initial appointment in our clinic. Follow-up questionnaires are mailed to patients 6 months and 1 month after their initial appointment. Additional questionnaires are sometimes sent to patients years later.

Clinician-initiated contact at regular intervals after the initial appointment is important for several reasons:

♦ To let patients know that we are committed to helping them

♦ To address patients' questions or concerns

♦ To check patients' compliance with our recommendations

♦ To modify recommendations or to suggest different strategies when necessary

♦ To assess the effectiveness of our tinnitus management program.

We remind patients that recommendations made to them at the conclusion of their initial appointment in our clinic are starting points. If a patient follows all of the initial recommendations, yet the severity of his or her tinnitus does not improve over the course of 6 months, we either suggest different strategies to try or ask the patient to return to our clinic for reevaluation and additional counseling. Different devices and tinnitus management strategies might be described or demonstrated during the follow-up appointment. Particular recommendations will then be reinforced or modified.

♦ Summary

If patients can be motivated to implement recommendations such as those described in this chapter, their overall condition will improve, and the severity of their tinnitus will decrease. The key word in this process is *implementation*: patients need to make concrete efforts to follow specific recommendations formulated by health care professionals. Patients should be encouraged to take responsibility for their own improvement. For chronic conditions such as tinnitus, much of the healing must come from within.

Appendix 21–1

Tinnitus Severity Index Questions

Directions: For the questions below, please CIRCLE the number that best describes you

Does your tinnitus:	Never	Rarely	Sometimes	Usually	Always
1. Make you feel irritable or nervous?	1	2	3	4	5
2. Make you feel tired or stressed?	1	2	3	4	5
3. Make it difficult for you to relax?	1	2	3	4	5
4. Make it uncomfortable to be in a quiet room?	1	2	3	4	5
5. Make it difficult to concentrate?	1	2	3	4	5
6. Make it harder to interact pleasantly with others?	1	2	3	4	5
7. Interfere with your required activities (work, home, care, or other responsibilities)?	1	2	3	4	5
8. Interfere with your social activities or other things you do in your leisure time?	1	2	3	4	5
9. Interfere with your overall enjoyment of life?	1	2	3	4	5
10. Interfere with your ability to sleep?	1	2	3	4	5
11. How often do you have difficulty ignoring your tinnitus?	1	2	3	4	5
12. How often do you experience discomfort from tinnitus?	1	2	3	4	5

References

Adams, P. F., Hendershot, G. E., & Marano, M. A. (1999). Current estimates from the National Health Interview Survey, 1996. Hyattsville, MD: National Center for Health Statistics.

Andersson, G. (2003). Tinnitus loudness matchings in relation to annoyance and grading of severity. Auris, Nasus, Larynx, 30(2), 129–133.

Andersson, G., Vretblad, P., Larsen, H. C., & Lyttkens, L. (2001). Longitudinal follow-up of tinnitus complaints. Archives of Otolaryngology–Head and Neck Surgery, 127, 175–179.

Arnold, W., Bartenstein, P., Oestreicher, E., Römer, W., Schwaiger, M. (1996). Focal metabolic activation in the predominant left auditory cortex in patients suffering from tinnitus: A PET study with F]deoxyglucose. ORL: Journal for Oto-rhino-laryngology and Its Related Specialties, 58, 195–199.

Beck, A. T., & Beck, R. W. (1972). Screening depressed patients in family practice: A rapid technic. Postgraduate Medicine, 52, 81–85.

Budd, R. J., & Pugh, R. (1995). The relationship between locus of control, tinnitus severity, and emotional distress in a group of tinnitus sufferers. Journal of Psychosomatic Research, 39(8), 1015–1018.

Budd, R. J., & Pugh, R. (1996). Tinnitus coping style and its relationship to tinnitus severity and emotional distress. Journal of Psychosomatic Research, 41(4), 327–335.

da Costa, S. S., deSousa, L. C., & Piza, M. R. (2002). Meniere's disease: Overview, epidemiology, and natural history. Otolaryngologic Clinics of North America, 35, 455–495.

Dauman, R. (2000). Electrical stimulation for tinnitus suppression. In R. S. Tyler (Ed.), Tinnitus handbook (pp. 377–398). San Diego, CA: Singular Publishing Group.

Drew, S., & Davies, E. (2001). Effectiveness of ginkgo biloba in treating tinnitus: Double blind, placebo-controlled trial. British Medical Journal, 322(7278), 73–75.

Drukier, G. S. (1989). The prevalence and characteristics of tinnitus with profound sensori-neural hearing impairment. American Annals of the Deaf, 134, 260–264.

Duckro, P. N., Pollard, C. A., Bray, H. D., & Scheiter, L. (1984). Comprehensive behavioral management of complex tinnitus: A case illustration. Biofeedback and Self-Regulation, 9, 459–469.

Folmer, R. (2002). Long-term reductions in tinnitus severity. BMC Ear Nose and Throat Disorders, Retrieved August 31, 2007 from http://www/biomedcentral.com 1472-6815/2/3.

Folmer, R. L., & Carroll, J. R. (2006). Long-term effectiveness of ear-level devices for tinnitus. Otolaryngology–Head and Neck Surgery, 134(1), 132–137.

Folmer, R. L., & Griest, S. E. (2000). Tinnitus and insomnia. American Journal of Otolaryngology, 21, 287–293.

Folmer, R. L., Griest, S. E., & Martin, W. H. (2001). Chronic tinnitus as phantom auditory pain. Otolaryngology–Head and Neck Surgery, 124, 394–400.

Folmer, R. L., Griest, S. E., Meikle, M. B., & Martin, W. H. (1999). Tinnitus severity, loudness and depression. Otolaryngology–Head and Neck Surgery, 121, 48–51.

Folmer, R. L., & Shi, Y. B. (2004). SSRI use by tinnitus patients: Interactions between depression and tinnitus severity. Ear, Nose, and Throat Journal, 83, 107–117.

Folmer, R. L., Stevens, A. A., Martin, W. H., et al. (2002). Functional magnetic resonance imaging (fMRI) of brain activity associated with tinnitus severity and residual inhibition. In R. Patuzzi (Ed.), Proceedings of the Seventh International Tinnitus Seminar (pp. 131–135). Crawley: University of Western Australia.

Graham, J. (1981). Paediatric tinnitus. Journal of Laryngology and Otology 95(Suppl), 117–120.

Hain, T. C. (2004). Autoimmune inner ear disease. Chicago: American Hearing Research Foundation.

Hallam, R. S., Jakes, S. C., & Hinchcliffe, R. (1988). Cognitive variables in tinnitus annoyance. British Journal of Clinical Psychology, 27, 213–222.

Heller, M. F., & Bergman M. (1953). Tinnitus aurium in normally hearing persons. Annals of Otology, Rhinology and Laryngology, 62, 73–83.

House, P. R. (1981). Personality of the tinnitus patient. Ciba Foundation Symposium, 85, 193–203.

Ito, J. (1997). Tinnitus suppression in cochlear implant patients. Otolaryngology–Head and Neck Surgery, 117(6), 701–703.

Johnson, R. M. (1998). The masking of tinnitus. In J. A. Vernon (Ed.), Tinnitus treatment and relief (pp. 164–186). Boston: Allyn & Bacon.

Kirsch, C. A., Blanchard, E. B., & Parnes, S. M. (1989). Psychological characteristics of individuals high and low in their ability to cope with tinnitus. Psychosomatic Medicine, 51, 209–217.

Meikle, M. B. (1997). Electronic access to tinnitus data: The Oregon Tinnitus Data Archive. Otolaryngology–Head and Neck Surgery, 117, 698–700.

Meikle, M. B., Griest, S. E., Stewart, B. J., & Press, L. S. (1995). Measuring the negative impact of tinnitus: A brief severity index. Abstracts of the Association for Research in Otolaryngology, 18, 167.

Meikle, M. B., Vernon, J., & Johnson, R. M. (1984). The perceived severity of tinnitus. Otolaryngology–Head and Neck Surgery, 92, 689–696.

Neher, A. (1991). Tinnitus: The hidden epidemic; a patient's perspective. Annals of Otology, Rhinology, and Laryngology, 100(4, Part 1), 327–330.

Newman, C. W., Wharton, J. A., & Jacobson, G. P. (1997). Self-focused and somatic attention in patients with tinnitus. Journal of the American Academy of Audiology, 8, 143–149.

Norlen, M. (1999, October 25). Healing myself with the power of work. Newsweek, p. 12.

Pampallona, S., Bollini, P., Tibaldi, G., et al. (2004). Combined pharmacotherapy and psychological treatment for depression: A systematic review. Archives of General Psychiatry, 61(7), 714–719.

Physicians' desk reference. (2007). Montvale, NJ: Thomson PDR.

Porter, W. G., & McBride P. (1916). Diseases of the throat, nose and ears for practitioners and students. Bristol, UK: Wright.

Quirk, W. S., Avinash, G., Nuttall, A. L., & Miller, J. M. (1992). The influence of loud sound on red blood cell velocity and blood vessel diameter in the cochlea. Hearing Research, 63(1–2), 102–107.

Rizzardo, R., Savastano, M., Maron, M. B., et al. (1998). Psychological distress in patients with tinnitus. Journal of Otolaryngology, 27(1), 21–25.

Roy, D., & Chopra, R. (2002). Tinnitus: An update. Journal of the Royal Society of Health, 122(1), 21–23.

Saltzman, M., & Ersner, M. S. (1947). A hearing aid for the relief of tinnitus aurium. Laryngoscope, 57, 358–366.

Seidman, M. D., & Jacobson, G. P. (1996). Update on tinnitus. Otolaryngologic Clinics of North America, 29, 455–465.

Spaulding, J. A. (1903). Tinnitus, with a plea for its more accurate musical notation. Annals of Otology, 32, 263–272.

Spielberger, C. D. (1998). State-Trait Anxiety Inventory for Adults (Form Y). Palo Alto, CA: Mind Garden.

Spielberger, C. D., Gorsuch, R. L., Lushene, R., et al. (1983). State-Trait Anxiety Inventory for Adults: Sampler set, manual, test, scoring key. Palo Alto, CA: Mind Garden.

Stephens, S. D. G. (1987). Historical aspects of tinnitus. In J. W. P. Hazell (Ed.), Tinnitus (pp. 1–19). London: Churchill Livingstone.

Stouffer, J. L., Tyler, R. S., Booth, J. C., & Buckrell, B. (1992). Tinnitus in normal-hearing and hearing-impaired children. In J.-M. Aran & R. Dauman (Eds.), Tinnitus 91: Proceedings of the Fourth International Tinnitus Seminar (pp. 255–258). Amsterdam: Kugler Publications.

Sullivan, M., Katon, W., Russo, J., et al. (1994). Coping and marital support as correlates of tinnitus disability. General Hospital Psychiatry, 16, 259–266.

Tyler, R., Haskell, G., Preece, J., & Bergan, C. (2001). Nurturing patient expectations to enhance the treatment of tinnitus. Seminars in Hearing, 22(1), 15–21.

Urbantschitsch, V. (1883). Über die Wechselwirkungen der innerhalb eines Sinnesgebietes gesetzten Erregungen. [The reciprocal effects of excitations within a sensory modality.] Pflügers Archiv für die gesamte Physiologie des Menschen und der Tiere, 31, 280–309.

U.S. Preventive Services Task Force. (2002). Screening for depression: Recommendations and rationale. Annals of Internal Medicine, 136, 760–764.

Wilson, H. (1893). Vibratory massage of the middle ear by means of the telephone. New York Medical Journal, 57, 221, 222.

Index

Page numbers followed by *f* or *t* indicate material in figures or tables, respectively.